MEDICATION THERAPY MANAGEMENT

A Comprehensive Approach

Second Edition

Karen Whalen, PharmD, BCPS, CDE
Assistant Dean for Clinical Education
Clinical Professor
Department of Pharmacotherapy and Translational Research
University of Florida College of Pharmacy
Gainesville, Florida

Heather C. Hardin, PharmD, BCACP
Clinical Assistant Professor
Medication Therapy Management Center
Department of Pharmacotherapy and Translational Research
University of Florida College of Pharmacy
Gainesville, Florida

Mc Graw Hill Education

New York Chicago San Francisco Athens London Madrid Mexico City
Milan New Delhi Singapore Sydney Toronto

Medication Therapy Management: A Comprehensive Approach, Second Edition

1 2 3 4 5 6 7 8 9 DSS 23 22 21 20 19 18

ISBN 978-1-260-10845-3
MHID 1-260-10845-7

Notice

Medicine is an ever-changing science. As new research and clinical experience broaden our knowledge, changes in treatment and drug therapy are required. The authors and the publisher of this work have checked with sources believed to be reliable in their efforts to provide information that is complete and generally in accord with the standards accepted at the time of publication. However, in view of the possibility of human error or changes in medical sciences, neither the authors nor the publisher nor any other party who has been involved in the preparation or publication of this work warrants that the information contained herein is in every respect accurate or complete, and they disclaim all responsibility for any errors or omissions or for the results obtained from use of the information contained in this work. Readers are encouraged to confirm the information contained herein with other sources. For example and in particular, readers are advised to check the product information sheet included in the package of each drug they plan to administer to be certain that the information contained in this work is accurate and that changes have not been made in the recommended dose or in the contraindications for administration. This recommendation is of particular importance in connection with new or infrequently used drugs.

This book was set in Adobe Jenson Pro by Cenveo® Publisher Services.
The editors were Michael Weitz and Peter J. Boyle.
The production supervisor was Catherine H. Saggese.
Project management was provided by Smriti Joinwal and Kritika Kaushik, Cenveo Publisher Services.
The designer was Mary McKeon.

Cataloging-in-Publication data for this book is on file at the Library of Congress.

Contents

Contributors

Shawn D. Anderson, PharmD, BCACP
Clinical Pharmacy Specialist-Cardiology
Veterans Affairs
Gainesville, Florida

Katherine Vogel Anderson, PharmD, BCACP
Clinical Associate Professor
University of Florida College of Pharmacy
Gainesville, Florida

David M. Angaran, MS, FCCP, FASHP
Clinical Professor of Pharmacy (retired)
Communication Prescription LLC
University of Florida
Gainesville, Florida

Angel L. Ballew, MBA, PharmD, BCPP
Vice President
Pharmacy Clinical Programs
WellCare Health Plans, Inc.
Tampa, Florida

Daniel E. Buffington, PharmD, MBA
Associate Professor
University of South Florida
Tampa, Florida

Joshua Caballero, PharmD, BCPP, FCCP
Professor, Chair
Department of Clinical and Administrative Sciences
Larkin University
Miami, Florida

Charles F. Caley, PharmD, BCPP
Clinical Professor
University of Connecticut
School of Pharmacy
Storrs, Connecticut

Katie E. Cardone, PharmD, BCACP, FNKF, FASN
Associate Professor of Pharmacy Practice
Albany College of Pharmacy and Health Sciences
Albany, New York

Juan Hincapie Castillo, PharmD
Graduate Research Assistant
University of Florida
Gainesville, Florida

Jenna S. Clemons, PharmD
PGY-2 Geriatric Pharmacy Resident
Virginia Commonwealth University
Richmond, Virginia

Amber M. Connelly, PharmD
Clinical Pharmacist
Center for Quality Medication Management at the University of Florida
Gainesville, Florida

Kevin Cowart, PharmD, MPH
Assistant Professor of Pharmacy
Nova Southeastern University College of Pharmacy
Fort Lauderdale, Florida

Stacey D. Curtis, PharmD
Clinical Assistant Professor
University of Florida
Gainesville, Florida

Jeffrey C. Delafuente, MS, FCCP, FASCP
Professor Emeritus
Virginia Commonwealth University School of Pharmacy
Richmond, Virginia

Marvin A. Dewar, MD, JD
Senior Associate Dean and Associate Professor
Community Health and Family Medicine
University of Florida College of Medicine

Eric Dietrich, PharmD
Clinical Assistant Professor
University of Florida College of Pharmacy
Gainesville, Florida

Krista L. Donohoe, PharmD, BCPS, BCGP
Assistant Professor of Pharmacotherapy and Outcomes Science
Virginia Commonwealth University School of Pharmacy
Richmond, Virginia

Megan J. Ehret, PharmD, MS, BCPP
Behavioral Health Clinical Pharmacist
Fort Belvoir Community Hospital
Fort Belvoir, Virginia

Alexandre Endiakov, PharmD
Clinical MTM Pharmacist
Enhanced Medication Services, LLC.
Orlando, Florida

Anna Hall, PharmD, BCACP
Director of Quality Services
Enhanced Medication Services, LLC
Orlando, Florida

Heather C. Hardin, PharmD, BCACP
Clinical Assistant Professor
Medication Therapy Management Center
Department of Pharmacotherapy and Translational Research
University of Florida College of Pharmacy
Gainesville, Florida

Carol J. Hermansen-Kobulnicky, PhD, RPh
Associate Professor
School of Pharmacy
Adjunct Faculty
Fay W. Whitney School of Nursing
University of Wyoming
Laramie, Wyoming

Sarah E. Honaker, PharmD
Clinical Assistant Professor
Marshall University School of Pharmacy
Huntington, West Virginia

Andrew Y. Hwang, PharmD, BCPS
Assistant Professor of Clinical Sciences
High Point University
Fred Wilson School of Pharmacy
High Point, North Carolina

Jamie Kisgen, PharmD, BCPS-AQ ID
Pharmacotherapy Specialist-Infectious Diseases
Sarasota Memorial Health Care System
Sarasota, Florida

Robin Moorman Li, PharmD, BCACP, CPE
Assistant Director-Jacksonville Campus
Clinical Associate Professor
University of Florida College of Pharmacy
Jacksonville, Florida

Maria Maniscalco-Feichtl, PharmD
Associate Director
Interaction Design and Professional Development
Optum Care Services
Miramar, Florida

Karen D. McLin, PharmD
Regional Pharmacy Director
SinfoniaRx

Kyle Melin, PharmD, BCPS, AE-C
Assistant Professor of Pharmacy Practice
School of Pharmacy
University of Puerto Rico Medical Sciences Campus
San Juan, Puerto Rico

Alexander Miguel, PharmD, BCGP
Senior Director of Operations
Enhanced Medication Services
Orlando, Florida

Shannon A. Miller, PharmD, BCACP
Clinical Associate Professor
Department of Pharmacotherapy and Translational Research
University of Florida College of Pharmacy
Orlando, Florida

Cynthia R. Nacin, PharmD, MS, BCACP, CPh
Senior MTM Clinical Pharmacist
Center for Quality Medication Management at the University of Florida
University of Florida College of Pharmacy
Gainesville, Florida

David P. Nau, PharmD, PhD, RPh, CPHQ, FAPhA
Assistant Dean
College of Pharmacy
Nova Southeastern University
Ft. Lauderdale, Florida

Robert Navarro, PharmD
Clinical Professor
Department of Pharmaceutical Outcomes & Policy
University of Florida College of Pharmacy
Gainesville, Florida

Katie Neff-Golub, PharmD, BCGP, CPh
Director, Medication Therapy Management (MTM)
WellCare Health Plans, Inc.
Tampa, Florida

Kelechi C. Ogbonna, PharmD, MSHA, BCGP
Associate Dean of Admissions & Student Services
Associate Professor, Geriatrics
Virginia Commonwealth University
Richmond, Virginia

Kristyn M. Pardo, PharmD, BCPS, CACP
Clinical Pharmacy Specialist
North Florida/South Georgia Veterans Health System
Gainesville, Florida

Aditi V. Patel, PharmD
MTM Clinical Pharmacist
University of Florida
Gainesville, Florida

Jason G. Powell, PharmD
Assistant Clinical Professor College of Pharmacy
Pharmacotherapy and Translational Research
Assistant Clinical Professor College of Medicine
Family Medicine
University of Florida
Gainesville, Florida

Teresa E. Roane, PharmD, BCACP
Associate Director
Center for Quality Medication Management (CQM)
Clinical Assistant Professor
Department of Pharmacotherapy and Translational Research
University of Florida College of Pharmacy
Gainesville, Florida

Jennifer Salo, PharmD, BCACP, CPh
Director of Quality and Compliance
Center for Quality Medication Management and the University of Florida
Gainesville, Florida

Karen R. Sando, PharmD, BCACP, BC-ADM
Associate Professor of Pharmacy Practice
Nova Southeastern University College of Pharmacy
Davie, Florida

Jordan Sedlacek, PharmD, BCACP
Assistant Professor, Department of Clinical and Administrative Sciences
Larkin University College of Pharmacy
Miami, Florida

Kathryn J. Smith, PharmD
Clinical Assistant Professor
University of Florida
Gainesville, Florida

Kathleen J. Vieson, PharmD
Affiliated Assistant Professor
University of South Florida College of Pharmacy
Tampa, Florida

Kristin W. Weitzel, PharmD, FAPhA
Clinical Professor of Pharmacotherapy and Translational Research
University of Florida
Gainesville, Florida

Karen Whalen, PharmD, BCPS, CDE
Assistant Dean for Clinical Education
Clinical Professor
Department of Pharmacotherapy and Translational Research
University of Florida College of Pharmacy
Gainesville, Florida

Michelle Zeigler, PhD, PharmD, BCACP
Clinical Assistant Professor
Center for Quality Medication Management
University of Florida
Orlando, Florida

Preface

Medication therapy management (MTM) represents the first major, pharmacy-wide, reimbursable cognitive pharmacy service. In the years since MTM was implemented, it has gained momentum as a comprehensive method to address the safety, appropriateness, and effectiveness of medications. Provision of MTM services allows pharmacists to identify omissions in therapy as well as address issues with polypharmacy. MTM follows the steps of the Pharmacists' Patient Care Process: collect patient-specific information, assess the information to identify medication-related problems, create a patient-centered care plan, implement the care plan, and follow up with monitoring and evaluation. While MTM began as a Medicare-funded service, Medicaid and private health plans have also adopted the concepts of MTM. The services within the MTM scope are now integrated into mainstream healthcare in a variety of settings, including community pharmacies, hospitals, health plans, ambulatory care clinics, and university clinical practices. This text is our effort to provide information and an approach to MTM services that prepares the pharmacist to practice MTM in any setting.

As reimbursement models have transformed, pharmacists are now delivering MTM services in an efficient and effective way, providing patient care in a financial model that allows sustainability. MTM services can play an even larger role as the healthcare system evolves toward a pay-for-performance model that requires more value-based care. In some cases, MTM services have shown improved patient care and decreased healthcare costs. The next challenge is to continue to prove the cost savings and value that MTM practitioners bring to patients and the healthcare system.

The second edition has been updated to reflect current practice, yet it is a snapshot of MTM and therapeutics at one moment in time. We realize that the medication-use system is changing at a faster pace than therapeutics. However, the principles found in this text are applicable regardless of the practice setting or the introduction of new drugs, guidelines, or payment methods.

Our hope is that this text will be a useful resource that promotes the development of successful MTM services and more widespread adoption of MTM. As the medication-use system and therapeutics evolve, we will continue to update and refine the text to best meet the needs of MTM providers and the patients they serve.

Acknowledgments

We would like to thank several individuals for valuable contributions to this manuscript. The authors who contributed to the text spent countless hours away from family and friends to assure that the book provides the most accurate, thorough, and current information regarding the vast realm of MTM. We appreciate their considerable effort and time devoted to the success of this comprehensive edition.

In addition, we would like to acknowledge David Angaran (the "MTM Frontiersman") for the ingenuity, innovation, and imagination that led to the conceptualization of this text. As the editor of the original edition of the text, he provided guidance and inspiration to many authors and readers, empowering them with the confidence and knowledge to explore, engage in, and expand MTM services to new and enhanced levels. His endless enthusiasm and energy for the continued success of pharmacists and pharmacy practice continues to this day, especially within the realm of MTM.

1

Introduction to Medicare and Medicaid

Robert Navarro, PharmD

KEY POINTS

- Medicare and Medicaid are two of the three largest medical insurance programs in the United States, with each program comprising approximately 60 million enrollees. The largest health insurance programs are employer group insurance programs (commercial), with about 150 million members.
- Medicare and Medicaid have unique roles and influence in US healthcare financing and delivery. Both are government programs, and thus quite complex, with arcane, changing policies, regulations, and procedures.
- Medicare and Medicaid are heavily monitored for quality and cost outcomes, and both may impose significant financial penalties if providers or participating private insurers violate required compliance policies.
- The Centers for Medicare & Medicaid Services[1] (CMS) Innovation Center is actively testing novel payment and delivery models and concepts, and other patient access and quality initiatives.
- The CMS establishes payment standards for medical benefit drugs, bundled-payment models, preventive care, and quality programs that, if successful, are often adopted, or influence, private health insurance programs. Thus, although Medicaid and Medicare programs are each one-half the size of the employer group private insurance market, the state and federal regulatory authority and compliance penalties influence commercial employer group insurance, hospital, and all other healthcare delivery program operations.
- Although Medicaid is a state-administered program, the CMS has both financial investment and regulatory oversight, and can monitor and promulgate recommendations and requirements on all 54 state and US territory Medicaid programs, thus ensuring standardized and consistent minimum benefit coverage, although states can apply for waivers and benefit coverage.
- Both Medicaid and Medicare have been significantly altered through the Patient Protection and Affordable Care Act (PPACA) provisions, including benefit changes and expansion, as discussed in the following text. Today, both Medicare and Medicaid include inpatient and outpatient prescription drug benefits, but they are quite different in terms of drugs covered, access rules, and financial structure.

MEDICARE

INTRODUCTION TO MEDICARE

Medicare was established in 1965 under Title XIX in the Amendment to the Social Security Act (SSA). Medicare was originally created to provide healthcare benefits for citizens 65 years of age and above. As with most government programs, it has evolved and expanded over the past 50 years, adding younger enrollees with disabilities, skilled nursing and hospice care, home healthcare, and preventive services to the core inpatient and outpatient medical services. Outpatient prescription drug benefits were added in the 2003 Medicare Modernization Act. Medicare provides services to almost 70 million people, most over 65 years old, and about 10 million dual eligible disabled, who may be younger patients. The CMS Innovation Center has used Medicare to test innovative reimbursement models and benefits that have been adopted, with modification, by private insurance programs. Examples are development of various value-based programs,[2] the average sales price (ASP) medical benefit (Part B) specialty drug reimbursement,[3] the Oncology Care Model,[4] the Quality Payment Program,[5] and the Medicare Access and CHIP Reauthorization Act (MACRA).[5]

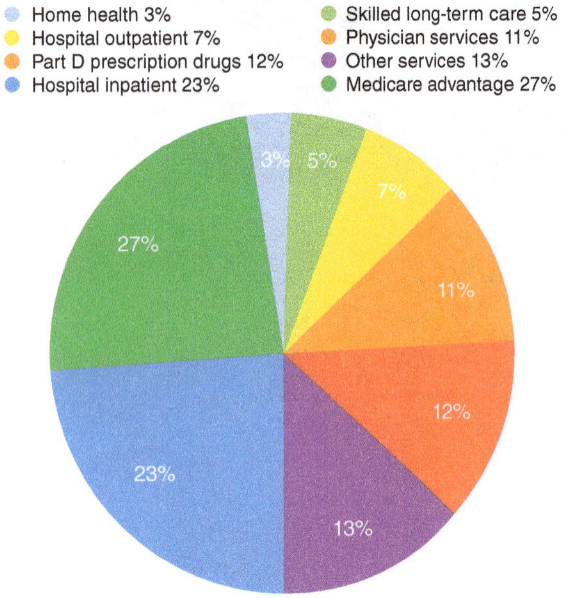

FIGURE 1-1 Medicare service expenditures, 2015.
* Other Services include hospice, durable medical equipment, Part B (physician administered) drugs, outpatient dialysis, ambulance, lab services, and other Part B services. Source: Kaiser Family Foundation webpage, Figure 2, "Medicare Benefit Payments by Type of Service, 2015." Available at http://kff.org/medicare/issue-brief/an-overview-of-medicare/. Accessed 29 December 2016.

Medicare recipients, who are older, are more likely to have multiple medical conditions (66% have 3 or more comorbidities), 17% are permanently disabled, 31% have cognitive impairment, and 21% have functional impairment in activities in daily living and use multiple medications. Of Medicare beneficiaries, 5% (2 million) reside in long-term-care facilities, and in 2014 one-half of Medicare recipients had annual incomes below $25 000 and savings below $64 000.[6] Figure 1-1 illustrates the percent of Medicare expenditures on various benefit services.

Medicare Advantage is the greatest expense, as it includes Medicare Part A inpatient and Part B outpatient medical services and often Part D outpatient prescription. As separate segments, outpatient prescription drug benefits (Part D) consume the second largest expense segment after inpatient hospital services (Part A), and greater than outpatient medical services (Part B). Medicare expenditure trends slowed during 2012 to 2015 due to provider payment reforms included in the PPACA that began implementation in 2011.[7,8] Medicare benefit expenditures in 2016 were $689 billion,[9] representing approximately 15% of total federal spending in 2015, and over 3% of the Gross Domestic Product.[10] Medicare benefit costs are now expected to grow to $708 billion in 2018, $839 billion in 2020, and over $1 trillion by 2015.[11]

DEVELOPMENT AND EVOLUTION OF MEDICARE BENEFITS

The SSA was passed in 1935 and signed into law by President Franklin Delano Roosevelt. The SSA established "old age" financial benefits (Old-Age Reserve Account financial benefits), financial aid to the blind and to dependent and crippled children, state public health services, and other benefits, as well as formation of the Social Security Board. Despite the social benefits, the 1935 SSA did not establish healthcare benefit programs for the elderly or other citizens.

President Theodore Roosevelt had an idea for national health insurance in 1912, but the idea did not gain serious consideration until 1945, just after the conclusion of World War II, when President Harry S. Truman asked Congress to consider formation of a national health insurance fund for all Americans. He was unsuccessful in getting his health insurance bills passed at that time. The American Medical Association (AMA) lobbied against President Truman's proposal, which it labeled as "socialized medicine," and the proposal died in Congress.[12,13] It would take another 20 years for the United States to have the first national health insurance programs.

President John F. Kennedy was also unsuccessful in passing national health insurance, partly due to the AMA's continuing negative lobbying. After Kennedy's assassination, President Lyndon B. Johnson announced his determination to pass Medicare, which became law as an amendment to the SSA in 1965.

On January 4, 1965, the 89th Congress of the United States of America passed HR 6675, the Social Security Amendments of 1965, which established a hospital insurance program for citizens 65 years and older, supplementary medical benefits, an expanded program of medical assistance, disability insurance, healthcare for low-income citizens, and other programs. The amendments were signed into law by President Lyndon B. Johnson as part of his Great Society agenda on July 30, 1965. Title XVIII of the Act became known as Medicare, which included Part A (hospital insurance for the "aged") and Part B (supplemental medical insurance). Title XIX of the Act became known as *Medicaid*, which provided funding for states to finance healthcare for individuals "at or close to public assistance level" with matching federal funds.

In 1972, President Richard M. Nixon signed into law a major update to Medicare. Severely disabled individuals younger than 65 years of age, and patients with end-stage renal disease (ESRD), became eligible for Medicare coverage. The Omnibus Reconciliation Act of 1980 expanded home health services. Hospice services were added in 1982, an upper limit on a Medicare recipient's out-of-pocket expenses was added to Parts A and B in 1988, and Part C (originally known as *Medicare + Choice*, now called *Medicare Advantage*) and quality measurements were introduced. Medicare has continued to slowly evolve with additional benefits passed by various administrations over the past 50 years as described above. Medicare would be immutably improved by two other significant healthcare acts passed in 2003 and 2010.

Medicare Modernization Act of 2003

The Medicare Modernization Act (MMA) of 2003 added outpatient prescription drug benefits, in addition to other important benefits. Older citizens are more likely to have comorbidities that require multiple prescriptions, and the absence of a pharmacy benefit seems to be an obvious deficit of the SSA Amendment of 1965, which included optional outpatient prescription drug benefits for Medicaid but not for Medicare recipients. This was corrected in 2003, when the MMA (Medicare Part D, outpatient drug benefits) was passed. Part D also required Medicare plans to provide Medicare Therapy Management (MTM) Program services to all recipients, and interventional individualized pharmacotherapy counseling, to specific Medicare recipients, based on the number of targeted medical conditions, the number of Part D prescriptions, and the total Part D prescription annual drug spend.

Today, Medicare covers almost 70 million Americans, about 60 million over 65 years of age, and about 10 million severely disabled, younger recipients who are also Medicaid-eligible ("dual eligible"). Medicare also covers specific chronic, severe medical conditions, including chronic kidney disease. About 10 000 Americans turn 65 years old every day, resulting in a significant expansion of citizens in the postwar "baby boomer" generation, challenging Medicare resources and financial stability.

Patient Protection and Affordable Care Act of 2010

Finally, the Patient Protection and Affordable Care Act (PPACA; ACA) of 2010 provisions expanded Medicare benefits, improved the Part D prescription affordability, and included additional low-income subsidies. The ACA expanded access to Medicare preventive services, and is credited with an 8% increase in the diagnosis of colorectal cancer due to prevention services and lower patient cost share.[14] Medicare continues to evolve and improve, most recently by testing innovative quality measurement programs and provider reimbursement models using bundled payments and incentives for quality of care.

MEDICARE BENEFITS PARTS A, B, C, AND D

The Medicare health insurance program has been amended over the past 50 years and has added healthcare benefit services, which are categorized into 4 primary "parts." The original Medicare program from the 1965 Amendments to the SSA included Part A (hospital inpatient) and Part B (outpatient medical). Part C (Medicare Advantage) and Part D (outpatient prescription services) were added through the 2003 Medicare Modernization Act (MMA).

1. *Medicare Part A* covers inpatient hospitalizations, care in skilled nursing facilities, hospice care, and some home healthcare services. Basic Part A is available at no cost for US citizens who enroll on their 65th birthday to later. Basic Part A covers only about 80% of the costs of covered benefits; the beneficiary is responsible for personally paying the remaining 20% up to the maximum out-of-pocket amount. However, insurance companies sell Medicare supplements that cover most of the remaining 20%, although the Medicare recipient must pay monthly premiums and a portion of the costs through an affordable cost share.
2. *Medicare Part B* covers outpatient medical services (such as physician services and injectable drugs administered or supervised by physicians), medical supplies and durable medical equipment (DME), and preventive services. Part B medications are often injectable drugs administered in an outpatient clinic or infusion center, or through home healthcare services. In general, Part B covers outpatient medical services except prescriptions dispensed by pharmacies (there are exceptions). Medicare recipients pay a monthly premium for Part B services directly to Medicare, or as members of a private Medicare health insurance plan, and pay a cost share when covered benefits are accessed according to their benefit coverage. Medicare Part B prescription drug coverage is addressed in a separate section, later in the chapter.
3. *Medicare Part C* (Medicare Advantage; MA) was authorized by the 2003 MMA, and includes comprehensive inpatient and outpatient medical services, often including outpatient prescription drug benefits (Part D). These plans are referred to as *Medicare Advantage-Prescription Drug* (MA-PD) plans. Medicare plans that offered a combination of inpatient and outpatient benefits were originally known as *Medicare + Choice*. MA plans are discussed below.
4. *Medicare Part D* began with the 2003 MMA and provides outpatient prescription drug benefits. Part D drugs are generally dispensed by a pharmacy (community, mail, or specialty pharmacy), are self-administered by patients or caregivers, and may include oral, subcutaneous, inhaled, transdermal, and topical medications not requiring physician supervision. As described above, Part D benefits are often packaged with Part C as an MA-PD (Medicare Advantage-Prescription Drug) program. Part D stand-alone prescription drug benefits are also sold alone (without medical benefits) by health plans and by pharmacy benefit managers (PBMs), and are termed *prescription drug plans* (PDPs). See the section on Part D, later in the chapter.

Medicare members may select how they will obtain, and pay, for various parts. Members may enroll in free Basic Part A, and purchase a Part D PDP; they may purchase a Part C + Part D (MA-PD) plan; or they obtain Part A free, and purchase Parts B and D separate supplements. However, purchasing a MA-PD plan likely provides the most comprehensive medical and prescription drug benefit coverages at an affordable cost, especially in highly competitive Medicare enrollment areas.

Medicare Prescription Drug Benefit Summary

To summarize, Medicare provides prescription drug benefits to almost 60 million Medicare recipients through four parts:

1. *Part A* covers all drugs administered while a patient is an inpatient in a medical facility, such as a hospital.
2. *Part B* includes drugs administered under physician supervision in medical offices, outpatient infusion centers, or home healthcare services. Part B drugs are often intravenously (IV) infused medications.
3. *Part C* includes Part A comprehensive inpatient benefits and Part B outpatient medical benefits (which includes Part B drugs), and may include Part D, outpatient prescription drug benefits.
4. *Part D* provides outpatient prescription drug benefits and covers drugs generally dispensed directly to patients or caregivers through community, mail, or specialty pharmacies.

Medicare benefits continue to evolve in terms of benefits offered, provider reimbursement approaches, and expanded preventive and lifestyle programs. The competitive private Medicare insurance market, especially in high-density Medicare geographic areas, offers high-benefit and low-cost Medicare benefit program options to attract and keep Medicare beneficiaries.

MEDICARE PART B PRESCRIPTION DRUG COVERAGE AND SITE-OF-CARE MANAGEMENT

Medicare Part B covers medical services such as outpatient physician visits, diagnostic tests, and some other medical procedures; some medical supplies and equipment; and certain prescription drugs.

Part B drugs are often IV-infused medications, and the IV route of administration generally limits and dictates the site of administration or site of care. The IV route of administration generally requires physician administration (or supervision), and thus the site of care is usually a medical office, an outpatient infusion center, or a home healthcare service. Physician administration or supervision or nurse home healthcare administration generally adds provider and facility administration costs and fees, which increase total drug costs. More information on site-of-care management is presented later in the chapter.

Medicare prescription drug expenditures were 97% billion, or 16% of total Medicare expenditures of $613.3 billion in 2014. Part B drugs represent 3% of total Medicare expenditures in 2014, compared with 13% for Part D drugs.[15] Common drugs covered under Medicare Part B are as follows:

- Drugs infused through a durable medical device, such as a nebulizer or an infusion pump
- Injectable drugs for treating postmenopausal osteoporosis
- Erythropoietin by injection for end-stage renal disease or for some other types of anemias
- Blood-clotting factors to treat hemophilia
- Other injectable or infused drugs administered under the supervision of a physician
- Intravenous nutrition
- Intravenous immune globulin
- Vaccinations, including for pneumonia and hepatitis B
- Immunosuppressive drugs following a transplant
- Some oral cancer drugs
- Oral antinausea drugs related to chemotherapy
- Some home healthcare services infused drugs

Part B versus Part D coverage may be confusing. For example, the oral antinausea drug ondansetron is covered under Part B if the patient is being treated for chemotherapy or radiation-induced nausea, but under Part D for other indications as an outpatient. Medicare Part B recipients may pay 20% of the Medicare-approved cost, and a deductible may apply. Some Medicare recipients have purchased a Part B insurance supplement, or have Part B drugs covered under their comprehensive Medicare Advantage Plan, which may reduce the recipient cost share.

Site-of-Care Management

The *route of administration* (RoA) often determines the site of administration, usually termed the *site of care* (SoC). Thus, drugs with an infusion RoA generally have a SoC of an physician-supervised infusion center or medical office. Part B drugs with a SoC of an outpatient healthcare facility are generally more expensive, and health plans and PBM often attempt to move the SoC to the lowest-cost facility, such as out of a hospital-owned infusion centers, and to a community-based infusion center or a physician-staffed medical clinic. As a result, Medicare insurance companies generally try to manage the SoC as an important cost-containment strategy, and require IV administration at the lowest-cost facility in their provider network. Another tactic is to convert the patient from a Part B drug to a Part D (outpatient pharmacy–dispensed) alternative drug, such as a Part D oral or subcutaneous self-injectable pen device rather than a Part B IV infusion. For example, a Medicare plan may require the use and failure of a Part D self-injectable subcutaneous anti-tumor necrosis factor (TNF) drug for rheumatoid arthritis before infused Part B drug infliximab is authorized for coverage. See the "Managing Medicare Pharmacy Benefits" section, below. In one survey, medical and pharmacy directors of health plans and PBMs managing Part B prescription drug benefits stated that SoC management was a very high cost management priority, and in 2015, 79% of surveyed health plans use, or plan to use this management activity.[16] SoC management is a critical cost management component of specialty pharmacy benefit management for all insurance programs, and especially for Medicare to reduce the enrollee cost share.

MEDICARE ADVANTAGE (PART C)

Medicare Advantage (MA) is a comprehensive medical health insurance program that provided benefits to over 30% of Medicare beneficiaries in 2015. MA began as Medicare + Choice through the Balanced Budget Act of 1997.[17] This was the "managed" Medicare, developed and administered by private health insurance plans, such as Humana, United Health Care, Aetna, and other regional plans. Prior to Medicare + Choice "managed" Medicare plans, Medicare was financed and benefits were delivered through direct provider contracts with CMS Medicare office. This "nonmanaged" Medicare is termed "traditional" Medicare. MA programs generally offer outpatient prescription drug benefit (Part D), but many plan options exist in competitive markets.

Medicare + Choice was renamed as *Medicare Advantage* through the Medication Modernization Act of 2003. MA is a combination of Parts A and B, with inpatient, outpatient medical, home healthcare, and required preventive services. If the MA plan also includes Part D outpatient prescription drug benefits, the plan is termed a "MA-PD" plan (Medicare Advantage-Prescription Drug plan). In 2016, Medicare provided benefits to 57 million people, with about 18 million through a MA plan, with MA membership tripling from 2004-2016.[17]

Initially, Medicare + Choice was more expensive per Medicare recipient than traditional Medicare, but payment reform in the PPACA has reduced the cost of Medicare Advantage to the level of traditional Medicare. The heavy competition among MA plans causes plans to introduce added benefits and reduce premiums to gain and retain Medicare members. The PPACA also provided for bonus payments to high-quality Medicare plans on the basis of 5-Star Quality Ratings, and large Medicare plans are required to spend at least 85% of all premiums and payments on the delivery of healthcare (known as the *medical loss ratio* [MLR]).

The average Medicare beneficiary is able to select from 19 different plans, although about one-quarter of beneficiaries will have a choice of three or fewer plans, depending on geography.[18] Plans compete to gain and keep Medicare members, and often offer low or no premium plans, although cost shares have been increasing. On average, premiums increased from 2016 to 2017 by 4%, representing about one-fourth of the premium increase in commercial plans.[19] Out of a possible five stars, 41% of MA plans are rated four stars or higher in 2017 (see "Medicare 5-Star Quality Rating Program" section). In 2016, average Medicare Advantage premiums were $38, up $1.00 from 2015, but the average out-of-pocket (OoP) expenditure per recipient increased to an average of $5223, up almost $1000 over 2011. One-third of recipients were enrolled in MA-PDs with a maximum OoP expenditure.[20] In highly competitive markets, almost one-half of MA-PD plans have "zero premiums" for monthly Part B premiums.

MODERNIZATION ACT AND PART D PRESCRIPTION DRUG BENEFITS

The MMA of 2003 was signed by President George W. Bush, and added Medicare Part D, the first optional outpatient prescription drug benefit for Medicare recipients, although a few Medicare plans had previously and voluntarily offered limited (often generic only) outpatient prescription drug benefits. The Final Rule that enacted the Medicare Part D prescription drug benefit of the SSA is 42 CFR Parts 400, 4003, 417, and 423 under the Department of Health and Human Services (HHS) for Center for Medicare & Medicaid Services (CMS). The Final Rule was enacted into law on December 8, 2003 in Section 101 of Title 1 of the Medicare Prescription Drug, Improvement, and Modernization Act of 2003.[21]

Part D is a fully managed prescription drug benefit similar to employer-based programs in terms of benefit components and management strategies. Part D is a voluntary program for which Medicare recipients enroll and pay a monthly premium (some plans in competitive areas have no premiums) and usually requires recipients to pay a cost share when covered prescription benefits are accessed. Some programs require no cost share for certain generic prescriptions. Part D also added the Medicare Therapy Management (MTM) Program benefit that required Part D plans to provide individualized and ongoing comprehensive pharmacotherapy counseling for eligible Medicare recipients, based on the number of targeted medical conditions, number of Part D prescriptions, and total Part D prescription annual drug expenditure.

Medicare Part D Prescription Drug Benefit Availability

Part D is available to recipients as part of an MA-PD, or as a stand-alone prescription drug program (termed a *prescription drug plan* [PDP]) through a Medicare health insurance plan or a PBM. Health plans may sell MA, MA-PD, or PDP programs; PBMs do not offer medical benefits, and can offer only PDP programs. Organizations approved to market and sell Part D plans are often termed *Part D plan sponsors*. The average recipient has a choice of 22 PDPs in 2017 (range of 18-24 per region). There were 746 PDPs offered in the United States in 2017, down from 886 in 2016 due to consolidation or some plans leaving the market due to unprofitability. This number is about one-half of the peak number of PDPs (1875) in 2007, at the start of the Medicare Part D program.

Part D Prescription Drug Benefits

Part D prescription drug benefits include outpatient prescription drugs (drugs dispensed by community, mail, or specialty pharmacies) that are self-administered by patients or caregivers. Part D drugs include oral, self-injectable subcutaneous, inhaled, transdermal, and topical medications. Part D expenditures were almost $80 million or 13% of total Medicare expenditures of $613.3 billion in 2014. Part D costs increased substantially in 2014 when new highly effective and very expensive hepatitis C virus (HCV) medications became available. Part D HCV drug costs in March 2015 more than doubled to $864 million, in 4 months, compared to November 2014.[15]

CMS Manual System Publication 100-18, *Medicare Prescription Drug Benefit Manual*, provides a complete explanation, as well as policies and procedures of the Part D benefit. The manual is divided into several chapters. Chapter 6 describes the drug formulary requirements, and Chapter 7 describes the MTM and Quality Improvement Programs.[22]

Chapter 5 of the *Medicare Prescription Drug Benefit Manual* describes MA-PD Part D benefits. MA-PD and PDP Part D sponsors must provide "qualified" (approved by CMS) prescription drug coverage directly (by the Part D sponsor) or indirectly through a contracted entity, such as a separate Part D sponsor (eg, a contracted PBM PDP) via either of the following options:[23]

1. Standard prescription drug coverage (as described in Chapter 5, Section 20.3 of the manual), which includes both defined standard coverage (as described in Section 20.3.1) and actuarially equivalent standard coverage (as described in Section 20.3.2)
2. Alternative prescription drug coverage (as described in Chapter 5, Section 20.4 of the manual), which includes both basic alternative coverage (as described in Section 20.4.1) and enhanced alternative coverage (as described in Section 20.4.2)

Pharmaceutical Manufacturer Price Concessions

Pharmaceutical manufacturers are required a minimum 50% rebate on brand drugs covered in the coverage gap. As of 2020, Medicare recipients will pay no more than 25% coinsurance for either brand or generic drugs in the coverage gap. If plan sponsors negotiate price concessions with pharmaceutical manufacturers (discounts or rebates), these discounted costs must be passed on to Medicare recipients. Figure 1-2 illustrates the coverage gap closure schedule from the PPACA.

Marketing Medicare Part D Plans to Medicare Recipients

Medicare recipients may voluntarily enroll in a Part D plan when they initially turn 65 years of age and enroll in Medicare Part A (anytime, throughout the year), or during the annual fall open-enrollment period. Medicare recipients may also enroll in Part D anytime throughout the year if they lose their employer insurance, or have a significant change in their lifestyle or income status. Medicare Part D members may also enroll or change plans once a year during the open-enrollment period.

Medicare recipients enroll or make changes in Part D plans through the government Medicare member portal at www.medicare.gov Plan Finder webpage. Recipients may select from several plans in their zip code area that meets their affordability and drug coverage needs using the Plan Finder web tool at www.medicare.gov. Health plan and PBM Part D sponsors are required to submit accurate benefit and drug information to CMS for posting in the patient enrollment Part D portal to allow Medicare recipients to find a Part D plan in their zip code regions that meets their affordability needs by offering a low-income subsidy and that covers the recipient medications. Part D sponsors face a substantial fine if their Plan Finder information is incorrect. Market competition has

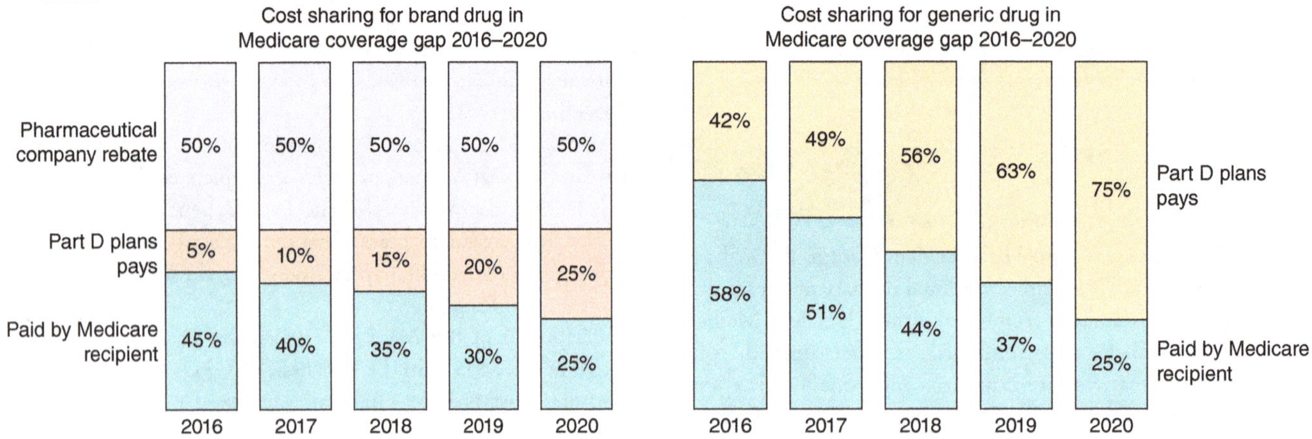

FIGURE 1-2 Cost sharing for brand and generic drugs in the Medicare Part D coverage gap (2016-2020) and coverage gap closure schedule.

Source: Kaiser Family Foundation Medicare website. Focus on Health Reform, Figure 3. Available at http://kaiserfamilyfoundation.files.wordpress.com/2013/01/8059.pdf. Accessed 2 January 2017.

driven down patient premiums, although cost shares for covered benefits have increased, as have the maximum out-of-pocket costs borne by Medicare recipients.

Medicare sponsors must also communicate their 5-Star Quality Rating program rating (see discussion below). Medicare recipients may select or change their plans during the annual open-enrollment period (during specific dates in the fall of each year). Plans of any star rating may advertise during the open-enrollment period. However, 5-Star plans may advertise throughout the year. Therefore, any citizen reaching her/his 65th birthday anytime during the year (including outside of the fall open-enrollment period) may enroll in Medicare, and because of year-around advertising, is likely to select a higher-quality 5-Star Medicare plan.

Medicare is highly regulated by CMS, which must approve all plans developed and sold by health plans and PBMs. CMS also actively monitors Part D performance and Medicare recipient satisfaction, and will fine or decertify Part D members or plans that do not comply with regulations or have shown consistently poor performance.

Part D PDP Plans and Premiums

Medicare Part D enrollment is optional and voluntary. Medicare recipients may select one of several options in their geographic regions. There are 746 PDPs in the United States in 2017, with an average of 22 PDPs per region (34 total regions). SilverScript Choice, sponsored by the PBM CVS Caremark, is the largest single PDP, with over 4 million members (20.6% of the total PDP enrollment).[24] The AARP Medicare Rx Preferred PDP (enhanced plan) has 3.14 million members (15.6% of the total), and the AARP Medicare Rx Saver (basic plan) has over 1 million members. Three Humana PDPs (Preferred Rx basic, Humana-Walmart Rx (basic), and the Humana Enhanced) include 4.6 million members.[25]

Medicare recipients usually pay a monthly Part D subscription fee (premium) that is contingent on the richness of plan benefits and market competition. Certain highly competitive areas (eg, Florida) may have zero-dollar premiums to attract members. The average national PDP premium in 2017 is estimated to be $42.17 per month, but this is highly variable (ranging from $0.00 to over $100 per month), depending on market competition and benefit richness. This represents a 9% increase in the average premium in 2017 over 2016. The Humana-Walmart Rx PDP has the lowest premiums in most regions ($16.81 per month) in 2017; 16% of recipients pay a monthly premium of less than $20, 37% pay $20 to $40, 44% pay $40 to $100, and 3% pay $100 or more per month premium. Compared to 2016, 25% of all Medicare Part D enrolled experienced a decrease in premium (competitive market areas with high Medicare-eligible members) and 65% experience a premium increase.[25]

Low-income subsidies (LISs) are available for recipients who will pay no or low premiums. 33% of LIS recipients pay zero premiums, 13% pay $1 to <$20, 24% pay $20 to $40, and 22% pay $100 or more. Recipients selecting Part D plans with enhanced benefits (richer than that required standard benefit) will pay an average of $57.13 monthly premium.

The Defined Standard Benefit Levels

The standard Part D prescription drug plan structure includes 4 levels or phases, as described below. Medicare recipients move through the levels according to the total Medicare-eligible drug expenditure and the true out-of-pocket (TrOoP) expenditure by Medicare recipients during the contract period (typically annually).

The following four Part D benefit levels are described in the CMS Part D manual, Chapter 5, Section 20.3.1:

1. The 2017 standard average annual PDP deductible is $400. The deductible is paid by the Medicare enrollees, and then the individual enrollee pays a 25% coinsurance for actual covered costs above the annual deductible.
2. The coinsurance is the initial coverage limit ($3700 in 2017).
3. Coinsurance is required within the coverage gap, which changes each year until 2020, when the coinsurance will be fixed 25% for all drugs. In 2015, the brand drug coinsurance was 40% and the generic drug coinsurance was 51%; the coinsurance on both brand and generic drugs will be 25% by 2020.
4. Catastrophic coverage with nominal cost-sharing (5% in 2015) begins once a recipient's TrOOP for covered drugs exceeds the annual OoP threshold ($4950 in 2017).[26]

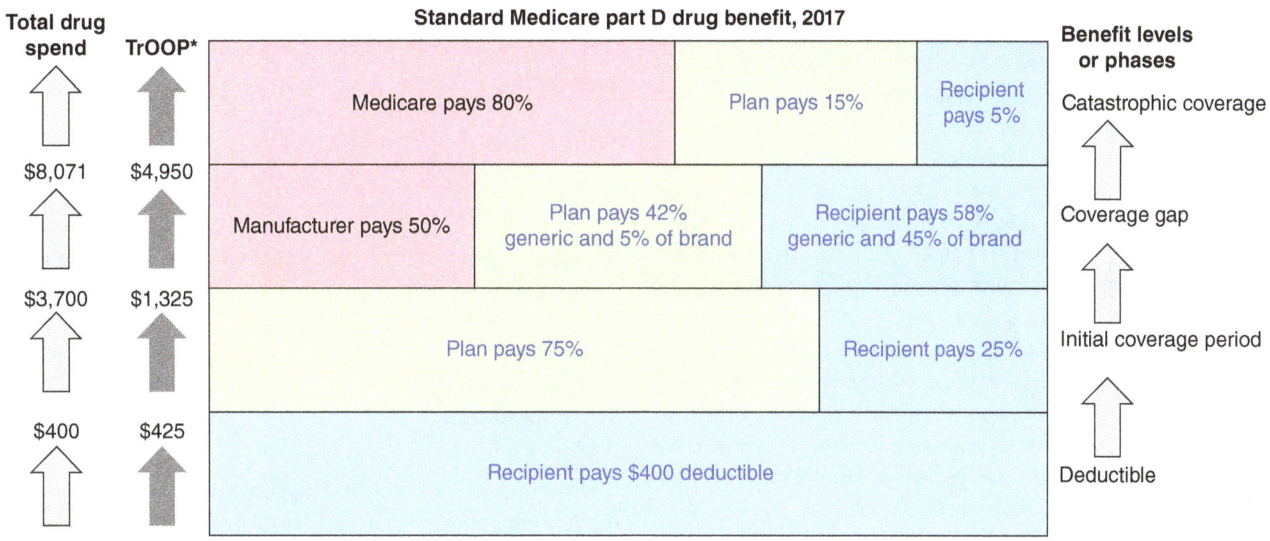

FIGURE 1-3 Standard Medicare Part D drug benefit, 2017.
* True out-of-pocket enrollee expenditures on eligible Part D drugs. At $4,950 of TrOOP, the enrollee enters catastrophic coverage.
Source: Kaiser Family Foundation. Medicare webpage. The Medicare Part D Prescription Drug Benefit, Figure 5. Available at http://kff.org/medicare/fact-sheet/the-medicare-prescription-drug-benefit-fact-sheet/. Data source: CMS Medicare Part D benefit, 2017. CMS Medicare Prescription Drug Benefit Manual. Available at https:// www.cms.gov/Regulations-and-Guidance/Guidance/Manuals/downloads/Pub100_18.pdf. Accessed 1 January 2017.

Figure 1-3 illustrates the phases (or levels) of the Medicare Part D Standard Defined Benefit and the total spend and recipient TrOOP spend that determines the benefit level of the recipient.

Actuarial Equivalence of Plans

Part D sponsors may offer variations to the standard coverage, but plan modifications must have actuarial equivalence (AE) as determined by the CMS.[26] Variations may include the annual deductible, prescription cost share, coinsurance for drugs in the coverage gap and in catastrophic coverage, and if all costs borne by Medicare recipients are actuarially equivalent. The concept of actuarially equivalent means that the recipient will, on average, pay no more than using the standard CMS Part D benefit and, on average, have similar benefit richness. Usually, variations in coverage can be no more than the costs provided in the standard coverage, or benefits at least as rich as in the standard coverage. For example, plan sponsors can offer copayments and coinsurance lower than the standard coverage. Actuarially equivalent benefits can be less expensive, or have greater benefits to the recipient than the standard benefit, but cannot be more expensive or have more restrictive benefits compared with the standard coverage.

A deductible (which must be paid out of pocket by the recipient before Part D benefit coverage begins) is included in 63% of PDPs programs, down from 67% in 2016. This is an example of the AE flexibility among PDP programs to improve the richness (or lowering costs) above the Standard Defined PDP Benefit. The standard Part D deductible is $400 in 2017 (included in 48% of PDPs), a $40 increase over 2016. However, PDP programs with no or very low deductibles often make up for costs in prescription high cost shares. Therefore, nearly 50% of Part D enrollees are in plans that are increasing their deductibles. About 15% of enrollees have a deductible less than the $400 average deductible.[27]

Common methods that plan sponsors use to enhance benefits, that satisfy actuarial equivalence, are to offer a zero-dollar copayment for generic drugs, to waive the deductible for generic drugs, and to offer reductions in cost-sharing in the coverage gap. The PPACA calls for closure of the coverage gap enrollee cost share by 2020. At that time, enrollees will pay 25% cost share for both brand and generic drugs. Pharmaceutical manufacturers must pay a minimum 50% rebate to have brand drugs covered in the coverage gap.

True Out-of-Pocket (TrOOP) Costs

The amount of total out-of-pocket costs paid by Medicare recipients for Part D–eligible prescription drugs is added from the first day of the beginning of the contract period (such as January 1 of a renewing annual contract). The running total of these out-of-pocket costs for eligible Part D drug expenses (TrOOP) determine when a recipient moves to a higher benefit phase within the Medicare Part D benefit structure. TrOOP costs include the annual deductible and prescription cost sharing, but not the monthly premium (if any). Cash payments for drugs not Medicare eligible are not included in the TrOOP. The TrOOP benefit level threshold amounts may change from year to year as determined by CMS, and are lower for recipients receiving low-income subsidies.

As shown in Figure 1-3, when the total Medicare-eligible drug spend reaches $3700, the enrollee enters the coverage gap, and has a 40% coinsurance for brand drugs (decreasing to 25% in 2020). This often leads to poor adherence due to lack of affordability. When the total Medicare drug spend reaches $8071, the recipient enters catastrophic coverage, and pays 5% coinsurance. This is a $556 increase in total expenditure over 2016. Although 5% cost share seems a small percent, patients who reach the coverage gap often have serious or multiple diseases that require expensive specialty medications. In addition to other healthcare and lifestyle costs, 5% of a $5000/month drug ($250 cost share) may be a barrier to affordability and adherence. The dollar amounts for Medicare benefit levels may change each year. For example, the deductible for 2018 has increased from $400 to $405, and the initial coverage limit has increased from $3700 to $3750.[28]

Part D Drug Formulary Structure and Cost Share

Part D sponsors develop and management drug formularies similar to commercial formularies in general management approach, structure, use of cost shares, and use of prescribing and dispensing edits, limitations, and restrictions. The drug formulary drug inclusions and management approaches must be approved by CMS prior to use. Typically, plan sponsors submit their initial formularies to CMS in the spring preceding the calendar year of use. CMS returns the formulary to the plan with approval or recommendations for remedy, and the plan sponsor can make final edits or additions in the fall before the contact period. The formulary is approved prior to fall open enrollment and is accurately loaded into the www.medicare.gov Plan Finder webpage to avoid a compliance violation and fine. Medicare PDP drug formularies usually have four to seven tiers, with a five-tier plan the most common for the initial coverage period. The five tiers and common cost share amounts are illustrated in Figure 1-4.

Plan sponsors use a Pharmacy & Therapeutics (P&T) Committee process similar to commercial P&T Committees, except that the Medicare Committees must include a physician and a pharmacist who are experienced in caring for the disabled or elderly, or include a geriatrician. The committee must review a new drug within 90 days of being on the open market, although a final formulary coverage decision may be delayed for another ≤90 days (180 days total before a final P&T Committee decision on a new drug).

Medicare Part D program P&T Committees must meet regularly to review new and current formulary drugs and make decisions on the basis of scientific evidence and pharmacoeconomic considerations. All meeting actions must be documented. CMS generally does not allow drug removals from the formulary other than at contract renewal (eg, January 1) unless there is a clinical reason to do so, although plan sponsors may add a drug anytime during the contract period.

Part D drug formularies must observe *US Pharmacopeia* and cover at least two chemically distinct drugs in each therapeutic category (if two are available) and cover dosage forms commonly used in long-term-care facilities. Plan sponsors may use a tiered formulary structure, variable cost shares, step edits, prior authorization (PA), quantity limits, maximum allowable cost (MAC) lists, and other reasonable edits. All edits, restrictions, and limitations must be approved by CMS. Plan sponsors may use more than one formulary if they are substantially different and approved by CMS.

High-cost drugs (eg, specialty drugs) may be managed but not excessively restricted. Sponsors may implement quantity limits and other reasonable controls on opioid products as safety edits.

Formulary Tier	Drug Type	Cost Share Example
Tier 1	Preferred (lowest-cost) generic drugs	$2 copay
Tier 2	Nonpreferred (higher-cost) generic drugs	$7 copay
Tier 3	Preferred (medium-cost) brand drugs	$40 copay or 20% coinsurance
Tier 4	Nonpreferred (higher-cost) brand drugs	40% coinsurance
Tier 5	Specialty and highest-cost drugs	25%-33% coinsurance

FIGURE 1-4 Example of a five-tier Medicare Drug Formulary and cost share examples.

Plan sponsors may use specialty drug tiers with a maximum of 25% coinsurance (or ≤33%) for sponsors with decreased or no deductible.

Formulary-Protected Classes

Part D formularies must include "all or substantially all" drugs in the following six classes:[29]

1. Immunosuppressants (for prophylaxis of organ transplant rejection)
2. Antidepressants
3. Antipsychotics
4. Anticonvulsants
5. Antiretrovirals
6. Antineoplastics

Coverage of all or most drugs in these classes is required to ensure that Medicare beneficiaries using drugs in these classes will not be discouraged from enrolling in Part D plans and to ensure continuity of therapy for vulnerable patient subgroups. Medicare explains "substantially all" as meaning all drugs and unique dosage forms in these six classes. Part D plans may use formulary edits (eg, step edits and PAs), but not to steer recipients away from the drugs that they have been taking or drugs that are required. In general, step edits and PAs are not widely used for HIV/AIDS drugs; plans are encouraged to be conservative in use of dispensing edits for patients taking drugs within these six classes.

Part D Excluded Drug Coverage

Medicare excludes certain drugs from Part D coverage, including drugs for weight loss or weight gain (except that drugs for AIDS wasting are not excluded); drugs for cosmetic purposes (eg, hair growth); nonprescription cough and cold drugs; drugs used to treat erectile dysfunction; multivitamins; and OTC smoking cessation drugs.[30]

MEDICARE MEDICATION THERAPY MANAGEMENT (MTM) PROGRAMS

The 2003 MMA authorized the requirement for Part D program sponsors to establish an MTM program to optimize therapeutic outcomes for targeted Medicare beneficiaries by improving medication use, reducing adverse drug events and interactions.[31] Additionally, MTM programs are expected to improve beneficiary medication understanding and appropriate use, increase adherence, and periodically reassess high-risk patients who satisfy one of three criteria: number of Medicare drugs used, total Medicare drug spend, and number of targeted medical conditions. CMS provides an annual Fact Sheet review of MTM criteria, activity, and outcomes.[32] A *comprehensive medication review* (CMR) is the process and report used to document MTM interventions and plans, which includes a portion of the individualized CMR provided to the beneficiary. A CMR is updated with subsequent MTM interventions leading to interactive, dynamic medication care plans for beneficiaries and their healthcare providers. The ACA includes amendments to the MTM process with minimum requirements for an annual CMR, and provides for a standardized format for MTM documents to improve the quality and consistency of MTM interventions and CMRs. MTMs may be performed by pharmacists or other appropriate healthcare professionals, depending on the intensity and frequency of MTM beneficiary interventions, CMS provides for reimbursement.

MEDICARE 5-STAR QUALITY RATING PROGRAM

The CMS developed the Parts C and D Star Quality Rating Program to measure, promote, and improve the quality of care for Medicare beneficiaries. The 5-Star Rating program provides an objective, transparent process to rank and rate the quality of care offered by Medicare plans, and assist beneficiaries in comparing and selecting their Medicare plan. The Star Rating program supports the CMS' Quality Strategy of optimizing health outcomes by improving quality and transforming the healthcare system. The CMS Quality Strategy goals reflect the six priorities described in the National Quality Strategy, which include the following:[33]

1. Safety
2. Person- and caregiver-centered experience and outcomes
3. Care coordination
4. Clinical care
5. Population/community health
6. Efficiency and cost reduction

Medicare plan quality ratings range from 1-Star to 5-Star (highest-quality performance). The benefit to plans for achieving high Star Ratings is to compare their quality ratings with other plans, receive a financial incentive from CMS (up to 5% of Medicare revenue), and attract Medicare beneficiaries to their plan. High-quality 5-Star plans may advertise to the public throughout the year, whereas other plans may advertise only during the fall open-enrollment period. Therefore, individuals achieving 65 years of age anytime during the year may sign up for Medicare and are more likely to be aware of, and select, a 5-Star plan. Over the past few years, CMS has eliminated financial incentives for lower star plans (less than 4-Star), and plans not improving a low Star Rating over time may be terminated from Medicare participation. CMS periodically publishes updates to the Star Rating Program Technical Notes,[34] as well as lists of Rating and Displays measures.[35] CMS collects Stars measure data from four data sources:

1. Medical and prescription drug plans
2. CMS contractors (data and research entities)
3. Survey of Medicare beneficiary experiences
4. CMS administrative data

5-Star Quality Rating Data Sources and Measurement Domains

CMS has identified, and collects measurement data, for specific quality domains that reflect different opportunities for Medicare beneficiaries to receive high-quality healthcare. The number of domains and constituent measures within each domain is adjusted by CMS periodically, and is specific to plan type and Medicare services included. To receive a domain rating, a plan must meet or exceed the minimum number of rated measures required for the domain.

The Star Rating program includes ≤47 measures in nine care domains. The number of measures applicable depends on the type of Medicare insurance product. For example, PDPs are measured in four domains with a maximum of 15 measures. MA-PD programs include all nine domains with a maximum of 47 measures, 44 of which are unique (see discussion below). Plan performance in the measures is used to calculate the organization's overall Medicare 5-Star Quality Rating. There is a 2-year lag in data collection and measurement, and Star Ratings published in 2018 will reflect plan performance using 2016 data.

Health plan overall Star Ratings measure healthcare services in five domains:[34]

1. Staying healthy: screenings, tests, and vaccines
2. Managing chronic (long-term) conditions
3. Member experience with health plan, primarily Consumer Assessment of Healthcare Providers & Systems (CAHPS) survey results[36]
4. Member complaints and changes in the health plans' performance
5. Health plan customer service

The Medicare Part D Prescription Drug Plan (PDP) is measured on four domains:[37]

1. Drug plan customer service
2. Member complaints and changes in their drug plan's performance
3. Member experience with plan's drug services
4. Drug safety and accuracy of drug pricing

Measures are assigned different weighting according to their importance as a quality indicator. Measures weighted as 3 have triple the rating value of a measure with a weight of 1.

Medicare Part D 5-Star Quality Rating Medication Measures

The Quality Rating includes several measures specifically intended for prescription drug use and outcomes, and the experience of Medicare recipients when they access prescription drug benefits. The Pharmacy Quality Alliance reports these 2016 measures as follows:[38]

1. High-risk medications (HRMs; drugs that should not be administered to the elderly) have a weight of 3, and plans with low use of drugs on the Beers List are rated more highly. HRM has been on and off the display measure list (CMS considers the Beers criteria for potentially inappropriate medication use in older adults[39] ("Beers List") when developing the HRM list).
2. Medication adherence for certain oral drugs each have a weight of 3
   a. Renin angiotensin system antagonists ("ACEs and ARBs")
   b. Drugs to reduce hypercholesterolemia ("statins" primarily)
   c. Antidiabetes medications (insulin excluded)
3. MTM comprehensive medication review (CMR) completion rate with a weight of 1

Medication adherence is measured by calculating the proportion of days covered (PDC), as shown in the Pharmacy Quality Alliance website.[40] CMS recognizes a Medicare beneficiary as fully adherent if the PDC is ≥80%. Therefore, beneficiaries who are adherent to specifically included chronic care medications (listed above) and are at last 80% adherent are counted as "adherent" for Star Ratings calculations. As the drug adherence measures are weighted as 3, plans and PBMs dedicate enormous resources in patient adherence interventions to improve adherence measurements.

Pharmacist-directed adherence improvement interventions commonly include brand-to-generic switches, prescription synchronization, conversion from a 30-day to a 90-day supply (through community or mail service pharmacy), distribution of free "pillboxes," automated reminder phone calls, and a combination of interventions based on specific beneficiary needs learned during in-person telephone motivational interviews. Plans and PBMs develop internal adherence intervention programs, or may contract with an external entity, such as a MTM company, a PBM (for plans), provider chain pharmacies, and often use a combination of intervention programs. Plans, PBMs, and other entities involved in adherence interventions often use predictive analytical programs that assess past beneficiary prescription history data to predict patients for whom adherence interventions are most appropriate, such as providing positive feedback to adherent members to continue their behavior, or identify and intervene with nonadherent members. Chronically nonadherent members, who, by July of a measurement period have missed four refills, and have no chance of reaching 80% adherence for the measurement period, may be ignored as not salvageable. Intervention resources are directed to Medicare recipients who are adherent, or are mostly already adherent, and will contribute to a positive Star adherence for the measurement period.

Stars Display Measures

The CMS system also introduces "test" measures, termed "Display Measures." Performance for Display Measures are collected, but only for research purposes, and do not contribute to the organization quality measurement rating. CMS may transition a Display Measure to a regular active measure from one year to the next, and may retire an active measure and move it to a Display Measure or eliminate the measure from the quality rating program. For example, the MTM CMR completion rate was a Display Measure and is now transitioned to a full measure with a weight of 1. High-risk medications (HRMs) use was an active measure, but CMS announced that this measure will be retired to a Display Measure in 2018.

CMS announced the following 2018 Display Measures as the following:[41]

1. Asthma measures
2. Formulary administration analysis
3. High-risk medications (HRMs)
4. Drug-drug interactions (DDIs)
5. Antipsychotic use in persons with dementia
6. Use of opioids from multiple providers and/or at high dosage in persons without cancer
7. Statin use in persons with diabetes

In summary, the Medicare 5-Star Quality Rating program provides competition and incentives for plans to continuously improve the quality of care for Medicare beneficiaries, and holds Medicare plan sponsors accountable for their care provided to their Medicaid members through their participating physicians, hospitals, pharmacies, and other healthcare providers. Each year the Star Rating measure sets evolve toward being more responsive to measuring quality of care.

MANAGING MEDICARE PHARMACY BENEFITS

Medicare prescription drug benefit coverage is complex and dynamic. CMS periodically publishes *Advance Notice of Methodological Changes* for various Medicare programs.[41] These notices, termed "Call Letters," provide a proactive notification by CMS of the planned changes in Medicare programs. For example, some changes in the CMS 2018 Advance Call Letter included updates in the methodology for calculating quality bonus payments and reimbursement rates for Parts C and D, Part D benefit structure, Part D risk-sharing, beneficiaries' subsidies, prescription drug benefit coverage gap coinsurance, and other benefit and payment changes.

As with all health insurance programs, Medicare is highly regulated, and all programs, fees, and reimbursements are subject to CMS oversight and approval. Pharmacists practicing in Medicare plans and PDPs develop and manage the Medicare prescription drug benefit (through Part C or Part D) using standard prescription drug management strategies used for commercial pharmacy programs, but developed to meet or exceed all CMS Medicare benefit compliance requirements. General pharmacy management strategies are summarized in Figure 1-5.

Community Pharmacy Practice and Medicare Beneficiaries

Pharmacists practicing in committee pharmacies will encounter Medicare beneficiaries, and will rely on the pharmacy management online real-time claims adjudication system to provide accurate information for specific Medicare beneficiary drug eligibility and successful claims adjudication. The computer system will provide up-to-date guidance for dispensing pharmacists on cost share, if any, to be collected from the beneficiary, as well as coverage guidance from the claims processor (usually a PBM) on beneficiary and drug coverage eligibility, and other necessary coverage information. Medicare MTM also provides an opportunity for pharmacists as a professional practice option and a source of additional income and patient loyalty. As the number of US citizens eligible for Medicare enrollment increases, pharmacists and other healthcare professionals must be increasingly capable

Pharmacy Benefit Management Strategy	Strategy Objectives
1. Benefit design specific for Medicare	Manage access; control costs and utilization
2. Community, mail, and specialty pharmacy network	Provide access and control costs
3. Online, real-time claims adjudication	Enforce eligibility and formulary controls
4. Tiered drug formulary with mandatory generics	Manage utilization, manage and share costs
5. Manufacturer price concessions	Manage drug costs and access
6. Clinical quality assurance programs, MTM	Optimize drug outcomes and patient health

FIGURE 1-5 Standard pharmacy benefit management strategies and objectives.

of providing the best, most appropriate care, and in conformance with complex and continually evolving CMS Medicare benefit regulations.

ACCOUNTABLE CARE ORGANIZATIONS

The ACA established *shared savings programs* (SSPs) as an important movement toward provider reimbursement and quality improvement reformation. The CMS programs stimulate the provider reimbursement mechanism from fee-for-service to a quality or outcomes-based reimbursement and incentive model. Shared savings programs later became known as *accountable care organizations* (ACOs). The ACOs, as briefly described in the ACA, were specifically intended for Medicare providers, although the "accountable care" reimbursement models are being implemented by health insurance plans for non-Medicare programs. In this section, only Medicare ACOs shall be discussed. SSP goals include better care for beneficiaries, better health for communities, and lower Medicare costs through innovative delivery and reimbursement models.[42] Accountable care organizations support quality performance standards that align with other CMS quality initiatives in four key domains:

1. Patient experience
2. Care coordination and patient safety
3. Preventive health
4. At-risk populations

Accountable care organizations are also aligned with Medicare electronic health record incentive programs, physician value modifiers, and the physician quality reporting system. All related activities improve the ability of ACO providers to have access to necessary data at the point of care, and change practice patterns based on incentives to achieve the best-quality patient outcomes. Accurate point-of-care patient information, incentivized reimbursement, and quality-based treatment protocols all contribute to improving the quality of care, reducing cost, and increasing provider reimbursement.

The ACA and CMS describe ACOs as groups of physicians and other healthcare professionals providing care to a minimum of 5000 Medicare beneficiaries, who apply to become a CMS-approved ACO. In 2017, CMS reported 480 ACOs were providing care to 9 million assigned beneficiaries in 50 states, Washington DC, and Puerto Rico.[43] ACOs are not Medicare health insurance plans, but are innovative incentive-based reimbursement models for Medicare providers who pay to participate in various Medicare health and prescription drug insurance programs.

Accountable care organizations are shared-risk models to incentivize ACO providers to provide high-quality and cost-efficient care. The ACOs share financial risk and savings with CMS according to defined performance requirements within risk corridors. CMS offers ACOs two risk-sharing options. Option 1 is a one-sided risk model where an ACO may receive shared savings if it meets performance requirements, but will not be liable for any shared losses. Option 2, a two-sided model, provides for a greater upside shared benefit or savings, but also includes sharing in potential financial losses with CMS.

Accountable care organizations are a form of coordinated care, and are consistent with the concept of patient-centered medical or health homes (PCMHs), a concept that has existed for over a decade.[44] The CMS Innovation Center continues to experiment and deploy new payment and service delivery models with the goals of improving patient care, more efficient healthcare resource use, and healthier communities. See the "CMS Innovation Center" section, below, for more information on the Medicare Medical Home Demonstration.[45]

Pharmacists are not specifically named as reimbursed healthcare providers in ACA ACO legislation. However, appropriate use of cost effective medications will assist ACO providers in achieving economic and patient quality of care objectives, which may result in increased financial income. Several ACOs include pharmacists specifically for this reason. One ACO reported the use of pharmacists employing MTM strategies to improve patient understanding of medications, increase adherence, and improve patient outcomes.[46]

CMS INNOVATION CENTER

The regulatory authority of CMS, and growing size of Medicare and Medicaid, provides an opportunity to guide the evolution of two of the nation's three largest health insurance programs, but also strongly influences program evolution in commercial and other healthcare delivery systems. The CMS Innovation Center (IC) tests new models of healthcare delivery and provider reimbursement to advance payment for quality outcomes, rather than traditional fee-for-service. The official mandate of the IC was to develop "'innovative payment and service delivery models to reduce program expenditures'...while preserving or enhancing the quality of care" for recipients of Medicare, Medicaid, or the Children's Health Insurance Program (CHIP).[47]

The Innovation Center mandate was authorized by Section 1115A of the SSA to develop and test novel quality payment and service delivery models. The Innovation Center is involved in implementing the Quality Payment Program as part of the Medicare Access and CHIP Reauthorization Act of 2015 (MACRA) to replace Medicare's Sustainable Growth Rate formula with incentive payments for providers participating in advanced alternative payment models (APMs) by which clinicians accept some risk for their patients' quality and cost outcomes and other criteria.

The PPACA authorized the Medicare shared savings programs (ACOs), which allow ACOs to accept upside or up/downside risk. Most recently, in 2015 Congress authorized CMS to implement an innovative physician reimbursement model to be implemented starting in 2017 and expanded through 2019. The new program, the Medicare Access and CHIP Reauthorization Act of 2015 (MACRA) updates physician fee schedules, a merit-based incentive payment system (MIPS), and introduces new alternative payment models (APMs). MACRA, ACOs, and other innovated bundled payments have the potential to significantly change the manner in which Medicare programs are financed, but more importantly, as Medicare providers and ACOs are partially reimbursed with performance incentives, their approach to selecting and utilizing procedures, programs, devices, and drugs may shift to consider not only cost alone, but medical resource long-term value, or economic utility, in terms of total costs, patient satisfaction, clinical, and economic outcomes.

MACRA describes expanding reimbursement for other healthcare professionals, but does not specifically include pharmacist reimbursement. CMS and MACRA include two measures that recognize the role of pharmacists: postdischarge medication reconciliation quality measures, and population-based clinical practice improvement activities (CPIAs). Overall, MACRA is another bold step toward value-based care. Physicians understand that appropriate use of cost-effective medications will contribute to cost-efficient and high-quality patient outcomes, which, theoretically, should contribute to improve provider reimbursement. Pharmacists play a natural role in selecting cost-effective drugs for Medicare and other program formularies, and by working with provider groups, contribute to CMS Innovation Center economic and quality of care goals.[48]

CONCLUSION

In summary, Medicare is a critical publicly sponsored health insurance program for approximately 70 million citizens, or over 20% of the population. Medicare continues to evolve and additional benefits are included to improve access, care affordability, and healthcare outcomes, but also test innovative reimbursement models to encourage providers as well as recipients to pursue the most cost-effective use of medical resources. As the population ages, Medicare will continue to grow and increase its importance. Because of the novel policies from the CMS Innovation Center, and CMS oversight and compliance enforcement, healthcare plans, and PBMs providing Medicare programs often implement similar benefit and reimbursement procedures for their commercial and exchange populations. Therefore, the influence and importance of Medicare exceed those of the current 70 million beneficiaries. Medicare has an unknown but broad influence over the entire US healthcare financing and delivery system.

MEDICAID

INTRODUCTION TO MEDICAID

Medicaid is one of the largest health insurance programs in the United States, providing healthcare benefits for almost 70 million recipients in 50 states and 4 US possessions and territories. Medicaid is the nation's primary health insurance program for low-income individuals and families, including children, pregnant women, adults without children, and individuals of all ages with severe disabilities. About 10 million Medicaid recipients are also eligible for Medicare benefits because of severe disabilities (dual-eligibility recipients). Medicaid provides health insurance to more than 32 million children, 20 million nonelderly adults (including parents), 7 million elderly adults, and more than 10 million individuals with disabilities. About 50% of Medicaid recipients are children.

Medicaid is primarily a state-administered and funded program, with some federal funding and CMS oversight. States establish and administer their own Medicaid programs and determine the type, amount, duration, and scope of services within broad federal guidelines. Federal law requires certain mandatory Medicaid benefits, including hospital services, outpatient physician services, diagnostic services, and home healthcare. States may augment the federally mandated benefits with prescription drug benefits, physical therapy, occupational therapy, and other services. Therefore, unlike the single Medicare benefit applied to all Medicare plans, individual state Medicaid programs may vary in the benefits covered, and healthcare delivery system that provides the services. States also vary in the income requirements (percent of the *federal poverty level* [FPL]) and duration of eligibility of Medicaid recipients.

DEVELOPMENT, EVOLUTION, AND EXPANSION OF MEDICAID

Medicaid was authorized by Title XIX of the SSA of 1965 along with Medicare. Medicaid has been continuously updated and amended at the federal level, such as mandated minimum benefits, pharmaceutical manufacturer rebate sharing, and federally funded expansion through the 2010 PPACA. Although the CHIP was enacted separately 35 years after the formation of Medicaid, the CHIP has become functionally related to Medicaid programs. The CHIP provides federal matching funds to states to provide coverage to children in families with incomes too high to qualify for Medicaid, but who cannot afford private insurance coverage, up to at least 200% of the FPL.

The Center for Medicaid and CHIP Services (CMCS) is the center for all national program policies and operations related to Medicaid, the CHIP, and the Basic Health Program (BHP).[49] The BHP was enacted as part of the ACA and provides states options to develop benefits for low-income individuals as an alternative to purchasing lower-cost insurance through the Health Insurance Marketplace (Insurance Exchange). BHP is forecast to expand as previously uninsured individuals seek insurance, and realize that Exchange programs are much more expensive, despite the low-income subsidies.

The 2009 Children's Health Insurance Program Reauthorization Act (CHIPRA) increased children's coverage by expanding coverage eligibility and improving the administrative processes, and included coverage for uninsured pregnant women, and provided financial resources for states to continue providing benefits to low-income children. Also, CHIPRA authorizes the Connecting Kids to Coverage national campaign to expand community awareness to this Medicaid health insurance benefit option. CHIRPA was reauthorized in 2015.[50]

Through the federal funding available in the ACA, 31 states and the District of Columbia have expanded their Medicaid programs, which have grown Medicaid by 17 million recipients, mostly working families, including 3 million children. Medicaid expansion helped reduce the percent of uninsured Americans to <9% in 2016 (about 28 million people). The ACA also helped standardize Medicaid eligibility requirements among states, including expanding coverage for low-income adults with incomes of ≤133% of the FPL in 2014. As a result, many states consider Medicaid as the de facto health insurance program for individuals and families that do not quality for other insurance programs and meet income or disability eligibility requirements (below 138% of the FPL in 2017).[51]

Medicaid will continue to evolve and expand because of new legislation and successful demonstration projects within the states that identify more efficient delivery systems of providing care access and program financial viability.

MEDICAID BENEFITS AND PROGRAMS

Medicaid is a federal-state partnership originally established as a health insurance program established initially for low-income individuals and children and families and disabled individuals. Many states had eligibility requirements requiring periodic eligibility reverification, causing Medicaid to be health insurance for individuals temporarily without access to employer health insurance, as well as long-term disabled beneficiaries and children. Medicaid has undergone continual evolution, especially through the PPACA, which increased benefit mandates, and provided federal funds to incentive states to expand Medicaid eligibility. In these 31 expansion states, Medicaid has grown through temporary federal funding, which gradually diminishes as states accept the financial burden to pay for expanded Medicaid programs. PPACA Medicaid expansion is discussed below.

The relationship between federal CMS and state Medicaid administration involves establishing minimum benefits as well as funding.[52] States fund Medicaid programs through state budgets and federal medical assistance percentages (FMAPs) used to calculate matching federal funds that vary by year, state Medicaid membership and needs, and other conditions.[53]

States establish and administer their own Medicaid programs and determine the type, amount, duration, and scope of healthcare, but must do so within federal minimum benefit guidelines for states to qualify for federal funding. Federal law requires states to provide certain mandatory benefits and allows states the choice of covering other optional benefits. Mandatory Medicaid benefits include inpatient and outpatient hospital services, physician services, laboratory and diagnostic tests, and home health services, among others.[51] Optional benefits include dental services, speech and hearing disorder services, podiatry services, optometry services, hospice facilities, prosthetics, prescription drugs (although all states include some level of drug benefits), case management, physical therapy, and occupational therapy.[54] Despite the optional nature of many of these important services, many states have elected to offer most optional benefits to some degree. Alternative Benefit Plans (ABPs, discussed below) may be offered by states as an optional to standard, minimum Medicaid benefits. ABPs include additional benefit requirements, such as prescription drug coverage as part of the Essential Health Benefits (EHBs) that are mandated by Qualified Health Plans (QHPs) through the PPACA.

Medicaid programs have the option to charge beneficiaries monthly enrollment premiums according to FPL requirements, and a cost share when covered prescription benefits are accessed. For example, pregnant women and infants with family income above 150% of the FPL may be charged a monthly premium. Premiums, if any, vary by state and FPL. Prescription cost shares, if any, are typically low (eg, $1.00 to $5.00) and often for brand drugs only. Some states grant Medicaid recipients the ability to obtain the prescription if they are unable or refuse to pay the cost share. Generic drug cost shares are typically $0.00 or $1.00.

Alternative Benefit Plans (ABP) Coverage

Medicaid regulations allow states the option to establish ABPs to provide specific, alternative benefits specifically tailored to the needs of certain Medicaid population groups, such as the medically vulnerable or frail, chronic substance abusers, or other patient groups. All ABPs include the 10 EHBs as described in PPACA Section 1302(b). These 10 required essential benefits include the following:[55]

1. Ambulatory patient services
2. Emergency services
3. Hospitalization
4. Maternity and newborn care
5. Mental health and substance abuse services
6. Prescription drugs
7. Rehabilitative and habilitative services and devices
8. Laboratory services
9. Preventive and wellness services and chronic disease management
10. Pediatric services including oral and vision care

The list of alternative benefit plan delivery system and coverage requirements is substantial and allows states to customize their alternative programs on the basis of CMS guidance.[56] CMS is developing a Medicaid and CHIP quality rating system (QRS), analogous to the Medicare 5-Star Quality Rating Program, that allows states to develop their own QRS that minimally complies with CMS requirements.[57]

Basic Health Plan (BHP)

Section 1331 of the ACA provides states the option of creating a BHP, which offers healthcare benefits to low-income or individuals who are otherwise unable to purchase medical coverage through the Health Insurance Marketplace ("Insurance Exchange"). A BHP allows states to provide an alternative, affordable insurance programs to individuals with fluctuating income above and below the FPL eligibility requirements (between 133% and 200% of the FPL).[58,59] Medicaid has specific income eligibility requirements, and individuals with fluctuating incomes may have and then lose Medicaid eligibility and disrupt healthcare access and their continuity of care.

Consistent with other Qualified Health Plans (QHPs), BHPs must minimally cover the 10 EHBs, specified in the ACA, including prescription drug benefits. A state that operates a BHP will receive federal funding equal to 95% of the amount of the premium tax credits and the cost-sharing reductions that would have otherwise been provided to (or on behalf of) eligible individuals if these individuals enrolled in QHPs through the Health Insurance Marketplace.

Behavioral Health and Substance Use Services

Medicaid is the largest single payer for mental health services in the United States and is increasingly expanding mental health and substance abuse disorder services. The Mental Health Parity and Addiction Equality Act[60] provides for mental health services in Medicaid beneficiaries receiving care from Managed Medicaid programs, the state ABPs, and the CHIP. Severe mental disorders, such as schizophrenia, often prevent an individual from maintaining employment and employer health insurance, and without an income, such individuals are often homeless. Homelessness presents multiple challenges in obtaining and accessing healthcare services. Drugs related to mental health conditions are often among the most commonly prescribed drugs in Medicaid programs. The ACA has expanded the application of the Mental Health Parity and Addiction Equity Act through improved access and more substance abuse and mental health services.[61] Medicaid has provided a series of resources and informational bulletins to state Medicaid programs to address prescription opioid overdose, misuse, and addiction, which are problems within Medicaid.[62]

State Medicaid Waivers and 1115 Demonstrations

Section 1115 of the SSA provides for experimental demonstration projects to promote the fundamental objectives and principles of the Medicaid and CHIP programs through approved waivers. The demonstration projects must be budget neutral and should improve Medicaid care through expanding eligibility or services, strengthening provider networks, improving outcomes, and with cost-efficient care delivery systems.[63] Multiple examples of state's waiver and demonstration projects are available on the Medicaid website.[64]

Several states have tested or experimented with alternative delivery systems and payment options as well as innovative benefit programs. The SSA allows states to apply for waiver authority to test the cost-effectiveness of innovative programs. A list of state waivers and demonstration projects under Sections 1115 and 1915 of the SSA is available on the Medicaid website.[64] The Maine Medicaid Health Care Reform Demonstration for Individuals with HIV/AIDS is one example of an approved state Medicaid waiver.[65]

Preventive and Enhanced Medicaid Benefits

Medicaid insurance benefits include preventive benefits, including immunizations, disease and cancer screening programs, behavioral health services, and counseling on healthy lifestyle, and self-management programs. Preventive services have been expanded through the ACA to include required preventive services and vaccines without cost-sharing requirements. Medicaid offers specific benefits for children, including Early and Periodic Diagnostic and Treatment (EPSDT), dental care, youth behavior health services, and innovative approaches to provide data-driven transparency to document services and costs.[66] Additional enhanced and expanded health benefits include the Maternal and Infant Health Initiative, the Strong Start for Mothers and Newborns, CMS Text4baby pilot project, family planning services and supplies, maternal depression screening and treatment, and home visiting services.[67]

Traditional and Managed Medicaid Programs

States have traditionally contracted directly with community healthcare systems, provider groups, and pharmacies to provide Medicaid services to eligible beneficiaries. Providers were paid and reimbursed on the basis of a specific state-determined fee schedule on a fee-for-service basis. Today, almost 80% of Medicaid benefits are provided through Medicaid managed-care programs as reported by CMS.[68] Every state, except Arkansas, Connecticut, and Wyoming, provide Managed Medicaid program options. The primary motivation for the growth of Managed Medicaid is the ability of states to predictably manage costs through shared-risk arrangements with the managed-care organizations.

Socially Security Act Section 1902 provides states with authority to subcontract with state-licensed and eligible health insurance programs and health plans to provide a Medicaid managed-care program.[69] Later, PBMs were included to provide only Medicaid prescription drug benefit programs. Health plans and PBMs compete on quality of service delivery and costs to be awarded a Medicaid Managed shared-risk-based contract, which may be full- or shared-risk arrangements that allows states to budget a fixed amount to pay on a per-capita basis for Medicaid services, and allows the Medicaid Managed plan to employ standard managed-care benefit management strategies and principles to manage benefits and costs, and be in compliance with both state and federal minimum benefit and access requirements.

MEDICAID PRESCRIPTION DRUG BENEFITS

Although pharmacy coverage is an optional benefit under federal Medicaid laws, all states currently provide coverage for outpatient prescription drugs to all categories of eligible individuals and most other enrollees within their state Medicaid programs. Medicaid states publish lists of covered drugs (drug formularies) usually termed *preferred drug lists* (PDLs), which are updated from time to time to account for new-drug availability, pharmaceutical manufacturer rebate contracts, new-drug information, and brand drug patent expirations. The Medicaid Covered Outpatient Drug Final Rule was published in the *Federal Register* in 2016, although states may expand coverage or apply for waiver coverage benefits.[70]

Medicaid Preferred Drug Lists (PDLs) and Formularies

State Medicaid agencies determine the drugs eligible for Medicaid coverage through a committee of physicians, pharmacists, and other healthcare professionals. The process is similar to evidence-based drug evaluation and decision processes employed by health plans, PBMs, and other healthcare systems. States develop their own drug formularies according to data provided by their own formulary committees.

The dynamic list of covered drugs is commonly termed a *drug formulary*, or, more commonly for Medicaid programs, a PDL. The drug literature and data collection, analysis, and evaluation process is initially conducted by one or more clinical pharmacists within, or contracted by, the Medicaid agency, or the contracted health plan or PBM providing the Managed Medicaid prescription drug benefit. This preliminary analysis and recommendations are provided to the formulary selection committee (termed a *Formulary Committee* or *Pharmacy & Therapeutics Committee*). Because Medicaid is a public government program, the final drug coverage decisions are often made in formulary committee meetings open to the public, at which pharmaceutical manufacturer representatives are provided an opportunity to provide verbal testimony supporting coverage of their drugs.

PDLs reflect the prescription drug benefits needs of Medicaid recipients. For example, about 50% of Medicaid recipients are children or young adults, which require appropriate pediatric drugs, including vaccinations and antibiotics. Medicaid also provides mental healthcare to many recipients, and antidepressants, antipsychotics, and related drugs must be included in PDLs. Other commonly covered categories include drugs for HIV/AIDS, HCV, cancers, and other geographically common illnesses and disabling diseases.

States also exclude certain drugs from coverage, such as nonprescription drugs, vitamins, barbiturates, and others that may vary by state.[71]

In general, Medicaid PDLs heavily promote and prefer generic drugs whenever possible, and many states impose a PA requirement on many expensive brand drugs, high-risk specialty drugs, or drugs with an abuse potential. Medicaid programs claims over a 90% generic fill rate for covered prescriptions, typically about 5% to 10% higher than commercial generic prescription use. The concept of formulary, or PDL drugs, arrayed in "tiers" based on drug type and patient cost-share incentives, generally does not apply to Medicaid, which often offers no or a very low-cost share, and often has a single tier that includes all drugs, or a two-tier formulary (tier 1 are preferred generics, and all other drugs are on tier 2). The CMS allows states to charge prescription drug copayments of $4.00 for brand drugs for recipients at any FPL, and an $8.00 copayment for nonpreferred drugs for recipients from 100% to150% of the FPL, and a coinsurance of ≤20% of the Medicaid drug cost for recipients receiving a nonpreferred drug if they are above 150% of the FPL.[72]

Express Scripts, Inc. (the PBM for many state Medicaid programs) publishes a *National Preferred Formulary* (ie, a PDL) of the most commonly prescribed drugs that indicates no tier designation, but states, "...you are encouraged to ask your doctor to prescribe generic drugs whenever appropriate."[73] Medicaid PDLs prefer generic drugs and employ a PA to limit the use of most brand drugs.

The PA process requires a prescriber to contact the Medicaid agency (or PBM providing the pharmacy benefit) to request a patient-specific exception to use the restricted drug according to the patient's prior drug use, drug failures, and unique medical conditions. If approved, a PA must be renewed periodically, such as every 6 to 12 months. An example of PDLs of some states with the largest Medicaid enrollment and some Managed Medicaid pharmacy program providers are provided to illustrate coverage policies, and the use of tiers, cost shares, and PA restrictions:

- Florida PDL (administered by the Florida Agency for Health Care Administration)[74]
- Texas Medicaid PDL and PA criteria[75]
- New York State Medicaid PDL[76]
- California Medi-Cal PDL[77]
- Molina Healthcare of South Carolina PDL[78]
- Amerigroup PDLs for various Medicaid programs[79]
- WellCare Health Plans Kentucky Medicaid PDL.[80]
- Express Scripts, Inc. PDL Exception List[73]

Drug Utilization Review (DUR) Programs

Medicaid regulations require states to perform utilization management tools and systems to promote patient safety and monitor inappropriate or dangerous drug use. DUR programs monitor for drug interactions, drug disease contraindications, drug allergies, and other forms of drug misuse or abuse. DUR programs also monitor and identify drug fraud, and gross overuse, and medically unnecessary drug use.[81] States are required to submit a summary of their DUR activities, findings, and remedial actions to the CMS Central Office by June 30 of each year for the previous October 1 through September 30 period.[82] The CMS publishes a Medicaid state DUR summary report annually for fee-for-service (non-Managed Medicaid), although Managed Medicaid programs are also expected to comply with this DUR requirement.[83]

Branded Prescription Drug Fee Program and Manufacturer Rebates

The 2010 PPACA Section 9008 described the *Branded Prescription Drug Fee Program* (BPD), which defines the requirements for government programs, including Medicaid, to report drug sales to the Department of Treasury to accurately calculate the fees paid by pharmaceutical manufacturers on the basis of drug sales to all government programs.[84]

Pharmacies are usually reimbursed on a discounted *average wholesale price* (AWP) basis for prescription drugs dispensed through Managed Medicaid prescription drug benefit programs. CMS allows states to use alternative pharmacy reimbursement methods, such as those based on the drug *actual acquisition cost* (AAC) or *national average drug acquisition cost* (NADAC), which can fluctuate weekly.[85]

Through the Medicaid Drug Rebate Program,[86] pharmaceutical manufacturers have been required to pay rebates on drugs covered by state Medicaid programs, based on Section 1927 of the SSA.[87] At that time, manufacturers were required to pay a minimum 15.1% rebate on drugs covered in a state Medicaid program, although many manufacturers paid higher rebates to gain preferable access on the states' PDLs. Some states passed regulations requiring manufacturers to pay additional supplemental fees on top of the standard 15.1% rebate. The PPACA increased the minimum brand drug rebate to 23.1% of the average manufacturer price (AMP) on innovator drugs, 17.1% of the AMP on blood-clotting factors, and a minimum of 17.1% of drugs administered exclusively for pediatric indications, with a variable formula for new formulations of existing products ("line extensions") based on the AMP and other rebates paid on the original brand drug.[86] The Government Accountability Office (GAO) found that Medicaid paid the lowest average net prescription prices compared to the Department of Defense and Medicare due to Medicaid prescription drug reimbursement discounts, formulary controls, including maximum allowable cost on most multisource generics, and mandatory rebates on brand drugs.[88]

Approximately 600 drug manufacturers participate in the Rebate Program through a national rebate agreement with the Secretary of the Department of Health and Human Services, and must also submit product pricing data through the Medicaid Drug Data Reporting (DDR) system.[89] These rebates are paid by drug manufacturers on a quarterly basis to states, which share rebates with the federal government to offset the overall cost of prescription drugs under the Medicaid program. Manufacturers must also participate in the 340B Drug Pricing Program, which requires manufacturers to provide discounted prices to healthcare systems providing services to Medicaid and Medicare recipients, state AIDS drug assistance centers, Ryan White clinics, disproportionate share hospitals, children's hospitals, and other safety net providers.[90]

Pharmacy Medicaid Prescription Reimbursement

Pharmacies dispensing drugs for Medicaid recipients are reimbursed directly through a state provider contract for traditional, or fee-for-service Medicaid programs, usually based on a discounted *average wholesale price* (AWP; eg, AWP −16%) plus a dispensing fee, or a reimbursement calculation based on pharmacy *actual acquisition cost* (AAC) or the *national average drug acquisition cost* (NADAC), as determined on a state basis. The drug cost must be below the *federal upper limit* (FUL), if calculated for a specific drug. CMS must approve the drug pricing metrics and pharmacy reimbursement methods used.[91] Pharmacies generally favor the NADAC, which is calculated using actual pharmacy-submitted acquisition cost data, and is updated weekly to reflect market prices.[92] The *Federal Register* includes a thorough discussion on Medicaid drug price calculations, AMP, FUL, and the rebate program.[93]

Most managed prescription drug benefit drug cost calculations employ a method that calculates the drug ingredient cost reimbursement at the lower of three pricing metrics: (1) the calculated ingredient cost based on the pharmacy contract with the reimbursing entity (usually a PBM), (2) the pharmacy calculated "usual & customary" (U&C) price (price charged to noninsured cash patients), or (3) the maximum allowable cost (MAC) for multisource generic drugs calculated by the PBM. This is termed "lower of" drug ingredient cost calculation logic and is automatically determined by the processing entity (often a PBM) on the basis of the contract and data, published drug cost, and drug U&C data submitted by the pharmacy.[94] Most Medicaid agencies have issued guidance documents to pharmacies that they must include all discount programs, discount cards, and other special pricing as the pharmacy's U&C.[95]

PPACA EXPANSION OF MEDICAID AND CHIP

The Patient Protection and Affordable Care Act (ACA; Public Law 111-148) and the Health Care and Education Reconciliation Act (Public Law 111-152), both passed in 2010, together expand Medicaid coverage to millions of low-income Americans and make numerous improvements in care delivery to both Medicaid and the CHIP. Thirty-one states accepted federal funding to expand Medicaid following CMS benefit policy requirements. Federal funding will be steadily reduced. As a result, expansion states showed reductions in Medicaid expenditures in 2015 and 2016, but forecast an increase in Medicaid spending in 2017 of 5.9% (compared to nonexpansion state Medicaid program growth of 4.0%) as federal funding diminishes from 100% to 95%.[96]

The ACA extends Medicaid coverage to all individuals between ages 19 and 64 with 2017 incomes up to 138% of the federal poverty level, or $16 643 for an individual. Additionally, enrollment processes were simplified and coordinated with the Health Insurance Marketplace (Insurance Exchanges). For the first time, states can provide Medicaid coverage for low-income adults without children and be guaranteed coverage through Medicaid in every state without need for a waiver.[97]

The ACA established a new methodology for determining eligibility for Medicaid, which is based on *modified adjusted gross income* (MAGI) to determine financial eligibility for Medicaid, CHIP, and premium tax credits and cost sharing reductions available through the Health Insurance Marketplace. Through one set of income determination rules and a single application across programs, the ACA made it easier for people to apply and enroll in the appropriate program.

Other Medicaid benefit and eligibility enhancements from the ACA include the following:[98]

1. Improved and expanded eligibility, as described above
2. Federal funding for state Medicaid expansion activities (to be phased down to 90% by 2020)
3. Coordinated, single-application processes for all programs
4. Expanded minimum benchmark of Essential Health Benefits (EHBs)
5. Community-based long-term-care services
6. Quality Rating System to measure and improve quality of care
7. Expanded prevention and wellness services
8. Extended CHIP funding through 2019
9. Improved efficiency for dual-eligibility benefit coordination
10. 100% matching federal funding to increase provider reimbursement
11. Increased transparency in policies
12. Several initiatives to improve program integrity and compliance with regulations

Medicaid Expansion Impact on the Uninsured

States that expanded their Medicaid programs with federal funding under the ACA experienced increases in Medicaid enrollment, driven by enrollment of adults made newly eligible for Medicaid as well as individuals who were previously eligible but not enrolled in Medicaid. Expansion states showed a reduction in the number of uninsured individuals. Expansion states also claim reductions in uninsured hospitalizations and uncompensated care.[99]

Access to healthcare, possible by Medicaid expansion for many previous uninsured, provides many benefits beyond medical treatment. Access to healthcare alleviates individual anxiety and financial stress and provides access to disease prevention programs, vaccinations, and diagnostic tests, and social and other supportive services.

MEDICAID HEALTHCARE OUTCOMES

Medicaid provides care to almost 80 million recipients, about 50% children, vulnerable, disabled, and high-risk low-income individuals. About 70% of US physicians participate in traditional fee-for-service or Managed Medicaid programs, although more specialists than primary care physicians are likely to accept new Medicaid patients (pediatricians are more likely; psychiatrists are less likely to participate).[100] Access to necessary healthcare resources and services for Medicaid recipients is similar to access for private insurance members; however, approximately 5% of children in the Medicaid CHIP program experienced difficulty in accessing healthcare, compared to approximately 2% of children with private insurance.[101]

Access to prescription drug benefits through Medicaid expansion had a positive impact on drug access and adherence. One study found a 30% reduction in uninsured prescription users, as well as a 58% reduction in out-of-pocket personal spending on prescriptions through Medicaid.[102] Medicaid expansion and increase in coverage produced an improvement in four of eight quality measures: asthma treatment, Pap (Papanicolaou) testing, body mass index assessment, and hypertension control, but did not show an improvement in colorectal cancer screening, diabetes control, or lipid lowering in patients with coronary artery disease.[103] Another study on the impact of the Medicaid expansion on drug use and costs revealed that implementation of the expansions may have increased the number of Medicaid drug prescriptions but had no significant immediate impact on drug spending growth.[104]

CONCLUSION

Medicaid has evolved, expanded, and increased eligibility requirements, as well as mandated preventive and treatment benefits to provide healthcare access and quality at least as good as that provided by private insurance. Medicaid provides a full suite of preventive and medical treatment, pediatric and adult benefits, and special services for recipients with unique and severe healthcare needs. Medicaid may become the de facto state health insurance program for citizens, especially in expansion states, and may be a prototype of a single government payer health insurance. Medicaid prescription drug benefits heavily emphasize the use of generic drugs, even more than the private insurance, although generics drugs represent over 85% of all outpatient prescriptions dispensed. Medicaid includes specialty programs and protection for highly medically needy, medically vulnerable, and medically frail subgroups, because, by definition, Medicaid recipients have low income and may be unable to represent themselves and their unique needs. Because of the ACA, Medicaid covers over 70 million members, and is a healthcare source for individuals who do not qualify for, or cannot afford, other healthcare program options. Because of these facts, Medicaid remains an important health insurance program that will continue to expand and provide healthcare for medically vulnerable, frail, and severely disabled children and low-income individuals.

REFERENCES

1. CMS website. Available at http://cms.gov. Accessed January 17, 2017.
2. CMS. "What are the value-based programs" webpage. Available at https://www.cms.gov/Medicare/Quality-Initiatives-Patient-Assessment-Instruments/Value-Based-Programs/Value-Based-Programs.html. Accessed April 3, 2017.
3. CMS. "Medicare Part B drug average sales price" webpage. Available at https://www.cms.gov/Medicare/Medicare-Fee-for-Service-Part-B-Drugs/McrPartBDrugAvgSalesPrice/index.html?redirect=/mcrpartbdrugavgsalesprice/10_vaccinespricing.asp. Accessed April 3, 2017.
4. CMS. "Oncology care model" webpage. Available at https://innovation.cms.gov/initiatives/oncology-care/. Accessed April 3, 2017.
5. CMS. "Quality payment program" website. Available at https://qpp.cms.gov. Also "Health Affairs Blog MACRA Final Rule: CMS strikes a balance; will docs hang on?" Available at http://healthaffairs.org/blog/2016/10/17/macra-final-rule-cms-strikes-a-balance-will-docs-hang-on/. Both Accessed April 3, 2017.
6. Kaiser Family Foundation. *Analysis of the CMS Medicare Current Beneficiaries 2011 Cost and Use File and the Urban Institute and Kaiser Family Foundation Analysis, 2015.* Stated in http://kff.org/report-section/an-overview-of-medicare-issue-brief/ (Figure 1).
7. Congressional Budget Office. *Budget and Economic Outlook: 2016 to 2026, pages* 16, 67. Available at https://www.cbo.gov/sites/default/files/114th-congress-2015-2016/reports/51129-2016outlookonecol-2.pdf. Accessed August 28, 2017.
8. Kaiser Family Foundation webpage. *Health Care Reform Pulling it Together: Implementation.* Available at http://www.kff.org/health-reform/perspective/pulling-it-together-implementation/. Accessed August 28, 2017.
9. Congressional Budget Office. *Medicare June 28, 2017 Baseline.* Available at https://www.cbo.gov/sites/default/files/recurringdata/51302-2017-06-medicare.pdf. Accessed August 28, 2017.
10. Kaiser Family Foundation webpage. *The Facts on Medicare Spending and Financing, July 18, 2017, figures 3 and 4.* Available at http://www.kff.org/medicare/issue-brief/the-facts-on-medicare-spending-and-financing/?gclid=Cj0KCQjw_o7NBRDgARIsAKvAgt25jYA2GujP5O0ZJreTYS_r9DHq4Bv8YzOBKAMYndADQWE3i0UdkwgaAvf0EALw_wcB. Accessed 28 August 2017.
11. Congressional Budget Office. *Medicare June 28, 2017 Baseline.* Available https://www.cbo.gov/sites/default/files/recurringdata/51302-2017-06-medicare.pdf. Accessed August 28, 2017.
12. Navarro RP, 2016; adapted from Kaiser Family Foundation webpage, "Medicare benefit payments by type of service, 2015" (see Figure 2). Available at http://kff.org/medicare/issue-brief/an-overview-of-medicare/. Accessed December 29, 2016.
13. The *New York Times* webpage, "How Medicare was made." Available at http://www.newyorker.com/news/news-desk/medicare-made. Accessed December 27, 2016.
14. Lissenden B, Yao N. "Aaron." Affordable Care Act changes to Medicare led to increased diagnosis of early-state colorectal cancer among seniors. *Health Affairs.* 2017;36(1):101-107. Accessed March 25, 2017.
15. Kaiser Family Foundation Medicare webpage, "10 essential facts about Medicare and prescription drug spending." Available at http://kff.org/infographic/10-essential-facts-about-medicare-and-prescription-drug-spending/. Accessed December 30, 2016.
16. *EMD Serono* (biopharmaceutical division of Merck KGaA) *Specialty Digest,* 12th ed., 2016, p. 28.
17. Kaiser Family Foundation. *Medicare Advantage Fact Sheet,* May 2016. Available at http://kff.org/medicare/fact-sheet/medicare-advantage/. Accessed April 21, 2017.
18. Kaiser Family Foundation Medicare website, "Turning the spotlight on Medicare Advantage for 2017." Available at http://kff.org/medicare/press-release/turning-the-spotlight-on-medicare-advantage-for-2017. Accessed December 22, 2016.
19. Kaiser Family Foundation website, "Medicare Advantage plans in 2017: Short-term outlook is stable." Available at http://kff.org/medicare/issue-brief/medicare-advantage-plans-in-2017-short-term-outlook-is-stable/. Accessed December 22, 2016.
20. Kaiser Family Foundation webpage, "Medicare Advantage 2006 spotlight: Enrollment market update." Available at http://kff.org/medicare/issue-brief/medicare-advantage-2016-spotlight-enrollment-market-update/. Accessed December 23, 2016.
21. CMS. *Medicare Prescription Drug Benefit Final Rule.* Available at https://www.cms.gov/Medicare/Prescription-Drug-Coverage/PrescriptionDrugCovGenIn/Downloads/CMS-4068-F3Column.pdf. Accessed December 29, 2016.
22. CMS. "Medicare Part D prescription drug benefit" website. Available at https://www.cms.gov/Medicare/Prescription-Drug-Coverage/PrescriptionDrugCovContra/Downloads/Part-D-Benefits-Manual-Chapter-6.pdf. Accessed December 29, 2016.
23. CMS. *Medicare Part D Prescription Drug Benefit Manual,* Chapter 5. Available at https://www.cms.gov/Medicare/Prescription-Drug-Coverage/PrescriptionDrugCovContra/Downloads/MemoPDBManualChapter5_093011.pdf. Accessed December 30, 2016.
24. SilverScript website. Available at https://www.silverscriptonline.com/ps/2017/brand03?infinity=ict2~net~gaw~ar~171298532376~kw~silverscript~mt~e~cmp~Brand%2BUS%2BENG%2BSPART~ag~SilverScript%2BEXACT&utm_medium=cpc&click=sem&gclid=Cj0KEQiAgJTGBRDLr5_az_Ouk44BEiQAIxaA4tulifmYbFUoBCZoDfxcTxAmg99qPlYeUEm3qsMqxeUaApSj8P8HAQ&gclsrc=aw.d. Accessed March 12, 2017.
25. Kaiser Family Foundation Medicare webpage. *Medicare Part D: A First Look at Prescription Drug Plans in 2017.* Available at http://files.kff.org/attachment/Issue-Brief-Medicare-Part-D-A-First-Look-at-Prescription-Drug-Plans-in-2017. Accessed January 1, 2017.
26. CMS. *Medicare Part D Manual,* Chapter 5, Section 20.3.2, "Actuarial equivalent standard coverage." Available at https://www.cms.gov/Medicare/Prescription-Drug-Coverage/PrescriptionDrugCovContra/Downloads/MemoPDBManualChapter5_093011.pdf. Accessed January 2, 2017.

27. Kaiser Family Foundation website. *Medicare Part D: A First Look at Prescription Drug Plans in 2017.* Available at http://files.kff.org/attachment/Issue-Brief-Medicare-Part-D-A-First-Look-at-Prescription-Drug-Plans-in-2017. Accessed March 10, 2017.
28. CMS. *Medicare Advantage and Part D Advance Notice and Draft Call Letter.* Available at https://www.cms.gov/Newsroom/MediaReleaseDatabase/Fact-sheets/2017-Fact-Sheet-items/2017-02-01.html. Accessed March 12, 2017.
29. CMS. *Medicare Part D Manual*, Chapter 6, Section 30.2.5, "Protected classes." Available at https://www.cms.gov/Medicare/Prescription-Drug-Coverage/PrescriptionDrugCovContra/Downloads/Part-D-Benefits-Manual-Chapter-6.pdf. Accessed January 7, 2017.
30. CMS Medicare Part D Prescription Drug Benefit website. Available at https://www.cms.gov/Medicare/Prescription-Drug-Coverage/PrescriptionDrugCovContra/Downloads/Part-D-Benefits-Manual-Chapter-6.pdf. Accessed December 29, 2016.
31. CMS Innovation Center. "Part D Enhanced Medication Therapy Management Model" webpage. Available at https://innovation.cms.gov/initiatives/enhancedmtm. Accessed March 12, 2017.
32. CMS. *2016 Medicare Part D MTM Programs Fact Sheet.* Available at https://www.cms.gov/Medicare/Prescription-Drug-Coverage/PrescriptionDrugCovContra/Downloads/CY2016-MTM-Fact-Sheet.pdf. Accessed March 11, 2017.
33. National Quality Strategy website. Available at https://www.ahrq.gov/workingforquality/nqs/nqs2011annlrpt.pdf. Accessed March 11, 2017.
34. CMS. "2017 Medicare Part C & D Star Rating Technical Notes" webpage. Available at https://www.cms.gov/Medicare/Prescription-Drug-Coverage/PrescriptionDrugCovGenIn/Downloads/2017_Technical_Notes_preview_1_2016_08_03.pdf. Accessed March 10, 2017.
35. CMS. "Part C and D performance data" webpage. Available at https://www.cms.gov/Medicare/Prescription-Drug-Coverage/PrescriptionDrugCovGenIn/PerformanceData.html. Accessed March 10, 2017.
36. CMS. "Consumer assessment of healthcare providers & systems (CAHPS)" webpage. Available at https://www.cms.gov/Research-Statistics-Data-and-Systems/Research/CAHPS/. Accessed March 12, 2017.
37. CMS. "Pharmacy Quality Alliance" webpage http://pqaalliance.org/measures/cms.asp. Accessed 10 March 2017.
38. CMS. "Pharmacy Quality Alliance proportion of days covered as a preferred method of measuring medication adherence" webpage. Available at http://pqaalliance.org/measures/default.asp. Accessed March 10, 2017.
39. "American Geriatric Society beers criteria" webpage. Available at http://www.americangeriatrics.org/files/documents/beers/2012AGSBeersCriteriaCitations.pdf. Accessed April 4, 2017.
40. CMS. "Pharmacy Quality Alliance proportion of days covered as a preferred method of measuring medication adherence" webpage. Available at http://www.pqaalliance.org/images/uploads/files/PQA%20PDC%20vs%20%20MPR.pdf. Accessed March 10, 2017.
41. CMS. *2018 Medicare Advantage and Part D Advance Notice and Advance Call Letter.* Available at https://www.cms.gov/Newsroom/MediaReleaseDatabase/Fact-sheets/2017-Fact-Sheet-items/2017-02-01.html. Accessed March 11, 2017.
42. CMS. "Accountable Care Organizations (ACO) webpage. Available at https://www.cms.gov/Medicare/Medicare-Fee-for-Service-Payment/ACO/index.html. Accessed March 12, 2017.
43. CMS. "ACO fast facts" webpage. Available at https://www.cms.gov/Medicare/Medicare-Fee-for-Service-Payment/sharedsavingsprogram/Downloads/All-Starts-MSSP-ACO.pdf. Accessed March 11, 2017.
44. Agency for Healthcare Research and Quality (AHRQ). "Patient-centered medical home resource center" webpage. Available at https://pcmh.ahrq.gov. Accessed March 12, 2017.
45. CMS. "Medicare medical home demonstration" webpage. Available at https://innovation.cms.gov/Medicare-Demonstrations/Medicare-Medical-Home-Demonstration.html. Accessed March 12, 2017.
46. Brumel A, Lustig A, et al. Best practices: Improving patient outcomes and costs in an ACO through comprehensive medication therapy management. *J Manage Care Pharm.* 2014;20(12):1152-1158. Available at http://www.jmcp.org/doi/abs/10.18553/jmcp.2014.20.12.1152. Accessed March 11, 2017.
47. CMS. Innovation Center website. Available at https://innovation.cms.gov/. Accessed March 11, 2017.
48. Academy of Managed Care (AMCP) webpage. Joint Pharm. Org. comments to CMS on MACRA proposed rule final. Available at http://www.amcp.org/WorkArea/DownloadAsset.aspx?id=21186. Accessed March 11, 2017.
49. Medicaid program history website. Available at https://www.medicaid.gov/about-us/program-history/index.html. Accessed March 16, 2017.
50. Medicaid CHIPRA (Children's Health Insurance Program Reauthorization Act) website. Available at https://www.medicaid.gov/chip/chipra/chipra.html. Accessed April 3, 2017.
51. Medicaid. Medicaid & CHIP report. Available at https://www.medicaid.gov/medicaid/program-information/downloads/accomplishments-report.pdf. Accessed March 24, 2017.
52. CMS. Medicaid Federal Policy Guidance webpage. Available at https://www.medicaid.gov/federal-policy-guidance/federal-policy-guidance.html. Accessed March 23, 2017.
53. Assistant Secretary for Planning and Evaluation (ASPE). "Federal medical assistance percentages for federal financial participation in state assistance expenditures" website. Available at https://aspe.hhs.gov/federal-medical-assistance-percentages-or-federal-financial-participation-state-assistance-expenditures. Accessed March 23, 2017.
54. CMS. "Medicaid list of Medicaid benefits." Available at https://www.medicaid.gov/medicaid/benefits/list-of-benefits/index.html. Accessed March 23, 2017.
55. CMS. Center for Consumer Information & Oversight webpage. Available at https://www.cms.gov/CCIIO/Resources/Fact-Sheets-and-FAQs/ehb-2-20-2013.html. Accessed March 23, 2017.
56. Medicaid and CHIP Implementation Guides webpage. Available at https://wms-mmdl.cdsvdc.com/MMDLDOC/abpIG.html. Accessed March 23, 2017.
57. Medicaid and CHIP Managed Care Final Rule (CMS-2390-F), April 25, 2016. Available at https://www.medicaid.gov/medicaid/managed-care/downloads/improving-the-quality-of-care-for-medicaid-beneficiaries-fact-sheet.pdf. Accessed March 24, 2017.
58. Medicaid Basic Health Program website. Available at https://www.medicaid.gov/basic-health-program/index.html. Accessed March 16, 2017.
59. CMS. Medicaid Basic Health Program website. Available at https://www.medicaid.gov/basic-health-program/index.html. Accessed March 23, 2017.
60. CMS. The Center for Consumer Information & Insurance Oversight webpage. Available at https://www.cms.gov/cciio/programs-and-initiatives/other-insurance-protections/mhpaea_factsheet.html. Accessed March 23, 2017.
61. *Federal Register* Medicaid and Children's Health Insurance Programs, May 31, 2016, *Final Rules.* Available at https://www.federalregister.gov/documents/2016/03/30/2016-06876/medicaid-and-childrens-health-insurance-programs-mental-health-parity-and-addiction-equity-act-of. Accessed March 24, 2017.
62. CMS. *CMCS Information Bulletin.* Available at https://www.medicaid.gov/federal-policy-guidance/downloads/CIB-02-02-16.pdf. Accessed March 24, 2017.
63. *Medicaid Section 1115 Demonstrations.* Available at https://www.medicaid.gov/medicaid/section-1115-demo/about-1115/index.html; also CMS Medicaid State Waivers List website. Available at https://www.medicaid.gov/medicaid/section-1115-demo/demonstration-and-waiver-list/waivers_faceted.html. Accessed March 23, 2017.
64. CMS. Medicaid State Waivers List website. Available at https://www.medicaid.gov/medicaid/section-1115-demo/demonstration-and-waiver-list/waivers_faceted.html. Accessed March 23, 2017.
65. MaineCare Services webpage. Available at https://www.medicaid.gov/Medicaid-CHIP-Program-Information/By-Topics/Waivers/1115/downloads/me/me-hiv-pa.pdf. Accessed March 23, 2017.
66. *Federal Register* Medicaid Programs. *Methods for Assuring Access to Covered Medicaid Services*, January 4, 2016. Available at https://www.federalregister.gov/documents/2015/11/02/2015-27697/medicaid-program-methods-for-assuring-access-to-covered-medicaid-services, and, Medicaid & CHIP Report, January 2016. Available at https://www.medicaid.gov/medicaid/program-information/downloads/accomplishments-report.pdf. Accessed March 24, 2017.

67. *Medicaid & CHIP Report*, January 2017. Available at https://www.medicaid.gov/medicaid/program-information/downloads/accomplishments-report.pdf. Accessed March 24, 2017.

68. CMS. "Medicaid managed care enrollment and programs characteristics 2014" webpage. Available at https://www.medicaid.gov/medicaid-chip-program-information/by-topics/data-and-systems/medicaid-managed-care/downloads/2014-medicaid-managed-care-enrollment-report.pdf. Accessed March 23, 2017.

69. Social Security. "Compilation of the Social Security laws" webpage. Available at https://www.ssa.gov/OP_Home/ssact/title19/1902.htm. Accessed March 23, 2017.

70. *Federal Register* Medicaid Program. "Covered outpatient drug; Delay in changing definitions of states and United States" webpage. Available at https://www.federalregister.gov/documents/2016/11/15/2016-27423/medicaid-program-covered-outpatient-drug-delay-in-change-in-definitions-of-states-and-united-states. Accessed March 21, 2017.

71. "Medicaid excluded drug coverage" website. Available at https://www.medicaid.gov/medicaid/prescription-drugs/excluded-drug-coverage/index.html. Accessed March 23, 2017.

72. "Medicaid cost sharing out-of-pocket costs" webpage. Available at https://www.medicaid.gov/medicaid/cost-sharing/out-of-pocket-costs/index.html. Accessed April 3, 2017.

73. Express Scripts, Inc. webpage, *2017 National Preferred Formulary* (preferred drug list [PDL]). Available at https://www.express-scripts.com/art/open_enrollment/GASHBPRXPDFS_PrefDrugListherap.pdf. Accessed March 25, 2017.

74. *Florida PDL*. Available at http://www.fdhc.state.fl.us/medicaid/Prescribed_Drug/pharm_thera/pdf/PDL.pdf. Accessed March 23, 2017.

75. *Texas Medicaid PDL*. Available at https://www.txvendordrug.com/sites/txvendordrug/files/docs/formulary/2016-0721-preferred-drug-list.pdf. Accessed March 23, 2017.

76. *New York State Medicaid PDL*. Available at http://www.coalitionny.org/news_resources/prescription_drug_benefits/documents/NYRx_PDP_PDL.pdf. Accessed March 23, 2017.

77. *California Medi-Cal Drug Formulary*. Available at http://www.dhcs.ca.gov/services/pages/ff.html. Accessed 23 March 2017.

78. *Molina Healthcare of South Carolina PDL*. Available at http://www.molinahealthcare.com/providers/sc/medicaid/PDF/Preferred-Drug-List-2017.pdf. Accessed March 23, 2017.

79. *Amerigroup Medicaid Formularies*. Available at https://providers.amerigroup.com/QuickTools/Pages/FormularyCaid.aspx. Accessed March 23, 2017.

80. *WellCare Health Plans Medicaid Providers Preferred Drug List*. Available at https://www.wellcare.com/Kentucky/Providers/Medicaid/Pharmacy/Preferred-Drug-List. Accessed March 23, 2017.

81. *Medicaid Drug Utilization Review* webpage. Available at https://www.medicaid.gov/medicaid/prescription-drugs/drug-utilization-review/index.html. Accessed March 21, 2017.

82. *Medicaid Drug Utilization Review* annual report form. Available at https://www.medicaid.gov/medicaid/prescription-drugs/drug-utilization-review/index.html. Accessed March 21, 2017.

83. CMS. *Medicaid Drug Utilization Review State Comparison/Summary Report FFY 2015* annual report. Available at https://www.medicaid.gov/medicaid-chip-program-information/by-topics/prescription-drugs/downloads/2015-dur-summary-report.pdf. Accessed March 23, 2017.

84. Medicaid Branded Prescription Drug Fee Program webpage. Available at https://www.medicaid.gov/medicaid/prescription-drugs/branded-prescription-drug-fee-program/index.html. Accessed March 23, 2017.

85. National Average Drug Acquisition Cost (NADAC) Data Field Definitions webpage. Available at https://www.medicaid.gov/medicaid-chip-program-information/by-topics/prescription-drugs/ful-nadac-downloads/nadacdatadefinitions.pdf. Accessed March 23, 2017. See also Medicaid data webpage. Available at https://data.medicaid.gov. Accessed March 23, 2017.

86. Medicaid Drug Rebate Program website. Available at https://www.medicaid.gov/medicaid/prescription-drugs/medicaid-drug-rebate-program/index.html. Accessed March 23, 2017.

87. Social Security. "Compilation of the Social Security laws payment for covered outpatient drugs" webpage. Available at https://www.ssa.gov/OP_Home/ssact/title19/1927.htm. Accessed March 23, 2017.

88. US Government Accountability Office. *GAO Prescription Drugs. Comparison of DOD, Medicaid, and Medicare Part D Retail Reimbursement Prices*. GAO-14-578, 2014 (June).

89. *Federal Register* Medicaid Program; Announcement of Medicaid Drug Rebate Program National Rebate Agreement. Available at https://www.federalregister.gov/documents/2016/11/09/2016-26834/medicaid-program-announcement-of-medicaid-drug-rebate-program-national-rebate-agreement. Accessed March 23, 2017.

90. Health Resources and Services Administration (HRSA) 340B Drug Pricing Program website. Available at https://www.hrsa.gov/opa/index.html. Accessed March 23, 2017.

91. CMS. Covered Outpatient Drug Final Rule with Comment (CMS-2345-FC) FAQs webpage. Available at https://www.medicaid.gov/federal-policy-guidance/downloads/faq070616.pdf. Accessed March 23, 2017.

92. Medication NADAC webpage. Available at https://data.medicaid.gov/Drug-Pricing-and-Payment/NADAC-National-Average-Drug-Acquisition-Cost-/a4y5-998d. Accessed March 23, 2017.

93. *Federal Register* CMS 42 CFR Part 447 Medicaid Program. *Covered Outpatient Drugs; Final Rule*. Available at https://www.gpo.gov/fdsys/pkg/FR-2016-02-01/pdf/2016-01274.pdf. Accessed March 23, 2017.

94. US Pharmacist. *Understanding Drug Pricing*. Available at https://www.uspharmacist.com/article/understanding-drug-pricing. Accessed March 23, 2017.

95. Oregon Health Authority Health Systems Division: Medical Assistance Programs Division webpage. Available at http://arcweb.sos.state.or.us/pages/rules/oars_400/oar_410/410_121.html. Accessed March 23, 2017.

96. The Kaiser Family Foundation. *Medicaid Enrollment & Spending Growth: FY 2016 & 2-17*. Available at http://files.kff.org/attachment/Issue-Brief-Medicaid-Enrollment-&-Spending-Growth-FY-2016-&-2017. Accessed March 24, 2017.

97. Medicaid Eligibility webpage. Available at https://www.medicaid.gov/medicaid/eligibility/index.html. Accessed March 24, 2017.

98. *Medicaid Affordable Care Act*. Available at https://www.medicaid.gov/affordable-care-act/index.html. Accessed March 24, 2017.

99. The Kaiser Family Foundation website. *The Effects of Medicaid Expansion Under the ACA: Findings from a Literature Review*. Available at http://files.kff.org/attachment/Issue-brief-The-Effects-of-Medicaid-Expansion-under-the-ACA-Findings-from-a-Literature-Review. Accessed March 24, 2017.

100. Centers for Disease Control and Prevention website. *Acceptance of New Patients with Public and Private Insurance by Office-Based Physicians: United States, 2013*. Available at https://www.cdc.gov/nchs/products/databriefs/db195.htm. Accessed March 24, 2017.

101. Medicaid and CHIP Payment and Access Commission (MACPAC) 2015. *Analysis of the National Health Interview Survey 2014*. Available at https://www.macpac.gov/wp-content/uploads/2016/06/Children's-difficulties-in-obtaining-medical-care.pdf. Accessed March 24, 2017.

102. Mulcahy AW, Eisner C, Finegold K. Gaining coverage through Medicaid or private insurance increase prescription use and lower out-of-pocket spending. *Health Affairs*. 2016;35(9):1725–1733.

103. Cole MB, Galarraga O, Wilson I, et al. *Health Affairs*. 2017;36(1):40-48.

104. Wen H, Borders T, Druss B. Number of Medicaid prescriptions grew, drug spending was steady in Medicaid expansion states. *Health Affairs*. 2015;35(9):1604-1607. Available at http://content.healthaffairs.org.lp.hscl.ufl.edu/content/35/9/1604.full.pdf+html?sid=e126daeb-6fb6-432e-9ff4-332fd53b5768. Accessed March 25, 2017.

Review Questions

1. Which of the following is true regarding the role of the Center for Medicare and Medicaid (CMS)?
   a. Both Medicare and Medicaid are federal programs managed directly by CMS.
   b. CMS has no role in regulating or managing either Medicare or Medicaid.
   c. CMS manages Medicaid from a federal perspective, but each state develops and manages its own Medicare insurance programs with no involvement of CMS.
   d. CMS plays a regulatory and financial role in Medicaid and Medicare programs, although Medicaid is primarily a state-administered program.

2. Select the best answer below regarding the drug program authorized by the Medicare Modernization Act of 2003.
   a. Part B medical benefit prescription outpatient drug coverage
   b. Part C home healthcare prescription drug benefits
   c. Part D outpatient prescription drug benefit coverage
   d. Part A inpatient prescription drug benefit coverage

3. Select the best answer below regarding Medicare and Medicaid programs.
   a. Medicare was developed as health insurance primarily for low-income individuals and families, mostly children and single parents. Medicaid is only for severely disabled individuals.
   b. Medicaid provides coverage only for individuals and families classified as *dual eligibles*, meaning that one member of the family is above 65 years old, and one is below 65 years.
   c. Medicaid is intended primarily for citizens 65 years and older, and Medicaid is for low-income individuals, families, and children. About 10 million disabled individuals are eligible for both programs.
   d. Medicare and Medicaid eligibility requirements are identical, and individuals can choose from either program (but not both) according to the states in which they reside.

4. Please select the best answer below regarding the various Medicare parts.
   a. Medicare Part A includes inpatient medical services; Part D covers outpatient prescription drugs.
   b. Medicare Part C includes inpatient medical services; Part B covers outpatient prescription drugs, and home healthcare drugs.
   c. Medicare Part D includes home healthcare medical benefit drugs, and Part A includes inpatient medical services, but excludes home healthcare drugs.
   d. Specialty drugs (high-cost, often injectable drugs) are covered under Part B if inpatient, but under Part B if outpatient pharmacy-dispensed drugs.

5. Select the best answer below regarding Medicaid and Medicare drug formularies.
   a. Medicaid formularies are often named *preferred drug lists* (PDLs), and Medicare formularies typically have a single tier and no patient cost share.
   b. Medicare formularies are often multitiered, often with a cost share for brand drugs, and Medicaid formularies often have a single or no tier, with no or low-cost share.
   c. According to the PPACA, both Medicaid and Medicare formularies must be identical as both are subject to Qualified Health Plan (QHP) and Essential Health Benefits (EHB) requirements.

6. Pharmacy Benefit Managers (PBMs) generally offer what type of Medicaid prescription drug benefit programs, and why? Select the best answer below.
   a. PBMs may offer medical and pharmacy benefits and are authorized to offer Part D benefits through Part C Medicare Advantage plans.
   b. PBMs are prohibited from developing and offering Medicare PDP prescription drug plans except through a subcontract with a health plan Part A Medicare Advantage plan.
   c. PBMs are exempt from PPACA Part D regulations and compliance requirements, and may develop and sell any type of unregulated prescription drug benefit to Medicare recipients.
   d. PBMs do not offer medical benefits, and therefore may offer Medicare Part D benefits through a PDP.

7. Pharmaceutical manufacturers may offer price concessions on brand drugs to health plans and PBMs. Select the best answer below regarding rebates, one type of price concession.
   a. In many Medicare and Medicaid prescription drug benefit programs, rebates are often offered by pharmaceutical manufacturers in exchange for a brand drug preferred formulary position.
   b. Rebates are illegal per the PPACA for Medicaid programs, although a minimum of 23.1% is required for brand drugs in Medicare programs.
   c. Rebates reduce the net prescription cost of contracted products for Medicaid programs, but are illegal for Medicare programs due to the use of coupons for government programs.
   d. As a result of the Pricing Transparency amendment to the 2003 MMA, rebates have been completely replaced by drug cost share offset and discount coupons.

8. Select the best answer below regarding Medicare standard Part D defined benefit levels.
   a. The standard Medicare benefit includes (1) an initial Coverage Gap, (2) Catastrophic Coverage, and (3) Initial Coverage. The Catastrophic Coverage gap will be closed by 2020.
   b. The Coverage Gap following Initial Coverage, and is following by Catastrophic Coverage. By 2020, the Coverage Gap between branded generic drug cost shares will be closed.
   c. Per the PPACA, the Coverage Gap is now closed and Medicare recipients pay zero-dollar cost share for brand and generic drugs. Home healthcare drugs are always covered in the Coverage Gap.
   d. Catastrophic Coverage covers only injectable high-cost cancer specialty medications, whenever prescribed, independent of any other coverage level, but will be closed by 2020.

9. CMS regulations require Medicare prescription drug programs to cover "all or substantially all" drugs in six protect classes. Select the best answer below regarding this fact.
   a. Drugs in the six protected classes are all on the high-risk medication (HRM) list and must be covered but also must be monitored closely.
   b. Drugs in the six protected classes are used by medically vulnerable individuals and plans must not use lack of coverage to discourage enrollment.
   c. Drugs in the six protected classes are investigational and experimental, but have shown promise in orphan diseases for older patients, and thus, must be covered, regardless of cost.
   d. Drugs in the six protected classes have zero-dollar cost share according to the PPACA, and must be included in formulary tier 1 with other generics to ensure affordability and promote adherence.

10. Select the best answer below regarding the Medicare 5-Star Quality Rating Program.
   a. Medicare plan participation in the Medicare 5-Star Quality Rating Program is voluntary and results in no financial incentive for plans.
   b. The Medicare 5-Star Quality Rating Program allows every Medicare plans to advertise their star ratings throughout the year.
   c. The financial reward for plans that achieve four and five stars in the Quality Rating Program concludes in 2020 with closure of the coverage gap.
   d. The Medicare 5-Star Quality Rating Program identifies and rewards high quality plans, may include a financial reward, and 5-Star plans may advertise throughout the year.

ANSWERS

1. d	2. c	3. c
4. a	5. b	6. d
7. a	8. b	9. b
10. d		

2

Medicare Part D's Medication Therapy Management and Other Related Services

Alexander Miguel, PharmD, BCGP, and Cynthia R. Nacin, PharmD, MS, BCACP, CPh

KEY POINTS

- Participation in Part D medication therapy management (MTM) programs is lower than predicted, and this has frustrated Part D plan sponsors and the federal government, especially considering MTM's success in some Medicaid and private-sector programs.
- The Centers for Medicare and Medicaid Services (CMS) defines MTM as a patient-centric and comprehensive approach to improve medication use, reduce the risk of adverse events, and improve medication adherence.
- The MTM scope of services within Part D is evolving. This requires constant surveillance of the literature and CMS communications.
- Under Part D, free MTM services are generally reserved for enrollees who meet criteria related to their annual Part D drug costs, number of prescription drugs, and prevalence of certain chronic diseases.
- The Centers for Medicare and Medicaid Innovation (CMMI) have developed the Enhanced MTM Model to allow sponsors regulatory flexibility and financial resources to design MTM programs that best fit their beneficiaries' needs. The goal of this innovative MTM model is to align the interest of Part D sponsors and CMS.
- MTM is showing promise in other non-Medicare drug benefit programs.
- The Patient Protection and Affordable Care Act (PL 111-148) authorized grants for "medication management services" in all practice settings (Section 3503), noting that such services will help manage chronic disease, reduce medical errors, and improve patient adherence to therapies while reducing acute-care costs and hospital readmissions. However, funds were never appropriated for this section.
- Part D's inherent structure makes it particularly challenging to create and sustain robust MTM programs. However, CMS research (2013) identified effective MTM practices of highly effective drug plans.

BACKGROUND AND PROGRAM EXPECTATIONS

Federal law requires Medicare Part D drug plan sponsors to offer MTM programs to help targeted enrollees avoid drug-related problems and optimize medication benefits. In 2006, such programs were hailed as a "win-win" proposition for plans, pharmacists, and beneficiaries.[1] However, today, MTM participation is lower than predicted, and it is still not possible to evaluate whether Part D MTM programs are working as intended. This has frustrated Part D plan sponsors and the federal government, especially considering MTM's success in some Medicaid and private-sector programs. This chapter describes policy strategies implemented by CMS to increase MTM participation and improve health outcomes while reducing Medicare expenditure. Additionally, other medication management services beyond standard Part D MTM are profiled.

For most people, the term "pharmacists' services" may conjure up traditional pill-counting and -dispensing functions and nothing more. Since 2006, however, Medicare's voluntary prescription drug benefit, Part D, has played an important role in expanding the scope of such services. Part D plans must provide MTM programs to help eligible enrollees avoid drug-related problems and achieve desired clinical benefits from medications.[2]

In 2016 CMS defined MTM as a patient-centric and comprehensive approach to improve medication use, reduce the risk of adverse events, and improve medication adherence.[3] Historically, MTM services represent a bundling of "pharmaceutical care" interventions. *Pharmaceutical care* is a patient-centered practice model in which a pharmacist works directly with patients, as well as prescribers and other clinicians, to help patients achieve intended drug therapy outcomes.[4]

This model formed the backbone of what was expected to be an effective MTM benefit. Many observers might have anticipated the creation of a well-defined MTM program, with on-target participation by enrollees who truly benefited from enhanced pharmaceutical care. This would likely be undergirded by a comprehensive network of MTM-providing pharmacists, whose education and training distinguishes them as logical (but not necessarily exclusive) MTM providers. Under Part D, MTM programs must be developed in cooperation with practicing pharmacists and physicians, and the MTM services must be administered by a pharmacist or other qualified healthcare professional.[3] In 2016 all Part D sponsors utilized pharmacists as providers of MTM services. Other practitioners providing MTM services included pharmacist interns, nurse practitioners, registered nurses, licensed practical nurses, physicians, and physician assistants (Figure 2-1).[5] However, some key program results remain a mystery, and participation is much lower than expected, from both enrollees and community-based clinicians who could provide MTM services. Pharmacists who have successfully integrated MTM services into their workflows (including being compensated for Part D MTM services—a discretionary payment from drug plans) are the exception rather than the norm.[6] Moreover, the government's original evaluation of Part D MTM found "limited evidence to determine which beneficiaries would benefit most from MTM, which features achieved the desired outcomes, and which outcomes should be measured to compare MTM program performance."[7] Their 2013 report examining MTM in chronically ill patients[8] was more instructive, and is discussed later in this chapter.

This chapter examines current program requirements, shifting program parameters, and success in several MTM programs conducted outside of Part D. It also describes CMS' enhanced MTM pilot and other applications of MTM to pharmacists' clinical practice.

SCOPE OF SERVICES

Medication therapy management's scope of services within Part D has evolved over time. Initial regulations established "a general framework that allowed sponsors flexibility to promote best practices."[9] Thus, CMS did not limit the provision of MTM services to pharmacists alone, nor did CMS specify how to provide services.

Originally, drug plans could satisfy the law's intent by mailing letters to targeted patients about their drug therapy, legally bypassing any real-time provider-to-patient communication. Such low-tech interventions helped plans minimize MTM program costs, which must be incorporated into plan sponsors' annual prospective bids to CMS. Further, MTM services must be provided to eligible enrollees at no charge.

These fundamental administrative elements were set prior to 2006, yet the scope of MTM services—defined annually by CMS—has expanded since then. Presently, Part D MTM programs must provide these service elements:

1. Interventions for both beneficiaries and prescribers.
2. Annual comprehensive reviews for beneficiaries that (a) are conducted by a pharmacist or other "qualified provider," (b) are performed face to face or by telephone, and (c) feature written summaries with medication action plans and personal

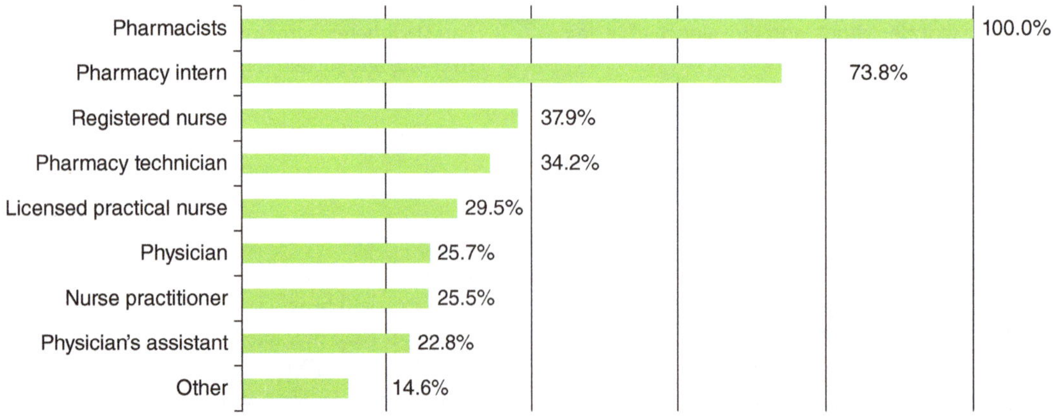

FIGURE 2-1 Provider of MTM services: percent of 2016 MTM programs.
Source: Centers for Medicare and Medicaid Services (CMS). *2016 Medicare Part D Medication Therapy Management [MTM] Programs Fact Sheet Summary of 2016 MTM Programs*, May, 4, 2016. Available at https://www.cms.gov/Medicare/Prescription-Drug-Coverage/PrescriptionDrugCovContra/Downloads/CY2016-MTM-Fact-Sheet.pdf. Accessed February 1, 2016.

medication lists. Such reviews assess use of prescribed medicines, nonprescription products, and dietary supplements. The structure and length of such reviews are at the plan's discretion.

3. Quarterly, targeted medication reviews with follow-up interventions when necessary.

The extent to which patient data gleaned during MTM, and the methods by which plans communicate with prescribers, are variable. CMS reported that in 2012, while 100% of MTM programs communicated with prescribers about resolving drug problems or possibly optimizing drug therapy, 84% did so by fax, 78% did so by telephone, and 69% mailed consultations. Only about one-fifth (21%) of MTM programs shared with prescribers a patient's medication list.[10]

These results do not reveal the extent to which MTM clinicians' recommendations may have generated desired therapy changes—something that plans must report to CMS annually, but that had not been reported publicly at time of publication. Moreover, reliance on fax, postal mail, and telephone may delay timely—or risk lack of relevant—feedback to prescribers (eg, with few programs sharing a comprehensive list of medicines that a patient is using). With quarterly medication reviews, feedback could be at least 3 months old by the time a prescriber receives it. More timely and robust data exchange between prescribers and MTM providers proved to be a key element in MTM programs outside of Part D. Currently the Pharmacy Quality Alliance (PQA) is working on developing a *MTM: medication therapy problem resolution* measure. The measure development team is working on a *systematized nomenclature of medicine–clinical terms* (SNoMED-CT) crosswalk that will help standardize how medication therapy problems are categorized and reported.[11] If the measure is finalized and adopted by CMS, the ability for MTM programs to identify and resolve medication therapy problems will be measurable across Part D sponsors. In fact, in the 2017 *MTM Program Guidance and Submission Instructions to Medicare Part D Sponsors*, CMS emphasizes using MTM services to promote coordination of care. CMS recommends plans coordinate the annual CMR prior to beneficiaries' annual wellness visit so that the medication action plan and personal medication list can be shared with providers at the annual wellness visit. Additionally, CMS encourages plan sponsors to adopt standardized health information technology (HIT) through the use of SNoMED-CT codes to document MTM services and to ease information transfer between providers.[3]

As for Part D enrollees' acceptance of some key MTM services, new data are not promising. In 2013, CMS reported that in 2011, only 11% of MTM enrollees (who were not in long-term-care facilities) received comprehensive medication reviews (CMRs)—a service that must have been offered to all MTM participants in 2010.[12] (Effective in 2013, CMRs must be offered at least annually to long-term-care beneficiaries, too.) The rate in 2011 for standalone prescription drug plans (PDPs), which attract a large majority of Part D enrollees, was even lower, just 7.3%. Since 2012 CMS has placed increased pressure on Part D sponsors to increase beneficiary participation in CMRs and in 2016 adopted the CMR completion rate as a Star Measure.[13]

Interestingly, two-thirds of people aged ≥65 years who responded to a national poll in 2012 reported that their physician "or healthcare provider" had performed a CMR.[14] Whether these respondents were eligible for Part D MTM is unknown, as is who extended the offer, how their reviews might have differed in scope from a Part D review, and what, if any, therapy changes resulted following review.

TABLE 2-1 • Part D Medication Therapy Management Eligibility Criteria, 2017

Annual drug costs ≥ $3919, representing the total of plan's costs and enrollee's costs, plus annual percentage increase specified in 42 *CFR* §423.104(d)(5)(iv)
Minimum threshold for number of different prescription medicines ranges from two to eight
Enrollees must have at least two or three multiple chronic diseases Target beneficiaries with any chronic diseases; or target SPECIFIC chronic diseases If targeting persons with SPECIFIC diseases, they must choose at least five of nine core chronic conditions: Alzheimer, chronic heart failure, diabetes, dyslipidemia, end-stage renal disease, hypertension, respiratory disease, bone diseases-arthritis, or mental health
Frequency for targeting beneficiaries for MTM enrollment: at least quarterly
Qualified enrollees are automatically enrolled and must opt out of participating
Annual CMR must be offered to MTM enrollees who reside in long-term care settings

Source: Centers for Medicare and Medicaid Services (CMS). *Memo: CY 2017 Medication Therapy Management Program Guidance and Submission Instructions*, April 8, 2016.

Eligibility

Under Part D, free MTM services are generally reserved for enrollees who meet criteria related to their annual Part D drug costs, number of prescription drugs, and prevalence of certain chronic diseases. These criteria, set by CMS with some flexibility for plans, have changed since 2006. For example, eligible enrollees originally had to opt in to the MTM program; they would be solicited for MTM services only annually; and prior to 2010 eligible enrollees had to be taking 2 to 15 drugs. Today, enrollment is opted out; plans must target enrollees at least quarterly, and they must take two to eight drugs. The dollar threshold, originally $4000, has also changed: CMS dropped it to $3000 in 2010. Since 2012 the threshold is $3000 plus a mandatory annual percentage increase.[15] For 2017, the cost threshold is $3919.[3] These changing criteria have limited methodologically sound research on Part D MTM's effectiveness over time. Table 2-1 details eligibility criteria.

CENTERS FOR MEDICARE AND MEDICAID SERVICES CONCERNED BY LOWER-THAN-EXPECTED MEDICATION THERAPY MANAGEMENT PARTICIPATION

In 2010, CMS predicted that reducing the dollar eligibility threshold (to 3000) in annual Part D–covered drug expenditures would result in 25% of Part D enrollees qualifying for MTM programs.[16]

TABLE 2-2 • Percent of 2016 MTM Programs With Expanded Eligibility Criteria

Eligibility Criteria	# of Programs	% of Programs
Target only enrollees who meet the specified targeting criteria per CMS requirements	468	75.1
Use expanded criteria: Target both enrollees who meet the specified targeting criteria per CMS requirements and enrollees who meet other plan-specific targeting criteria	155	24.9
Total	623	100

Source: Centers for Medicare and Medicaid Services (CMS). *Fact Sheet: 2016 Medicare Part D Medication Therapy Management (MTM) Programs Fact Sheet Summary of 2016 MTM Programs*, May 4, 2016. Available at https://www.cms.gov/Medicare/Prescriptions-Drug-Coverage/PrescriptionDrugCovContra/Downloads/CY2016-MTM-Fact-Sheet.pdf. Accessed February 1, 2016.

Instead, the eligibility rate dropped from 11% in 2008 to 9.1% in 2009, to 8.2% in 2010, to 7.9% in 2011.[12,17] The actual number of participants appears to has not increased significantly over the years and averaged about 10% among Part D plans in 2013.[18] CMS expressed concern that sponsors are restricting MTM eligibility criteria to limit the number of qualified enrollees. In 2016, for example, only 25% of MTM programs used expanded criteria for MTM eligibility beyond the CMS minimum requirements (Table 2-2).[5] Additionally, CMS is concerned that establishing utilization as a criterion for MTM participation has created racial and ethnic disparities in MTM eligibility. Two studies by Wang and colleagues found that Hispanic and African-American beneficiaries could be less likely to meet MTM eligibility criteria due to being traditionally lower utilizers of healthcare.[19,20]

The CMS data released in 2012 reveal a comprehensive portrait of Part D MTM-eligible enrollees versus those who are not MTM-eligible. Between these two groups, in 2010 there was a 2.5-fold variation in average annual drug costs, more than a 2-fold variation in total prescriptions filled, and almost a 3-fold difference in the percentage of enrollees who entered the Part D coverage gap. In 2010, this "doughnut hole" gap left enrollees who did not receive the low-income subsidy (LIS) fully exposed to their drug costs. This gap is being closed gradually, from 2011 to 2020, with discounts on brand and generic prescriptions. About half (51.3%) of all MTM-eligible enrollees received the LIS in 2010.[21] This subgroup tends to use the most prescription drugs.

These data characterize people eligible for MTM (Figure 2-2), but how closely they resemble actual recipients of MTM services has not been shared publicly. For example, CMS is studying the relationship between MTM-eligible LIS enrollees and those who received MTM in 2010, but their actual participation has not been reported.[22] In 2013, CMS published its final report examining the effect of MTM on certain Part D enrollees in 2010 with congestive heart failure, chronic obstructive pulmonary disease, or diabetes.[8] For those who received CMRs, congestive heart failure patients had hospital savings of $526 for the year; and diabetes patients had hospital savings that averaged $399 for the year, compared to similarly matched Part D enrollees who did not receive MTM.

The report described above did not identify subsidy status of MTM enrollees, however, so it is undetermined whether its projected cost savings would apply to the LIS population. Understanding clinical and economic effects of MTM services provided to LIS enrollees could prove strategic, as the Medicare Payment Advisory Commission reported that their drug costs represent 55% of total Part D expenditures.[23] Other research has found that LIS enrollees and those who are dually eligible for Medicare and Medicaid with common chronic conditions are more likely to incur a hospitalization than non-LIS/non-dual-eligibility persons.[24]

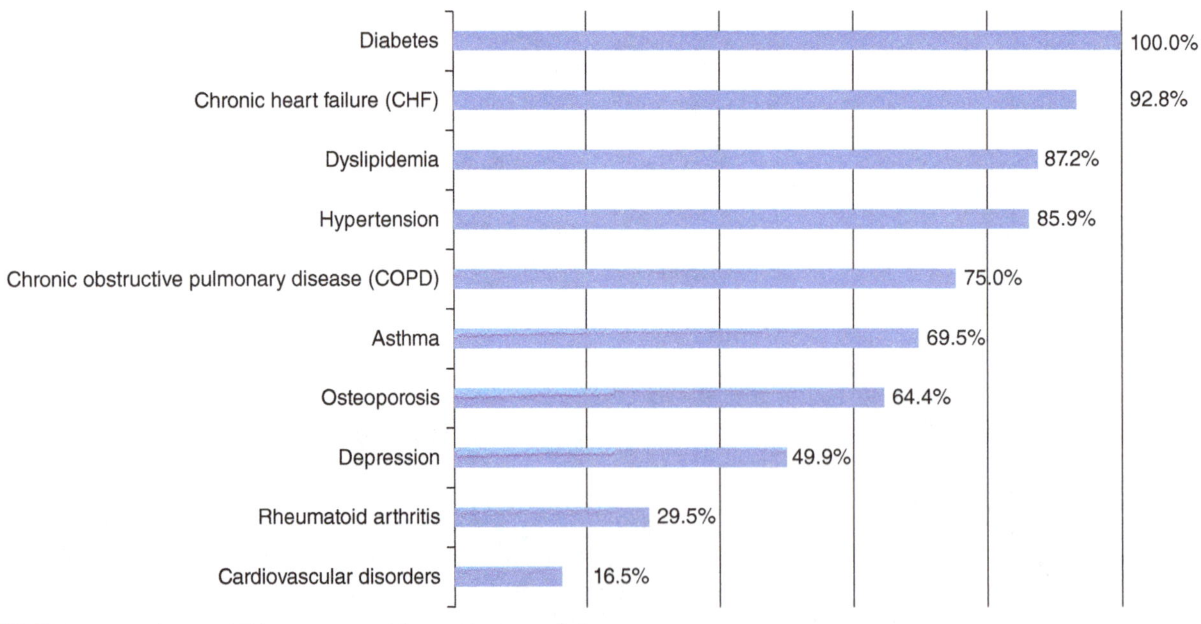

FIGURE 2-2 Percent of 2016 MTM programs with top 10 targeted diseases.
Source: Centers for Medicare and Medicaid Services (CMS). *Fact Sheet: 2016 Medicare Part D Medication Therapy Management (MTM) Programs Fact Sheet Summary of 2016 MTM Programs*, May 4, 2016. Available at https://www.cms.gov/Medicare/Prescription-Drug-Coverage/PrescriptionDrugCovContra/Downloads/CY2016-MTM-Fact-Sheet.pdf. Accessed February 1, 2016.

Given the success of some Medicaid MTM programs in reducing overall program costs through robust prevention of drug-related problems (see discussion below), it is unfortunate that the verdict is still out for Part D MTM.

ENHANCED MTM MODEL

Currently, CMS continues to promote innovative strategies for Part D MTM to improve health outcomes while reducing net Medicare expenditures. In September 2015, the Centers for Medicare and Medicaid Innovation (CMMI) announced the Part D Enhanced MTM Model. The Enhanced MTM Model, which was to be conducted across five Part D regions, began in January 2017 and will run for a total of 7 years.[25] The model is designed to test changes to the Part D MTM program that achieve better alignment between interests of Part D sponsors and CMS by allowing for regulatory flexibility with regard to targeting and interventions. Participating Part D sponsors also will be given a prospective per-member per-month payment for the enhanced services and will be eligible for a performance-based incentive payment earned via a reduction in Medicare costs of care. This incentive payment will be in the form of a lower beneficiary premium through an increase in government contribution to the plan premium.

Through the removal of the standard Part D MTM program requirements, CMS is giving Part D sponsors the ability to design MTM programs that they believe will best fit their beneficiary populations. Under the Enhanced MTM Model, Part D sponsors will have the flexibility to offer more expansive MTM services, a variety of MTM services aimed at tackling the medication-related risks of individual beneficiaries, and to test different communication strategies to improve coordination of care between beneficiaries, their pharmacists, and medical providers. CMS is also giving the Part D sponsors access to their beneficiaries' Medicare Parts A and B data to sharpen their targeting and care coordination.

As part of the Enhanced MTM Model, participating plans must submit enhanced MTM encounter data to CMS on a quarterly basis. Part D sponsors will have to submit encounter data for any of the following MTM encounters: referral, procedure, issue, and outcome. The encounter data will include 17 unique data elements per record. This will allow CMS to ensure that sponsors are implementing their approved enhanced MTM programs and to measure the success of the Enhanced MTM Model.

MEDICATION THERAPY MANAGEMENT: BEYOND MEDICARE PART D

Standard Medicare Part D MTM has been discussed throughout this chapter. However, Part D MTM is not the only outlet for delivering medication management services. In 2010, the Patient Centered Primary Care Collaborative (PCPCC) named comprehensive medication management (CMM) as a new patient approach that includes review and evaluation of the complete patient profile. In 2012, California began actively implementing CMM as part of the California Wellness Plan (CWP). The California Wellness Plan successfully demonstrated a positive impact when medication management services were provided. In 2011, the University of California San Diego (UCSD) provided a transitions-of-care program to inpatient and outpatient heart failure patients by board-certified pharmacists. Patients who received services were found to have a 18.9% less likely rate of hospital remittance within 30 days of initial discharge and a 7% increase in comprehension of medication use.[26] Medication-related problems are among the highest reason for increasing healthcare costs.[27] Thus, it is essential to continuously improve both patient care and healthcare professionals' knowledge for care.

The American College of Clinical Pharmacy (ACCP) defines CMM as "the standard of care that ensures [that] each patient's medications (ie, prescription, nonprescription, alternative, traditional, vitamins, or nutritional supplements) are individually assessed to determine that each medication is appropriate for the patient, effective for the medical condition, safe given the comorbidities and other medications being taken, and able to be taken by the patient as intended." CMM includes collaboration between pharmacists, physicians, nurses, and the patient to determine a treatment plan to achieve the goals of each individual.[28] The goal of CMM is to decrease both the burden of chronic disease states and healthcare expenses while improving patient outcomes. Therefore, high-risk patients who are suboptimally utilizing their medications and have high healthcare costs, and patients with multiple comorbidities are generally the most valuable population for providing CMM services.[26]

Collaboration practice agreements between pharmacists, physicians, nonphysician providers (NPPs), and the patient are essential in CMM.[27] Depending on the laws of each state and physician's criteria, collaborative practice agreements may allow pharmacists to perform various clinical privileges such as monitoring, titrating doses of medications, and adjusting therapies. Implementation of collaborative practice agreements allows a physician to focus on diagnosing patients, rather than routine monitoring.[26]

Pharmacists are responsible for reviewing the clinical-physical status for each patient prior to making clinical interventions. For this reason, the ACCP recommends residency, postlicensure experience, and/or board certification as qualifications for pharmacists to provide services of comprehensive medication management.[27] Additional training may be required on behalf of the pharmacist, to perform duties of CMM such as identifying gaps in therapy, potentially inappropriate medications (Beer's List), therapeutic substitutions, laboratory values, and clinical goals.[29] Therefore, pharmacists should perform CMM within their scope of practice and training. Without the appropriate knowledge, patients may not be adequately evaluated, ultimately leading to clinical inaccuracies.

Initially, the patient is seen by a primary-care physician (PCP) for diagnosis and is then referred to the clinical pharmacist. During an evaluation by a pharmacist for CMM, the guidelines state that there are four components to review: (1) an assessment of the patient's medication-related needs, (2) identification of the patient's medication-related problems, (3) development of a care plan with individualized therapy goals and personalized interventions, and (4) follow-up evaluation to determine actual patient outcomes.[30] As a result, the patient must agree to be an actively engaged participant for a CMM to be complete.[26]

It is important to recognize the different opportunities that each medication management program provides. While CMM and MTM appear to share many commonalities, there are distinguishing characteristics of each one. Since CMS provides guidelines for eligibility requirements for general MTM services, there are a number of restrictions. MTM may focus directly on a specific disease state or list of medications, while CMM includes factors such as age, underlying disease state(s), and number of medications may either include or exclude a patient's eligibility for a medication review.[26,27] However, a benefit of MTM services is the accessibility for both the patient and the pharmacist, since these services may be provided in any appropriate setting. Important distinctions among CMM and MTM is the availability of the patient chart to evaluate clinical status. Some main differences are both the ability and expectation for collaboration with healthcare providers and the patient when practicing CMM, as well as patient follow-up.[26]

Disease state management is a privileged relationship built between the patient and the pharmacist. Patients with asthma, diabetes, hypertension, hypercholesterolemia, heart failure, and kidney disease are common target populations that have the potential to benefit the most from this type of program.[26] Since these disease states are often complex and difficult to manage, it is essential to assist patients in setting and reaching their personal goals. Improving adherence, enhancing patient understanding, and improving patient costs are all ways in which pharmacist may impact patient care. Pharmacists are frontline healthcare professionals in which a patient often has the most open access to care.

As medication management becomes a more integrative and collaborative effort, pharmacists have a greater opportunity to improve patient health outcomes. The benefits of practicing CMM have been demonstrated by improving quality of life, access to caregivers and healthcare providers, continuity of care, and a better understanding of health literacy, paving the path for pharmacists to demonstrate unsurpassed value as providers within the healthcare community.[26]

MEDICATION THERAPY MANAGEMENT SHOWING PROMISE IN OTHER DRUG BENEFIT PROGRAMS

Parallel to Part D implementation, several MTM programs outside of Part D have yielded positive results. For example, Minnesota Medicaid started providing MTM in 2006, reimbursing pharmacists to provide and document MTM to people taking four or more prescription drugs to treat two or more chronic diseases or when a recipient's drug therapy problem caused, or was likely to cause, significant nondrug program costs. A 2007 evaluation found that more than one-third (36%) of Medicaid MTM recipients with diabetes achieved optimal care standards versus the statewide average of diabetes performance standards of 6%.[31]

Also in Minnesota, a 10-year evaluation of MTM provided to patients in an integrated health system estimated a return on investment (ROI) of \$1.29 per \$1.00 in MTM administrative costs. This was based on estimated cost savings for avoided visits to physician offices, urgent-care facilities, and emergency departments that MTM intervention helped prevent. MTM services, paid out of pocket by the patient or reimbursed by insurance, were delivered face to face only. Evidence-based clinical goals of therapy helped determine patient-specific targets.[31]

In 2000, Iowa implemented a 9-month pharmaceutical case management program for Medicaid recipients who were taking four or more prescription medications. Pharmacists met with over 900 patients, two-thirds of whom were 45 years of age or older. They found an average of 2.6 medication-related problems per person. Pharmacists' most frequent recommendations were to: add a drug (52% of patients), change a medication (36% of patients), or discontinue a medication (33% of patients). Across the program, physicians accepted just under half (49.2%) of pharmacists' recommendations. Even so, Medicaid patients aged ≥60 years still benefited from pharmacists' case management services; these patients realized a decrease in use of medications considered to be inappropriate for the elderly.[32]

Iowa's present Medicaid MTM-like program relies on pharmacist-physician teams; either team member can recommend a patient for interventions, and physicians must approve or modify medication action plans. Under this program, both pharmacists and physicians can be reimbursed for drug therapy management services.[32]

Patients in the above mentioned examples benefited from elements that may differ from current Part D MTM practice: (1) interventions delivered face to face by pharmacists; (2) regular and frequent visits, often monthly; (3) timely access by MTM providers to patients' complete medical, hospital, and laboratory data; (4) standardized documentation of MTM interventions, follow-up, and tracking of patient progress toward clinical goals; (5) standardized billing process and reimbursement of MTM providers; (6) eligibility independent of patient's annual prescription drug costs; and (7) program success that could be gauged by documented systemwide savings, rather than a singular focus on pharmaceutical expenditures.

These elements represent a sample of those that are reportedly critical to the success of some non-Part D MTM programs.

FEDERAL REGULATORY ACTION SUPPORTING MEDICATION THERAPY MANAGEMENT

The Patient Protection and Affordable Care Act (PPACA, PL 111-148) authorized grants for "medication management services" in all practice settings (Section 3503), noting that such services will help manage chronic disease, reduce medical errors, and improve patient adherence to therapies while reducing acute-care costs and hospital readmissions. The goal of this provision is to produce measurable MTM results and to replicate them in Medicare, Medicaid, state health insurance exchanges, and other programs. The Agency for Healthcare Research and Quality (AHRQ) is the lead implementing agency, but no funds were appropriated. Nevertheless, an important first step came in 2011, when AHRQ published a detailed MTM research agenda that closely parallels the intent of Section 3503.[33]

Meanwhile, through AHRQ's Effective Health Care Program, a multicenter trial was conducted to test the effectiveness of MTM interventions. The trial enrolled 600 participants 65 years of age and older who were at high risk of adverse drug events. One-third received no MTM (representing usual care or the control group); one-third received MTM based on information gleaned solely from patient interviews (this "mirrors the scenario encountered by most community-based pharmacists"); and one-third received MTM from pharmacists who had access to prescribers' clinical data. The standard intervention was two face-to-face MTM visits from a pharmacist over 6 months. Recommendations included recruiting patients during an existing clinical visit and delivering the MTM intervention on the same day (to reduce the patient's need for an extra trip). They also identified as an ideal situation locating a clinical pharmacist within a primary care clinic, so that MTM can be delivered at the point of care.[34]

CONCLUSION

To date, Medicare Part D policy debates have centered largely on the benefit's principal goal of enhancing access to prescription drugs. This includes the PPACA provision to close the Part D coverage gap, which continues through 2020. Meanwhile, secondary goals of optimizing the quality of medication therapy and preventing drug-related problems are gaining traction, bolstered in part by adoption of new clinical quality measures (such as adherence to drug therapy) for determining CMS Star Ratings. Another example of drug therapy management challenges is research that found that just four medications or drug classes were responsible for 67% of adverse-drug-event-related hospitalizations of elderly adults.[35]

Since 2006, Part D MTM programs have evolved slowly, with many programmatic changes, no dedicated budget, and no opportunity for shared savings. This has resulted in a conglomerate of MTM programs facing increasing challenges to demonstrate success and an increasing need to enhance Part D's value across the full Medicare program benefit.

The PPACA reaffirmed MTM's value by authorizing grants for "medication management services" in multiple settings, a related assessment with which AHRQ is proceeding. As patient-centered care matures alongside quality metrics, there is a growing recognition that "more powerful solutions are necessary to promote overall medication quality, not just adherence to a checklist at discharge."[36] MTM has the potential to represent just such a solution.

With the announcement of the Enhanced MTM Model, CMS is sending a message that while the current Part D MTM programs may not be optimal, there is still momentum within the federal government to find strategies for success. Plans will have financial incentives and the regulatory freedom to develop optimal MTM programs that deliver a measurable improvement for healthcare outcomes.

REFERENCES

1. MaCallan M. Testimony before the US Congress, House Ways and Means Committee, Subcommittee on Health, May 3, 2006. Available at https://waysandmeans.house.gov/Media/transcript/10205.html. Accessed February 11, 2017.
2. Public law 108-173, December 8, 2003. *Medicare Prescription Drug, Improvement, and Modernization Act of 2003*. Available at https://www.gpo.gov/fdsys/pkg/PLAW-108publ173/pdf/PLAW-108publ173.pdf. Accessed February 11, 2017.
3. Centers for Medicare and Medicaid Services. Memo: CY 2017 medication therapy management program guidance and submission instructions. April 8, 2016. Available at https://www.cms.gov/Medicare/Prescription-Drug-Coverage/PrescriptionDrugCovContra/Downloads/Memo-Contract-Year-2017-Medication-Therapy-Management-MTM-Program-Submission-v-040816.pdf. Accessed February 1, 2016.
4. Hepler C, Strand L. Opportunities and responsibilities in pharmaceutical care. *Am J Hosp Pharm*. 1990;47(3):533-543.
5. CMS. *Fact Sheet: 2016 Medicare Part D Medication Therapy Management (MTM) Programs Fact Sheet Summary of 2016 MTM Programs*, May, 4, 2016. Available at https://www.cms.gov/Medicare/Prescription-Drug-Coverage/PrescriptionDrugCovContra/Downloads/CY2016-MTM-Fact-Sheet.pdf. Accessed February 1, 2016.
6. Mitchell P, Hall L, Gaines M. A social compact for advancing team-based high-value health care, *Health Aff*. 2012. Available at http://healthaffairs.org/blog/2012/05/04/a-social-compact-for-advancing-team-based-high-value-health-care/. Accessed February 11, 2017.
7. Shoemaker S, Hassol A. Understanding the landscape of MTM programs for medicare Part D: Results from a study for the centers for Medicare & Medicaid Services. *J Am Pharm Assoc*. 2011;51(4):520-526.
8. Perlroth D, Olinger L, et al. *Medication Therapy Management in Chronically Ill Populations: Final Report*. CMS. August 2013;242. Available at http://innovation.cms.gov/Data-and-Reports.
9. CMS. *2012 Medicare Part D MTM Programs, Fact Sheet*, November 2012. Available at http://www.cms.gov/Medicare/Prescription-Drug-Coverage/PrescriptionDrugCovContra/Downloads/CY2012-MTM-Fact-Sheet.pdf.
10. Ahern V. CMS presentation at Pharmacy Quality Alliance annual meeting, May 2013. Slides available at http://www.pqaalliance.org.
11. Pharmacy Quality Alliance. *PQA Measure Development Update*, October 2016. Available at http://files.constantcontact.com/e9a15233201/41eab207-63bc-4d14-a5c2-45c940a3780b.pdf?ver=1475544366000). Accessed February 1, 2016.
12. John A. Hartford Foundation. *How Does It Feel? The Older Adult Health Care Experience*, April 2012. Available at http://www.johnahartford.org/events/view/john-a.-hartford-foundation-public-poll-how-does-it-feel-the-older-adult-he. Accessed February 11, 2017.
13. CMS. *Medicare 2016 Part C & D Star Rating Technical Notes*, August 2015. Available at https://www.cms.gov/Medicare/Prescription-Drug-Coverage/PrescriptionDrugCovGenIn/Downloads/2016-Technical-Notes-Preview-1-v2015_08_05.pdf. Accessed February 1, 2016.
14. 42 *Code of Federal Regulations* §423,104(d)(5)(iv).
15. CMS. *2010 Medicare Part D MTM Programs, Fact Sheet*, June 2010. Available at https://www.cms.gov/PrescriptionDrugCovContra/Downloads/MTMFactSheet_2010_06-2010_final.pdf. Accessed February 11, 2017.
16. Tudor C. State of Part D:2006-2012. Powerpoint presentation presented at CMS Medicare Prescription Drug Benefit Symposium, March 20, 2012. Available at http://www.cms.gov/Medicare/Prescription-Drug-Coverage/PrescriptionDrugCovGenIn/ProgramReports.html.
17. CMS. *Advance Notice, Part D Payment Policies and 2013 Call Letter*. February 17, 2012. Available at 105-107. http://www.cms.gov/Medicare/Health-Plans/HealthPlansGenInfo/Downloads/2013-Call-Letter.pdf.
18. CMS. *2013 Medicare Part D MTM Programs, Fact Sheet*, September 2013. Available at https://www.cms.gov/medicare/prescription-drug-coverage/prescriptiondrugcovcontra/downloads/cy2013-mtm-fact-sheet.pdf.
19. Wang J et al. Disparity implications of Medicare eligibility criteria for medication therapy management services. *Health Serv Res*. 2010;45(4):1061-1082 (PMC, web Feb. 3, 2017).
20. Wang J et al. Historical trend of disparity implications of Medicare MTM eligibility criteria. *Res Social Adm Pharm*. 2012;9(6):758-769.
21. Medicare Payment Advisory Commission. *Report to the Congress: Medicare Payment Policy*, Chapter 13, Table 13-9, March 2012; 354. Available at http://www.medpac.gov/docs/default-source/reports/mar13_entirereport.pdf?sfvrsn=0. Accessed February 11, 2017.
22. Medicare Payment Advisory Commission. *Health Care Spending and the Medicare Program: A Data Book*, June 2011. Available at http://www.medpac.gov/documents/Jun11DataBookEntireReport.pdf.
23. Priest J, Buikema A, et al. Quality of care, health care costs, and utilization among Medicare Part D enrollees with and without low-income subsidy. *Popul Health Manage*. 2012;15(2).
24. Isetts B. *Evaluating Effectiveness of the Minnesota Medication Therapy Management Care Program. Final Report*, December 14, 2007. Available at http://archive.leg.state.mn.us/docs/2008/mandated/080113.pdf.
25. CMMI. *Announcement of Part D Enhanced Medication Therapy Management Model Test*, September 2015. Available at https://innovation.cms.gov/Files/x/mtm-announcement.pdf. Accessed February 1, 2016.
26. Butler A, Dehner M, et al. *California Department of Public Health. Comprehensive Medication Management Programs: Description, Impacts, and Status in Southern California*, Sacramento, CA, 2015. Available at http://www.cdph.ca.gov/programs/cdcb/Documents/CMMWhitePaperCDPH2015Dec23FINALrev.pdf. Accessed February 11, 2017.

27. Mcbane, SE, Dopp AL, et al. Collaborative drug therapy management and comprehensive medication management—2015. *Pharmacotherapy*. 2015; 35(4):E39-E50 (web Jan. 20, 2017).

28. American College of Clinical Pharmacy (ACCP). *Comprehensive Medication Management in Team-Based Care*. Available at https://www.accp.com/docs/positions/misc/CMM%20Brief.pdf. Accessed January 20, 2017.

29. American Society of Health-System Pharmacists (ASHP). *ASHP Guidelines: Minimum Standard for Ambulatory Care Pharmacy Practice*. Available at http://www.ashp.org/doclibrary/bestpractices/settingsgdlminamb.aspx. Accessed January 20, 2017.

30. Patient-Centered Primary Care Collaborative. 2012. *The Patient-Centered Medical Home: Integrating Comprehensive Medication Management to Optimize Patient Outcomes*, 2nd ed. Available at http://www.pcpcc.org/guide/patient-health-through-medication-management. Accessed January 20, 2017.

31. Ramalho de Oliveira D, Brummel A, Miller D. Medication therapy management: 10 years of experience in a large integrated health care system. *J Manage Care Pharm*. 2010;16(3): 185-195. See also Brummel A. Fairview MTM. Webinar, patient-centered primary care collaborative, July 26, 2012. Available at https://www.ncbi.nlm.nih.gov/pubmed/20331323. Accessed February 11, 2017.

32. ASHP. *Pharmaceutical Case Management Helps Iowa Medicaid Patients*. Available at http://www.ashp.org/menu/News/PharmacyNews/NewsArticle.aspx?id=1207. Accessed February 11, 2017.

33. Dolor R, Masica A, Touchette DR, et al. Patient safety-focused MTM: Challenges affecting future implementation. *Am J Manage Care*. 2012;18(7): e238-e244. Available at https://www.ncbi.nlm.nih.gov/pubmed/22823552. Accessed February 11, 2017.

34. Tudor C. *CY 2013 Part D Reporting Requirements–Request for Comments*. CMS, January 13, 2012. Available at https://www.cms.gov/Medicare/Prescription-Drug-Coverage/PrescriptionDrugCovContra/downloads/ReqforCommentson2013ReportingRequirements_01102012.pdf. Accessed February 11, 2017.

35. Wynia M, Classen D. Improving ambulatory patient safety: Learning from the last decade, moving ahead in the next. *JAMA*. 2011;306(22):2504-2505.

36. Stuart B, Loh E, et al. Increasing Medicare Part D enrollment in medication therapy management could improve health and lower costs. *Health Aff*. 2013;1212-1220. Available at http://content.healthaffairs.org/content/32/7.toc.

Review Questions

1. Which of the following apply to Part D MTM services?
   a. They are required for all transition-of-care patients.
   b. Prescriber approval is required to provide services.
   c. It is required that services be face to face.
   d. The use of telehealth is required.
   e. Set selection criteria must be used to identify MTM-eligible patients.

2. Which of the following is true about a Part D MTM comprehensive medication review?
   a. It is done on all Medicare members enrolled in a PDP or MA-PD plan.
   b. It is done for MA-PD plans only.
   c. It addresses prescriptions, nonprescriptions, herbals, and dietary supplements.
   d. It requires access to medical records.
   e. Low-income subsidy recipients are excluded.

3. Medication therapy management eligibility criteria include which of the following?
   a. The number of chronic brand drugs
   b. Evidence of nonadherence
   c. Part B usage
   d. Selected chronic disease states
   e. An out-of-pocket spending limit

4. Which of the following statements best characterizes Part D MTM?
   a. Overall member participation has been below CMS expectations.
   b. Part D MTM has been proved to improve member outcomes.
   c. ACOs are required to provide Part D MTM to all members.
   d. Plans have no flexibility in choosing Part D MTM eligibility criteria.
   e. Prescribers are prohibited from conducting Part D MTM.

5. Unanswered questions for Part D MTM include which of the following?
   a. What information and data are useful for enhancing beneficiary awareness of MTM programs and services?
   b. What is the best method for evaluating the quality of an interactive, person-to-person comprehensive medication review (CMR) and other interventions?
   c. Which Part D MTM program eligibility criteria are most useful to beneficiaries in selecting a health plan?
   d. Which beneficiaries may derive the greatest benefit from a CMR and other MTM services or interventions?
   e. All of the above.

6. One of the major Part D MTM changes for 2016 is
   a. Access to complete medical records is required.
   b. Adoption of the CMR completion rate as a Star Measure is required.
   c. Physician approval of MAP is required.
   d. Fifty percent of all plan members must receive a CMR.
   e. Prescribers must receive and endorse copies of PMLs.

7. Features of the Part D Enhanced MTM Model include all of the following EXCEPT:
   a. Enhanced MTM is being conducted across five Part D regions.
   b. Part D sponsors also will be given a prospective per-member per-month payment for the enhanced services and will be eligible for a performance-based incentive payment.
   c. Each plan will have access to its beneficiaries' Medicare Part A and B data.
   d. Plans must submit enhanced MTM encounter data to CMS on a quarterly basis.
   e. The plan must target those with adherence issues no matter how many drugs they take.

8. Which of the following apply to enrollment in Part D MTM?
   a. A patient who declines MTM is disenrolled from the Part D plan.
   b. More than one method must be used to recruit a member.
   c. Eligibility criteria are applied once a year.
   d. Soliciting participation by mailings is prohibited.
   e. Enrollment strategies must include a face-to-face visit.

9. Which of the following apply to targeting Part D MTM members?
   a. Eight or more Part D drugs are required.
   b. All nine core disease states are required.
   c. Alzheimer patients are excluded because of their inability to do the CMR.
   d. The annual drug cost calculation includes Parts D and B drugs.
   e. The member must meet all three criteria: disease state, drugs, and drug spending.

10. To increase member involvement in Part D MTM, CMS
   a. made opt-out optional.
   b. eliminated the dollar qualification.
   c. plans to use percentage of MTM-eligible members who completed a CMR as a performance measure.
   d. eliminated the disease criteria requirement.
   e. eliminated the minimum number of required drugs.

ANSWERS

1. e	2. c	3. d
4. a	5. e	6. b
7. e	8. b	9. e
10. c		

3

Considerations for Establishing a MTM Service Practice Model

Teresa E. Roane, PharmD, BCACP, and Karen D. McLin, PharmD

KEY POINTS

- Medication therapy management (MTM) practice models should strive to be safe, timely, efficient, effective, equitable, and patient-centric.
- The chronic-care model provides a comprehensive view of the provision of care that is applicable to MTM.
- There are many different models of MTM and little evidence supporting a best practice for providing MTM services.
- The various MTM practice settings have differing MTM models.
- The successful provision of MTM will require an outline of the roles and responsibilities of the various people involved.
- Barriers to the provision of MTM exist and vary by the entity involved.

INTRODUCTION

Chronic Care Model

The measurement of quality in providing care is expanding rapidly throughout the US healthcare system. The 2001 Institute of Medicine report *Crossing the Quality Chasm: A New Health System for the 21st Century* defines *quality* as the degree to which health services for individuals as well as populations increase the likelihood of desired health outcomes and are consistent with current professional knowledge. The report targets for improvement of six fundamental attributes of effective healthcare:[1]

1. *Safety*: Care should be directed toward helping the patient and should not cause injury.
2. *Effectiveness*: Care and services should be based on the current accepted scientific knowledge.
3. *Patient-centeredness*: Care should be responsive and provided in a respectful manner.
4. *Timeliness*: The healthcare provider should ensure that the patient receives care without harmful delays.
5. *Efficiency*: The healthcare provider should ensure that the patient receives care without waste.
6. *Equitable patient care*: Care received should not vary in quality according to geographic location or patient characteristics such as socioeconomic status, race, or ethnicity.

With a rapidly aging population and the increasing longevity of people with chronic conditions, there is a significant push to improve not only the quality of care but also how that care is delivered. Data projections indicate that by 2020 more than 157 million people, over 50% of the American population, are expected to be living with a chronic condition that requires ongoing management and interaction with a healthcare team.[2] Among those, almost half have multiple conditions that are not being effectively managed.[2,3] Various deficiencies hindering the treatment of these patients include increased demands and time constraints on practitioners, which affect their ability to follow established practice guidelines; lack of coordination among healthcare teams; the data-sharing paradox; lack of ongoing follow-up with patients to ensure optimal outcomes; and inadequately trained patients to self-manage their own conditions.

TABLE 3-1 • Key Elements of the Chronic-Care Model (CCM)

Organization of healthcare	Clinical information system
Delivery system design	Patient self-management
Decision support	Community resources

The fundamental problem at the root of these challenges is the design of the total healthcare system, which has focused mostly on reacting to the acute needs of the patient versus being proactive about the prevention of such problems in the first place. Thus, a multidimensional solution for changing the system was defined by the Group Health Research Institute called the *chronic-care model* (CCM), which identifies six essential elements (Table 3-1, Figure 3-1) necessary for high-quality chronic disease care. Four important considerations include:[3-7]

1. An effective healthcare organization includes strong leadership to provide motivation, secure required resources, and remove any barriers that may affect or delay quality improvement. It also includes a delivery system that provides effective, efficient care focusing on proactive visits and follow-up, in which the patient is an integral part of the team.
2. The second important element is decision support that incorporates the latest evidence-based treatment guidelines for the care and management of chronic conditions and encourages practitioners to stay up-to-date on such standards through continuous educational outreach.
3. Clinical information systems that provide real-time patient data along with comprehensive clinical information are essential for patient care planning, information exchange with patients as well as other providers, performance monitoring of the treatment plan, and aid with follow-up requirements.
4. Finally, patient self-management is one of the most critical elements of the entire model. Patients need to be active managers of their own health, and healthcare providers need to empower patients by helping them develop self-management skills. Such support strategies include assisting the patient in accepting the reality of living with a chronic illness, setting realistic goals, establishing action plans, identifying barriers, and developing problem-solving skills to overcome those barriers. This is not a single action but rather a fluid process that persists throughout the continuum of a patient's care. Access to healthcare, along with utilization of community resources, can further support and enhance a patient's self-management of a chronic illness. These resources may include educational offerings, exercise programs, support groups, or other self-help-type support systems.

The CCM provides an evidence-based foundation for improving care for people with chronic illnesses, and it has been shown to be a successful strategy in guiding quality improvement in numerous settings. In fact, research-based evidence has shown that components of the CCM can not only improve quality but also reduce costs.[8,9] A Cochrane Review of ambulatory care diabetes management programs identified 39 studies involving more than 200 practices and 48 000 patients that included one to four CCM elements as part of each study's intervention.[8] These components included self-management, decision support, delivery system design, and clinical information systems. Studies were also evaluated on the basis of whether they detected significant improvements in care (measuring of hemoglobin A1c, urine albumin, serum lipid profiles) or patient outcomes (lowering hemoglobin A1c, improving organ problems). Table 3-2 groups the studies according to the CCM elements that were utilized. Of the 39 studies, 32 showed the intervention improved at least one process or outcome measure for diabetes.[9]

Pharmaceutical Care

Hepler and Strand[10] define *pharmaceutical care* as the provision of drug therapy in order to achieve definite outcomes that improve a patient's quality of life. It is a patient-centric way of delivering medication management services. Positive outcomes include cure of a disease, elimination or reduction of a patient's symptoms, arresting or slowing a disease process, and prevention of disease or symptoms. The process includes pharmacist collaboration with other healthcare professionals in designing, implementing, and monitoring a therapeutic care plan for a patient. Pharmaceutical care focuses on the pharmacist's role in achieving therapeutic goals to improve the patient's quality of life. It also stresses a pharmacist's responsibility for a patient's medication-related needs, with the pharmacist

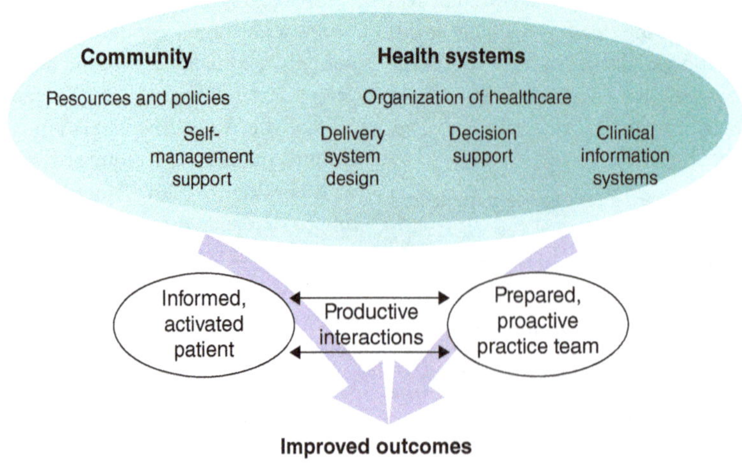

FIGURE 3-1 The chronic-care model.
Source: Reprinted with permission from Wagner EH. Chronic disease management: What will it take to improve care for chronic illness? *Effect Clin Pract.* 1998;1:2-4.

TABLE 3-2 • Summary of Studies of Chronic-Care Model Component Interventions for Diabetes Mellitus According to Components Included in Study

Chronic-Care Model Components	No. of Studies			
	Overall	Positive Outcomes[a]	Positive Process[a]	Positive Outcomes or Process
4 components				
SM, DS, DSD, CIS	5	5/5	2/2	5
3 components				
SM, DS, DSD	2	1/1	1/1	2
DS, DSD, CIS	4	0/3	1/2	1
SM, DS, CIS	3	3/3	2/2	3
SM, DSD, CIS	3	2/2	1/2	3
2 components				
DS, CIS	7	1/1	5/7	6
DS, DSD	2	2/2	0/0	2
SM, DSD	5	5/5	0/0	5
SM, DS	2	1/2	0/0	1
DSD, CIS	1	0/1	1/1	1
1 component				
DS	2	0/2	1/1	1
CIS	2	0/0	2/2	2
DSD	1	0/1	0/0	0
Total	**39**	**20/28**	**16/20**	**32**

[a] Figures indicate the number of studies with at least one positive finding divided by the number of studies that examined outcome or process measures. Denominators in these columns may sum to more than the total number of studies in each row because some studies examined outcome and process measures.

Abbreviations: CIS = clinical information system; DS = decision support; DSD = delivery system design; SM = self-management.

held accountable for patient outcomes along with ensuring that all of the patient's medication therapy is indicated, effective, and safe, and that the patient is willing as well as able to adhere to necessary instructions.[10]

Medication Therapy Management

The Medicare Modernization Act (MMA) of 2003 established the concept MTM. The law, fully implemented in 2006, recognized the need for the provision of MTM services to Medicare patients at high risk for problems related to their medication use. The law also indicated that these services should be provided by a pharmacist or other qualified healthcare provider. MTM is defined as a distinct service or group of services that optimize therapeutic outcomes for individual patients. The goal of MTM programs is to ensure that medications provided to patients are appropriately utilized to optimize therapeutic outcomes through improved medication use, and to reduce the risk of adverse events.[11] MTM services are distinct from medication dispensing and focus on a patient-centric process of care with an assessment, as well as evaluation, of the patient's entire medication therapy regimen rather than an individual medication product.[12]

Pharmacists' Patient Care Process

As healthcare continues to evolve, pharmacists are becoming increasingly recognized as members of the healthcare team. Their focus is also moving away from solely dispensing medications toward expanded clinical services for optimizing patient care. With this evolution, a need for a consistent means of care delivery and promotion of consistency has been a concern, and has been a focus of the Joint Commission of Pharmacy Practitioners (JCPP). To meet this need, JCPP worked to develop the *patient care process*, which is essentially a framework for the collaborative approach between the pharmacist and other healthcare providers in providing patient-centric care with a goal of optimizing patients' health and medication outcomes while building a supportive and engaging patient-pharmacist relationship.[13]

The patient care process contains concepts that are supported by evidence-based practice and include four basic elements: collection, assessment, planning, implementation, and follow-up in the form of monitoring and evaluation. In a little more detail, the process outlines the following pharmacist responsibilities: (1) collecting the necessary subjective and objective information, (2) assessing and analyzing the gathered information collected, (3) using a collaborative approach for developing a plan of care, (4) implementing the plan in collaboration with the patient and other providers, and (5) monitoring and evaluating how well the plan works as well as making adjustments as necessary. The process is ongoing and allows for the pharmacist to consistently cycle through the concepts to help ensure continuity of care, outcome evaluation, and ongoing care improvement. It is important to note that the basic foundation for the patient care process can be recognized within the pharmaceutical care model as well as the core elements that make up the framework of providing medication therapy management services.[13]

Incorporating Concepts of the CCM, Pharmaceutical Care, and the Pharmacists' Patient Care Process into MTM

The basic premise of the CCM, pharmaceutical care, and the patient care process can easily be incorporated into providing MTM services. In fact, many of the CCM elements and pharmaceutical care concepts are already included in MTM programs, as well as the ideals presented in the patient care process. These elements and concepts include establishing an efficient delivery system that consists of a framework for the consistent provision of services with a practice team led by a pharmacist that focuses on collaborating with patients and healthcare providers and establishes a clear delineation of required clinical and nonclinical tasks. For the best program efficiency, support staff should be utilized. Support staff includes a nonpharmacist team member who can be trained for many of the nonclinical tasks involved in providing MTM services (Table 3-3). Support staff can increase the efficiency of the pharmacist, allowing her/him to focus on clinical aspects of individualized comprehensive health assessments through interactive dialogs with patients. Access to a clinical information system that can ensure real-time patient data and record comprehensive clinical information is essential in facilitating comprehensive MTM services. This provides the foundation for patient care planning, information exchange with patients and other providers, assessment as well as documentation of the treatment plan, and follow-up reminders.

Elements of the comprehensive medication review (CMR) are summarized in Table 3-4. Decision support is a critical step in this process to ensure that the latest evidence-based disease management treatment guidelines are being followed, and are incorporated into the patient's care plan and medication action plan.

The interactive dialogue with the patient often consists of collecting information as well as providing education on disease management, and prevention, with a focus on empowering the patient with various tools to manage their chronic illnesses. The medication action plan that is completed as part of the CMR is specifically designed to be a collaborative effort with the patient, to outline the patient's responsibilities in helping to solve various identified problems. This format mandates the patient's active participation in the management of her/his chronic conditions. Providing information on community or national resources to enhance a patient's education, provide additional support, or aid in attainment of the patient's goals is also a part of the CMR process as well as the individualized care plan.

TABLE 3-3 • Nonclinical Services That Can Be Provided by Support Staff

Explain benefits of MTM
Coordinate appointments and follow-up appointments
Collect medication history or refill history
Gather responses to lifestyle questions
Other administrative tasks:
Billing
Filing paperwork
Faxing/mailing patients/providers

TABLE 3-4 • Elements of the Comprehensive Medication Review (CMR)

Review of all medications, including but not limited to
Prescription medications
Over-the-counter medications
Herbals
Samples
Review of all conditions to identify medication therapy problems (MTPs)
Development of interventions to reduce risk of MTPs, diseases, and disease progression

Incorporating aspects of the CCM and patient care process into MTM programs may help ensure implementation of a collaborative health plan using an evidence-based approach to improve patient's medication-related outcomes (Figure 3-2). This also allows a strategic approach to achieving the overall goals of MTM as outlined in Table 3-5 as well as measuring goal attainment and health outcomes. It is also beneficial in the continual cycle of care and modification of the care plan as necessary.

So, what is the best way to ensure that MTM programs meet these defined program goals? In addition, what is the best practice model to ensure that these goals are met? The American Pharmacists Association (APhA) in coordination with the National Association of Chain Drug Stores (NACDS) developed a model framework that describes elements for the delivery of MTM services in pharmacy practice.[11] Each element of the framework is essential to the provision of MTM services and meeting goals of the MTM program. In addition, the fundamental steps of the pharmacists' patient care process provide a means for ensuring consistency among pharmacists when providing MTM services. Even with both of these incorporated into the framework of MTM services, the Centers for Medicare and Medicaid Services (CMS) have chosen not to issue a strict definition of what constitutes an acceptable MTM program, and there is not one universally accepted gold-standard MTM practice model.

This chapter provides information pertinent to devising a MTM practice model and the delivery of MTM services. This includes an overview of current practice models, various practice types in diverse practice sites, staffing requirements, patient eligibility requirements, determining who may be involved in providing such services, prescriber and payer expectations, and documentation software, as well as identifying barriers that may arise in providing MTM services.

CURRENT MEDICATION THERAPY MANAGEMENT PRACTICE MODELS

Because of the lack of a universally accepted, gold-standard practice model, various MTM practice models or programs are currently in place (Table 3-6). Some practice models focus on face-to-face interactions with patients, other models utilize telephonic communications, and some provide a combination of both face-to-face and telephonic encounters. In a majority of

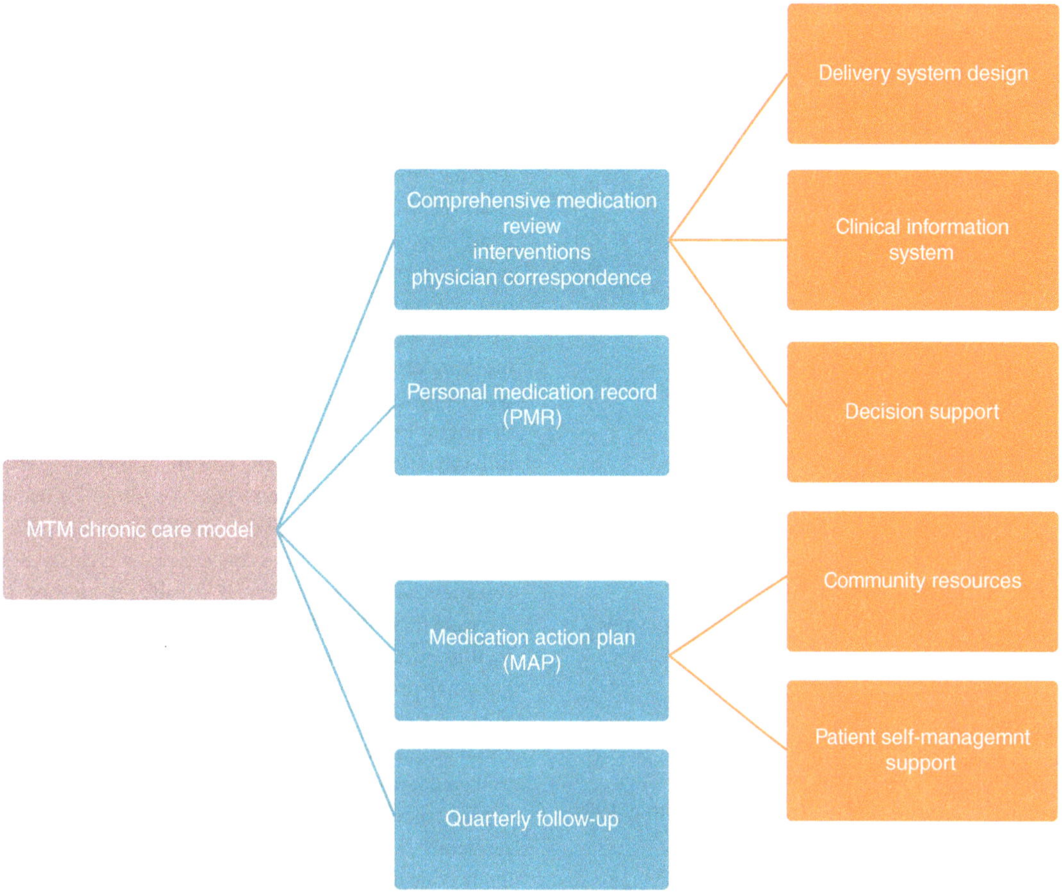

FIGURE 3-2 MTM chronic-care model.

practice models, pharmacists are the main providers of MTM services, although other models employ nurses or physicians to provide these services. A number of models have narrowed their focus to target specific chronic conditions or medications, while other programs allow for numerous chronic disease states and all chronic medications. Various programs incorporate a multitude of information for the MTM provider, such as access to the patient's electronic health record that includes prescriber notes and laboratory values, while other programs are limited to only prescription claims information. A number of programs, mainly those that offer face-to-face services, include additional services such as point-of-care testing for diabetes, cholesterol, and other risk factors. Many programs even allow for coordination with other patient care programs such as disease management or case management (Table 3-7). Regardless of the type of MTM practice model, the endpoint and goals of providing MTM services will always be the same (see Table 3-5).

TABLE 3-5 • Goals of Medication Therapy Management

Ensure optimal therapeutic outcomes
Reduce the risks of medication-related adverse events
Ensure collaboration among all healthcare providers
Increase percentage of CMRs
Provide potential cost savings (direct and indirect costs)
Improve adherence

MODE OF DELIVERING MEDICATION THERAPY MANAGEMENT

There is much debate regarding the optimum service delivery mode for providing MTM services: face-to-face or telehealth.[14] As of 2015, Medicare MTM program payers reported that 96% of MTM services were being delivered using telecommunications (including phone, 86% and web-based or videocommunications, 10%), while 71% reported services being delivered face to face or in person with 62% using both approaches.[15] There are obvious pros and cons to the various modes of communication (Table 3-8); however, currently there are insufficient data to suggest that any delivery method is superior to the other, although multiple approaches may be the most optimal to fully engage patients.

PRACTICE SETTINGS

Medication therapy management services are currently being provided in a number of different practice settings including call centers, community pharmacies, specialty pharmacies, physician offices, ambulatory care clinics, hospitals, long-term-care (LTC) facilities, and even within the patient's home.

Telehealth/Call Center

Telehealth is the use of electronic information and telecommunication technologies to support long-distance clinical healthcare,

TABLE 3-6 • Various Modifiable Components of MTM Practice Models

Mode of delivery	Face-to-face Telephonic Combination of face-to-face and telephonic
Setting	Call center Clinics Community pharmacy Physician offices LTC facilities Patient's home
Provider	Pharmacist Physicians Nurses Other
Qualifying conditions	All chronic conditions Limited by certain chronic conditions
Information source	Claims data Medical charts ± laboratory values Patient Caregiver
Additional point-of-care services (mainly in face-to-face model)	Diabetes Blood pressure Cholesterol International normalized ratio (INR)
Working as a team	Coordination of care Case management Disease management

patient and professional health-related education, public health, and health administration.[16] Telehealth technologies include videoconferencing, interactive websites, streaming media, and wireless communications. Telehealth also includes using telephonic interactions to provide effective medication therapy through an easily accessible model. Calls to initiate and/or conduct a person-to-person comprehensive medication review (CMR) are made by pharmacists, pharmacy technicians, and pharmacy interns typically located in call centers. During the call, information is gathered including lifestyle habits; allergies; disease conditions; current medications, including prescription and over-the-counter (OTC) products; vitamins, herbal supplements, and physician samples; as well as vaccination history, medical history, and any problems experienced with current medications. Patient-reported information is then incorporated into the patient's profile and reviewed by a pharmacist prior to the MTM session. The CMR consultation with the pharmacist (or supervised pharmacy intern) includes an evaluation of the patient's medications to identify opportunities to improve safety, reduce cost, and optimize pharmacotherapeutic treatment by identifying deviations from clinical practice guidelines and a general assessment of their various disease conditions. Call center pharmacy staff are primarily employed by health maintenance organizations (HMOs), pharmacy benefit management (PBM) companies, medication management vendors, and individual health plans; however, they also work in other environments as well.

Telehealth may also include the use of social media to not only engage patients to participate in MTM services but also provide a means to educate and interact with patients and caregivers. Social media has become part of the modern landscape of medicine, providing a means for patients to acquire health information instantaneously, connect or reconnect with others affected by similar conditions, and to actively participate in their treatment decisions. The use of social media within healthcare has risen dramatically from 41% in 2010 to 90% in 2011.[17,18] Social media is used by healthcare providers as a tool to share practice challenges, information, promote health behaviors, develop professional networks, increase personal awareness of news and discoveries, motivate patients, and provide health information to communities. These tools are also being used to improve clinical education.[19] "The overwhelming use of social media by clinicians falling into the youngest demographical segments has motivated adapting clinical curriculums to reflect the changing culture of incoming students."[20] However, there are certain concerns regarding the use of social media in medicine and the delivery of MTM services via these methods of communication. These concerns may include: breaching patient confidentiality and potential Health Insurance Portability and Accessibility Act (HIPAA) violations as well as distributing poor-quality information, publicizing unprofessional content, exceeding personal-professional boundaries, and licensing issues. Although these concerns are valid, technologies are rapidly evolving to enhance privacy controls, and guidelines are being development by healthcare institutions to safely and effectively integrate social media processes into healthcare, including the provision of MTM services.[18,21] This means the use of social media in medicine will likely continue to increase over the next few years as younger clinicians come into the workforce.

Community Pharmacy

Pharmacists in a community pharmacy setting typically provide MTM services through face-to-face encounters. Some of the largest national Medicare plans contract with community pharmacists directly, or through an MTM vendor, to provide face-to-face services to patients.[14] MTM services may be performed by the pharmacist on duty or by a different pharmacist who is scheduled for the specific task of providing MTM services. MTM services typically occur during scheduled appointment times, but can also be performed on a walk-in basis if the MTM pharmacist has adequate time, such as during slow hours of operation or if there is overlap in pharmacist coverage. Often a pharmacist specifically trained in providing MTM services will travel from one location to another to meet with patients. Community pharmacists also have the ability to incorporate additional services such as vaccination clinics, smoking cessation initiatives, and point-of-care testing to enhance their MTM services.

Prescriber's Office/Clinic

Medication therapy management services are being performed within some prescribers' offices often by the prescribers themselves, a pharmacist, or a nurse. Most prescribers have the training and experience to manage medications effectively within their general or specialized area of practice and many of them feel competent to provide MTM services.[15,22] Prescribers may; however, seek additional consultation in managing medications outside their usual scope of care, when patients do not reach clinical therapeutic goals,

TABLE 3-7 • Practice Model Components/Dimensions

MTM Practice Models	Primary Focus	MTM Providers	Intervention Frequency	Telephone Calls To/ From Patient Homes	Face-to-Face Sessions With Patients	Mailings to Patients	Additional Patient Education and Support	Rx Reconciliation With Prescribers	Disease State Monitoring (eg, Lab Results)
Hybrid MTM-disease management	MTM as one element, also lifestyle change and other DM	Pharmacists	Monthly or per refill or as needed	No call centers. some make refill reminder calls	Yes	Yes; educational materials	Yes	Yes	Yes Lab tests available to MTM providers at clinics or in charts
Care teams	MTM as one element, also lifestyle change and other DM	Pharmacists collaborating with physicians and nurse teams	Monthly or per refill or as needed	No call centers, Veterans Administration (VA) mails refills—no reminders needed; some others make refill reminder calls	Yes	VA no; some others mail educational materials	Yes; group support, education, case management	Yes	Yes; lab tests available to MTM providers at clinics or in charts
Required collaboration	Medication therapy Management only	Collaboration required between pharmacists and physicians	Driven by patient need (usually monthly or quarterly)	No call centers. May make telephone follow-up calls	Yes	No	No	Yes	Lab tests may be available to MTM providers
Multimode, comprehensive MTM	Medication therapy management only	Pharmacists	Driven by patient need (usually monthly or quarterly)	Some have call centers; others use telephone only for brief follow-up	Yes	Some (Medicare Part D plans)	Some	Yes	Some health plans monitor lab results and revise prescriptions
Pharmacy-based disease monitoring	Medication therapy Management with lab monitoring (usually single disease focus)	Pharmacists	Monthly or quarterly	Use telephone for brief follow-up.	Yes	No	Yes	Yes	Yes; pharmacists perform tests (eg, lipids, HbA1C)
Telephonic MTM	Medication therapy management only	Pharmacists, nurses for some patients education and reminder functions	Some annual, some more frequent	All MTM conducted by phone, usually from call centers	No	Most do not; a few send educational materials	No	Some yes, some no	Some health plan MTM programs monitor lab results and revise prescriptions
Medication regimen review (MRR) for nursing home patients	MRR	Consultant pharmacists	Monthly	No	N/A	N/A	N/A	Notes in charts with recommendations for prescribers	Yes

Source: Copyright American Pharmacists Association (APhA). Reprinted by permission of APhA.

TABLE 3-8 • Pros and Cons of Face-to-Face and Telephonic Models

Face-to-Face		Telephonic	
Pros	**Cons**	**Pros**	**Cons**
Physical assessment of the patient	Difficult to schedule with pharmacy	Patient in comfortable environment (ie, own home)	Physical assessment not possible
Possible to leverage existing relationships with pharmacy staff	Lack of dedicated space (eg, in the pharmacy)	Patient has access to information such as labs and other medical history	Pharmacist may not have ongoing relationship with the patient
Patients can bring in their prescription bottles and pharmacist can perform a brown-bag procedure	Pharmacy staffing is a challenge when there are few patients to sustain service delivery business model	Scheduling consultation is easier as visits can be coordinated for a clinician regardless of patient location	Lack of data (eg, prescription claims, medical chart, labs)
Counsel patients on administration techniques, especially for inhalers, insulin, and glucose monitors	Privacy can be an issue when dedicated space is open	Consultations can be recorded for oversight and auditing	
	Pharmacy may not have complete information on the patient's medical conditions or prescription claims	Cases can be centralized to the pharmacists, with increase in the volume of completed cases/ interactions	
	Pharmacists may be interrupted by other distractions (eg, phone calls, other patients, staff members)	Pharmacists can focus and deliver patient interactions without interruptions from other pharmacy staff	
		Provides opportunities to reach home-bound or nonambulatory patients	

or when their available time is limited.[22] MTM services within the prescriber's office or clinic setting is typically through face-to-face interactions with the patient, although some follow-up appointments may be handled telephonically for minor concerns, problem resolution, or when patients have transportation issues.

Hospital Setting/Outpatient Clinic

The provision of MTM services in hospital settings appear to be on the rise, although medication reconciliation has existed for years.[15] There are more than 34 million hospital discharges each year, and about 20% of those are complicated by a postdischarge adverse event, almost two-thirds of which are medication-related.[15] According to the Agency for Healthcare Research and Quality (AHRQ), "medication reconciliation is a process to decrease medication errors and patient harm by comparing the patient's current medication regimen against the physician's admission, transfer and/ or discharge orders to identify discrepancies."[23] APhA indicates that "medication reconciliation...is a critical, if not the primary, element in MTM."[24] The increased focus on providing MTM services within the hospital setting may suggest that pharmacists within the hospital are being incorporated into integrated-care models as well as care transition activities. *Integrated care* is a fairly new trend in healthcare that focuses on the coordination and integration of care provision. Transition-of-care activities, or encounters, occur at the time of hospital discharge and center around patients who may be vulnerable to medication-therapy problems when experiencing a change in their care settings (eg, when the patient enters, or is discharged from, a hospital or LTC facility; if the patient changes prescribers; or if the patient has a change in health insurance coverage). These types of transitions often result in medication therapy changes that may lead to medication-therapy problems or events. It is important that systems be established so that MTM services can ensure the provision of appropriate medication management during these points of transitions.[11]

Long-Term-Care Facility

The term *long-term-care* (LTC) encompasses pharmacy practice in skilled nursing facilities, intermediate-care facilities, assisted-living facilities, psychiatric centers, rehabilitation centers, and sub-acute-care settings. LTC facilities employ consultant pharmacists as a result of a 1974 federal mandate stipulating that pharmacists must conduct medication regimen reviews at least monthly for all residents of skilled nursing facilities. This regulation was extended to include intermediate-care facilities in 1987, and further expanded in 1990 to ensure the appropriate use of psychoactive medications and that residents' medication regimens are optimized. In 1999, the Beers Criteria were added to the medication therapy guidelines for nursing facility residents to ensure avoidance of certain medications that are inappropriate, or potentially unsafe, for use by seniors.[25] In addition to meeting these requirements, pharmacists are also providing MTM services to residents in LTC settings, when possible. These MTM services may be provided by the consultant pharmacist through face-to-face interactions; however, telehealth technology may be used when a pharmacist other than the consultant pharmacist is providing the MTM services.

STAFFING REQUIREMENTS

Pharmacists

Pharmacists, because of their training and expertise in medications, are in the unique position to be recognized as the optimal health-care professional for providing MTM services. According to the MMA of 2003, MTM services should be provided by "a pharmacist or other qualified healthcare provider."[26] As indicated by the Health Resources and Services Administration (HRSA), "clinical services are best provided by a pharmacist or by another healthcare professional in collaboration with a pharmacist."[26]

Studies have demonstrated the clinical and economic benefits of MTM services provided by pharmacists.[22] "MTM encompasses a broad range of professional activities and responsibilities within the licensed pharmacist's scope of practice." Pharmacists have the ability to obtain accurate disease and medication histories, along with a thorough understanding of the primary medical problem, comorbidities, and pharmacologic effects of an individual's medication regimen. In cases where patients are taking multiple medications, an in-depth understanding of drug interactions is necessary. In the area of medication-therapy problems, pharmacists have developed expertise in monitoring the pharmacologic effects of medications for certain disease states, including diabetes, asthma, hypertension, seizures, hyperlipidemia, anticoagulation, and infectious diseases.[25] These initiatives provide an early-warning system that identifies patients with suboptimal treatment responses and patients who may experience interactions, excessive medication effects, adverse medication effects, or medication toxicities.

Pharmacists have assumed an expanded role in medication safety, prevention of medication-therapy problems, disease management, and wellness programs. Pharmacists have also developed practices in the area of disease prevention and health promotion; specialties include reducing morbidity from obesity, osteoporosis, heart failure, hypertension, diabetes, and other chronic medical conditions, as well as helping improve patient habits and behaviors, such as smoking cessation and adherence. The rapid, dramatic advances in medication therapy over recent decades have also created a niche for pharmacy practitioners who specialize in specific kinds of treatment and aspects of care.[25]

On the basis of data from the 2013 MTM trend report, and also described in the 2016 CMS fact sheet for Part D MTM programs, pharmacists are currently the leading provider of MTM services across all MTM programs.[27,28] Pharmacists provide MTM services in various environments, and many have advanced training, in total, 75% have a doctor of pharmacy degree, 28% have completed a residency, 21% have participated in APhA's MTM Certificate Training Program, 5% are board-certified pharmacotherapy specialists, and 2% are board-certified ambulatory-care pharmacists.[15]

A topic that is currently at the forefront for pharmacy is the concept of pharmacists being able to obtain classification and recognition as a healthcare provider or receiving "provider status." Currently, pharmacists and the services that they provide are not included in the key sections of the Social Security Act, and this act determines a providers' eligibility to participate in healthcare programs such as Medicare Part B.[29] Not being recognized as a healthcare provider, through the Social Security Act, is often a source of contention as pharmacists are not able to receive compensation directly for providing comprehensive patient-centered care. Lack of provider status also impacts pharmacists from participating in integrated care delivery models that are promoted by the government in the Affordable Care Act (ACA). "Attaining provider status means coverage for pharmacists' patient care services and value recognition of those services."[29] It should also mean an improvement in a patient's access to pharmacist-provided care as well as an increase in the professional satisfaction of pharmacists.

Pharmacy Technicians

In its Model Act, the National Association of Boards of Pharmacy (NABP) defines *pharmacy technicians* as "personnel registered with the board who may, under the supervision of the pharmacist, assist in the pharmacy and perform such functions as assisting in the dispensing process, processing medical coverage claims, stocking medications, cashiering but excluding drug regimen review, clinical conflict resolution; prescriber contact concerning prescription drug order clarification or therapy modification; patient counseling, dispensing process validation, prescription transfer, and receipt of new prescription drug orders from prescribers."[25] NABP also indicates pharmacy technicians are skilled, valuable members of the pharmacy team who assist pharmacists in providing quality patient services.[25] Pharmacy technicians are a critical part of the pharmacy team, and their role has evolved over the years to assist the pharmacist in a variety of settings and responsibilities. The pharmacy technician is accountable to the supervising pharmacist, who, in turn, is legally responsible for the care and safety of patients served by the pharmacy. Many states are require technicians to meet high standards of practice and demonstrate mastery of knowledge through certification by passing a national exam and registering with the state board.

Pharmacy technicians work in a wide variety of practice settings, including community pharmacies, hospitals, military, home healthcare, LTC, prescription mail-order facilities, managed healthcare facilities, and educational settings as well as training programs.[30] According to the Bureau of Labor Statistics, about 70% of pharmacy technicians in the United States work in a retail setting such as community pharmacy or in mail-order or online pharmacies, while 13% of technicians work in hospitals and the remaining 17% working in other areas.[31] Other areas where technicians may work include nursing homes, pharmaceutical wholesalers, the federal government, health plans, and PBMs, as well as MTM vendors.[28]

With the proper training, technicians can assist in tasks that do not require the professional or clinical judgment of the pharmacist, freeing the pharmacist to focus on clinical activities and enabling an MTM program to be more sustainable. Technicians are valuable in many areas, including scheduling patient appointments and making reminder calls. Technicians can also provide education to patients regarding the MTM program as well as gather data and information, such as lifestyle attributes along with allergies, and identify questions that the patient may have for the pharmacist. Technicians can also assist the pharmacist with data collection, including medication use with health histories as well as creating charts, filing, gathering release forms, and documenting the information received by the patient. There are also new programs available that will assist in the training of pharmacy technicians specifically in the area of MTM as well as medication safety. These expanded functions of the technician allow the pharmacist more time to focus on the clinical aspects of the patient encounter.[31]

Student Pharmacists (Interns)

Student pharmacists in their third and fourth years of education begin to apply their knowledge by attending classes in advanced pharmacy practice experiences (APPEs), known as *rotations* or *clerkships*.[32] Some APPEs focus on direct patient care through face-to-face or telehealth encounters. Direct patient care experience is an important aspect of preparing student pharmacists for the challenges and opportunities that they will face in their professional careers. Like pharmacy technicians, student pharmacists work under the direct supervision of a pharmacist; however, student pharmacists have an expanded role in providing direct patient care because of their extensive training and education and clinical knowledge. Student pharmacist responsibilities vary by state; nevertheless, student pharmacists can be a valuable asset when providing MTM services. According to the 2016 CMS fact sheet for Part D MTM programs, student pharmacists (interns) are the second leading provider of MTM services across all MTM programs.[28] Data also indicate that student pharmacists have the opportunity to gain confidence in their ability to provide MTM services to patients, as well as develop skills that will be useful in overcoming barriers in the provision of MTM.[32] Another study indicates that student pharmacists in the community pharmacy setting were able to make significant patient-centric MTM interventions, with the majority of patients feeling better about their medications after speaking with a student pharmacist.[33]

Other Professionals

According to the MMA of 2003, MTM services should be provided by a pharmacist or other qualified healthcare provider.[26] Although pharmacists continue to be the leading providers in most MTM programs, some programs utilize other healthcare professionals, including nurses, nurse case managers, physicians, and support staff. Support staff can include pharmacy technicians, student pharmacists, pharmacy case coordinators, case workers, social workers, and MTM assistants (Figure 3-3).[28]

PATIENT ELIGIBILITY REQUIREMENTS

Medication therapy management programs were originally created in response to requirements set forth by the MMA of 2003, and centered around Medicare Part D participants and CMS requirements.[26] Since 2006, patient eligibility requirements for inclusion into MTM programs have been modified. Currently, to qualify for enrollment into a Medicare MTM program, the patient must have a certain number of chronic conditions, fill a predetermined number of prescription medications covered by Medicare Part D, and meet a minimum annual cost threshold. Patients who meet all eligibility criteria are automatically enrolled in the MTM program unless they request otherwise. Also, the MTM program must meet certain obligations to maintain compliance with CMS requirements.[28]

The number of MTM programs for non-Medicare patients is also on the rise, but the eligibility requirements are not so straightforward. Non-Medicare MTM programs include those offered by state Medicaid plans; employer groups, both self-insured as well as non-self-insured; the Department of Veterans Affairs; and programs that target cash-paying patients or caregivers of patients. In general, non-Medicare MTM programs have less restrictive eligibility criteria. For example, although some non-Medicare MTM programs focus on high-cost patients, several other non-Medicare MTM programs (eg, Project ImPACT, Asheville Project) target patients with specific chronic conditions.[14] However, most non-Medicare MTM programs lack explicit eligibility criteria and instead offer services to any patient whom clinicians or pharmacists believe would benefit from MTM services (Table 3-9).[14]

PAYER PERSPECTIVE

Medication therapy management programs are a requirement of a Medicare Part D prescription drug plan sponsor or health plan. These Medicare plans receive funding from the government in the form of administrative fees, which help cover the cost of establishing and maintaining an MTM program. Non-Medicare plans, such as state Medicaid MTM programs, receive funding from the state. Employer-sponsored programs are fully funded by the employer if self-funded; others may be funded through health insurance premiums.

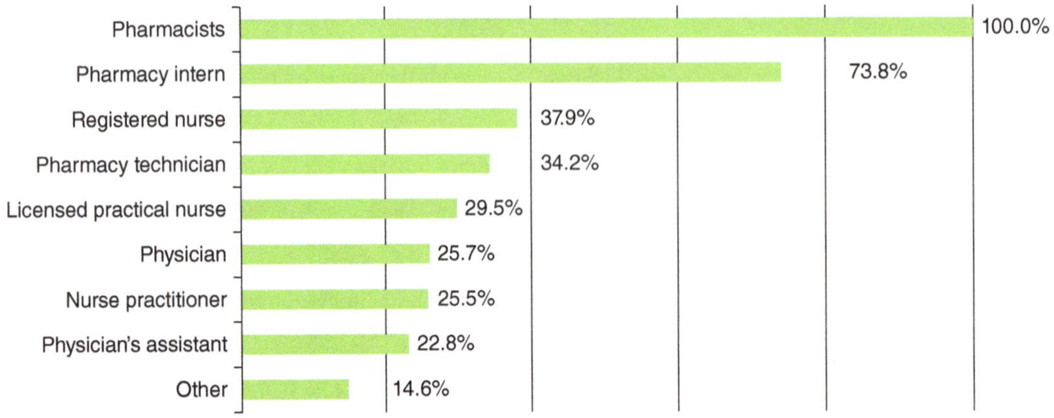

FIGURE 3-3 Provider of MTM services, showing percent of 2016 MTM programs.

Source: Centers for Medicare and Medicaid Services (CMS). *2016 Medicare Part D Medication Therapy Management (MTM) Programs: Fact Sheet: Summary of 2016 MTM Programs, May 4, 2016*. http://www.cms.gov/Medicare/Prescription-Drug-Coverage/PrescriptionDrugCovContra/Downloads/CY2016-MTM-Fact-Sheet.pdf.

TABLE 3-9 • Medicare Prescription Drug Plans Interviewed: MTM Eligibility Criteria

Number and Type of Conditions				Number and Type of Medications
Large, national PDP and its PBM	≥5 conditions, 2 of which are Diabetes Asthma (Soon will decrease to ≥2 of these conditions)	CHF COPD	Hypertension Dyslipidemia	Any 6+ Part D drugs
Plan with 1 PDP in 4 states	≥2 of 3 conditions: Diabetes	Asthma	Dyslipidemia	≥2 Part D drugs related to specified chronic conditions
Large, national PDP	≥2 of 6 conditions: Diabetes Hypertension Rheumatoid arthritis	Heart failure Atrial fibrillation	Dyslipidemia	≥6 Part D Drugs related to chronic disease
Plan with 1 PDP, over 1 million enrollees	≥4 of 5 chronic conditions: Diabetes Asthma	Hypertension Chronic pain	Dyslipidemia	Any ≥10 Part D drugs
Single-state MA-PDP	≥2 of 5 conditions: Diabetes COPD	Heart failure CAD	Asthma	Any ≥7 Part D drugs
Plan with 1 MA-PD	Both of the following: Heart failure	COPD		4 of ACE inhibitors, β-lockers or nebulizer; and oxygen in home
Regional MA-PDP	≥3 of most chronic conditions including the following: Diabetes Asthma	Heart failure COPD	Hypertension Dyslipidemia	Any ≥5 Part D drugs
Plan with 2 PDPs and 2 MA-PD plans	All of the following: Diabetes	Hypertension	Dyslipidemia	≥3 drugs for treatment of 3 identified chronic conditions
Plan with 1 PDP and 1 MA-PD plan	≥5 chronic conditions, including ≥2 of the following: Diabetes Asthma	Heart failure COPD	Hypertension Dyslipidemia	≥12 Part D drugs related to chronic disease
Plan with 1 PDP and 2 MA-PD plans	≥2 of 6 conditions: Diabetes Asthma	Heart failure COPD	Hypertension Dyslipidemia	Any ≥5 Part D drugs related to chronic disease
Plan with 1 PDP and 6 MAPD plans	≥4 of the following: Chronic pain Diabetes Dyslipidemia Asthma	Angina CAD COPD Hypothyroidism	Migraine headaches Anticoagulation Rheumatoid arthritis	≥12 Part D drugs
Large, national MA-PDP	≥2 chronic medical conditions			≥5 Part D drugs related to chronic disease
Large, national PDP	4 out of 10 diagnoses: Asthma Diabetes Heart failure Alzheimer's disease/ dementia	COPD ESRD Dyslipidemia	Angina/arrhythmia Rheumatoid Arthritis Hypertension	Any ≥10 Part D drugs

(Continued)

TABLE 3-9 • Medicare Prescription Drug Plans Interviewed: MTM Eligibility Criteria (*Continued*)

Number and Type of Conditions				Number and Type of Medications
Large, multistate MAPD plan (case study)	2 or more of the following: Diabetes CAD Pulmonary embolism CVA DVT	Dyslipidemia	Hypertension Atrial Fibrillation Peripheral Artery Disease Mechanical Heart Valve	≥2 medications from the following: Anticoagulants Antihyperlipidemics Antihypertensives Hematopoietic agents Insulin Oral hypoglycemics
	≥5 chronic conditions, with ≥2 of the following: Asthma/COPD CHF Hyperlipidemia	Diabetes	Hypertension	Any ≥9 Part D drugs

Abbreviations: ACE = angiotensin-converting enzyme; CAD = coronary artery disease; CHF = congestive heart failure; COPD = chronic obstructive pulmonary disease; CVA = cerebrovascular accident; DVT = deep-vein thrombosis; ESRD = end-stage renal disease.

Source: Copyright American Pharmacists Association (APhA). Reprinted with permission from APhA.

Some MTM programs receive funding based on a capitated rate, some programs offer a performance guarantee, and other programs use a fee-for-service model. Capitated rates are monies paid to the provider for a set number of patients enrolled in the program over a certain period of time, regardless of whether the patients receive services. Capitation is typically described in terms of "per-member per-month" rates. In the performance guarantee model, the program offers a targeted return on investment (ROI) that is calculated on the basis of the care that was avoided because of pharmacist intervention. In the fee-for-service model, used by the majority of community pharmacists, the provider is paid for services, with preestablished rates for different services.[14]

Regardless of the payment model, the payers of MTM programs have certain expectations for both providers and programs. Payers expect value—economic, clinical, or humanistic—from the MTM services being provided. Increased quality of care and performance measure outcomes, such as Star Ratings, have been primary focal points for payers, followed by interventions that reduce costs, for both medical care and total healthcare. Other services considered valuable by payers include improved patient outcomes, high patient satisfaction, enhanced interdisciplinary care, optimizing medication use along with increase in medication adherence, avoidance of adverse events as well as drug interactions, and retaining patients in the health plan.[15]

In addition, payers are concerned with the quality of their MTM programs and are evaluated by CMS utilizing a 5-Star Rating system. Star Ratings are created from performance measures that contribute to the overall rating for individual health plans, where 5 Stars is the highest rating. One of the performance measure elements that has most recently been included in this Star Rating system is the completion rate for comprehensive medication reviews (CMRs). The CMR completion rate as defined by CMS is calculated by dividing the number of beneficiaries from the denominator who received a CMR during the reporting period by the total number of nonhospice beneficiaries who were aged ≥18 years at the beginning of the reporting period. Beneficiaries must meet specified targeting criteria, and be enrolled in the MTM program for at least 60 days during the reporting period."[34] The ultimate goal of the health plan or payer is to achieve and maintain a high Star Rating on specific performance measures as well as an overall high rating. To learn more about the payer perspective, please see Chapter 5 of this text for more detailed information.

PRESCRIBER PERSPECTIVE

Physician or prescriber understanding of MTM services, and the acceptance of MTM provider recommendations, are important to the success of a MTM program. Although evidence has shown that pharmacist-provided services are beneficial, physician acceptance rates of pharmacist recommendations are relatively low and often depend on the relationship between the prescriber and the recommending pharmacist.[1] Although many colleges (of pharmacy, medicine, nursing, etc) encourage interdisciplinary healthcare with collaboration between health professional students as a component of the curriculum, there is still a huge void and push for collaboration among different healthcare providers in everyday practice. This is evidenced in the provision of MTM services.

The literature suggests that physicians often consider "pharmacists to be on the periphery of the healthcare team," which becomes a challenge when providing MTM services.[1] Often MTM services are provided telephonically, so the MTM provider making the recommendations may have no previous relationship with the prescriber, and may not even be located in the same state, providing a further challenge. Prescribers have concerns regarding the amount of time required to follow up with pharmacist recommendations, and also express dissatisfaction with not being paid for the additional responsibility. They also do not like to feel as though their prescribing decisions are being second-guessed. In addition, some prescribers may feel as though they are the most qualified to provide MTM services.[35]

The literature; however, also shows that prescribers acknowledge the benefits of collaborating with pharmacists, and recognize the value of a pharmacist identifying medication-therapy problems.[1,35] Prescribers appreciate having a completed medication list, including OTC products, provided to them following an MTM encounter, and expect that the pharmacist will notify the prescriber when the patient does not adhere to medication regimens. Prescribers also feel a strong preference for practice models that support the pharmacist working within the physician's office, which for obvious reasons is the most ideal scenario.[35] To learn more about the physician's perspective, please see Chapter 6 of this text for more detailed information.

BARRIERS TO PROVIDING MTM SERVICES

Despite the fact that pharmacists and other qualified healthcare professionals have the necessary skills and opportunities to provide MTM services, many providers cite barriers for being able to implement a successful program (Table 3-10). Data show that pharmacists overwhelmingly agree that they are best positioned (99.3%), have the clinical knowledge necessary (95.7%), and have the clinical experience required to deliver effective MTM services.[14] Pharmacists also agree that barriers prevent or hinder them from adopting MTM services in ambulatory settings. The most common barriers include health plans having different eligibility requirements for MTM services, reimbursement issues, and high workloads, as well as lack of time, staffing, access to patient records, and acceptance by prescribers.[15,36] Finding software to meet the needs of an MTM program was another barrier indicated by pharmacists.[15]

TABLE 3-10 • Barriers to Providing MTM Services

Pharmacist-identified barriers	Different eligibility requirements across plans (eg, number of medications required and types of disease states covered) Lack of time with high workload demands Lack of staffing Reimbursement issues Lack of access to patient records Lack of acceptance by prescribers Lack of access to ideal software
Payer-identified barriers	Lack of patient and prescriber awareness of MTM Engaging patients (members) and getting the member to participate in MTM programs Achieving scalability for MTM programs Conducting outcome assessments Lack of optimum software platform Lack of standardized documentation Lack of ideal billing mechanisms
Service-related barriers	Cultural sensitivity issues Language barrier difficulties (translator) Health literacy problems (patient may not be able to read or write) Privacy disclosure concerns Technology problems (software or internet connectivity not working properly) Contact information challenges (wrong/no phone number or address) Scheduling conflicts (no-show appointments) Cognitive impairment of the patient Fraud/waste/abuse concerns Crisis situations Location to conduct such private encounters

Payers also face challenges with barriers when attempting to provide MTM services: raising patient and prescriber awareness, engaging patients (members) to actually participate in MTM programs, achieving scalability for MTM programs, and conducting outcomes assessments.[15] Payers also feel that finding the optimum software platform is a barrier, as well as the lack of standardized documentation and billing mechanisms.[15,36]

Other barriers that may appear include cultural sensitivity issues, language barrier difficulties, literacy problems, privacy disclosure concerns, technology issues, absence of or incorrect patient contact information, scheduling conflicts and no-show appointments, cognitive impairment of the patient, fraud/waste/abuse concerns, crisis situations, and the availability of a suitable location to conduct such private discussions. Although these barriers exist, many can be overcome with the proper consideration of the issues, and applications of procedures and protocols outlining how to handle such events.

OTHER CONSIDERATIONS

Return on Investment

Many MTM programs have been able to demonstrate that the program improves patient outcomes and decreases overall medical costs, although calculating the ROI can be challenging. The ROI is defined as how much value the services add compared to the overall cost of delivering the service; basically a ratio of savings to costs.[37] Components that are captured in calculating ROI include determining the number of patients that are successfully engaged to participate in MTM services; the financial value of the impact those services demonstrate, which includes cost avoidance such as decreases in hospital admissions, physician visits, along with emergency room admissions, and actual cost savings, such as a reduction in or discontinuation of unnecessary as well as inappropriate medications; retention time during which patients successfully participate in the program; total number of staff required to provide such services; and the direct and indirect cost for the resources needed to deliver those services.[38-45] ROI is frequently difficult to calculate and may vary depending on the patient population being evaluated, the limited availability of data (medical and pharmacy costs), and varying healthcare costs across practice sites; however, the ROI of medication management services has been established through various models.[22] Outcome data captured from the delivery of these services across various patient populations have been very positive, with a demonstrated ROI as high as 12:1 and an average of 3:1 to 5:1.[38-45] ROI values may be somewhat conservative because of practitioners routinely underestimating the impact of the outcome of these services on a patient's quality of life. Likewise, it is difficult to put a value on high patient satisfaction and physician acceptance rates.[37] Although ROI has not been calculated directly by CMS, Acumen reports have indicated that "MTM programs within the Medicare setting consistently helped enrollees with heart failure and chronic obstructive pulmonary disease improve adherence to their evidence-based regimens and discontinue the use of high-risk medications" and that a CMR "appeared to exert a strong effect on outcomes, as beneficiaries who received CMRs were more likely to benefit from MTM program participation across almost all outcomes relative to those in MTM programs who did not receive CMRs."[46] As healthcare services continue to evolve away from a fee-for-service model to a pay-for-performance model, it is critical to ensure that ROI is being effectively captured for all MTM services being provided regardless of the practice environment in order to substantiate the value it brings to patient care.

Balancing Efficiency and Effectiveness

In business, there is always a concern about having employees productive and efficient in order to meet the needs of both the business model and the practice model. Effectiveness "is the degree to which the goals and objectives are successfully met" and is often measured in terms of performance outcomes.[47] For example, in providing MTM services, productivity could be measured by the number of CMRs that a pharmacist performs in a typical day, while *efficiency* would equate to the pharmacist exceeding those productivity goals, and *effectiveness* would be how well the pharmacist is identifying clinical issues while conducting the CMRs.

Balancing efficiency and effectiveness is not always an easy task, and in some instances a tradeoff must occur. Time is a variable that affects efficiency when providing MTM services. In most settings, the pharmacist often has a number of responsibilities and has to engage in many different tasks. The amount of time allotted for the pharmacist-patient interaction during a CMR is often limited in efforts to maintain efficiency; therefore, a tradeoff occurs. The pharmacist must try to completely assess the patient's medication use while addressing as many issues as possible in a relatively short amount of time. Although the pharmacist may want to spend more time with the patient, allowing this would negatively affect productivity and efficiency. Attempting to increase efficiency and/or productivity by requiring the pharmacist to complete more CMRs in a shorter amount of time may also affect the quality of care the patient receives.[47]

TECHNOLOGY, STANDARDIZATION, AND SNoMED CT CODES

Documentation is one of the core elements of the model framework for providing MTM services.[11] Some MTM providers may choose to document patient encounters using pen and paper, while most others use an electronic documentation system that has its obvious advantages. The use of technology for electronic documentation may improve efficiency, foster continuity of care, aid in billing of services, facilitate the reporting of outcomes, and ease the burden of record retention. The documentation systems currently being used to provide MTM services vary dramatically, and often depend on the setting.[48] Some of the systems are web-based, requiring limited training, and are relatively easy to use; however, they may pose a barrier for providers who have limited or no internet access in their work environments. Some systems are incorporated into the technology already being used for certain functions of the provider's daily activities, such as an electronic medical record (EMR), while other systems are totally separate and require the provider to learn and work in two different documentation platforms. Some systems facilitate interaction and data exchange between the health plan and the MTM provider, while other systems do not allow for such interoperability.

There are proponents for the standardization of documentation systems in the same way that CMS has standardized the format of the MAP and personal medication list (PML). Proponents say that standardization could help promote collaboration, and help address most of the barriers that MTM providers face with current technology.[15] A goal of standardization would be for the software system to be interoperable, allowing for the exchange of information between two or more systems. Interoperability and "health information technology (HIT) are expected to assist in the delivering of effective, efficient, coordinated care as health professionals strive to improve the quality of care and outcomes for the individual patient."[48]

Systematized Nomenclature of Medicine–Clinical Terms (SNoMED CT) codes is a universal clinical coding system developed for use in documenting patient care. This system has been in place for many years and covers a broad range of health-related topics. As a component of HIT and a means of helping improve documentation and reporting of outcomes when providing MTM services, the use of SNoMED-CT codes specific for MTM have been developed. "Ensuring that pharmacists establish the same clinical coding foundation as other health care providers will help ensure the integration of MTM services documentation into the [electronic health record] and the national HIT interoperable framework." SNoMED-CT codes are ready and available for use. To alleviate issues and facilitate use, pharmacists are not required to remember or even select the codes during their documentation process; the codes are embedded into the computer programming system and automatically assigned to the documentation options that would be available to the pharmacist.[49] The use of these codes will help with consistency and tracking of various services provided by the pharmacist, and problems identified during the provision of MTM services, as well as ease of outcome reporting, which will allow for improvement in patient care.

Affordable Care Act Implications on the Practice Model

Making progress in healthcare has often been proposed in government throughout the years, although rarely would change come to fruition. With enactment of the Patient Protection and Affordable Care Act (PL 111-148) and the Health Care and Education Reconciliation Act of 2010 (PL 111-152), change did occur and became what is now known as *legislated healthcare reform*.[50] Many elements of the Patient Protection and Affordable Care Act will have a direct impact on the pharmacy profession and provide opportunities for pharmacists to be more involved in direct patient care. The ACA also indicates the need for the provision of MTM services to those outside of the high-risk Medicare population. These include patients not eligible or enrolled in an MTM program but who have been identified as being at risk, such as those who have experienced a transition in care (eg, recent hospitalization or stay in a skilled nursing facility transitioning to an alternate location). At a minimum, MTM services must include strategies to improve medication adherence and patient health outcomes. The services and strategies include the following:[50]

1. Performing or obtaining necessary assessments of the health and functional status of each patient who receives MTM services
2. Formulating a medication treatment plan according to therapeutic goals agreed on by the prescriber and the patient or caregiver (or authorized patient representative)
3. Selecting, initiating, modifying, recommending changes to, or administering medication therapy
4. Monitoring, which may include access to, ordering, or performing laboratory assessments, and evaluating the response of the patient to therapy, including safety and effectiveness
5. Performing an initial CMR using either person-to-person or telehealth technologies (telephones, videoconferencing) by a licensed pharmacist or other qualified provider to identify, resolve, and prevent medication-therapy problems, including adverse drug events; quarterly targeted medication reviews for ongoing monitoring; and additional follow-up intervention on a schedule developed collaboratively with the prescriber
6. Providing education and training to enhance the understanding and appropriate use of the medications by the patient, caregiver, or other authorized representative
7. Providing information, support services, resources, and strategies to enhance services provided to the patient
8. Coordinating and integrating MTM services within the broader healthcare management services provided to the patient
9. Other patient care services allowed under pharmacist scope of practice in use in other federal programs that have implemented MTM services

The ACA also emphasizes integrated-care models to improve the quality of care while managing costs. Accountable care organizations (ACOs), patient-centric medical homes, community health teams, and home-based primary-care teams are among the models included in the ACA. The provision of MTM services within ACOs, medical homes, and other team-based clinical groups could help manage or prevent medication-therapy problems.[26,51,52]

CONCLUSION

Getting an MTM business up and running may be a daunting task—there are quite a few things to consider in order to establish a successful practice model. Many of the items covered in this chapter need to be taken into account for an MTM business to succeed. Goals for the business should be established initially but often need adjustment throughout the year as business requirements change or as regulations are amended. Policy and procedures need to be written to guide decisions and help ensure that services are being provided according to established business protocols. Staffing requirements ought to be assessed and may need alteration to accommodate business needs or as performance measures dictate. The readiness of the staff being employed should be measured prior to the provision of MTM services as well ensuring continual and ongoing training of staff as new clinical information emerges. Technology should be capable of handling the initial requirements of the business and have the capacity to adapt to changes in regulations or the practice model. Incorporating these various elements into a practice model will ensure that the overall values of MTM services to enhance patient care are being met.

REFERENCES

1. Institute of Medicine. *Crossing the Quality Chasm: A New Health System for the 21st Century*. Washington, DC: The National Academy Press; 2001.
2. Robert Wood Johnson Foundation. *Chronic Conditions: Making the Case for Ongoing Care*. Baltimore, MD: Johns Hopkins University; 2004. Available at http://www.partnershipforsolutions.org/DMS/files/chronicbook2004.pdf. Accessed December 28, 2016.
3. Bodenheimer T, Chen E, Bennett H. Confronting the growing burden of chronic disease: Can the U.S. health care workforce do the job? Available at http://content.healthaffairs.org/content/28/1/64.full. Accessed December 28, 2016.
4. Wagner EH, Austin BT, Davis C, et al. Improving chronic illness care: Translating evidence into action. *Health Aff*. 2001;20(6):64-78.
5. Wagner EH, Austin BT, Von Korff M. Organizing care for patients with chronic illness. *Milbank Q*. 1996;74:511-544.
6. Wagner EH. Chronic disease management: What will it take to improve care for chronic illness? *Effect Clin Pract*. 1998;1(1):2-4.
7. NCHC-IHI. *Accelerating Change Today (ACT) for America's Health; Curing the System: Stories of Change in Chronic Illness Care*. Washington, DC: The National Coalition on Health Care and the Institute for Healthcare Improvement (NCHC-IHI); May 2002. Available at http://www.improvingchroniccare.org/downloads/act_report_may_2002_curing_the_system.pdf. Accessed December 29, 2016.
8. Renders CM, Valk GD, Griffin S, et al. Interventions to improve the management of diabetes mellitus in primary care, outpatient and community settings. *Cochrane Database Syst Rev*. 2001;(1):1-3.
9. Bodenheimer T, Wagner E, Grumbach K. Improving primary care for patients with chronic illness: The chronic care model, Part 2. *JAMA*. 2002;288(15):1909-1914.
10. Hepler CD, Strand LM. Opportunities and responsibilities in pharmaceutical care. *Am J Hosp Pharm*. 1990;47:533-543.
11. American Pharmacists Association and National Association of Chain Drug Stores Foundation. Medication therapy management in pharmacy practice: core elements of an MTM service model (version 2.0). *J Am Pharm Assoc*. 2008;48:341-353.
12. Academy of Managed Care Pharmacy. *Sound Medication Therapy Management Programs*, version 2.0. Available at http://www.amcp.org/sound_mtm_program/. Accessed December 22, 2016.
13. Joint Commission of Pharmacy Practitioners. *Pharmacists' Patient Care Process*; 2014. Available at https://www.pharmacist.com/sites/default/files/files/PatientCareProcess.pdf. Accessed December 22, 2016.
14. Shoemaker S, Hassol A. Understanding the landscape of MTM programs for Medicare, Part D: Results from a study for the centers for Medicare and Medicaid services. *J Am Pharm Assoc*. 2011;51:520-526.
15. American Pharmacists Association. Pharmacists emerging as interdisciplinary health care team members. *Medication Therapy Management Digest*; March 2013. Available at http://www.pharmacist.com/sites/default/files/files/MTMDigest_2013.pdf. Accessed December 22, 2016.
16. National Academy of Sciences: Institute of Medicine of the National Academies. *The Role of Telehealth in an Evolving Health Care Environment*; November 2012. Available at http://www.ic4n.org/wp-content/uploads/2014/06/IoM-Telehealth-2012-Workshop-Summary.pdf. Accessed January 27, 2017.
17. Bosslet G, Torke A, Hickman S, Terry C, Helft P. The patient-doctor relationship and online social networks: Results of a national survey. *J Gen Intern Med*. 2011;2:1-7.
18. Modahl M, Tompsett L, Moorhead T. *Doctors, Patients & Social Media*; September 2011. Available at http://www.quantiamd.com/q-qcp/DoctorsPatientSocialMedia.pdf. Accessed December 28, 2016.
19. Ventola CL. Social media and healthcare professionals: benefits, risks, and best practices. *P&T (Pharmacy and Therapeutics)*. 2014;39(7):491-499, 520.

20. Von Muhlen M, Ohno-Machado L. Reviewing social media use by clinicians. *J Am Med Inform Assoc*. 2012;19(5):777-781.
21. George D, Rovniak L, et al. Dangers and opportunities for social media in medicine. *Clin Obstet Gynecol*. 2013;56(3).
22. Patient-Centered Primary Care Collaborative. *The Patient-Centered Medical Home: Integrating Comprehensive Medication Management to Optimize Patient Outcomes. Resource Guide*. Washington, DC; 2012. Available at http://www.accp.com/docs/positions/misc/CMM%20Resource%20Guide.pdf. Accessed December 18, 2016.
23. Martin C. Avoiding errors during transitions of care: Medication reconciliation. *Consult Pharm*. 2012;27:764-769.
24. ASHP. *Improving Care Transitions: Optimizing Medication Reconciliation*. American Pharmacists Association, American Society of Health-System Pharmacists; March 2012. Available at https://www.pharmacist.com/sites/default/files/files/2012_improving_care_transitions.pdf. Accessed January 27, 2017.
25. Council on Credentialing in Pharmacy Practice. Scope of contemporary pharmacy practice: Roles, responsibilities, and functions of pharmacists and pharmacy technicians. *J Am Pharm Assoc*. 2010;50:e35-e69.
26. Medicare Prescription Drug, Improvement and Modernization Act of 2003. Public Law 108-173, 108th Congress. Available at https://www.congress.gov/108/plaws/publ173/PLAW-108publ173.pdf. Accessed January 27, 2017.
27. Bartholomew B, Tice B, Ansel M. *PharmMD 2011 MTM Industry Trend Report*. Available at http://amcp.org/pharmmd_mtm_trend_report/. Accessed December 18, 2012.
28. CMS. *2016 Medicare Part D Medication Therapy Management (MTM) Programs Fact Sheet*; May 4, 2016. Available at https://www.cms.gov/Medicare/Prescription-Drug-Coverage/PrescriptionDrugCovContra/Downloads/CY2016-MTM-Fact-Sheet.pdf. Accessed December 28, 2016.
29. American Pharmacist Association. *The Pursuit of Provider Status: What Pharmacists Need to Know*; September 2013. Available at https://www.pharmacist.com/sites/default/files/files/Provider%20Status%20FactSheet_Final.pdf. Accessed December 28, 2016.
30. Powers M, Bright D. Pharmacy technicians and medication therapy management. *J Pharm Technol*. 2008;24:336-339.
31. Bureau of Labor Statistics. *Occupational Outlook Handbook: Pharmacy Technicians*; December 2015. Available at https://www.bls.gov/ooh/healthcare/pharmacy-technicians.htm#tab-3. Accessed January 1, 2017.
32. Hardin H, Hall A, Roane T, Mistry R. An advanced pharmacy practice experience in a student-staffed medication therapy management call center. *Am J Pharm Educ*. 2012;76(6):110.
33. Hata M, Klotz R, Sylvies R, et al. Medication therapy management services provided by student pharmacists. *Am J Pharm Educ*. 2012;76(3):51.
34. Miller D, Roane TE, Salo JA, Hardin H. Evaluation of comprehensive medication review completion rates using 3 patient outreach models. *J Manag Care Spec Pharm*. 2016;22(7):796-800.
35. McGrath SH, Snyder M, Duenas GG, et al. Physicians perceptions of pharmacist-provided medication therapy management: qualitative analysis. *J Am Pharm Assoc*. 2010;50:67-71.
36. Gruber J. Medication therapy management: A challenge for pharmacists. *Consult Pharm*. 2012;27:782-796.
37. Lenz TL, MS Monaghan. Pay-for-performance model of medication therapy management in pharmacy practice. *J Am Pharm Assoc*. 2011;51:425-431.
38. Cobb CD. Optimizing medication use with a pharmacist-provided comprehensive medication management service for patients with psychiatric disorders. *Pharmacotherapy*. 2014;34(12):1336-1340.
39. Zeiger RS, Schatz M, Dalal AA, Qian L, et al. Utilization and costs of severe uncontrolled asthma in a managed-care setting. *J Allergy Clin Immunol Pract*. 2016;4(1):120-129, e3.
40. Bunting BA, Smith BH, Sutherland SE. The Asheville Project: Clinical and economic outcomes of a community-based long-term medication therapy management program for hypertension and dyslipidemia. *J Am Pharm Assoc*. 2008;48(1):23-31.
41. Isetts BJ, Schondelmeyer SW, Artz MB, et al. Clinical and economic outcomes of medication therapy management services: The Minnesota experience. *J Am Pharm Assoc*. 2008;48(2):203-211.
42. Barnett MJ, Frank J, Wehring H, et al. Analysis of pharmacist-provided medication therapy management (MTM) services in community pharmacies over 7 years. *J Manag Care Pharm*. 2009;15(1):18-31.
43. Chisholm-Burns MA, Graff Zivin JS, Lee JK, et al. Economic effects of pharmacists on health outcomes in the United States: A systematic review. *Am J Health Syst Pharm*. 2010;67(19):1624-1634.
44. Ramalho de Oliveira D, Brummel AR, Miller DB. Medication therapy management: 10 years of experience in a large integrated health care system. *J Manag Care Pharm*. 2010;16(3):185-195.
45. Lada P, Delgado G Jr. Documentation of pharmacists' interventions in an emergency department and associated cost avoidance. *Am J Health Sys Pharm*. 2007;64:63-68.
46. Marrufo G, Dixit A, Perlroth D, et al. *Medication Therapy Management in a Chronically Ill Population: Interim Report. Acumen, LLC*. Available at http://innovation.cms.gov/Files/reports/MTM-Interim-Report-01-2013.pdf. Accessed December 28, 2016.
47. Flood A, Shortell S, Scott WR. Organizational performance: Managing for efficiency and effectiveness. In: *Essentials of HealthCare Management*. Albany, NY: Delmar. 1997;381-420.
48. Millonig M. Mapping the route to medication therapy management documentation and billing standardization and interoperability within the health care system. *J Am Pharm Assoc*. 2009;49:372-382.
49. Pharmacy Health Information Technology Collaborative. *Documenting Comprehensive Medication Management in Team-Based Models Using SNoMED CT Codes*; August 2014. Available at http://pharmacyhit.org/pdfs/workshop-documents/WG2-Post-2014-03.pdf. Accessed January 2, 2017.
50. National Conference of State Legislatures (NCSL). *The Patient Protection and Affordable Care Act* ("PPACA"; Public Law 111-148). Available at http://www.ncsl.org/documents/health/ppaca-consolidated.pdf. Accessed March 3, 2013.
51. Lofton JC. APhA pharmacy law matters 2010: Focused on selected provisions of the affordable care act. *Pharm Today*. 2010;16(12):72-78.
52. Matzke GR. Health care reform 2011: Opportunities for pharmacists. *Ann Pharmcother*. 2012;46(Suppl 1):S27-S32.

Review Questions

1. The IOM Report definition of *quality* includes which of the following?
   a. *Safe*: Care should be without injuries and should be helping the patient.
   b. *Effective*: Care and services should be based on the current accepted scientific knowledge.
   c. *Patient-centered*: Care should be responsive and provided in a respectful manner.
   d. *Time-appropriate*: Drug administration should be based on effectiveness.
   e. *Efficient*: Care should include reducing waste.

2. The chronic-care model can best be described as
   a. most useful for physician practice.
   b. too limited in scope for Part D MTM.
   c. indicating that there are many aspects of patient care beyond those that healthcare providers can supply.
   d. applying only to care of chronic diseases such as diabetes.
   e. limited, because it does not include the pharmacist.

3. The pharmacy technician's role in Part D MTM services includes
   a. creating the contents of the MAP.
   b. collecting medication history.
   c. contacting physicians about interventions.
   d. counseling patients about drug interactions.
   e. establishing causality of adverse drug reactions.

4. Which of the following are true about the current Part D MTM practice models?
   a. Pharmacists are the only Part D MTM providers.
   b. Community pharmacies and call centers are the only MTM practice settings.
   c. Long-term-care residents are excluded from Part D MTM services.
   d. Access to the complete medical record is not required.
   e. Point-of-care services such as blood pressure and HgBA1C are required.

5. Which of the following is true about providing Part D MTM regulations for face-to-face meetings in community pharmacies without private counseling rooms?
   a. Physical assessments must be recorded.
   b. Visual inspection of prescription bottles is required.
   c. Cognitive impairment is not an issue.
   d. Health literacy must be tested.
   e. No maximum or minimum time limit is specified.

6. Comparison of a Part D MTM call center to face-to-face sessions in a community pharmacy reveals that:
   a. Face-to-face sessions are more effective than call center MTM sessions.
   b. The MTM method preferred by Medicare is face-to-face.
   c. Both meet the criteria for interactive.
   d. Patients are not as truthful over the phone.
   e. Call center CMRs must be completed more quickly than face-to-face CMRs.

7. Which of the following is a barrier to the provision of Part D MTM services?
   a. More patients demand Part D MTM than can be accommodated.
   b. CMS dictates what type of Part D MTM software must be used.
   c. PDPs opt out of participating in the Part D MTM program.
   d. MA-PD plans substitute disease management and case management for MTM.
   e. None of the above.

8. Which of the following could be useful training principles for the provision of Part D MTM?
   a. being efficient and effective with CMRs and consultations
   b. defining how to provide a safe and effective CMR given limited time and patient information
   c. motivating and supporting pharmacy staff to do clinical problem solving
   d. balancing clinical problem solving with nonclinical activities
   e. all of the above

9. Current Part D MTM practice models can best be characterized as which of the following?
   a. dependent on medical record access
   b. using the CMS-standardized PML and MAP
   c. having uniform pharmacist experience and certification requirements
   d. requiring a collaborative agreement with physicians
   e. operating independently of state pharmacy regulations

10. A practice model may be composed of which of the following?
   a. roles, responsibilities, and expectations for each professional and patient involved
   b. care process description
   c. performance measures
   d. business model requirements
   e. all of the above

ANSWERS

1. d	2. c	3. b
4. d	5. e	6. c
7. e	8. e	9. b
10. e		

4

Medication Therapy Management Quality and Performance Improvement

Anna Hall, PharmD, BCACP, and David P. Nau, PharmD, PhD, RPh, CPHQ, FAPhA

KEY POINTS

- The US healthcare system is moving from a fee-for-service payment model to one of value-based purchasing, with provisions set forth in legislation for accountable-care organizations, medical homes, bundled payments, and a focus on quality.
- *Value-based payment* is a payment method that provides financial incentives to providers who meet certain quality standards in order to foster clinical and financial accountability.
- Measurement of quality is expanding rapidly throughout the US healthcare system. Quality in healthcare is usually measured through the use of performance indicators, also known as *performance measures*.
- It is essential for Medication Therapy Management (MTM) providers to understand the quality metrics that apply to medication therapy management, which will influence the focus of their practice models.
- The Medicare Advantage and Medicare Prescription Drug Plan Quality Strategy provide a framework for measuring quality performance for both Medicare Advantage and Medicare Prescription Drug (Medicare Parts C and D) plans. The Centers for Medicare and Medicaid (CMS) measures the quality of Medicare Parts C and D plans with the Star Ratings system.
- By publicly reporting the ratings, CMS encourages Parts C and D sponsors to improve service quality to attract enrollees to their plans. The measures are also used to determine quality bonus payments (QBPs) for Medicare Advantage (MA) organizations.
- Medicare Part D ratings include measures for medication use under the domain of patient safety and accuracy of drug pricing. MTM program providers should be mindful of the medication use, safety, and adherence measures as they provide MTM services on behalf of Medicare Part D plans.
- Starting with the 2016 Star Ratings, CMS has included an MTM-specific quality measure, which evaluates the percentage of MTM-eligible beneficiaries who received a comprehensive medication review. The measure was developed, and is maintained, by the Pharmacy Quality Alliance.
- CMS intends to adopt further process and outcomes measures for MTM once they are developed and endorsed.
- Beyond the Star Ratings and quality measures reported by CMS, MTM programs and vendors, like all healthcare providers, should ensure the quality of the services that they provide. Payers should be able to rely on the accuracy, completeness, and appropriateness of patient interactions, written communications to patients and providers, and MTM encounter records.

INTRODUCTION

A Focus on Quality

The 2003 Medicare Modernization Act began to move the United States toward a value-based healthcare system. This was echoed in the Patient Protection and Affordable Care Act (PPACA) of 2009, in which the word *value* is mentioned at least 214 times.[1] The act reforms Medicare payments, with a shift from a fee-for-service model to one of value-based purchasing, with provisions for accountable-care organizations, medical homes, and bundled payments. There is also a focus on quality, exemplified by programs such as the Hospital Value-Based Purchasing Program and updates to the Physician Quality Reporting Program, including financial incentives (Table 4-1).[1-3]

Value is defined as a balance between quality and cost. Value is optimized by improving quality at the same time as reducing costs.[4] *Value-based payment* is a payment method that provides financial incentives to providers who meet certain quality standards in order to foster clinical and financial accountability.[5] This incentivized payment plan is termed *pay for performance* and abbreviated *P4P*. In this value-driven system, quality is determined by attaining certain benchmarks for performance set forth by the CMS as well as showing performance improvement overtime.[5] Two of the four cornerstones of the US Value-Driven Health Care Initiative (Table 4-2) include measuring and publishing quality information, as well as promoting quality and efficiency of care. These cornerstones are designed to provide consumers with the information necessary to make informed decisions about their providers and treatment options. This not only drives consumer choice but also allows providers to see how the quality of care that they deliver compares to others. These arrangements are intended to reward both those who offer and those who purchase high-quality, competitively priced healthcare.[6]

Quality measurement is expanding rapidly throughout the US healthcare system. The 2001 Institute of Medicine report, *Crossing the Quality Chasm: A New Health System for the 21st Century*, defines *quality* as the degree to which health services for individuals and populations increase the likelihood of desired health outcomes and are consistent with current professional knowledge.[7] The report lays forth six objectives for healthcare improvement (Figure 4-1).

The Institute for Healthcare Improvement's Triple Aim framework promotes three dimensions of healthcare:

1. *Better care*—improving the patient experience of care (including quality and satisfaction)
2. *Healthier people/healthier communities*—improving the health of populations
3. *Lower costs*—reducing the per capita cost of healthcare[8]

The US Value-Driven Health Care Initiative is founded on transparency, provided to consumers through data collected on performance of provider-specific quality measures (Figure 4-2).[9] This has led to the availability of public performance data on many providers, including hospitals, physicians, long-term-care facilities, and health plans.[10] Many accrediting bodies require providers to collect data on performance measures to maintain deemed status.

TABLE 4-1 • Examples of Current CMS Pay-for-Performance Initiatives

Initiative	Provider Type	Incentives/Penalties
Hospital Value-Based Purchasing Program[a]	Hospitals	Incentive payments to hospitals for inpatient acute-care services are based on hospital quality reporting for quality measures through the Hospital Inpatient Quality Reporting Program
Hospital Readmissions Reduction Program[b]	Hospitals	Medicare can reduce payments to hospitals that have high rates of avoidable readmissions for patients experiencing acute myocardial infarction, heart failure, or pneumonia
Merit-based Incentive Payment System (MIPS)[c]	Physicians, physician assistants, nurse practitioners, clinical nurse specialists, and certified registered nurse anesthetists	One of 2 tracks for providers in the Medicare Quality Payment Program; providers that bill Medicare >$30 000 a year and provide care for >100 Medicare patients a year and participate in MIPs earn a performance-based payment adjustment on Medicare payments; the adjustment is based on quality, improvement activities, advancing care information, and cost
Advanced Alternative Payment Models (AAPMs)[c]	Networks of physicians and other providers such as hospitals	One of 2 tracks in the Medicare Quality Payment Program; in 2017 certain alternative payment models are eligible to be considered advanced AMPs and earn a 5% Medicare Part B incentive payment for taking on a certain amount of financial risk, performing on quality measures, and using electronic health technology
Medicare Advantage Plan Bonuses[d]	Medicare Advantage plan sponsors	Bonus payments to Medicare Advantage plans that achieve at least a 3-Star Rating on the 5-Star Quality Rating scale; plans with a 4- or 5-Star Rating will receive even greater bonus payments

[a] *Hospital Quality Initiative*. Available at: http://www.cms.gov/Medicare/Quality-Initiatives-Patient-Assessment-Instruments/HospitalQualityInits/index.html?redirect=/hospitalqualityinits.

[b] *Readmissions Reduction Program*. Available at: http://www.cms.gov/Medicare/Medicare-Fee-for-Service-Payment/AcuteInpatientPPS/Readmissions-Reduction-Program.html.

[c] *MACRA Delivery System Reform, Medicare Payment Reform*. Available at: https://www.cms.gov/Medicare/Quality-Initiatives-Patient-Assessment-Instruments/Value-Based-Programs/MACRA-MIPS-and-APMs/MACRA-MIPS-and-APMs.html

[d] *CMS Fact Sheet*. Available at: http://www.cms.gov/apps/docs/Fact-Sheet-2011-Landscape-for-MAe-and-Part-D-FINAL111010.pdf.

TABLE 4-2 • Four Cornerstones for Healthcare Improvement

Goals	Description
Interoperable health information technology (health IT standards)	Interoperable health information technology has the potential to make healthcare delivery more efficient. Significant progress has been made to develop standards that enable health information systems to communicate and exchange data quickly and securely to protect patient privacy. Additional standards must be developed, and all healthcare systems and products should meet these standards as they are acquired or upgraded.
Measure and publish quality information (quality standards)	To make confident decisions about their healthcare providers and treatment options, consumers need quality-of-care information. Similarly, this information is important to providers who are interested in improving the quality of care that they deliver. Quality measurement should be based on measures that are developed through consensus-based processes involving all stakeholders, such as the processes used by the AQA (a multi-stakeholder group focused on physician quality measurement) and the Hospital Quality Alliance.
Measure and publish price information (price standards)	To make confident decisions about their healthcare providers and treatment options, consumers also need price information. Efforts are underway to develop uniform approaches for measuring and reporting price information for the benefit of consumers. In addition, strategies are being developed to measure the overall cost of services for common episodes of care and the treatment of common chronic diseases.
Promote quality and efficiency of care (incentives)	All parties—providers, patients, insurance plans, and payers—should participate in arrangements that reward both those who offer and those who purchase high-quality, competitively priced healthcare. Such arrangements may include implementation of pay-for-performance reimbursements for providers or the offering of consumer-directed health plan products, such as account-based plans for enrollees in employer-sponsored health benefit plans.

Source: Institute of Medicine. *Crossing the Quality Chasm: A New Source*: Institute of Medicine. Rona Briere, ed. Health System for the 21st Century. Washington, DC: National Academy Press; 2001.

The Joint Commission and CMS report performance data on hospitals and other institutional providers.[11–13] The National Committee for Quality Assurance (NCQA) maintains the Healthcare Effectiveness Data and Information Set (HEDIS) and composite ratings for managed-care organizations, which include performance for medical services such as those involved with managing diabetes and hypertension.[14] Table 4-3 provides examples of public reports on healthcare providers. The demand for quality report cards is growing, and the shift to value-based payment has accelerated with the implementation of the Medicare Access and CHIP Reauthorization Act (MACRA) of 2015.[15]

In the past, retail or community pharmacy practice was largely unaffected by demands for quality measurement data and value-based payment. Some states now require community pharmacies to provide quality assurance and improvement programs, which focus primarily on medication errors. However, the focus on pharmacy quality is now expanding to quality of medication use and performance measures that align with physician and health plan measures.[4] CMS facilitated the formation of The Pharmacy Quality Alliance (PQA) in 2006 to develop pharmacy quality measures and coordinate the efforts of pharmacy stakeholders in developing such measures.[4,16] In 2007, PQA tested an initial set of quality measures focusing on medication adherence, safety, and appropriate medication use. The organization continues to develop new measures.[16,17]

The Center for Pharmacy Practice Accreditation (CPPA) and Utilization Review Accreditation Commission (URAC) have

Safe—avoiding injuries to patients from the care that is intended to help them
Effective—providing services based on scientific knowledge to all who could benefit and refraining from providing services to those not likely to benefit
Patient-Centered—providing care that is respectful of and responsive to individual patient preferences, needs, and values and ensuring that patient values guide all clinical decisions
Timely—reducing waits and sometimes harmful delays for both those who receive and those who give care
Efficient—avoiding waste, including waste of equipment, supplies, ideas, and energy
Equitable—providing care that does not vary in quality because of personal characteristics such as gender, ethnicity, geographic location, and socioeconomic status

FIGURE 4-1 Institute of Medicine's six objectives for healthcare improvement.

Source: Adapted from Rona Briere, ed. *Crossing the Quality Chasm: A New Health System for the 21st Century*. Washington, DC: National Academy Press, Institute of Medicine; 2001.

(1) The federal government, individual private employers, and health plans commit to sharing information on price and quality in healthcare. Together, the government and major employers provide healthcare coverage for some 70% of Americans.

(2) The federal government and individual private employers commit to quality and price standards developed with the medical community. This will help guarantee a fair and accurate view of the quality of care delivered by individual providers, as well as providing consistent measures for quality.

(3) The federal government and individual private employers commit to standards for health information technology (IT). Health IT will be important for gathering and using the best information for consumers. These standards are also crucial to the goal of achieving electronic health records for all Americans.

(4) The federal government and individual private employers commit to offering plans that reward consumers who exercise choice based on high quality of care and competitive price for healthcare services.

FIGURE 4-2 Steps to transparency in healthcare.

Source: US Department of Health and Human Services (HHS). *Value-Driven Health Care Home*. HHS.government archive. Available at http://archive.hhs.gov/valuedriven/. Accessed April 17, 2014.

TABLE 4-3 • Examples of Public Reports on Quality of Healthcare Providers

Program Name	Provider Type	Public Display Site (URL)
Hospital Compare	Hospitals	http://www.medicare.gov/hospitalcompare/
Nursing Home Compare	Long-term-care facilities	http://www.medicare.gov/NHCompare
National Committee for Quality Assurance (NCQA) Health Plan Report Card	Health plans	http://reportcard.ncqa.org/plan/external/plansearch.aspx
Center for Medicare and Medicaid (CMS) 5-Star Quality Rating System	Medicare Advantage and Medicare Prescription Drug Plans	https://www.medicare.gov/find-a-plan/questions/home.aspx
Massachusetts Health Quality Partners	Physicians	www.mhqp.org

launched accreditation programs for community pharmacies that will increase demands for quality-related information from pharmacies. While neither of these programs currently requires public reporting of quality metrics to maintain accreditation, both programs require pharmacies to be actively engaged in quality improvement.[18,19] With the cost of drug-related morbidity and mortality estimated to exceed $177 billion per year, there is no doubting the importance of a focus on quality for the medication use system.[20]

Medicare Advantage and Medicare Part D Quality Strategy

Recognizing the need to ensure appropriate and effective medication use with the development of Medicare Part D, Congress required that Medicare plans provide certain beneficiaries with MTM services.[21] CMS has developed the CMS Quality Improvement Strategy to further ensure the quality of Medicare Advantage (MA) and Medicare Part D (PDP) plans.[22] This framework is based on the 2001 Institute of Medicine report and the Triple Aim. The expanded strategy (2011) reflects the Department of Health and Human Services National Strategy for Quality Improvement in Health Care, referred to as the *National Quality Strategy* and *National Prevention Strategy*, which were developed in accordance with the Affordable Care Act.[22] The strategy requires all MA organizations to develop a quality improvement program to coordinate the care of plan members. Part D plans are required to develop quality assurance measures for safe and effective medication use; there are seven domains that CMS uses for defining quality and the requirements of these quality improvement programs.[22] Figure 4-3 depicts components of the MA and PDP Quality Strategy. With the goals set forth in the MA and PDP Quality Strategy, CMS

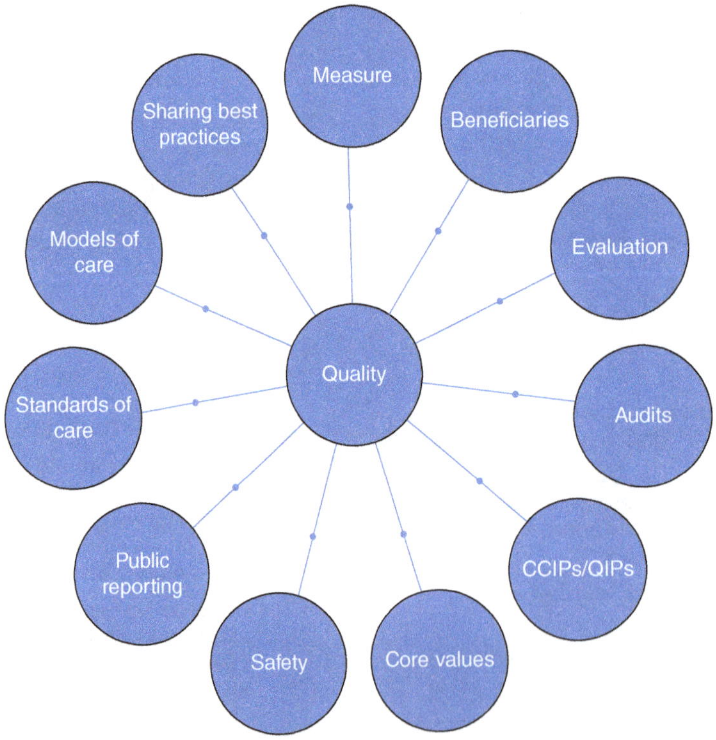

FIGURE 4-3 Components of the MA and PDP Quality Strategy and QI Program that contribute to the quality of care for Medicare beneficiaries enrolled in MA and PDP programs.

Notes: Core Values = MA and PD Quality Strategy core values: 1—robust; 2—consumer-friendly; 3—comparable; 4—comprehensive; 5—transparent. Abbreviations: CCIP = Chronic Care Improvement Program for Medicare Advantage organizations [a set of interventions designed to improve the health of individuals who live with multiple or sufficiently severe chronic conditions, including patient identification and monitoring]; QIP = Quality Improvement Program for Medicare Advantage organizations [MA sponsors must have an ongoing quality improvement program for each of their plans].

Source: Centers for Medicare and Medicaid Services (CMS). Quality assessment. In: *Medicare Managed Care Manual*, Chapter 5. Available at http://www.cms.gov/Regulations-and-Guidance/Guidance/Manuals/downloads/mc86c05.pdf.

makes clear that its ongoing efforts will include continued implementation of strategies for improving quality and metrics for monitoring MA and PDP progress in attaining quality strategy goals.

The MA and Medicare Prescription Drug Plan Quality Strategy provides a framework for measuring quality performance of MA and PDP plans. By working with organizations such as NCQA and PQA, CMS has established and reports on performance measures for MA and PDP plans in order to provide consumers with information on plan quality and to ensure efficient, high-quality Medicare plans.[22] PQA methods for measuring the quality of medication use are applied by Medicare for Part D plans. This publicly reported performance measurement rating system is described in detail in this chapter. CMS does not collect or publicly report on the quality of individual pharmacies, and there is currently only one Part D performance measure specific to MTM programs. However, the pressure on Part D plans to perform well on ratings measures will likely drive them to require network pharmacy participation in quality measurement.[4] It will also likely require that patient and provider interactions resulting from MTM services focus on plan rating quality measures related to medication use.

Impact of Value-Driven Healthcare and Quality Initiatives on MTM Service Providers

Medication therapy management providers must be aware of the US healthcare system's move toward value-driven healthcare. They must also understand the quality metrics used in Star Ratings of Medicare plans, which ought to influence the focus of their MTM practice model. The practice of pharmacy throughout the healthcare system is likely to experience new mandates for quality improvement, public reporting, and pay-for-performance incentives.[4] PQA's MTM Part D Workgroup is dedicated to developing MTM-specific performance measures, which will focus on the effectiveness and quality of MTM interventions as well as programs. MTM programs will soon see an increased demand for evidence of quality and effectiveness as they operate within the framework of value-driven healthcare. MTM programs will need to develop their own practice-specific quality assurance and improvement programs to ensure that they are consistently meeting the requirements for MTM delivery, including regulations set forth in the *Medicare Prescription Drug Benefit Manual*, providing quality customer service, and effective clinical services.

FOUNDATIONS OF QUALITY MEASUREMENT

This section provides a brief overview of the foundational concepts and tools of quality measurement. (For an in-depth discussion, please refer to the textbook *Quality and Safety in Pharmacy Practice*, Chapters 5-8.[23-26]) Understanding these foundations will help pharmacists. Health plans create an optimal culture for quality measurement as well as assurance in medication use.

The Purpose of Measuring Quality

As mentioned previously, *quality* in a health system as defined by the Institute of Medicine is the degree to which health services for individuals and populations increase the likelihood of desired health outcomes and are consistent with current professional knowledge.[7] The purpose of measuring quality is to identify problems within a system which can be considered opportunities for improvement. Improvements can then be monitored as the system is modified. Performance data are used to measure quality and thus improve healthcare services. Data from performance measurement can be used in many different ways by various stakeholders to encourage performance and quality improvement. Healthcare organizations such as hospitals and long-term-care facilities use data to identify areas that need improvement and guide policy as well as procedure. Accrediting bodies use the data to determine eligibility for accreditation. Most recently in the United States, performance data is being used for pay-for-performance wherein a portion of payment to a provider or healthcare facility is dependent on the quality of care delivered.[4]

Quality Measurement of Healthcare

The fundamental method for measuring healthcare quality was created by Donabedian and is known as the *structure, process, outcome* (SPO) model.[27] Within healthcare, *structure* refers to systems, resources, physical or organizational settings, electronic systems, policies and procedures, even philosophy—all of the things that make up a particular environment of care.[4,28]

Processes, which depend on structure, are the activities that take place in the form of services and products or procedures provided to patients. Processes can be evaluated from technical and interpersonal perspectives. The technical perspective is usually evaluated by comparing the process against clinical guidelines or by their impact on outcomes. Outcomes can be clinical in nature, referring to the effect on a patient's health status, economic or humanistic. This is referred to as the *economic, clinical, and humanistic outcomes* (ECHO) model.[29] Outcomes may be intermediate or long-term.[4] For example, medication adherence rates are considered an intermediate outcome because they mediate the connection of the care process to clinical outcomes. Donabedian theorized that processes are influenced by the structure of the healthcare environment and outcomes are influenced by the care provided.[27]

How Quality Is Measured: The Use of Performance Indicators

Quality in healthcare is most often measured through the use of performance indicators, also known as *performance measures*.[30] Performance indicators may screen for quality in structure, processes, or outcomes. Ideally, indicators should be clearly defined, quantitative, reliable, clinically meaningful, and actionable.[4] Common sources of data for performance measurement include medical records, prescription records, medical claims or prescription claims data, operational records, and patient reports. Performance data must be collected and organized in order to be interpreted as well as used for evaluating or comparing quality and identifying potential areas for improvement. Data may be presented as, for example, charts, diagrams, graphs, or regression analyses to allow for comparison and visualization of performance. In order to determine a benchmark for quality performance, a comparison or frame of reference is necessary. Performance may be compared over time or to an external criterion.[4] Indicators may be sentinel or aggregate. As described by Nau, sentinel indicators signal the need for further investigation or

(1) Identify an area of concern.
(2) Select the process, or segments of a process, to study.
(3) Determine what can be measured to evaluate the process.
(4) Define the numerator for your indicator.
(5) Define the denominator for your indicator.
(6) Determine the method for data collection.
(7) Select tools to display the indicator data.

FIGURE 4-4 Steps to constructing rate-based process indicator.
Source: Nau DP. Measuring pharmacy quality. *J Am Pharm Assoc.* 2009;492:154-163.

root-cause analysis; these are sometimes referred to as *never events* or events that are not expected to happen. Aggregate indicators provide a summary of frequency or timeliness of numerous cases of the same event and may be continuous or rate-based.[4] The measures for drug safety used by CMS to evaluate performance of PDP plans are all rate-based measures. Nau describes the steps for constructing a rate-based process indicator (Figure 4-4).[4]

Although outcomes (eg, cost of care, hospitalization rates, clinical endpoints) may seem to be the ideal indicators of healthcare quality, they are often difficult to measure. Outcomes can be complex and multidimensional; they can encompass longevity and quality of life, as pointed out recently by Uwe Rinehardt.[31] Process indicators must be used when outcome is difficult to measure, removed from the process, or influenced by factors other than the process, or when the process itself is of interest.[4] Some would argue that healthcare quality can never be defined and measured properly, to which Rinehardt applies the common aphorism, "Let not the perfect become the enemy of the good!"[31]

Measuring Quality of Medication Use and Medication Therapy Management

As focus is placed on quality and value-driven healthcare, pharmacy services, including MTM, will need to demonstrate quality and value. Quality improvement efforts can be stimulated in three ways: regulation, public reporting, and financial incentives.[32] Hospital and retail pharmacies have traditionally been regulated by state boards of pharmacy, many of which have begun to require pharmacies to implement quality assurance or improvement programs. Each year CMS presents a call letter for MA and Medicare PDP plans with new or redefined regulations for the upcoming plan year. As performance is compared across plans and best practices are identified, plans are required to adopt these modified regulations. There have been recent strides in public reporting of pharmacy performance measures that align with provider and health plan measures.[17] As described in this chapter, CMS is publicly reporting plan data on performance measures for MA and PDP plans. Quality measures for nursing homes, home health agencies, hospitals, and kidney dialysis facilities are also publicly reported.

As part of the value-driven healthcare initiative, providers are rewarded financially for high-quality performance. CMS provides bonus payments to MA plans that score high on performance measure ratings, described later in this chapter. As hospitals are seeing with the CMS value-based purchasing program, pay-for-performance incentives can come in the form of bonus payments for high quality or in the form of funds withheld if quality falls below a certain threshold. The Physician Quality Reporting System allowed physicians to report publicly on quality measures about services they provide for certain medical conditions and obtain bonus payments for high-quality care.[33] With the implementation of MACRA, CMS has further accelerated the financial consequences for physicians relative to quality-related performance. The CMS goal for 2019 is that at least 90% of Medicare fee-for-service payments will be adjusted for quality and value.[15] It is clear that CMS will use regulation, public reporting, and financial incentives to encourage quality in Medicare plans and MTM programs.

MEDICARE ADVANTAGE AND PART D PLAN PERFORMANCE MEASURES

The Star Rating Program

In keeping with the Triple Aim for better care, healthier populations, and lower costs, CMS measures the quality of MA and Medicare prescription drug plans (Medicare Parts C and D) with its Medicare Plan Ratings Program, also known as the *Star Rating Program*.[34] CMS continues to reiterate its commitment to improving MA and Part D plan quality by creating accountability through publicly reporting performance data:[34]

> We are committed to continuing to improve the Parts C and D quality performance measurement system to increase the focus on improving beneficiary outcomes, beneficiary satisfaction, population health, and efficiency of healthcare delivery. To that end, we have been working to develop a more robust system to measure quality and performance of MA and Prescription Drug Plan (PDP) contracts. As new measures are developed and adopted, CMS incorporates them into the Plan Ratings published each year on the Medicare Plan Finder website to assist beneficiaries in finding their plan and used to determine Star Ratings for QBPs.

These performance measures hold Medicare Part C and D sponsors accountable, not only for the services they provide to consumers, but also for the care provided by physicians, hospitals, and other providers.[34]

Medicare uses a 5-Star system to evaluate plans in order to provide beneficiaries information on plan quality and performance. The rating system is commonly referred to as *Star Ratings*. A rating of 3 stars is considered to indicate average performance (Figure 4-5).[35] Plans receiving a 5-Star Rating have received the highest rating possible and are referred to as *5-Star contracts*. Medicare Advantage plans without prescription drug coverage are rated on 32 measures (Table 4-4), and stand-alone prescription drug plans are rated on 15 measures (Table 4-5) for the 2017 plan year.[35] Medicare Advantage plans that include prescription drug coverage (MA-PD plans) are rated on 44 unique performance

*means poor performance
**means below-average performance
***means average performance
****means above-average performance
*****means excellent performance

FIGURE 4-5 Star Rating performance levels.
Source: Centers for Medicare and Medicaid Services (CMS). *Plan Quality and Performance Ratings*. Available at https://www.medicare.gov/find-a-plan/(S(1hp4zh45baqbl52pt1blig2m))/results/planresults/planratings/compare-plan-ratings.aspx?PlanType=MAPD&AspxAutoDetectCookieSupport=1. Accessed January 17, 2017.

TABLE 4-4 • 2017 Medicare Advantage (Part C) Plan Ratings and Measure Weights

Measure Name	2017 Weighting Category	Measure Weight
Breast Cancer Screening	Process measure	1
Colorectal Cancer Screening	Process measure	1
Annual Flu Vaccine	Process measure	1
Improving or Maintaining Physical Health	Outcome measure	3
Improving or Maintaining Mental Health	Outcome measure	3
Monitoring Physical Activity	Process measure	1
Adult BMI Assessment	Process measure	1
Care for Older Adults—Medication Review	Process measure	1
Care for Older Adults—Functional Status Assessment	Process measure	1
Care for Older Adults—Pain Screening	Process measure	1
Osteoporosis Management in Women Who Had a Fracture	Process measure	1
Diabetes Care—Eye Exam	Process measure	1
Diabetes Care—Kidney Disease Monitoring	Process measure	1
Diabetes Care—Blood Sugar Controlled	Intermediate-outcome measure	3
Diabetes Care—Cholesterol Controlled	Intermediate-outcome measure	3
Controlling Blood Pressure	Intermediate-outcome measure	3
Rheumatoid Arthritis Management	Process measure	1
Reducing the Risk of Falling	Process measure	1
Plan All-Cause Readmissions	Outcome measure	3
Getting Needed Care	Patients' experience and complaints measure	1.5
Getting Appointments and Care Quickly	Patients' experience and complaints measure	1.5
Customer Service	Patients' experience and complaints measure	1.5
Overall Rating of Healthcare Quality	Patients' experience and complaints measure	1.5
Overall Rating of Plan	Patients' experience and complaints measure	1.5
Care Coordination	Patients' experience and complaints measure	1
Complaints About the Health Plan	Patients' experience and complaints measure	1.5
Beneficiary Access and Performance Problems	Measures capturing access	1.5
Members Choosing to Leave the Plan	Patients' experience and complaints measure	1.5
Health Plan Quality Improvement	Outcome measure	5
Plan Makes Timely Decisions About Appeals	Measures capturing access	1.5
Reviewing Appeals Decisions	Measures capturing access	1.5
Call Center—Foreign Language Interpreter and TTY/TDD Availability	Measures capturing access	1.5

Source: Centers for Medicare and Medicaid Services (CMS). *Part C and D Performance Data: 2017 Part C and D Performance Data Technical Notes.* Available at http://www.cms.gov/Medicare/Prescription-Drug-Coverage/PrescriptionDrugCovGenIn/PerformanceData.html. Accessed September 20, 2017.

measures for 2017.[35] Three measures—complaints about a health/drug Plan (CP), beneficiary access and performance problems (BAPPs), and members choosing to leave the plan (MCLP)—are reported for both MA and Part D plans and share the same data source; therefore, they are counted only in the overall plan rating for MA plans that include prescription drug coverage. The exclusion of these and the aforementioned duplicate measures results in the 44 measures for MA-PD plans.

Annual ratings of Medicare plans are made available on the Medicare Plan Finder and CMS website.[31,36] By publicly reporting the ratings, CMS encourages Part C and D sponsors to improve the quality of services provided in order to attract enrollees to their plan.[22] The measures are also used to determine QBPs for MA organizations. Data to determine plan scores are collected through several sources: HEDIS, the Consumer Assessment of Healthcare Providers and Systems (CAHPS), and Health Outcomes Survey (HOS), as well as administrative and claims data.[35]

Plan Rating Structure

The Star Ratings are multifaceted in that they include performance measures related to customer service, complaints, appeals, health outcomes, and member satisfaction.[22] There are five measure

TABLE 4-5 • 2017 Medicare Prescription Drug Plan (Part D) Plan Ratings and Measure Weights

Measure Name	2013 Weighting Category	Measure Weight
Call Center—Foreign Language Interpreter and TTY/TDD Availability	Measures capturing access	1.5
Appeals Auto-Forward	Measures capturing access	1.5
Appeals Upheld	Measures capturing access	1.5
Complaints About the Drug Plan	Patients' experience and complaints measure	1.5
Beneficiary Access and Performance Problems	Measures capturing access	1.5
Members Choosing to Leave the Plan	Patients' experience and complaints measure	1.5
Drug Plan Quality Improvement	Outcome measure	5
Rating of Drug Plan	Patients' experience and complaints measure	1.5
Getting Needed Prescription Drugs	Patients' experience and complaints measure	1.5
MPF Price Accuracy	Process measure	1
High Risk Medication	Intermediate-outcome measure	3
Part D Medication Adherence for Oral Diabetes Medications	Intermediate-outcome measure	3
Part D Medication Adherence for Hypertension (RAS Antagonists)	Intermediate-outcome measure	3
Part D Medication Adherence for Cholesterol (Statins)	Intermediate-outcome measure	3
CMR Completion Rate	Process measure	1

Source: Centers for Medicare and Medicaid Services (CMS). *Part C and D Performance Data: 2017 Part C and D Performance Data: Technical Notes*. Available at http://www.cms.gov/Medicare/Prescription-Drug-Coverage/PrescriptionDrugCovGenIn/PerformanceData.html. Accessed September 20, 2017.

domains for MA plans and four measure domains for Medicare Prescription Drug Plan ratings.[35] The MA domains include

1. Staying healthy—screenings, tests, and vaccines
2. Managing chronic and long-term conditions
3. Member experience with health plan
4. Member complaints, problems getting services, and improvement in the health plan's performance
5. Health plan customer service

The Medicare Prescription Drug Plan domains include

1. Drug plan customer service
2. Member complaints, problems in obtaining services, and improvement in the drug plan's performance
3. Member experience with the drug plan
4. Patient safety and accuracy of drug pricing

TABLE 4-6 • Star Ratings Measure Categories

Outcomes	Outcome measures focus on improvements to a beneficiary's health as a result of the care that is provided.
Intermediate outcomes	Intermediate-outcome measures are closer to true therapeutic outcome measures. Controlling blood pressure is an example of an intermediate-outcome measure where the related outcome of interest would be better health status for beneficiaries with hypertension.
Patient experience	Patient experience measures represent beneficiaries' perspectives about the care that they have received.
Access	Access measures reflect issues that may create barriers to receiving needed care.
Process	Process measures capture the method by which healthcare is provided.

Source: Centers for Medicare and Medicaid Services (CMS). *Announcement of Calendar Year (CY) 2013 Medicare Advantage Capitation Rates and Medicare Advantage and Part D Payment Policies and Final Call Letter.* Available at http://www.cms.gov/medicare/health-plans/healthplansgeninfo/downloads/2013-call-letter.pdf. Accessed April 17, 2014.

Within the rating domains, there are five categories of measures: outcomes, intermediate outcomes, patient experience, access, and process (Table 4-6). A Star Rating is calculated for each measure as well as each domain and a summary plan rating for Part C and for Part D. For MA-PD plans, the Part C and Part D summary ratings are combined for an overall Star Rating.[35]

Medicare Parts C and D Measure Selection

The CMS Measures Management System (MMS) provides a set of business processes and decision criteria allowing for a standardized approach for developing and maintaining quality measures.[37] When selecting measures for Medicare Parts C and D, CMS works with independent developers of performance measures, such as NCQA and PQA. As they develop new measures, they may be adopted by CMS for the plan ratings. The performance measure sets for Medicare are reviewed and updated each year "taking into consideration the reliability of the measures, clinical recommendations, feedback received from stakeholders, and data issues."[33]

Weighting of Star Measures

The CMS determines the thresholds to achieve each level of Stars for each measure, and these thresholds (or cutpoints) are available in the technical specifications published on the CMS website.[35] For most measures, CMS evaluates the distribution of performance rates across all contracts and uses a statistical methodology for determining the most appropriate cutpoints for each measure. When calculating the summary ratings, the individual measures are weighted differentially so that some measures have a greater impact on the summary rating. Process measures are assigned a weight of 1. All new measures are assigned a weight of 1 for the first implementation year; the weighting is based on category for subsequent years. Outcomes and intermediate outcome measures are given a weight 3 times that of process measures. Patient experience and access measures are weighted 1.5 times the weight of process measures (see Tables 4-4 and 4-5). The improvement measures receive a weighting of 5 since CMS views improvement from year to year as highly important.

Display Measures

Display Measures are performance measures that are reported on the CMS website but do not count toward a plan's Star Rating. Display measures consist of measures that were plan ratings in the past but have been transitioned to display measures or new measures that are being tested before being included in the plan ratings. Although not part of the plan ratings, display measures are collected, monitored, and publicly reported, and CMS states that poor scores will be subject to compliance actions.[36] These measures are important for MTM programs because they encompass drug safety issues, such as the occurrence of drug-drug interactions, excessive doses of oral diabetes medications, or overuse of opioid medications.

Impact on Plans

Star Ratings carry significant implications for Medicare plans. Plans that receive high ratings are rewarded, while plans that score below average may face administrative sanctions and/or removal from the Medicare program. As mandated in the Affordable Care Act, CMS began a QBP demonstration for Medicare Advantage plans in 2012.[38,39] The 3-year project, which awarded QBPs to Medicare Advantage plans on the basis of Star Ratings, provided scaled bonuses for MA plans with ≥3 Stars and allowed a smooth transition to the high-stakes rewards that are currently in place. As of 2014, Medicare Advantage contracts that achieve a 4-Star overall rating receive a QBP award of 5%. The bonus is incorporated into the plan's bid for the following contract year.[34]

Plans that have higher-quality scores also receive a higher percentage of rebates from CMS. *Rebates* are the share of the difference between a plan's bid and the county benchmark that CMS pays for a plan to provide Medicare Part A and B benefits.[39] Receiving a higher percentage rebate based on Star Ratings provides incentive to high-scoring plans to keep their plan bids below the county benchmark.

Since the Star Rating for a Medicare contract is based on historical data, and since the QBP is applied to the contract bid for the year following the achievement of the 4-Star Rating, a considerable time lag exists between the performance period and the "reward" for the contract. For example, administrative claims data from 2014 were used to calculate the 2016 Star Ratings. Medicare plan sponsors that received a 4-Star Rating for 2016 were able to apply the QBP within their bids for the 2017 contract year. Thus, a 3-year lag occurs between performance and reward.

The CMS considers plans that do not achieve at least a 3-Star summary rating for 3 straight years to be "substantially out of compliance" with Medicare contracts. CMS issues formal compliance notices to all sponsors that achieve less-than-average ratings each year with the expectation that they will take corrective action to come into compliance. CMS scrutinizes these plans' operations and notifies members of the low rating. CMS makes clear that its intention is to terminate contracts with low ratings. To this end, poorly performing plans are subject to several actions that hinder obtaining membership. To encourage beneficiary enrollment in plans with higher plan ratings, CMS notifies beneficiaries enrolled in noncompliant plans of the low rating and offers them the chance to request a special enrollment period in order to move to a higher-quality plan.[34]

The CMS also uses the Medicare Plan Finder (MPF) website as a means to discourage enrollment in low-performing plans. During the 2011 open-enrollment period, CMS began using a low-performing plan icon as a visual symbol to identify plans receiving less than 3-Star summary ratings for 3 consecutive years. In 2012, CMS added messages to warn beneficiaries about enrolling in a low performing plan.[38] Starting with the 2013 open-enrollment period, online enrollment through MPF was disabled for plans with a low-performing icon, thus requiring beneficiaries to contact the plan directly for enrollment.

Medicare Part D Medication Use Measures

The Medicare Part D plan ratings under the domain of patient safety and accuracy of drug pricing include measures for medication use. The domain includes one measure of price accuracy, one measure of medication safety, one measure related to MTM activity, and three measures of medication adherence.[35] The measures of medication adherence and safety carry a weight 3 times that of process measures, and thus they account for a large percentage of the Medicare Part D summary rating. MTM program providers should be mindful of the measures related to safety and adherence as they provide MTM services on behalf of Medicare Part D plans. The measures for MTM, medication safety and adherence were developed by PQA (and also endorsed by the National Quality Forum) and include high-risk medications, medication adherence for oral diabetes medications, medication adherence for hypertension (renin angiotensin system [RAS] antagonists), and medication adherence for cholesterol (statins).[35]

The high-risk medication measure calculates the percentage of Medicare Part D beneficiaries aged ≥65 years who receive two or more prescription fills for a medication that carries a high risk of serious side effects in the elderly.[35] The current list of medications used to calculate the rate for this measure is maintained jointly by PQA and NCQA and is based on clinical recommendations from the American Geriatric Society.[35,40] A lower rate indicates higher-quality performance.

The three medication adherence measures assess the proportion of plan members who maintain at least an 80% adherence rate (measured as a proportion of days covered) to prescribed medications in the following classes: oral diabetes medications, antihypertensive medications (RAS antagonists), and cholesterol-lowering medications (statins).[35] The adherence measures were all developed and endorsed by PQA. A higher rate for each of the adherence measures indicates better performance.

Table 4-7 defines the numerators and denominators of each of these rate-based measures. The HRM and proportion of days covered (PDC) measures are calculated strictly with data from prescription claims for Medicare Part D plans (also known as prescription drug event [PDE] data).[35] CMS accounts for members who are enrolled in the plan for only part of the year by reporting rates based on member-years of enrollment. *Member-years* are

TABLE 4-7 • Medicare Part D Star Ratings Measures Related to Medication Use

High-risk medications (HRMs)	*Numerator*: number of member-years[a] of enrolled beneficiaries aged ≥65 years with ≥2 fills of the same HRM *Denominator*: number of member-years[a] of enrolled beneficiaries aged ≥65 years
Adherence	*Numerator*: number of member-years[a] of beneficiaries aged ≥18 years enrolled during measurement period with a proportion of days covered (PDC)[b] of ≥80% *Denominator*: number of member-years[a] of beneficiaries aged ≥18 years enrolled during measurement period with ≥2 fills of medications within specified measure class
CMR completion rate	*Numerator*: number of beneficiaries in denominator who received a CMR during their period of MTM enrollment *Denominator*: number of adult beneficiaries who were enrolled in an MTM program for ≥60 days during reporting period and who were not in hospice at any point during that period

[a] Member-years: for each beneficiary, the number of months enrolled divided by 12. Overall member-years is the total of individual member-years for each patient.

[b] PDC: the percent of days in measurement period covered by prescription claims for the same medication (or another in its therapeutic category).

Source: Centers for Medicare and Medicaid Services (CMS). *Part C and D Performance Data: 2017 Part C and D Performance Data Technical Notes*. Available at http://www.cms.gov/Medicare/Prescription-Drug-Coverage/PrescriptionDrugCovGenIn/PerformanceData.html. Accessed September20, 2016.

calculated for each beneficiary by dividing the number of months a member has been enrolled for the benefit year by 12.[35] The adherence rate, based on PDC, is also adjusted to account for members who have inpatient facility stays during the measurement period, since the plan is not responsible for prescription drug coverage during inpatient stays.[35] The PDC rate is not adjusted by any information collected from patients during MTM encounters or reported to CMS as a result of an MTM encounter. The method for calculating PDC is shown in the current measure technical notes on the CMS website.[35]

In fall 2012, CMS publicly reported data on the first MTM-specific quality measure. On the basis of 2011 MTM program data, the measure was a display measure for the 2013 ratings and became a Star Ratings measure for 2016 (based on 2014 program data). The measure was developed, tested, and endorsed by PQA to gauge the percentage of MTM-eligible beneficiaries who received comprehensive medication reviews (CMRs).[41] The numerator of this rate-based measure includes beneficiaries from the denominator who received a CMR during the reporting period. The denominator includes non-long-term-care (non-LTC) beneficiaries who were at least 18 years old at the beginning of the reporting period and who were enrolled in the MTM program for at least 60 days during the reporting period. Eligibility for enrollment in the MTM program is determined by each contract according to CMS guidelines, and beneficiaries must meet the MTM eligibility criteria for the contract to be included in the CMR measure rate.[35] This measure serves to promote CMR delivery to those who are eligible for MTM services. A higher rate on the measure indicates higher-quality performance (Table 4-8).[35]

Significantly, this is the first quality measure for MTM. CMS intends to adopt other MTM process and outcomes measures once they are developed and endorsed.[34] PQA has a measure development team dedicated to developing quality measures for Medicare Part D MTM programs.[41] The draft technical specifications for potential measures are reviewed by the PQA Quality Measurement Expert Panel, and pilot-testing of the potential measures is conducted prior to endorsement consideration by the PQA membership.[41]

Medicare Part D Plan Strategies for Improvement

Medicare Advantage and Part D sponsors can monitor their performance on quality measures monthly by viewing reports

TABLE 4-8 • 2017 Cutpoints for Selected Star Rating Measures

Plan Type	1 Star	2 Stars	3 Stars	4 Stars	5 Stars
2017 Measure D15 MTM Program Completion Rate for CMR					
MA-PD	<33.2%	≥33.2% to <47.8%	≥47.8% to <58.1%	≥58.1% to <76.8%	≥76.8%
PDP	<12.6%	≥12.6% to <20.3%	≥20.3% to <33.9%	≥33.9% to <51.6%	≥51.6%
2017 Measure D12 Medication Adherence for Diabetes Medications					
MA-PD	<70%	≥70% to <76%	≥76% to <79%	≥79% to <83%	≥83%
PDP	<74%	≥74% to <78%	≥78% to <82%	≥82% to <86%	≥86%
2017 Measure D13 Medication Adherence for Hypertension (RAS Antagonists)					
MA-PD	<71%	≥71% to <75%	≥75% to <79%	≥79% to <83%	≥83%
PDP	<77%	≥77% to <80%	≥80% to <83%	≥83% to <85%	≥85%
2017 Measure D14 Medication Adherence for Cholesterol (Statins)					
MA-PD	<66%	≥66% to <73%	≥73% to <77%	≥77% to <82%	≥82%
PDP	<70%	≥70% to <74%	≥74% to <80%	≥80% to <84%	≥84%

Source: Centers for Medicare and Medicaid Services (CMS). *Part C and D Performance Data: 2017 Part C and D Performance Data Technical Notes*. Available at http://www.cms.gov/Medicare/Prescription-Drug-Coverage/PrescriptionDrugCovGenIn/PerformanceData.html. Accessed December 30, 2016.

prepared by a CMS contractor (Acumen, LLC) on the Patient Safety Analysis website. Plan sponsors are granted access for up to five users by the Medicare Compliance Officer.[42] The reports provide contract-level, provider-level, beneficiary-level, and claims-level performance analyses on quality measures for each of a plan's contracts. The contract-level analysis provides overall, contract-level, and contract-type (MA or PDP) measures to monitor performance across a plan's contracts. Service provider analysis provides data that allow a contract to monitor service providers (prescribers and pharmacies) that influence their plan ratings. Providers are identified by their provider identifier such as National Provider Identifier or NCPDP number. Claim-level analysis provides the individual prescription drug event data for each prescription claim, including beneficiaries that are in the ratings numerator, thus allowing plans to identify individual beneficiaries influencing the rating score.

These reports enable plans to evaluate their performance across their own contracts and against other sponsors' contracts. Plans can identify outlier prescribers, pharmacies, and members that influence their quality ratings. Plans can monitor their performance month to month throughout the measurement period, allowing them to monitor their progress in improving their final rate for the measurement period. CMS expects that plans will use these reports and the data provided through the website for performance monitoring and to initiate quality improvements for plan measures.[42] In the following paragraph we see an example of how a plan might use the Patient Safety Analysis Report for the adherence measures to initiate improvement efforts.

A plan might use the Patient Safety Analysis Report for Adherence to identify the number of beneficiaries with improved adherence needed to achieve 4- and 5-Star levels and specific beneficiaries to target for adherence interventions.

1. The contract-level analysis provides the overall levels of adherence rates by contract type (MA or PDP). Plans can determine the number of beneficiaries who would need to achieve improved adherence (a proportion of days covered of at least 0.8 for the medication class at hand) in order to increase the plan's rating in comparison to other contracts (Table 4-9) and to a 4- or 5-Star level (see Table 4-8). On basis of the CMS cutpoints for 2017 Stars (which were based on 2015 data) (see Table 4-8), our hypothetical PDP (Plan X) currently has a 3-Star Rating for this measure.[35] In order to earn a 4-Star Rating (PDC-diabetes > 82%), the plan would need 123 000 member-years of adherent beneficiaries before the end of the plan year (December 2015). Therefore, Plan X needs an additional 5250 member years of adherent beneficiaries to be at a 4-Star level of performance. The actual number of nonadherent members (rather than "member-years") required to achieve 4-Star performance will be somewhat different from 5250 and will depend on the number of beneficiaries with partial-year enrollment in Plan X. Additionally, it is almost certain that no intervention deployed by a plan for increasing adherence will be 100% successful, so Plan X should plan to target more than 5250 nonadherent members, based on the predicted success of the intervention.
2. Beneficiary-level analyses will enable the plan to further refine its target population for adherence interventions by determining which members will be able to achieve a PDC of at least 0.80 before the end of the year. (Table 4-10). Assuming that these are the data as of September 30, 2015, there are 92 days left in the plan year (January to December 2015). If beneficiary 1 remains in the plan for the rest of the plan year, she or he will have a total of 348 days in the measurement period. In order to obtain a proportion of days covered of at least 0.80, the member would need to have medication in his possession (per prescription drug event data) for at least 86 of the remaining days in the plan year.

The PDC for beneficiary 2, however, will never be 0.80 or above for the current plan year. Assuming the member is enrolled in the plan for the remaining 92 days of the plan year, for a total of 332 days in measurement period, she/he would need 266 covered days to obtain a PDC of 0.80. That would require 118 more covered days, but as of September 30, 2015, there are only 92 days left in the plan year. By analyzing the beneficiary-level Patient Safety Analysis Report, the plan can determine which members to target at various points throughout the plan year, with interventions aimed at improving adherence in order to increase their overall adherence score.

The assigned measure weights (see Tables 4-4 and 4-5) can be used to estimate the contribution of each measure to the overall plan rating each year. For an MA-PD plan rated on 44 measures in 2017, the five medication use measures from PQA account for approximately 42% of the Part D summary rating and 17% of the overall MA-PD rating. Although these measures represent less than one-fifth of the overall Star Rating, they are often the measures with which plans struggle the most. It is unlikely that a Part D contract would reach a 5-Star Rating without doing well on these measures. Furthermore, it is likely that adherence measures for diabetes, cholesterol, and blood pressure medications will correlate to the plan's performance for outcomes-related Part C measures: diabetes care—blood sugar controlled, diabetes care—cholesterol controlled, and controlling blood pressure. It is likely that individual quality improvement measures will affect other measures.[43] Therefore, interventions for medication adherence may have positive impacts beyond PDC rates.

Medicare plan sponsors use a number of methods to improve quality of care. Through formulary management, prior authorization, disease management, drug utilization review, targeted

TABLE 4-9 • Example of Contract-Level Adherence Rates from Patient Safety Report

Contract	Member-Years of Enrolled Beneficiaries	Member-Years of Adherent Beneficiaries	Adherence Rate (%)
All contracts	10 000 000	8 000 000	80.0
PDPs	2 000 000	1 620 000	81
Plan X	150 000	117 750	78.5

TABLE 4-10 • Sample Beneficiary-Level Data for a Hypothetical Plan[a]

Beneficiary Number	DoB	Gender (M/F)	Diabetes Medications: Days in Measurement Period	Diabetes Medications: Covered Days	Diabetes Medications: Proportion of Days Covered
1	1/1/1940	M	256	192	0.75
2	2/23/1932	F	240	148	0.61

[a] Date of report, October 2015; period measured, January to September 2015; Contract No. 1234; contract name, Hypothetical Plan.

interventions to prescribers, pay-for-performance plans, and MTM programs, plans work to decrease healthcare costs while ensuring high quality of care. As the demand for value-driven care and high-quality performance increases, plans are also using a number of performance improvement solutions—such as predictive analytic and quality improvement platforms—which will allow them to address quality improvement needs effectively and efficiently.[44-46] Plans will need to implement multifaceted strategies to maintain high-quality performance.

QUALITY ASSURANCE FOR MEDICATION THERAPY MANAGEMENT PROGRAMS

Beyond the Star Ratings and quality measures reported by CMS, MTM programs and vendors, like all healthcare providers, will need to ensure the quality of the services that they provide. Payers need to be able to trust the accuracy, completeness, and appropriateness of patient interactions, written communications to patients and providers, and MTM encounter records.

Patient Interactions

For MTM to be successful, providers must be able to convince patients to participate in a CMR. Without successful patient engagement, an MTM program will not be effective. From the moment when patient outreach begins, MTM providers must offer extraordinary customer service and provide patients with experiences that are useful to them as consumers. With the new Medicare MTM quality measure for CMR participation, it is essential that providers find ways to overcome barriers to participation. MTM providers will need to measure and evaluate the success of different outreach methods. They will need to evaluate each aspect of customer contact for effects on overall patient engagement, such as how patient materials are worded, modes of communication, preparedness to answer patient questions, promotional and informational materials, length of time required to complete a CMR, and patient satisfaction. MTM programs will need to measure their ability to engage patients in services over time. When a decrease in a program's ability to engage patients is noted, the plan will be able to investigate both possible causes and potential steps to remedy it.

During a CMR, the MTM provider must coordinate several tasks while providing skillful customer service. The provider must obtain a complete and accurate medication list, including, but not limited to, medication name, strength, indication, prescriber, dose, frequency, side effects, and adherence. A list of 15 medications may result in over 120 items for the provider to collect, just for the medication list alone. The provider must also identify, assess, and prioritize medication-related problems and make recommendations that take into account the social, financial, and emotional needs of each patient. The provider must listen, provide empathy, and overcome communication barriers. In order to ensure quality patient interactions, MTM programs will need to audit patient interactions. This may require direct observation, audio recordings, or videorecordings to evaluate provider-patient interactions. An audit of a CMR may capture the accuracy of information stated versus what was recorded and ultimately provided to the patient. Beyond accuracy, a plan may wish to audit the appropriateness of information provided by its MTM providers to ensure quality patient encounters.

Written Communications

In 2013, CMS implemented a standardized format for cover letters, personal medication records, and medication action plans sent to Medicare Part D recipients following a CMR. MTM programs must make certain that these written materials consistently meet CMS requirements. Audits of materials sent to patients are a critical component of an MTM quality assurance program. Examples of items that might be included on such an audit include whether the format adheres to CMS requirements, whether the medication action plan exceeds the CMS-suggested length of one page front and back, the accuracy of the personal medication record (spelling, dosing, etc), and completeness of personal medication record (allergies, medication names, medication strength, instructions for medication use, prescriber, etc).

In order to communicate medication-related problems and opportunities, communications from an MTM provider to a prescriber must be clear, credible, and concise. An MTM program that wishes to ensure the quality of prescriber communications may audit these materials for items such as clearly stated medication names, doses, problems and opportunities, clear recommendations, the inclusion of patient-specific information related to a problem or opportunity, appropriate as well as accurately referenced recommendations, along with the absence of spelling and typographic errors.

Documentation and Reporting

Documentation and reporting may arguably be the most critical area for an MTM program to focus on in the efforts to ensure quality. In order to be paid, MTM programs providers must audit their documentation for billing of services for accurate claims transmission and appropriate payment. All MTM recommendations and interventions must be documented consistently by MTM providers, particularly if a program is billing based on estimated cost avoidance.[47]

Documentation must capture all services provided, recommendations along with interventions made, and ultimately be reportable to payers as well as regulatory bodies such as CMS. An audit of documentation and billing elements for an MTM program may include verification that there is evidence of services billed; for example, if a CMR is billed a personal medication list, medication action plan and patient interaction (if recorded) should be accessible for audit. There should be evidence that recorded recommendations to prescribers were actually made, such as through the verification of a fax including a documented recommendation or by documenting a phone conversation with a prescriber.

As one of the core elements of MTM, documentation is also critical for continuity of care and appropriate follow-up within the program and among other healthcare professionals. Because of the comprehensive nature of MTM services, providers will be flooded with an excess of information. This information will need to be organized as well as summarized in order to be useful to other healthcare professionals and for follow-up patient encounters. In contrast, noting that studies regarding clinical summarization are nearly absent from the literature, Feblowitz et al offer a model for synthesizing and recording patient information to produce a subset of patient data that will be useful for healthcare service provision.[48] Regardless of an MTM practice model's format for documentation, the program must ensure that users are following a consistent method of recording information and including all required elements. Programs may use a combination of manual chart auditing and software that can produce reports to catch potential sources of error in documentation.

REFERENCES

1. GPO. *Patient Protection and Affordable Care Act*, PL 111-148; 2010. Available at http://www.gpo.gov/fdsys/pkg/PLAW-111publ148/pdf/PLAW-111publ148.pdf. Accessed March 10, 2013.
2. Quality Net. *Hospital Value-Based Purchasing Program Overview*. Available at http://www.qualitynet.org/dcs/ContentServer?c=Page&pagename=QnetPublic%2FPage%2FQnetTier2&cid=1228772039937. Accessed March 10, 2013.
3. CMS. *Statute Regulations Program Instructions*. Available at http://www.cms.gov/Medicare/Quality-Initiatives-Patient-Assessment-Instruments/PQRS/StatuteRegulationsProgramInstructions.html. Accessed March 10, 2013.
4. Nau DP. Measuring pharmacy quality. *J Am Pharm Assoc*. 2009;49(2):154-163.
5. CMS. *Roadmap for Implementing Value Driven Healthcare in the Traditional Medicare Fee-for-Service Program*. Available at http://www.cms.gov/Medicare/Quality-Initiatives-Patient-Assessment-Instruments/QualityInitiativesGenInfo/downloads/vbproadmap_oea_1-16_508.pdf. Accessed March 10, 2013.
6. HHS. *Value-Driven Health Care: Four Cornerstones*. Available at http://archive.hhs.gov/valuedriven/fourcornerstones/index.html. Accessed March 10, 2013.
7. Briere R, ed. Institute of Medicine. *Crossing the Quality Chasm: A New Health System for the 21st Century*. Washington, DC: National Academy Press; 2001.
8. Berwick DM, Nolan TW, Whittington J. Triple aim: Care, health and costs. *Health Aff*. 2008;27(3):759-769.
9. HHS. *Value-Driven Health Care Home*. Available at https://archive.hhs.gov/valuedriven/. Accessed January 17, 2017.
10. Moore T, Nau DP. Reporting on health care quality. In: Nau DP, ed. *Quality and Safety in Pharmacy Practice*. New York, NY: McGraw-Hill; 2010. Available at http://www.accesspharmacy.com/content.aspx?aID=6496430. Accessed March 13, 2013.
11. The Joint Commission. *Quality Check*. Available at http://www.qualitycheck.org/. Accessed March 10, 2013.
12. *Hospital Compare*. Available at http://www.medicare.gov/hospitalcompare/. Accessed March 10, 2013.
13. *Nursing Home Compare*. Available at http://www.medicare.gov/NHCompare/. Accessed March 10, 2013.
14. NCQA. *HEDIS and Performance Measurement*. Available at http://www.ncqa.org/tabid/59/dealut.aspx. Accessed March 10, 2013.
15. CMS. *MACRA, MIPS and APMs*. Available at https://www.cms.gov/Medicare/Quality-Initiatives-Patient-Assessment-Instruments/Value-Based-Programs/MACRA-MIPS-and-APMs/MACRA-MIPS-and-APMs.html. Accessed September 27, 2016.
16. PQA. Report available at www.pqaalliance.org. Accessed September 17, 2016.
17. Pillittere-Dugan D et al. Development and testing of performance measures for pharmacy services. *J Am Pharm Assoc*. 2009;49(2): 212-219.
18. Center for Pharmacy Practice Accreditation Community Pharmacy Practice Standards. Report available at https://pharmacypracticeaccredit.org/. Accessed January 17, 2017.
19. Utilization Review Accreditation Commission (URAC). *Accreditation Programs*. Available at http://www.urac.org. Accessed September 27, 2016.
20. Ernst FR, Grizzle AJ. Drug-related morbidity and mortality: Updating the cost-of-illness model. *J Am Pharm Assoc*. 2001;41:192-199.
21. *The Medicare Prescription Drug, Improvement, and Modernization Act*, PL 108-173; 2003. Available at http://www.gpo.gov/fdsys/pkg/PLAW-108publ173/html/PLAW-108publ173.htm. Accessed March 10, 2013.
22. *Medicare Advantage and Medicare Prescription Drug Plan Quality Strategy: A Framework for Improving Care for Beneficiaries*; June 2012. Available at http://www.healthlawyers.org/Members/PracticeGroups/PPMC/MAPD/Documents/HPMS%20Memoranda/June%202012/Final%20Quality%20Strategy%20June%202012.pdf. Accessed March 10, 2013.
23. Scott GG, Legner D. Health care quality improvement. In: Nau DP, ed. *Quality and Safety in Pharmacy Practice*. New York, NY: McGraw-Hill; 2010. Available at http://www.accesspharmacy.com/content.aspx?aID=6494971. Accessed March 11, 2013.
24. Nau DP. Recognizing and defining quality problems. In: Nau DP, ed. *Quality and Safety in Pharmacy Practice*. New York, NY: McGraw-Hill; 2010. Available at http://www.accesspharmacy.com.lp.hscl.ufl.edu/content.aspx?aID=6495158. Accessed April 7, 2013.
25. Hincapie A. Identifying causes of quality problems. In: Nau DP, ed. *Quality and Safety in Pharmacy Practice*. New York, NY: McGraw-Hill; 2010. Available at http://www.accesspharmacy.com.lp.hscl.ufl.edu/content.aspx?aID=6495257. Accessed April 7, 2013.
26. Moczygemba LR. Statistical process control. In: Nau DP, ed. *Quality and Safety in Pharmacy Practice*. New York, NY: McGraw-Hill; 2010. Available at http://www.accesspharmacy.com.lp.hscl.ufl.edu/content.aspx?aID=6495445. Accessed April 7, 2013.
27. Donabedian A. Explorations in quality assessment and monitoring. In: *The Definition of Quality and Approaches of its Assessment*. Ann Arbor, MI: Health Administration Press; 1980:79-128.
28. Skledar SJ, Weber RJ. Measuring medication safety and quality. In: Nau DP, ed. *Quality and Safety in Pharmacy Practice*. New York, NY: McGraw-Hill; 2010. Available at http://www.accesspharmacy.com/content.aspx?aID=6495526. Accessed March 11, 2013.
29. Kozma CM, Reeder CE, Schulz RM. Economic, clinical and humanistic outcomes: A planning tool for pharmacoectonic research. *Clin Ther*. 1993;15:1121-1132.
30. Angaran DM. Selecting, developing and evaluating indicators. *Am J Hosp Pharm*. 1991;48:1931-1937.
31. Reinhardt U. Measuring the "quality" of health care. *New York Times*; February 1, 2013. Available at http://economix.blogs.nytimes.com/2013/02/01/measuring-the-quality-of-health-care/. Accessed March 10, 2013.
32. Nadkarni A, Nau DP. Is regulation the key to quality improvement? *Mich Pharm*. 2005;4:4-7.
33. CMS. *Physician Quality Reporting System*. Available at https://www.cms.gov/Medicare/Quality-Initiatives-Patient-Assessment-Instruments/PQRS/index.html. Accessed September 27, 2016.
34. CMS. *Announcement of Calendar Year (CY) 2013 Medicare Advantage Capitation Rates and Medicare Advantage and Part D Payment Policies and Final Call Letter*. Available at http://www.cms.gov/medicare/health-plans/healthplansgeninfo/downloads/2013-call-letter.pdf. Accessed September 27, 2016.

35. CMS. *Medicare 2017. Parts C and D Star Rating Technical Notes*. Available at http://www.cms.gov/Medicare/Prescription-Drug-Coverage/PrescriptionDrugCovGenIn/PerformanceData.html. Accessed September 27, 2016.
36. CMS. *Part D and D Performance Data*. Available at https://www.cms.gov/Medicare/Prescription-Drug-Coverage/PrescriptionDrugCovGenIn/PerformanceData.html. Accessed September 27, 2016.
37. CMS. *A Blueprint for the CMS Measures Management System*. Available at https://www.cms.gov/Medicare/Quality-Initiatives-Patient-Assessment-Instruments/MMS/Downloads/BlueprintVolume1-combined-v90.pdf. Accessed September 27, 2016.
38. CMS. *Announcement of Calendar Year (CY) 2012 Medicare Advantage Capitation Rates and Medicare Advantage and Part D Payment Policies and Final Call Letter*. Available at http://www.cms.gov/Medicare/Prescription-Drug-Coverage/PrescriptionDrugCovContra/downloads/Announcement2012final.pdf. Accessed September 27, 2016.
39. Kaiser Family Foundation. *Medicare Advantage Plan Star Ratings and Bonus Payments in 2012*. Data brief; November 2011. Available at http://kaiserfamilyfoundation.files.wordpress.com/2013/01/8257.pdf. Accessed September 27, 2016.
40. Fick D, Semla T, Beizer J, et al. American Geriatric Society updated Beers criteria for potentially inappropriate medication use in older adults. *J Am Geriatr Soc*. 2012;60(4):616-631.
41. Pharmacy Quality Alliance. *Information for Measure Development*. Available at http://pqaalliance.org/mdg/default.asp. Accessed September 27, 2016.
42. Tudor C. *Memo to All Part D Sponsors. Request for Comments Regarding Enhancements to the Patient Safety Analysis Website*; October 2012. Available at http://www.cms.gov/Medicare/Prescription-Drug-Coverage/PrescriptionDrugCovContra/Downloads/PatientSafetyWebsiteAnalysis.pdf. Accessed March 10, 2013.
43. Ta JT, Erickson SC, Qiu W, et al. Is there a relationship between Part D medication adherence and Part C intermediate outcomes Star Ratings measures? *J Manag Care Pharm*. 2016;22(7):787-795.
44. EQuIPP website. Report available at https://www.equipp.org/default.aspx. Accessed September 27, 2016.
45. RxAnte website. Report available at http://www.rxante.com/. Accessed September 27, 2016.
46. Inovalon website. Report available at http://www.inovalon.com/pages/default.aspx. Accessed September 27, 2016.
47. Barnett MJ, Frank J, Wehring H, et al. Analysis of pharmacist-provided medication therapy management (MTM) services in community pharmacies over 7 years. *J Manag Care Pharm*. 2009;15(1):18-31.
48. Feblowitz JC, Wright A, Singh H, Samal L, Sittig D. Summarization of clinical information: A conceptual model. *J Biomed Informatics*. 2011;44:688-699.

Review Questions

1. The Institute of Medicine strategies for healthcare improvement include
   a. paying for injuries resulting from unsafe care.
   b. applying the Medicare Star Ratings to community pharmacy practice.
   c. prescribing the role of each profession.
   d. requiring the use of telehealth technology.
   e. none of the above.

2. CMS MTM-related Star Ratings:
   a. are based on pharmacy adverse drug reaction detection and resolution.
   b. are focused primarily on Part D MTM.
   c. are used to inform the public about diagnostic error rates.
   d. may change from year to year.
   e. are used for healthcare organization accreditation purposes.

3. Star Rating underperformance by an MA-PD plan can result in
   a. civil monetary fines for underperformance.
   b. members being automatically disenrolled from the plan.
   c. loss of quality bonus payment.
   d. the MA-PD plan being required to switch to a PDP.
   e. all of the above.

4. The CMS MA-PD PDP Star performance measures system is best characterized as
   a. a rate-based measure system.
   b. proven to improve patient outcomes.
   c. including diagnostic accuracy measures.
   d. including physician acceptance rates of suggested therapeutic changes.
   e. focused primarily on formulary design.

5. Improving the MA-PD medication Star Measures for an individual plan from 4 to 5 guarantees:
   a. overall Star Ratings will be 4.
   b. overall Star Ratings will be 4.5.
   c. overall Star Ratings will be 5.0.
   d. a quality bonus of 5%.
   e. nothing, as the rating depends on other performance measures.

6. Which of the following are included in the CMS quality improvement framework?
   a. Beneficiaries
   b. Standards of care
   c. Public reporting
   d. Core values
   e. All of the above

7. Medicare Advantage Star Rating domains include all of the following EXCEPT:
   a. staying healthy: screenings, tests, and vaccines
   b. generic drug use rate
   c. managing chronic (long-term) conditions
   d. member experience with health plan
   e. health plan customer service

8. Medication-related Star Measures in the PDP ratings are
   a. under the domain of patient safety and accuracy of drug pricing.
   b. five measures of drug price accuracy and stability.
   c. focused on adherence to all chronic medications.
   d. setting an acceptable rate of adverse drug events.
   e. weighted by a factor of 5 for each measure.

9. PDC is
   a. percentage of days that a patient consumes her/his medication appropriately.
   b. acceptable at 0.8 for all drugs.
   c. something that requires a patient interview to calculate.
   d. calculated from prescription claims data over time.
   e. probability of detecting compliance.

10. The CMS Star performance measures
    a. eliminate the need for an MTM CQI program.
    b. depend on an accurate MAP.
    c. influence the focus of the comprehensive medication review.
    d. are integrated with NCQA and JCAHO measures.
    e. do not apply to Medicare patients who are not MTM-eligible.

ANSWERS

1. a	2. d	3. c
4. a	5. e	6. e
7. b	8. a	9. d
10. c		

5

Payer Perspective

Angel L. Ballew, MBA, PharmD, BCPP, and Katie Neff-Golub, PharmD, BCGP, CPh

KEY POINTS

- Plan sponsors are approached about medication therapy management (MTM) from various players for a variety of reasons.
- Some plans offer MTM to some or all of their members due to contractual agreements, while others provide MTM to improve patient outcomes and reduce healthcare costs.
- Medicare Part D sponsors are mandated to provide MTM to beneficiaries who meet certain requirements as outlined by the Centers for Medicare & Medicaid Services (CMS).
- CMS' Center for Medicare & Medicaid Innovation (Innovation Center) announced a model test spanning 5 years to further explore benefits of MTM for stand-alone Part D sponsors.
- A Medicare Advantage Plan may choose to use MTM programs to supplement efforts to improve quality measures.
- When establishing an MTM program, plan payers must determine membership criteria, service offerings, and service delivery methods as well as whether to insource or outsource the program to meet the desired outcomes.
- Plans can use national pharmacy organizations, MTM vendors, pharmacy benefit managers, and individual MTM providers as sources for determining program services and potential outcomes.
- MTM service providers should respond to plan requests for information and requests for proposals in order to be considered as a potential vendor for the plan.
- Plans may contract for reimbursement of MTM services through a variety of methods.
- Vendors of MTM services should be prepared for required audits by plan payers (eg, delegation audits, data validation audits, etc).
- Quality assurance is a key component of any MTM program and should be implemented by every MTM provider.
- All clinical programs, including MTM, should be continuously evaluated to ensure that desired outcomes are achieved and that improvements are implemented.

INTRODUCTION

Plan sponsors are often approached by internal and external parties to consider medication therapy management (MTM) as a plan service to improve patient outcomes. A payer must determine which members to enroll, what services to provide, what service providers to use, and how to measure success.

A plan's perspective on the establishment, oversight, and management of an MTM program will vary depending on the reasons it was initiated. Commercial, employer group, and government-sponsored plans tend to establish MTM programs to either satisfy regulatory requirements or to manage healthcare outcomes for an anticipated return on investment (ROI).

The 2003 Medicare Modernization Act (MMA) mandated that all Medicare Part D plan sponsors offer MTM services.[1] Under guidelines set by the states, Medicaid sponsors can be contractually obligated to perform MTM through state contracts. Based on expected ROIs, plan sponsors may identify population-specific parameters that may warrant drug therapy interventions through MTM.

The value of MTM in stand-alone Part D plans is being further evaluated through the Part D Enhanced Medication Therapy Management (EMTM) model test. Announced by the Centers for Medicare & Medicaid Services (CMS) Center for Medicare & Medicaid Innovation (Innovation Center), this model test will run for a 5-year performance period and aims to "identify innovative strategies to optimize medication use, improve care coordination, and strengthen system linkages."[2]

DETERMINING MTM CRITERIA

Determining membership criteria is an essential step for any payer establishing an MTM program. The 2003 MMA mandated that all Part D plan sponsors offer MTM services to beneficiaries who meet certain requirements[a]:

1. Multiple chronic disease states
2. Multiple medications covered by Part D
3. Annual costs for Part D medications exceeding a specified threshold determined by the United States Secretary of Health and Human Services[1]

State requirements are defined separately by each state and are often driven by programs spawned by state pilots, but they may also be based on common principles established by national pharmacy organizations. Beyond required enrollment criteria set by either CMS or state players, plans often choose who receives MTM services based on population factors that drive plan costs. Employer groups may also look at factors that drive missed work days. Plan population characteristics are unique, so plans focus on members with certain disease states and the use of certain therapeutic classes to maximize the benefit received for the costs spent on MTM services. Beyond those who meet the CMS-mandated Part D criteria, members may be enrolled in an MTM program at the plan's discretion. These members may be identified similarly to those who are enrolled in a commercial or employer plan, where set identification criteria are not mandated. Suggestions for additional populations to consider enrolling may be provided to plans by government agencies. For example, in the 2014 Call Letter, CMS suggested enrolling opioid over utilizers and those meeting the Million Hearts™ initiatives.[3] A Medicare Advantage Plan may wish to use MTM programs to supplement other quality-improvement efforts on both the Part C and Part D side of the equation by enrolling additional members into an MTM program. Part C measures are heavily influenced by the Healthcare Effectiveness Data and Information Set (HEDIS®), a tool used by the National Committee for Quality Assurance (NCQA) to measure quality of care in health plans.[4] Part D patient safety measures are heavily influenced by endorsed measures from the Pharmacy Quality Alliance (PQA).[5] Table 5-1 indicates a subset of measures that CMS used to assess health plan quality for the 2017 Plan Ratings that may directly or indirectly be influenced by MTM services.[6] Additional Part C and D Medicare Plan Ratings Display Measures could also be influenced by MTM services (Table 5-2).[7]

TABLE 5-1 • Medicare 2017 Part C and D Plan Ratings Performance Measures—Star Ratings

Measure ID	Individual Measure Name
C01	Breast Cancer Screening
C02	Colorectal Cancer Screening
C03	Annual Flu Vaccine
C07	Adult BMI Assessment
C09	Care for Older Adults—Medication Review
C11	Care for Older Adults—Pain Assessment
C12	Osteoporosis Management in Women Who Had a Fracture
C13	Diabetes Care—Eye Exam
C14	Diabetes Care—Kidney Disease Monitoring
C15	Diabetes Care—Blood Sugar Controlled
C16	Controlling Blood Pressure
C17	Rheumatoid Arthritis Management
C18	Reducing the Risk of Falling
D11	High Risk Medication
D12	Part D Medication Adherence for Diabetes Medications
D13	Part D Medication Adherence for Hypertension (RAS Antagonists)
D14	Part D Medication Adherence for Cholesterol (Statins)
D15	MTM Program Completion Rate for CMR

Source: Adapted from Part C and D performance data: 2017 Part C and D performance data technical notes. Centers for Medicare & Medicaid Services website. Available at http://www.cms.gov/Medicare/Prescription-Drug-Coverage/PrescriptionDrugCovGenIn/PerformanceData.html. Accessed January 30, 2017.

Enhanced MTM

The Centers for Medicare & Medicaid Services (CMS) Center for Medicare & Medicaid Innovation Center announced that the EMTM model test will begin January 1, 2017 with a 5-year performance period. In the past, standard Part D MTM programs have required uniform services and single program criteria. However, the uniform one-size-fits-all approach may not be identifying or providing services that have the most positive effect on patient outcomes.

The EMTM model test offers an opportunity for stand-alone Part D prescription drug plans, those with prescription coverage only, to offer an innovative MTM program that would replace the standard CMS MTM model. The purpose of the model is to allow Part D sponsors to identify and implement innovative MTM programs in which enrollment criteria and services are determined by the sponsor. Services selected by sponsors had to be enrollee-specific. The EMTM programs' identification criteria as well as enrollee-specific services had to be reviewed and approved by CMS. Six Part D sponsors that operate a total of 22 plan benefit packages were selected to participate in the model across five Part D regions: Region 7 (Virginia), Region 11 (Florida), Region 21 (Louisiana), Region 25 (Iowa, Minnesota, Montana, Nebraska, North Dakota, South Dakota, and Wyoming), and Region 28 (Arizona).[2]

DETERMINING MEDICATION THERAPY MANAGEMENT PROGRAM SERVICES

A payer must also decide which services will be required for members enrolled in the MTM program. For Part D sponsors, CMS provides guidance in Chapter 7 of the Part D *Prescription Drug Benefit Manual* (PDBM),[8] the yearly Call Letter, and other CMS materials. During MTM's infancy, CMS gave plan sponsors free reign to decide which services constituted MTM. In 2010, CMS increased guidance, requiring the comprehensive medication review (CMR) as the central component of an MTM program.[9] In 2013, CMS

[a] Enhanced Medication Therapy Management (EMTM) is exempt from these requirements. As part of the Innovation Center model test, plan sponsors participating in EMTM submit their plan specific program for CMS approval, including all identification criteria.

TABLE 5-2 • Medicare 2017 Part C and D Medicare Plan Ratings Display Measures

Measure ID	Individual Measure Name
DMC01	Follow-up Visit After Hospital Stay for Mental Illness (within 30 days of discharge)
DMC02	Antidepressant Medication Management (6 months)
DMC03	Continuous Beta Blocker Treatment
DMC04	Appropriate Monitoring for Patients Taking Long-term Medications
DMC05	Osteoporosis Testing
DMC06	Testing to Confirm Chronic Obstructive Pulmonary Disease
DMC09	Pneumonia Vaccine
DMC10	Access to Primary Care Doctor Visits
DMC12	Pharmacotherapy Management of COPD Exacerbation—Systemic Corticosteroid
DMC13	Pharmacotherapy Management of COPD Exacerbation—Bronchodilator
DMC14	Initiation of Alcohol or Other Drug Initiation of Alcohol or Other Drug Treatment
DMC15	Engagement of Alcohol or Other Drug Treatment
DMC16	Reminders for Appointments
DMC17	Reminders for Immunizations
DMC18	Reminders for Screening Tests
DMC22	Improving Bladder Control
DMC23	Medication Reconciliation Post Discharge
DMC25	Statin Therapy for Patients With Cardiovascular Disease
DMC26	Medication Management for People With Asthma
DMC27	Asthma Medication Ratio
DMD05	Drug-Drug Interactions
DMD06	Diabetes Medication Dosing
DMD09	Rate of Chronic User of Atypical Antipsychotics by Elderly Beneficiaries in Nursing Homes
DMD15	Reminders to Fill Prescriptions
DMD16	Reminders to Take Medications
DMD17	Statin Use in Persons With Diabetes (SUPD)

Source: Adapted from Part C and D performance data: 2017 display measures technical notes. CMS website. Available at http://www.cms.gov/Medicare/Prescription-Drug-Coverage/PrescriptionDrugCovGenIn/PerformanceData.html. Accessed January 30, 2017.

began requiring a standardized form for documentation, given to members following a CMR.[10] Despite the additional requirements to Part D sponsors over the last decade, plans still have some discretion on the provision of MTM services. In 2017, Part D sponsors selected to participate in the EMTM model test are required to provide services as outlined in their approved program application.[2]

Outside of Part D, however, MTM services are not compulsory, and guidance is limited to recommendations from national pharmacy organizations and information conveyed by MTM vendors. The most important manual for MTM services, *Medication Therapy Management in Community Pharmacy Practice: Core Elements of an MTM Service*, was developed in consensus by 11 national pharmacy organizations with the aim of creating a model that would "maximize both effectiveness and efficiency of MTM service delivery across pharmacy practice settings in an effort to improve continuity of care and patient outcomes."[11,12] In addition to this document and other resources from national pharmacy organizations, MTM services may be described to plans by those who are currently performing MTM services for other clients. This can include, for example, MTM vendors, pharmacy benefit managers (PBMs), and individual providers of services in clinic-based or retail settings.

The Medication Review

Whether federally mandated or not, the services a plan concludes to be the most beneficial for its membership will typically involve medication review. For Part D sponsors, this is termed the *comprehensive medication review* (CMR).

There is debate in the industry regarding the most effective mechanism for MTM service delivery, both from the standpoint of plan members agreeing to and completing the service as well as from the standpoint of quality and patient satisfaction. Because the plan is paying for MTM services, it must consider these and other factors, such as patient population mix, to determine the best delivery mechanism—this may include a hybrid approach that includes both face-to-face and telephonic services. When determining the method of delivery, it is important to consider the distinct benefits of both face-to-face and telephonic MTM.

Face-to-Face Delivery

- Ability to leverage the established relationship with the member's retail or consultant pharmacists
- Ability to engage the member at the time of prescription pickup for medication review completion or to schedule an appointment to conduct the medication review
- Ability to engage the member at the long-term care facility and coordinate recommendations with the members' healthcare team
- Ability to physically review medication bottles or the members' chart to clarify prescriptions
- Ability to assess a patient's nonverbal cues that occur during the encounter
- Ability to demonstrate appropriate techniques for medication delivery (eg, inhalers, insulin)
- Can occur in conjunction with dispensing, thus eliminating additional appointments in the retail setting
- Outreach is not dependent on correct member contact information (eg, address and telephone number)
- Ability to leverage support staff or vendors going into a member's home during in home assessment outreach or other case management type functions (eg, case management nurses, nurse practitioners, physicians doing home visits)

Telephonic Delivery

- Ability to record MTM interactions for oversight and quality assurance
- Distractions that may be present in a retail pharmacy setting are limited or eliminated (eg, no dispensing functions, drive-thru, or waiting patients)

- Ability to reach members unable to travel to a pharmacy (ie, nonambulatory members)
- Can complement mail-service pharmacy services as members do not typically have a relationship with a retail or community pharmacist
- Can provide an alternative if a member has a nonexistent relationship with retail or community pharmacist
- Elimination of judgment, real or perceived, on the part of either the provider or the member based on physical and cultural attributes
- Members can be in their own familiar surroundings when they receive MTM services

As telehealth continues to gain traction as a way of delivering clinical services, it is not surprising that MTM services would also be delivered this way. But whether provided in person or remotely, services must be documented in order to comply with regulations as well as to report outcomes to plan leadership, prove ROI, and provide oversight to determine quality and prevent fraud, waste, and abuse.

Beyond the Medication Review: Add-on Services

Although the staple of most MTM programs, regardless of the plan type, is some type of medication review, plans may also explore add-on services. These can be used to increase membership in the MTM program and member uptake of MTM services, as well as to provide additional resources to MTM members to help them effectively manage their conditions and medication regimens. Program hotlines, member or provider educational materials, and plan-branded tools are a few examples of add-on services. Toll-free hotlines enable members to access pharmacists or other clinicians with questions regarding their medications or disease states. Some hotlines are accessible to members 24 hours a day, 365 days a year, while others maintain specific operational hours. Member newsletters, flyers, and pamphlets can help remind members of their enrollment in the MTM program and the services offered. In addition, they can reinforce medication-related concepts and provide education about conditions. Seasonal topics, such as a flu shot reminder in the fall, can also be included as an extra layer of support for managing a member's well-being. Other materials can educate providers about the purpose and goals of the MTM program, the services offered to enrolled members, and why their patients would benefit from participating in services. If applicable per plan enrollment criteria, this is also a method for informing prescribers on how to enroll and refer members to the MTM program. Plans that provide both medical and pharmacy benefits to their members may find it beneficial to coordinate with their disease state management, case management, and other wellness services. This allows for the dissemination of consistent information across business units, and more importantly, coordination of care among MTM and other providers. Through engagement with MTM staff, members may opt-in to education-related services like email or text alerts as prescription refill reminders. Lastly, branded items can provide members with additional support regarding medication management and reminders to use MTM program services. Examples of branded items include pillboxes, blood glucose logs, and calendars to track healthcare provider appointments.

INSOURCING VERSUS OUTSOURCING

Medication therapy management services can be managed entirely in-house or partially or entirely outsourced. The type of program desired by the plan, the anticipated membership, and the allocated budget are a few of the factors that will determine whether insourcing, outsourcing, or a hybrid approach is most beneficial. No matter what route the plan decides upon, it will be reevaluated as member outcomes are reviewed. If the selected approach is proven effective, additional dollars maybe allocated, opening the opportunity for additional internal and external resources. In addition, as MTM evolves, new opportunities for partnerships may arise, even in areas that did not align in the past.

If choosing a hybrid approach, a plan must determine how to maintain continuity of care. Ideally, every member will have the opportunity to receive the same level of quality service, whether from an in-house provider or from an outsourced vendor. Quality assurance programs can help maintain consistency among providers.

When MTM is provided in-house, the plan's branding is prominent in all communications, and MTM providers are often well versed not only in the MTM program but also in the plan itself. This may allow for more effective communication between the MTM provider and member when plan-related questions arise during a medication review, providing a less fragmented experience. Health plan branding, however, can be maintained even when services are outsourced, as long as this is stipulated in the contract.

Insourcing Medication Therapy Management

Plans that insource fully or maintain a portion of their MTM program in-house must identify staffing and space needs and define the structure of the program. Staffing metrics must be developed to see whether additional resources are needed or if they can be absorbed by other clinical programs. Initial metrics may be gleaned from estimates of the number of members projected to enroll, the percentage of members expected to uptake the various service offerings, and an estimation of the average time needed for each service. Established clinical service metrics within the plan (ie, case management or quality initiatives involving clinicians) can also be used as guidance. Policies and procedures must be developed to ensure that program services are being provided consistently and that the program's structure is sound.

Once policies and standard operating procedures are in place, allocated staff should be trained. Some plans may require staff to obtain certain credentials or certifications or pass competency tests in order to perform MTM services.

Plans that insource will not only have to consider staffing metrics and procedures, they will also need to determine a method for documenting the services provided in order to report to regulatory agencies, states, employer groups, and senior leadership. Plans may choose to track services in preexisting documentation systems, such as case management software, or build a documentation tool specifically for tracking MTM services. Plans may also choose to purchase licenses for MTM-specific software. The tracking system a plan chooses will depend on many factors, including the volume of data it is expected to house, the number of staff using the system, the ability to capture necessary data for reporting, as well as security and back-up capabilities.

Utilizing the same systems or having direct links from MTM-specific software to other systems utilized by health plan resources not only helps show a complete picture of the member to internal associates, but it also allows alignment of recommendations, care plans, etc, among resources servicing members and their providers. Consistent communication from the plan to members and their providers should strengthen the program results by avoiding duplication of work or misaligned messages.

A sound documentation system will ensure that data is retrievable and reportable, but it will not guarantee the quality of the information entered. For this reason, plans will likely perform quality assurance on the documentation of services provided. Quality assurance reviews typically ensure compliance with standard operating procedures, but some may also include clinical quality assessments. For programs offering a telephonic or telehealth delivery model, opportunities to listen to calls or watch screens in real time during medication reviews can ensure successful communication between the MTM service provider and the member. MTM programs offering face-to-face MTM could monitor encounters at periodic intervals to ensure that services are being provided in a private setting without interruption and that communication is successful. Quality assurance programs will identify areas of improvement for individual MTM providers, among groups of providers, and with the MTM program overall.

Outsourcing Medication Therapy Management

Plans that choose to outsource the entire, or a portion of their MTM programs will most likely determine which vendors to contract with through a selection process managed by the plan's procurement and legal teams. This is typically commenced through either a request for information (RFI) or a request for proposals (RFP). Vendors then submit the appropriate documentation for initial review and provide additional documentation to satisfy any of the health plan's questions; potential vendors may also make a presentation to showcase their product and services. In many cases, the potential vendors and the plan will sign nondisclosure agreements to protect confidential and proprietary information from being shared by either party at any time during and after the selection process. Standard RFI and RFP documents do not exist for MTM in the Medicare, Medicaid, or commercial spaces at the time of publication. However, sections that are typically covered in an RFI or RFP may include:

- Organization profile (ie, important statistics about the organization, affiliation with other organizations)
- Account management (ie, key support staff for the plan)
- Service offerings and methods (ie, member identification, documentation systems, types of reviews)
- Staffing credentials (ie, certifications, licensure, training)
- Network or service regions (ie, where the plan's members can receive services)
- Quality assurance and oversight (ie, policies and procedures, prevention of fraud, waste and abuse, policies on safeguarding protected health information (PHI), policies on handling complaints)
- Documentation and billing (ie, data elements captured and association to billing practices, reimbursement practices)
- Reporting and data validation (ie, data elements reported, frequency, data validation procedures to ensure accuracy of data reported to the plan)
- Outcome measurement processes (ie, data elements for measuring success, including calculations)
- Information technology (IT) and data transfer processes (ie, how to securely transfer data, back-up procedures in the event of a disaster, data retention, server security)

Plans may forgo the vendor selection process and outsource through other mechanisms, such as through its PBM's MTM program, particularly if the PBM is able to prove positive outcomes and ROI. Plans may also contract directly with pharmacies independently or through the PBM, if the PBM is contracted to develop the pharmacy network.

Plans may also form relationships with other entities outside traditional MTM vendor relationships. These include relationships with the member's providers through accountable care organizations (ACOs) or patient-centered medical homes (PCMHs). Other vendors are entering the MTM space, such as vendors that support plan efforts through in-home assessment type services. These vendors are completing CMRs along with health risk assessments (HRAs), offering preventative services and closing HEDIS and CMS Star Measure gaps.

Contracting

Many payment methods exist currently that align in structure with those of other healthcare services. The typical methods of payment are through a capitated rate, a per-member-per-month (PMPM) or per-member-per-year (PMPY) rate, and a transactional fee-for-service approach. Some contracts may specify a hybrid approach, with a PMPM fee for housing membership or developing a case for review, plus fees-for-service upon completion of certain services.

The payment structure a plan chooses depends on multiple factors, but can include the plan's experience with an MTM program's metrics (ie, percent membership, percent uptake, and completion of services), the willingness of the vendor to assume risk or offer a performance guarantee for all or portions of the provided services, and the budget for the MTM program.

When initially launching an MTM program, plans may find that capitation or PMPM/PMPY approaches may be easier to budget for because the total cost of the program does not depend on the number of services provided. Conversely, a plan may decide that service uptake or completion was low and that paying for services under a capitation model would be costlier than a fee-for-service model. Therefore, plans may request a performance guarantee from a vendor to ensure a service completion rate in order to make a capitated or PMPM/PMPY approach more attractive. The use of CMR completion rate in the CMS Star Ratings has likely increased the utilization of this quality measure as a driving variable in payment.

A fee-for-service approach prevents budget dollars from being applied to members who do not participate in the MTM program. In this case, plans will negotiate a certain fee to be paid upon completion of each service, and fees are usually based on the level of clinical effort needed for each service. Plans may also choose to allow submission of Current Procedural Terminology (CPT) codes for payment of MTM program services. Developed by the Pharmacist

TABLE 5-3 • Current Procedural Terminology (CPT) Codes for MTM Services

CPT Code	Description
99605	Medication therapy management services provided by a pharmacist, individual, face-to-face with patient, initial 15 minutes, with assessment, and intervention if provided; initial 15 minutes, new patient
99606	Initial 15 minutes, established patient
99607[a]	Each additional 15 minutes (list separately in addition to code for the primary service)

[a] Use 99607 in conjunction with 99605, 99606.

Source: Medication therapy management service codes. Pharmacist Services Technical Advisory Coalition (PSTAC) website. http://www.pstac.org/services/mtms-codes.html. Accessed December 14, 2016.

Services Technical Advisory Coalition (PSTAC), these three codes (Table 5-3) became effective on January 1, 2008.[13] Since these codes bill by time to complete services versus a standard transactional fee, budgeting for the use of CPT codes may be more complicated than other routes. As CPT codes become more widely used, however, plans may use this form of payment more readily.

When outsourcing, the payer must also keep in mind the capability of systems to deliver and receive data from the vendors. Requiring MTM vendors to have their own software might limit the amount of participation the payer and vendor could expect. The current trend is for payers to contract with a national MTM vendor, which then supplies the pharmacies with a web-based program that allows the payer to review a member's complete up-to-date pharmacy claims and allows the pharmacy to send information about the MTM encounter in a format that the payer can use for billing and reporting.

Delegation

Choosing to outsource may limit the day-to-day operational undertaking of an MTM program, but it does not supplant the need for oversight. Plans should ensure that the MTM services for which they are paying are provided in a cost-effective manner, that a certain level of quality is maintained, and that potential problems are addressed in a timely manner. Plans must have mechanisms to respond to member grievances, including those resulting from an outsourced MTM provider. In addition, plans should have an avenue to monitor potential fraud, waste, and abuse stemming from outsourced service providers.

Providers of government-sponsored MTM services (ie, Medicare Part D) must not be among those on the U. S. Department of Health and Human Services Office of Inspector General's list of excluded individuals and entities, and a plan must have a process in place to address this situation should it arise. The Office of Inspector General maintains this list to track individuals and entities that have committed fraud against any health and human services program, including Medicare and Medicaid. Those on the list are prohibited from being reimbursed from the federal budget for any services provided to recipients of these programs. A searchable and downloadable list of excluded individuals and entities is publicly available: https://oig.hhs.gov/exclusions/index.asp.[14]

A plan's oversight of an MTM vendor and providers typically begins during the contracting period with a process known as *delegation*, a method in which plans authorize others to perform services on their behalf.

Plans must ensure that delegated entities meet minimum requirements to provide services through a predelegation audit. Once an entity has been delegated to perform services and contracts have been signed, plans perform periodic audits of the delegated entity to ensure that they are continually able to perform the contracted services. Audit timelines are dependent upon the plan's operational guideline, which may or may not be determined by regulatory agencies or plan contracts with customers. Audits of delegated entities typically occur yearly at minimum.

Audits encompass far more than simply gauging an entity's ability to perform services. They also evaluate an entity's compliance with government-mandated regulations such as the Health Insurance Portability and Accessibility Act (HIPAA)[15] and determine the entity's ability to recover data during a disaster. A standard audit document for MTM does not exist at the time of publication; however, MTM-specific requirements that a plan may review during a delegation audit may include the following:

- Entity's Global Policies
  - Compliance (ie, what the entity does if a compliance issue arises)
  - HIPAA privacy and security (ie, how the entity safeguards PHI)
  - Record retention (ie, how the entity retains data and documentation for future need, including length of record retention)
  - Fraud, waste, and abuse (ie, what the entity does to identify and report suspected cases)
  - IT (ie, recovery plan including business continuity assurance during a disaster)
- MTM Administrative Documents
  - MTM program descriptions, policies with procedures, and operational documents for each service provided to the plan
  - Job descriptions, training programs, and credentialing as well as licensing verification for MTM service providers
  - Sampling of documentation of MTM services to prove reported data elements and support service billing

Entities that do not meet certain requirements may be removed as a delegated entity or placed on a corrective action plan (CAP) to remediate any problems. The time that a delegated entity has to satisfy a CAP and whether services can be continued during this period will depend upon the nature and severity of the problems identified during the audit.

Quality Assurance

Quality assurance must be undertaken for delegated entities performing services on behalf of a plan, just as it is for internal MTM programs. For outsourced programs, quality assurance may be delegated to the entity itself (and be included in the delegation audit), or it may be performed by the plan in order to provide continuous feedback to the delegated entity. The process to ensure both operational and clinical quality, however, is consistent regardless of whether MTM is outsourced or sourced internally. In the event that the plan operates with a hybrid approach, quality assurance can be performed similarly to provide an opportunity to benchmark and leverage successes and failures across both groups of providers. This also allows the ability to determine differences seen with utilization of different disciplines conducting the service.

Whether insourcing or outsourcing an MTM program, plans must also consider the IT necessary to ensure success. Beyond the documentation platform, at minimum, eligibility and pharmacy data will be used to determine eligibility and as a resource while conducting services. If a plan is utilizing external services, standardized data feeds may be required, which means that the plan's IT department will need time to coordinate and develop the essential infrastructure. Non-Part D sponsors may wish for medical and lab data to be included to aid in member identification or to provide patient context for MTM providers. There may also be opportunities for plans to share formularies or plan benefits via data feeds to arm the provider with even more customized information.

REPORTING OUTCOMES OF A MEDICATION THERAPY MANAGEMENT PROGRAM

Outcomes will ultimately determine whether a plan continues or expands its current MTM programs. Part D-mandated programs and state contracts may still need to be fulfilled, but unless there are demonstrable positive outcomes from MTM services, the mechanism by which the requirements are met may change drastically. When positive outcomes in healthcare expenditure are realized, plans may decide to expand MTM services to members for whom it is not a requirement.

The CMS requires reporting elements for Part D MTM program services. These are currently reported annually at a beneficiary level. Requirements for Part D reporting have changed over the years in an effort not only to track services provided but to also to showcase the positive impact that MTM has on recipients. The CMS reporting requirements for 2016 Part D MTM programs included the following items[16]:

- Plan Contract Number
- Beneficiary Information
  - Beneficiary Health Insurance Claim Number (HICN) or Railroad Retirement Board (RRB) Number
  - First name, middle initial, last name
  - Date of birth
- Program Enrollment Information
  - Beneficiary's cognitive impairment status at time of CMR offer or delivery
  - Date beneficiary enrolled
  - Date beneficiary met CMS criteria (if enrolled due to targeting criteria)
  - Date beneficiary opted out and reason for opt out
- MTM Program Service Information
  - Date beneficiary was initially offered a CMR
  - Number of CMRs received by the beneficiary and dates the CMRs were provided
  - Date of CMR delivery
  - Method of delivery for the CMR (ie, face-to-face, telephonic, etc)
  - Qualified provider who performed the CMR
  - Recipient of the CMR (ie, beneficiary, caregiver, etc)
  - Number of targeted medication reviews provided
  - Number of drug therapy problem recommendations made
  - Number of drug therapy problem resolutions

State contracts may also require particular reporting elements, but these are not standard across states. As a payer for MTM services, a plan must ensure that data requested from regulatory agencies is accurate and can be validated as such. Regardless of the need for certain required data elements, plans must receive data on the MTM program in order to report to senior plan leadership—continuous review of the MTM program is necessary in order to maintain effectiveness. The plan should ensure that the investment in MTM services is producing desired savings in total healthcare costs and improvements in plan member outcomes. The plan should also ensure appropriate documentation of services to analyze productivity metrics and perform quality assurance. Plans must guard against paying for clinical services that have not occurred, and regular reviews are necessary to prevent this as well as identify fraud, waste, and abuse.

Positive member outcomes as a demonstration of MTM success will lead to greater pharmacy revenue, professional satisfaction, and expansion of MTM services. Furthermore, outcomes data will be an important component of the EMTM model test as it seeks to provide further evidence of the role of MTM in improving quality of care and reducing costs.

CONTINUOUS IMPROVEMENT OF THE MEDICATION THERAPY MANAGEMENT PROGRAM

Clinical programs should be continuously evaluated to ensure that they are achieving the desired outcomes. This has several benefits in addition to quality assurance. Evaluations help the plan understand where improvements can be made, from minor tweaks to full overhauls. Evaluations also help ensure that the maximum number of members are receiving services without sacrificing quality. MTM operations that use scheduled appointments similar to a physician's office should assess the number of appointments available by the provider and factor in missed appointments to ensure that providers operate at maximum capacity. Plans should monitor completion times to see if technological upgrades or additional staff training can make providers more efficient in the delivery of services without sacrificing quality. Quality assurance procedures should be continuously reviewed to ensure they are consistent with the most recent industry best practices. This should include not only operational consensus on the delivery of MTM, but also clinical consensus updates on evidence-based medicine.

Endorsed quality metrics should also be leveraged to drive continuous improvement. Measuring the completion rates of comprehensive medication reviews has become increasingly important in the Medicare Part D space. Endorsed by the PQA and adopted by CMS as a Star Rating after spending time as a display measure, this quality measure speaks directly to an MTM provider's ability to engage members and promote the key service offering of an MTM program.[5,17]

Internal reviews are essential for improvement, but it is also important to seek feedback from external sources, such as prescribers and, most importantly, the members enrolled in the MTM program. Prescribers can offer insight regarding the types of recommendations they receive and the extent to which they are valuable in modifying patient care. Members can rate their satisfaction with the current service offerings, the service providers, and the value they perceive from the service. Prescriber and member experience surveys are a common method for obtaining feedback and are conducted in various ways. Some assess the entire member population or the full panel of contracted prescribers; others may use a randomized sample that can be generalized to the entire population (of prescribers or members). These types of surveys offer a global picture of an MTM program but can sometimes be skewed by individuals who choose not to participate in MTM services or be hindered by recall bias if a large amount of time has lapsed between the service and the survey. Another method is a transactional approach, which asks for immediate feedback following a service such as a medication review. These can be included with take-away materials provided to the member for later completion and returned to the plan or offered directly at the conclusion of the service. The transactional approach helps reduce recall bias and limits the responses to individuals who actually participated in the service. This approach does have limitations because it does not give insight into individuals who are not participating, which could be due to flaws in the MTM program's engagement processes.

As the MTM program evolves, it will be important to continually analyze the initial ROI calculations; they may need to be modified to showcase actual results, changes in costs for services and technology, or new methods used to calculate healthcare costs. Various calculations can be used, but the most common utilize cost avoidance to estimate the healthcare costs that have been avoided through MTM services. Other methods use actual healthcare costs and utilization, pre- and postservice offering (pharmacy claims, medical claims), by analyzing a plan's actual claims data. Payers or MTM service providers may modify these or use other proprietary methods to calculate the estimated or actual ROI.

PROGRAM AUDITING

Just as payers may audit entities providing MTM services, plans may be audited on their MTM program. Part D sponsors currently participate annually in a data validation audit of the reporting requirements, and CMS also performs program audits on Part D sponsors to ensure they are compliant with their CMS contract. In 2016, as part of the program audit, MTM programs were included as a pilot audit.[18]

As plans choose vendors to partner with, services to provide, and methods of delivery, it is important that they keep in mind the items that may be audited to ensure appropriate documentation and oversight of the program.

CMS MTM Program Pilot Audit

The CMS announced the release of the MTM pilot audit protocol beginning in 2016 and requested data sets (or universes) to evaluate whether health plans are accurately identifying and enrolling targeted beneficiaries in MTM programs, appropriately disenrolling beneficiaries, and offering required services to the MTM program enrollees. As part of this audit, CMS utilizes 3 data universes, spanning 2 calendar years.[b] Plans must supply the requested universes to CMS within 15 days of being notified of the impending program audit. After reviewing the supplied universes, CMS selects sample cases from the universe for specific review with the health plan.[18]

The purpose of the audit will likely remain the same, and findings during the pilot will drive future determination of data elements collected to ensure compliance with guidance around MTM in the coming years.

Audit Preparation

Plans typically perform mock audits to identify risks and gaps in documentation, process flow, data integrity, and outcomes prior to receiving word of an impending audit. Where possible, plans should request audit materials to review in advance. This enables plans to prepare the materials that will be required as well as turnaround times. Internal audits can also aid in preparation. In this case, the plan hires a vendor to audit particular aspects of the plan. An internal audit should be treated as if it were the real thing, meaning that the same time constraints and requirements should be set. If the auditor finds opportunities for improvement, the plan should immediately begin to take remedial steps. If MTM services are outsourced, the vendor should also be informed of audit requirements as it may need to provide information when an audit occurs.

During the audit, providing clear, up-to-date documents is essential for showcasing the program. Having a dedicated team to respond to questions and a point person to relay additional information requests can be beneficial in giving the auditors the information they need. Payers will expect any delegated entities performing services to provide documents and assist in answering auditor questions.

At the completion of the audit, it is important that payers conduct a debriefing to document any missteps. Auditor comments should be reviewed, and similarly to the steps taken after an internal audit, opportunities for improvement should be evaluated and remedial steps put in place.

PREDICTING THE FUTURE OF MEDICATION THERAPY MANAGEMENT

As health plans continue to strive to provide cost-mitigating, quality-driven MTM solutions, they must keep pace with ever-changing MTM regulations as well as evolving expectations on how and where MTM is provided.

Part D sponsors must keep abreast of CMS memorandums, Federal Register notifications, the Annual Advanced Notification, and most importantly the Annual Call Letter. Other plan providers may gain insight by reviewing various state RFI and RFP questions regarding MTM to monitor potential new requirements. All plans should maintain continuous survey of the clinical literature and participate in professional organizations that shape the landscape of MTM.

---

[b] Specific data elements are outlined in the memo and include unique patient identifiers, enrollment status, service offerings and completion, and prescription drug events (PDEs) to ensure appropriate identification related to the submitted program description. This universe, therefore, is already supplied to CMS and not required to be supplied again by the sponsor at time of MTM program audit.

MTM providers will not only have to adapt to new requests and expectations from payers of MTM services but will also have to adjust to service delivery methods, documentation requirements, and expected outcomes that may arise due to inclusion of these services in new arenas, such as accountable care organizations.

Since its introduction in the Medicare Modernization Act of 2003, MTM has continuously evolved, leaving plans searching for ways to comply with regulatory and state contractual requirements. It has also opened the door for plans to improve outcomes in patients not mandated to receive it. In order to do this, however, plans have been faced with proving the value of MTM services on healthcare outcomes. They have also been faced with determining the most cost-effective way to provide a quality MTM program that allows for an appropriate level of oversight and the opportunity to make continuous program improvements. With many touting MTM as the wave of the future for pharmacists, payers will be continuously faced with opportunities for engagement and undoubtedly unique models in which to perform MTM. It will be up to MTM vendors along with providers to prove to plan payers that their service offerings as well as delivery modes are cost effective, quality driven, compliant, and produce outcomes that reduce healthcare costs and improve outcomes for plan members.

REFERENCES

1. The Medicare Prescription Drug, Improvement, and Modernization Act, Pub. L. No. 108-173; 2003. Available at https://www.gpo.gov/fdsys/pkg/PLAW-108publ173/pdf/PLAW-108publ173.pdf. Accessed January 30, 2017.
2. Participants selected for Part D Enhanced Medication Therapy Management model. October 2016. CMS website. Available at https://www.cms.gov/Newsroom/MediaReleaseDatabase/Fact-sheets/2016-Fact-sheets-items/2016-10-03.html. Accessed December 28, 2016.
3. Announcement of calendar year (CY) 2014 Medicare Advantage capitation rates and Medicare Advantage and Part D payment policies and final Call Letter. April 2013. CMS website. Available at https://www.cms.gov/Medicare/Health-Plans/MedicareAdvtgSpecRateStats/Downloads/Announcement2014.pdf. Accessed December 28, 2016.
4. HEDIS and performance measurement. NCQA website. Available at http://www.ncqa.org/tabid/59/dealut.aspx. Accessed January 30, 2017.
5. PQA measures used by CMS in the Star Ratings. PQA website. Available at www.pqaalliance.org. Accessed January 30, 2017.
6. Part C and D performance data: 2017 Part C and D performance data technical notes. CMS website. Available at http://www.cms.gov/Medicare/Prescription-Drug-Coverage/PrescriptionDrugCovGenIn/PerformanceData.html. Accessed January 30, 2017.
7. Part C and D performance data: 2017 display measures technical notes. CMS website. Available at http://www.cms.gov/Medicare/Prescription-Drug-Coverage/PrescriptionDrugCovGenIn/PerformanceData.html. Accessed January 30, 2017.
8. *Prescription Drug Benefit Manual.* Medication therapy management and quality improvement program. CMS website. Available at http://www.cms.gov/Medicare/Prescription-Drug-Coverage/PrescriptionDrugCovContra/Downloads/Chapter7.pdf. Accessed December 14, 2016.
9. Announcement of calendar year (CY) 2010 Medicare Advantage capitation rates and Medicare Advantage and Part D payment policies. CMS website. Available at http://www.cms.gov/Medicare/Health-Plans/MedicareAdvtgSpecRateStats/Downloads/Announcement2010.pdf. Accessed January 30, 2017.
10. Announcement of calendar year (CY) 2013 Medicare Advantage capitation rates and Medicare Advantage and Part D payment policies and final Call Letter. CMS website. Available at http://www.cms.gov/medicare/health-plans/healthplansgeninfo/downloads/2013-call-letter.pdf. Accessed January 30, 2017.
11. American Pharmacists Association; National Association of Chain Drug Stores Foundation. Medication therapy management in community pharmacy practice: core elements of an MTM service (Version 1.0). *J Am Pharm Assoc.* 2005;45(5):573-579.
12. American Pharmacists Association; National Association of Chain Drug Stores Foundation. Medication therapy management in pharmacy practice: core elements of an MTM service model (Version 2.0). *J Am Pharm Assoc.* 2008;48(3):341-353.
13. Pharmacist Services Technical Advisory Coalition (PSTAC). Current procedural terminology (CPT) codes for MTM services. Available at http://www.pstac.org/services/mtms-codes.html. Accessed December 14, 2016.
14. U.S. Department of Health and Human Services. Office of Inspector General (OIG) website. Available at https://oig.hhs.gov/. Accessed December 14, 2016.
15. Health Insurance Portability and Accountability Act, Pub. L. No. 104-191; 1996. Available at http://www.gpo.gov/fdsys/pkg/PLAW-104publ191/html/PLAW-104publ191.htm. Accessed December 14, 2016.
16. Medicare Part D reporting requirements. CMS website. Available at https://www.cms.gov/Medicare/Prescription-Drug-Coverage/PrescriptionDrugCovContra/Downloads/CY2016_Part-D-Reporting-Requirements-06092016.pdf. Accessed December 14, 2016.
17. Part C and D performance data: 2016 Part C and D performance data technical notes. CMS website. Available at http://www.cms.gov/Medicare/Prescription-Drug-Coverage/PrescriptionDrugCovGenIn/PerformanceData.html. Accessed January 30,2017.
18. CY 2016 pilot audit protocol release and updates: medication therapy management (MTM) and provider network accuracy [memorandum]. March 16, 2016. CMS website. Available at https://www.cms.gov/Medicare/Compliance-and-Audits/Part-C-and-Part-D-Compliance-and-Audits/Downloads/HPMS_Memo_MTM_Protocols_PNA_Update.zip. Accessed Dec 29 2016.

Review Questions

1. MTM may be sponsored by
   a. CMS Medicare.
   b. employers.
   c. Medicaid.
   d. managed care organizations.
   e. all of the above.

2. Part C performance measures are heavily influenced by
   a. HEDIS, which was developed by NCQA.
   b. HEDIS, which was developed by JCAHO.
   c. HEDIS, which was developed by PQA.
   d. HEDIS, which was developed by CMS.
   e. HEDIS, which was developed by the pharmacy group that created the MTM consensus document.

3. Reasons to select telephonic over face-to-face MTM delivery include all of the following EXCEPT
   a. ability to record each communication service for oversight and quality assurance of MTM providers.
   b. limited distractions that may be present in a retail pharmacy setting (ie, no dispensing functions, drive-thru, or waiting patients).
   c. ability to reach members unable to travel to a pharmacy (ie, nonambulatory members).
   d. they are proven more effective than busy retail pharmacy setting.
   e. elimination of judgments on the part of the provider or patient, based on the physical attributes of the other.

4. MTM services provided to patients who are not enrolled in Part D are
   a. not required to follow CMS guidelines.
   b. required to follow HEDIS measures.
   c. required to be part of an ACO.
   d. required to use pharmacists as providers.
   e. required to provide a medication action plan.

5. Complementary programs to MTM can include
   a. a newsletter.
   b. a toll-free pharmacy hotline.
   c. educational materials.
   d. pill boxes.
   e. all of the above.

6. When deciding between MTM program insourcing versus outsourcing, consideration must be given to all of the following EXCEPT
   a. quality assessment process.
   b. branding requirements.
   c. interoperability of information technology.
   d. requirement that CPT codes be used for billing.
   e. internal patient capacity.

7. Payment methods for MTM may include all of the following EXCEPT
   a. per-member-per-month charges.
   b. capitated charges.
   c. CPT codes.
   d. fee for service.
   e. sliding scale for changes in prescription volume.

8. An RFP for Part D MTM services would include all of the following EXCEPT
   a. service offerings and methods (ie, member identification, documentation systems, types of reviews).
   b. Local Effective Interventions Efficiency (LEIE) rating.
   c. staffing credentials (ie, certifications, licensure, training).
   d. network or service regions (ie, where plan members can receive service).
   e. policies on safeguarding protected health information (PHI).

9. A delegation audit would contain all of the following EXCEPT
   a. MTM program descriptions, policies as well as procedures, and operational documents for each service provided to the plan.
   b. PHI and HIPAA practices, policies, and procedures.
   c. record retention, including length of record retention.
   d. employees who have committed fraud, waste, and abuse.
   e. disaster recovery capability.

10. CMS Part D MTM reporting requirements do not include
    a. method of delivery for the CMR (ie, face-to-face, telephonic, etc).
    b. qualified providers who work for the company.
    c. number of targeted medication reviews provided.
    d. number of drug therapy problem recommendations made.
    e. number of drug therapy problem resolutions.

ANSWERS

1. e	2. a	3. d
4. a	5. e	6. d
7. e	8. b	9. d
10. b		

6

Perspectives: Patient, Pharmacist, and Physician Views of MTM

Michelle Zeigler, PhD, PharmD, BCACP, Anna Hall, PharmD, BCACP, Alexandre Endiakov, PharmD, and Marvin A. Dewar, MD, JD

KEY POINTS

- Achieving high patient participation rates in medication therapy management (MTM) services for Medicare Part D plans has been challenging since the inception of MTM.
- Patient barriers to participating in MTM services include lack of familiarity with what the services include and benefits of participation.
- Health plans are measured on MTM comprehensive medication review (CMR) completion rate, so overcoming barriers to MTM provision is essential to improve patient participation.
- Pharmacists often face barriers to providing MTM services, including compensation, time, staffing issues, and collaboration.
- Key stressors in the current physician practice environment include dealing with increasing administrative burdens, integrating electronic health records into practice workflows, and downward pressures on physician income.
- Payer value-based purchasing programs increasingly score physicians on clinical and efficiency metrics and tie reimbursement to those metrics.
- Survey data indicate that physicians have an incomplete understanding of MTM programs.
- Physicians respond most favorably to MTM services such as general patient medication education, identifying prescribing errors, assisting patients with obtaining refills, developing accurate medication lists, working to increase patient adherence, and detecting medication adverse effects. Physicians express concerns about MTM programs creating ambiguity about professional roles, imposing new and additional administrative or time burdens on physicians, and the sufficiency of pharmacist training for disease state education and specific medication recommendations. More high quality evidence is needed on the impact of MTM programs on ultimate health outcomes and cost reduction.
- Key opportunities for pharmacists and physicians to work together in the MTM arena include supporting more research into MTM effectiveness, promoting innovations that integrate MTM services into electronic health records (EHRs), and establishing adequate reimbursement for MTM.

INTRODUCTION

Pharmacist-provided MTM is delivered in collaboration with physicians and other healthcare providers with the goal of optimizing therapeutic outcomes for individual patients. MTM services typically involve direct pharmacist-patient interaction and include an ala carte menu of discrete services including, but not limited to, the following:

- Individual patient medication therapy review
- Creating a personal medication record
- Developing an individualized medication-related action plan
- Recommending intervention and referral where appropriate
- Documentation of services and arranging follow-up[1]

MTM programs were established in recognition of the critical role that safe and effective medication management plays in optimizing medical outcomes. To illustrate this point, note that more than 1.5 million preventable medication adverse events occur in the United States each year, resulting in an excess of $177 billion in health-related costs.[2,3] And to highlight the potentially modifiable nature of this excess morbidity and cost, up to two-thirds of all medication-related hospital admissions are the result of medication nonadherence, which is clearly subject to improvement with intervention.[4] The clear hope and intent is that MTM services will improve outcomes such as these.

Recognizing individual pharmacists as key participants in the patient's health team, strategically positioned to assist with medication-related outcomes, has a long and venerable history. The creation of MTM services took this value that pharmacists already provided in a somewhat ad hoc basis and incorporated the services into a program that could be systematically applied to larger patient cohorts. Initially integrated into private managed care insurance plans, as well as in academic and safety net medical practice settings, MTM services became even more formally entrenched into healthcare delivery when they were included as a mandatory component of the Medicare Part D program in 2006. It is fair to say that Medicare Part D MTM services have not thus far produced all of the outcomes that some had expected. The reasons for this are multiple: the variable implementation of MTM services by different Part D Medicare providers; the incomplete acceptance of MTM services by patients who have an incomplete understanding of the programs, yet bear some of the cost; the reality that Part D MTM eligibility criteria do not perfectly define the population of patients most likely to benefit from the programs; and the regulatory restrictions around Part D MTM services that often preclude tailoring services to local circumstances.

Despite the challenges, MTM programs aimed at optimizing medication outcomes are firmly entrenched in population healthcare management programs, both public and private. MTM services are included in most Medicare Advantage programs, over half of state Medicaid programs, and in over a third of private health insurance payer plans.[5] Although higher quality research and evidence is still needed, reports of positive health outcomes from individual MTM program efforts continue to accumulate.[4] The Centers for Medicare & Medicaid Services (CMS) is currently testing continuing enhancements of Part D MTM services that should improve the effectiveness and efficiency of those programs. The 2016 Part D Enhanced Medication Therapy Management Model Test will pilot program enhancements that include additional regulatory flexibility to allow programs to better match local needs, additional prospective payments to cover services that are outside the previous Part D MTM scope, and performance payments for MTM plans that meet specified outcomes. Taken together, it seems likely that MTM programs will continue to evolve and improve to better impact health outcomes in both private and public settings.[6]

HISTORICALLY LOW PARTICIPATION IN MTM SERVICES

The comprehensive medication review (CMR) is a key MTM service defined as "an interactive, person-to-person or telehealth medication review and consultation of a beneficiary's medications ... by a pharmacist or qualified provider that is intended to aid in assessing medication therapy and optimizing patient outcomes."[7] The original goal was to offer CMRs to patients with multiple chronic medications and comorbidities to help improve patient care due to their complexity. Research shows that member participation (in CMRs) is low compared to other MTM services. Barnett et al analyzed 50 MTM programs over 7 years that used community pharmacies to analyze trends in MTM services from 2001 to 2006.[8] They found that only 3.3% of all MTM claims processed through these MTM programs were for CMRs. In 2012, an analysis performed by Avalere Health found that only about 11% of eligible Part D enrollees were enrolled in MTM programs. The analysis showed low rates of members completing CMRs, ranging from 2.4% to 9.6% of eligible MTM enrollees receiving a CMR.[9] CMR rates in the study population of the 2013 Acumen report on MTM in chronically ill populations were 11% to 14%.[4,10] The National Committee for Quality Assurance (NCQA) surveyed 20 MTM programs and found that PDPs had an average participation rate of 14% in programs that required opting-in, such as with CMRs, while Medicare Advantage Prescription Drug (MA-PD) plans reported an 18% average participation rate.[10] In 2016, CMS announced that CMR completion rate would become a Star Rating for health plans.[11] CMS uses a 5-Star Rating system to help consumers compare health plans, with one star being the lowest rating and five stars being the highest rating.[12] The 2017 Star Ratings showed that the average CMR participation rate for MA-PD plans was about 45%; for PDPs it was about 25%.[13] Even though the completion rate for MA-PD plans is higher than for PDPs, a 45% completion rate is rated as two out of five stars for MA-PD plans, and a 25% completion rate falls in the three-star category for PDPs, so there is ample room for improvement.[13] Given that CMS has been more focused on MTM program eligibility rates and CMR participation rates, the remaining discussion will explore how patients, pharmacists, and physicians perceive MTM services and how to overcome barriers regarding knowledge and delivery of these services to improve patient care.

PATIENT BARRIERS TO RECEIVING MTM SERVICES: "WHAT IS MTM ... DID YOU SAY 'ATM'?"

Research has shown that the general population is not familiar with MTM services and what benefits MTM offers. One survey completed in community pharmacies and an internet survey of Medicare Part D enrollees, found that between 60% and 93% of respondents were unfamiliar with or never heard of the term *MTM*.[14,15] The term MTM itself may be confusing or unfamiliar to patients who are unaware of the benefits of the service. One survey participant noted an issue with the abbreviation for MTM after being educated on MTM services: "Not abbreviated, maybe? That might confuse people. MTM, like an ATM."[16] In fact, 70% of patients surveyed did not believe that they would need MTM services even after hearing a description about it, and 40% did not believe they would benefit from these services.[15] Patients may decline MTM services if they already feel comfortable with their current medication regimen.[17] Others may not think they need the service because they only understand it as medication information and education, not necessarily an opportunity to coordinate care with a physician.[18]

In addition, patients may not view pharmacists as professionals, and one survey identified responses that associated the filling of prescriptions to filling orders at a fast food restaurant: "Have it ready quickly," "when told," "fill my 'order,'" and "get it right."[15] While the majority of participants trusted their pharmacist (54%), about 75% said they would prefer to ask their physician about any medication-related problems.[15] Patients are also concerned with overstepping their physicians, betraying their trust, or that recommendations made by the pharmacist may contradict what their physician has recommended for them.[16,19] One participant responded, "I kind of like the physician deciding what medications that I would want to be on."[20] Aside from the lack of knowledge of MTM and apprehension of pharmacists as providers of clinical services, the literature also shows that patients are concerned with the amount of time it takes to complete a CMR and being a nuisance on the pharmacist's time.[16,19]

The location of the CMR may also influence the patient's comfort level in discussing health and medications with a pharmacist. Maintaining privacy and apprehension of discussing health conditions and medications are concerning to patients considering MTM services.[16] Patients may prefer to complete a CMR at their usual pharmacy,[21] while others are highly satisfied with clinical phone interventions and telephonic CMRs.[22] Patients that complete telephonic reviews have also reported they would be willing to complete a face-to-face CMR.[21,22] Thus, it is important to offer multiple avenues for patients to complete CMRs to account for individual preferences or other barriers, such as transportation issues.

IMPROVING PATIENT UNDERSTANDING OF MTM SERVICES—A PERSONAL TOUCH

The CMS has taken steps to ensure that health plans are promoting and increasing awareness of MTM programs. In the 2015 MTM Program Submission instructions, CMS made it clear that health plans should make sure their customer service agents are familiar with the plan's MTM program.[23] Plans were also held accountable for including specific information in plain language about their MTM program on their website such as eligibility requirements, who to contact, program description, how members will be contacted, and a blank copy of the Personal Medication List. Additionally, the Medicare Plan Finder website now provides links to the health plans' MTM program details. CMS is attempting to increase awareness of MTM programs at the health plan level to help improve patient care.

Although CMS is making an effort to improve awareness of MTM services on a health plan level, encouraging individuals to participate in the service is another challenge in itself. When building scripts to offer the CMR, MTM providers should describe what the service involves so patients understand what is actually being offered. Patients do find several benefits to MTM services, and these are points to highlight when explaining MTM services to patients. Personalized attention may appeal to patients, as one survey participant preferred to hear "something with a more personal kind of feeling to it" when learning about an MTM service.[16] A positive association was found between CMR participation and use of a Medication User Self-Evaluation (MUSE) tool to engage beneficiaries by communicating their personal likelihood of benefiting from a CMR.[24] Patients were sent a letter by the MTM provider and received a follow-up phone call. During the phone call, patients were asked seven questions pertaining to medication use and health history. At the end of the call, patients were told the likelihood they would benefit from receiving a CMR. Patients that completed the MUSE tool were 3 times more likely to accept the CMR than those who did not receive the MUSE tool intervention. Additionally, using standardized scripting on call offers has also proven to be a successful strategy. In one study, a CMR script was modified to explain the CMR process, how the member can benefit from the CMR, and offering the CMR earlier in the dialogue. Patients who were offered a CMR using the updated script were 58% more likely to participate in a CMR than those offered a CMR with the original script.[19] Health plans are responding to the expectation of increasing CMR participation by creating strategies to increase patient engagement.

Patients who have received a CMR appreciate what the service offers, such as receiving a personal medication list,[17,21,22] answering questions and providing personalized information about medications,[17,21,22] coordinating care with their other providers,[18,21] wanting to improve overall health, and finding cost-reduction opportunities.[17,18] These are all points that should be emphasized when explaining MTM services to patients during a one-on-one interaction. Patients have also reported feeling more empowered regarding their health[21] and that completing a CMR gave one survey participant "reassurance that they were 'doing the right thing' regarding their medications, and receive(d) the expert opinion of the pharmacist."[16] Incorporating this personal touch into the CMR engagement process may help individualize a patient's expectations of MTM services.

PHARMACIST BARRIERS TO IMPLEMENTING MTM SERVICES

Each year the American Pharmacists Association (APhA) conducts an environmental scan of providers and payers regarding MTM services and reports them. The 2010 survey cited the most significant barriers of providing MTM services included: billing for MTM services, time, and documentation of services.[25] Money, time, and staffing have remained consistent themes in subsequent years, with lack of insurance coverage for MTM services, time, low reimbursement, lack of support staff, and patients not keeping appointments as the most significant challenges.[5,26] In 2016, lack of collaboration with physicians was also listed as a significant barrier in addition to challenges with engaging patients to participate in the services and lack of access to complete medical records.[27] Pharmacists have indicated that they would be interested in training regarding billing and documentation in previous surveys.[28]

BILLING AND COMPENSATION

Perhaps one of the largest concerns that pharmacists have is getting compensated for the MTM services they provide. From 2001 to 2007, "pharmacist-provided MTM interventions changed from primarily education and monitoring for new or changed prescription therapies to prescriber consultations regarding cost-efficacy management."[8] As mentioned earlier, pharmacist duties have been traditionally viewed as being focused on medication education, while MTM services may typically require more time and training to assess medication-related issues and make recommendations to prescribers. Due to the variability of billing and fee structures by different payers, it can be very confusing for pharmacists to understand exactly how they will be compensated for the services they provide. Please see Chapter 10 for more details on how MTM services are billed. A payer may also have requirements for compensation, including clinical training. In the most recent APhA survey of MTM providers, 30% of pharmacists in the community setting and 23% of pharmacists in IHOs (integrated health organizations) are required to obtain certifications or advanced training to deliver MTM services by payers.[27] Specific credentials may include residency training or board certification beyond the PharmD degree. These training programs and certifications lay the foundation for pharmacists to adapt their practice to the wide range of MTM services.

Billing challenges and concerns with low reimbursement rates for patient-care services are a recurring theme for pharmacists involved in MTM services.[27,29] For those pharmacists that were already being compensated for MTM, a pharmacist survey reported that the most common barriers were lack of compensation, ability to obtain that compensation, an unstructured billing process, and lack of recognition as a provider.[29] This shows that even the pharmacists who were getting paid for MTM services still felt that the compensation was not enough and that they were not receiving recognition as a healthcare provider. Many states have taken actions to support provider status and expand pharmacists' scope of practice, including California, Oregon, North Dakota, and Washington State.[27]

TIME, STAFFING, AND SPACE

Time, staffing, and space are major concerns for pharmacists who are already under a strict work schedule. Both the APhA and Lounsbery et al pharmacist surveys reported significant concerns regarding work setting for pharmacists such as: time constraints, staffing deficiencies, inadequate physical space to perform MTM services, lack of access to medical information, and lack of collaborative practice agreements with providers.[27,29] Over 80% of the 194 responding pharmacists agreed upon all 4 of these issues as being a concern.[29] Having to allocate time and staff attention to providing MTM can prove very difficult, especially if the pharmacist is not being compensated for doing so. Pharmacists surveyed in the Wisconsin Pharmacy Quality Collaborative (WPQC) MTM program rated a lack of confidence in providing MTM services if their time was limited.[30] If the pharmacy does not have a designated booth or area for counseling and talking to patients, providing appropriate MTM services can be very difficult. Lack of access to medical information also makes delivering comprehensive MTM services challenging for pharmacists.[27] Despite these challenges, pharmacists have reported feeling confident in their abilities to rely on their coping skills to successfully deliver MTM services when multiple patient issues are occurring at the same time.[30] In addition, pharmacy technician roles are expanding, with pharmacy technicians listed as collaborators by 28% of pharmacists,[27] which may help with time constraints.

ACCESS TO MEDICAL DATA AND COLLABORATION

Access to a patient's medical chart varies among different settings—from clinical, to retail, to call centers. It may not be possible for an MTM provider to have access to medical data such as disease states, lab values, or other pertinent medication information, which can make it difficult for a pharmacist to get the whole picture when assessing a patient's profile for MTM services. Pharmacists may also feel that there is a lack of collaboration with primary care providers depending on their practice site. To improve collaboration with MTM services, CMS published "A Physician's Guide to Medicare Part D Medication Therapy Management (MTM) Programs" in 2012 that provided a description of MTM services and examples of the standardized formatting of the documentation that patients receive, such as the cover letter, Medication Action Plan, and Personal Medication List.[31] Pharmacists in IHOs receive a significantly higher number of referrals for MTM services from physicians (47%) than those in community settings (9%, $P < 0.001$),[27] likely due to the proximity of the healthcare team. Pharmacists surveyed in the WPQC MTM program mentioned previously were relatively confident in their clinical abilities even if physicians did not accept their clinical recommendations.[30] Patient participation and buy-in to the benefits to the services is also important for pharmacists to be able to provide MTM services. The WPQC study also showed that pharmacists were lacking confidence in their ability to offer MTM services to patients who had recently rejected the offer.[30]

Some of the more challenging aspects of collaboration include defining the roles of practitioners in the healthcare team, reimbursement for pharmacist services, and reimbursement for the physician to coordinate care.[28] Physicians may be open to pharmacists adjusting drug dosages, but not necessarily initiating medication therapies.[28] Physician surveys have shown that physicians view the complete patient medication list as the most important benefit of MTM services, and they also value the pharmacist's role in educating patients about their medications and Medicare Part D services.[28] The practice setting can influence the number of patients referred to MTM services and openness for collaboration with patients as well as other providers, as discussed in the next section.

MTM PROGRAMS AND THE CURRENT PHYSICIAN PRACTICE ENVIRONMENT

Establishing a collaborative working relationship between physicians and pharmacists to maximize the impact of MTM services requires an understanding of their individual practice environments and challenges. For physicians, the current practice environment is characterized by increasing administrative burdens and pressures on revenue streams. This results in longer work hours and the need to see more patients in order to maintain steady income levels. In addition, the physician workforce is becoming more diverse over time with an appropriate increased level of attention payed to work–life balance and issues of physician burnout.[32]

The widespread introduction of electronic health records (EHRs) in physician offices is another disruptive influence in the physician work environment. Although EHRs carry great promise for improving the reliability and safety of care delivery, specifically including medication management, the early experience with EHR implementation has been limited by immature current product design, frequent incompatibility of EHR processes with existing practice clinical workflows, and the widespread impression that EHRs decrease the efficiency of many providers. Medication record keeping and prescribing using the EHR does promote a more reliable prescription of standard medication dose forms, facilitates medication allergy checks, and helps providers identify medication interactions that may have previously gone unsuspected. In addition, some EHRs include formulary support to help clinicians identify preferred drugs in an individual patient's health plan. But even in the arena of medication prescribing support, there is a significant need for substantial improvement in the current generation of EHR design. Medication interaction checking is often overly sensitive, inundating clinicians with potential interactions they deem of no clinical significance. And the connection of EHR prescribers to pharmacies through a very limited network of national electronic clearinghouses creates a rigid system that is not responsive to local needs and slow to implement needed improvements. Finally, very few EHR systems include meaningful decision support for prescribers.

Despite these shortcomings, EHRs will continue to be the platform for medication management in the future and should serve as a focal point for delivery of MTM services. Physicians will likely respond most effectively to MTM services that can be deliver through their EHR platform, which will save them time by delivering messages and tasks in the same space where they are already working. Working with national prescription clearinghouses and EHR vendors on safe medication refill and duplicate medication reduction protocols, medication adherence monitoring, and evidence-based medication decision support is fertile ground for collaboration and joint advocacy between MTM providers and physicians.

One of the most dramatic recent changes in the physician practice environment is the proliferation of value-based purchasing (VBP) programs, which evaluate the effectiveness and efficiency of a physician's practice by measuring both the clinical health outcomes and resource use of a population of patients whose care is attributed to the physician, and then tying some aspect of the provider's reimbursement to the metrics. VBP programs often go by names such as "accountable care" or "volume to value" programs and are sponsored by private insurers, self-insured employers, and public payers. Adoption of the Medicare Access and CHIP Reauthorization Act of 2015 (MACRA) moved the clinical practice world much further down this path by making VBP the organizing reimbursement principle for all physician-delivered Medicare services going forward. Many of the clinical quality metrics tracked in VBP programs relate to medication management, and optimal medication management is certainly pivotal to maximizing both clinical and resource use outcomes for patient populations. The increasing prevalence and prominence of VBP programs creates a prime opportunity for MTM programs and providers to collaborate with physicians, since successful MTM efforts should help physicians improve their performance on VBP metrics.

MTM SERVICES: EXAMPLES OF POSITIVE OUTCOMES

A key factor affecting enthusiastic adoption of MTM services by physicians is the degree to which those programs demonstrably improve clinical outcomes for patients. Although there are many reports of the positive clinical impact of MTM services, there is also a consensus that the quality of the evidence base supporting the effectiveness of MTM programs in improving ultimate clinical and efficiency outcomes needs to be expanded and improved.[33] This is certainly an area where active collaboration between MTM providers and physicians should be mutually beneficial.

Some recent reports of the positive clinical impact of MTM programs include:

- Randomized trial of clinical pharmacist-enhanced services for children affected by β-thalassemia demonstrated significant reduction of serum ferritin levels and significant improvement in patient satisfaction and quality of life measures.[34]
- MTM program telephone reminder calls significantly improved medication adherence measures in a Medicare Advantage patient population.[35]
- MTM services significantly reduced medication problems and improved adherence in a before-and-after study of 70 patients with Parkinson's disease.[36]
- Randomized trial of MTM services in 166 hypertensive patients found a significantly lower blood pressure in the study group at 6 months, but not at 9 months.[37]
- MTM program was associated with A1c reduction of 0.27 and a blood pressure reduction of 6.0 systolic and 4.2 diastolic in a pre-post longitudinal study of 101 diabetic patients who were part of an employee health program.[38]

PHYSICIAN ACCEPTANCE OF MTM

Physicians increasingly express frustration about the bureaucratic burdens associated with delivering patient care. To the degree MTM programs are perceived as yet another administrative hassle for physicians, they will likely be resisted. One recent study found that 54% of physicians have symptoms of physician burnout, and one of the major contributors is thought to be nonpatient-centered administrative work.[39,40] The author noted:

> *Although extensive literature suggests that contributors include excessive workload, loss of autonomy, inefficiency due to excessive administrative burdens, a decline in the sense of meaning that physicians derive from work, and difficulty integrating personal and professional life, few interventions have been tested.*[40]

Physician engagement with MTM programs will be driven by their assessment of a mixture of clinical, administrative, economic, and professional issues. To the extent that MTM programs deliver positive clinical outcomes in a way that does not increase physician administrative work, recognize the distinct roles of the different professional members of the health care team, and do not negatively affect physician practice economics, physicians should support MTM programs with enthusiasm. On the other hand, to the degree that MTM services create ambiguity about professional roles, impose new and additional administrative or time burdens on physicians, or reduce provider income, it will not be surprising if physicians are less than fully supportive. Given the current care gaps in medication therapy, and the potential role MTM programs can play to close those gaps, it behooves both MTM providers and physicians to find ways to work together to their mutual benefit and to the benefit of patients.

A 2008 mail survey of 500 physicians found them more comfortable with certain MTM services, such as general patient education about their medications, identification of prescribing errors, and assisting patients obtain refills on time. Physicians were less enthusiastic about pharmacists assisting in designing drug therapy treatment plans, suggesting new prescription medications to patients or physicians, and providing specific disease state education. About 60% of the surveyed physicians supported collaborative practice agreements with pharmacists.[41] A different focus group study involving primary care physicians (PCP) found little general understanding of MTM. The positive aspects of MTM identified by the PCPs were developing complete and accurate medication lists, working to increase patient adherence to medication regimens, and detecting medication adverse effects. PCPs raised concerns about the potential for role confusion among patients related to pharmacists and physicians, pharmacists not knowing patients well enough to offer specific clinical recommendations, potential overstepping of professional boundaries while delivering MTM services, and pharmacists needing more clinical training before offering specific disease state education. The study emphasized the key role played by an established, trusting relationship between pharmacist and the physician in the success of their joint efforts.[42]

Maintaining clarity around professional roles will be important in fostering joint pharmacist and physician advocacy for MTM programs. Pharmacists are expert in drug therapy, administration, and distribution. Physicians are expert in patient evaluation, diagnosis, and disease management. Although there is certainly some overlap in these skill sets, they are distinct, and a beneficial collaboration has evolved over time where pharmacists and physicians both contribute to patient care in a complementary way. MTM services will likely experience the greatest degree of physician support when they extend that collaboration to an even greater positive clinical result for patients. On a cautionary note, to the extent that either pharmacists or physicians focus on threats to or expansion of professional roles, collaborative efforts become more challenging.[5,43] Indeed, integrating pharmacists and MTM efforts more directly in existing clinical practice structures is consistent with the focus on team-based care currently embedded in the patient-centered medical home concept widely advanced as a best practice in contemporary health care delivery design.[44] Promoting team-based care, optimal patient outcomes, and cost-effective health care benefits patients and society and are values that physicians and pharmacists can universally support.

RECOMMENDATIONS

Based upon the current state of MTM program evolution and the potential for MTM services to make important contributions to improved clinical outcomes and cost-effective care, the following recommendations apply to both physicians and MTM providers. Ideally, pharmacists and physicians should jointly advance each recommendation.

1. Continue to promote MTM programs as a component of contemporary healthcare delivery design.
2. Support high quality research that continues to validate MTM outcomes. A moderate level of current evidence supports the conclusion that MTM services improve clinical outcomes. Evidence that MTM services reduce health costs is less extensive.
3. Promote strong professional collaboration and linkages between physicians and pharmacists that recognize the complementary professional roles of each. Avoid creating structures that may confuse patients by making professional roles ambiguous and accountability for different aspects of care unclear.
4. Refine MTM services so that they can be delivered with the minimal amount of administrative or time burden on physicians.
5. Promote portable electronic personalized medication records and the integration of MTM services into electronic health records.
6. Advocate to national prescribing clearinghouses for improved electronic prescribing interfaces.
7. Leverage emerging telemedicine platforms for providing MTM services.
8. Incorporate collaborative practice arrangements between physicians and pharmacists in the next generation of patient-centered medical homes.
9. Establish payment structures for MTM services that facilitate the delivery of services and create alignment between pharmacists and physicians.

To the extent that physicians and pharmacists support and accomplish these goals together, the beneficiaries will be both patients and payers.

REFERENCES

1. American Pharmacists Association; National Association of Chain Drug Stores Foundation. Medication therapy management in pharmacy practice: core elements of an MTM service model (version 2.0). *J Am Pharm Assoc.* 2008;48(3):341-353.
2. Ernst FR, Grizzle AJ. Drug-related morbidity and mortality: updating the cost-of-illness model. *J Am Pharm Assoc.* 1001;41(2):192-199.
3. Committee on Identifying and Preventing Medication Errors; Aspden P, Wolcott JA, Bootman JL, Cronenwett LR, eds. *Preventing Medication Errors.* Washington, DC: National Academies Press; 2007. *Quality Chasm Series.*
4. Perlroth D, Marrufo G, Montesinos A, et al. Medication therapy management in chronically ill populations: final report. CMS website. Available at https://innovation.cms.gov/files/reports/mtm_final_report.pdf. Accessed July 19, 2017.
5. American Pharmacists Association. *Medication Therapy Management Digest: The Pursuit of Provider Status to Support the Growth and Expansion of Pharmacists' Patient Care Services.* Washington, DC: American Pharmacists Association; March 2014. Available at https://www.pharmacist.com/sites/default/files/MTM%20Digest_2014%20FINAL.pdf. Accessed July 23, 2017.
6. CMS. Announcement of Part D Enhanced Medication Therapy Management Model Test [memorandum]. Available https://innovation.cms.gov/Files/x/mtm-announcement.pdf. Published September 28, 2015. Accessed July 19, 2017.
7. CMS. MTM program standardized format revisions (v07.15.14). Available at https://www.cms.gov/medicare/prescription-drug-coverage/prescriptiondrugcovcontra/mtm.html. Accessed July 19, 2017.
8. Barnett MJ, Frank J, Wehring H, et al. Analysis of pharmacist-provided medication therapy management (MTM) services in community pharmacies over 7 years. *J Manag Care Pharm.* 2009;15(1):18-31. doi:10.18553/jmcp.2009.15.1.18.
9. Pearson CF. Few Medicare beneficiaries receive comprehensive medication review services [press release]. http://avalere.com/expertise/managed-care/insights/few-medicare-beneficiaries-receive-comprehensive-medication-management-serv. Published August 7, 2014. Accessed July 19, 2017.
10. Academy of Managed Care Pharmacy. Sound medication therapy management programs; version 2.0 with validation study. *J Manag Care Pharm.* 2008;14(1 Suppl B):S2-44.
11. CMS. Announcement of calendar year (CY) 2016 Medicare Advantage capitation rates and Medicare Advantage and Part D payment policies and final Call Letter. Available at https://www.cms.gov/medicare/health-plans/medicareadvtgspecratestats/downloads/announcement2016.pdf. Published April 6, 2015. Accessed July 20, 2017.
12. CMS. Five-Star Quality Rating System. Available at https://www.cms.gov/medicare/provider-enrollment-and-certification/certificationandcomplianc/fsqrs.html. Updated June 28, 2017. Accessed July 20, 2017.

13. CMS. 2017 Part C and D Medicare Star Ratings data (v11 02 2016). Available at https://www.cms.gov/Medicare/Prescription-Drug-Coverage/PrescriptionDrugCovGenIn/PerformanceData.html. Accessed July 20, 2017.

14. Truong HA, Layson-Wolf C, de Bittner MR, Owen JA, Haupt S. Perceptions of patients on Medicare Part D medication therapy management services. *J Am Pharm Assoc.* 2003;49(3):392-398. doi:10.1331/JAPhA.2009.08008.

15. Law AV, Okamoto MP, Brock K. Perceptions of Medicare Part D enrollees about pharmacists and their role as providers of medication therapy management. *J Am Pharm Assoc.* 2003;48(5):648-653. doi:10.1331/JAPhA.2008.07084.

16. Garcia GM, Snyder ME, McGrath SH, Smith RB, McGivney MS. Generating demand for pharmacist-provided medication therapy management: identifying patient-preferred marketing strategies. *J Am Pharm Assoc.* 2003;49(5):611-616. doi:10.1331/JAPhA.2009.08089.

17. Huet AL, Frail CK, Lake LM, Snyder ME. Impact of passive and active promotional strategies on patient acceptance of medication therapy management services. *J Am Pharm Assoc.* 2003;55(2):178-181. doi:10.1331/JAPhA.2015.14091.

18. Schultz H, Westberg S, Ramalho de Oliveira D, Brummel A. Patient-perceived value of Medication Therapy Management (MTM) services: a series of focus groups. *Inov Pharm.* 2012;3(4). Available at https://conservancy.umn.edu/handle/11299/145818. Accessed July 20, 2017.

19. Miguel A, Hall A, Wei L, et al. Improving comprehensive medication review acceptance by using a standardized recruitment script: a randomized control trial. *J Manag Care Spec Pharm.* 2017;23(1):13-21. doi:10.18553/jmcp.2017.23.1.13.

20. Witry M, Chang E, Mormann M, Doucette W, Newland B. Older adult perceptions of a self-reported medication risk questionaire: a focus group study. *Inov Pharm.* 2011;2(3). Available at http://pubs.lib.umn.edu/cgi/viewcontent.cgi?article=1049&context=innovations. Accessed July 20, 2017.

21. Doucette WR, Zhang Y, Chrischilles EA, et al. Factors affecting Medicare Part D beneficiaries' decision to receive comprehensive medication reviews. *J Am Pharm Assoc.* 2003;53(5):482-487. doi:10.1331/JAPhA.2013.12233.

22. Moczygemba LR, Barner JC, Brown CM, et al. Patient satisfaction with a pharmacist-provided telephone medication therapy management program. *Res Social Adm Pharm.* 2010;6(2):143-154. doi:10.1016/j.sapharm.2010.03.005.

23. CMS. CY 2015 medication therapy management program guidance and submission instructions [memorandum]. Available at https://www.cms.gov/Medicare/Prescription-Drug-Coverage/PrescriptionDrugCovContra/Downloads/MemoContractYear2015MedicationTherapyManagementProgramSubmission050714.pdf. Published May 7, 2014. Accessed July 20, 2017.

24. Doucette WR, Pendergast JF, Zhang Y, et al. Stimulating comprehensive medication reviews among Medicare Part D beneficiaries. *Am J Manag Care.* 2015;21(6):e372-378.

25. American Pharmacists Association. *Medication Therapy Management Digest: Tracking the Expansion of MTM in 2010: Exploring the Consumer Perspective.* Washington DC: American Pharmacists Association; March 2011. Available at http://www.pharmacist.com/sites/default/files/files/mtm_2011_digest.pdf. Accessed July 22, 2017.

26. American Pharmacists Association. *Medication Therapy Management Digest: Pharmacists Emerging as Interdisciplinary Health Care Team Members.* Washington DC: American Pharmacists Association; March 2013. Available at https://www.pharmacist.com/sites/default/files/files/MTMDigest_2013.pdf. Accessed July 22, 2017.

27. American Pharmacists Association. *Pharmacists' Patient Care Services Digest: Building Momentum. Increasing Access.* Washington DC: American Pharmacists Association; March 2016. Available at http://media.pharmacist.com/documents/APhA_Digest.pdf. Accessed July 22, 2017.

28. Oladapo AO, Rascati KL. Review of survey articles regarding medication therapy management (MTM) services/programs in the United States. *J Pharm Pract.* 25(4):457-470. doi:10.1177/0897190012442715.

29. Lounsbery JL, Green CG, Bennett MS, Pedersen CA. Evaluation of pharmacists' barriers to the implementation of medication therapy management services. *J Am Pharm Assoc.* 2003;49(1):51-58. doi:10.1331/JAPhA.2009.017158.

30. Martin BA, Chui MA, Thorpe JM, Mott DA, Kreling DH. Development of a scale to measure pharmacists' self-efficacy in performing medication therapy management services. *Res Social Adm Pharm.* 2010;6(2):155-161. doi:10.1016/j.sapharm.2010.05.001.

31. CMS. A physician's guide to Medicare Part D medication therapy management (MTM) programs (10.12.12). Available at https://www.cms.gov/medicare/prescription-drug-coverage/prescriptiondrugcovcontra/mtm.html (2012). Accessed July 20, 2017.

32. Zimlich R. 5 things for you to worry about in 2013. *Med Econ eConsult.* December 11, 2012.

33. Ai AL, Carretta H, Beitsch LM, Watson L, Munn J, Mehriary S. Medication therapy management programs: promises and pitfalls. *J Manag Care Spec Pharm.* 2014;20(12):1162-1182.

34. Bahnasawy SM, El Wakeel LM, El Beblawy N, El-Hamamsy M. Clinical pharmacist-provided services in iron overloaded beta-thalassemia major children; a new insight to patient care. *Basic Clin Pharmacol Toxicol.* 2017;120(4):354-359. doi:10.1111/bcpt.12695.

35. Park H, Adeyemi A, Wang W, Roane TE. Impact of a telephonic outreach program on medication adherence in Medicare Advantage Prescription Drug (MAPD) plan beneficiaries. *J Am Pharm Assoc.* 2003;57(1):62-66.e62. doi:10.1016/j.japh.2016.07.006.

36. Foppa AA, Chemello C, Vargas-Peláez CM, Farias MR. Medication therapy management service for patients with Parkinson's disease: a before-and-after study. *Neurol Ther.* 2016;5(1):85-99. doi:10.1007/s40120-016-0046-4.

37. Hirsch JD, Steers N, Adler DS, et al. Primary care-based, pharmacist-physician collaborative medication-therapy management of hypertension: a randomized, pragmatic trial. *Clin Ther.* 2014;36(9):1244-1254. doi:10.1016/j.clinthera.2014.06.030.

38. Pinto SL, Kumar J, Partha G, Bechtol RA. Pharmacist-provided medication therapy management (MTM) program impacts outcomes for employees with diabetes. *Popul Health Manag.* 2014;17(1):21-27. doi:10.1089/pop.2012.0124.

39. Shanafelt TD, Hasan O, Dyrbye LN, et al. Changes in burnout and satisfaction with work-life balance in physicians and the general US working population between 2011 and 2014. *Mayo Clin Proc.* 2015;90(12):1600-1613. doi:10.1016/j.mayocp.2015.08.023.

40. Shanafelt TD, Boone S, Tan L, et al. Burnout and satisfaction with work-life balance among US physicians relative to the general US population. *Arch Intern Med.* 2012;172(18):1377-1385. doi:10.1001/archinternmed.2012.3199.

41. Alkhateeb FM, Unni E, Latif D, Shawaqfeh MS, Al-Rousan RM. Physician attitudes toward collaborative agreements with pharmacists and their expectations of community pharmacists' responsibilities in West Virginia. *J Am Pharm Assoc.* 2009;49(6):797-800. doi:10.1331/JAPhA.2009.08111.

42. McGrath SH, Snyder ME, Dueñas GG, Pringle JL, Smith RB, McGivney MS. Physician perceptions of pharmacist-provided medication therapy management: qualitative analysis. *J Am Pharm Assoc.* 2010;50(1):67-71. doi:10.1331/JAPhA.2010.08186.

43. American Medical Association letter to CMS's Dr. McClellan, providing comment on the Medicare Prescription Drug Benefit proposed rule. October 4, 2004.

44. Agency for Healthcare Research and Quality. Defining the PCMH. US Department of Health & Human Services. Available at https://pcmh.ahrq.gov/page/defining-pcmh. Accessed July 20, 2017.

Review Questions

1. Physicians tend to respond favorably to all of the following MTM services EXCEPT
   a. medication education.
   b. identifying adverse medication reactions.
   c. formulation of an independent medication treatment plan.
   d. ensuring the accuracy of medication records.
   e. monitoring and evaluation of the patient's response to therapy, including safety and effectiveness.

2. Which of the following are factors in physicians' attitudes toward MTM?
   a. declining reimbursement
   b. increasing administrative burdens
   c. electronic health records
   d. clarity regarding professional roles
   e. all of the above

3. Which statement is true regarding increasing patient acceptance rate of comprehensive medication reviews (CMRs)?
   a. The scripting and explanation of a CMR has no impact on whether or not a patient decides to participate in the MTM service.
   b. Medicare Part D plans do not need to increase the acceptance rate of CMRs since participation is over 90% according to Star Ratings reports.
   c. Patients are already familiar with MTM services, so pharmacists do not need to explain the benefits of a CMR.
   d. Pharmacists can increase the acceptance rate of CMRs by offering medication reviews in a face-to-face setting as well as over the telephone according to patient preference.

4. Which of the following are barriers for pharmacists to provide MTM services?
   a. time
   b. reimbursement
   c. staffing
   d. space
   e. all of the above

5. The Patient-Centered Medical Home is not designed to
   a. enhance access and continuity.
   b. identify and manage patient populations.
   c. provide self-care and community support.
   d. track and coordinate care.
   e. eliminate the need for MTM.

6. MTM has the potential to help with transformational change and improvement in
   a. coordinated care.
   b. medication adherence.
   c. reducing healthcare costs.
   d. being patient-centric.
   e. all of the above.

7. With regard to Part D Medicare MTM services, all of the following are true EXCEPT
   a. all Part D Providers must offer MTM services.
   b. Part D MTM eligibility criteria do not completely identify those patients who might benefit from MTM services.
   c. the MTM services offered by different Part D providers are identical.
   d. ongoing collection of high quality evidence documenting the impact of MTM services is needed.
   e. MTM programs are firmly established in the Part D program.

8. Physicians' concerns about pharmacist-provided MTM include all of the following EXCEPT
   a. the ability of pharmacists to be paid for MTM services.
   b. lack of clinical training.
   c. lack of complete patient understanding.
   d. limited view of the complete therapeutic plan.
   e. incomplete information about the patient's conditions.

9. Value-based purchasing programs
   a. tie aspects of physician reimbursement to patient care metrics.
   b. are increasingly used by public and private payers.
   c. score performance using a balanced score card that looks at clinical and resource utilization parameters.
   d. are an opportunity for MTM providers and physicians to work together.
   e. all of the above.

10. Physician acceptance of MTM programs could be enhanced by
    a. elimination of EHRs.
    b. pharmacist-physician professional collaborative agreements.
    c. elimination of value-based purchasing programs.
    d. less contact between physicians and pharmacists.
    e. making patients pay for MTM services.

ANSWERS

1. c	2. e	3. d
4. e	5. e	6. e
7. c	8. a	9. e
10. b		

7

Conducting the Comprehensive Medication Review

Heather C. Hardin, PharmD, BCACP, and Jennifer Salo, PharmD, BCACP, CPh

KEY POINTS

- The comprehensive medication review (CMR) is an essential element of Medicare Therapy Management (MTM). The CMR involves an interactive face-to-face or telehealth medication review and is a systematic process of collecting patient-specific data, assessing medication therapies to identify medication-related problems, prioritizing a list of medication-related problems, and creating a plan to resolve them with the patient, caregiver, and prescriber.
- Good clinical decisions require good data; before making recommendations to prescribers, the MTM provider should attempt to collect the most accurate drug use information using all available resources.
- Discrepancies and inaccuracies can occur in any setting in which the medication review takes place; it is helpful to understand what discrepancies can occur during the CMR and be prepared to take action to collect the most accurate medication list.
- Preparation of both the patient and the MTM pharmacist is necessary.
- Before performing the CMR, the MTM pharmacist should gather a potential medication list, determine potential disease states, identify healthcare providers, and identify potential medication-related problems.
- Efficiency is important when conducting the CMR as the MTM pharmacist must address the objectives of all parties involved, as well as collect all required data necessary to make accurate and helpful recommendations with the patient's healthcare team.
- Documenting a care plan creates a record of the patient interaction and rationalization for the MTM decision-making process. It also allows for continuity of care and is usually required for reimbursement.
- The personal medication list (PML) is patient-directed and should contain any prescription medications, over-the-counter (OTC) medications, and medical supplies.
- The medication action plan (MAP) is the patient's guide to medications as well as disease states and should include empowering actions to assist him or her in reaching the agreed-upon health goals.
- When communicating with a physician, it is important to be informative and suggestive as well as concise and respectful.
- Follow-up allows the MTM pharmacist to monitor the resolution of issues and identify any new medication-related problems.

INTRODUCTION TO MEDICATION THERAPY MANAGEMENT AND THE COMPREHENSIVE MEDICATION REVIEW

Definitions

The American Pharmacists Association, the National Association of Chain Drug Stores, and the Centers for Medicare & Medicaid Services (CMS) have defined five core elements of MTM:

1. A CMR
2. A personal medication list (PML), which is a record of all of the patient's medications (including prescriptions, over-the-counter medications, herbals, and dietary supplements)
3. A medication action plan (MAP), which is a patient-centered document that empowers the patient to take personal action and track their progress of self-management
4. Intervention and referral to other healthcare professionals as appropriate
5. Documentation and follow-up[1]

An essential element of MTM is the CMR, described by CMS as a systematic process of collecting patient-specific information, assessing medication therapies to identify medication-related problems, developing a prioritized list of medication-related problems, and creating a plan to resolve them with the patient, caregiver, and prescriber. The CMR involves an interactive person-to-person or telehealth medication review and consultation conducted in real time between the patient or other authorized individual, such as a prescriber or caregiver, and the pharmacist or other qualified MTM provider. It is designed to improve patients' knowledge of their prescriptions, OTCs, herbal therapies, along with dietary supplements; identify as well as address problems or concerns that patients may have; and empower patients to manage their medications and health conditions.[1-2]

The five core elements of MTM each require time and attention. CMS estimates that the time required to complete all of these activities is 40 minutes, including time to search data resources, gather data, as well as complete and document all aspects of the review.[3] Depending on the complexity of a given case, it may require less time, or it could take considerably longer. Organization along with time management becomes imperative; it becomes important to strike a balance between patient care and meeting the goals of productivity as well as quality.

Comprehensive Medication Reviews and Other Medication Reviews

Many medication reviews occur within the healthcare system. During hospital admittances, medication reconciliation is used to detect whether drug-related problems are the cause for admission and to ensure appropriate drug therapy during hospitalization.[4] Medication reconciliation is an active process that occurs at points of transition, including admissions, transfers in levels of care, and discharge. Its aim is to capture an accurate medication list for the patient and compare current medications to the drug regimen being considered at the next location. Like a CMR, medication reconciliation can identify medication-related problems; in contrast to a CMR, the goal is to focus primarily on patients' medication use while they are in transition from one setting to another. When patients experience a transition of care, there may be additional situations to consider such as the potential risk of duplicate therapies, gaps in therapy, adverse drug events, and confusion. MTM can be a useful tool to help patients understand all of their medications especially at any transition of care as well as at discharge when they are faced with how and when to take their medications on their own. MTM pharmacists may also be contracted to perform medication reconciliations to address specific CMS performance measures.

Physicians and nurses conduct medication reviews during regular office visits. These medication histories assist the physician in identifying polypharmacy and multiple prescriptions, clarifying any differences in administration of drugs compared to the way they are prescribed along with identifying adherence issues. The result is a medication list that assists the prescriber in addressing issues in the patient's continuum of care. Accurate and complete CMRs can take up to 45 minutes. For a physician with numerous important duties, this may not be feasible.[5-6] Medication therapy management can be an additional source of information to prescribers, providing additional data that can aid in medication therapy decisions.

CMRs are required for qualifying MTM members of any Medicare Part D prescription drug plan. The CMR helps create an accurate and complete medication list, including OTCs and herbal medications, which can be used to update the patient's medication history in other settings. Communication is key, and CMRs can assist with coordination of care by ensuring communication among all prescribers and healthcare providers in the patient's scope of care. CMRs also empower patients to engage in their own health and quality of life.

ACCURACY AND COMPLETENESS

Good clinical decisions require good data. Different medication profiles can have varying degrees of accuracy. Table 7-1 presents differing types of medication records with their respective strengths and weaknesses. Each medication record has a specific purpose, and a narrow focus may limit the scope and completeness. In addition, errors can exist in any type of medication database. The relative accuracy inherent to the medication data may not be sufficient for decision-making and may not reflect the patient's actual medication usage. Being cognizant of the particular limitations of medication data when providing MTM services will prepare the provider for inaccuracies and discrepancies. Before making recommendations to prescribers, the MTM provider should make every attempt to collect the most accurate medication utilization information.

COMPREHENSIVE MEDICATION REVIEWS DISCREPANCIES

Regardless of setting, discrepancies and inaccuracies can occur.[4,7] Being aware of these discrepancies is important when making MTM interventions; acting on inaccurate data only leads to having a recommendation disregarded and could possibly lead to patient harm. Medication information can be collected from many sources during a CMR, including from the patient. Patient-reported information can have limitations regarding accuracy.[8] Patients may have personal barriers such as visual or language impairments that prevent them from providing accurate information. They may also have disease states that can limit their ability to self-report their drug usage. For example, a patient with Alzheimer disease may not be able to accurately recall his or her medication use. Discrepancies can also stem from the physician. Prescribers may give patients verbal instructions but not write an updated prescription. Prescribers can distribute samples, which may lead to inaccuracies in medication data. Table 7-2 lists discrepancies that can occur during a CMR, how these can be detected, and what action can be taken to remedy them. During a CMR, an MTM provider aims to collect the most comprehensive and accurate medication use history possible in order to make helpful recommendations to the patient's healthcare team.

PREPARING FOR THE COMPREHENSIVE MEDICATION REVIEW

Figure 7-1 presents the general flow of the process of a CMR. Once a patient who may benefit from MTM is identified, he or she should be scheduled for a CMR at a time that is convenient for both the patient and the MTM provider. Depending on the

TABLE 7-1 • Medication Databases

Type of Medication Record	Information Strengths	Information Weaknesses
Medical record: inpatient	• Medication reconciliation during hospital admittance, transfers in levels of care, and at discharge • Provides medication, indications, adverse reactions, and problems • Part B and Part D medications included • Readmissions prevention program should facilitate integration of inpatient medications and home medications • All healthcare providers included	• Limited scope: focuses on hospital medication use • Hospital formulary may lead to changes in the patient's usual medication brand and generic or therapeutic substitution • Medications started for hospital-only conditions not discontinued • OTCs, herbals, dietary supplements may be missing • Lacks outpatient prescription claims data; unable to detect unfilled prescriptions or refill frequency

Medical record: outpatient	• Knowledge of:
	  • Prescriber
	  • New drug replacing a current drug or added to therapy
	  • Verbal changes in administration directions
	  • Medication indications and problems
	  • Part B and Part D medications
	  • Office-based drug administration
	  • Samples
		• May not contain all OTC, herbal, dietary supplements
		• Patients may not bring all medications to the physician's office for the review (refrigerated medicines, eye drops, inhalers)
		• Lack prescription claims data; unable to detect unfilled prescriptions or refill frequency
		• May represent only one of many prescribers caring for patient

Independent pharmacy	• Knowledge of:
	  • Medications dispensed
	  • Medications filled, but not picked up
	  • Refill patterns
	• PDC calculation is possible
		• Medication records limited to single pharmacy
		• May lack:
		  • OTC, herbal, dietary supplements
		  • Indications of medications
		  • Prescription not filled
		  • Internet/Canadian medications
		  • Borrowed medications
		  • Limited Part B medication exposure
		  • Non-PDC adherence issues
		  • Specialty pharmacy drugs
		  • Verbal changes in administration directions

Retail chain pharmacy	• Medication list from all chain pharmacies in the retail network
	• Knowledge of:
	  • Medications dispensed
	  • Medications filled, but not picked up
	  • Refill patterns
	  • Prescriptions not purchased through insurance
	• PDC calculations possible
		• May lack:
		  • OTC, herbal, dietary supplements
		  • Indications of medications
		  • Prescriptions not filled
		  • Internet/Canadian medications
		  • Borrowed medications
		  • Limited Part B medication exposure
		  • Non-PDC adherence issues
		  • Specialty pharmacy drugs
		  • Verbal changes in administration directions

Pharmacy benefit manager	• Knowledge of:
	  • All medications filled through insurance plan, regardless of filling location
	  • Medications dispensed
	  • Medications filled, but not picked up
	  • Refill patterns
	• PDC calculations possible
		• May lack:
		  • OTC, herbal, dietary supplement record
		  • Indications of medications
		  • Prescriptions not filled
		  • Internet/Canadian medications
		  • Borrowed medications
		  • Cash prescriptions
		  • Part B medications
		  • Non-PDC adherence issues
		  • Patient interview
		  • Verbal changes in administration directions

(Continued)

TABLE 7-1 • Medication Databases (*Continued*)

Type of Medication Record	Information Strengths	Information Weaknesses

Personal medication list (MTM CMR)	• Interactive interview provides patient-subjective information
	• Includes all prescription medications including OTCs, herbals, and dietary supplements
	• Compares patient report to claims data or other medical information
	• Relies on patient to update accurately and completely on an ongoing basis
	• May discover:
	  • Prescriptions not filled
	  • Internet/Canadian medications
	  • Borrowed medications
	  • Cash prescriptions
	  • Part B medications
	  • Non-PDC adherence issues
	  • Verbal changes in administration directions
		• Self-reported data
		• Accuracy and completeness have not been systematically investigated
		• Once a year, can become out of date
		• Relies on patient to update accurately and completely on an ongoing basis

Abbreviations: CMR = comprehensive medication review; MTM = medication therapy management; OTC = over the counter; PDC = proportion of days covered.

TABLE 7-2 • Reasons for Discrepancies in CMR

Problem	Detection	Action

Language barriers (see Chapter 8, Oral and Nonverbal Communication in Medication Therapy Management)	• Look/sound of confusion at time of interaction; confers with another person, in foreign language, before responding
	• Saying a response repeatedly that may not always coincide with question (repeatedly saying "yes" to every question)
	• Strong accent
	• Difficulty creating complete sentences
		• Patient may need a translator
		• Training the translator may be necessary
		• Ensure the translator is HIPAA trained and compliant
		• Confirm CMR content with other providers
		• Understand that information through a translator may not be as accurate or complete as with an English-speaking patient
		  • Information may be lost in translation
		  • Empathy, emotion, and minor details may not be communicated well

Low health literacy (see Chapter 8, Oral and Nonverbal Communication in Medication Therapy Management)	• Unable to read or spell from the prescription labels and not visually or cognitively impaired
	• Suspect low health literacy in the following groups:
	  • Patients with English as a second language
	  • Lower incomes
	  • Poorer health
	  • Limited English proficiency
	  • Age 65 and older
		• Assess your pharmacy for its ability to present information in a well-understood fashion
		• AHRQ tool: Is our pharmacy meeting patients' needs? Pharmacy Health Literacy Assessment Tool[a]
		• Use the "teach back" method to assess understanding
		• Use visual presentations and demonstrate products, if appropriate
		• Assure written patient communications are at an appropriate communication level (fourth-to-eighth grade level)
		• Determine if PML and MAP need to be sent to a designated person
		• Confirm CMR contents with other providers

Mental health	• Diagnosis of mental illness (depression, bipolar, schizophrenia, etc)
	• Medications that indicate mental illness
	• Patient seems:
	  • Hyperexcited and goes from one idea to another, not focused on medication review
	  • Delusions or hallucinations
		• Have patient or caregiver bring in medications for review
		• Ask if someone else helps the patient with medications
		• Reschedule the CMR if there is a temporary issue
		• Consider alternate healthcare provider source for CMR
		• Determine if PML and MAP need to be sent to another person
		• Notify prescriber of inability to conduct CMR
		• Confirm CMR content with other provider

(*Continued*)

TABLE 7-2 • Reasons for Discrepancies in CMR (*Continued*)

Problem	Detection	Action
Cognitive impairment (dementia, Alzheimer disease, postchemotherapy cognitive impairment, etc)	• Medications for cognitive impairment (such as cholinesterase inhibitors and memantine) may signify potential memory impairment • Drugs that can affect cognitive function (eg, anticholinergic burden, chemotherapeutic agents, etc) • Medical conditions (eg, depression, heart failure, pain, withdrawal, stroke) • Recent surgery • Difficulty concentrating • Difficulty finding words or losing train of thought • Patient may state he or she is not taking a medication that is clearly being filled regularly • Repeating information or asking the same questions frequently	• Have the patient bring bottles of medications to the review along with any lists or documentation regarding their health • Ask if someone else helps with medications or provides care • Consider healthcare provider source for CMR • Determine if PML and MAP need to be sent to another person
Visual impairment	• Legally blind • Asks if font size can be increased • Asks for help in reading prescriptions and labels • Patient is very concerned with any changes in drug color or shape	• Ask if anyone assists the patient with medications • Determine if magnification will help • Suggest change in font size for PML, MAP • Determine if the PML and MAP need to be sent to another person

OTCs/herbals/dietary supplements are often overlooked	• Reports use of prescription medications only
	• Has disease states or symptoms where CAM use is high:
	  • Obesity
	  • Insomnia
	  • Pain
	  • Allergies
	  • GERD
	  • Cold/Flu
		• Ask every patient if there are any nonprescription medications used for health
		• Use a system approach during the CMR, with specific examples for each system:
		  • Headache
		  • Allergies
		  • Cold/Flu
		  • Stomach
		  • Bowels
		  • Pain
		  • Sleep
		  • Health and well-being
		• OTCs that are commonly used and forgotten about include:
		  • Daily aspirin
		  • Vitamins
		  • Pain medications
		  • Herbals and other supplements

Samples	• Patient states that he or she is using medications that are not visible in claims data • Patient displays medications without any pharmacy label • Patient has unexplained side effects or change in therapeutic status • Prescriber is known to provide samples • Patient goes to clinic that uses samples	• Determine if prescription cost is a factor • Determine if patient qualifies for free or reduced price medication programs • Explain to patient the necessity of making sure the pharmacist and other providers know about the sample medications because of the possibility of misdiagnosed drug interactions or side effects

(*Continued*)

TABLE 7-2 • Reasons for Discrepancies in CMR (*Continued*)

Problem	Detection	Action

Free or cash pay medications	• Patient states that he or she is using medications that are not visible in claims data
	• Patient's bottles have pharmacy labels but the medications are not visible in claims data
	• Patient has unexplained side effects or change in therapeutic status
		• Explain to patient the necessity of making sure the pharmacist and other providers know about free or cash medications because of the possibility of misdiagnosed drug interactions or side effects
		• Determine if:
		  • Prescription cost is a factor
		  • Condition being treated carries stigma
		  • Patient has privacy concerns
		  • Abuse is a possibility

Online/Canadian medications	• Patient states that he or she is using medications that are not visible in claims data
	• Patient presents medication bottles with labels from an out-of-state pharmacy
	• Patient has unexplained side effects or change in therapeutic status
		• Document where these medications are being filled
		• Counsel the patient on the importance and value of having all of the medications filled at one pharmacy
		• Counsel the patient on risks of counterfeit medications
		• Determine if:
		  • Prescription cost is a factor
		  • Condition being treated carries stigma
		  • Patient has privacy concerns
		  • Abuse is a possibility

Drugs administered at prescriber's office	• Patient mentions medications that are not in prescription claims data
	• Patient's profile is missing recommended injectable medications
	• Conditions:
	  • Rheumatoid arthritis
	  • Osteoporosis
	  • Multiple sclerosis
		• Inquire about any medications that are administered in the physician's office; documenting all details
		  • These are processed through medical claims, not prescription claims, and may not be apparent if prescription data is the only source of medications

Borrowed drugs	• Patient presents bottles that are not in prescription data, perhaps even containing someone else's name (family member or other)
	• Late refill but still has medication supply
	• Patient has unexplained side effects or change in therapeutic status
		• Explaining the importance of the medication review and medication list containing all medications used by the patient
		• Determine if:
		  • Prescription cost is a factor
		  • Condition being treated carries stigma
		  • Patient has privacy concerns
		  • Abuse is a possibility

Unfilled prescriptions	• Indication without corresponding medication
	• Prescriber believes patient is receiving medication
	• Just-in-case prescription (ie, prednisone for asthma flare)
	• Prescriptions may appear in claims data without any fills being processed (prescription "on hold" at pharmacy)
	• Patient sorts through a number of written prescriptions when presenting a prescription to fill
		• Inquire at every CMR if the patient has any medications that the physician has prescribed, but the patient has decided not to fill
		• Notify prescriber
		• Determine if:
		  • Prescription cost is a factor
		  • ADR previously
		  • Lack of understanding about indication
		  • Does not believe necessary
		  • Condition being treated carries stigma
		  • Patient has privacy concerns

Filled prescriptions/never picked up	• Lack of therapeutic response	• During the medication review, make a point to ask the patient if there are any prescriptions that he or she has not picked up from the pharmacy
		• Notify prescriber
		• Determine if:
		  • Prescription cost is a factor
		  • ADR previously
		  • Lack of understanding about indication
		  • Does not believe necessary
		  • Condition being treated carries stigma
		  • Privacy concerns

(*Continued*)

TABLE 7-2 • Reasons for Discrepancies in CMR (*Continued*)

Problem	Detection	Action
Picked up medications/never taken	• Lack of therapeutic response • Late on refills	• Clarify adherence to all medications assessed during the CMR • Document all adherence issues; address any barriers
Part B medications	• Patient is a transplant recipient or cancer patient and mentions drugs that do not appear in Part D claims data • Patient claims to be using nebulizer solutions that do not appear in claims data	• Document all details of transplant or cancer medications in the medication list • Document all details of nebulizer solutions in medication list, clarifying pharmacy of record for all Part B medications in patient's record

[a] O'Neal K, Crosby K, Miller M, et al. Assessing health literacy practices in a community pharmacy environment: experiences using the AHRQ pharmacy health literacy assessment tool. *Res Social Adm Pharm.* 2013;9(5):564-596.

Abbreviations: HIPAA = Health Insurance Portability and Accountability Act; CAM = complementary and alternative medicine; CMS = Centers for Medicare & Medicaid Services; PML = personal medication list; MAP = medication action plan; AHRQ = Agency for Healthcare Research and Quality; CMR = comprehensive medication review; OTC = over the counter; ADR = adverse drug reaction.

business practice of the MTM provider and the preparedness of the patient, the CMR could be offered immediately instead of being scheduled for a future date.

Preparing the Patient

It is essential that patients know when the CMR appointment is scheduled. Providing reminder tools, such as a sticker for the calendar, and making reminder calls may be helpful in reducing missed appointments. Patients also need to be informed of what to bring to the appointment such as medications, physcians' names, and recent lab work if possible. It is important to ask whether a family member or caregiver should attend the CMR with the patient and to coordinate with these people as well. Having the patient complete any paperwork—HIPAA forms,

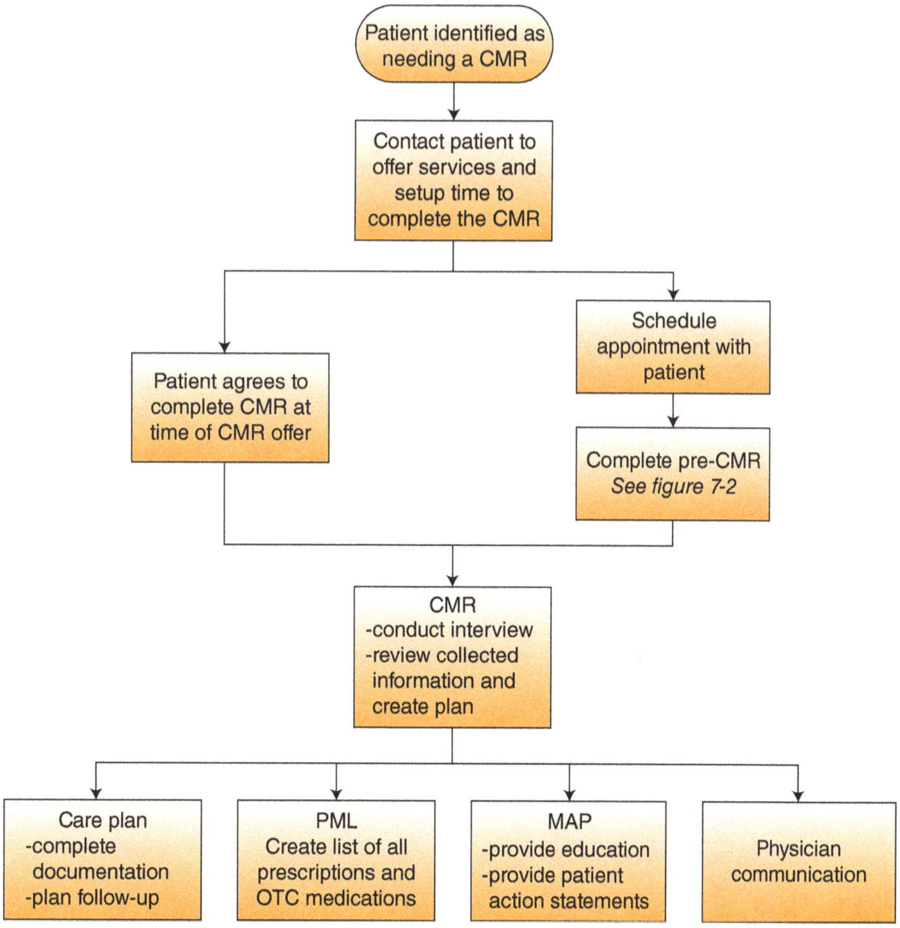

FIGURE 7-1 General flow of CMR process.

a complete initial medication record, and preliminary data form (including allergies, immunizations, smoking status, etc)—prior to the CMR can help save time. The patient should also be told what the CMR is, how and where it will be conducted, and a general idea of what to expect.

Preparing the Medication Therapy Management Pharmacist

MTM is performed in a variety of settings, which means that the amount and quality of information available to the MTM pharmacist prior to the CMR is also variable. Table 7-3 shows the challenges and benefits to preparation inherent in the various CMR settings. In addition to understanding the setting, MTM providers must prepare their own clinical knowledge. Pharmacists performing MTM can stay up-to-date on disease state guidelines through continuing education programs and by studying the various medication therapy databases. References such as the updated Beers Criteria, the Screening Tool of Older Person's Prescriptions (STOPP), and the Screening Tool to Alert doctors to Right Treatment (START) can be helpful in identifying specific issues for assessment and discussion during the CMR.[9-10] The University of Iowa has created *TIMER: Tool to Improve Medications in the Elderly via Review*, which may be helpful.[11] If a patient presents with a disease state that is unfamiliar to the MTM provider, he or she should take the time to research and prepare for the CMR encounter.

Understanding the goals of every entity involved in MTM can influence how the pharmacist prepares for the CMR, how the CMR is conducted, and how the workflow will be organized. The goals of CMS for all MTM programs are clear; CMRs are expected to:

- Be designed to ensure that covered Part D drugs prescribed to targeted beneficiaries are appropriately used to optimize therapeutic outcomes through improved medication use
- Be designed to reduce the risk of adverse events, including adverse drug interactions, for targeted beneficiaries
- Be furnished by a pharmacist or other qualified provider
- Distinguish between services in ambulatory and institutional settings
- Be developed in cooperation with licensed and practicing pharmacists and physicians[2]

TABLE 7-3 • Advantages and Disadvantages of Various CMR Settings

Situation	Advantages	Disadvantages
Access to full medical chart	Should provide: • More efficient and accurate CMR • Better identification of drug-related problems • Detection of prescriptions written but not filled • Detections of disease indications not being treated • More appropriate interventions • Physician practice patterns • Progress toward therapeutic goals	• One chart may not provide information from all providers • More data may require greater preparatory time • May lack prescription claims data and thus lack refill history
Claims data only	• Filled prescriptions documented • Refill patterns and PDC calculations	• Questionable accuracy of drug-inferred diagnoses • Is the data current and complete or only from one pharmacy? • Lack of administration directions
Patient-provided data only	• Establish a relationship • Face-to-face; read body language • Symptom report • Adverse drug reaction detected • Therapeutic goals assessment • Values communicated	• Accuracy and completeness may be an issue • Literacy and disease understanding • Imprecise terminology (eg, heart failure; is it systolic or diastolic?)

Via telephone	• CMR in the home where the majority of medications are
	• Potentially more privacy and controlled environment for both parties
	• Comfort with surroundings
	• Lack of visual cues that might inhibit conversation
	• Easier to ask embarrassing questions
	• Do not have to travel
		• No physical assessment
		• Lack visual cues to direct conversation
		• Visual assessment of device use (ie, inhaler)
		• Mobile phone
		  • Minute limitations
		  • Dropped calls
		  • Unsafe conditions (driving)
		  • Privacy concerns in a public setting
		• Risk of losing concentration on long calls
		• Tone of voice very important

Face-to-face	• Read body language • More customary form of interaction • Brown bag viable option • Inspect prescription bottle labels and contents	• Need private area • Visual appearance of either party may be off-putting • Travel; unless home visit

Payers have their own goals and objectives for CMR encounters. Payers are typically concerned with specific performance measures (eg, number of patients who do not adhere to chronic medications, number of patients who take high-risk medications; see Chapters 4 and 5 for more details). Additionally, employers may have specific productivity expectations for the MTM pharmacist. For example, the employer may require a certain number of CMRs to be completed each day. These productivity expectations may influence how much time can be allotted to the patient interview and administrative duties. Understanding the priorities and goals of all entities involved will help structure the CMR so that all these objectives can be accomplished.

The payment of MTM services will also influence how the CMR is conducted. Being paid a fee-for-service for the completion of a CMR versus getting paid per intervention can lead to two different business practices and affect the focus of the CMR. More information on reimbursement can be found in Chapter 10. These nonpatient factors can drive how the MTM session is performed and influence how the MTM pharmacist prepares for the CMR.

PERFORMING A PRELIMINARY COMPREHENSIVE MEDICATION REVIEW

In order to understand the patient's medical history, prescriptions, and disease states and to identify potential medication-related problems, the MTM provider should conduct a preliminary medication review prior to the interaction. Documenting potential issues before the CMR can help prepare the pharmacist for issues that are likely to arise during the patient interaction. Specific MTM software can assist the MTM provider by automatically identifying certain medication-related problems, such as drug-drug interactions and duplicate therapies. Figure 7-2 is a template for conducting pre-CMR, CMR, and post-CMR work. This template will be referenced throughout this text. Before beginning the pre-CMR, performance measures of the various entities involved should be considered. Table 7-4 presents many factors that can influence the focus of the CMR. Because the goals of all parties involved with the MTM service may affect the priorities of the CMR, they should be identified early in the pre-CMR process.

Gathering a Medication List

The patient's current medication use can be inferred by prescription data. Prescription claims data provides a good indication of what the patient may currently be taking and what he or she may not be taking.[12] Prescription information is available from pharmacy claims, medical records, and managed care records. This data allows the MTM provider to review medication use before speaking with the patient in order to identify possible drug-drug interactions, duplications of therapy, gaps in therapy, high-cost medications, combination possibilities, and high-risk drugs (if the patient is elderly).

Determining Disease States

The MTM provider should attempt to identify the patient's disease states prior to the CMR. Some software can report a patient's disease state information via International Classification of Diseases (ICD) diagnostic codes. This information may be directly available through electronic medical records. Some MTM software programs assimilate ICD information from outside sources for the MTM provider to review prior to the CMR. Should this specific information not be available, disease states can oftentimes be inferred from the patient's current medications. Some medications provide a clear indication of a patient's disease states, such as diabetes and hypercholesterolemia, while other disease states may be difficult to identify by medications alone—some medications can be used for multiple conditions, such as antidepressants and seizure medications.

Having lab values available during the pre-CMR process can be helpful in assessing the outcomes of the current disease state management program. If medication reviews are performed in a closed clinical or hospital setting where the MTM provider has full access to the patient's records, attaining current lab values prior to the CMR can be quite simple. However, not all CMRs are performed in an arena where there is full access to patient data. If this is the case, a quick call to the primary care provider may elicit the lab information needed. The patient may also know this information.

Identifying Healthcare Providers

It is also important to identify the patient's current healthcare providers prior to the CMR so that the MTM provider knows whom to contact if he or she finds medication-related problems. Compile a list of prescribers, including physicians, nurse practitioners, and physician assistants, identifying their specialties, addresses, phone numbers, and fax numbers. This will allow for efficient communication with a prescriber after the CMR is complete and can be helpful in identifying "doctor hopping."

Identifying Potential Medication-Related Problems

Next, the patient's data should be reviewed thoroughly to identify and document potential medication-related problems. A tool, such as that in Figure 7-2, can aid in the documentation of this pre-CMR assessment. The pre-CMR should encompass many aspects of the patient's medication use.

Medication adherence is an important factor that should be monitored in all patients, as nonadherence to drugs can causes unnecessary suffering and death. In the United States, adherence rates are estimated to be at 50%.[13] Adherence to oral diabetes, hypertension, and cholesterol medications are current quality measures used by CMS to assign Star Ratings to Part D prescription drug plans. Improving adherence rates in patients is a goal of these Part D payers, as these Star Ratings are tied to financial bonus payments to the plan. A percentage of days covered (PDC) calculation can help identify patient adherence for chronic medications. A PDC equal to or greater than 0.8% is often used as an indication of adherence, except for HIV medications for which 0.95% is the recommended adherence rate.[14,15] If a patient is not adhering to his or her medication, it is likely that the full benefit of the drug is not being realized. If a physician is unaware of an adherence problem, he or she may prescribe additional unnecessary therapy to further treat a still-unmanaged condition.

Indication-based medication problems should be analyzed: Is the medication therapy appropriate for the patient's disease states, as well as current guidelines and therapeutic goals? The MTM provider

Pre-CMR			
Potential concern		Details	Priority
Performance Measures			
• Payer			
• Employer			
Adherence/Nonadherence			
• Does not understand instructions			
• More cost effective medication available			
• Prefers not to take (does not perceive need or effectiveness, excess pill burden, complicated regimen)			
• Forgets to take			
• Medication product not available			
• Cannot swallow/administer medication			
• PDC calculations			
• Medications overused			
Indication/Therapeutic Goal			
Untreated Indication			
Needs Additional Therapy			
	Potential gap		
Diabetes	ACE inhibitor or ARB		
Diabetes	Statin		
Heart failure	ACE inhibitor or ARB		
Heart failure	BB (or HF appropriate BB)		
CAD	Statin		
CAD	BB		
CAD	SLNTG		
CAD	ASA/Antiplatelet		
Stroke	ASA/Antiplatelet		
A Fib	Anticoagulant		
Asthma/COPD	Controller		
Asthma/COPD	Rescue		
Osteoporosis	Bisphosphonate		
Osteoporosis	Calcium/Vitamin D		
Long-term steroid use	Bisphosphonate		
Preventative Medication Therapy Needed			
Lack of Immunization			
Unnecessary Medication Therapy			
• Duplicate therapies			
• No medical indication			
• Drugs treating avoidable adverse medication events			
• Addictive/recreational medication use			
Safety			
Adverse Medication Event			
• Drug-drug interaction			
• Drug-disease interactions			
• Drug-age interactions			
• Drug-food/alcohol interaction			
• Drug-pregnancy interaction			
• Allergic reaction			
• Undesirable effect (adverse reaction)			
• Unsafe medication for the patient			
• Incorrect administration			
• Dose increase/decrease too fast			

FIGURE 7-2 CMR template.

Dosage Too High		
• Dose too high		
• Frequency inappropriate		
• Duration inappropriate		
• Medication interaction (including renal dosing issue)		
Needs Additional Monitoring		
Effectiveness		
Ineffective Medication		
• More effective medication available		
• Condition refractory to medication		
• Dosage form inappropriate		
• Contraindication present		
• Medication not effective for condition		
Dosage Too Low		
• Dose too low		
• Frequency inappropriate		
• Duration inappropriate		
• Incorrect storage		
Incorrect Administration		
Needs Additional Monitoring		
CMR		
Identify Patient Concerns		
Collect Details on Confirmed and Newly Identified Concerns (above)		
Post-CMR		
Prioritize (above) Identified Concerns Based on:		
• Performance measures		
• Patient expectations		
• Seriousness of concern		
Determine Plan for Patient Take-Away (Medication Action Plan)		
Determine Concerns to Communicate to Prescriber(s)		

CMR = comprehensive medication review; PDC = percentage of days covered; ACE inhibitor = angiotensin-converting enzyme inhibitor; ARB = angiotensin II receptor blocker; BB = beta blocker; HF = heart failure; CAD = coronary artery disease; SLNTG = sublingual nitroglycerin; ASA = aspirin; A Fib = atrial fibrillation; COPD = chronic obstructive pulmonary disease

FIGURE 7-2 *(Continued)*

should document potential untreated conditions, lack of recommended therapies, lack of immunizations, and unnecessary therapies. For example, a patient may have both diabetes and hypertension and not have a prescription for an angiotensin-converting enzyme (ACE) inhibitor or angiotensin receptor blocker (ARB), as recommended by current guidelines. It would be important to note this on the pre-CMR and assess the reason for the lack of therapy during the interaction.

Safety of current medications should be noted prior to the CMR. Inappropriate medication use may lead to patient harm. For example, the medications can be analyzed for drug-drug interactions, excessive dosages, etc. Discussion with the patient during the CMR will provide further information as to whether there are any clinically relevant safety issues.

The effectiveness of the current drug regimen should be documented during the pre-CMR process in order to assess it further during the CMR. An MTM pharmacist can access the refill history of medications, which is helpful. Current dosing frequency can be noted; refill history can provide information about how often a patient uses "as needed" medications. Prescribers write prescriptions, but they may not have contact with the patient for many months, and the CMR can facilitate the identification and communication of this important information.

If possible, collect information from previous drug and medical histories, along with prior medication reviews as well. These reports could provide helpful information regarding past failed therapies and will allow for more accurate recommendations for any interventions noted during the CMR.

Assessing the global picture of the patient prior to the CMR will help the MTM provider know what to expect. Knowing what questions to ask to assess each condition is vital. The disease-specific

TABLE 7-4 • Factors That Can Affect the Choices Made During a CMR

Entity	Considerations

Patient	• Life goals
	• Therapeutic goals
	• Financial goals
	• Quality of life goals
	• Definition of quality care
	• Social support
	• Respect for personal values and needs
	• Perception of:
	  • Value of care
	  • Risk
	  • Reward
	• Healthcare beliefs
	• Socioeconomic status
	• Cultural expectations
	• Healthcare literacy
	• Involved in care and decision-making to the level they desire
	• Trust in system and providers
	• What the illness means to them

Payers	• How they make money
	• Competition
	• Members
	  • Age
	  • Medicare
	  • Dual eligible
	  • Medicaid
	  • Ethnic and racial composition
	  • Socioeconomic status
	  • Education levels
	  • Disease prevalence
	  • Multiple chronic conditions
	• MTM selection criteria
	  • Disease selection
	  • Drug selection
	  • Cost
	• MTM performance measures
	• ROI expectations
	• Quality bonus payments
	• Star Ratings; current and goal
	• Member retention and satisfaction
	• Detection of fraud, waste, and abuse
	• Business plan and performance measures
	• Other care programs (ie, disease management, case management)
	• Payer type: employer, self-insured, MA plan, MA-PD plan, PDP, MCO, SNPs
	• Geographical variation in care

Family/caregiver	• Role of family in making therapeutic decisions • Effect of disease states on family/caregivers • Therapeutic benefits/harms on family and caregivers

Prescriber	• Prescriber qualifications/expertise
	  • Specialty
	  • Professional designation (eg, MD, ARNP, DO, etc)
	• Practice model
	  • PCMH
	  • Fee for service
	  • Bundled payment
	  • ACO
	  • Capitated/bundled payments
	• Practice/prescribing patterns
	• MTM knowledge/awareness/opinions
	• Prescriber-pharmacist relationship
	• Prescriber's pharmacy views
	• Communication preferences

Individual conducting CMR	• Professional standards • Pharmacotherapy expertise • Time • Technology • MTM experience • Practice site experience • Team work • Performance measures and feedback

Employer expectations	• MTM
	  • Business goals
	  • Priority in relation to overall business
	  • Performance measures
	• Employee overall productivity measures

Abbreviations: ACO = accountable care organization; ARNP = advanced registered nurse practitioner; DO = doctor of osteopathic medicine; MD = doctor of medicine; MTM = medication therapy management; MA = Medicare Advantage plan; MA-PD = Medicare Advantage-Prescription Drug plan; MCO = managed care organization; PCMH = patient-centered medical home; PDP = prescription drug plan; ROI = return on investment; SNP = special needs plan.

Minimum Data Set chapters within this publication can assist in preparing the proper words and disease-specific questions to ask during the CMR. At times, a CMR session may go in a direction that was not clear at the pre-CMR stage—expecting the unexpected can be a challenge. For example, prior to the call, it may appear that the patient is overusing a rescue inhaler; the focus at the outset of the CMR may be improving the patient's asthma control. The MTM provider may be fully prepared with questions and counseling tips for asthma, but upon speaking with the member, it becomes immediately clear that he is overwhelmed with depression because his spouse has recently died. Depression will now become the primary focus of the session. Being prepared for the expected and adapting to the unexpected are crucial for successfully conducting CMRs with patients.

CONDUCTING THE COMPREHENSIVE MEDICATION REVIEW

Objectives and Time Management

Time management and efficiency are concerns when completing the CMR; the MTM provider must be concise, thorough, and caring. Meeting the objectives of the payer and the employer, while still assessing the issues identified during the pre-CMR assessment, can be a challenge. The patient's goals will also need to be addressed. The MTM provider must ensure that the required activities are completed while still showing care and concern for the patient and his or her needs. The core of the CMR is the patient; the primary focus of the CMR should be the patient's concerns regarding his or her conditions and medications. If the patient's concerns are not addressed, he or she may not be receptive to the MTM provider's interventions. Acknowledging the patient's concerns can help establish rapport and respect during the CMR.

The aim of the patient interview, the CMR, is to gain direct information from the patient that will allow for clear identification and assessment of medication-related problems to help the MTM provider make recommendations to others on the patient's health-care team for improving the health and well-being of the patient.

Informed Consent

At the beginning of a CMR, MTM providers should introduce themselves, their job titles, and their roles in collecting patient information. A brief description of the reason for the interview and how it will be conducted should be provided to the patient. Once the patient understands the method and rationale of the CMR, the patient's identity should be verified via date of birth, mailing address, and unique identification numbers. It is important to be sure that all documentation is consistent with HIPAA regulations and that the patient is informed of such protection as well as any type of information recording. Once the patient consents and understands how the information will be used, recorded, documented, and protected, the interviewer may proceed to collect data. This is also the time for the MTM provider to set expectations for the patient or the person completing the CMR on the patient's behalf. It can be explained that once the medication list is obtained, other questions about clinical status, lifestyle, and side effects may be asked. This information will be assessed to determine an action plan to increase the patient's understanding of drug therapy, help manage disease states, and improve the patient's overall health.

Documenting Medication Usage

When obtaining the medication list, the MTM provider should confirm the medication strength, time(s) of day it is taken, dosage form, indication, and prescriber. Medication usage should be collected for all prescription medications (including samples and free or no-cost prescriptions), all OTCs (including vitamins, herbals, and supplements), and all other items used to support the patient's health. This information will be compiled into a PML to be given to the patient after the CMR. Depending on the payer, there may be specific formatting requirements for documenting the medications in the PML. For example, for Medicare Part D MTM members, there is a very specific standardized format for the PML.[3] Most medications are given in a consistent dosing pattern and are simple to document. Table 7-5 provides a list of medications that have frequent dosage changes and provides suggestions on how to document these.

TABLE 7-5 • Drugs With Frequent Dose Changes

Medication	Reason for Changes	Suggestions/Examples for Directions in PML
Coumadin (warfarin)	INR results	Take 1 tablet (__ mg) by mouth on Monday, Wednesday, and Friday. Take one-half tablet (__ mg) on Tuesday, Thursday, Saturday, and Sunday. Dose may change based on INR.
Insulin	Sliding scale adjustments	Inject under the skin per sliding scale for blood sugar levels above __ mg/dL.
	Adjustments to basal insulin when blood glucose is too low	Inject __ units under the skin at bedtime. Hold if blood sugar is less than 70 mg/dL.
Prednisone	Maintenance versus flares	Take 1 tablet (__ mg) by mouth once daily. Dose may change during asthma flares.
	Tapers	Take as directed on package, tapering down as instructed.
Blood pressure medications	Low blood pressure readings	Take 1 tablet (__ mg) by mouth every morning. Hold dose if systolic blood pressure (top number) is less than 90 mm Hg.
Colcrys (colchicine)	Maintenance versus flares	Take 1 tablet (0.6 mg) by mouth once daily. May take 2 tablets (1.2 mg) by mouth at first sign of gout flare, then wait at least 12 hours before starting regular daily dose again.
Nebulizer solutions (such as DuoNeb)	Maintenance versus acute exacerbation	Inhale contents of 1 vial using nebulizer twice daily. Inhale contents of 1 vial using nebulizer every 4-6 hours as needed for shortness of breath.
Medications initiated with a taper	Doses fluctuate over time	Provide complete dosing taper, or if too complex, include current dosing and add "continue adjusting dose as directed by your doctor."

Abbreviation: INR = international normalized ratio.

Using open-ended questions can help assess a patient's understanding of medications. Gaps in the patient's knowledge are opportunities for counseling and patient education. The medication listing is also a great platform for assessing potential medication-related problems noted during the pre-CMR process. Creating a workflow that addresses disease state concerns while assessing the medications involved can aid in conciseness and efficiency, as well as create an organized environment conducive to open dialogue.

Collecting Health-Related Details: The Comprehensive Medication Review Template

The medication list can be created in tandem with the CMR template (see Figure 7-2). MTM software can also help in the collection of medication data. Collecting medication information typically results in other aspects of a patient's health status being communicated. This is an opportune time to collect and document additional information offered by the patient, including disease states; surgeries or procedures; the need or use of pacemakers, pain pumps, intravenous supplies, syringes, insulin pumps, and defibrillators; mobility issues; use of durable medical equipment [oxygen, wheelchairs, canes, Continuous Positive Airway Pressure (CPAP)]; and the social and economic support systems that may or may not be available to the patient.

Additional information that can be obtained during a CMR may include clinical aspects of care, such as whether the patient performs home monitoring of blood pressure or glucose. If so, the patient may be able to provide specific values or state whether the conditions are stable. Documentation, including details and information from the patient regarding potential issues, can be made during the CMR with the assessment template.

Adherence

Adherence problems should be noted during the CMR, and barriers—such as cost, transportation challenges, forgetfulness, difficulty or complexity of medication regimen, and lack of knowledge or lack of belief in the importance/effectiveness of therapy—should be assessed. Medications that appear to be overused should also be noted and evaluated.

Indications and Therapeutic Goals

In order to assess any indication-related issues noted in the pre-CMR, the MTM pharmacist can ask about previous drug usage. For example, if a gap in therapy was noted for a patient with hypertension and diabetes who lacks a current prescription for an ACE inhibitor or ARB, the pharmacist could ask the patient if he or she has ever used a medication "such as lisinopril or Diovan." The MTM pharmacist could also inquire about disease states or conditions that would explain the lack of therapy. For example, the patient may have severe renal insufficiency, a contraindication for ACE inhibitors and ARBs.

During the CMR, untreated indications may be noted and should be communicated afterward to the patient's care team. Additionally, medications lacking a clear indication should be analyzed. An example would be a patient taking omeprazole that was prescribed as prophylaxis while in the hospital who continues the medication with no indication of gastric reflux or esophagitis.

An MTM pharmacist can also be an advocate to patients when there are indications requiring specific immunizations. During the CMR, the patient can be educated about the value of immunizations, and the pharmacist can either provide the immunization immediately as part of the MTM service or can advocate to the doctor.

Lifestyle

Lifestyle issues can affect and be affected by indications as well as disease states. Identifying any special diets that the patient is following is an important component of a CMR. This information will allow the MTM provider to provide dietary counseling and to reinforce as well as congratulate the patient for adhering to diet recommendations. The patient's ability or willingness to exercise should also be assessed as well as whether mobility or physical condition limits daily activities, such as getting to and from appointments or the pharmacy. Documenting and assessing tobacco and illicit drug use (for medical or recreational purposes) is important as well.

Safety

MTM providers should inquire about adverse drug effects, any symptoms that can be attributed to drug–drug, drug–disease, or drug–food interactions, and any signs of dosing problems (eg, excessive dosing, incorrect administration). Any severe medication safety problems should be communicated immediately to the prescriber.

Effectiveness

The CMR should assess the patient's perceptions on whether the medication regimen is effective and should include clinical observations that may indicate the need for improved efficacy. During the CMR, the patient may say that certain disease states are not being treated to his or her satisfaction. For example, the patient may say that nerve pain continues despite treatment with low dose of gabapentin. Or the patient may merely share self-measured biometric values (eg, fasting blood glucose) that indicate more effective treatment is needed.

Concluding the Comprehensive Medication Review

Every patient interaction is unique. Situations may arise during the CMR that call for special attention or lead to the early conclusion of the CMR. Circumstances may arise in which the patient must be referred immediately to another provider, transferred to a crisis line, or rescheduled for a CMR at another time. Table 7-6 lists various scenarios that can occur during a CMR and includes suggestions for remedying those situations.

At the end of the review, the patient should be offered a chance to express additional questions or concerns. Once the medication review is completed, it is important to summarize the information with the patient or caregiver. The MTM provider should encourage the patient's continued relationship with local pharmacists and physicians for continuity of care. The patient should be referred to outside resources (including financial support, social services, and crisis counselors) for any needs that have come up during the CMR, and follow-up appointments should be discussed. The MTM pharmacist can provide a PML and MAP at the conclusion of the CMR. If these cannot be provided immediately, the provider should give the patient a timeframe for their delivery.

TABLE 7-6 • Situations Requiring Special Attention During a CMR

Scenario	Action
Patient does not speak English (see Chapter 8, Oral and Nonverbal Communication in MTM)	• Enlist a family member who understands medical and pharmacy terms • Use a translator or a telephonic medical translator service • Consider whether MAP and PML need to be in English, for providers, or the patient's spoken language
Patient is deaf or hard of hearing (see Chapter 8, Oral and Nonverbal Communication in MTM)	• Ask if the patient has a signing relative who can help with the CMR • Address privacy issues for "loud" conversations • Take extra care to avoid miscommunication due to hearing deficiencies • Keep facing patient to facilitate lip reading • Adjust phone volume • Utilize Telecommunications Device for the Deaf Service • Obtain permission to speak with member's caregiver or relative

Patient has medically related crisis during the CMR	• Pre-CMR may provide information on those patients who are predisposed to crisis (ie, COPD, Angina, etc)
	• Immediately call 911 and assist as well as provide medical attention until emergency services arrive
	• Patient out of 911 area: It is not possible to dial out-of-area 911 numbers. If possible:
	  • Keep patient on the phone; ascertain crisis situation
	  • Find out if there is another person with the patient or nearby
	  • Contact patient's local law enforcement agency
	  • Stay on the phone until help arrives and to provide assistance

Patient expresses suicidal ideation, thoughts, or plans	• Identify family member or friend who can provide immediate support and monitoring • If no one else is available, contact a local suicide crisis line for immediate assistance; directly transfer the call if speaking with patient on the phone: • 1-800-273-8255 is the nationwide hotline • If patient is not currently having suicidal thoughts, but has in the past, provide the crisis hotline number in the MAP for future reference • Notify physician

Patient needs financial or benefits assistance	• Do an internet search to identify:
	  • Social Security Office's contact information for patient to apply for low-income subsidy
	  • State and local financial assistance programs www.needymeds.org/state_programs.taf
	  • Coupons for specific expensive medications
	  • Use www.medicare.gov to select best PDP or MA-PD plan

Patient requests using email for CMR or transmission of PML and MAP (see Chapter 9, Documentation, for further detail)	• Email policy must address:
	  • Access control
	  • Audit controls
	  • Authentication
	  • Transmission security
	• Have patient sign informed consent regarding the use of email
	• Establish the guidelines for email use:
	  • Content
	  • Appropriate subject manner
	  • Response time expectations
	  • Privacy expectation

Long-term care resident[a]	• Drug regimen review does not replace the CMR
	• Must provide CMR, PML, and MAP
	• Must be interactive with beneficiary unless cognitively compromised
	  • Physical and cognitive impairment may require using surrogate or LTC provider
	  • Enlisting the LTC consultant pharmacist may be beneficial
	  • The nursing staff may be a good resource of information (cognitive status, caregiver, and medications)
	• Coordinate and integrate with the LTC healthcare providers and care plan
	• Adherence is less an issue in this environment
	• Focus on overuse, medications without a clear indication, suboptimal dosing, and polypharmacy
	• Align medication use to the beneficiary's goals and wishes in addition to the care team's

(*Continued*)

TABLE 7-6 • Situations Requiring Special Attention During a CMR (*Continued*)

Scenario	Action
Patient misses CMRs because of convenience issues or erratic schedule	• Schedule CMR when medication refills are due • Synchronizing all medication refills may be helpful to the patient • Make reminder calls • Probe for privacy or embarrassment concerns; use telephone if preferred • Identify if convenience issues can be remedied by a telephonic review (be mindful of cell phone minutes)
Patient refuses to share all or part of gathered information with physician	• Attempt to explain the importance of creating and maintaining a complete health record
Determining when to contact physician directly, rather than fax or email	• Serious ADR detected • Suicidal ideation or plan • Opioid abuse • Evidence of fraud, waste, and abuse • Addiction admission • Obvious deterioration in physical, mental, or behavioral symptoms • Recommended patient seek immediate medical assistance • Physical or psychological abuse • 911 called/emergency care

[a] CMS. CY 2014 Medication therapy management program guidance and submission instructions [memorandum]. April 5, 2013. Available at http://www.cms.gov/Medicare/Prescription-Drug-Coverage/PrescriptionDrugCovContra/Downloads/Memo-Contract-Year-2014-Medication-Therapy-Management-MTM-Program-Submission-v040513.pdf. Accessed April 17, 2013.

Abbreviations: ADR = adverse drug reaction; CMR = comprehensive medication review; LTC = long-term care; MAP = medication action plan; MA-PD = Medicare Advantage-Prescription Drug plan; PDP = prescription drug plan; PML = personal medication list.

AFTER THE COMPREHENSIVE MEDICATION REVIEW: CARE PLAN

Without documentation, there will not be a complete record of the patient interaction and rationalization for the decision-making processes. Thorough documentation allows for continuity of care and is usually required for obtaining reimbursement. After concluding the patient interview, any identified medication-related issues should be documented. When documenting the assessment of the patient, objective language should be used (eg, "the patient reported that he lives a very sedentary lifestyle, spending much of the day on the couch watching television" rather than "the patient seemed lazy"), and judgmental words should be avoided in describing the patient or medication.[16] There are many techniques for documentation; the Subjective, Objective, Assessment, and Plan (SOAP) format is one example. Specific MTM software may present unique methods of documentation.

During the CMR, some medication-related issues identified during the pre-CMR stage will likely be nullified. Other medication-related problems may have been clarified as being clinically significant, and newly discovered medication-related issues may become evident. The remaining clinically relevant medication-related issues should be prioritized, and the MTM provider should determine which require immediate action and which can be deferred until the next follow-up with the patient (see Figure 7-2, far right column). In addition, it must be determined which medication-related issues need to be brought to the attention of the physician and which could be resolved with the patient through the MAP. If there are issues that need to be addressed with the prescriber, the pharmacist should determine whether the issue requires an immediate call to the pharmacy or prescriber or if the issue is nonurgent and can be communicated via fax, email, or letter. Once the issues have been prioritized and the method of intervention identified, it is time to document the plan of action and follow-up for each of these issues in the care plan.

PERSONAL MEDICATION LIST

The PML should contain all prescription medications, OTCs, and medical supplies. Information that should be included for each item on the PML is as follows: medication name, dose of medication, indication, prescriber name, directions for use, and special instructions.

If the patient is unaware of the indication for any medication, the provider should make every effort to determine the condition being treated in order to maintain the accuracy of the PML. The patient can be told about the common indications for the medication and asked if he or she has a history of those conditions. If this technique does not help, the MTM pharmacist should call the physician's office to obtain the correct indication. The provider can also include a note in the PML stating, "Please speak with your doctor about why you are taking this medication." Patient-directed statements may remind patients to educate themselves on why they are using medications.

The directions for the medications on the PML should follow the same format as that ordered by the prescriber—which may be different from what the patient says. For example, a patient may say that he or she takes the medication every other day to offset expense; the directions should still be consistent with how the prescriber wrote the prescription, and the nonadherence issue should be communicated to the prescriber. There are some medications whose dosing can change frequently based on lab values or during acute flares, which may cause the information in the PML to be incorrect at times. To prevent confusion regarding these medications on the

PML, specific dosing information can be included (see Table 7-5). Other information that may be included in the PML can include date of birth, phone number, emergency contact information, primary care physician and contact information, pharmacy name and contact information, and allergies.[1]

MEDICATION ACTION PLAN

The MAP is the patient's guide regarding any potential medication-related problems, disease-related problems, or general counseling provided by the MTM provider during the CMR encounter. During the interview, disease states may have been discussed and future health goals set; it is important that the goals are ones that the patient can realistically attain on his or her own. The MAP should only include information and goals that are within the pharmacist's scope of practice, not issues that require prescriber approval or guidance.[1] Based on the CMS guidelines, a MAP created for a Medicare Part D member should include action items that were discussed with the member, and it is recommended to limit the length to two pages. The most important counseling points should be prioritized, and this counseling can take place as early as the patient interview. Such knowledge can allow the MTM pharmacist to focus the CMR on the areas of most importance and reserve less critical issues for future encounters.

Refer to Chapter 9 (Documentation) regarding the additional CMS requirements for the MAP and PML. The MAP and PML should be checked for word choice, spelling, and grammar to ensure that the information is clear and useful for the patient. It is important that the information be at an appropriate reading level for the patient, yet currently, there are no specific rules regarding which reading level is most appropriate. The average reading level in the United States is estimated to be at eighth grade. The standard of practice is to write medical information at a fourth- or fifth-grade reading level.[17] If the patient speaks a language besides English, it is important that the information is in the native language, if possible.

PRESCRIBER COMMUNICATION

Prescriber communication can take place in many formats. The MTM pharmacist should determine whether an issue is urgent and requires a phone call, or nonurgent and able to be handled via fax, email, or letter. Situations that may require immediate communication with the prescriber can include a patient who has excessive bleeding from warfarin or a severe drug interaction. Other issues may be appropriately communicated by a letter or fax. These may include a patient who is missing a recommended medication for a particular disease state (eg, heart failure without a beta blocker), a patient who is taking a medication that is cautioned/contraindicated with a disease state (eg, nondihydropyridine calcium channel blocker in a patient with heart failure), or a potential cost-saving opportunity that has been identified. Refer to Chapter 8 for information on telephone communication with prescribers and to Chapter 9 regarding physician communication.

When communicating with a physician, it is important to be concise yet thorough. Enough detail about the issue should be provided (including a clear definition of the problem, patient symptoms as well as complaints, and documented references), and yet it should be concise enough that the doctor can review the information within the course of a busy workday. Providing the prescriber with specific suggestions can assist the physician in acting quickly to remedy the issue. For example, providing the specific formulary alternative for a nonformulary drug will save the patient and the prescriber the time as well as frustration of trial and error. Another example is providing a specific generic drug recommendation in the appropriate strength as an alternative to expensive brand medication. Communication with the prescriber should never be condescending or accusatory. Having a respectful, collaborative attitude with a prescriber will help build rapport and respect. This can lead to more collaborative relationships in the future.

FOLLOW-UP

The final component of the CMR is follow-up. The time between follow-ups may vary depending on the patient population and the severity of medication-related issues. For Medicare Part D patients, follow-ups are required at least quarterly.[3] The follow-up may include a phone call, personal interview, or at minimum, a review of the patient's current health record and prescription refill history (if available). In the care plan for the CMR, actions were determined for pertinent medication-related issues; at follow-up these should be reviewed and reassessed for resolution or further action. New medication-related problems arising from newly added or discontinued medications may also be identified; the MTM pharmacist should document these and take appropriate action. Refer to Chapter 9 for further guidance regarding documentation of follow-ups to CMRs.

CONCLUSION

The CMR is the core of the MTM process; all other factors of MTM center around, or depend upon, patient interactions. A CMR should be focused on gleaning important details from the patient to confirm or alleviate potential medication-related issues and communicating this important information to the patient's healthcare team. The patient should be empowered to engage in his or her own healthcare and well-being.

The comprehensiveness of the patient-centered CMR makes the practice of MTM unique and adds another layer of support to the patient's overall healthcare. This comprehensiveness requires time and attention. The MTM provider must strike a balance between making the CMR patient-focused and comprehensive, while addressing the requirements as well as goals of the payer and the MTM provider's employer. Having a clearly defined process can help the provider accomplish the CMR in an effective and efficient manner.

REFERENCES

1. American Pharmacists Association; National Association of Chain Drug Stores Foundation. Medication therapy management in pharmacy practice: core elements of an MTM service model (version 2.0). *J Am Pharm Assoc (2003)*. 2008;48(3):341-353.

2. CMS. CY 2017 Medication Therapy Management program guidance and submission instructions [memorandum]. April 8, 2016. Available at https://www.cms.gov/Medicare/Prescription-Drug-Coverage/PrescriptionDrugCovContra/Downloads/Memo-Contract-Year-2017-Medication-Therapy-Management-MTM-Program-Submission-v-040816.pdf. Accessed August 4, 2016.

3. CMS. MTM Program standardized format revisions (v07.15.14) [ZIP file]. Medication Therapy Management Program standardized format—English form CMS-10396 (07/14). Available at https://www.cms.gov/Medicare/Prescription-Drug-Coverage/PrescriptionDrugCovContra/MTM.html. Accessed August 4, 2016.
4. Cornish P, Knowles S, Marchesano R, et al. Unintended medication discrepancies at the time of hospital admission. *Arch Intern Med*. 2005;165(4): 424-429.
5. Hardin H, Hall A, Roane T, et al. An advanced pharmacy practice experience in a student-staffed medication therapy management call center. *Am J Pharm Educ*. 2012;76(6):110.
6. Tarn D, Paterniti D, Kravitz R, et al. How do physicians conduct medication reviews? *J Gen Intern Med*. 2009;24(12):1296-1302.
7. Fitz Gerald R. Medication errors: the importance of an accurate drug history. *Br J Clin Pharmacol*. 2009;67(6):671-675.
8. Wang P, Benner J, Glynn R, et al. How well do patients report noncompliance with antihypertensive medications? A comparison of self-report versus filled prescriptions. *Pharmacoepidemiol and Drug Saf*. 2004;13(1):11-19.
9. Fick D, Cooper J, Wate W, et al. Updating the Beers criteria for potentially inappropriate medication use in older adults: results of a US consensus panel of experts. *Arch Intern Med*. 2003;163(22):2716-2724.
10. Gallagher P, Ryan C, Byrne S, et al. STOPP (screening tool of older person's prescriptions) and START (screening tool to alert doctors to right treatment). Consensus validation. *Int J Clin Pharmacol Ther*. 2008;46(2):72-83.
11. Lee S, Schwemm A, Reist J, et al. Pharmacists' and pharmacy students' ability to identify drug-related problems using TIMER (tool to improve medications in the elderly via review). *Am J Pharm Educ*. 2009;73(3):52.
12. Caskie G, Willis S. Congruence of self-reported medications with pharmacy prescription records in low-income older adults. *Gerontologist*. 2004;44(2):176-185.
13. Haynes R, McDonald HP, Garg AX. Helping patients follow prescribed treatment: clinical applications. *JAMA*. 2002;288(22):2880-2883.
14. Pharmacy Quality Alliance. PQA measures used by CMS in the Star Ratings. Update on Medication Quality Measures in Medicare Part D Plan Star Ratings—2016. Available at http://pqaalliance.org/measures/cms.asp. Accessed September 2, 2016.
15. Gross R, Yip B, Lo Re V 3rd, et al. A simple, dynamic measure of antiretroviral therapy adherence predicts failure to maintain HIV-1 suppression. *J Infect Dis*. 2006;194(8):1108-1114. Epub 2006 Sep 12.
16. American Pharmacists Association. Medication therapy management services: documenting pharmacy-based patient care services. July 30, 2012. Available at http://www.pharmacist.com/sites/default/files/files/mtm_services_documenting_pharm_based_pcs_CPE.pdf. Accessed September 2, 2016.
17. U.S. Department of Health and Human Services Food and Drug Administration Center for Drug Evaluation and Research (CDER). Guidance for industry label comprehension studies for nonprescription drug products. August 2010. Available at http://www.fda.gov/downloads/Drugs/GuidanceComplianceRegulatoryInformation/Guidances/UCM143834.pdf. Accessed September 2, 2016.

Review Questions

1. All of the following statements are true regarding the CMR EXCEPT
   a. CMRs can be performed in various settings.
   b. CMRs are only effective if provided face-to-face.
   c. Pharmacists performing CMRs should assess prescription medications, OTC medications, herbals and vitamins, and any other products used by the patient for their health.
   d. The medication list produced after a CMR can be communicated with the patient and the prescriber in order to help with the coordination of care.
   e. CMRs involve direct patient interaction.

2. Which of the following may contribute to inaccuracies and discrepancies in medication use information?
   a. Mental issues or cognitive impairment.
   b. Language barriers.
   c. Low health literacy.
   d. Vision problems.
   e. All of the above.

3. Which information is important to keep in mind when preparing the patient for the CMR?
   a. Reminding the patient to bring in any lab results to the CMR appointment can save time and help the pharmacist make more sound clinical judgements during the review.
   b. The CMR should always be scheduled during a time that is most convenient for the pharmacist.
   c. Reminders are not recommended to assist the patient in attending their CMR appointment.
   d. The pharmacist should not inform patients of what to expect during the CMR, as it will only lead to them having unrealistic expectations.
   e. In order to protect the patient's privacy, caregivers should not be included in the CMR interview.

4. When preparing for the CMR, the pharmacist could benefit from gathering
   a. the patient's diseases states, either from medical/pharmacy records or inferred from drug listings.
   b. the patient's medication list from claims data or other medical databases.
   c. a listing of all of the patient's healthcare providers.
   d. a list of potential medication therapy problems that may need assessing during the CMR.
   e. all of the above.

5. Many entities have goals and objectives for the CMR. Which statement is LEAST accurate?
   a. CMS hopes that CMRs ensure that covered Part D medications prescribed to targeted beneficiaries are appropriately used to optimize therapeutic outcomes through improved medication use.
   b. Payers (health plans) expect that CMRs will help them increase their profit margin.
   c. Employers of the MTM pharmacist set goals for productivity and aim for efficiencies in providing the CMR.
   d. All of the above are true.
   e. None of the above are true.

6. A pharmacist is managing an MTM business and is training new pharmacists on documentation. What information is important to convey to them?
   a. Documentation is required for payment of MTM services.
   b. MTM software exists that makes documentation efficient.
   c. SOAP notes are sometimes used to document CMRs.
   d. Pharmacists should be explicit in subjective notes, for example: "Mrs. Smith seemed a little crazy."
   e. Documentation of the CMR helps show the pharmacist's rationale for clinical decision-making.

7. Which statement is TRUE regarding the PML?
   a. The PML for Medicare patients has to conform to specific formatting requirements.
   b. The PML should contain all prescription medications, OTC medications, vitamins, herbals, and supplements.
   c. The PML is created as a document for the patient.
   d. All of the above are true.
   e. None of the above are true.

8. A managing pharmacist is explaining the MAP to new pharmacists. The managing pharmacist explains that
   a. the MAP is created to empower the patient to impact his or her own health and well-being.
   b. the MAP will be sent over to the physician.
   c. the MAP gives the patient driving directions to the pharmacy.
   d. the MAP is a listing of all of the patient's medications.
   e. the MAP is a bill for the MTM services.

9. Communication to physicians should be all of the following EXCEPT
   a. informative.
   b. suggestive.
   c. condescending.
   d. respectful.
   e. concise.

10. At the follow-up for the CMR, a medication therapy problem is noted that was not addressed by the pharmacist at the CMR. What is the MOST LIKELY reason for this?
   a. The MTM pharmacist did not adequately perform the CMR.
   b. Another pharmacist went into the patient's profile after the CMR and deleted the intervention.
   c. The problem is from a new drug that was started in between the CMR and the follow-up and was not visible to the MTM pharmacist; it should now be assessed.
   d. The physician that needs to be contacted for this problem never accepts pharmacists' interventions anyway, so the CMR pharmacist decided not to address the issue.
   e. The MTM software is faulty.

ANSWERS

1. b	2. e	3. a
4. e	5. b	6. d
7. d	8. a	9. c
10. c		

8

Oral and Nonverbal Communication in Medication Therapy Management

Carol J. Hermansen-Kobulnicky, PhD, RPh

KEY POINTS

- Good communication is a key requirement of patient-centered care that addresses patients' needs and wants.
- Nonverbal communication contributes to how individuals understand each other, especially when feelings are expressed.
- Each mode of communication, eg, in-person, telephone, and telehealth, have unique communication requirements.
- Building rapport with patients is critical for helping them feel comfortable with medication therapy management (MTM) services and providers.
- Asking patients both open-ended and closed-ended questions helps elicit the information needed to understand their perspectives and conditions.
- To listen well, the listener must be engaged, noticing nuances of what is said, observing and attending to nonverbal cues, and providing useful responses to the speaker.
- Choosing to listen to patients in order to understand them and then communicating that understanding back to them is patient-centered.
- Empathic responding explicitly acknowledges the emotional aspect of what has been said and the reason for such emotion.
- A service script can be a very useful tool for any pharmacy service activity requiring standardization for quality assurance purposes.
- When you are personally selling your MTM service, believing in the service and being confident are key.
- The way in which an interview or consultation is organized can be improved by using transitions, orientation, cues, and summarizing.
- According to a 2003 nationwide study (the National Assessment of Adult Literacy), only 12% of the over 19 000 adults surveyed were found to be "proficient" in health literacy, and only 3% of those 65 years and older demonstrated proficiency.
- Motivational interviewing (MI) is a communication technique and philosophy of helping individuals with behavioral change.
- Screening, Brief Intervention, and Referral to Treatment (SBIRT) is a successful technique for addressing alcohol and other substance use with patients. SBIRT stands for screening, brief intervention, and referral to treatment.
- Working effectively with people who have lower incomes and who experience generational poverty takes a deep appreciation for, and knowledge of, the characteristics of this group as well as those who experience situational poverty and members of the middle class.
- The mnemonic Situation, Background, Assessment, Recommendation (SBAR) is a useful framework when speaking with prescribers. It stands for situation, background, assessment, and recommendation.
- Developing a working collaborative relationship with a physician is a multistage process.

INTRODUCTION

Good communication is important for patient-centered care that addresses patients' needs and wants.[1] A whitepaper by the Joint Commission Public Policy Initiative presents a call to action to improve patient-professional communication and cites patient safety concerns as well as the need to communicate effectively with patients and to improve health outcomes across the continuum of care.[2] Taking time to reflect on and improve personal communication skills as part of the medication therapy management (MTM) program can help providers deliver the highest level of patient-centered care. This chapter gives an overview of how to effectively and efficiently communicate when providing MTM services, including data gathering, discussion, and responding to difficult situations; it is not intended to substitute for active, hands-on learning.

The material in this chapter is primarily geared toward helping pharmacists communicate effectively with patients; however, it also includes topics relevant for pharmacy technicians and other pharmacy employees who work with patients, as well as the topic of pharmacist-physician communication. First, general communication topics of nonverbal communication, building rapport, question asking and listening are presented. Next, nuances of three key communication opportunities within MTM are discussed: information gathering, patient education, and discussion to promote behavioral change. Insights are included regarding differences to consider when communicating in-person, via telephone, and face-to-face over the internet (also known as online video). The chapter concludes with information on how to effectively communicate with patients about sensitive issues and with members of special populations, including other healthcare professionals. Online resources are cited for many of these topics for further study.

GENERAL COMMUNICATION TOPICS

Nonverbal Communication

Nonverbal communication contributes significantly to how individuals understand each other, especially when expressing feelings.[3] Except for words, it includes every aspect of interpersonal communication, including body language and proximity to the other person, tone of voice, facial expressions, silence, and rate of speech. Figure 8-1 describes a simple activity that can help you become more aware of your own nonverbal communication. Figure 8-2 provides a second activity to help determine the rate at which you speak. How a person interprets and understands nonverbal communication is in part related to cultural background, a topic that extends beyond this chapter. For more information about cultural competency, see eChapter 2 "Cultural Competency" in DiPiro et al, eds, *Pharmacotherapy: A Pathophysiologic Approach*, ninth edition (McGraw-Hill Education, 2014). Other useful references include the Cultural Competency section of the U.S. Department of Health and Human Services Office of Minority Health (https://minorityhealth.hhs.gov/omh/browse.aspx?lvl=1&lvlid=6) and the National Center for Cultural Competency at Georgetown University (http://nccc.georgetown.edu/resources/publicationstitle.html).

> A simple exercise to become more aware of your nonverbal communication while listening is to have another person speak to you without interruption for about two minutes about something important to them. Respond to them using body language and facial expressions only, without using any words. Then break to discuss what you did to convey you were listening and consider how to improve, if needed. Repeat this exercise in person and over online video (if relevant to your pharmacy practice) to discern any differences. If you attempt the exercise via telephone, you will find the need to use words of course, or "passive listening" such as uttering "mmhmm" because there is no way for the speaker to discern you, as listener, are attending to their message without this.

FIGURE 8-1 Listening without saying a word.

> **Am I speaking too fast?**
> For that matter, am I speaking too slowly? The following paragraph is 156 words long. By reading it aloud at your normal rate of speech, you will be able to gauge your rate of speech against the average of 125-150. Test yourself briefly...the results may surprise you!
>
> **One Minute Statement**
> Most experts agree that the ideal rate of speech is between one hundred and twenty-five and one hundred and fifty words per minute. At this rate, people who are listening to you will be able to understand you easily. Over the telephone your voice carries eighty-five percent of the message you wish to convey. Therefore, it is important to speak at an acceptable rate. Since the remaining fifteen percent of the message is conveyed by the actual content, choose your words wisely. With every telephone call, you create an image of you and your organization. Be sure the image you create is favorable so that your customers will want to call again. You know what other people sound like on the telephone. How do you sound? Sincere or insincere? Interested or indifferent? Take the time to evaluate how you come across. "If you read this statement in one minute, your speech rate is excellent."

FIGURE 8-2 An exercise to measure rate of speech.

Source: From Melanson MS. *Effective Telephone Communication Skills*. Colorado Springs, CO: Help Desk Institute; 2003:18 (Figure 3-2), with permission.

Congruence and Incongruence. A person's nonverbal communication may or may not be congruent with the words he or she speaks. An example of incongruence between verbal and nonverbal communication would be to say, "Take two tablets," while holding up one finger to make the point. When verbal and nonverbal communication are incongruent—that is, when they are not conveying the same message—confusion tends to result. Nonverbal communication is believed to have up to 5 times more impact than spoken words.[4] Being conscious of one's own nonverbal messages can help ensure that the message the listener receives is the same as the one he or she intends to deliver. However, nonverbal communication may be difficult to control because it is not always conscious. Various lie detector tests are based on the assumption that congruent nonverbal and verbal communication must originate from a speaker who believes what he or she says. If a person asks something using polite words but honestly finds the other person annoying, there is likely to be incongruence; the "kind" message may not be interpreted as kind due to the tone of voice, facial expression, level of eye contact, and body language. If the receiver of the message notices the incongruence, he or she is likely to believe the nonverbal message and determine that the speaker is insincere. This may be especially true for female message receivers; research shows women tend to be more accurate readers of facial expressions and body language.[4]

So, it is important to believe in your message—whether it be your confidence in the benefits of MTM or truly caring about a patient's well-being when encouraging behavioral change. If you do not believe in your message, you need to ask yourself why. If possible, revise your message so that it is still effective, but not contrary to what you believe. If you follow a service script, you may need to modify the wording to stay true to the message, while tailoring it to your own approach or style.

One way to increase the likelihood of communicating congruently with patients is to use an *open stance* and to smile when appropriate. An open stance includes sitting squarely in front of the person, leaning in slightly, and giving the person 50% to 75% eye contact. This stance tells the other person that you are listening and engaged in the conversation. In contrast, a *closed stance* communicates inattentiveness and lack of concern by leaning away or turning away from the other person, limited eye contact, folding your arms across your chest, or supporting the back of the neck with the hands, elbows out. Computer use can cause practitioners to turn away from patients when communicating in person. Keeping a small laptop between the pharmacist and patient, with the screen open at an angle that does not create a substantial visual barrier, may help address this. It may also be helpful to simply tell the patient that you would like to take notes by typing while she speaks but that you are listening and will look up as often as possible, noting the situation is less than optimal.

MTM services are frequently provided via telehealth, including over the telephone or online using video. When communicating via online video, people can often see a display of themselves as well as the person with whom they are communicating.[5] When providing MTM via online video, minimize your own picture, place it on the screen as close to the camera as possible and resist the temptation to look at it. Also, tell the patient that you have the patient's profile or documents on the screen or in front of you and that you will be looking at him or her at times during the call. Aside from looking at documents, be aware of the messages that your facial expressions send. As you listen, do you often furrow your brow in a way that could be construed as being confused or skeptical? Do you vary your expressions to include the furrowed brow when concerned, with occasional nodding and smiling as the patient relates his or her story to show interest and receptivity? Ask a colleague to monitor an MTM video call visually to provide feedback later about the nonverbal communication presented.

Smiling raises the pitch of one's voice and is easily discernible over the telephone, especially because there are no visual cues for the other person to use.[6] Research confirms listeners can discern when speakers are smiling or not without visual cues (eg, talking via telephone).[7] Obviously, smiling is not always appropriate; however, smiling when appropriate, such as during the greeting and the goodbye and when working to explicitly assist the patient can communicate a high level of engagement rather than irritation or annoyance.

Some recommend using video calling only when the visual component is urgently needed. This is because internet video calls have certain drawbacks, including mismatched video and audio, the inability to truly make eye contact, and the "interference with the natural flow of communication."[5] Examples where the benefits may outweigh the drawbacks include needing to demonstrate medication use (eg, an inhaler) or either party wanting to show the other a medication vial, for example, or the size of a tablet. Otherwise, telephone calls may suffice, especially when working with patients who do not have private internet access or when providing follow-up care. Keep in mind that when communicating via telephone, nonverbal communication is limited to tone of voice, rate of speech, and the use of silence. For an in-depth analysis of the role of telehealth, please refer to the Institute of Medicine's *The Role of Telehealth in an Evolving Health Care Environment: Workshop Summary*.[8]

Whenever possible, face-to-face consultations are preferred. Beyond the ability to physically assess patients, significant advantages include having all nonverbal and verbal communication available, as well as the opportunity for informal interactions[5] that can help build rapport. When arranging the space for face-to-face consultation, consider the level of privacy needed, the size of the room, and the distance between you and the patient. The typical distance for personal communication is 1.5 to 4 feet. Allow for patients to move within that range as they feel comfortable. Culture and how positive or negative the conversation is can affect a person's space preferences.[9] Also, experimental research suggests that too small of a room may actually limit patients' willingness to self-disclose.[9] Having the perception of enough space while ensuring privacy may provide for greater comfort.

While an open stance and showing receptivity to others through nonverbal communication can be learned and refined to improve effective and congruent communication, what we ultimately communicate with both our words and our actions is our attitude toward, and beliefs about, the other person. Treating patients as people, and not as "objects," is critical.[10,11] For more in-depth discussion about how we can deceive ourselves into thinking that our negative attitudes and behaviors toward others can be justified, read *Leadership and Self-Deception*[10] or "Choosing to See Patients as People," a pharmacist version of the Arbinger Institute's book condensed into a chapter of a communications text.[11] The bottom line is that thinking poorly of, or judging patients, (eg, for their negative attitudes or unhealthy lifestyle choices) is rarely, if ever, justifiable. In addition, a provider's negative attitudes certainly can be discerned by patients, even if neutral or positive words are used. You may detect this if patients with whom you speak are unresponsive to or defensive toward your words, even when those words are chosen extremely carefully. The patient may even react in the opposite way we would prefer. In these instances, it is possible that the patient has determined, from the delivery of the message, that what is said is untruthful, insincere, or rude. Again, this is likely due to the simultaneous use of positive words and negative nonverbals, thus creating message incongruence.

It is also important to notice when others' nonverbal and verbal communications are incongruent. When a patient says that she is taking her medication as prescribed but her nonverbal communication suggests otherwise (eg, the patient hesitates significantly or her voice suddenly changes), a different approach for discussion may be needed. Nonadherence and behavioral change should be discussed so as to not force a patient to feel as if he or she needs to lie to make you happy. It is beyond the scope of this chapter to explore how to determine whether a person is lying, and of course it is not necessary to become an expert in lie detection to provide good MTM. Suffice it to say that if what a person says leaves you wondering if he or she was sincere, it is possible your subconscious picked up on incongruent communication.[4] Pursuing discussion about that topic, if important, requires a nonaccusatory approach. Examples of this will be presented when behavioral change is addressed later in this chapter.

Building Rapport

Building rapport with patients is critical to helping them feel comfortable with the MTM service and providers. Building rapport is not just for the pharmacist, but also the technician and any other employees who arrange for the first encounter or interact with the patient at other times. A first impression is critical for a patient new to an MTM service, and simple attempts to build rapport can help ensure that it is a positive impression. Because everyone has his or her own personalities, preferences, and levels of comfort, building rapport cannot be standardized. A workplace culture where patients are treated as individuals will make it easier to build rapport in the context of MTM. Good places to start are being friendly and unhurried, inviting the patient to ask questions, and using the patient's name, erring on the side of formality to start (full name or Mr. or Ms.). Use the patient's first name only after receiving permission to do so. Showing the patient that you are concerned about him or her and explicitly taking his or her preferences into account shows that you think of the patient as an individual and not a number. This could be as simple as asking at the beginning of a telephone call, "Is this still a good time for you?" or, in a face-to-face encounter, asking if the patient would like a glass of water.

Last, humor is considered by some a way to build rapport, and yet there are significant considerations when using it. Patients' use of humor to build their relationship with providers may help to create a more relaxed atmosphere if the provider acknowledges the humor (eg, laughing). On the other hand, the use of humor by patients to speak about serious topics must be responded to carefully by providers so as not to miss a key opportunity to address that serious topic. Responding in a way that is not "face-threatening" is key; the provider needs to help the patient maintain his or her desired image of themselves (eg, a fun person) while transitioning well to a more overt discussion of the serious topic (eg, "This is difficult to talk about, but it's really important").[12] When providers initiate humor, they risk creating culturally-based misunderstandings or appearing unprofessional, and therefore, it is less advised.

Asking Questions

Open-ended and closed-ended questions.

Asking good questions is one of the most important aspects of communicating well during MTM. Both open-ended and closed-ended questions help elicit the information needed to understand the patient's perspective and to gain necessary information. Open-ended questions are those that evoke more than just a one- or two-word statement. Open-ended questions typically begin with "what" or "how." Examples include: "What difficulties have you had with your diabetes?" or "How did you fit your new medication into your schedule?" Using starter words like "how" and "what" can be deceiving, however. "How many tablets do you take?" is a closed-ended question. Asking a patient "How are you doing?" can easily result in the predictable one-word answer of "fine"—which *is* fine if the question was meant to help build rapport and not aid in symptom identification. "What over-the-counter medications are you taking?" may elicit a list from one patient and a short, closed response of "Tylenol" from another. That question still offers the opportunity for the patient to give a broader answer, as opposed to the question, "Do you take any over-the-counter medications?" which could result in a "yes" without elaboration.

Topics that more obviously require open-ended questions rather than closed include needing to hear about the patient's experience. Instead of asking a series of specific questions about a patient's reaction to a medication, one could begin with, "How have you been feeling since starting the new medication?" Depending on the patient, the patient's relationship with the provider, and the situation at hand, he or she may elaborate to differing degrees. Additional questions can always be used for follow-up. For example, if the patient talks about side effects, at some point, you can easily ask "How can you tell if it's working?" to check for effectiveness, "How have you been taking it?" to discuss adherence, and "What are your thoughts about taking the medicine?" to address patient acceptability.

Open-ended questions are especially beneficial for truly hearing a patient's perspective, especially when the answer is not predictable or simple. Asking the open-ended question can provide a wealth of unexpected and valuable information about the patient, in addition to the answer itself. It can help determine how well the patient hears and understands you and the language you are speaking and whether the patient is engaged and actively participating in the conversation. A provocative example of an open-ended question is to ask, "What matters to you?" (rather than another open-ended question: "What's the matter?") to pursue "the essence of patient-centered care."[13] In addition to asking open-ended questions, using follow-up prompts encourages reticent patients to provide more detail. Examples of prompts include: "Tell me more"; "Can you give me an example?"; and repeating a word or phrase the patient used as a question, such as asking, "You're feeling 'different'?"

Closed-ended questions are needed to complement open-ended questions during any comprehensive medication review (CMR) or follow-up MTM consultation. Closed-ended questions are more focused, resulting in a one- or two-word answer. Examples include: "How often this past week did you take the medication?" or "Did you have any nausea?" Closed-ended questions help get to the exact information needed, increasing efficiencies and targeting specifics. Drawbacks to using too many close-ended questions is less rapport building and a choppy line of questioning that actually can take more time than if an effective open-ended question had been used to start. When using closed-ended questions, it is important to avoid narrowing the focus of questioning too early, precluding an unanticipated variable from being elicited and explored.

Leading, loaded, and "why" questions.

Closed-ended questions that are leading or loaded should be avoided. A leading question is one that steers the recipient to a particular answer, which is often what the person asking is hoping or expecting to hear. Asking a person who has experienced a possible heart attack whether pain radiated up to his jaw can lead the patient to recall the incident differently. A common leading question in pharmacy is: "Is the medication working alright?" This type of question makes it easy for a patient who had not planned to admit to deviating from a regimen or having possible side effects to respond affirmatively rather than honestly. Because leading questions are typically asked inadvertently and benevolently, becoming aware of one's tendency to ask them is critical to obtaining accurate and complete information. This tendency may be increased in working environments where time limitations are palpable because the shortest response is for the patient to say "Yes [I'm doing fine]." In this example, asking about efficacy via an open-ended question is more effective. Preferable questions would be, "How have you felt since starting the medication?" (open-ended) or "Have you had any problems while taking this medication?" (closed-ended). One common trap to avoid is asking the open-ended question that is quickly followed up with an unnecessary (closed) leading question. The question "How has the medication been working for you?" if not answered immediately can too easily be followed up with a well-meaning, "Is it better now that we changed it?"

A loaded question is a leading question that communicates judgment. An example of a loaded question would be: "Are you taking your medication like we told you to?" It not only leads the respondent to a desired answer, it also makes the person feel like she will be looked down upon if she gives any answer other than what is desired by the person asking. It is difficult for some people to develop an awareness of their own tendencies toward leading and loaded question-asking. Reviewing recordings of MTM consultations for quality assurance can help.

It is best to avoid "why" questions because they can cause the recipient to feel defensive. Instead, reword the question so that you ask for the same information without any judgment. For example, instead of asking, "Why are you taking it differently than prescribed?" use "How did you decide to take your medication differently than prescribed?"

Question order. Asking open-ended questions followed by a mix of closed- and open-ended questions is a useful structure for an MTM encounter. This allows the patient to express things in his or her own words and helps the pharmacist to focus the conversation when needed. Asking less sensitive questions first before moving on to more personal questions provides more time to build rapport before delving into more difficult subject matter. This approach can increase the likelihood of a patient responding honestly. For example, it is important to wait to ask about using substances such as tobacco, alcohol, and recreational drugs until closer to the end of an interview unless the topic is key to the entire consultation.

LISTENING SKILLS

Perhaps the most important aspect of good communication is effective listening. To listen well, the listener must be engaged, noticing nuances of what is said, observing and attending to nonverbal cues, and contributing useful responses. Basic tips for good listening within the broader realm of customer service are listed in Table 8-1. In addition, there are different types of listening, including passive listening, providing affirmations, and listening for understanding. Passive listening includes listening without words or with minimal verbal responses such as "uh-huh." Listening for understanding is the emphasis in this section because it is typically the more difficult.

Listening for Understanding

Choosing to listen to patients to understand them and then communicating that understanding back to them is patient-centered. It is not enough to listen passively, although allowing patients to speak without interruption is a good start. There are different ways to respond to a person when listening for understanding. Terms such as "active listening" and "reflective listening" are used with different nuances and sometimes interchangeably. Suffice it to say that if patient-centered care is the intent, then the focus should be on understanding patients and letting them know you heard them and understand (or are trying to understand) them. Listening for understanding can be done with the use of repeating, paraphrasing, summarizing, empathic responding, and reflective listening.

TABLE 8-1 • Listening Do's and Don'ts

Do	Don't
1. Pay attention 2. Listen for ideas 3. Take notes 4. Assess the customer's emotional state 5. Assess the customer's level of expertise 6. Read between the lines 7. Listen for "unspoken" service requests	1. Interrupt 2. Finish a customer's sentence 3. Make assumptions

Source: Reproduced, with permission, from Melanson MS. *Effective Telephone Communication Skills*. Colorado Springs, CO: Help Desk Institute; 2003:19, 22 (see Figures 3-3, 3-4).

Repeating, paraphrasing, and summarizing. Three types of active listening are presented here. *Repeating* is the simplest form of reflective listening. Sometimes using the exact words the patient has used can be especially poignant and stirring. An example would be to repeat "it may be possible" to a patient who earlier expressed resistance to change, but who later admitted the possibility of making the change. Another example is to repeat "*every* time" if that is a key phrase the patient has used that you wish to acknowledge and address. *Paraphrasing* involves the listener lending interpretation to what has been said. This is a form of reflective listening that can help the listener to hear what he or she has said in a slightly different way. Taking this approach may acknowledge some emotional content if that was originally conveyed. If a patient said, with some level of frustration, "My physician changed me from this cheaper medicine to one that is so much more expensive; I don't know what he was thinking," an example of paraphrasing could be: "Your physician prescribed something more expensive and you don't understand why." *Summarizing* involves the listener, in this case the pharmacist, communicating the main points back to the patient. When skillfully done, it can even help to reveal discrepancies in the patient's thinking, if needed, to help them think through a decision. For example, if a patient shares a lengthy explanation as to why she decided to stop a medication, including reasons she considered not to, the pharmacist can use summarizing to juxtapose the two different sides of the decision saying, "So you didn't like the side effects and found taking the medicine to be cumbersome, but on the other hand, you realize you ultimately need to treat your condition and diet alone isn't working ... so this was a difficult decision for you."

Empathic responding and reflective listening. *Empathic responding* explicitly acknowledges the emotional aspect of what the patient says and the reason behind such emotions. While open nonverbal communication may help the patient know you are listening and attending to what has been said, a truly empathic response *makes it clear you have heard what has been said* and *understand the emotion behind it.* In response to the patient with the more expensive medication, an empathic response would be to say, "You're frustrated because you have to pay more for the new medication." Imagine a patient with arthritis who expresses extreme dismay at not being able to open his or her eye drop bottle, slamming the bottle on the table and exclaiming, "I can't even open my eye drops anymore!" If a pharmacist were to reply with, "You can't open the bottle," it would show that you have *heard* and *observed* part of what was expressed, but it could be perceived as cold and unfeeling. It is a paraphrase that fails to acknowledge the emotion behind the statement. Instead, a statement such as, "It really aggravates you that you can't open the bottle," is more likely to cause the patient to feel understood. This latter response is empathic because it: (1) acknowledges the emotion (aggravation); and (2) states the reason for it (the physical limitation). Another response that captures the emotion and the reason for it considers what is unspoken, but implied, and therefore is a higher-level reflection. The listener/observer might realize the real problem is not opening the bottle, but rather the increasing limitations of progressive arthritis. An example of this type of response would be: "The worsening of your arthritis is really affecting your life."

Regarding awareness, a rule of thumb is that empathic responses are appropriate when the listener experiences a higher level of cognitive demand—greater mental effort is required to know how to respond. Higher levels of cognitive demand on the part of the listener result from high self-disclosure on the part of the speaker.[14] This can cause listeners to feel awkwardness, discomfort, or not knowing what to say. This higher level of self-disclosure may be commonly referred to as "too much information," and yet as healthcare professionals, this information can help explain a patient's reluctance to accept treatment, his or her inability to follow through with recommendations, or myriad other health-related attitudes or behaviors. By responding empathically, the speaker may feel reassured that his or her self-disclosure was not inappropriate or for naught.

Final Words About Listening Well

Avoid Roadblocks. Active listening lets the speaker know you understand what he or she has said and allows the speaker to continue in his or her train of thought. When talking with patients who are explaining something to you, helping them to continue and showing you are fully engaged as the listener can make a huge difference regarding the quantity and quality of information, not to mention building rapport. In contrast, "roadblocks" can detour the speaker's train of thought or cause him or her to stop talking altogether.[15] Examples of roadblocks include expressing judgment ("That wasn't fair to you!"); saying something that outdoes the speaker ("I've seen a lot worse than that."); or asking probing questions before the person is done explaining and before the experience being described is acknowledged. As problem-solvers, pharmacists typically like to ask questions, so this last roadblock may be especially common when providing MTM. The idea is to not jump into probing and clarifying questions without first communicating that you have heard what the patient has said: listen before helping. It is possible that glossing over a patient's emotional state before jumping into problem-solving may result in the patient not feeling heard. As a result, he or she may be less receptive to suggestions or less likely to share honestly next time.

Responding to anger. What if you are speaking with an individual (eg, a patient, caregiver, or other healthcare professional) who is angry? If that is the case, listen first without speaking. Let him or her tell his or her story. Make sure the first words out of your mouth are nondefensive.[16] Begin to defuse the person's anger by quietly listening and by then responding with an empathic response. Only then, should you attempt to address the problem. Additional suggestions for responding to angry individuals are listed in Figure 8-3.

Practitioner self-disclosure. While listening to a patient, there may be a temptation to share one's own experience as a means

- Listen, giving your full attention (this includes having an open stance)
- Unless he or she is verbally abusing you, allow the person to completely tell his or her story until he or she are done.
- Do not interrupt. Silence shows respect *and* it is difficult for a person to yell for a long period of time without realizing the commotion he or she is making and the silence around them. Silence can be *very* effective over the telephone because at some point, the individual will stop and wonder if you are still on the line, listening.
- When the person stops speaking or yelling. Respond empathically. Acknowledge the persion's heightened emotion and the reason for it. For example, "You're *really* upset about the way your problem was handled." A common default of using the word "frustrated" is not intense enough to capture anger!
- Keep your voice and tone at normal levels. Do not raise your voice to match the other person no matter how tempting.
- Always "stay above the drama" and stay professional.
- If the person does not stop yelling, get paper and a pen and proceed to write down what he or she is telling (yelling at) you. Tell the person you are writing to ensure you remember all that he or she is telling you. This communicates to him or her how important the information is to you. Doing this can help to de-escalate the situation if the person is yelling. You can reasonably ask him or her to slow down as you cannot write down things as quickly as he or she can when yelling at you. Slowing them down will naturally bring the volume down. If you have to leave the person's presence to get the paper and pen, it can quiet someone's yelling even faster; if you step away for a moment to pursue the writing materials with quick explanation, there is no one standing in front of the person at which to yell.
- If the person becomes verbally abusive to you or too disruptive for the patient care environment, it is your right and responsibility to tell the person it is unacceptable. If needed, speak up (not as loudly as them, but loudly enough to be heard), use the person's name. If in person, inform him or her that if the verbal abuse or disruption does not stop, he or she will need to leave or you will seek means to have them removed from the premises. If speaking on the telephone, calmly tell the person you will hang up if he or she does not stop yelling (and then do so if needed).

FIGURE 8-3 Ways to defuse an angry person.

Source: Umiker W. Hostile People. In Coping with Difficult People in the Health Care Setting. Chicago, IL: American Society of Clinical Pathologists; 1994:215-224.

to better relate to the patient and build rapport. Practitioner self-disclosure occurs frequently in medical practice; there are no guidelines regarding it, and patient impact is not well understood.[17] Self-disclosure by a practitioner may risk detracting from the patient's experience or provoke too much curiosity about the practitioner's personal life, and yet in some cases, it may improve patient support or improve the patient-practitioner relationship.[18] Therefore, if using self-disclosure when speaking with patients, do so carefully, weighing the pros and cons. Simply acknowledging that you have also had a difficult time with a similar experience may help the patient to feel understood. Avoid generalizing or making the patient feel like his or her experience or reaction is not legitimate. You also certainly would not want to communicate that your own experience was more significant. Keep the focus on the patient. Even if self-disclosing, never fully liken a patient's experience to your own, as there will always be different variables to consider, whether apparent or not.

Do you really understand? One phrase that is easily used when intending to empathize is "I understand." This is unlikely to be true. What may be true is that you are *trying* to understand. It is better to avoid "I understand" altogether unless you clearly separate the phrase, "I understand you're angry" (meaning you are recognizing the anger) from "I understand your situation." It is highly unlikely that anyone can truly understand a person's stage in life, illness experience, difficulty with barriers to receiving good healthcare, family situation, background, and experiences. A young, healthy, educated, or wealthy person is not going to understand what it is like to be older, infirm, uneducated, or poor. Ultimately, when in doubt, it is best to leave "I understand" out of your lexicon to avoid inadvertently communicating something that is not true and that could offend the other person.

COMPRENSIVE MEDICATION REVIEW: CONDUCTING THE INTERVIEW

Arranging for the Interview

After MTM eligibility has been determined, it is time to arrange for the CMR. If affiliated with patients' physicians, the CMR or follow-up MTM services should be scheduled together with other clinic appointments to lower cancellation rates.[19] The experience between the service provider and the patient begins with the first contact, which is often a telephone call. Whether with a pharmacy technician, pharmacist, or other trained employee, listening and responding well to patients' concerns even at this early time is critical to securing their commitment to complete the CMR. Before addressing a patient's medication-related needs, motivational interviewing (MI) can help patients realize for themselves the benefit of MTM services. (Refer to "Addressing Behavioral Change" within this chapter.)

A service script can be useful for any pharmacy activity that requires standardization for quality assurance purposes.[20] Service scripts should be written in detail, tested, taught, and rehearsed. Practice among pharmacy employees will make the script seem natural and unscripted, while ensuring the same level of service quality is provided every time to every patient, no matter who is providing the service. The same questions will be asked, and the same type of information will be gained and recorded. Use of an MTM script should include branching in order to provide options to anticipated responses, such as when a patient hesitates, appears unreceptive, or does not appear to understand the importance of the service. An example of a script used at the University of Florida MTM Call Center is provided in Figure 8-4.

When a patient agrees to receive MTM services and sets the first scheduled appointment, which will likely include a CMR, it is important to give your expectations for the visit, telephone call, or online video call. When patients are first contacted, they may have little knowledge of what MTM entails. For this reason, they may not perceive the value of participating. Using basic principles of personal selling, you can help patients to better realize their need for the service. Asking probing questions in the context of a patient care encounter may incorporate the SPIN model.[21] This mnemonic stands for Situation, Problem, Implication, and Need-Payoff questions. Examples are included in Figure 8-5.

Once need is established, personal selling includes communicating the features and benefits of the service.[21] Features may include the length of time, the qualifications of the staff, and a description of how the encounter will proceed. Benefits may include helping the patient to better understand his or her medications, possibly eliminating unnecessary medications, saving the patient money, or reducing or better managing side effects of medications. Should objections be raised, they should first be acknowledged, but without apology or excuse by the pharmacist. Second, you might probe for further information that can help you better understand the objection. Last, you respond to the objection, using the features and benefits of the service to explain to the patient how the service can address his or her unique needs. An example of responding to an objection is also shown in Figure 8-5.

Promoting your MTM service may require personal selling on your part, direct marketing (mailing directly to eligible patients), and advertising. When personally selling your MTM service, believing in the service and being confident are essential. These require a clear understanding of what the service entails, how it is provided, and what it is intended to achieve. Making sure all involved understand these principles and subscribe to them is critical. Learning how to personally sell a service can start with reading a reference geared toward pharmacists who sell their services.[21] Practice is also needed to do this effectively.

Beyond personal selling, direct mailings can be useful and should be accessible to the reader. See the Patient Education section in this chapter for resources on making your printed materials readable. Last, advertising could take the form of a video embedded in your organization's website. A video can make a new service more tangible by showing patients what the service looks like and clarifying frequently asked questions. An example of a video-based advertisement is shown on the Fairview Pharmacy MTM website (http://www.fairview.org/Pharmacy/MedicationTherapyManagement/About/index.htm).

Openings and Introductions

Regardless of its purpose, an MTM appointment should begin with a friendly greeting as well as the common elements recommended when counseling a patient on a new medication. The opening can be most effective when it includes: (1) introductions in which you confirm the other person's identity and identify yourself by name

Intro-duction

- Hello, May I please speak to *<Mr./Ms.> <Member's first name> <Member's last name>*?
- This is *<your first name>*, **a Student Pharmacist, calling from the University of Florida, College of Pharmacy on behalf of WellCare's Healthy Living Program.**
- IF PATIENT NOT AVAILABLE: *See instructions for leaving a message and missed appointment procedures.*
- ONCE PATIENT IS ON PHONE: **I am calling regarding our appointment for your comprehensive medication review today.** *If patient wishes to reschedule - see rescheduling procedures.*

Recording Statement

- Well before we begin I want to let you know that **any information you provide to us today will not affect your plan with WellCare in any way. Also, this call may be recorded for quality assurance and training purposes.**

Verification

- Since I *may* be sending you something in the mail, **I need to verify your address and date of birth to ensure that this information is only received by you** (*See Phone Verification Procedure if talking with someone other than the member*).
- Could you please provide me with your address so I can verify it matches what we have on file?
- Could you please provide me with your DOB so I can make sure it matches what we have?
- Also is your primary physician Dr*<insert MD name>* and your pharmacy *<insert pharmacy name>*?
- Thank you for that information.

About the CMR...

- I'll explain a little about how this review will go...
- We will start by going through your medications and I'll ask a little bit of information about each.
- *I'd like to know...*
  - *which doctor gave you the medicine,*
  - *what you are taking the medication for,*
  - *how you take it,*
  - *if you are having any problems with the medication.*
- I want to make sure you feel your medications are helping you, and answer any questions you have about your medications.
- Afterward I'll review some information that you told my technician earlier.
- And I **may** send you information in the mail regarding what we speak about today and we **may** fax your doctor with any concerns you have.

Review of medica-tions

- So now that we are ready to begin, do you have your medications in front of you now? (If not, allow time for member to get their medications, remember a list is okay)

Ending the call

- Thank you for all the information...
- I have enjoyed speaking with you today...
- **Before I end this call, do you have any questions for me, I do have time?**
- **I will be sending you information in the mail regarding what we have talked about today, and I will fax your doctor with any concerns about your medications.**
- Well, thank you for your time and have a great day!

FIGURE 8-4 Example service script from the University of Florida MTM call center.
Source: From the University of Florida College of Pharmacy MTM Call Center Reference Manual, MTM Exchange Version 2.0, p. 56, with permission.

and title; (2) an explanation of what is to occur (in terms of benefit to the patient); (3) the expected time; (4) request for oral consent; and (5) an assurance of confidentiality. Regardless of the context and role of the employee, introducing yourself and giving your title or role is critical for developing good rapport with the patient. Also, without identification, patients could assume it is a pharmacist when it actually is a technician, or vice versa. This identification matters when it comes to developing a trusting relationship not only with the pharmacist, but also with the entire staff. Trust influences the level of a patient's commitment to follow through and honestly disclose important information. Within the explanation of what is to occur, it is useful to include the expected (and needed)

Use Probing Questions (SPIN Model) to Clarify the Problem That Could Be Addressed With an MTM Service

Situation: (to help the pharmacist know more about the patient's background and possible needs)

- How are you feeling?
- What current medical conditions do you have?

Problem: (to help uncover issues the patient may have that could be addressed with MTM)

- What side effects have you been experiencing?
- How has your arthritis been since starting this medication?

Implication: (to help the patient think about the impact of the problem(s) identified; these may be leading)

- Has your arthritis been preventing you from doing what you really enjoy?
- Have the side effects been keeping you from attending social engagements you used to look forward to?

Need-payoff: (to aid the patient in realizing and stating their needs explicitly)

- Would it be worthwhile to have your arthritis medications possibly changed if it meant having greater use of your hands?
- What would you say if we could work to minimize these medication side effects to get you back to doing what you enjoy?

Respond to an Objection

Patient: I don't have time for this MTM service.

Pharmacist or pharmacy staff: And your time is valuable [Acknowledge objection]. Have you considered the amount of time and energy it takes for you to deal with such a complicated medication regimen every day? [Probe with a question] Taking part in this MTM service has the potential to help you simplify your medication regimen, and to help you better organize and manage all of your medication needs [Respond].

FIGURE 8-5 Using personal selling to sell an MTM service.

Source: Material summarized and adapted from McDonough RP, Doucette WR. *Using Personal Selling Skills to Promote Pharmacy Services.* 2003;43(3):363-374.

role of the patient. For example, an opening for a CMR may include a request that the patient be as honest and thorough as possible to ensure the most complete gathering of information. Another expectation would be to request that the patient ask questions to make sure his or her concerns are addressed.

When conducting a CMR, it is important to remember that it is an interview and structure it as such. The pharmacist should maintain control of the conversation, while considering and balancing the needs of the patient. Needs of the patient may include sharing complaints or wanting to be "heard" or vindicated. The patient's needs may also relate to interruptions, especially if the interview is held via telephone or video conferencing.

Professional judgment and experience will help determine how to handle inquiries that are tangential to the interview. One courteous and assertive approach to tangents that are not pertinent to the interview itself is to respectfully say: "I appreciate you sharing this with me. I want to make sure that we get through all of the information (or questions) without taking too much of your time. If we have time at the end, you can tell me more about that." Suggested approaches to responding to patients' tangents that are pertinent to the interview include acknowledging the importance of the topic by noting, "That is really important" or "I'm glad you told me that." What follows depends on the professional judgment of the pharmacist. If needed, the patient can be told the topic will be covered within the interview. In some cases, the tangent should be pursued immediately to ensure the moment of patient self-disclosure is not lost. Further questioning should be used to elicit any details about the patient's experience that are relevant to the CMR. It is likely that a more experienced MTM provider will feel more comfortable pursuing this tangent, remaining aware of the need to return to the line of questioning afterward. At some point, redirecting will likely be needed. Again, it is important to remember that the pharmacist must remain in control of the interview.

Organization and Flow

The way in which an interview or consultation is organized can be improved by using transitions, orientation, cues, and summarizing. Using transitions helps the patient know that the line of questioning is going to change. An example would be to signal to the patient that now you would like to transition from nonprescription therapies to prescription medications. Any time a topical question has the potential to surprise the patient or be off-putting, use some form of orientation to prepare him or her. This might be as simple as using some transitional statement to let the patient know the line of questioning is about to change. In some cases, it may require assuring him or her that the next question or line of questioning is asked of everyone. For some, it can provide explanation regarding the reason for the question. For example, "Because you are a woman of childbearing age, I need to ask you a few other questions." Another approach is to affirm the patient by stating the information to be gained will help determine the best medication regimen. Cues include letting the patient know when you are close to completing an interview, for example. Last, summarizing is one way to let the patient know you are listening and can serve as a signal that the line of questioning is changing or ending. It also, of course, helps you ensure you have complete information. Scripting well-timed summaries can be a formal means of structuring an interview or consultation for quality assurance purposes.

Closing the Interview

Providing for proper closure during any encounter with a patient leaves an impression and serves an important purpose. For interviews (and consultations), closure should include the next steps for you and for the patient. These next steps may include further scheduling of an appointment or consultation, instructions for taking medication, or detailed steps for follow through. Letting patients know what you plan to do with the information you have gathered is important in order to increase the likelihood of their future engagement with MTM. After-visit summaries (AVS) are used in primary care and could present unique opportunities with MTM. A recent study of the usefulness of AVS supports the potential to customize patient education regarding follow-up care and to use the AVS as a teaching tool when wrapping up the visit.[22]

PATIENT EDUCATION

Techniques to Improve Understanding and Recall

Giving information and educating are not equivalent activities. Techniques that can help in the transition from simply feeding information to patients to educating them are provided in Table 8-2.

TABLE 8-2 • Improving Recall and Understanding

Strategy	Examples
Be specific	• Instead of simply saying "take plenty of water," state how big of a glass of water. • Instead of saying "take on an empty stomach," detail the exact timing in relation to a meal.
Use categorizing or chunking	If giving a lot of information, use pertinent categories to help the patient remember. For example, if teaching a patient how to use an inhaler, categorize information based on how to actuate the inhaler, how to breathe in relation to inhaler use, and how to care for the inhaler. The Indian Health Service PRIME questions are an example of categorizing information about a medication. Categories include purpose, directions, and monitoring. When using categorizing, refer to the categories by using prefacing questions like the Indian Health Service or by introducing the categories.
Use the active voice	Avoid the passive voice. Instead of telling a patient, "It's important that the tablets be taken with food," say "Take the tablets with food."
Avoid left-handed clauses	Do not include the left-handed clause as it is used here: "Because food can decrease the effectiveness of the medicine, take this about 45 minutes before you eat breakfast." Instead provide the explanation contained in the clause at the end of the sentence: "Take this about 45 minutes before you eat breakfast because food can decrease the effectiveness of the medicine."
Use summarizing	Summarizing is used as a form of active listening; however, it is also used to improve recall. Use it to highlight important points for the patient to remember. When using online video with document sharing, consider showing the patient the summary as a visual aid.
Offer information in writing	Basic principles to aid understanding and improve readability include the following: • Use few words with three or more syllables • Use short sentences • Use the active voice • Use bullet points or question/answer format • Leave whitespace on the page; dense text is more difficult to read
Ask patients to demonstrate	• Ask patients with complex regimens to show how many doses they use to ensure they understand a label's directions. • Ask the patient to demonstrate how he or she uses an inhaler or eye drops, for example. • Ask the patient to talk through the steps he or she takes when using his or her blood glucose monitor or when applying a transdermal patch.
Use emphasizing	• Highlight especially important pieces of information by saying, "This is really important ..." or "Really pay attention to ..." • If using printed information, highlight or circle critical information on the printed sheet to draw the patient's attention to it during a consultation and afterward.
Avoid or limit medical or pharmacy jargon	• Avoid jargon and define it when used. • Whenever possible, translate complex medical concepts into lay terms. • Develop culturally relevant analogies that you can use regarding commonly complex topics. Two examples would be to explain blood pressure using a garden hose analogy or to explain arthrosclerosis using a clogged sink analogy.
Use teach-back to verify a patient has heard and understood the information	• There are different ways to use teach-back, and it is best used scattered throughout consultations rather than at the end. This can promote two-way dialogue and prevent the teach-back from appearing to be a "quiz." Use prefacing to introduce the idea of teachback to the patient who is new to the technique: • "To make sure I was clear ..." • "That was a lot of information I just gave you ..." Open-ended questions that provoke more than just a one- or two-word answer are likely to be more effective: • How will you fit that into your schedule? • How will you know the medication is working? • What side effects will you especially watch out for? • What information was especially important to you? • When would you contact us or your physician? Closed-ended questions that provoke a one- or two-word answer may be useful if you are especially concerned about a specific piece of information the patient needs to remember: • What time will you take your first dose? • What will you do before using your inhaler, to make sure it is ready to be used?

They represent ways to improve recall and understanding. Some also help engage the patient, making the CMR a dialogue rather than a monologue.

Communicating Risk Information

Talking with patients about side effects and precautions of medications can be difficult. While it is important not to overwhelm the patient with information, there is no definitive recommended approach on how much or how little to give. Although research in risk communication acknowledges that pharmacists indeed believe they are responsible for communicating the risks of taking medications, patients typically perceive it is the responsibility of the physician.[23] Talking with patients about the risks of medication use therefore may create an added challenge of convincing patients that discussing the risks of medication-taking is one of the pharmacist's roles.[23] Techniques for discussing medication side effects in particular are included in Table 8-3. These techniques include making the information more understandable, memorable, useable, and accessible.[1] Acknowledging prospect theory, it may be wise to use both a negative and positive frame when presenting risks, as the former can result in higher risk-acceptance and the latter in lower risk-acceptance.[24]

Health Literacy

Health literacy correlates to self-assessment of overall health[25]; the lower one's health literacy, the lower the self-reported rating of overall health. According to a 2003 nationwide study (the National Assessment of Adult Literacy), only 12% of the over 19 000 adults surveyed were found to be "proficient" in their health literacy, and only 3% of those 65 years and older demonstrated proficiency.[25] These figures are distressing, considering that proficiency in health literacy is necessary for navigating the healthcare system as well as for forming the habits that promote health and prevent disease.[26] Patients who are likely to need more intense MTM services are also likely to have lower health literacy, which presents a significant challenge.

Formal written tests to assess health literacy have been anecdotally reported as degrading to patients, who may feel humiliated because of poor literacy skills.[27] Formal written tests are also impractical. Possible behavioral clues to lower health literacy are listed in Figure 8-6. In addition, several questions can be asked of patients to assess their health literacy. The Single Item Literacy Screener (SILS)[28] performs moderately well and reads: "How often do you need to have someone help you when you read instructions, pamphlets, or other written material from your physician

TABLE 8-3 • Strategies for Communicating Risk Information (Focus on Side Effects)

Strategy	Examples
Present in a balanced manner; do not present side effect-information in isolation.	"What did the physician tell you to expect?" Discuss both the benefits and the possible side effects of the medications.
Use both positive and negative framing to provide a balanced perspective for the patient.	Positive frame: "Taking this medication will reduce your chance of stroke..." Negative frame: "Not taking this medication will increase your chance of stroke..."
Reinforce intended benefits of therapy and consider indirect benefits as well as direct.	"The flu shot decreases your likelihood of getting influenza, which means you're less likely to miss work and expose your friends and family to flu."
Discuss opportunities for self-monitoring.	"Take note of how you're feeling now, before the change in therapy. Once the change is made, if you notice anything unusual or unexpected, call us..." "How will you know the medication is working?"; "May I suggest some things you can keep track of?" "How do you think you could keep track of this until I see you again?"
Give information by categorizing side effects.	• Those the patient may grow to tolerate • Those that may worsen over time • Those more severe versus more benign • Those more common versus very rare
Explain risks stated as percentages in terms that are better understood.	"0.1% means that 1 out of 1000 people taking this medication will experience this side effect"; "If everyone in this city of 100 000 people were taking this medication, 100 people would experience this side effect (and 99 900 would not)."
Provide information and suggestions on how to prevent side effects or to effectively manage them.	"Do not drink alcohol with this medication, because the combination can hurt your liver." "It's really important to call us or your physician if you experience any muscle weakness." "It's okay to take it with food to avoid having an upset stomach."
When describing side effects, unless dangerous, using the word "bother" or "bothersome" is typically understood by most patients.	"Pay attention to how you feel after you start the new medication. Let us know if something starts to bother you."
Present risk on an individual level (not just population-based) when possible. Advances in pharmacogenomics will provide greater opportunity for this. Until this is more common, knowledge of the patient variables that can increase risk should inform your advice and information given.	"...because of your age." "...in light of your other conditions." "...because you tend to be more sensitive to the drowsiness effects of medicines like this one..."

• Filling out forms incompletely or incorrectly • Handing written materials to a relative or other person accompanying the patient • Making excuses when asked to read or fill out forms such as, "I'll read it later at home" • Frequently missing appointments • Making frequent errors when applying medication or self-care instructions, and consequently being considered chronically "noncompliant" • Pointing to the text with a finger while reading	• Letting their eyes wander over a page to be read without having a central focus • Showing signs of nervousness, confusion, frustration, and even indifference when faced with needing to read • Withdrawing or avoiding situations where complex learning is required • Giving incorrect answers when questioned about what they've read • Identifying medications by looking at the pills for color, size, and shape rather than identifying them based on the container's label content

FIGURE 8-6 Possible behavioral clues to lower health literacy.

Source: Cornett S. Assessing and Addressing Health Literacy. *Online J Iss Nurs.* 2009;14(3):2. Signs of Low Health Literacy. Physicians and Other Providers. Pfizer. http://www.pfizerhealthliteracy.com/physicians-providers/SignsOfHealthLiteracy.aspx. Accessed 14 March 2014.

or pharmacist?" The suggested response range is "1" (never) to "5" (always). Anyone responding with a 2 or higher should be considered in need of greater assistance. Due to its prevalence, some advocate for assuming lower health literacy and to make accommodations for it, regardless of assessment.

Figure 8-7 suggests strategies for addressing low health literacy, including creating a supportive environment and modifying written materials. Many of these ideas are drawn from a helpful online article by Cornett.[29] Taking a comprehensive perspective, the Agency for Healthcare Research and Quality (AHRQ) provides the "Health Literacy Universal Precautions Toolkit, 2nd edition." It contains a variety of tools to help individual professionals and organizations to improve oral and written communication and to help empower patients for self-management. It also highlights specific actions to take when providing "brown bag medication reviews" that are intended to increase the likelihood of obtaining an accurate medication history. This free toolkit is accessible online (https://www.ahrq.gov/sites/default/files/publications/files/healthlit-toolkit2_4.pdf). Additional information about health literacy, information, and resources are available at the Health Literacy website (http://nnlm.gov/outreach/consumer/hlthlit.html) of the National Network of Libraries of Medicine. Advice on writing educational materials in plain language is available at http://www.plainlanguage.gov/ and at the Centers for Disease Control website under "Plain language promotional materials" (http://www.cdc.gov/healthliteracy/developmaterials/PlainLanguage.html).

- Offer patients help in completing forms, preferably in a confidential manner.
- Simplify all forms using clear language.
- Advocate for the patient whenever possible.
- Use nonmedical terms when possible.
- Develop and use low jargon explanations for common disease states and medications.
- Review instructions with patients and check understanding. Have them tell you in their own words.
- Supplement oral and written instructions with pictorial and video-based instructions (Ex: www.videomd.com). (Note, do not rely on pictograms that can be misinterpreted.)
- Encourage patients to ask questions. (See https://www.ahrq.gov/topics/topic-questions-are-the-answer.html for useful video resources under the title of "Questions are the Answer" at the Agency for Health care Quality.)
- Use yellow or light colored paper with black ink.
- DO NOT USE ALL CAPITAL LETTERS.
- Use serif fonts rather than nonserif fonts.
- Provide plenty of "white space" on each page (less dense text).
- Use easy-to-read formats including Questions and Answers and bullet points.

FIGURE 8-7 Strategies for supporting patients with lower health literacy.

Source: Cornett S. Assessing and Addressing Health Literacy. *Online J Iss Nurs.* 2009;14(3):2.

ADDRESSING BEHAVIORAL CHANGE

Focus on Adherence

Within MTM services, behavioral change may include adherence to medication regimens, tobacco cessation, dietary changes, activities that result in weight loss, and more. A typical approach to addressing behavioral change is to educate a patient about the need to change and to try to motivate them to do it. Although various behaviors may be addressed by pharmacists to help patients with their medication-related health, medication adherence is the predominant behavior and will be the primary focus of this section.

Most patient education around medication use is intended to improve adherence, whether explicitly stated or not. Discussions with patients already taking prescribed medications would normally begin with some form of assessment to determine the extent to which adherence is occurring and reasons for nonadherence. Table 8-4 provides an overview of tools available for assessing adherence to medications. Other tools include laboratory tests (to check serum concentrations of medications) and therapeutic markers (eg, reduction in blood pressure), although the latter may be affected by other patient behaviors. In addition, simple questions regarding adherence can be asked to begin the conversation. Examples include: "How many times did you miss a dose this past week?" and "What difficulties have you had taking your medication this past month?" Notably, these questions allow the patient to not have been completely adherent. Simply stated, they are not loaded (ie, they are not leading and are free from judgment).

It is important to remember that adherence can be intentional or unintentional. For unintentional medication nonadherence, where patients inadvertently deviate from a prescribed regimen, a simplified regimen and better instructions tailored to the patient may solve the problem. If intentional, patients have made the choice to deviate from the prescribed regimen. From the patient's perspective, this deviation may be perfectly rational; it may be the result of unwanted side effects, not perceiving adequate benefits of the medication, or needing to save money. These decisions may or may not be made on the advice of a prescriber. Changes that are sanctioned by a prescriber without a formal change to the prescription of course will not be evident until discussed with the patient and/or prescriber. Regardless of the type of nonadherence, a constructive response omits judgment and condescension from both oral and nonverbal communication. Reprimanding patients will result

TABLE 8-4 • Positive Elements of Medication Adherence Scales

	Number of Questions	Reliability[a] (Cronbach alpha)	Barriers to Medication-taking Behavior Identified	Validated in Patients With Low Literacy[b]	Assess Self-efficacy?	Simple Scoring at Bedside?[c]
MAQ	4	0.61	Forgetfulness, adverse effects	Yes	No	Yes
SEAMS	13	0.89	Identify specific problem areas	Yes	Yes	No
BMQ	3[d]	NA; 95% overall accuracy reported	Evaluates regimen and recall	No	Yes	No
Hill-Bone Compliance Scale	14[e]	0.65	Forgetfulness, adverse effects	No	Yes	No
MARS	10	0.75	Forgetfulness, adverse effects, value of medication	No	No	Yes

[a] Internal consistency reliability is the ability to judge consistency across results of survey items; high internal consistency reliability is defined as Cronbach alpha = 0.7.

[b] Examples of low-literacy populations include individuals with less than a high school education or a sixth-grade reading level or less.

[c] Simple scoring at bedside is defined as requiring a calculation of 10 or fewer numbers to determine the score and the lack of requirement of a scoring tool.

[d] Three main question headings with multiple questions in subheading.

[e] Only nine questions relate to medication adherence specifically.

Abbreviations: BMQ = brief medication questionnaire; MAQ = medication adherence questionnaire; MARS = medication adherence rating scale; NA = not applicable; SEAMS = Self-efficacy for Appropriate Medication Use Scale.

Source: Reproduced, with permission, from Lavsa SM, Holzworth A, Ansani NT. Selection of a validated scale for measuring medication adherence. *J Amer Pharm Assoc.* 2011;51(1):92 (Table 1).

in patient embarrassment, annoyance, or lying in attempt to "save face," therefore severely compromising communication.

In most instances of nonadherence, whether unintentional or intentional, effective interventions are needed. A 2013 report by the Agency for Healthcare Research and Quality summarizes existing literature regarding medication adherence intervention effectiveness and concludes that education and case management were the two most effective types of interventions. Self-management-based interventions also were determined to be successful for patients with certain symptomatic diseases.[30] Based on these findings, MTM-based approaches to improving patient medication adherence need to extend beyond patient education to include a more intensive case-based or self-management approach. Patient education is not enough when addressing intentional nonadherence, where patients consciously decide to take their medications differently than prescribed. The patient's motivations may not be consistent with healthy behaviors (in this case, medication adherence). It is in these situations that motivational interviewing (MI) can be especially helpful when speaking with patients about changing their approach to medication-taking.

Motivational Interviewing

The spirit of motivational interviewing. MI is a communication technique and philosophy of helping individuals with behavioral change. It is not a way to manipulate people into changing. See Table 8-5 for a comparison of MI with traditional counseling approaches.

MI was originally developed to work with people struggling with alcohol addiction, but it has since been applied successfully to many different health-related behavioral applications. MI techniques are used to guide individuals to find and activate their own motivation to change and to help them identify and mobilize resources to assist with the change. The "spirit" of MI is collaborative and evocative, and it honors the other person's autonomy.[31] It is collaborative in that the practitioner forms a cooperative partnership with the patient, leading to a shared decision-making process regarding an identified behavior. It is evocative in that the intent is to activate the patient's own motivation and resources to change his or her behaviors by evoking from the patient what he or she thinks, knows, and has. Honoring the patient's autonomy means to truly accept that the patient makes his or her own choices. By actually caring about

TABLE 8-5 • Comparison of Motivational Interviewing With Traditional Counseling

Traditional Counseling	Motivational Interviewing
Practitioner is the healthcare expert, assumes patient lacks knowledge, tells patient what to do, and hopes patient follows instructions.	Practitioner develops partnership with patient and exchanges information to facilitate an informed decision. Patient has the right to decide own care.
Practitioner provides information to patient.	Practitioner provides information to patient for the purpose of developing discrepancy.
Practitioner dictates healthcare behavior.	Practitioner and patient negotiate behavior and reach agreement.
Goal is to motivate the patient.	Goal is to access motivation and inspire commitment to change behavior.
Practitioner persuades patient to change behavior.	Practitioner understands and accepts patient's action.
Practitioner expects respect from patient.	Practitioner must earn respect from patient.
Practitioner saves patient.	Patient saves self.

Source: Reproduced, with permission, from Possidente CJ, Bucci KK, McClain WJ. Motivational interviewing: a tool to improve medication adherence? *Amer J Health-Sys Pharm.* 2005;62:1312 (Table 1).

the patient's choices, the practitioner guides the patient to think constructively about the behavior, rather than telling the patient what to do in a directive manner, which is often counterproductive.[31] To do this successfully, health professionals must avoid the "expert trap," which is defined as an error of the professional who assumes and then communicates that he or she is best able to solve the patient's problems.[32] Stated differently, the professional should facilitate an "exchange of expertise" between self and the patient so as not to undermine the patient's own expertise, abilities, and autonomy, and to increase the likelihood that the professional use a guiding approach.[33]

Decisional balance and readiness to change. Motivational interviewing aligns well with the transtheoretical model, which explains behavioral change as a process involving five stages (precontemplation, contemplation, preparation, action, and maintenance). Embedded within this model is the concept of decisional balance, which reflects the weighing of pros and cons involved in making any type of change.[34] A person whose decisional balance shows more cons (reasons not to change) compared to pros (reasons to change) is likely to be *resistant* to change. He or she will not be ready to change. A person whose decisional balance shows about equal pros and cons is likely to be *ambivalent* to change. The *changing* individual likely has a decisional balance where the pros outweigh the cons. MI techniques provide guidance on to how to speak with individuals who are resistant, ambivalent, and changing.

Readiness to change, a key consideration within motivational interviewing, includes two key dimensions to assess and address: the patient's perceived importance to change and the patient's self-efficacy (confidence and ability) to change. For a person to change a behavior, that person must view it as important and also feel capable and confident in his or her ability to make the change. In practice, it is helpful to discuss importance first—if a person does not feel the change is important, his or her level of confidence is secondary to addressing importance. Indeed, resistant patients may feel very confident about their ability to change, but see no reason why they should. This is revealed in the statement, "I could if I wanted to." It is typically believed that most people are ambivalent about making healthy changes. Most of us do not spend much time deliberating about changing our unhealthy behaviors. These individuals' decisional balances reveal nearly equal reasons for and against changing unhealthy behaviors. But, when approached in a nonjudgmental way, they are likely to be open to discussing behavioral change; they are on the proverbial "fence" in terms of making the change. A practitioner skilled in MI is skilled to help them think about more reasons to make the change and help them consider first steps without it seeming too overwhelming.

Improving the likelihood that individuals will seriously consider changing—and access the resources needed to do it—requires "change talk" and discussion of what the patient values.[31] Change talk is a critical component of MI because it provides the opportunity for the individual to speak words that support making a behavioral change. It is critical that people, themselves, speak the need to change and the reasons for it, rather than being told to change and the reasons for it. This requires skillful question-asking and reflective listening on the part of the practitioner. When needed, the practitioner can provide information using techniques that are respectful of the patient's knowledge and encourage reflection as well as a response to the information (Figure 8-8). Summarizing change talk can also help reveal discrepancies in thinking, showing both the pros and cons within the decisional balance.[31] Doing so can help develop cognitive dissonance in the individual's mind, which results from believing one thing and doing the other. For example, if a patient shares his clear love for his grandchildren, but admits he has not been making healthy choices that can help extend his life, summarizing this for the patient highlights the discrepancy making it easier to address. In this sense, the patient is guided to be reminded of his own values—rather than the clinician's—which should always be the focus of the discussion.

Elicit-Provide-Elicit[a]

Pharmacist: What is your understanding of why it's important to take your warfarin exactly as prescribed? [Elicit]

Patient: I know it's to keep my blood from clotting too much. To keep me out of the hospital.

Pharmacist: Yes, and may I share with you a few more reasons? [Respectfully offer information]

Patient: Okay.

Pharmacist: (proceed with patient education) [Provide] What are your thoughts about that? [Elicit]

Patient: Well, I didn't really realize how this one is different than other medicines I take....

FIGURE 8-8 An "Informing" Tool in MI applied to MTM.

[a] Tool cited in Rollnick S, Miller WR, Butler CC. *Motivational Interviewing in Health Care: Helping Patients Change Behavior.* New York, NY: The Guilford Press; 2008:95-98.

Motivational interviewing techniques applied to medication therapy management. MI may help patients to eventually choose to change their behaviors. Tools use the principle of *guiding* rather than directing or following. Taken together, they are intended to include equal amounts of asking questions, listening to the patient, and informing the patient through education.[31] The *guiding* approach is in contrast to the directing approach, where the practitioner focuses on providing high levels of informing rather than listening. It also contrasts to a following approach where the practitioner focuses on listening rather than on providing information.

The guiding approach helps patients to think more about their behaviors and realize the benefits to changing their behaviors based on the values they hold dear. Some guiding tools pose thought-provoking questions, some include key follow-up questions, and others emphasize a respectful approach for offering the practitioner's own perspectives. Reflective listening and empathic responding are crucial to motivational interviewing because a great deal of question-asking requires good, active listening and the acknowledgement of the patient's feelings.

Examples of tools presented within the context of a conversation are included in Figures 8-8 and 8-9. One informing tool, "Elicit-Provide-Elicit," is shown in Figure 8-8. Ways to ask about a patient's typical day, how to include the patient in setting the agenda, and how to use a "ruler" to encourage change talk are included in Figure 8-9. The ruler can be used to initiate talk about how important the change is to the patient, how confident the patient feels about making the change, or both—addressing the patient's readiness to change. By discovering perceived *importance*, the practitioner can help the patient to reflect on the reasons for positive change. The ruler also can be used to help the patient consider what it would take to make the change more important to him or her. By facilitating discussion about *confidence*, the patient's ability and belief in his

Typical Day[a]

Instead of asking a series of focused questions, invite the patients to describe one of their typical days for you. For example: "Tell me what a typical day looks like for you and how you fit your medication in." Such a request may need prompting to elicit needed information; however, as time allows, stay curious and ask for details, but resist the desire to start solving the patient's, problems. If used via the telephone where visuals do not give clues to listening, it is necessary to use "passive listening" sounds and statements such as "mmhmm" or "yes, continue." Disclosure that is emotionally laden is likely to demand an empathic response to help the patients feel understood and to encourage them to continue, without detracting them from their explanation. Again, asking for details about matters important to the pharmacist is appropriate; however, jumping into problem-solving without allowing the patients to finish their description is typically disruptive and less effective. Allowing elaboration by the patients can uncover the unexpected, valuable piece of information.

Agenda-Setting[a]

One trap with talking about behavioral change is to prematurely focus the conversation onto what the professional believes is most important. With motivational interviewing, the strategy is to recognize that the patients are most willing to change what they are most willing to discuss. Therefore, it helps to invite the patients into the agenda setting of the consultation. One idea is to use a menu of possible discussion topics presented visually or just in spoken words. The idea is to acknowledge what topics are available and to ask what they are ready to discuss. One approach is to include what you, as pharmacist, want to discuss, but to invite their choice and offer it as the first point of discussion. For example:

Pharmacist: "I realize you may have some things you'd like to talk about today. I'd like to make sure we go over your inhaler, to make sure you are using it correctly, but what would you like to talk about first?"

Patient: "I want to talk about the side effects from the new pill my doctor gave me."

Pharmacist: "Okay, let's talk about those first and then we'll look at your inhaler."

Another example is to note the many problems that need to be addressed and to ask the patient what it is s/he is willing to work on or even just discuss.

Pharmacist: "I'm concerned about your blood sugar and what you've told me about your diet. I also am still concerned that you are smoking cigarettes. Of those three, your blood sugar, diet and smoking, what are you willing to talk with me about today?"

The Ruler[a] **(Focus on Importance)**

Pharmacist: "How important is it to you to take your medication, on a scale from 1-10 with 1 being "not at all important" and 10 being "very important"? [Use the ruler to assess readiness to change, focusing on importance]

Patient: "About a 6."

Pharmacist: "And what made you say a 6 instead of a 3 or 4?" [Use a follow-up question as part of the ruler to elicit arguments for adhering to the prescribed regimen]

Patient: "They said it helps to prevent strokes by keeping my blood pressure down."

Pharmacist: "So, you have a good reason to take it, to avoid having a stroke. What do you think it would take to move from a 6 to an 8 in terms of importance?" [Use affirmation followed by a follow-up question to elicit information to help the pharmacist assess what is preventing the patient from adhering more closely to the regimen]

Patient: "Well, I don't think my blood pressure is all that high, really—I'm not having any bad headaches or anything like that. And no one in my family has ever had a stroke."

Pharmacist: "So on one hand, you know that the medicine can help to prevent strokes by keeping your blood pressure down, but on the other hand, you don't think you're really at risk for a stroke because you don't have bad headaches or feel bad." [Use summarizing and begin to identify possible discrepancies in the patient's thinking.]

The Ruler[a] **(Focus on Confidence)**

Pharmacist: "So increasing your exercise is really important to you, but you're not so sure you can do it. On a scale from 1-10 with 1 being "not at all confident" and 10 being "very confident," how confident are you to increase your exercise to help with your weight loss?"

Patient: "I'm about a 5 for confidence."

Pharmacist: "Why a 5 and not a 1?"

Patient: "Well, I used to exercise a lot more but I had knee surgery so I stopped my morning workout at the gym."

Pharmacist: "Your knee surgery has gotten in the way of your normal exercise routine." [Use of paraphrasing as one form of active listening]

Patient: "Yes, exactly."

Pharmacist: "How is your knee now?" [Use open-ended question to explore]

Patient: (hesitating) "It's better, the physical therapist said it's okay to start exercising again, but my friends don't go to the mall to walk anymore."

Pharmacist: "So it's safe to exercise, and to use your knee more, but you don't have anyone to go with to the mall, and you enjoyed having the company." [Use of paraphrasing with reflective listening noting the enjoyment factor] "What do you think you could do about that?" [Use open-ended question to invite problem-solving by the patient rather than imposing your own ideas]

Patient: "Well, I guess I could call them up and see if anyone would meet me there again."

Pharmacist: "That sounds reasonable. What if no one else is willing to go back to the mall walking?" [Use open-ended question to prompt further reflection]

Patient: "I don't know. I guess I could still go."

Pharmacist: "Are you willing to commit to walking at the mall once or twice a week, even if no one joins you?" [Move to secure commitment that is doable, moving from "I could" to "I will"]

Patient: "Yeah, I'll try it twice a week. The mall opens at 6 am for walkers. That's when the others used to go. Maybe I can get at least one of them to start coming again."

Pharmacist: "That sounds great."

FIGURE 8-9 "Asking" Tools in MI applied to MTM.

[a] Tools cited in Rollnick S, Miller WR, Butler CC. *Motivational Interviewing in Health Care: Helping Patients Change Behavior.* New York, NY: The Guilford Press; 2008:52-61.

ability to change or perform the new behavior can be assessed and resources can be discussed. Figures 8-10 and 8-11 provide example dialogues using the MI tools of "Typical Day" and "Elicit-Provide-Elicit" as well as active listening.

Working with the resistant patient and the changing patient. Resistant patients do not want to talk about behavioral change, and their oral and nonverbal communication will tell you

> Pharmacist: [smiling] "Mr. Jones, thank you again for agreeing to participate in this important telephone call. My name is Virginia, and I am one of the pharmacists here at the Medication Therapy Management Service. We're scheduled now to complete what is known as a Comprehensive Medication Review or CMR. This involves me asking you various questions to gather information from you about the medications you take. I will keep all of this information we discuss confidential. With you sharing what you know and your experience with your medications, we will be able to look in detail to see if there are recommendations I can make to help improve your health, the quality of your life or even the money you spend on medications. This will take about 45 minutes to complete. Are you ready to begin?" [Patient name used, friendly, introduction of self, expectations for the phone call given, confidentiality assured, expectation for patient offered, benefits explained and consent sought]
>
> Mr. Jones: [hesitating] "I don't know if I want to take the time now."
>
> Pharmacist: "You're concerned about the time this will take." [Paraphrasing]
>
> Mr. Jones "Well, yeah."
>
> Pharmacist: "I know we scheduled this telephone call last week. What is your understanding about why you were referred to us for this service?" [Elicit patient's thoughts without judgment; start of "Elicit-Provide-Elicit" tool]
>
> Mr. Jones: "I don't think I'm so sick that I need it."
>
> Pharmacist: "You feel like you don't have enough health problems to make it worthwhile." [Reflective listening]
>
> Mr. Jones: "I guess so."
>
> Pharmacist: "May I share with you some information about what this service is designed to do for you and others like you?" [Respectfully asking to give information rather than forcibly sharing it]
>
> Mr. Jones: "Yeah, okay."
>
> [Pharmacist provides education about what MTM is and does to improve patient care, relating it to the patient's expressed concern about eligibility, using words that are accessible to the patient.]
>
> Pharmacist: "What do you think about all that?" [Open-ended question to non-judgmentally elicit patient's response; end of "Elicit-Provide-Elicit" tool]
>
> Mr. Jones: "Well, I didn't realize this helps my physician too, for when I go to see him."
>
> Pharmacist: "It helps to have a little more information about what this phone call is for. What do you think about completing this interview with me today?" [Affirmation followed by an open-ended question to pursue consent]
>
> Mr. Jones: "Hmm, yeah, I guess that's okay. I did set this time aside, and I guess it's important."
>
> Pharmacist: "Should we proceed then with the first set of questions?" [Gain consent]
>
> Mr. Jones: "Yeah, go ahead."

FIGURE 8-10 Scenario 1: gaining consent at the start of a comprehensive medication review.

> Mrs. Green: "Sometimes I just forget to take my medicine. I keep a pretty busy schedule for someone my age."
>
> Pharmacist: "Mrs. Green, would you be willing to tell me about what your typical day looks like, and how you fit your medicine-taking into it?" [Asking about a typical day to help diagnose issues surrounding presumably unintentional medication adherence]
>
> Mrs. Green: "Well, on most mornings I get up early and go walking with my friend Ruth. She and I have been walking most mornings for years. If the weather is bad, we usually meet for coffee at the shop down the street. When I get home I take my morning doses of everything—that's usually around 8 am. I tried taking them before I go out, but for some reason, it upsets my stomach too much, so I wait until I get home and have a bit of breakfast.... Some evenings we go watch my grandson play basketball or we like to go to the performances at the nearby community college. I take my evening doses somewhere between 5 and 9 pm because I'm not always home you see. And sometimes I do forget."
>
> Pharmacist: "So you have a regular routine most mornings, but your evenings are more irregular which makes it harder to remember to take your evening doses."
>
> Mrs. Green: "Yes."
>
> Pharmacist: "May I offer a couple of ideas to help you to remember those evening doses...?"

FIGURE 8-11 Scenario 2: discussing unintentional medication adherence during a follow-up consultation.

this clearly. They might change the subject, turn away, or show offense. Knowing how to respond appropriately takes a great deal of skill. Remember to focus on building a (professional) relationship with resistant patients. Communicate that you care about their situation and that you are not going to force the topic. One basic approach is to acknowledge their dismissal or offense (eg, "You don't want to talk about quitting smoking right now"), express your concern (eg, "I'm very concerned about what smoking is doing to your asthma"), and let patients know the opportunity to talk with you is always available (eg, "When you're ready to talk about this, I'm here").

Working with patients who are already making positive changes or who are on the cusp of making a change should involve supporting their self-efficacy and helping them with goal-setting. Instead of imposing your ideas about goals, ask the patient what he or she would like to achieve. Help the patient to set a goal that is SMART (specific, measurable, attainable, rewarding, and timed). For example, a goal may be to lose 10 pounds in the next 4 months. Help the patient to think through how he will achieve the goal and to develop a step-wise plan. Continuing the example, the patient may choose to add exercise to his daily routine. He may first need to locate the nearest recreational center, then establish membership, tour the facility, purchase walking shoes, and designate a time of day to use the walking track before he can truly begin an exercise routine. Supporting patients' self-efficacy can simply include encouragement when they are doing well or providing examples of others like them who have accomplished what they have set out to do. Another way is to provide friendly reminders using prearranged and agreed upon text messaging.[35]

Training for skilled motivational interviewing. The material presented here is a brief introduction to MI. There is much more to the technique and philosophy. To become skilled at using MI with patients in difficult situations, training and practice is required. Numerous MI resources (commercial and governmental) can be found on the internet, including those at http://www.motivationalinterviewing.org/motivational-interviewing-training, http://www.integration.samhsa.gov/clinical-practice/motivational-interviewing and http://www.mihcp.com/.

SPECIAL TOPICS AND SPECIAL POPULATIONS

Discussing Difficult Topics

Substance use and abuse. Screening, Brief Intervention, and Referral to Treatment (SBIRT) is a successful technique for addressing alcohol and other substance use with patients. Information about it is available on the Substance Abuse and Mental Health Services Administration (SAMHSA) website at http://www.integration.samhsa.gov/clinical-practice/sbirt. Screening tools available include the Alcohol, Smoking, and Substance Involvement Screening Test known as ASSIST.[36] More information about ASSIST is also available on the World Health Organization website under Management of Substance Abuse at http://www.who.int/substance_abuse/activities/assist/en/. Other screening tools, including CAGE, TWEAK, and AUDIT-C, have varying levels of sensitivity sometimes by gender and ethnicity.[37] None is intended to be used for diagnosis.

Excellent resources are available for clinicians who need to address issues related to alcohol overconsumption on the National Institute for Alcohol Abuse and Alcoholism (NIAAA) website, including an online training program with clinician's guide and video vignettes (available at http://www.niaaa.nih.gov/guide). The screening process to identify heavy alcohol consumption in patients is provided in a convenient pocket guide by NIAAA (http://pubs.niaaa.nih.gov/publications/Practitioner/PocketGuide/pocket.pdf). The approach taught in this program integrates MI principles to help patients move toward behavioral change.

Discussing weight and weight loss. Talking with patients about weight presents a sensitive yet important topic that many avoid. This is despite increasing national obesity trends.[38] One helpful approach is to begin the conversation by asking, "What is your current weight?" If patients hesitate or refuse to answer, briefly explain the importance of knowing their weight for accurate medication dosing. A follow-up question can be: "Is this your preferred weight?" If the patient simply responds with a "yes" or "no," invite him or her to tell you more, if you would like to discuss it further. If he or she says something akin to "I could lose a few pounds" or "I know I should lose some weight," use that as an opening and pursue it carefully. A helpful open-ended question consistent with MI is, "What have you done to successfully lose weight before?" This helps focus on positive behaviors and successes. If the patient has not had any success in the past, ask, "What do you think it would take to work toward losing 5 pounds?" This helps the patient to start thinking about small, achievable goals.[39]

In addition to questions, the words you use to talk about an overweight person's weight may make a difference as well. A recent study examined how patients who were seeking physician care regarding weight loss rated their preference for terms describing excess weight. Terms deemed *more acceptable* by those in the study were "weight," "BMI," "unhealthy body weight," "unhealthy BMI," "weight problem," and "excess weight." The terms deemed *least acceptable* by these patients were "fatness," "excess fat," "large size," "obesity," and "heaviness."[40]

Sexual health. With so many medications being implicated in sexual dysfunction, it may be helpful to speak with patients during an MTM consultation about their sexual health. (For one reference, see "Drugs That May Cause Impotence" in MedLine Plus available at http://www.nlm.nih.gov/medlineplus/ency/article/004024.htm.) Addressing this quality-of-life issue may be dealt with carefully by first obtaining permission to discuss sex.[41] Once permission is granted, four assessment questions are recommended as per Figure 8-12. These questions present opportunities for identifying medication changes, deletions, or additions.

Because some medications can cause sexual side effects, may I talk with you about your sexual health?

- Can you tell me how you express your sexuality?
- What concerns or questions do you have about fulfilling your continuing sexual needs?
- In what ways has your sexual relationship with your partner changed as you have aged?[a]
- What interventions or information can I provide to help you to fulfill your sexuality?

FIGURE 8-12 Sexuality assessment.

[a] Question applicable for older adults in particular.

Source: The Hartford Institute for Geriatric Nursing, College of Nursing, New York University.

Special Populations

Non–English-speaking patients. Resources available for interpreting over the telephone include Language Line Solutions available at https://www.languageline.com/interpreting, CTS Language Link available at http://www.ctslanguagelink.com/ and Network Interpreting Service available at https://networkinterpretingservice.com/. Interpreting service resource listings are sometimes available at the state level, and while many interpreting services include a huge variety of languages, some specialize solely in sign language.

Working with an interpreter, whether in-person, via video, or telephone requires forethought and correct orientation among you, the interpreter, and the patient. A great resource for learning how to work with an interpreter in healthcare is available at the website for the University of British Columbia, Division of Health Care Communication (http://www.chd.ubc.ca/dhcc/videos). The video has an accompanying toolkit that includes guidelines that feature general comments about the use of interpreters, how to orient the interpreter for the patient encounter, how to effectively communicate with the patient via the interpreter, and how to follow-up with the interpreter after the patient encounter. A potentially promising innovation that omits the need for an interpreter is an earpiece that works by translating between two users who are speaking different languages (https://www.indiegogo.com/projects/meet-the-pilot-smart-earpiece-language-translator-headphones-travel#/).

Patients in poverty. Working effectively with people who experience generational poverty takes a deep appreciation for, and knowledge of, the differences between this group and people who

Relationships	Find ways to build a trusting relationship, working to overcome their likely distrust of organizations. Attempt to overcome any workplace barriers that can prevent pharmacist-patient relationship development. Understand that the primary motivation for success lies in their relationships. Respect the priorities and demands of their relationships.
Goal-setting	Help them to set goals. Do not tell them what goals they need to achieve with their health and/or behavioral change.
Resources	Help them to identify resources and options. Do not judge them for not valuing or not having available resources.
Humor and story-telling	Appreciate their humor and the importance of individual personality. Realize that story telling is a common means of communication. Listen to their story-telling to help you learn about them, their health-related experiences. Listen for what is not said, and accept the fact that they may not want to share certain details with you about their situation. Use stories to educate and to help guide patient behavior.

FIGURE 8-13 How to better assist and work with patients in generational poverty?

Source: Payne RK, DeVol PE, Smith TD. In: *Bridges Out of Poverty: Strategies for Professionals and Communities.* Highlands, TX: aha! Process, Inc., 2001.

experience situational poverty along with members of the middle class. Generational poverty occurs when two sequential generations have lived in poverty or when a family lives with others in generational poverty.[42] This is in contrast to situational poverty, which occurs as the result of a particular event (eg, illness or divorce). One major difference between these two types of poverty is that while situational poverty typically leads to a proud response of not wanting to accept charity, generational poverty is characterized by an attitude of society owing the person a living. Discussing different forms of language and hidden rules that differentiate societal groups is beyond the scope of this chapter; however, the reference by Payne et al is recommended for further reading.[42] Figure 8-13 presents several considerations to improve your ability to successfully help and work with patients who are in generational poverty.[42]

An important resource for talking with individuals with various social needs is a newer publication called the "Social Needs Screening Toolkit" (https://healthleadsusa.org/wp-content/uploads/2016/07/Health-Leads-Screening-Toolkit-July-2016.pdf). Its content addresses several social determinants of health, providing screening tool options (various question sets) to be used to ask individuals about topics including food insecurity, housing instability, transportation needs, and financial resource strain among others.

Intergenerational communication and working with older adults. MTM services are likely to involve older adult patients. Considerations should be made for intergenerational communication. This includes avoiding ageist remarks, attitudes, and behaviors; adjusting one's speech to accommodate; and recognizing patients' age-related strengths. Ageism is revealed in part by the many derogatory terms used for older adults. Ageist terms such as "old fogey" or "geezer" are unlikely to be used by professionals, but terms like "senior citizen" and "retired person" are deemed to be stronger, progressive, as well as more acceptable by older and younger alike than "aged" or "elderly."[43] When approaching older adults with a line of questioning, be mindful of ageist information-seeking that may cause you to skip questions that you believe are irrelevant. The temptation may be to include or gloss over questions pertaining to substance use or sexual health, when in reality, both questions are as important to ask of older adults as of any other person.

When speaking with older adults (and really all patients, if possible), reduce the number of "left branch" clauses (like the one in this sentence).[43] Instead of saying, "Because of your past history ..., we'll need to ... ." say, "We'll need to ... because of your past history ... ." Prefacing the main statement with a lengthy clause can make it more difficult to follow. Also, pay attention to the speed with which you speak. Reduce the speed as well as incorporate pauses for the patient to have time to process and reflect. This will help cognitive processing, something that can help older adults, but again, most other people as well. If reducing your speaking pace, be aware not to overaccommodate, which is the "overplaying of a particular language or communication style relative to the needs, wishes, or desires of the listener."[43] Overaccommodation can lead to patronizing speech that treats the listener as a child, instead of an adult. Overaccommodation may result when an older adult's deficits are heavily emphasized. It is important to acknowledge the strengths of older adults, which include a vast array of experiences, knowledge, and resiliency.

An interesting caveat is older patients may respond differently than younger patients to seemingly benign questions. Asking, "How are you doing?" or "How is your health?" can trigger emotionally-laden, high-level self-disclosure in the form of painful stories that may simultaneously cause discomfort to the younger listener and a sense of empowerment to the older adult speaker.[44] Realizing this possibility can help the younger practitioner be prepared for the patient's response. High self-disclosure requires appropriate active listening. Empathically responding to these stories shows understanding of the emotional content and is likely to be well received by the patient. Doing so may help the patient not to feel self-conscious about the disclosure, while the practitioner may realize that the disclosure answers a plethora of unasked questions about the patient's response to therapy.

Hard-of-hearing and deaf patients. According to the National Institute on Deafness and Other Communication Disorders, about 36 million (17%) American adults have some degree of hearing loss and the likelihood of having hearing loss increases with age. Thirty percent of adults aged 65 to 74 and nearly half of all adults 75 years old or older have hearing loss. Notably, only 1 in 5 people who could benefit from a hearing aid actually use one.[45] For these reasons, consider how you can better communicate with people who have hearing loss.

Providing MTM services to patients who have diminished hearing capability may require face-to-face communication, text telephone (TTY) services, or document-sharing if using video calling. TTY services can be used by hard-of-hearing and deaf people, but the individuals themselves have to instigate their use. For explanations on how to use TTY, see the 711 for Telecommunications Relay Service webpage on the Federal Communications Commission webpage at https://www.fcc.gov/consumers/guides/711-telecommunications-relay-service.

Direct or indirect assessment of hearing difficulties can be made by asking, "Are you having trouble hearing me?" or noticing an inappropriate "yes" or "no" answer to an open-ended question. Ultimately, how you respond is best negotiated with the patient. With telephone-based MTM calls, you may be able to ask the patient to turn off the television or to minimize other sources of background noise at home. On the telephone or when using video calling it may be possible for them to increase their listening volume or for you to increase the volume on your microphone so that you do not have to raise your voice. Do not speak so loudly as to be yelling, of course. With women's voices, especially, it is important to keep the pitch lower, which is easier for many people to hear.

Communicating with patients who are deaf requires interpreting, as a deaf person's first (and possibly only) language is likely to be American Sign Language. Writing back and forth is impractical for a lengthy interview or consultation. When communicating face-to-face for a shorter consultation, do not assume a deaf patient can lip read, and take care to not use gestures that could be misunderstood. If your clientele includes deaf individuals, learn how to fingerspell for occasional use. Without an interpreter, if the patient can read and write in English, you may negotiate with the patient to write back and forth. This process can be facilitated, if in person, using an UbiDuo 2, a portable device designed to help deaf patients communicate in real time with another person without the need for Wi-Fi. It has a built-in wireless network for confidential face-to-face (typed) communication. If speaking over the telephone, in addition to TTY, deaf individuals may use video relay services because they allow the deaf person to use American Sign Language to sign to an interpreter who then speaks to you via the telephone. This is faster and simpler than typing text, making communication more fluid. For more information, refer to the Federal Communications Commission Guide to Video Relay Services online (http://transition.fcc.gov/cgb/consumerfacts/videorelay.pdf).

LGBTQ patients. LGBTQ stands for lesbian, gay, bisexual, transgender, and queer (and/or questioning). It represents a diverse subset of the population with differing health care-related needs and documented health disparities. Recent research indicates that transgender and queer or questioning individuals, in particular, may face greater denial of access to healthcare and more disrespect in healthcare settings.[46] A resource guide provided by the Human Rights Campaign Foundation exists for pharmacists and pharmacy staff that provides useful information to improve understanding of the LGBTQ population with suggested areas pharmacists can help (http://hrc-assets.s3-website-us-east-1.amazonaws.com//files/assets/resources/LGBTQ_Pharmacy_Guide_2016.pdf). In addition, a published online document is available which provides strategies for communicating with individuals in the healthcare setting who are transgender and gender nonconforming (http://www.lgbthealtheducation.org/wp-content/uploads/13-017_TransBestPracticesforFrontlineStaff_v6_02-19-13_FINAL.pdf).

Communicating with caregivers. Caregivers often are informal family members or friends. Activities of informal caregivers are many and include maintaining a continuous supply of administering, managing, and making judgments about often complex regimens on behalf of a loved one,[47] and research shows they, themselves, use more healthcare than noncaregivers, a result partially attributable to the stresses of caregiving.[48,49] One notable stressor in regards to communicating with caregivers is the changing nature of the caregiver–patient relationship as the patient becomes more dependent on the caregiver. For example, conflict can ensue if the caregiver is perceived as undermining the patient's autonomy.[47] For individuals caring for patients with dementia, unique strategies for managing medication use are reported and should be acknowledged and discussed. These include establishing more regular and simplified medication routines, using various dose administration aids and using liquid oral medications when possible.[47]

Communicating with other healthcare professionals. *Assertiveness* is needed to effectively communicate with other healthcare professionals. Simply stated, assertive communication respects the rights of both the message sender and receiver. In contrast, passive communication is less self-respecting, and aggressive communication ignores the rights of the message receiver. Assertive interprofessional communication keeps the patient's well-being central. To be assertive is to avoid unneeded apologies and excuses. Thanking a prescriber for calling you back and acknowledging that his or her time is important is a professional courtesy. Apologizing for interrupting a prescriber's work when it is the right thing to do to ensure a timely solution is usually unnecessary and considered to be passive. Using the word "I" and using clear statements is also assertive. For example, telling a pharmacy staff member, "I need you to call the patient back to schedule his CMR" is more assertive than asking, "Could you possibly call the patient back to schedule his CMR?"

Inappropriate Behaviors and Intimidation. In 2009, The Joint Commission issued a sentinel event alert regarding inappropriate and disruptive behaviors by healthcare professionals that "undermine a culture of safety."[50] A new standard was established that requires accredited organizations to have a code of conduct defining this type of inappropriate behavior and requiring that they implement ways to manage such behaviors.

Intimidation and disruptive behaviors have been defined to include disrespect and micromanagement as well as belittling, bullying, and using force or aggression to get one's way.[51,52] Such behaviors can cause dislike, aversion, workplace turnover, and unsafe practices to go unreported.[52] Instead of silence in the face of these behaviors, professional confrontation is advocated; however, many have an aversion to confrontation, especially in the context of hierarchy and fear of retaliation.[50,52] To prevent or limit intimidation by and of healthcare professionals, protective factors have been advocated including a flattened hierarchy, clear roles as well as responsibilities, the integration of team training, and a consistently enforced zero-tolerance policy for intimidation and disruptive behaviors.[53] The Joint Commission Alert contains additional suggested actions for institutions.[50] In addition to organization-wide changes, remaining assertive in the face of such intimidation is needed to ensure safe and high quality patient care.

Clinical communication with other healthcare professionals, including prescribers, is an important consideration when providing MTM services. Nonwritten communication highlighted here includes tools presented as part of the Agency for Healthcare Research and Quality TeamSTEPPS: National Implementation including SBAR and Check-Back,[54] assertive communication, developing a collaborative working relationship with prescribers, and calling on prescribers to personally sell an MTM service idea to them.

The mnemonic SBAR is useful when speaking with prescribers.[54] It stands for situation, background, assessment, and recommendation. It is a clear, concise, and complete way to communicate information in nonemergent patient care situations. Check-Back is another useful tool when communicating with prescribers as a means of verification.[54] See Table 8-6 for explanation of these tools with an example of each.

TABLE 8-6 • SBAR Framework[a] With Check-Back[a] for Communicating With Prescribers

Component	Content	Example Text
Situation	What is going on with the patient? What is happening?	"Hello, Dr. Green. This is Vanessa Strauss, one of the pharmacists at Community Pharmacy. I'm calling in regard to George Jones. He's a 72-year-old African-American patient of yours who began receiving services from us through our medication therapy management program in January. I saw him today and he complained of…."
Background	What is the clinical background and context?	"Mr. Jones has a diagnosis of…and is taking…. He expressed concern about his medication regimen…His symptoms include…He has also experienced unexplained weight gain of…"
Assessment	What do you think is the problem?	"I believe his weight gain could be…and also…due to…."
Recommendation	What would you suggest or ask the prescriber to consider changing?	"Based on his clinical presentation and the guidelines for treating…I would like to suggest that we change the dose of his…and consider adding…. What are your thoughts?"
Check-Back	After the sender (here, the prescriber) speaks, the receiver (pharmacist) accepts the message and provides feedback confirmation. The sender then verifies the message was received accurately.	Prescriber: "Let's increase his…and have him come in to see me this week…." Pharmacist: "Okay. We'll increase his…and I'll tell him to schedule an appointment with you this week…" Prescriber: "Yes, that's right. Thank you."

[a] Agency for Healthcare Research and Quality (AHRQ). Teams EPPS®: National Implementation. Available at http://teamstepps.ahrq.gov/. Accessed November 7, 2012.

Developing a working collaborative relationship with a physician. Forming a collaborative working relationship with physicians in your area is likely needed when building a community MTM practice. The physicians of choice are generalists, those physicians you may find easier to talk to and those who appear to have a significant number of eligible patients. A model for developing a collaborative relationship with physicians in the community setting is detailed by McDonough and Doucette.[55] The model begins with stage 0 (professional awareness), where a pharmacist's contact with a physician is in discrete exchanges only. It culminates with stage 4, in which a collaborative practice agreement or other protocols are established. The basic premise of the model lies in the reality that a pharmacist must work to gain the trust of a physician in the community, exceeding expectations by providing excellent services to the physician and his or her patients to gain professional recognition. The pharmacist is the professional to explicitly offer a higher level of service to the physician in stage 1 (professional recognition) and, if accepting of the offer, the physician in stage 2 (exploration and trial) proceeds to test the pharmacist's ability and commitment to providing the level of service the physician needs and expects. The time of trial eventually leads to a time of growth in the relationship (stage 3: professional relationship expansion), where the unilateral communication becomes more bilateral. Conflicts naturally arise, and if moving "upward," they help redefine the roles. The last stage of the relationship model is stage 4 (commitment to the collaborative working relationship), where protocols and practice agreements are established.

Moving from stage 1 to stage 2 of the model will likely require a pharmacist to "sell" MTM services to the physician.[21] Although this communication tool was presented earlier in the context of selling to a patient, the same principles can be applied and adapted to selling one's service to the physician with the goal of obtaining a referral. In this context, selling includes arranging to meet with the physician. Focus your message on how your MTM service is able to address the physicians' needs. This requires learning what those needs are and what problems they experience in medication management. As with patients, this means asking open-ended questions and listening well.

As discussed earlier, apply the SPIN model to help define the problem (for you and the physician). In addition, communicate the features as well as benefits of the service, and be ready to respond to objections. Keep in mind that the features along with benefits of the service should be tailored specifically to the physician, and cite benefits that are especially relevant to him or her, such as adherence to prescribed medication regimens. In a study of physician views of collaborating with community pharmacists, the authors concluded that pharmacist-provided services may be better received if aimed at helping patients to be more adherent to prescribed regimens.[56] At the end of a personal selling encounter with a physician, an offer should be made—in this example, to welcome the future referral opportunity to improve medication adherence among the physicians' patients.

COMMUNICATING IN AN AGE OF CHANGING TECHNOLOGY

While not all changes in technology show promise for improved communications, a few deserve mention. Adherence technology continues to develop to provide more accurate measurement of adherence, as well as reminders and notifications to individuals other than the patient. An example of this technology is Medacheck (www.medacheck.com). Electronic communications provide more opportunities for healthcare systems and professionals to be in contact with patients. An example is to email patients in regards to their health, including forwarding their personal health information. In spite of the risks, encryption is not necessary, though safeguards are required.[57] With MTM services relating more to transitions of care, it is noteworthy to consider transition care management communications. In a white paper, highlighted best practices include automated outreach via voice call, email, or text and smart reminder messaging that is bidirectional and allows for contacted patients or caregivers to be transferred to the organization's call center for rescheduling purposes as needed.[58] In May 2016, the Joint Commission began allowing text messaging of medical orders, including prescription drugs, for all accredited programs as long as a secure platform is used.[59] Further specification of expectations for such text messaging beyond the initial update is being assessed.

Last, a unique approach to using technology to improve communications with patients in the context of medication use is to create a "communication prescription." Such a communication is intended to take advantage of emerging technologies to provide a patient-centered "communication care plan that enhances the efficiency and effectiveness of achieving the designated therapeutic objectives at the personal and population level."[60] Such a prescription or care plan for communication can be tailored to patient's health needs and capabilities while using technologies available and preferred by the patient and the population.[60]

CONCLUSION

This chapter provides an overview of communication principles, both general and those unique to providing MTM services. Included are resources in the form of references, links to online resources, tools, scripts, and examples for improving your communication with the patients and professionals with whom you will work. As the healthcare environment, technologies, and patient needs continue to change, the need to be an effective communicator will always remain. As a motivational speaker and author once said, "The way we communicate with others and with ourselves ultimately determines the quality of our lives."[61] May the quality of your communication foster a quality work environment and quality outcomes for your patients.

REFERENCES

1. Institute of Medicine. *Envisioning the National Health Care Quality Report*. Washington, DC: National Academies Press; 2001.
2. The Joint Commission. "What did the doctor say?": improving health literacy to protect patient safety. Available at http://www.jointcommission.org/What_Did_the_Doctor_Say/2007. Accessed March 8, 2013.
3. Mehrabian A. *Nonverbal Communication*. Chicago, IL: Aldine Transaction; 2007.
4. Pease B, Pease A. *The Definitive Book of Body Language*. New York, NY: Bantam Dell; 2004.
5. Kappas A, Kramer NC, eds. *Face-to-Face Communication Over the Internet: Emotions in a Web of Culture, Language and Technology*. Cambridge: Cambridge University Press; 2011.
6. Juslin PN, Laukka P. Communication of emotions in vocal expression and music performance: different channels, same code? *Psychol Bull*. 2003;129(5):770-814.
7. Drahota A, Costall A, Reddy V. The vocal communication of different kinds of smile. *Speech Comm*. 2008;50(4):278-287.
8. Institute of Medicine. *The Role of Telehealth in an Evolving Health Care Environment: Workshop Summary*. Washington, DC: The National Academies Press; 2012. Available at http://www.iom.edu/Reports/2012/The-Role-of-Telehealth-in-an-Evolving-Health-Care-Environment.aspx
9. Okken V, Van Rompay T, Pruyn A. Exploring space in the consultation room: environmental influences during patient-physician interaction. *J Health Comm*. 2012;17(4):397-412.
10. The Arbinger Institute. *Leadership and Self-Deception*. San Francisco, CA: Berrett-Koehler Publishers; 2010.
11. Berger BA, Smith RE. Choosing to see patients as people. In: Berger BA, ed. *Communication Skills for Pharmacists*, 3rd ed. Washington DC: American Pharmacists Association; 2009;33-47.
12. Schöpf AC, Martin GS, Keating MA. Humor as a Communication Strategy in Provider–Patient Communication in a Chronic Care Setting. *Qual Health Res*. 2017;27(3):374-390.
13. Kebede S. Ask patients "What matters to you?" rather than "What's the matter?" *BMJ*. 2016; 354:i4045.
14. Weisel JJ, King PE. Involvement in a conversation and attributions concerning excessive self-disclosure. *South Comm J*. 2007;72(4):345-354.
15. Miller WR, Rollnick S. *Motivational Interviewing: Helping People Change*. 3rd ed. New York, NY: The Guilford Press; 2013.
16. Umiker W. Hostile people. In: *Coping with Difficult People in the Health Care Setting*. Chicago, IL: American Society of Clinical Pathologists; 1994;215-224.
17. Arroll B, Allen ECF. To self-disclose or not self-disclose? A systematic review of clinical self-disclosure in primary care. *Brit J Gen Pract*. 2015;Sept:e609-e616.
18. Lussier MT, Richard C. Self-disclosure during medical encounters. *Canad Fam Phys*. 2007;53(3):421-422.
19. Dolor RJ, Masica AL, Touchette DR, Smith SR, Schumock GT. Patient safety-focused medication therapy management: challenges affecting future implementation. *Am J Manag Care*. 2012;18(7):e238-e244.
20. Holdford DA. *Designing Pharmacy Services in Marketing for Pharmacists*. Washington, DC: American Pharmaceutical Association; 2003;75-99.
21. McDonough RP, Doucette WR. Using personal selling skills to promote pharmacy services. *J Am Pharm Assoc*. 2003;43(3):363-374.
22. Lyles C, Gupta R, Tieu L, Fernandez A. Primary care implementation of after-visit summaries for patients with limited health literacy. National Academies Commissioned Paper. Available at http://www.nationalacademies.org/hmd/~/media/Files/Activity%20Files/PublicHealth/HealthLiteracy/Commissioned-Papers/AVS%20for%20Patients%20with%20Limited%20Health%20Lit.pdf?la=en. Accessed February 19, 2017.
23. Schommer JC, Pederson CA, Worley MM, et al. Provision of risk management and risk assessment information: the role of the pharmacist. *Res Soc Admin Pharm*. 2006;2(4):458-478.
24. Tversky A, Kahneman D. The framing of decisions and the psychology of choice. *Science*. 1981;211(4481):453-458.
25. Kutner M, Greenberg E, Jin Y, Paulsen C. *The Health Literacy of America's Adults: Results From the 2003 National Assessment of Adult Literacy (NCES 2006-483)*.

Washington, DC: United States Department of Education, National Center for Education Statistics; 2006.

26. U.S. Department of Health and Human Services, Office of Disease Prevention and Health Promotion. *National Action Plan to Improve Health Literacy.* Washington, DC; 2010.
27. Osborne H. *Health Literacy from A to Z: Practical Ways to Communicate Your Health Message*. Boston, MA: Jones & Bartlett Publishers; 2005.
28. Morris NS, MacLean CD Chew LD, Littenberg B. The single item literacy screener: evaluation of a brief instrument to identify limited reading ability. *BMC Fam Prac*. 2006;721. doi:10.1186/1471-2296-7-21.
29. Cornett S. Assessing and addressing health literacy. *OJIN: Online J Iss Nurs.* 2009;14(3):2. Available at http://www.nursingworld.org/MainMenuCategories/ANAMarketplace/ANAPeriodicals/OJIN/TableofContents/Vol142009/No3Sept09/Assessing-Health-Literacy-.aspx. Accessed February 26, 2013.
30. McDonald KM, Chang C, Schultz E. Through the Quality Kaleidoscope: Reflections on the Science and Practice of Improving Health Care Quality. Closing the Quality Gap: Revisiting the State of the Science. Methods Research Report. Rockville, MD: Agency for Healthcare Research and Quality; February 2013.
31. Rollnick S, Miller WR, Butler CC. *Motivational Interviewing in Health Care: Helping Patients Change Behavior*. New York, NY: The Guilford Press; 2008.
32. Glossary of Motivational Interviewing Terms. Motivational Interviewing Network of Trainers. Available at http://www.motivationalinterviewing.org/sites/default/files/glossary_of_mi_terms-1.pdf. Accessed February 20, 2017.
33. Berger BA, Villaume WA. *Motivational Interviewing for Health Care Professionals: A Sensible Approach*. Washington, DC: American Pharmacists Association; 2013:16.
34. Prochaska JO, Redding CA, Evers KE. The transtheoretical model and stages of change. In: Glanz K, Lewis FM, Rimer BK, eds. *Health Behavior and Health Education: Theory, Research, and Practice*. 2nd ed. San Francisco, CA: Jossey-Bass Publishers; 1997;60-84.
35. Ybarra ML, Holtop JS Bosi ATB, Emri S. Design considerations in developing a text messaging program aimed at smoking cessation. *J Med Internet Res.* 2012;14(4):e103. doi:10.2196/jmir.2061.
36. World Health Organization ASSIST Working Group. The alcohol, smoking and substance involvement screening test (ASSIST): development, reliability and feasibility. *Addiction*. 2002;97(9):1183-1194.
37. Fagbemi K. Q: What is the best questionnaire to screen for alcohol use disorder in an office practice? *Cleve Clin J Med*. 2011;78(10):649-651.
38. Morbidity and Mortality Weekly Report. Vital Signs: State-Specific Obesity Prevalence Among Adults—United States, 2009. 59(30):951-955.
39. Ideas based on personal communications with Beth Martin, PhD, RPh, February 2013.
40. Dutton GR, Tan F, Perri MG, et al. What words should we use when discussing excess weight? *J Am Board Fam Med*. 2010;23(5):606-613.
41. Kazer MW. Sexuality assessment for older adults. *Try This: Best Practices in Nursing Care to Older Adults*. 2012;10.
42. Payne RK, DeVol PE, Smith TD. *Bridges Out of Poverty: Strategies for Professionals and Communities*. Highlands, TX: aha! Process, Inc; 2001.
43. Williams A, Nussbaum JF. *Intergenerational Communication Across the Life Span*. Mahwah, New Jersey: Lawrence Erlbaum Associates; 2001;108.
44. Gallois C. Group membership, social rules, and power: A social-psychological perspective on emotional communication. *J Pragmat*. 1994;22:301-324.
45. Quick Statistics. National Institute on Deafness and Other Communication Disorders. National Institutes on Health. Available at http://www.nidcd.nih.gov/health/statistics/Pages/quick.aspx. Accessed March 11, 2013.
46. Macapagal K, Bhatia R, Greene GJ. Differences in healthcare access, use, and experiences within a community sample of racially diverse lesbian, gay, bisexual, transgender, and questioning emerging adults. *LGBT Health*. 2016;3(6):434-442.
47. Gillespie R, Mullan J, Harrison L. Managing medications: the role of informal caregivers of older adults and people living with dementia. A review of the literature. *J Clin Nurs*. 2014;23:3296-3308.
48. Brodaty H, Green A. Defining the role of the caregiver in Alzheimer's Disease and treatment. *Drugs and Aging*. 2002;19:891-898.
49. Robison J, Fortinsky R, Kleppinger A, Shugrue N, Porter M. A broader view of family caregiving: effects of caregiving and caregiver conditions on depressive symptoms, health, work, and social isolation. *J Gerontol B Psychol Sci Soc Sci*. 2009;64(6):788-798.
50. Behaviors that Undermine a Culture of Safety. Sentinel Event Alert. The Joint Commission. 2008;40(July 9):1-3.
51. Lamontagne C. Intimidation: a concept analysis. *Nurs Forum*. 2010;45(1):54-65.
52. Maxfield D, Grenny J, McMillan R, Patterson K, Switzler A. *Silence Kills: The Seven Crucial Conversations for Healthcare*. VitalSmarts, L.C.; 2005.
53. Nadzam D. Nurses' role in communication and patient safety. *J Nurs Care Qual*. 2009;24(3):184-188.
54. Agency for Healthcare Research and Quality (AHRQ). TeamSTEPPS®: National Implementation. Available at http://teamstepps.ahrq.gov/. Accessed November 7, 2012.
55. McDonough RP, Doucette WR. Developing collaborative working relationships between pharmacists and physicians. *J Amer Pharm Assoc*. 2001;41(5):682-692.
56. Kucukarslan S, Lai S, Dong Y, Al-Bassam N, Kim K. Physician beliefs and attitudes toward collaboration with community pharmacists. *Res Soc Admin Pharm*. 2011;7:224-232.
57. West Healthcare. *White Paper: Six Communication Best Practices for Transitional Care Management*. Available at https://www.west.com/wp-content/uploads/2016/04/Six-Comm-Best-Practices-for-TCM.pdf. Accessed February 19, 2017.
58. Health and Human Services. Health Information Privacy. Does the HIPAA Privacy Rule permit health care providers to use e-mail to discuss health issues and treatment with their patients? Available at https://www.hhs.gov/hipaa/for-professionals/faq/570/does-hipaa-permit-health-care-providers-to-use-email-to-discuss-health-issues-with-patients/. Accessed February 19, 2017.
59. Update: Texting Orders. *Joint Commission Perspectives*. 2016;36(5):15. Available at https://www.jointcommission.org/assets/1/6/Update_Texting_Orders.pdf. Accessed February 19, 2017.
60. Angaran DM. MTM and the Communication Prescription. Presentation, Gainesville, FL, February 14, 2012.
61. BrainyQuote. Tony Robbins Quotes. https://www.brainyquote.com/quotes/quotes/t/tonyrobbin147783.html. Accessed February 19, 2017.

Review Questions

1. An open stance when talking with another person includes what body position?
   a. Arms folded comfortably in front of you.
   b. Leaning out (away), providing space.
   c. Head held still.
   d. Eye contact about 50% to 75% of the time.
   e. Hands clasped behind the neck with elbows out.

2. Which statement is TRUE about asking questions?
   a. "How are you doing?" (within the dominant United States culture) can best be classified as an open-ended question.
   b. "How did you decide to change the time you take your medicine?" is a way to ask a "why" question without using the word "why."
   c. "Are you able to infuse it by yourself, or is the visiting nurse still helping you?" is an open-ended question.
   d. "Are you doing alright?" is a loaded question.
   e. "Which side effect bothers you most?" is a double-barreled question.

3. Which statement is FALSE about listening to a patient?
   a. Asking probing questions is a means of active listening, as it effectively conveys to the patient that you have heard him or her.
   b. Empathic responses acknowledge the patient's emotional response as well as the reason for it.
   c. Active listening includes summarizing or paraphrasing what a patient has just told you.
   d. Reassuring the patient that everything will be fine is considered to be a "roadblock" because it can cause the patient to change what he or she is telling you.
   e. Listening quietly and saying only short utterances such as "mmhmm" and "uh-huh" is considered passive listening.

4. What is advised when initially responding to a patient's anger?
   a. Kindly tell the person he or she needs to calm down.
   b. Begin to problem solve to fix whatever is causing the anger.
   c. Defend your position.
   d. Empathically respond.
   e. Listen quietly.

5. What is TRUE about using a "service script" within MTM?
   a. A separate one should be written for each individual providing the same service.
   b. It uses the mnemonic "SPIN" to address patient inquiries about a service.
   c. It is a quality-assurance tool that helps ensure that the same service quality is provided to each patient every time.
   d. It requires motivational interviewing training to change the service recipient's behavior.
   e. Streamlining of what is asked and said is necessary to prevent too many needs for "branching."

6. Which statement is FALSE about the process of conducting a comprehensive medication review (CMR)?
   a. As an interview, it needs to be structured, which means the pharmacist should keep control of the conversation while acknowledging and working within the needs of the patient.
   b. The introduction to the CMR is recommended to contain a brief explanation of the role of the patient during the interview.
   c. It is recommended that pharmacists follow up an important patient-initiated tangential inquiry by first acknowledging the importance of the patient's inquiry.
   d. When organizing the interview, summarizing is used as a means to prepare a patient for a topic that is potentially surprising or off-putting.
   e. Effective closure of the CMR should include the next steps for the patient and for the pharmacist.

7. A motivational interviewing tool that provides an opportunity to respectfully give information to the patient during an MTM visit is referred to as
   a. agenda setting.
   b. elicit-provide-elicit.
   c. the ruler.
   d. typical day.
   e. none of the above.

8. Recommendations for effective communication with older adults includes all of the following EXCEPT
   a. avoiding over accommodation, which can lead to patronizing speech.
   b. reducing long left-branch clauses to improve understandability of speech.
   c. skipping over certain questions about sexual health or substance use to avoid embarrassment.
   d. being prepared for potentially high self-disclosure when asking how they are doing.
   e. recognizing their resiliency, knowledge, and experiences.

9. When communicating with other professionals, SBAR is
   a. used as a means of verification.
   b. most applicable in urgent patient care situations.
   c. characterized by its level of aggressiveness.
   d. advocated in the Code of Conduct to address inappropriate and disruptive behaviors by healthcare professionals.
   e. used to communicate a patient's situation and background and your own assessment and recommendation.

10. Which statement is TRUE in relation to the Collaborative Working Relationship Model (developed by McDonough and Doucette)?
    a. It is advocated that pharmacists target physicians who are specialists rather than generalists.
    b. The professional recognition stage (stage 1) is characterized by development of a collaborative practice agreement.
    c. Pharmacists and physicians are expected to work equally as hard to develop the working relationship.
    d. An intermediary stage is characterized by a time of trial in which the physician tests the pharmacist's commitment and ability.
    e. All of the above are true.

ANSWERS

1. d	2. b	3. a
4. e	5. c	6. d
7. b	8. c	9. e
10. d		

9

Documentation

Aditi V. Patel, PharmD, Amber M. Connelly, PharmD, and David M. Angaran, MS, FCCP, FASHP

KEY POINTS

- Knowing how to document is an essential part of being a member of the medical team. The old adage, "If you didn't document it, it didn't happen," still holds true.
- Pharmacists can deliver medication therapy management (MTM) services anywhere, including the pharmacy, clinic, hospital, or even inside the patient's home. This physical separation from prescribers creates unique barriers that need consideration prior to documentation.
- The Patient Protection and Affordable Care Act (PPACA) mandates that pharmacists should document MTM encounters; however, precise instructions on how to document have yet to be determined.
- The pharmacy community at large is still searching for ways to implement strategies that will allow a bidirectional flow of clinical and medication-related information.
- Barriers to documentation include, but are not limited to: where does MTM fit into work flow in retail pharmacies, how do pharmacists feel about documenting patient encounters, and how can a patient's complete medical record be used to document an MTM encounter?
- The documentation requirements that Medicare defines are: each patient who completes an MTM appointment must receive a personal medication list (PML) and medication action plan (MAP).
- CMS has not created a standardized way of communicating recommendations to prescribers. Eventually, the PML, MAP, and prescriber communication have to be integrated into a multidisciplinary care plan to coordinate patient care.
- In order to be recognized as a Medicare provider and bill for services, providers need to know how to document services appropriately, and pharmacists are no exception. In order to be MTM providers and bill Medicare, a documentation process needs to be established.
- Electronic health records (EHRs) improve continuity of care. MTM software should abide by similar standardization requirements.
- As patients gain more access to their health records, personal health records (PHR) need to be Health Insurance Portability and Accountability Act (HIPAA) compliant and user-friendly.
- Documentation evaluations traditionally focus on presence or absence of documentation and clinical accuracy. The challenge is establishing methods to measure the documentation efforts of individual providers.
- Pharmacists can minimize documentation errors by being: correct, complete, concise, consistent, and cautious.

INTRODUCTION

Documentation is inherent to most professions. Pharmacy has always been on the outside of the medical record looking in and treading lightly. The profession is now at the point where a convergence of law, regulation, performance measures, restructured care, financial realignment, and health information technology make adequate documentation essential for professional growth. The old statement, "If you didn't document it, you didn't do it," could be expanded to say, "If your documentation is not shared with the healthcare team, you are not a team member."

Becoming a deemed Medicare provider is going to require the pharmacist be able to follow Medicare rules on evaluation and management (E&M) to be reimbursed and avoid being fined for inadequate documentation. In addition, quality improvement requires that everyone's contribution, or lack of, be part of the record for evaluation. The pharmacist's verbal prescription counseling over the counter (OTC) are words lost in the wind and allow for no evaluation for improvement.

Another Information Silo

The typical pharmacy practice involves a professional operating at a physical distance and lacking real insight into the physician's overall therapeutic goals for the patient. The pharmacist has always dispensed advice to patients without documentation or communicating with the physician and other health team members. This separation, with its ensuing lack of information exchange and coordination of care, has not been conducive to professional relationships (see Chapter 6). MTM has now added a new layer of complexity. Some items to consider:

1. **Why didn't my patient tell me that?** The comprehensive medication review (CMR) interview is a unique event in pharmacy practice that will frequently uncover relevant facts unknown to the physician. While patients often confide in pharmacists about their symptoms or concerns that they have not shared with their physicians, this information is now documented in a permanent record. One can understand how a physician could be embarrassed about being presented with previously unknown information about a patient with whom he or she had a long-term and seemingly trusting relationship.
2. **I have not thought about this patient since the last visit.** The usual interaction between physician and pharmacist is tied to a single prescription-related issue and most often occurs just after the patient has come from the physician's office. MTM can take place weeks or months after the last physician visit and may require the prescriber to revisit the patient's chart to determine the appropriate course of action from the interventions suggested by the pharmacist. This constitutes rework (a reactive vs proactive approach)—precisely what every quality improvement program tries to eliminate. (Physicians are pressed for time and generate no revenue.) (See Chapter 6.)
3. **Why is this MTM fax important?** Physicians are inundated with phone calls and faxes about medication-related issues from pharmacists, insurers, and benefit managers, to name a few. Even though the MTM related communication represents more patient-centric information, separating it from the usual data alerts or theoretical drug interactions is a challenge.
4. **The Patient Protection and Affordable Care Act (PPACA).** The PPACA states that MTM should be coordinated and integrated with the broader healthcare management services provided to the patient.[1] Unfortunately, there is no concrete guidance on how this will be accomplished.

MEDICATION THERAPY MANAGEMENT AND DOCUMENTATION

The PPACA clearly states that the pharmacist, when providing MTM, should: "Document the care delivered and communicate essential information about such care, including a summary of the medication review, and the recommendations of the pharmacist to the patient's other health care providers in a timely fashion."[1] MTM is the pharmacist's marching orders to begin the documentation of care beyond prescription claims data and brief interventions associated with drug use evaluation. As pharmacists transition to being "cognitive providers" and expect to be paid for services above and beyond dispensing medications, we can learn by examining how our physician colleagues view the challenges and utility of documentation. Often, conversations on documentation center on obtaining reimbursement for cognitive services.

Koshy et al. provide a physician perspective regarding documentation for reimbursement but emphasize that documentation serves many important purposes beyond getting reimbursed for cognitive services:

> Documentation is key to accurate clinical coding, validating length of stay, resource utilization, physician profiling, case management, severity of illness, risk of mortality, quality management, risk management, clinical outcomes, critical pathways, regulatory compliance, Joint Commission accreditation, managed care, and reimbursement. Good documentation minimizes coding errors, reduces claim denials, and optimizes reimbursement. Implementing quality improvement strategies that make documentation and coding an organizational priority can positively influence operations, services, and revenue.[2]

Moving the Profession Toward Documentation

Documenting in an efficient and comprehensive manner is crucial. A 2008 American Pharmacists Association invitational conference addressed the need for a strategy to create a system to integrate MTM documentation into the healthcare system.[3] The ultimate goal for MTM documentation software is to allow pharmacists to have their choice of an integrated documentation-and-billing system for their practices that:

- Is integrated with dispensing systems where applicable.
- Operates using established industry standards to promote connectivity and interoperability.
- Is based on competition among systems regarding functionality—but not on proprietary data elements and limited interfaces.
- Promotes care to individual patients and improves outcomes.
- Improves efficiency as well as effectiveness for providers and the healthcare system for MTM service billing, documentation, standardization, along with interoperability that allows competition while following identified strategies (eg, systems should not compete on data elements and interfaces, but rather on functionality).

The most recent attempt to move the pharmacy profession to documentation and interoperability comes from the Center for Pharmacy Practice Accreditation (CPPA) programs. Their community pharmacy practice standards propose the following:

> Pharmacy practice information systems support effective and efficient documentation into the patient's medication (or pharmacy practice) and/or medical record. Pharmacy practice information systems allow for documentation of prescription medications, OTC medications, dietary supplements, laboratory values, diagnoses, and other information required to deliver available patient care services. Pharmacy practice implements strategies to facilitate bidirectional flow of clinical and medication-related information.
>
> Pharmacy practice is exploring strategies for interfacing with electronic health records (EHRs). The patient electronic medication/medical record is stored and accessible in a manner that facilitates

effective pharmacist communication with other pharmacists in the practice, patients, caregivers, prescribers, or other appropriate health care professionals or organizations.[4]

Barriers to Documentation

Table 9-1 provides a list of the challenges for implementing such a system and an overall game plan to move the profession toward documentation.[5] Unfortunately, CPPA does not address issues on how to reconfigure the current retail practice model, based on prescription volume. Challenges that still need to be addressed, but are not limited to:

1. Where would pharmacists incorporate evaluation and review of a complete patient medical record into their retail practice?
2. Would MTM pharmacists now be liable for drug-related problems because more information is available for the pharmacist to evaluate? (eg, QTc prolongation in the patient's EKG?)
3. Would the medical record be from the primary physician or every physician and provider who is involved in the care of the patient?

One of the most unfortunate oversights in the development of clinical pharmacy was not including time and training for adequate documentation of activities and findings as an essential component of the clinical pharmacist's tasks. The creation of the prescription record was automated and confined to a limited set of data. Therefore, it is unsurprising that documentation, billing confusion, inadequate staffing, and lack of time have become barriers to the provision of MTM services.[6]

Pharmacists are reluctant to document for various reasons, including fear of increased liability, desire to maintain professional relationships with prescribers, and lack of clinical confidence. Nearly 30 years ago, Broadhead and Facchinetti reported on pharmacists' angst and ambivalence regarding documenting pharmacy observations:

> I think documentation can be bad because, legally, it's terrible! Writing a note saying the dosage should be adjusted and then, after treatment, if the patient sues and there's a note from the pharmacist saying that the dosage was wrong... well, that's all it takes! You know it's frequently an academic point whether or not that dosage made a difference. That doesn't matter in a court of law these days. It's just so overwhelming what someone can do with a chart.
>
> I would like to talk to the physician face-to-face. You're trying to correct the mistake in a nonthreatening way. You know, "I'm not trying to put you down for making this mistake, but it's something that I want you to reconsider." It's not that I'm afraid to confront a physician, bending over backward because he's up there and I'm down here. It's just that I want to maintain a relationship and the way you interact is important .... The key thing, I think, is just trying to talk to the person, rather than leaving a note in the chart, which would be the last thing I want to do if I was trying to correct a mistake. Because, then, you are putting the world on notice, and everyone that looks at the chart knows there was a mistake made here and the person may be even more defensive.[7]

Pharmacy practice has come a long way since the aforementioned article. It is important to remember that as long as pharmacists are documenting their recommendations, even if the prescribers do not accept them, they are providing the patient with the best care possible. Whenever recommendations are not made and/or not documented out of fear of rejection, it could be argued that patient care was compromised. Ultimately, recommendations are suggestions that can be accepted or rejected by the prescriber. The profession has adopted the principles of pharmaceutical care and MTM, and pharmacy education now includes extensive pharmacotherapy education. There is extensive literature on successful integration of pharmacists into clinical care teams. Yet, the following was posted online in 2012: "We practice within a medical residency outpatient office. Our pharmacists do a comprehensive

TABLE 9-1 • Challenges for MTM Documentation

- Gaining permission to access records and obtaining information necessary to provide care can be difficult
- Availability of electronic health record systems using HL7 standards in practice
- Connectivity variability/barriers imposed for pharmacists to connect via health information exchanges
- Functionality of current pharmacy management systems
- Inconsistent documentation methods/procedures used by pharmacists
- Most community-based practices have not invested in the implementation of EHR systems built on HL7 standards
- Reasons for lack of implementation of EHR in community-based practice
    - Lack of adequate numbers of patients receiving patient care services
    - Insufficient payment for services/inadequate business model to support substantial capital investment
- Rather than installing EHR systems in practice some pharmacists are only relying on access granted to hospital/health-system EHR systems to provide care to their defined population of patients
- Practices may need to connect to multiple health information exchanges to provide care to their population of patients
- Requirements to enroll in exchanges may vary
- Time consuming
- Majority of community-based practices are using pharmacy management systems built on NCPDP standards systems originally designed for records management of prescription dispensing
- Systems offer variable levels of documentation for services
- Some practices have invested in pharmacy management systems that have been upgraded to permit varying levels of patient care documentation with or without ability to store and retrieve attachments
- Some practices have invested in EHR systems that interface with pharmacy management systems at varying levels
- Pharmacists not recognized by some exchanges as eligible providers
- Training on documentation is highly variable
- Standardized templated formats for concise documentation of patient care not commonly used in practice
- Structured electronic documents such as the Pharmacy Care Note not built into systems used by pharmacists for documenting care
- Community-based pharmacists documenting in multiple systems including paper-based, web portals, and pharmacy management systems
- Community-based pharmacists still relying on faxing information vs electronic exchange of information

Source: Reference 5.

review of patient medical charts prior to their office appointment and leave any pharmacotherapy recommendations to the medical residents **in a temporary "sticky note" section** for their review."[8] While we do not know all the reasons behind the practice of "sticky notes," one interpretation is that we have not come all that far and continue to defer our suggestions to the physician's discretion. Documentation is about taking responsibility. It says to the world, "Here is what I understand about the problem at hand, and here are my recommendations." Documentation implies confidence is clinical knowledge. It informs the reader about one's recommendations that can help optimize a patient's health. As pharmacists, we are asked to make clinical recommendations in every practice setting to ensure safe drug use, and part of doing this is documenting recommendations.

Content and Format

What precisely constitutes a complete MTM record has yet to be defined. The great majority of clinical pharmacy studies that have been conducted are in settings where there was ready access to traditional medical records. If the medical record was not available, the pharmacist's responsibilities were appropriately limited to what was known. As the pharmacist takes on more therapeutic decision-making responsibilities, there is no part of the traditional medical record that is "optional" or lacks importance. Being patient-centered means knowing and understanding the patient's family history, social history, race, culture, other providers' care plans, objective data (eg, lab values and x-rays), treatment history, etc. Now the issue is not about not having the information available, but instead it is about what to do with all that is known about the patient. It is hard to envision having access to a patient's complete medical record in a traditional dispensing pharmacy and incorporating those into the provisions of MTM.

MEDICARE PART D MEDICATION THERAPY MANAGEMENT PROGRAM STANDARDIZED FORMAT

Medicare has provided detailed guidance on the structure and content of the personal medication list (PML) and medication action plan (MAP) (Appendix 9-1).[9] The PML, MAP, and prescriber communication, alone, do not constitute as adequate documentation, as described in Tables 9-2 and 9-3.[10,11] Both tables provide a

TABLE 9-2 • Guidelines for Documenting the Comprehensive Medication Review

1. A record of the patient's medication experience (understanding, concerns, preferences, beliefs, behavior)
2. Medication allergies (along with a description of the allergy, time frame, and severity) and adverse reactions (separated into dose-related and preventable)
3. Medication history (including immunizations), complete with dates, effectiveness information, record of issues, problems, etc
4. Current medication record (including all medications regardless of source, mode of administration, or prescriber); indication for use, product, dose, and duration, and how the medication is actually being taken
5. Active drug therapy problem list, complete with the cause of each problem (associated with the medical condition and medications relating to the drug therapy problem)
6. Therapeutic treatment plans for the patient and practitioner (a patient and prescriber version of the treatment plan needs to be available, provided, and communicated). The following functionality must be available in the electronic therapeutic record to provide medication management services:
   (a) Connect indication for medication (reason for use) to specific drug product, dose, duration, and actual outcomes for each medical condition
   (b) Identify, resolve, and prevent drug therapy problems:
      Appropriateness:
      - Eliminate unnecessary medications
      - Initiate necessary medications not being taken
      Effectiveness:
      - Identify most effective medication in specific patient
      - Increase dosages to effective levels
      Safety:
      - Eliminate toxicities
      - Identify adverse reactions
      Adherence:
      - Increase patient's willingness to adhere to medication regimen
      The cause of each of the aforementioned drug therapy problems also needs to be documented.
   (c) Record and evaluate actual outcomes from drug therapy
      - Record personalized therapy goals and evaluate against outcome measures for each medical condition
      - Graph laboratory levels against changes in drug therapy and doses
      - Record outcome changes with changes in medication details
   (d) Provide postmarketing surveillance on appropriateness, effectiveness, safety, and adherence variables
   (e) Record drug therapy problems specific to drug product, medical condition, and patient parameters
   (f) Offer clinical decision support and analysis
   (g) Support patient participation and decision making in drug therapy (adherence tools, record keeping, etc)
   (h) Provide patients with medication information that is individualized and complements the therapeutic care plan

Source: Reference 10.

TABLE 9-3 • MTM Patient Documentation

Pharmacist must document each patient encounter.
Documentation must include but should not be limited to:

Patient Information
- First name
- Last name
- Middle initial
- Address
- Phone number
- Gender
- Date of Birth
- Current medical conditions
- Resolved medical conditions
- Allergies
- Primary physician and contact information

Other Information
- Date of encounter
- Date of documentation
- Time spent with patient
- List of all prescription and nonprescription drugs with their indications
- List drug doses, directions, and intended use
- List of all relevant medical devices
- List all dietary supplements, herbal products
- Alcohol and tobacco history
- List of environmental factors that impact the patient
- Drug problems identified; assessment of drug problems should include but is not limited to:
    - Determining that the medications are appropriately indicated
    - Determining if patient needs additional medications
    - Determining if the medications are the most effective products available for the conditions
    - Determining if the medications are dosed appropriately to meet goals of therapy
    - Identifying adverse effects caused by medications
    - Determining if the medications are dosed excessively and causing toxicities
    - Determining if the patient is taking the medications appropriately to meet goals of therapy
    - Evaluating effectiveness and safety of current drug therapy
- Written plan including goals and actions needed to resolve issues of current drug therapy
- Evaluation of success in meeting goals of medication treatment plan
- Information, instructions, and resources delivered to the patient
- Content of pharmacist's communications to patient's other healthcare providers

Billing

The level of payment is based on patient need and patient need is placed into 1 of 5 levels. The payment level is calculated to be at the lowest level where all the qualifying criteria are met:
- The number of medications the patient is currently taking
- The number of drug therapy problems the patient has at present
- The number of medical conditions for which the patient is currently being treated

Source: Reference 11.

comprehensive overview of the documentation content, but neither provide direction on just how the data should be summarized to be clear, concise, and credible. Various MTM platforms or programs do a great job at offering a place for medication lists to be entered, and some even capture adherence data and allow side effect information to be inputted with the medication list. Other platforms provide unique documentation spaces, but what should be included in that space is up to the pharmacist completing the MTM session. Medication therapy problems need to be identified, and if acted upon, (ie, recommendation is sent to the prescriber or the patient) documentation needs to happen. This blank canvas is used for pharmacists to efficiently summarize the encounter and rationalize clinical judgement to avoid any gaps in communication. The Subjective, Objective, Assessment, and Plan (SOAP) format is widely used (Table 9-4).[12] Another format is the situation, background, assessment, resolution (SBAR) method. The following is an example:

S: During her MTM interview, Mrs. Doe said that she has developed a dry hacking cough over the last 3 weeks.

B: She started taking lisinopril 10 mg daily for hypertension on March 17, 2013, which was 3.5 weeks ago. No other medication changes are noted, and she has no other complaints.

A: The cough may be associated with lisinopril. ACE inhibitor-induced cough most commonly occurs early in therapy and does not resolve on its own.

R: Consider substituting the lisinopril with an ARB, which is the recommended strategy for ACE inhibitor-induced cough. Losartan (Cozaar) is the formulary ARB of choice.

The CMS standardized form is silent on the content and organization of communications to a prescriber that arise from a CMR. The mode of communication between the prescriber and the pharmacist may influence the acceptance of the MTM interventions and the pharmacist's professional relationship with the prescriber. For example, a face-to-face communication with the prescriber be more effective than compared to faxing a recommendation to the

TABLE 9-4 • SOAP Documentation

1. **Subjective:** symptoms the patient or caregiver verbally expresses. These descriptions provide a clinician with insight into the severity of a patient's condition, the level of dysfunction, the illness progression, and the degree of pain.
2. **Objective:** measurements that are observed (seen, heard, touched, smelled) by the clinician. Examples include vital signs, pulse, temperature, skin color, edema, and diagnostic testing.
3. **Assessment:** a prioritized list of assessed patient conditions. This may consist of the level of control, differentials, potential confounders to control, pertinent positive or negative signs and symptoms related to the condition, reference to evidence-based medicine goals, considerations for pharmacotherapy, and adjunctive lifestyle measures.
4. **Plan:** care plan action steps for the patient and healthcare practitioners. These steps may include requests for laboratory or diagnostic assessments, alterations in pharmacotherapy, lifestyle recommendations, standards of care, special directions, referrals, self-monitoring, emergency contacts, and time to follow-up appointments.

Source: Reference 12.

prescriber's office. Most MTM services are undertaken without access to complete medical records and with variable patient prescriber relationships. This presents a challenge on how to communicate accurate information while simultaneously acknowledging the lack of a complete picture of the patient's conditions, care plan, and the physician's therapeutic strategies. (See examples of how lack of information may affect the choice of words and certainty of recommendations in the following section.)

Identifying drug-related problems from what the patient says and claims data presents a challenge regarding the degree of certainty that can be expressed in a written communication. Given an apparent drug-related problem, it would be prudent to avoid stating unequivocal causality, assuming the prescriber has made an error, or has neglected to provide information to the patient. Word choice can make all the difference:

- **Avoid "is caused by,"** eg, "The cough is caused by lisinopril."
  - **Instead, raise the possibility,** eg, "May be caused by," "Has been reported," "Is commonly associated with."
- **Avoid making determinations,** eg, "Your patient HAS NOT responded to X drug."
  - **Instead, report the facts,** eg, "The patient reports a BP of 150/100"; "The patient reports pain as 9 out of a possible 10."
- **Avoid using judgmental language,** eg, "The patient is INADEQUATELY being treated for diabetes."
  - **Instead, cite sources,** eg, "ADA guidelines give a grade A recommendation for the inclusion of HMG CO-A's for patients with type 2 diabetes."
- **Avoid appearing to question the physician's knowledge,** eg, "You may not be aware that your patient is taking OTC and herbal medications."
  - **Instead, report the facts,** eg, "Patient reported taking the following OTC and herbal medications."
- **Avoid a condescending tone,** eg, "Since your patient has heart failure, she requires an ACE inhibitor and beta blocker."
  - **Instead, cite sources,** eg, "The AHA guidelines on heart failure recommend the use of ACE inhibitors and beta blockers."
- **Avoid accusations,** eg, "Patient lacked information or was misinformed."
  - **Instead, relay the circumstances,** eg, "The patient couldn't relate an understanding of his disease state."
- **Avoid terms like *unnecessary drugs* and *polypharmacy*.**
  - **Instead, use patient-centered terms,** eg, "The patient expressed a desire to reduce his or her total number of drugs"; "The patient was unable to provide an indication for the following therapy."
- **Avoid the term *contraindicated*.**
  - **Instead, cite sources,** eg, "Use with caution; our source recommends avoiding this medication, if possible, for this condition or in this situation or with this allergy."
- **Avoid making diagnoses,** eg, "The patient is depressed."
  - **Instead, report the facts,** eg, "The patient reported being very sad, losing weight, not sleeping well, and having trouble concentrating."

Care Plan

Even if you have a complete PML, MAP, and prescriber communication, there still needs to be a summary and care plan to ensure follow-up and continuity of care. Table 9-5 provides an overview of the essential elements of a care plan.[13]

As of now, CMS does not require the PML and MAP to be shared among the patient's other healthcare providers. It is not hard to imagine the confusion and possible negative consequences that could result from the lack of coordination between the MTM PML, MAP, and the care plan proposed by the physician or other healthcare providers. Just how the PML, MAP, and prescriber communication will be integrated into the multidisciplinary care plan and coordinated among other health professionals has yet to be resolved.

Documentation for Billing

It is only recently, with the advent of pharmacy Current Procedural Terminology (CPT) codes, that proper documentation for the purpose of reimbursement has needed to be addressed. Pharmacist use of CPT codes is discussed in Chapter 10. If the pharmacist is going to become a qualified MTM provider and bill Medicare, he or she must adopt a sophisticated approach to billing.

TABLE 9-5 • Care Plan

The plan of care should be jointly created and managed by the patient, caregiver, and care provider according to their preferences and the accountable provider. Elements of the plan of care should include, but not be limited to:

- Patient's diagnosis or problem
- Updated list of medications
- Appointments for follow-up care
- Environmental or social factors that may contribute to the problem
- Other known factors that may contribute to the problem, including assets and strengths
- Plan of care to address the diagnosis or problem, including preventive care
- Documentation of the surrogate decision-maker for patient care
- Self-management training and skills identified by the patient
- Evaluation of participation and level of engagement in activities of daily living
- Existence of advance directives

Based on NQF Preferred Practice 22

Data elements should accompany the patient during all transitions of care and should be appropriate to the type of transition and accessible throughout the transition. These core data elements should include, but not be limited to:

- Medical diagnosis and significant health problems
- Clinical status
- Medication lists
- Treatments/procedures completed within the setting
- All treatments (durable medical equipment [DME], medications, therapies) including posttransitions treatments
- Relevant past medical history
- Functional status
- Communication skills
- Patient and caregiver priorities for care
- Preferences relevant to the transition
- Advance directive status

Source: Reference 13.

Edsall and Moore provide an overview from the physician perspective on how to document an encounter for Medicare billing. They address the appropriate level of complexity to justify the appropriate CPT code and payment:

> *The rationale is that any such step implies an increase in the complexity and volume of the data you need to win now. Specifically, they (CMS) ask that you make sure the documentation reflects the following:*

- The nature of any diagnostic service you order, plan, schedule or perform at the time of the encounter.
- Any review of diagnostic test results that you perform. An entry in the progress note such as "WBC elevated" or "chest x-ray unremarkable" is acceptable, as is your simply initialing and dating the reports of test results.
- Any decision to review old records or obtain history from sources other than the patient.
- Relevant findings from any review of old records or from any additional history you obtain—or a note to the effect that you carried out such a review but found no additional relevant information. "Old records reviewed" or "additional history obtained from family" is not enough. You need to give relevant findings or say explicitly that there were none.
- The results of any discussion you have with the physician who carried out or interpreted a diagnostic test or service. That the guidelines talk about "*discussion of contradictory or unexpected test results*" (emphasis added) at least suggests the possibility that carriers might question such a discussion of results unless they were contradictory or unexpected.
- Your "direct visualization and independent interpretation of an image, tracing or specimen" that has been or will be interpreted by another physician. Again, the guidelines suggest that such independent checking is not expected to be a regular thing, but rather something that happens only "on occasion."[14]

The Electronic Health Record

There is a remarkable lack of definition and guidelines for MTM software beyond providing the necessary forms and reports for CMS. Therefore, the Electronic Health Record (EHR) will be the focus of this section, with the anticipation that MTM and EHR will be interchangeable in a number of situations. According to HIMSS:

> The EHR is a longitudinal electronic record of patient health information generated by one or more encounters in any care delivery setting. Included in this information are patient demographics, progress notes, problems, medications, vital signs, past medical history, immunizations, laboratory data and radiology reports. The EHR automates and streamlines the clinician's workflow. The EHR has the ability to generate a complete record of a clinical patient encounter—as well as supporting other care-related activities directly or indirectly via interface—including evidence-based decision support, quality management, and outcomes reporting.[15]

The days of the paper medical chart are numbered. The EHR brings with it some great advantages as well as some challenges. One of the advantages is that it supports continuity of care and measurement of performance. Table 9-6 provides the elements necessary for an EHR to be legally compliant.[16] These criteria should apply equally to any MTM software.

Medicare recognizes that MTM is currently an information silo. CMS is raising awareness of coming changes by encouraging proactive integration of what will likely become required changes:

> Plan sponsors are encouraged to adopt standardized health information technology (HIT) for documentation of MTM services. Structured, universal codes are available for clinical coding of MTM services delivered to beneficiaries, such as findings, recommendations, and outcomes. The use of standardized coding systems improves the efficiency of documentation by the MTM provider, supports consistent clinical record keeping, facilitates the transfer of information between healthcare providers and beneficiaries, and will allow better collection and analysis of the impact of MTM services on beneficiaries' care. CMS is considering the expansion of the MTM reporting requirements to collect the findings and recommendations that were discussed during CMRs and listed in the beneficiary's MAP. Combining standardized coding systems (eg, SNOMED) and

TABLE 9-6 • The Basics of a Legal Electronic Health Record

Do not assume that a given EHR will meet all the requirements for a legal record. As the EHR marketplace increases awareness of these matters, products will continue to improve. Here are four areas to look at:

How is documentation created?
- Is the author of each element of documentation accurately recorded, including the author of vitals, chief complaint, history of present illness, orders, plans, and prescriptions?
- How are different, successive versions of the encounter (before signature) treated?
- Do signature procedures and tools meet your state's and your organization's requirements?

How is documentation managed and preserved over time?
- After signature, if a correction, clarification, or amendment is added, is it clear what is original and what is not, and can all original documentation be recovered if needed?
- How is documentation protected from being altered, in all parts of the system including the underlying database?
- How are new templates, guidelines, forms, etc, created, preserved, retired?
- Are all clinical messages and clinical behaviors (prompts, etc) reproducible and recoverable?
- Do other periodic and necessary tasks, such as report creation and auditing, also expose documentation to additional security risks?
- Are critical support functions, such as auditing, always operable and reasonably accessible, or do they require vendor supports or other extra costs?

How does documentation interact with billing?
- Does the system prompt users to add documentation for "improved revenue?"
- Does the system allow the sending of billing information without completion of documentation?
- Does the system send billing information for tests without means to ensure the tests were actually done?

How is documentation presented?
- When asked to produce a view or a printout of an encounter, does the system offer a view that conforms to your organization's definition of its legal record?
- If documentation has been amended or otherwise altered, is that clearly identified in the viewed and printed version?

Source: Reference 16.

industry-supported templates will also enable sponsors to update and print summaries of CMRs in a standardized format based on standard elements in databases and EHRs rather than manipulating free-form text documents.[17]

Imagine a healthcare record written composed of information written in Russian, English, and Chinese.

While an exaggeration, it represents the challenges for the electronic exchange of current information. Systematized Nomenclature of Medicine–Clinical Terms (SNOMED CT) codes, a standardized nomenclature set, allow electronic submission of data. This set of codes was developed by the National Library of Medicine and is now required as part of the enhanced medication therapy model.

The use of SNOMED CT codes to document patient care, will allow for the following:

Comprehensive Medication Management (CMM) documentation to be captured using structured data that can be easily retrieved, sorted, and analyzed to guide individual patient care.

CMM documentation to be captured using structured data that can be easily retrieved, sorted, and analyzed for reports and quality improvement. Further, these data can be correlated to patient care outcomes affected by these pharmacist-provided services.

CMM documentation to be captured in a format determined suitable for health information in order that patient data can be integrated into the EHR and be interoperable with other systems.[18]

Refer to SNOMED CT documents that address the development and use of the codes for MTM Services.[18] Table 9-7 provides an example of how the SNOMED CT codes would be used in the conduct of a CMM interview.

A challenge beyond the inner workings of the EHR is its influence on the practitioner-patient relationship and communication. Lown and Rodriguez note that:

EHRs introduce a "third party" into exam room interactions that reshapes the patient-physician encounter, alters the patient's narrative, and diverts physicians' attention away from the patients. This diminishes the patient-centeredness of interactions, which in turn affects the patient-physician relationship. As Marshall McLuhan said nearly 50 years ago, "The medium is the message." It changes how we think, how we act, and who we are. Through the new medium of EHRs, will compassionate, effective, patient-centered care get lost in translation?[19]

They go on to point out that "screen-driven" information and behavior may reduce a physician's awareness of the patient's psychosocial and emotional concerns, which are essential for compassionate, patient-centered care. In addition, multitasking between the patient and the screen can lead to errors.[19]

TABLE 9-7 • Exhibit 2: Comprehensive Documentation of Services (Example #1)

Beneficiary Sequence	Encounter Date	Encounter Code	Encounter Code Description
1	20170110	435411000124108	Patient notified of eligibility for medication therapy management service (situation)
2	20170117	448337001	Telemedicine consultation with patient (procedure)
3	20170201	432341000124108	Taking multiple medications for chronic diseases (finding)
4	20170201	448177004	Adverse drug interaction with drug (disorder)
5	20170201	408377007	Compliance issues discussed with patient (finding)
6	20170210	11429006	Consultation (procedure)
7	20170210	447871000124109	Medication therapy management recommendation accepted by prescriber (situation)
8	20170210	395006008	Medication stopped—interaction (situation)
9	20170215	435441000124107	Medication reminder device setup (procedure)
10	20170305	448337001	Telemedicine consultation with patient (procedure)
11	20170305	414059009	Drug therapy compliance observations (finding)
12	20170305	359746009	Patient's condition stable (finding)
13	20170507	1991000124105	Referred by self (finding)
14	20170507	448337001	Telemedicine consultation with patient (procedure)
15	20170507	448511000124101	Transition from acute care to self-care (finding)
16	20170507	6021000124103	Targeted medication therapy review (procedure)
17	20170507	473234001	Dyslipidemia medication review (procedure)
18	20170507	473226007	Heart failure medication review (procedure)
19	20170507	423167009	Chronic disease process education (procedure)
20	20170507	162667001	Patient's condition poor (finding)

Source: CMS. Medicare Part D Enhanced Medication Therapy Management (MTM) Model, Enhanced MTM Model Encounter Data Specification Plan. July 28, 2016 (version 1). https://innovation.cms.gov/files/x/mtm-encounterplan.pdf. Accessed December 22, 2016.

Personal Health Record

The role of patients in documenting their care continues to evolve as they become more active participants in the decision-making process. The internet has empowered patients to educate themselves about their disease states as well as treatments and to share experiences with others who have the same conditions. The last and possibly most important source of information was their medical record. CMS has given notice that the patient is going to be an active part of the documentation process:

> HIPAA specifies that an individual's right of access to personal health information, as it applies to health plans, includes the health plan's enrollment, payment, claims adjudication, and case or medical management record systems, as well as any records used in whole or in part by or for the health plan to make decisions about the individual (45 C.F.R. 164.501).[8] The Blue Button Initiative is Medicare's way of encouraging Medicare Advantage Organizations to allow beneficiaries to download PHI. The Blue Button was created by the Department of Veterans Affairs. It is available, at no cost, at expanding use of the Blue Button Initiative (http://www.va.gov/bluebutton/).[17]

The Blue Button and enabling beneficiaries to download their own health records is just a short step away from the personal health record, as discussed by CMS in the following section:

> In general, a Personal Health Record (PHR) is controlled by the individual, and can be shared with others, including caregivers, family members and providers. This is different from a provider's EHR, which is controlled by the provider just as paper medical records are today. Ideally, a Personal Health Record will have a fairly complete summary of an individual's health and medical history based on data from many sources, including information entered by the individual (allergies, OTC medications, family history, etc).[20]

Table 9-8 provides advice for consumers about what to expect from a PHR as well as questions to ask. These are relevant to all healthcare providers as they transition to working with PHRs. A major innovative effort to test giving patients access to their own medical records was named "Open Notes." While not conclusive, the study did provide support that shared notes may improve patient-practitioner communication, safety, relationships and stimulate greater patient involvement in their own care. The implications of this for all healthcare practitioners is of a great magnitude. One of the most interesting is the concept of a flipped clinic visit, where the patient reads his or her care notes prior to an office visit, allowing for more open time. The challenges would be manifold, including how would documentation change about sensitive topics or observations, what vocabulary would be appropriate, and how to settle disagreements about the interpretation of the record, to name a few. It would seem that this is the future, in which we really are committed to being transparent and patient-centric.[21]

Quality Improvement

There is very little in literature about assessing the quality of pharmacy documentation. It is the author's impression that while verbal communication is taught in every pharmacy school, the art and science of documentation is not part of the curriculum. Milchak et al described a peer review process in a managed care organization (Figure 9-1).[22] While their peer review data collection sheet

TABLE 9-8 • The Personal Health Record

Attributes of the PHR

The following attributes describe more completely the ideal PHR:

Functionality

- Aids the transition from paper to electronic record-keeping
- Allows the individual to refill prescriptions electronically
- Addresses the major issues of health literacy skills (reading and writing) in the context of culture and language
- Allows selective retrieval and formatting of information by individuals or agents
- Is portable (remains with the individual)
- Helps the individual organize personal health information
- Educates the individual about personal health information
- Assists the individual with decision making and health management and wellness (eg, reminders of health activities, health risk assessments, and public health and patient safety alerts)
- Is flexible and expandable to support evolving health needs of the individual and family

Format and Content

- Dynamic record that is continuously updated
- Standard format is electronic
- Incorporates paper documents and other media formats
- Linked with, or contains copies of, provider's legal or electronic records
- Original and immediate source of information is identifiable
- Includes dates of entry and occurrence of all information
- Contains lifelong health information
- Not considered a complete record
- Not restricted by any one format
- Not the legal record or electronic health record of a provider
- Not restricted by culture or language
- Providers use their professional judgment, as they do with any patient-supplied history, for clinical decision support or health management of the individual

Privacy Access and Control

- Private and secure
- Controlled by the individual
- Accessible any place and time by individual
- Accessible in an emergency
- Individual has primary responsibility for the information

Maintenance and Security

- Audit trail shows what information was viewed, by whom, and when
- Amendable by original source as a means of maintaining record integrity
- Individual decides what is incorporated into his or her record

Interoperability

- Achieves easy, accurate, and consistent exchange with others by using communication and health vocabulary standards
- Standard-driven to support evolving health information technology
- Supports structured data collection from individual and stores information using a defined vocabulary
- Links to supportive educational, management, productivity, and quality knowledge bases

Source: Reference 20.

QUARTER OF REVIEW: ________ CPS MEMBER: ________ SUPERVISOR: ________

PATIENT ID#: ________ DATE OF NOTE: ________

SECTION 1: Content (required)

1a. Is the source of the referral or rationale for being in the patient's chart clearly stated? Y ☐ N ☐

COMMENTS: ________

1b. Are the disease state (s) to be addressed or reason for the referral clearly stated? Y ☐ N ☐ NA ☐

COMMENTS: ________

1c. Is there a verbal or written order documented for any new, stopped or adjusted medication orders? Y ☐ N ☐ NA ☐

COMMENTS: ________

1d. Are the medications and labs ordered accurately? Y ☐ N ☐ NA ☐

COMMENTS: ________

1e. If appropriate or necessary, is follow-up addressed? Y ☐ N ☐ NA ☐

COMMENTS: ________

1f. Does the note have physician approval, either by comments or co signature? Y ☐ N ☐ NA ☐

COMMENTS: ________

1g. Is appropriate or necessary, are subjective, objective, and plan clearly stated? Y ☐ N ☐ NA ☐

COMMENTS: ________

1h. Is plan evidenced based and/or reasonable? Y ☐ N ☐ NA ☐

COMMENTS and OTHER POTENTIAL THERAPEUTIC OPTIONS: ________

SECTION 2: CDTM (as appropriate)

2a. Are medication changes and lab orders consistent with the corresponding CDTM protocol? Y ☐ N ☐ NA ☐

COMMENTS: ________

2b. Is the follow-up consistent with the corresponding CDTM protocol? Y ☐ N ☐ NA ☐

COMMENTS: ________

2c. Was the note sent to an appropriate provider within 24 hours? Y ☐ N ☐

COMMENTS: ________

2d. Was the CDTM referral appropriately documented in the FYI tab of KPHC (N/A, if CDTM is one-time only referral)? Y ☐ N ☐ NA ☐

COMMENTS: ________

2e. Did a PCCPS preceptor sign off on the PGY2 resident's automated medical chart note? Y ☐ N ☐ NA ☐

COMMENTS: ________

SECTION 3: Non-formulary Reviews (as appropriate)

3a. Is the statement of medical necessity from the provider clearly documented prior to proceeding with the non-formulary request?

COMMENTS: ________ Y ☐ N ☐

3b. Is the involvement of the Department Chief or designee clearly stated? ________ Y ☐ N ☐ NA ☐

COMMENTS:

3c. Is the non-formulary approval or denial documented in PIMS (census comment) and KPHC, including a notation in the KPHC Problem List?

COMMENTS: ________ Y ☐ N ☐

3d. Was the non-formulary time frame met?

COMMENTS: ________ Y ☐ N ☐

3e. Does the note include 3 options given to patient if request was denied?

COMMENTS: ________ Y ☐ N ☐ NA ☐

SECTION 4: PharmDoc (required)

4a. Is the referral source correctly documented?

COMMENTS: ________ Y ☐ N ☐

4b. Is the indication section appropriate?

COMMENTS: ________ Y ☐ N ☐

4c. Is the 'action taken' section appropriate?

COMMENTS: ________ Y ☐ N ☐

4d. Is the annual supply correctly calculated?

COMMENTS: ________ Y ☐ N ☐ NA ☐

Signature of Reviewer: ________ Date: ________

Abbreviations:
CDTM = collaborative drug therapy management; CPS = clinical pharmacy specialist; FYI = for your information; KPHC = Kaiser Permanente Health Care; N/A = not applicable; PCCPS = Primary Care Clinical Pharmacy Services; PGY2 = second postgraduate year; PharmDoc = Pharmacy documentation system; PIMS = pharmacy information management system.

FIGURE 9-1 Primary care clinical pharmacy peer review data collection sheet.

Source: Reproduced with permission from Milchak JL, Shanahan RL, Kerzee JA. Implementation of a peer review process to improve documentation consistency of care process indicators in the EMR in a primary care setting. *J Manag Care Pharm*. 2012;18(1)46-53.

provides an efficient way to cover those elements they deemed necessary, it leaves out some important aspects, such as word choice and risk management.

The documentation evaluations focus largely on the presence or absence of documentation and whether all the correct data elements were included. The challenge is how to measure, grade, and improve a practitioner's ability to document in a way that is clear, concise, credible, and complete. This oversight could be explained by the absence in the pharmacy curriculum of writing skills assessments and instruction. This, of course, reflects the lack of need for pharmacists to document beyond filling in rudimentary data fields connected to prescriptions or drug allergies.

The PML, MAP, and prescriber communication all benefit from an understanding of how to engage the audience, educate effectively, and inspire appropriate actions. While a complete discussion about writing is beyond the scope of this chapter, Table 9-9 provides some examples and a valuable reference.[23,24]

TABLE 9-9 • Patient-Centered Language

Plain Language	
Acute	Sudden start, short term, quick
Additional	Extra, added, more
Administer	Give, manage, take care of
Aggravate	Make worse, harm, anger, hurt

Write in a Conversational Style, Using Active Voice

Active voice is the most common sentence structure in English. It is the one we use the most often in conversation because it is clear and direct. It can take several forms, but the basic one has the subject of the sentence performing the verb: *authors write; children play; clients read*. It can take an object: *authors write books; children play games; clients read signs*. Use "Insulin can cause low blood sugar" rather than "Low blood sugar may be caused by insulin."

To make your message informal and appealing, use "we" and "you." To make it direct and easy to understand, write in the active voice. Use "you," "your," and "yours" to address the reader directly. Provide positive actions: "Get your flu shot."

Keep most of your sentences relatively short.

Use simple conjunctions (*or, but, and*).

Limit the number of explanatory or qualifying clauses in your sentences.

Clear and effective material accomplishes the following:

- Attracts the intended reader's attention. Within the MAP, can the patient easily find and understand the most important sentences?
- Holds the reader's attention. Is it in active voice and personalized to the patient and his or her situation?
- Acknowledges and respects the patient. Not everyone is health illiterate, and nobody likes being talked down to. Do you need to write your instructions at a sixth-grade level or medical school level?
- Helps the patient understand the message. This should help patients remember what was talked about in the CMR.
- Move the patient to action. Give clear and concise positive action steps.

Source: Reference 24.

Risk Management

The risk management aspects of documentation should become more important for pharmacists as they learn more about their patients. With MTM, pharmacists can no longer protect themselves by claiming they do not know enough about their patients to be responsible and have this claim supported by a corresponding dearth of information. A proper CMR will frequently uncover new facts that will be documented and require a response of some sort (whether that be patient education, or prescriber outreach, or combination of the two).

The Five C's of Risk Management-Sensitive Practice

1. **Be correct.** Accuracy of expression is essential. Most errors in recordkeeping and communicating result from failure to accurately convey information.
2. **Be complete.** Documents must contain a record and patients must be told all information that is necessary for a continuing high level of care for the patient.
3. **Be concise.** Verbal instructions and patient records should be efficient. Wordy responses are more likely to contain statements that can be misconstrued or that will trigger suspicion or blame.
4. **Be consistent.** Once a pattern of verbal comments or documented remarks develops, a break from that pattern can be interpreted in a way that was not intended.
5. **Be cautious.** Careless use of language can cause people to misinterpret the meaning of even the most innocuous comment or notation.

SUMMARY

MTM documentation is essential for the provision of safe, effective, efficient, and patient-centered care. Pharmacists must be proactive in developing business models and a culture that support the accurate and complete documentation of the care process. The current movement toward all forms of health information technology provides great opportunities and challenges to the pharmacy profession.

REFERENCES

1. The Patient Protection and Affordable Care Act, Pub. L. No. 111-148, §2702, 124 Stat; 2010. http://www.gpo.gov/fdsys/pkg/PLAW-111publ148/pdf/PLAW-111publ148.pdf. Accessed December 22, 2016.
2. Koshy S. Documentation tips for pulmonary medicine implications for the inpatient setting. *Chest.* 2012;14(2):1035-1038.
3. Millonig MK. Mapping the route to medication therapy management documentation and billing standardization and interoperabilility within the health care system: meeting proceedings. *J Am Pharm Assoc.* 2009;49:372-382.
4. Vision for Center for Pharmacy Practice Accreditation (CPPA) Programs. Community pharmacy practice standards: draft for public comment. American Pharmacists Association website. http://www.pharmacist.com/sites/default/files/files/DraftCPPAStandards.pdf. Accessed December 22, 2016.
5. PQA Quality Forum. The changing landscape of pharmacy HIT. CMS/PQA Webinar, PQA Quality Forum: The changing landscape of pharmacy HIT. April 28, 2016. Available at http://pqaalliance.org/images/uploads/files/Apr%202016%20Quality%20Forum_The%20Changing%20Landscape%20of%20Pharmacy%20HIT_Wilkins_Spiro_Owen.pdf. Accessed December 22, 2016.
6. American Pharmacists Association. *Medication Therapy Management Digest: Tracking the Expansion of MTM in 2010.* Washington DC: American Pharmacists Association; 2011.

7. Broadhead RS, Facchinetti NJ. Drug iatrogenesis and clinical pharmacy: the mutual fate of a social problem and a professional movement social problems. *Social Programs.* 1985;32:425-436.

8. American Society of Health-System Pharmacists. Student Association of Community Pharmacists. Ambulatory Care Practitioners Digest for Monday December 31, 2012. Janna Fett. Clinical intervention documentation tool. Available at http://connect.ashp.org/communities/all-discussions/discussions-moderation/message?MID=16490&ssopc=1&ct=36bfa6394ba8c82da8b57ab9c03b77832b0cba0d12ef32cead78bb9243c2d0960415347d38cb640faf51a7086c4c91230a88cb40d294430049d1d850fa203cb1. Accessed December 22, 2016.

9. CMS. Medicare Part D Medication Therapy Management Program. Standardized format. Effective as of January 1, 2013 Form CMS-10396 (01/12) Form Approved OMB No. 0938-1154. CMS website. https://www.cms.gov/Medicare/Prescription-Drug-Coverage/PrescriptionDrugCovContra/Downloads/MTM-Program-Standardized-Format-English-and-Spanish-Instructions-Samples-.pdf. Accessed December 22, 2016.

10. McInnis T, Webb E, Strand L. *The Patient-Centered Medical Home: Integrating Comprehensive Medication Management to Optimize Patient Outcomes.* 2nd ed. June 2012. Appendix A: guidelines. http://www.accp.com/docs/positions/misc/CMM%20Resource%20Guide.pdf. Accessed December 22, 2016.

11. Minnesota Department of Human Services. The 2005 Minnesota legislature directed the Minnesota Department of Human Services (DHS) to pay qualified pharmacist for medication therapy management services (MTMS) for Medicaid or general assistance medical care recipients. Revised August 8, 2015. Available at http://www.dhs.state.mn.us/main/idcplg?IdcService=GET_DYNAMIC_CONVERSION&RevisionSelectionMethod=LatestReleased&dDocName=dhs16_136889. Accessed December 12, 2016.

12. Zierler-Brown S, Brown TR, Chen D, Blackburn RW. Clinical documentation for patient care: models, concepts, and liability considerations for pharmacists. *Am J Health-Syst Pharm.* 2007;64(17):1851-1858.

13. McDonald KM, Schultz E, Chapman T, et al. Prospects for care coordination measurement using electronic data sources (Prepared by Stanford University under subcontract to Battelle on Contract No. 290-04-0020–AHRQ SQI-II.) AHRQ Publication No. 12-0014-EF. Rockville, MD: Agency for Healthcare Research and Quality; March 2012.

14. Edsall RL, Moore KJ. Thinking on paper: documenting decision making. *Fam Pract Manage.* July/August 2010;10-15.

15. Electronic health records. Available at http://www.himss.org/library/ehr/?navItemNumber=13261. Accessed December 22, 2016.

16. The Legal Electronic Health Record. http://www.himss.org/legal-electronic-medical-record-himss. Accessed December 22, 2016.

17. CMS. Advance notice of methodological changes for calendar year (CY) 2014 for Medicare Advantage (MA) Capitation Rates, Part C and Part D Payment Policies and 2014 Call Letter. https://www.cms.gov/Medicare/Health-Plans/MedicareAdvtgSpecRateStats/Downloads/Advance2017.pdf. Accessed December 22, 2016.

18. Pharmacy Health Information Technology Collaborative. Documenting Comprehensive Medication Management in Team-Based Models Using SNOMED CT Codes August 1, 2014. http://www.pharmacyhit.org/pdfs/workshop-documents/WG2-Post-2014-03.pdf. Accessed December 22, 2016.

19. Lown BA, Rodriguez D. Commentary: lost in translation? How electronic health records structure communication, relationships, and meaning. *Acad Med.* 2012;87(4):392-394.

20. Burrington-Brown J, Fishel J, Fox L, et al; AHIMA e-HIM Personal Health Record Work Group. Defining the personal health record. *J AHIMA.* 2005;76(6):24-25.

21. Sigall K, Bell MD, Deblanco T, Walker J. OpenNotes: how the power of knowing can change health care. Published October 27, 2016. http://catalyst.nejm.org/opennotes-knowing-change-health-care/?utm_campaign=Connect+Weekly&utm_source=hs_email&utm_medium=email&utm_content=36802887&_hsenc=p2ANqtz--yJlbu9cxdQrlEgMULK3QQzZqGarnRi-FjCnuiD7Kay2mHRLOkvU68VGqllEVg_BbK4fMKyQBFzbhIVWAjLQAqcnxkYw&_hsmi=36802887. Accessed December 22, 2016.

22. Milchak JL, Shanahan RL, Kerzee JA. Implementation of a peer review process to improve documentation consistency of care process indicators in the EMR in a primary care setting. *J Manag Care Pharm.* 2012;18(1):46-53.

23. Plain Language Thesaurus: National Center for Health Marketing Draft Version 10 2009. Available at http://www.plainlanguage.gov/populartopics/health_literacy/thesaurus_v-10.doc. Accessed December 22, 2016.

24. CMS. Toolkit for making written material clear and effective. ToolkitPart01-03Files.zip [ZIP, 3MB]. http://www.cms.gov/Outreach-and-Education/Outreach/WrittenMaterialsToolkit/index.html?redirect=/WrittenMaterialsToolkit/. Accessed December 22, 2016.

Review Questions

1. Barriers to pharmacist documentation include all of the following EXCEPT
   a. pharmacy culture and relationship to physicians.
   b. job descriptions do not include documentation as a primary responsibility.
   c. technology limitations.
   d. lack of documentation experience.
   e. that it is not required since pharmacists are not Medicare qualified providers.

2. MTM documentation challenges include all of the following EXCEPT
   a. varying documentation methods.
   b. that HIPAA prohibits pharmacists from documenting social and family histories.
   c. adoption of SNOMED terminology.
   d. pharmacy practice setting diversity.
   e. lack of MTM software interoperability.

3. Which statement is true about MTM-required documentation?
   a. The MAP must include all identified problems.
   b. The PML may only include Part D medications.
   c. The care plan is not part of MTM documentation.
   d. The physician communication must be sent by fax.
   e. The physician communication must be in the SOAP format.

4. Creating a MAP requires
   a. the patient must fill out the action part and return it to the MTM provider.
   b. writing in such a way to gain attention, hold attention, achieve understanding, and move to appropriate action.
   c. CMS-approved MAP content for disease conditions.
   d. the physician must sign off on the MAP.
   e. the MAP must include comments on medication adherence and access to low-cost medications.

5. Which of the following is a question that a patient using a personal health record (PHR) should ask?
   a. Can I allow my physicians or family members to look at my PHR for me?
   b. If a physician offers a PHR, can I use it to refill my prescriptions or make appointments?
   c. What are the PHR's privacy and security policies?
   d. What happens to my PHR information if I leave a health plan or change physicians?
   e. All of the above.

6. All of the following are risk-management-appropriate strategies for recording observations EXCEPT
   a. document all positive findings that are essential to an evaluation or to patient care.
   b. document positive findings that are customarily recorded in similar situations.
   c. avoid including negative findings because they make documentation too lengthy.
   d. continuous processes that are unchanged need not be recorded.
   e. any lists written in the record should either be complete or contain a general inclusive statement.

7. The PML, MAP, and physician letter do not meet the criteria for complete documentation of the MTM encounter because
   a. the physician's progress notes are not included.
   b. they are in the SOAP format.
   c. they are not written at the sixth-grade level.
   d. they are not included in the medical record.
   e. none of the above.

8. Which statement best describes the EHR?
   a. It improves patient-provider verbal communication.
   b. It makes the Blue Button initiative possible.
   c. It eliminates cultural barriers to pharmacist documentation.
   d. It eliminates time barriers for pharmacist documentation.
   e. It has achieved interoperability between systems.

9. What is a word choice that should be avoided when documenting a drug-related problem?
   a. The patient's edema may be caused by amlodipine 10 mg tablets.
   b. The patient reports needing to use his inhaler three times daily due to wheezing.
   c. The physician is not aware that the patient is depressed.
   d. The patient was unable to identify which inhaler is used for maintenance therapy and which is used for symptom management.

10. Which statement accurately describes an ideal MTM documentation software?
    a. The software is integrated with dispensing systems (if applicable).
    b. The software does not connect or communicate with other networks.
    c. Clinical decisions are standardized based on automatic responses; individualized care does not fit into the system.
    d. The interfaces are complex and prolong patient appointments.

ANSWERS

1. e	2. b	3. c
4. b	5. e	6. c
7. e	8. b	9. c
10. a		

Appendix 9-1

Medicare Part D Medication Therapy Management Program Standardized Format

INSTRUCTIONS FOR IMPLEMENTING THE STANDARDIZED FORMAT

Changes included in this revision (08/15/2012) apply to cognitively impaired beneficiaries and to the Spanish translation of the Standardized Format:

1. Recommendations for using the Standardized Format for summaries of CMRs performed for cognitively impaired beneficiaries are described on pages 144, 146, 152.
    a. The requirement to offer CMRs to all beneficiaries, regardless of setting, is described on page 144.
    b. Content for the *Inside Address* and the *Additional Space* fields are described on page 146.
    c. Use of the carbon-copy field is described on page 146.
    d. Adding the name of the person who represented the beneficiary as a data source in the PML is described on page 152.
2. Changes related to the Spanish translation appear in on page 161.
    a. Added an accent to the word "como" in second paragraph of the Cover Letter (CL).
    b. Adjusted the text to properly display small caps for the Titles and Date Prepared fields in the MAP and PML.
    c. Deleted the second occurrence of the word "la" in the third bullet of the instructions in the PML.
    d. Added additional spacing within the instruction section in the PML.
    e. Changed both words to title case in "Otra Information" in the PML.

INTRODUCTION

The Medicare Part D MTM Program Standardized Format (Format) is a written summary of a CMR. A CMR is an interactive, person-to-person, or telehealth medication review and consultation of a beneficiary's medications (including prescriptions, OTC medications, herbal therapies, and dietary supplements) by a pharmacist or qualified provider that is intended to aid in assessing medication therapy and optimizing patient outcomes. Part D sponsors must, at a minimum, offer a CMR annually for targeted beneficiaries and provide written summaries. The summaries must comply with requirements as specified by CMS for the Format as of January 1, 2013.

BACKGROUND

Section 10328 of the Affordable Care Act amended section 1860D-4(c)(2)(ii) of the Act to require prescription drug plan sponsors to offer, at a minimum, an annual CMR that may be furnished person-to-person or via telehealth technologies. The CMR must include a review of the individual's medications, which may result in the creation of a recommended MAP with a written or printed summary of the results of the review provided to the targeted individual. The Act further required the development of a standardized format for the action plan and summary. Standardization of the format of these documents is expected to improve the quality of the MTM program services and provide consistency in beneficiary communications across differing Medicare Part D programs.

As noted previously, a CMR is an interactive, person-to-person, or telehealth medication review and consultation of a beneficiary's medications (including prescriptions, OTC medications, herbal therapies, and dietary supplements) by a pharmacist or qualified provider that is intended to aid in assessing medication therapy and optimizing patient outcomes. Refer to Chapter 7—Medication Therapy Management and Quality Improvement Program—of the Prescription Drug Benefit Manual (http://www.cms.gov/Medicare/Prescription-Drug-Coverage/PrescriptionDrugCovContra/Downloads/Chapter7.pdf) and other related guidance to Part D plans for expanded information on the CMR (http://www.cms.gov/Medicare/Prescription-Drug-Coverage/PrescriptionDrugCovContra/MTM.html).

Use of the Format is subject to all applicable rules, regulations, and industry standards, including but not limited to the Health Insurance Portability and Accountability Act (HIPAA) of 1996 and Section 508 of the Rehabilitation Act.

PURPOSE

The purpose of this publication is to provide detailed instructions and examples on how to complete the MTM Program Standardized Format (Form CMS-10396 (01/12), Form Approved OMB No. 0938-1154), which at this time is provided in both English and Spanish.

A blank version of the Standardized Format can be found in Appendix A. Completed samples of the Standardized Format are provided in Appendix B, followed by a Spanish version of the Standardized Format in Appendix C.

COMPONENTS OF THE FORMAT

The Format for the written summary given to beneficiaries after a CMR includes three documents:

- CMR Cover Letter (CL)
- Medication Action Plan (MAP)
- Personal Medication List (PML)

The Format is not considered marketing material and should not include any marketing messages, marketing disclaimers, or other sales information.

LIMITED CUSTOMIZATION OF THE FORMAT

The Format provides a template for the written summary after a CMR. The Format cannot be modified, but the specific content to populate the Format must be tailored to the beneficiary and customized for the Part D plan and MTM program. There is limited variability in the Format for Part D plans to provide additional information, such as supplemental instructions and goals of therapy. This limited variability is provided to meet the unique needs of each beneficiary beyond the requirements of the basic Format and to promote innovation.

The Format should be considered a foundation upon which to innovate to improve healthcare outcomes of beneficiaries, increase quality, reduce costs, and implement new standards for healthcare technology. Part D plans are encouraged to provide supplemental materials in addition to the Format as needed to help beneficiaries manage their healthcare needs. The enclosure notations or postscript of the CL may be used to list or describe supplemental materials that will be included in the package with the Format.

COMMUNICATING WITH THE BENEFICIARY

Pharmacists or other qualified providers who conduct CMRs are encouraged to explain to beneficiaries that the Format, namely the MAP and PML, was created to help beneficiaries get the most benefit from their medications, as well as assist with keeping track of their medications.

The CMR provider should discuss the delivery options for the Format with the beneficiary, such as postal delivery service, transmission by email, or access through a secure Website. Part D plans may provide the Standardized Format to a beneficiary immediately following a CMR, or, if distributed separately, materials must be sent out within 14 calendar days.

Based on stakeholders' feedback and changing demographics of Medicare beneficiaries, there is a Standardized Format available in Spanish. Throughout the instructions booklet, there are unique requirements noted for this version.

GENERAL FORMATTING SPECIFICATIONS

- ***Orientation:*** Portrait orientation is required for all documents of the Format.

- *Paper stock:*
  - Standard letter-size paper stock measuring 8.5 inches by 11 inches.
  - Paper stock should be thick enough (20-22 lb) to keep information on the back from showing through.
  - Different color paper stock may be used, as long as there is high-contrast combination of light paper and dark font color. CMS recommends black text on white or cream-colored nonglossy paper.
- *Margins:* 0.9 to 1 inch on all sides.
- *Font:* 14-point font size is required except where another font size is specified below (eg, **DATE PREPARED** field, footers). Where a specific font is specified, an alternative, equivalent font with the same size, space, and serif specifications and appearance may be used (eg, 7-pt Arial substituted for 7-pt Helvetica). Text sections and field entries must be printed with a serif font, such as Times New Roman or Cambria. Headings and titles are printed in bold font, and a sans serif font, such as Arial or Calibri, may be used. Narrow, compressed, or condensed fonts are prohibited.
- *Justification:* All fields are left justified except where specified below (eg, **DATE PREPARED** field on the MAP and PML is right justified).
- *Header:* Part D plan/MTM program identification should be consistent with other Medicare publications of Part D plans/MTM programs. A header with MTM provider/Part D plan identification must be included on the first page of the CL, MAP, and PML and must not appear on the other pages.
- *Footer:*
  - The **CMS form number and OMB approval number** must appear in the footer of every page of the CL, MAP, and PML. Use Helvetica or equivalent, 7-point font for the CMS-required footer.

Form CMS-10396 (01/12)	Form Approved OMB No. 0938-1154

  - The **Paperwork Reduction Act (PRA) statement** must be included at the bottom of the last page of the PML above or within the CMS-required footer. Use Helvetica or equivalent, 7-point font for the PRA statement.

> According to the Paperwork Reduction Act of 1995, no persons are required to respond to a collection of information unless it displays a valid OMB control number. The valid OMB number for this information collection is 0938-1154. The time required to complete this information collection is estimated to average 37.76 minutes per response, including the time to review instructions, searching existing data resources, gather the data needed, and complete and review the information collection. If you have any comments concerning the accuracy of the time estimate(s) or suggestions for improving this form, please write to: CMS, Attn: PRA Reports Clearance Officer, 7500 Security Boulevard, Baltimore, Maryland 21244-1850.

  - **Page Numbers:** The CL, MAP, and PML forms have their own page numbers and should use 12-point serif font, the same font as the text sections of the documents. Page number sequences must restart at "Page **1** of **Y**" for each document.
  - **Privacy Statement:** Part D plan-specific privacy statements, if desired, may be included on the last page of any or each document, above the CMS-required footer and also above the PRA statement on the PML. Use 14-point serif font to match the text portions of the documents.
- *Form Sequencing:* The forms must be prepared and delivered in the following order: the CL comes first, followed by the MAP, and then the PML. The MAP and PML forms are designed to be used alone or in conjunction with the other forms in the Format. The first page of each form must begin on a new sheet of paper, with page number sequences restarting at Page **1** of **Y**.
- *Instructions in the Format:* Imbedded instructions shown as italicized text within < > symbols must be deleted prior to distribution to beneficiaries.
- *Language:* For ease of understanding, Part D plans and MTM providers are encouraged to use plain language, concrete nouns, and active voice and present the most important information first, where applicable, in each of the documents.

COGNITIVELY IMPAIRED BENEFICIARIES

Part D Plans are required to offer a CMR to all beneficiaries, regardless of setting. In the event the beneficiary is cognitively impaired and cannot make decisions regarding his or her medical needs, CMS recommends that the MTM provider reach out to the beneficiary's prescriber, caregiver, or other authorized individual, such as the beneficiary's health care proxy or legal guardian, to take part in the CMR. Throughout this instructions booklet, there are unique recommendations noted for the CMR summary prepared for cognitively impaired beneficiaries.

COMPLETING THE FORMAT

The following pages provide accompanying instructions below each extracted section of the Format. Always remove the type in italics (eg, *<insert date>*) prior to sending to the beneficiary. Entries in the blanks may be typed (preferred) or handwritten by the MTM provider but should be large enough (ie, approximately 14-point font) to allow ease in reading.

When conducting a CMR, CMS suggests a minimum look-back of 6 months to identify current medications and prescribers and for utilization review. Regardless of the lookback period or availability of historical data, the interactive CMR is an opportunity to capture, reconcile, and update data from the beneficiary, including current medications, OTCs, other unreported medications, and beneficiary concerns. Although the PML may be initially populated with information from claims data, EMRs, or other data files, there should be a verification step by the MTM provider with the beneficiary. This step may also identify adherence concerns to be addressed in the MAP.

Cover Letter (CL)

CL-1

< *MTM PROVIDER HEADER* >

CL-2

< *PLAN LOGO* >

CL-3

< *Insert date* >

< *Insert inside address* >

< *Insert salutation* >:

< *Additional space for optional plan/provider use, such as barcodes, document reference numbers, beneficiary identifiers, case numbers or title of document* >

CL-4

Thank you for talking with me on < *insert date of service* > about your health and medications. Medicare's MTM (Medication Therapy Management) program helps you make sure that your medications are working.

Along with this letter are an action plan (Medication Action Plan) and a medication list (Personal Medication List). **The action plan has steps you should take to help you get the best results from your medications. The medication list will help you keep track of your medications and how to use them the right way.**

- Have your action plan and medication list with you when you talk with your physicians, pharmacists, and other healthcare providers.
- Ask your physicians, pharmacists, and other healthcare providers to update them at every visit.
- Take your medication list with you if you go to the hospital or emergency room.
- Give a copy of the action plan and medication list to your family or caregivers.

CL-5

If you want to talk about this letter or any of the papers with it, please call < *insert contact information for MTM provider, phone number, days/times, TTY, etc.* >. < *I/We* > look forward to working with you and your physicians to help you stay healthy through the < *insert name of Part D Plan* > MTM program.

CL-6

< *Insert closing, MTM provider signature, name, title, enclosure notations, etc.* >

PURPOSE

The purpose of the CL is to remind the beneficiary of what occurred during the CMR, introduce the MAP and PML, and describe how the beneficiary can contact the MTM program.

The CL is not considered marketing material and should not include any marketing messages, marketing disclaimers, or other sales information.

Length: The length of the CL is limited to one piece of paper if printed double-sided, or two pieces of paper if printed singled-sided.

CL-1: < *MTM PROVIDER HEADER* >

- < *MTM PROVIDER HEADER* >: Include the MTM provider's identification information unless precluded by the structure of the Part D plan's MTM program, such as if MTM services are provided by in-house staff. Remove the italics type in the field that states "<*MTM PROVIDER HEADER* >."
- The < *MTM PROVIDER HEADER* > only appears on the first page of the CL.

CL-2: < *PLAN LOGO* >

- < *PLAN LOGO* >: Include the Part D plan logo. Remove the italics type in the field that states "<*PLAN LOGO* >."
- The < *PLAN LOGO* > only appears on the first page of the CL.

CL-3:

< *Insert date* > < *Insert inside address* > < *Insert salutation* >:	< *Additional space for optional plan/provider use, such as barcodes, document reference numbers, beneficiary identifiers, case numbers, or title of document* >

Part D plans can customize and personalize the inside address, salutation, closing, and other fields within the body of the letter.

- < *Insert date* >: Enter the date the letter is prepared in month, day, year format (eg, April 12, 2013). Remove the italics type in the field that states "<*Insert date* >."
- < *Insert inside address* >: Enter beneficiary's name and mailing address. Remove the italics type in the field that states "<*Insert inside address* >."

When the CMR is performed on the behalf of a cognitively impaired beneficiary with someone other than the beneficiary's legally authorized representative, such as a caregiver or prescriber, the MTM provider should discuss the delivery of summary materials with the beneficiary's representative to determine to whom and where they should be sent. CMS expects the CMR summary will be delivered to the beneficiary's authorized representative, such as the healthcare power of attorney, if known. When sending the CMR summary to the beneficiary's legally designated authorized representative, the inside address should include the beneficiary's name, c/o <name and address of their authorized representatives>.

- < *Insert salutation* >: Enter the greeting and beneficiary's name (eg, "Dear Mr. Smith"). Remove the italics type in the field that states "<*Insert salutation* >."
- < *Additional space for optional plan/provider use …* >: Additional space to the right of the date/address/salutation area is optional for Part D plan/provider use. This area may be used as an extension of the header area for Part D plan information or used for items such as barcodes, document reference numbers, beneficiary identifiers, case numbers, or title of document. This area may also be left blank. Remove the italics type in the field that states "<*Additional space for optional plan/provider use …* >."

When the CMR is performed with an authorized individual on the behalf of a cognitively impaired beneficiary, CMS recommends that sponsors include an explanatory note in the Additional Space section near the top right of the CL, such as the following:

NOTE: A review of your medications was done on <*date of CMR*> with <*name of beneficiary's representative*> who served on your behalf. Here is a summary of your medication review.

CL-4:

Thank you for talking with me on <*insert date of service* > about your health and medications. Medicare's MTM (Medication Therapy Management) program helps you make sure that your medications are working.

Along with this letter are an action plan (Medication Action Plan) and a medication list (Personal Medication List). **The action plan has steps you should take to help you get the best results from your medications. The medication list will help you keep track of your medications and how to use them the right way.**

- Have your action plan and medication list with you when you talk with your physicians, pharmacists, and other healthcare providers.
- Ask your physicians, pharmacists, and other healthcare providers to update them at every visit.
- Take your medication list with you if you go to the hospital or emergency room.
- Give a copy of the action plan and medication list to your family or caregivers.

- <*insert date of service* >: Enter the date the beneficiary interacted with the MTM provider in month, day, year format (eg, April 12, 2013). Remove the italics type in the field that states " <*insert date of service* >."

CL-5:

If you want to talk about this letter or any of the papers with it, please call <*insert contact information for MTM provider, phone number, days/times, TTY, etc* >. < *I/We* > look forward to working with you and your physicians to help you stay healthy through the <*insert name of Part D Plan* > MTM program.

- <*insert contact information for MTM provider, phone number, days/times, TTY, etc* >: Enter the name of the MTM provider (or Part D plan if administered in-house), contact information and method as appropriate, periods of availability, and other applicable information. CMS recommends that the name and contact information of the individual who conducted the CMR be included, unless precluded by the Part D plan's MTM program structure. Remove the italics type in the field that states "<*insert contact information for MTM provider, phone number, days/times, TTY, etc* >."
- < *I/We* >: Choose *I* or *We* as appropriate and remove the italics font. Remove the nonselected pronoun and "<>" symbols.
- <*insert name of Part D Plan* >: Enter name of the Part D plan. Remove the italics type in the field that states "<*insert name of Part D Plan* >."

CL-6:

< *Insert closing, MTM provider signature, name, title, enclosure notations, etc* >

- < *Insert closing, signature, name, title, enclosure notations, etc* >: Enter closing (eg, "Sincerely,"). The letter should be signed with a cursive signature, if possible, of the individual who performed the interactive CMR with the beneficiary, with printed annotation of name in order to be understood. A cursive font is recommended if a printed name is used in lieu of the signature. Enclosure notations, if appropriate, can be placed below the printed annotation. The postscript of the CL may be used to describe the availability of the materials by alternative methods, such as text telephones, Braille, or alternative languages, and the availability of language translation services. Remove the italics type in the field that states "<*Insert closing, signature, name, title, enclosure notations, etc*>."

When the CMR is performed on the behalf of a cognitively impaired beneficiary with someone other than the beneficiary's legally authorized representative, such as a caregiver or prescriber, the summary may also be cc'd to the beneficiary's proxy who participated in the CMR, if appropriate for treatment purposes.

MEDICATION ACTION PLAN (MAP)

MAP-1

< *MTM PROVIDER HEADER* >

MAP-2

< *PLAN LOGO* >

MAP-3

MEDICATION ACTION PLAN FOR < *Insert Member's name*, DOB: *mm/dd/yyyy* >

MAP-4

This action plan will help you get the best results from your medications if you:

1. Read "What we talked about."
2. Take the steps listed in the "What I need to do" boxes.
3. Fill in "What I did and when I did it."
4. Fill in "My follow-up plan" and "Questions I want to ask."

Have this action plan with you when you talk with your physicians, pharmacists, and other healthcare providers. Share this with your family or caregivers too.

MAP-5

DATE PREPARED:< *Insert date* >

MAP-6

What we talked about: < *Insert description of topic* >	
What I need to do: < *Insert recommendations for beneficiary activities* >	**What I did and when I did it:** < *Leave blank for beneficiary's notes* >

What we talked about:	
What I need to do:	**What I did and when I did it:**

What we talked about:	
What I need to do:	**What I did and when I did it:**

What we talked about:	
What I need to do:	**What I did and when I did it:**

What we talked about:	
What I need to do:	**What I did and when I did it:**

MAP-7

My follow-up plan (add notes about next steps):
< *Leave blank for beneficiary's notes* >

MAP-8

Questions I want to ask (include topics about medications or therapy):
< *Leave blank for beneficiary's notes* >

MAP-9

If you have any questions about your action plan, call < *insert MTM provider contact information, phone number, days/times, etc.* >.

Purpose

The MAP describes the specific action items resulting from the interactive CMR consultation, the beneficiary's responsibilities in the MAP, and healthcare provider activities that may affect the beneficiary's tasks.

The MAP is not considered marketing material and should not include any marketing messages, marketing disclaimers, or other sales information.

The MAP is a plan to assist the beneficiary with resolving issues of current drug therapy and to help achieve the goals of medication treatment. It may also include acknowledgement and reinforcement of favorable behaviors. The MAP should not include detailed action plans of the MTM provider and is not intended to be a template for communications with other healthcare providers. The MTM provider must determine the most important activities for the beneficiary based on the beneficiary's concerns, the therapeutic need, and the beneficiary's ability to understand and complete the recommended activities.

There may be CMRs that do not identify issues of current drug therapy or beneficiary-specific action items. The standardized format allows plan sponsors to enter other statements into a new MAP as appropriate for the beneficiary, such as reinforcing compliance, maintaining beneficiary's actions, and acknowledging beneficiary success in his/her medication therapy. Beneficiaries will best understand a consistent deliverable after their CMRs, including the MAP, even if there are no new beneficiary-specific action steps.

Order of action items: Part D plans may select the sort order for the action items to be listed, such as alphabetically by medication involved or by health condition. CMS recommends that the most important action item be presented first.

Number of action items and length: The number of action items is based on the needs of the beneficiary that were discussed during the CMR and the professional judgment of the MTM provider. CMS recommends no more than one piece of paper (either single- or double-sided) for the MAP. Blank action item sections may be deleted. Part D plans and MTM providers are encouraged not to separate or break action item sections or rows across pages.

Sizes of border lines and divider lines:

- Narrow lines around MAP titles and within rows are 0.5 pt.
- Wide lines around sections of the MAP are 2.25 pt.

Size and field descriptors: The number of characters in the fields within the Format is not limited to a maximum number of characters. Field sizes for Part D plan-reported information have a minimum height but may expand automatically, as necessary, to accommodate the information entered. Fields for beneficiary-entered data have static height and width requirements. See individual field descriptions in Table A9-1.

Spacing between sections of the MAP: The horizontal space between action plan sections of the MAP is 0.20 inch.

MAP-1: *< MTM PROVIDER HEADER >*

- *< MTM PROVIDER HEADER >*: Include the MTM provider's identification information, unless precluded by the structure of the Part D plan's MTM program, such as if MTM services are provided by in-house staff. Remove the italics type in the field that states "*<MTM PROVIDER HEADER >*."

TABLE A9-1 • Individual Field Descriptions

Medication Action Plan (MAP)	Requirements for Row Height/ Cell Width
What we talked about	Row height is at least 0.70 inch; cell width is 6.5-6.7 inches.
What I need to do	Row height is at least 0.90 inch; cell width is 3.25-3.35 inches.
What I did and when I did it	Row height is at least 0.90 inch; cell width is 3.25-3.35 inches.
My follow-up plan	Row height is 1.15 inches; cell width is 6.5-6.7 inches.
Questions I want to ask	Row height is 1.15 inches; cell width is 6.5-6.7 inches.

- The *< MTM PROVIDER HEADER >* only appears on the first page of the MAP.

MAP-2: *< PLAN LOGO >*

- *< PLAN LOGO >*: Include the Part D plan Logo. Remove the italics type in the field that states "*<PLAN LOGO>*."
- The *< PLAN LOGO >* header only appears on the first page of the MAP.

MAP-3: **Medication Action Plan For** < *Insert Member's name,* DOB: *mm/dd/yyyy* >

- **Medication Action Plan For:** This field title is 14-point bold font with small caps.
- < *Insert Member's name,* DOB: *mm/dd/yyyy* >: Enter the beneficiary's first and last names, and date of birth (DOB) in the format of *mm/dd/yyyy* (eg, 11/15/1925) in 14-point font. Remove the italics type in the field that states "<*Insert Member's name*" and "*mm/dd/yyyy*>."

MAP-4:

> This action plan will help you get the best results from your medications if you:
>
> 1. Read "What we talked about."
> 2. Take the steps listed in the "What I need to do" boxes.
> 3. Fill in "What I did and when I did it."
> 4. Fill in "My follow-up plan" and "Questions I want to ask."
>
> Have this action plan with you when you talk with your physicians, pharmacists, and other healthcare providers. Share this with your family or caregivers too.

- During the CMR, the MTM provider should discuss with the beneficiary the fours things to do when receiving the MAP.

MAP-5: **DATE PREPARED:** < *Insert date* >

- **Date Prepared:**< *Insert date* >: Enter the date the MAP (Medication Action Plan) was prepared in the format of *mm/dd/yyyy* (e.g., 12/14/2013). This date may be different from the date the beneficiary interacted with the MTM provider. This field is right-justified, with 16-point, bold font and small caps for field title and date. Remove the italics type in the field that states "*<Insert date >*."

MAP-6:

What we talked about: *< Insert description of topic >*	
What I need to do: *< Insert recommendations for beneficiary activities >*	**What I did and when I did it:** *< Leave blank for beneficiary's notes >*

- **What we talked about:** *< Insert description of topic >*: Enter a description of the topic that was discussed with the beneficiary, including the medication or care issue to be resolved or the behavior to be encouraged. The Part D plan or MTM provider has the discretion to choose how to make reference to the medication or care issue, such as to list the medication first in the box or add emphasis to that specific text. In some cases, it may be appropriate to tell the beneficiary that the MTM provider will follow up with the physician or other practitioner or to include goals of therapy. Row height is at least 0.70 inch; cell width is 6.5 to 6.7 inches. Remove the italics type in the field that states "*<Insert description of topic >*."
- **What I need to do:** *< Insert recommendations for beneficiary activities >*: Enter recommendations on what the beneficiary should be doing (eg, "Check your blood pressure every morning. Record your blood pressure reading in your log book."). In some cases, it may be appropriate to tell the beneficiary to take no action pending outcome of the MTM provider's follow up with the physician or other practitioner. Row height is at least 0.90 inch; cell width is 3.25 to 3.35 inches. Remove the italics type in the field that states "*<Insert recommendations for beneficiary activities >*."
- **What I did and when I did it:** This field is for the beneficiary to use after the CMR is complete. Remove the italics type in the field that says to "*<Leave blank for beneficiary's notes>*." Discuss with the beneficiary that the box is for his/her use and to write in this box as appropriate. For example, the MTM provider may educate the beneficiary to take the medication with a meal to increase absorption (eg, calcium carbonate) and then the beneficiary can note when they started doing this and the effects if any. Row height is at least 0.90 inch; cell width is 3.25 to 3.35 inches.

MAP-7:

My follow-up plan (add notes about next steps): *< Leave blank for beneficiary's notes >*

- **My follow-up plan** (add notes about next steps): This field is for the beneficiary's use. Discuss with the beneficiary that the box is for his/her use and to write in this box as appropriate. Row height is 1.15 inches; cell width is 6.5 to 6.7 inches. Remove the italics type that says to "*<Leave blank for beneficiary's notes >*."

MAP-8:

Questions I want to ask (include topics about medications or therapy): *< Leave blank for beneficiary's notes >*

- **Questions I want to ask** (include topics about medications or therapy): Discuss with the beneficiary that the box is for his/her use and to write in this box as appropriate. For example, the beneficiary may want to know if a symptom he/she is experiencing could be a side effect of a medication. Row height is 1.15 inches; cell width is 6.5 to 6.7 inches. Remove the italics type that says to "*<Leave blank for beneficiary's notes >*."

MAP-9:

If you have any questions about your action plan, call *<insert MTM provider contact information, phone number, days/times, etc >*.

- *<insert contact information for MTM provider, phone number, days/times, TTY, etc >*: Enter the name of the MTM provider (or Part D plan if administered in-house), contact information and method as appropriate, periods of availability, and other applicable information. CMS recommends that the name and contact information of the individual who conducted the CMR be included unless precluded by the Part D plan's MTM program structure. Remove the italics type in the field that states "*<insert contact information for MTM provider, phone number, days/times, TTY, etc >*."

PERSONAL MEDICATION LIST (PML)

PML-1 *< MTM PROVIDER HEADER >*

PML-2 *< PLAN LOGO >*

PML-3 PERSONAL MEDICATION LIST FOR *< Insert Member's name, DOB: mm/dd/yyyy >*

PML-4 **This medication list was made for you after we talked. We also used information from** *< insert source of information >*

- Use blank rows to add new medications. Then fill in the dates you started using them.
- Cross out medications when you no longer use them. Then write the date and why you stopped using them.
- Ask your physicians, pharmacists, and other healthcare providers to update this list at every visit.

Keep this list up-to-date with:
☐ Prescription medications
☐ Over the counter drugs
☐ Herbals
☐ Vitamins
☐ Minerals

PML-5 If you go to the hospital or emergency room, take this list with you. Share this with your family or caregivers too.

PML-6 DATE PREPARED: *< Insert date >*

Allergies or side effects: *< Insert beneficiary's allergies and adverse drug reactions including the medications and their effects >*

PML-7

Medication: *< Insert generic name and brand name, strength, and dosage form for current/active medications. >*	
How I use it: *< Insert regimen, including strength, dose and frequency (eg, 1 tablet [20 mg] by mouth daily), use of related devices and supplemental instructions as appropriate >*	
Why I use it: *< Insert indication or intended medical use >*	**Prescriber:** *< Insert prescriber's name >*
< Insert other title(s) or delete this field >: *< Use for optional product-related information such as additional instructions, product image/identifiers, goals of therapy, pharmacy, etc., and change field title accordingly. This field may be expanded or divided. Delete this field it not used.>* (PML-8)	
Date I started using it: *< May be estimated by plan or entered based upon beneficiary-reported data, or leave blank for beneficiary to enter start date >* (PML-9)	**Date I stopped using it:** *< Leave blank for beneficiary to enter stop date >*
Why I stopped using it: *< Leave blank for beneficiary's notes >*	

(*Continued*)

PERSONAL MEDICATION LIST FOR < *Insert Member's name,* DOB: *mm/dd/yyyy* >

Medication:	
How I use it:	
Why I use it:	Prescriber:
< *Insert other title(s) or delete this field* >:	
Date I started using it:	Date I stopped using it:
Why I stopped using it:	

Medication:	
How I use it:	
Why I use it:	Prescriber:
< *Insert other title(s) or delete this field* >:	
Date I started using it:	Date I stopped using it:
Why I stopped using it:	

Medication:	
How I use it:	
Why I use it:	Prescriber:
< *Insert other title(s) or delete this field* >:	
Date I started using it:	Date I stopped using it:
Why I stopped using it:	

Medication:	
How I use it:	
Why I use it:	Prescriber:
< *Insert other title(s) or delete this field* >:	
Date I started using it:	Date I stopped using it:
Why I stopped using it:	

Medication:	
How I use it:	
Why I use it:	Prescriber:
< *Insert other title(s) or delete this field* >:	
Date I started using it:	Date I stopped using it:
Why I stopped using it:	

PERSONAL MEDICATION LIST FOR < *Insert Member's name,* DOB: *mm/dd/yyyy* >

Medication:	
How I use it:	
Why I use it:	Prescriber:
< *Insert other title(s) or delete this field* >:	
Date I started using it:	Date I stopped using it:
Why I stopped using it:	

Medication:	
How I use it:	
Why I use it:	Prescriber:
< *Insert other title(s) or delete this field* >:	
Date I started using it:	Date I stopped using it:
Why I stopped using it:	

Medication:	
How I use it:	
Why I use it:	Prescriber:
< *Insert other title(s) or delete this field* >:	
Date I started using it:	Date I stopped using it:
Why I stopped using it:	

Other Information:

PML-10

PML-11

According to the Paperwork Reduction Act of 1995, no persons are required to respond to a collection of information unless it displays a valid OMB control number. The valid OMB number for this information collection is 0938-1154. The time required to complete this information collection is estimated to average 40 minutes per response, including the time to review instructions, searching existing data resources, gather the data needed, and complete and review the information collection. If you have any comments concerning the accuracy of the time estimate(s) or suggestion for improving this form, please write to: CMS, Attn: PRA Reports Clearance Officer, 7500 Security Boulevard, Baltimore, Maryland 21244-1850.

Purpose

The PML is a reconciled list of all the medications in use (ie, active medications) by the beneficiary at the time of a CMR. Information for this section may be prepopulated by the Part D plan and must be completed and updated with information provided by the beneficiary and/or caregiver during the consultation. Part D plans must also collect and report the purpose and instructions for the beneficiary's use of his/her medications. The use of OTC medications is important for drug utilization review and should be captured during the interactive CMR and reported in the PML by the Part D plan.

The PML is intended to help beneficiaries understand their medications and how they relate to their treatment plans; to engage beneficiaries in the management of their drug therapy; and to improve both communication about medications and tracking of all medications, including self-prescribed medicines, with their healthcare providers. The PML assists the beneficiary with managing his/her medications by allowing the beneficiary to add new medications and their start dates, redacting discontinued products, and indicating the stop dates and reasons for stopping.

The PML is not considered marketing material and should not include any marketing messages, marketing disclaimers, or other sales information.

The PML is not a wallet card. Some MTM programs may also provide supplemental wallet cards, such as the one prepared by AHRQ: http://www.ahrq.gov/consumer/safemeds/walletform.pdf.

Order of medications: MTM programs may select the sort order for the medications to be listed, such as alphabetically, by purpose, by prescriber, or by product type (eg, prescription, OTC, vitamin, herbal supplement).

Length: The number of pages of the PML is based upon the number of medications used by the beneficiary. The PML may be printed either single- or double-sided. At least three blank medication sections or enough to fill the last page of the PML, whichever is greater, must be included for use by beneficiaries to update the PML. Part D plans and MTM providers are encouraged not to separate medication sections or rows across pages.

Sizes of border lines and divider lines:

- Narrow lines around PML titles, text box on PML, and within rows are 0.5 pt.
- Wide lines around sections of the PML are 2.25 pt.

Size and field descriptors: The number of characters in the fields within the Format is not limited to a maximum number of characters. Field sizes for Part D plan-reported information have a minimum height but may expand automatically, as necessary, to accommodate the information entered. Fields for beneficiary-entered data have static height and width requirements. See individual field descriptions in Table A9-2.

Spacing between sections of the PML: The horizontal space between medication sections of the PML is 0.20 inch.

Paperwork Reduction Act (PRA): The PRA statement must be included at the bottom of the last page of the PML above or within the footer. Use Helvetica, 7-point font.

TABLE A9-2 • Individual Field Descriptions

Personal Medication List (PML)	Requirements for Row Height/Cell Width
Allergies or side effects	Row height is at least 0.45 inch; cell width is 6.5-6.7 inches.
Medication	Row height is at least 0.23 inch; cell width is 6.5-6.7 inches
How I use it	Row height is at least 0.23 inch; cell width is 6.5-6.7 inches.
Why I use it	Row height is at least 0.23 inch; cell width is 3.25-3.35 inches.
Prescriber	Row height is at least 0.23 inch; cell width is 3.25-3.35 inches.
< Insert other titles or delete this field >	This field may be expanded or divided. Delete this field if it is not used. Row height is at least 0.23 inch; cell width is 6.5-6.7 inches.
Date I started using it	Row height is 0.23 inch; cell width is 3.25-3.35 inches. [Allow 0.45-inch height for Spanish Format.]
Date I stopped using it	Row height is 0.23 inch; cell width is 3.25-3.35 inches. [Allow 0.45-inch height for Spanish Format.]
Why I stopped using it	Row height is 0.23 inch; cell width is 6.5-6.7 inches.
Other information	Row height is 1.15 inches; cell width is 6.5-6.7 inches.

According to the Paperwork Reduction Act of 1995, no persons are required to respond to a collection of information unless it displays a valid OMB control number. The valid OMB number for this information collection is 0938-1154. The time required to complete this information collection is estimated to average 37.76 minutes per response, including the time to review instructions, searching existing data resources, gather the data needed, and complete and review the information collection. If you have any comments concerning the accuracy of the time estimate(s) or suggestions for improving this form, please write to: CMS, Attn: PRA Reports Clearance Officer, 7500 Security Boulevard, Baltimore, Maryland 21244-1850.

Part D plans are also encouraged to post a blank PML on their website(s) or provide information to beneficiaries about how to obtain a blank copy.

PML-1: *< MTM PROVIDER HEADER >*

- *< MTM PROVIDER HEADER >*: Include the MTM provider's identification information unless precluded by the structure of the Part D plan's MTM program, such as if MTM services are provided by in-house staff. Remove the italics type in the field that states "*<MTM PROVIDER HEADER >*."
- The *< MTM PROVIDER HEADER >* only appears on the first page of the PML.

PML-2: *< PLAN LOGO >*

- < *PLAN LOGO* >: Include the Part D plan Logo. Remove the italics type in the field that states "<*PLAN LOGO* >."
- The < *PLAN LOGO* > header only appears on the first page of the PML.

PML-3: PERSONAL MEDICATION LIST FOR < *Insert Member's name,* DOB: *mm/dd/yyyy* >

- **Personal medication list for:** This field title is 14-point bold font with small caps.
- < *Insert Member's name,* DOB: *mm/dd/yyyy* >: Enter the beneficiary's first and last names and date of birth (DOB) in format of *mm/dd/yyyy* (e.g., 11/15/1925) in 14-point font. Remove the italics type in the field that states "<*Insert Member's name*" and "*mm/dd/yyyy* >."

PML-4:

> This medication list was made for you after we talked. We also used information from <*insert sources of information* >.
>
> - Use blank rows to add new medications. Then fill in the dates you started using them.
> - Cross out medications when you no longer use them. Then write the date and why you stopped using them.
> - Ask your physicians, pharmacists, and other healthcare providers to up date this list at every visit.
>
> If you go to the hospital or emergency room, take this list with you. Share this with your family or caregivers too.
>
> Keep this list up-to-date with:
>
> - ☐ Prescription medications
> - ☐ Over the counter drugs
> - ☐ Herbals
> - ☐ Vitamins
> - ☐ Minerals

- <*insert sources of information* >: Enter sources of information, such as prescription claims information, electronic medical records, pharmacy records, physician or caregiver, etc. If physician or caregiver, such as for a CMR of a cognitively impaired beneficiary, include the name of the person. Patients may also self-report their prescription and OTC medications. Remove the italics type in the field that states "<*insert sources of information* >."

PML-5: DATE PREPARED: < *Insert date* >

- **Date Prepared:**< *Insert date* >: Enter the date the PML (Personal Medication List) was prepared in the format of *mm/dd/yyyy* (eg, 12/14/2013). This date may be different from the date that the beneficiary interacted with the MTM provider. This field is right-justified, with 16-point, bold font and small caps for field title and date. Remove the italics type in the field that states "<*Insert date* >."

PML-6:

> **Allergies or side effects:** < *Insert beneficiary's allergies and adverse drug reactions including the medications and their effects.* >

- **Allergies or Side Effects:** Enter the beneficiary's allergies and adverse drug reactions in this field. There is only one section for this information, and it is not separated by allergic versus adverse drug reaction. Record the medication, and note what happened to the beneficiary. If the MTM provider is able to distinguish between allergy and adverse event, the MTM provider may label true allergies with the text "allergy" after the medication. Row height is at least 0.45 inch; cell width is 6.5 to 6.7 inches. Remove the italics type in the field that states "<*Insert beneficiary's allergies and adverse drug reactions including the medications and their effects* >."

PML-7:

Medication: < ***Insert generic name and brand name, strength, and dosage form for current/active medications.*** >	
How I use it: < *Insert regimen, including strength, dose and frequency (eg, 1 tablet [20 mg] by mouth daily), use of related devices and supplemental instructions as appropriate* >	
Why I use it: < *Insert indication or intended medical use* >	**Prescriber:** < *Insert prescriber's name* >

- **Medication:** Enter the medication's generic drug name (and brand name if applicable), strength, and dosage form for medications currently being used by the beneficiary, including starter supplies (eg, samples), prescription medications, OTC drugs, herbal products, vitamins, and minerals. For brand drugs and branded generics, list both generic and brand names, such as "Generic Name (Brand Name)." An example is Furosemide (Lasix). For generic drugs, list the medication name as "Generic Name" (eg, Furosemide). This would ensure a consistent format of: "Generic Name (Brand Name if applicable)." Information about medication-related devices should be included in the field for the applicable medication(s) where appropriate. Row height is at least 0.23 inch; cell width is 6.5 to 6.7 inches. Remove the italics type in the field that states "<*Insert generic name and brand name, strength, and dosage form for current/active medications.* >."
- **How I use it:** Enter the directions for use and supplemental instructions for using the medication. Directions must be specific and include the dose, frequency and route of administration (as ordered for prescribed products, or as being taken for self-selected products). For the dose that the beneficiary takes, it should, when appropriate and reasonable, include both the number of tablets/capsules/ teaspoonfuls, etc, and the strength (eg, 3 teaspoonfuls [27 mg] by mouth

every 8 hours). Enter supplemental and device-related instructions (eg, "Shake the bottle for one minute prior to measuring the dose"), if appropriate, or in the optional "*insert other titles...*" field. Row height is at least 0.23 inch; cell width is 6.5 to 6.7 inches. Remove the italics type in the field that states "*<Insert regimen, including strength, dose, and frequency (eg, 1 tablet [20 mg] by mouth daily), use of related devices and supplemental instructions as appropriate >*."

- **Why I use it:** Enter the reason for use, indication, or intended purpose. It may be appropriate to include a lay term (eg, high blood pressure) more easily understood by the beneficiary, rather than or in addition to the medical term (eg, hypertension). The MTM provider may also describe the goal(s) of therapy in this field. Row height is at least 0.23 inch; cell width is 3.25 to 3.35 inches. Remove the italics type in the field that states "*<Insert indication or intended medical use >*."
- **Prescriber:** Enter the name of the authorized practitioner who ordered the medication for the beneficiary. This field may also include other prescriber data, such as designation of practitioner type (eg, MD, PA, or NP), telephone number, address, site, etc, such as J. Johnson-Smith, NP. For nonprescribed OTCs, enter "self" or leave this field blank. Row height is at least 0.23 inch; cell width is 3.25 to 3.35 inches. Remove the italics type in the field that states "*<Insertprescriber's name >*."

PML-8:

< *Insert other title(s) or delete this field* >: *< Use for optional product-related information, such as additional instructions, product image/identifiers, goals of therapy, pharmacy, etc, and change field title accordingly. This field may be expanded or divided. Delete this field if not used. >*

- **< *Insert other titles or delete this field* >:** This is an optional field that can be used as appropriate by the Part D plan or MTM provider. This field is intended to capture other medication-related information that Part D plans and MTM providers prefer to include consistently in a medication list, such as images of medications, goals of therapy, other product identifiers, supplemental instructions, or comments. Therefore, the name of this field and its content are determined by the Part D plan or MTM program. Change the field title as appropriate for the information being provided in this customizable field. Row height is at least 0.23 inch; cell width is 6.5 to 6.7 inches. Remove the italics type that states "*<Use for optional product-related information, such as additional instructions, product image/identifiers, goals of therapy, pharmacy, etc, and change field title accordingly. This field may be expanded or divided. Delete this field if not used. >*." Font, size, and emphasis should match the other field titles. This field may be expanded or divided. Delete this field if it is not used.
- In the blank medication sections for the beneficiaries to use, this **< *Insert other titles...*>** field must be retitled or deleted consistent with the completed medication sections of the PML, or given a title that is useful for self-entry by the beneficiary, such as **"Notes."**

PML-9:

Date I started using it: *< May be estimated by Plan or entered based upon beneficiary-reported data, or leave blank for beneficiary to enter start date >*	**Date I stopped using it:** *< Leave blank for beneficiary to enter stop date >*
Why I stopped using it: < *Leave blank for beneficiary's notes* >	

- **Date I started using it:** The medication start date may be entered by the Part D plan if known or reasonably estimated, or entered based upon beneficiary-reported data; or the field may be left blank for the beneficiary to complete. The last prescription fill date should not be entered in this field. Row height is 0.23 inch; cell width is 3.25 to 3.35 inches. Remove the italics type in the field that states "*<May be estimated by Plan or entered based upon beneficiary-reported data, or leave blank for beneficiary to enter start date >*."
- **Date I stopped using it:** This field allows the beneficiary to record the date he/she stops using the medication. Remove the italics type that states "*<Leave blank for beneficiary to enter stop date >*." Leave this field blank for the beneficiary to enter the stop date. Discuss with the beneficiary that when a medication is no longer being taken, he/she should write the date that the medication was stopped and the reason why the medication was stopped. Row height is 0.23 inch; cell width is 3.25 to 3.35 inches.
- **Why I stopped using it:** This field allows the beneficiary to record the reason he/she stops using the medication. Remove the italics type that states "*<Leave blank for beneficiary's notes >*." Leave this field blank for the beneficiary's notes. Discuss with the beneficiary that when a medication is no longer being taken, he/she should write the date that the medication was stopped and the reason why the medication was stopped. Row height is 0.23 inch; cell width is 6.5 to 6.7 inches.

PML-10:

Other Information:

- **Other Information:** This field may be personalized for the beneficiary, such as including a list of the beneficiary's medical conditions, primary care provider, primary pharmacy provider, or emergency contact information. Row height is 1.15 inches; cell width is 6.5 to 6.7 inches.

PML-11:

If you have any questions about your medication list, call <insert MTM provider contact information, phone numbers, days/times, etc >.

- *<insert contact information for MTM provider, phone number, days/times, TTY, etc >*: Enter the name of the MTM provider (or Part D plan if administered in-house), contact information and method as appropriate, periods of availability, and other applicable information. CMS recommends that the name and contact information of the individual who conducted the CMR be included unless precluded by the Part D plan's MTM program structure. Remove the italics type in the field that states "*<insert contact information for MTM provider, phone number, days/times, TTY, etc >*."

MEDICATION THERAPY MANAGEMENT PROGRAM STANDARDIZED FORMAT—BLANK VERSION

< MTM PROVIDER HEADER > *< PLAN LOGO >*

< Insert date > *< Insert inside address >* *< Insert salutation >:*	*< Additional space for optional plan/provider use, such as barcodes, document reference numbers, beneficiary identifiers, case numbers or title of document >*

Thank you for talking with me on *<insert date of service >* about your health and medications. Medicare's MTM (Medication Therapy Management) program helps you make sure that your medications are working.

Along with this letter are an action plan MAP and a medication list PML. **The action plan has steps you should take to help you get the best results from your medications. The medication list will help you keep track of your medications and how to use them the right way.**

- Have your action plan and medication list with you when you talk with your physicians, pharmacists, and other healthcare providers.
- Ask your physicians, pharmacists, and other healthcare providers to update them at every visit.
- Take your medication list with you if you go to the hospital or emergency room.
- Give a copy of the action plan and medication list to your family or caregivers.

If you want to talk about this letter or any of the papers with it, please call *<insert contact information for MTM provider, phone number, days/times, TTY, etc >*. *< I/We >* look forward to working with you and your physicians to help you stay healthy through the *<insert name of Part D Plan >* MTM program.

< Insert closing, MTM provider signature, name, title, enclosure notations, etc. >

MEDICATION ACTION PLAN FOR *< Insert Member's name,* DOB: *mm/dd/yyyy >*

This action plan will help you get the best results from your medications if you:

1. Read "What we talked about."
2. Take the steps listed in the "What I need to do" boxes.
3. Fill in "What I did and when I did it."
4. Fill in "My follow-up plan" and "Questions I want to ask."

Have this action plan with you when you talk with your physicians, pharmacists, and other healthcare providers. Share this with your family or caregivers too.

	DATE PREPARED: < *INSERT DATE* >
What we talked about: *< Insert description of topic >*	
What I need to do: *< Insert recommendations for beneficiary activities >*	**What I did and when I did it:** *< Leave blank for beneficiary's notes >*
What we talked about:	
What I need to do:	**What I did and when I did it:**
What we talked about:	
What I need to do:	**What I did and when I did it:**
What we talked about:	
What I need to do:	**What I did and when I did it:**
What we talked about:	
What I need to do:	**What I did and when I did it:**
My follow-up plan (add notes about next steps): *< Leave blank for beneficiary's notes >*	
Questions I want to ask (include topics about medications or therapy): *< Leave blank for beneficiary's notes >*	

If you have any questions about your action plan, call *<insert MTM provider contact information, phone number, days/times, etc >*.

< *MTM PROVIDER HEADER* >	< *PLAN LOGO* >

PERSONAL MEDICATION LIST FOR < *Insert Member's name,* DOB: *mm/dd/yyyy* >

This medication list was made for you after we talked. We also used information from <*insert sources of information* >.

- Use blank rows to add new medications. Then fill in the dates you started using them.
- Cross out medications when you no longer use them. Then write the date and why you stopped using them.
- Ask your physicians, pharmacists, and other healthcare providers to up date this list at every visit.

If you go to the hospital or emergency room, take this list with you. Share this with your family or caregivers too.

Keep this list up-to-date with:

- ☐ Prescription medications
- ☐ Over the counter drugs
- ☐ Herbals
- ☐ Vitamins
- ☐ Minerals

	DATE PREPARED: < ***INSERT DATE*** >
Allergies or side effects: < *Insert beneficiary's allergies and adverse drug reactions including the medications and their effects* >	
Medication: < *Insert generic name and brand name, strength, and dosage form for current/active medications.* >	
How I use it: < *Insert regimen, including strength, dose and frequency (eg, 1 tablet [20 mg] by mouth daily), use of related devices and supplemental instructions as appropriate* >	
Why I use it: < *Insert indication or intended medical use* >	**Prescriber:** < *Insert prescriber's name* >
< Insert other title(s) or delete this field >: < *Use for optional product-related information, such as additional instructions, product image/identifiers, goals of therapy, pharmacy, etc, and change field title accordingly. This field may be expanded or divided. Delete this field if not used.* >	
Date I started using it: < *May be estimated by Plan or entered based upon beneficiary-reported data, or leave blank for beneficiary to enter start date* >	**Date I stopped using it:** < *Leave blank for beneficiary to enter stop date* >
Why I stopped using it: < *Leave blank for beneficiary's notes* >	
Medication:	
How I use it:	
Why I use it:	**Prescriber:**
< Insert other title(s) or delete this field >:	
Date I started using it:	**Date I stopped using it:**
Why I stopped using it:	
Medication:	
How I use it:	
Why I use it:	**Prescriber:**
< Insert other title(s) or delete this field >:	
Date I started using it:	**Date I stopped using it:**
Medication:	
How I use it:	
Why I use it:	**Prescriber:**
< Insert other title(s) or delete this field >:	
Date I started using it:	**Date I stopped using it:**
Why I stopped using it:	
Medication:	
How I use it:	
Why I use it:	**Prescriber:**

< Insert other title(s) or delete this field >:	
Date I started using it:	**Date I stopped using it:**
Why I stopped using it:	
Medication:	
How I use it:	
Why I use it:	**Prescriber:**
< Insert other title(s) or delete this field >:	
Date I started using it:	**Date I stopped using it:**
Why I stopped using it:	
Medication:	
How I use it:	
Why I use it:	**Prescriber:**
< Insert other title(s) or delete this field >:	
Date I started using it:	**Date I stopped using it:**
Why I stopped using it:	
Medication:	
How I use it:	
Why I use it:	**Prescriber:**
< Insert other title(s) or delete this field >:	
Date I started using it:	**Date I stopped using it:**
Why I stopped using it:	
Medication:	
How I use it:	
Why I use it:	**Prescriber:**
< Insert other title(s) or delete this field >:	
Date I started using it:	**Date I stopped using it:**
Why I stopped using it:	

Other Information:

If you have any questions about your medication list, call *<insert MTM provider contact information, phone numbers, days/times, etc >*.

According to the Paperwork Reduction Act of 1995, no persons are required to respond to a collection of information unless it displays a valid OMB control number. The valid OMB number for this information collection is 0938-1154. The time required to complete this information collection is estimated to average 37.76 minutes per response, including the time to review instructions, searching existing data resources, gather the data needed, and complete and review the information collection. If you have any comments concerning the accuracy of the time estimate(s) or suggestions for improving this form, please write to: CMS, Attn: PRA Reports Clearance Officer, 7500 Security Boulevard, Baltimore, Maryland 21244-1850.

MEDICATION THERAPY MANAGEMENT PROGRAM STANDARDIZED FORMAT—SAMPLES

Dr. Jane Doe
1500 Main Street
Anytown, MD 21201

Birchwood Medicare Plus

January 30, 2013
Mr. John Smith
999 Straight Road
Washington, DC 80008
Dear Mr. Smith:

Thank you for talking with me on January 14, 2013 about your health and medications. Medicare's MTM (Medication Therapy Management) program helps you make sure that your medications are working.

Along with this letter are an action plan (Medication Action Plan) and a medication list (Personal Medication List). **The action plan has steps you should take to help you get the best results from your medications. The medication list will help you keep track of your medications and how to use them the right way.**

- Have your action plan and medication list with you when you talk with your physicians, pharmacists, and other healthcare providers.
- Ask your physicians, pharmacists, and other healthcare providers to update them at every visit.
- Take your medication list with you if you go to the hospital or emergency room.
- Give a copy of the action plan and medication list to your family or caregivers.

If you want to talk about this letter or any of the papers with it, please call Dr. Jane Doe at 1-800-222-3333 between the hours of 9 am and 5 pm, Monday through Friday. I look forward to working with you and your physicians to help you stay healthy through the Birchwood Medicare Plus MTM program.

Sincerely,
Jane Doe
Jane Doe, PharmD
Pharmacy Manager

Dr. Jane Doe
1500 Main Street
Anytown, MD 21201

Birchwood Medicare Plus

If you have any questions about your action plan, call Dr. Jane Doe at 1-800-222-3333 between the hours of 9 am and 5 pm, Monday through Friday.

Dr. Jane Doe
1500 Main Street
Anytown, MD 21201

Birchwood Medicare Plus

Medication Action Plan For Mr. John Smith, DOB: 07/04/1940

This action plan will help you get the best results from your medications if you:

- Read "What we talked about."
- Take the steps listed in the "What I need to do" boxes.
- Fill in "What I did and when I did it."
- Fill in "My follow-up plan" and "Questions I want to ask."

Have this action plan with you when you talk with your physicians, pharmacists, and other healthcare providers. Share this with your family or caregivers too.

	Date Prepared: 01/14/2013
What we talked about: • High Cholesterol	
What I need to do: • Monitor diet; eat fewer high cholesterol foods (see dietary handout for healthier options). • Get your cholesterol checked.	**What I did and when I did it:**
What we talked about: • High Blood Pressure—at visit on 1/14/2013 it was 154/92 mm Hg	
What I need to do: • Check blood pressure at least 3 times a week and record on log. • Maintain blood pressure less than 130/80 mm Hg. • Monitor salt in my diet and increase daily exercise. • Make an appointment with physician to have blood pressure rechecked and share log.	**What I did and when I did it:**
What we talked about: • Diabetes	
What I need to do: • Continue to check blood sugar once a day. • Maintain fasting blood sugar less than 120 and greater than 70. • Make an appointment to see the podiatrist within one month.	**What I did and when I did it:**
What we talked about: • How to use your Metered Dose Inhaler—Albuterol	
What I need to do: • Refer to the attached handout on proper inhaler technique. • Always use spacer with inhaler. • Keep this medication with me at all times—"rescue inhaler."	**What I did and when I did it:**
My follow-up plan (add notes about next steps):	

Questions I want to ask (include topics about medications or therapy):

Personal Medication List For Mr. John Smith, DOB: 07/04/1940

This medication list was made for you after we talked. We also used information from Medicare Part D claims data.

- Use blank rows to add new medications. Then fill in the dates you started using them.
- Cross out medications when you no longer use them. Then write the date and why you stopped using them.
- Ask your physicians, pharmacists, and other healthcare providers to up date this list at every visit.

If you go to the hospital or emergency room, take this list with you. Share this with your family or caregivers too.

Keep this list up-to-date with:

- ☐ Prescription medications
- ☐ Over the counter drugs
- ☐ Herbals
- ☐ Vitamins
- ☐ Minerals

	Date Prepared: 01/14/2013
Allergies or side effects: Penicillin—hives and difficulty swallowing	
Medication: Simvastatin 20 mg tablet	
How I use it: Take one tablet (20 mg) by mouth every night	
Why I use it: High Cholesterol	**Prescriber:** Dr. Joe Anne
Goals: • LDL (Low Density Lipoproteins) <100 mg/dL • HDL (High Density Lipoproteins) >40 mg/dL	
Date I started using it: January 2009	**Date I stopped using it:**
Why I stopped using it:	
Medication: Glipizide XL (Glucotrol XL) 5 mg tablet	
How I use it: Take one tablet (5mg) by mouth once daily	
Why I use it: Type 2 Diabetes	**Prescriber:** Dr. Joe Anne
Date I started using it: June 2010	**Date I stopped using it:**
Why I stopped using it:	
Medication: Acetaminophen 325 mg tablet	
How I use it: Take one tablet (325 mg) by mouth as needed for pain (3-4 tablets usually each day)	
Why I use it: Knee Pain	**Prescriber:** Self
Reminder: • Taking more than 3000 mg of Acetaminophen a day can increase your chance of liver toxicity. • Do not drink alcohol with this medication. It can increase your risk of liver problems.	**Date I started using it:**
Date I stopped using it:	**Why I stopped using it:**
Medication: Albuterol Sulfate Inhalation Solution (Ventolin HFA)	
How I use it: Use 2 puffs every 6 hours as needed for shortness of breath	
Why I use it: Breathing	**Prescriber:** Dr. Joe Anne
Reminder: • Refer to leaflet on proper technique. • Keep with you at all times—"rescue inhaler."	**Date I started using it:** Early 2011
Date I stopped using it:	**Why I stopped using it:**
Medication:	
How I use it:	
Why I use it:	**Prescriber:**
< Insert other title(s) or delete this field >:	
Date I started using it:	**Date I stopped using it:**
Why I stopped using it:	
Medication:	
How I use it:	
Why I use it:	**Prescriber:**
< Insert other title(s) or delete this field >:	
Date I started using it:	**Date I stopped using it:**
Why I stopped using it:	

Medication:	
How I use it:	
Why I use it:	**Prescriber:**
< Insert other title(s) or delete this field >:	
Date I started using it:	**Date I stopped using it:**
Why I stopped using it:	
Medication:	
How I use it:	
Why I use it:	**Prescriber:**
< Insert other title(s) or delete this field >:	
Date I started using it:	**Date I stopped using it:**
Why I stopped using it:	
Medication:	
How I use it:	
Why I use it:	**Prescriber:**
< Insert other title(s) or delete this field >:	
Date I started using it:	**Date I stopped using it:**
Why I stopped using it:	

Other Information:

If you have any questions about your medication list, call Dr. Jane Doe at 1-800-222-3333 between the hours of 9 am and 5 pm, Monday through Friday.

MEDICATION THERAPY MANAGEMENT PROGRAM STANDARDIZED FORMAT–SPANISH VERSION

FORMATO ESTANDARIZADO PARA EL PROGRAMA DE CONTROL DE LA TERAPIA DE MEDICAMENTOS DE LA PARTE D DE MEDICARE

Vigente desde el 1 de enero de 2013

< MTM PROVIDER HEADER >

< PLAN LOGO >

< Fecha > *< Dirección >* *<Saludo >:*	*< Espacio adicional para uso optativo del plan/proveedor para códigos de barra, número de referencia del documento, título o número del caso >*

Le agradezco por el tiempo que me dedicó el *< ingrese la fecha >* para hablar sobre su salud y sus medicamentos. El Programa de Control de la Terapia de Medicamentos de Medicare (MTM en inglés) le ayuda a asegurarse de que sus medicamentos estén dando los resultados deseados.

Le adjuntamos a esta carta un plan de acción (Plan de medicamentos) y una lista de los medicamentos (Lista personal de medicamentos). **El plan de acción le indica los pasos que debe seguir para obtener los mejores resultados de su terapia de medicamentos. La lista de medicamentos le ayudará a monitorear sus medicamentos y le explicará cómo tomarlos correctamente.**

- Cuando hable con sus médicos, farmacéuticos y otros profesionales de la salud tenga a mano su plan de acción y la lista de medicamentos.
- Pídale a sus médicos, farmacéuticos y otros profesionales de la salud que los actualicen en cada visita.
- Si tiene que ir a la sala de emergencia o al hospital lleve su lista de medicamentos.
- Entréguele a sus familiares y a la persona que lo cuida una copia del plan de acción y de la lista de medicamentos.

Si tiene preguntas sobre esta carta o los documentos adjuntos, llame a *< ingrese la información de contacto delproveedor del MTM, el número de teléfono, fechas/horas, TTY, etc >*.*<Espero/amos>* trabajar con usted y sus médicos a través de *< nombre del plan de la Parte D>* del programa MTM, para mantenerlo saludable.

< Ingrese el párrafo de despedida, la firma del proveedor del programa MTM, el nombre, título, adjuntos, etc >

PLAN DE ACCIÓN PARA *< Nombre del beneficiario, fecha de nacimiento: mes/día/año >*

Este plan de acción le permitirá obtener los mejores resultados si:

1. Lee "Acerca de lo que hablamos."
2. Sigue los pasos mencionados en "Lo que debo hacer".
3. Anota "Lo que hice y cuándo lo hice."
4. Anota "Mi plan de seguimiento" y "Las preguntas que quiero hacer."

Cuando hable con sus médicos, farmacéuticos y otros profesionales de la salud, tenga a mano su plan de acción. Compártalo también con sus familiares y con la persona que lo cuida.

	PREPARADO EL: *< FECHA >*
Acerca de lo que hablamos: *< Describa el tema tratado >*	
Lo que debo hacer: *< Las actividades recomendadas al beneficiario >*	**Lo que hice y cuándo lo hice:** *< Deje el espacio en blanco para que lo use el beneficiario >*
Acerca de lo que hablamos:	
Lo que debo hacer:	**Lo que hice y cuándo lo hice:**
Acerca de lo que hablamos:	
Lo que debo hacer:	**Lo que hice y cuándo lo hice:**

Acerca de lo que hablamos:	
Lo que debo hacer:	**Lo que hice y cuándo lo hice:**
Acerca de lo que hablamos:	
Lo que debo hacer:	**Lo que hice y cuándo lo hice:**
Mi plan de seguimiento (escriba los pasos próximos): *< Deje el espacio en blanco, es para uso del beneficiario >*	
Las preguntas que quiero hacer (preguntas sobre los medicamentos o la terapia): *< Deje el espacio en blanco, es para uso del beneficiario >*	

Si tiene preguntas sobre el plan de acción, llame a *<ingrese la información de contacto del proveedor del MTM, el número de teléfono, fechas/horas, TTY, etc >*.

LISTA PERSONAL DE MEDICAMENTOS PARA *< Nombre del beneficiario, fecha de nacimiento: mes/día/año*

Después de hablar con usted preparamos esta lista de medicamentos. Para hacerlo también usamos la información de *< mencione las fuentes de información >*.

- Use las líneas en blanco para agregar medicamentos nuevos y ponga las fechas en las que comenzó a tomarlos.
- Tache los medicamentos que ya no toma, ponga las fechas y el motivo porel que dejó de tomarlos.
- Pídale a sus médicos, farmacéuticos yotros proveedores de la salud queactualicen la lista de medicamentos encada visita.

Si tiene que atenderse en la sala de emergencia o en el hospital, lleve con usted su lista de medicamentos. Compártala con sus familiares y con quien lo cuida.

Actualice la lista incluyendo:

- ☐ Los medicamentos recetados
- ☐ Los de venta libre
- ☐ Hierbas
- ☐ Vitaminas
- ☐ Minerales

	PREPARADO EL: *< FECHA >*
Alergias o efectos secundarios: *< Mencione las alergias del beneficiario así como los medicamentos que toma y los efectos secundarios >*	
Medicamento: *< Ingrese el nombre genérico y de marca del medicamento(s)que toma, la potencia y la dosis. >*	
Cómo lo toma: *< La terapia que le ordenaron, incluya la potencia, dosis y frecuencia (por ejemplo, 1 píldora (20 mg) diaria por boca), los aparatos para usarla e instrucciones adicionales si correspondiera*	
Para qué lo toma: *< Mencione las indicaciones o el uso médico >*	**Proveedor:** *< Nombre del médico >*
< Ponga otro título(s) o borre este casillero >: *< Ingrese información opcional sobre el medicamento, instrucciones adicionales, identificadores del producto, objetivos de la terapia, la farmacia, etc y cambie el título de este casillero según sea apropiado. Si no usa este casillero, bórrelo. >*	
Fecha en la que comencé a tomarlo: *< Tal vez sea una fecha estimada por el plan o informada por el beneficiario. Puede dejarlo en blanco para que lo llene el beneficiario >*	**Fecha en la que dejé de tomarlo:** *< déjelo en blanco para que lo llene el beneficiario >*
Dejé de tomarlo por: *< Déjelo en blancopara que lo llene el beneficiario >*	
Medicamento:	
Cómo lo toma:	
Para qué lo toma:	**Proveedor:**
< Ponga otro título(s) o borre este casillero>:	
Fecha en la que comencé a tomarlo:	**Fecha en la que dejé de tomarlo:**
Dejé de tomarlo por:	

Medicamento:	
Cómo lo toma:	
Para qué lo toma:	**Proveedor:**
< Ponga otro título(s) o borre este casillero>:	
Fecha en la que comencé a tomarlo:	**Fecha en la que dejé de tomarlo:**
Dejé de tomarlo por:	
Lista Personal De Medicamentos Para < *Nombre del beneficiario, fecha de nacimiento: mes/día/año* (Continuación)	
Medicamento:	
Cómo lo toma:	
Para qué lo toma:	**Proveedor:**
< Ponga otro título(s) o borre este casillero>:	
Fecha en la que comencé a tomarlo:	**Fecha en la que dejé de tomarlo:**
Dejé de tomarlo por:	
Medicamento:	
Cómo lo toma:	
Para qué lo toma:	**Proveedor:**
< Ponga otro título(s) o borre este casillero>:	
Fecha en la que comencé a tomarlo:	**Fecha en la que dejé de tomarlo:**
Dejé de tomarlo por:	
Medicamento:	
Cómo lo toma:	
Para qué lo toma:	**Proveedor:**
< Ponga otro título(s) o borre este casillero>:	
Fecha en la que comencé a tomarlo:	**Fecha en la que dejé de tomarlo:**
Dejé de tomarlo por:	
Medicamento:	
Cómo lo toma:	
Para qué lo toma:	**Proveedor:**
< Ponga otro título(s) o borre este casillero>:	
Fecha en la que comencé a tomarlo:	**Fecha en la que dejé de tomarlo:**
Dejé de tomarlo por:	
Medicamento:	
Cómo lo toma:	
Para qué lo toma:	**Proveedor:**
< Ponga otro título(s) o borre este casillero>:	
Fecha en la que comencé a tomarlo:	**Fecha en la que dejé de tomarlo:**
Dejé de tomarlo por:	

Otra Información:

Para preguntas sobre la lista de medicamentos, llame a <*ingrese la información de contacto del proveedor del MTM, el número de teléfono, fechas/horas, TTY, etc* >.

De conformidad con la Ley de reducción de los trámites burocráticos de 1995, nadie estará obligado a responder a una solicitud de información a menos que se identifique con un número de control válido de la Oficina de Administración y Presupuesto. El número de control válido de la Oficina de Administración y Presupuesto para esta recolección de información es 0938-1154. El tiempo necesario para completar esta solicitud es en promedio, 37.76 minutos incluido el tiempo necesario para revisar las instrucciones, buscar en las fuentes de datos existentes, seleccionar los datos necesarios y completarla. Si tiene comentarios sobre el tiempo estimado para responder o sugerencias para mejorar este formulario, sírvase escribir a: CMS, Attn: PRA Reports Clearance Officer, 7500 Security Boulevard, Baltimore, Maryland 21244-1850.

10

Reimbursement for Pharmacist Services

Daniel E. Buffington, PharmD, MBA, and Kathleen J. Vieson, PharmD

KEY POINTS

- Medical service billing is an essential process between a healthcare provider and a payer.
- In the United States, the medical service billing system is based on the American Medical Association's (AMA) Current Procedural Terminology (CPT) coding system.
- Pharmacist providers billing for patient care services must obtain and use a National Provider Identifier (NPI) number for both service documentation and claim forms.
- Medication therapy management services (MTMS) codes (99605, 99606, and 99607) were developed specifically to describe pharmacists' patient care services.
- "Incident to" billing is when a physician serves as the primary billing party to facilitate payment for patient care services provided by other healthcare professionals or staff members.
- The Transitional Care Management Services (TCMS) codes were added to the AMA CPT code-book in 2013 and reflect the importance of reducing hospital readmissions.
- The Complex Chronic Care Management Services (CCCMS) codes describe patient-centered management and clinical support services provided by a physician or other qualified healthcare provider and their staff on an outpatient basis on a per-month basis.
- It is imperative to identify and confirm whether the payer will pay for the services before the services or procedures are provided.

INTRODUCTION

Medical service billing is an essential process between a healthcare provider and a payer. There are many different models for payer-provider relationships, including fee for service (FFS), pay for performance, capitated rate schedules, bundled payments, and integrated health plans (employer model). As pharmacists have evolved their scope of patient care services, traditional medical billing processes (ie, the AMA Current Procedural Terminology codes) were developed similar to physician services to ensure viable revenue to support the delivery of these clinical services.[1] Medical service billing, including billing for pharmacists' services, is not limited to commercial insurance or government healthcare agencies. Healthcare providers commonly invoice patients directly for elective and specialty services or procedures. Payment for medical services may be obtained from many different entities, including

- Private payment (patient, family, caregivers)
- Health insurance
- Health plans
- Patient-centered medical homes
- Accountable-care organizations
- Medicare Part D (state prescription drug programs)
- Government health agencies (Medicare, Medicaid, Tricare, VA)
- Employer-based programs
- Retirement programs
- Self-insured companies
- Indigent health plans
- 340B prescription programs
- Charitable programs

It is important for pharmacists to understand the foundation of the medical billing process to ensure compliance prior to delivering patient care services. Pharmacists have made significant progress integrating into the national medical billing environment and are now recognized as healthcare providers who play an essential role in the healthcare system by optimizing medication therapy, improving health outcomes, and reducing risks associated with pharmacologic treatment.

Medical Services Billing Framework

In the United States, the medical service billing system is based on the AMA CPT coding system. CPT represents a master set of medical billing codes, descriptions, and guidelines for healthcare services and procedures. Historically the CPT codebook was physician-centric, but now it includes other healthcare professionals and healthcare facilities as well. The CPT codebook is divided into sections that include Evaluation and Management, Anesthesia, Surgery, Radiology, Pathology/Laboratory, Medicine, Category II Codes, Category III Codes, Appendix, and Index. These sections are reviewed and updated annually.[2]

The CPT codes are classified into three categories (Table 10-1). Category I codes have received full or permanent status within the CPT code set and are fully functional for billing purposes. Category II codes provide a mechanism to articulate performance or quality measurement purposes, but do not impact service or procedure reimbursement. Category III codes are often provided on a temporary basis and may be used to acknowledge new or emerging technologies, services, or products that have not been broadly implemented across the healthcare system. Category III codes may be converted to Category I status by the CPT editorial panel following demonstration that either the Category III service is currently being provided by many healthcare professionals and in many different healthcare settings or the Category III product/procedure has received FDA approval. Payers commonly delay adoption of Category III codes until the utility and benefits have been demonstrated to justify payment. Category I codes are more likely to receive global payer acceptance and reimbursement.

The AMA CPT organizational structure includes provider representatives from nearly all medical and allied healthcare specialties. The participants include a provider member and a staff representative from their professional specialty organization for each of the participating specialties. The CPT provider members are referred to as *CPT advisors*. A central executive panel of elected members, called the *CPT editorial panel*, is the central decision-making body. However, the CPT editorial panel operates with the input, guidance, and participation of the entire body of CPT Advisors who serve as subject matter experts.

TABLE 10-1 • Categories of CPT Codes

Category	Description
I	Primary codes
II	Supplemental tracking and performance measurement codes
III	Temporary or emerging technology

Pharmacists have been represented in the AMA CPT process through the Pharmacists Collaborative, a collective body representing many of the nation's leading pharmacist professional organizations.[3]

In 2006, pharmacists achieved the initial approval of Category III (temporary) codes that described MTMS. By 2008, following the demonstration of widespread use of the codes and delivery of services, the codes were converted to Category I (permanent) status. The current CPT MTMS codes are 99605, 99606, and 99607.[4]

Medical service billing codes may be submitted to payers either electronically or manually. If submitted manually (hardcopy), outpatient service and procedure codes are submitted via a Center for Medicare & Medicaid Services (CMS) form CMS-1500 (Figure 10-1), and inpatient service and procedure codes are submitted via form UB-04, also referred to as CMS-1450 (Figure 10-2).[5,6] Pharmacist providers billing for patient care services must obtain and use a National Provider Identifier (NPI) number for both service documentation and claim forms.[7]

Pharmacist Services Billing Codes

Pharmacists providing patient care services can use a variety of CPT codes for medical billing. Within the AMA CPT codebook, there are two main chapters, "Medicine" and "Evaluation and Management (E&M)," which are most applicable to pharmacists (Table 10-2). The "Medicine" chapter includes the MTMS codes (99605, 99606, and 99607) developed specifically to describe pharmacists' patient care services. The E&M chapter includes several medical billing codes that pharmacists also use depending on the circumstances and settings, including but not limited to office or other outpatient service (new patient, established patient), TCMS, and CCCMS.[8] The determination of which billing code to use may be affected by the patient's healthcare coverage and payer policy. Although the MTMS codes are specific to pharmacists, it does not preclude a payer from allowing pharmacists to utilize other CPT codes that may articulate certain other services or practice models (ie, physician and pharmacist combination services or "incident to"). The payer's payment processes and policies are the greatest determinant as to which billing codes should be used for MTM services.

Providers routinely use a practice-specific form that lists common services and codes, or superbill (Figure 10-3).[9] A *superbill* is an internal document that serves as the practitioner's encounter-specific billing record and provides an effective mode of communication with the practice's billing and accounting staff. The data elements on a medical superbill typically include patient information, provider information, date of service, place of service, diagnoses codes (ICD10), medical billing codes (CPT), and payer information. Superbills may focus on the scope of services as well as procedures provided by different providers and practice settings.[10] Pharmacists should also use a standard method to select accurate billing codes and level of service as part of a detailed and timely documentation process.

Following the initiation of Medicare Part D in 2006, there was an immediate need for the Medicare-approved Part D contracted plans (ie, prescription drug plans [PDPs]) to provide patient-specific support services for Medicare beneficiaries. These services are essential to ensuring improved health outcomes and avoidance of adverse drug events. Several healthcare companies serve as MTM

HEALTH INSURANCE CLAIM FORM

APPROVED BY NATIONAL UNIFORM CLAIM COMMITTEE (NUCC) 02/12

PICA PICA

CARRIER

1. MEDICARE (Medicare#) MEDICAID (Medicaid#) TRICARE (ID#/DoD#) CHAMPVA (Member ID#) GROUP HEALTH PLAN (ID#) FECA BLKLUNG (ID#) OTHER (ID#)

1a. INSURED'S I.D. NUMBER (For Program in Item 1)

2. PATIENT'S NAME (Last Name, First Name, Middle Initial)

3. PATIENT'S BIRTH DATE MM DD YY SEX M F

4. INSURED'S NAME (Last Name, First Name, Middle Initial)

5. PATIENT'S ADDRESS (No. Street)

6. PATIENT RELATIONSHIP TO INSURED Self Spouse Child Other

7. INSURED'S ADDRESS (No. Street)

CITY STATE

8. RESERVED FOR NUCC USE

CITY STATE

ZIP CODE TELEPHONE (Include Area Code) ( )

ZIP CODE TELEPHONE (Include Area Code) ( )

9. OTHER INSURED'S NAME (Last Name, First Name, Middle Initial)

10. IS PATIENT'S CONDITION RELATED TO:

11. INSURED'S POLICY GROUP OR FECA NUMBER

a. OTHER INSURED'S POLICY OR GROUP NUMBER

a. EMPLOYMENT? (Current or Previous) YES NO

a. INSURED'S DATE OF BIRTH MM DD YY SEX M F

b. RESERVED FOR NUCC USE

b. AUTO ACCIDENT? YES NO PLACE (State)

b. OTHER CLAIM ID (Designated by NUCC)

c. RESERVED FOR NUCC USE

c. OTHER ACCIDENT? YES NO

c. INSURANCE PLAN NAME OR PROGRAM NAME

d. INSURANCE PLAN NAME OR PROGRAM NAME

10d. CLAIM CODES (Designated by NUCC)

d. IS THERE ANOTHER HEALTH BENEFIT PLAN? YES NO *If yes,* complete items 9, 9a, and 9d.

READ BACK OF FORM BEFORE COMPLETING & SIGNING THIS FORM.

12. PATIENT'S OR AUTHORIZED PERSON'S SIGNATURE I authorize the release of any medical or other information necessary to process this claim. I also request payment of government benefits either to myself or to the party who accepts assignment below.

SIGNED DATE

13. INSURED'S OR AUTHORIZED PERSON'S SIGNATURE I authorize payment of medical benefits to the undersigned physician or supplier for services described below.

SIGNED

PATIENT AND INSURED INFORMATION

14. DATE OF CURRENT ILLNESS, INJURY, or PREGNANCY (LMP) MM DD YY QUAL.

15. OTHER DATE QUAL. MM DD YY

16. DATES PATIENT UNABLE TO WORK IN CURRENT OCCUPATION FROM MM DD YY TO MM DD YY

17. NAME OF REFERRING PROVIDER OR OTHER SOURCE

17a. 17b. NPI

18. HOSPITALIZATION DATES RELATED TO CURRENT SERVICES FROM MM DD YY TO MM DD YY

19. ADDITIONAL CLAIM INFORMATION (Designated by NUCC)

20. OUTSIDE LAB? YES NO $ CHARGES

21. DIAGNOSIS OR NATURE OF ILLNESS OR INJURY Relate A-L to service line below (24E) ICD Ind.

A. B. C. D.
E. F. G. H.
I. J. K. L.

22. RESUBMISSION CODE ORIGINAL REF. NO.

23. PRIOR AUTHORIZATION NUMBER

24.A. DATE(S) OF SERVICE From MM DD YY To MM DD YY	B. PLACE OF SERVICE	C. EMG	D. PROCEDURES, SERVICES, OR SUPPLIES (Explain Unusual Circumstances) CPT/HCPCS MODIFIER	E. DIAGNOSIS POINTER	F. $ CHARGES	G. DAYS OR UNITS	H. EPSDT Family Plan	I. ID. QUAL	J. RENDERING PROVIDER ID. #
1								NPI	
2								NPI	
3								NPI	
4								NPI	
5								NPI	
6								NPI	

PHYSICIAN OR SUPPLIER INFORMATION

25. FEDERAL TAX I.D. NUMBER SSN EIN

26. PATIENT'S ACCOUNT NO.

27. ACCEPT ASSIGNMENT? For govt. claims, see back YES NO

28. TOTAL CHARGE $

29. AMOUNT PAID $

30. Rsvd for NUCC Use

31. SIGNATURE OF PHYSICIAN OR SUPPLIER INCLUDING DEGREES OR CREDENTIALS (I certify that the statements on the reverse apply to this bill and are made a part thereof.)

SIGNED DATE

32. SERVICE FACILITY LOCATION INFORMATION

a. b.

33. BILLING PROVIDER INFO & PH # ( )

a. b.

NUCC Instruction Manual available at: www. nucc.org PLEASE PRINT OR TYPE APPROVED OMB-0938-1197 FORM CMS-1500 (02-12)

SAMPLE

FIGURE 10-1 CMS-1500 Outpatient Medical Service Claim Form.[5]

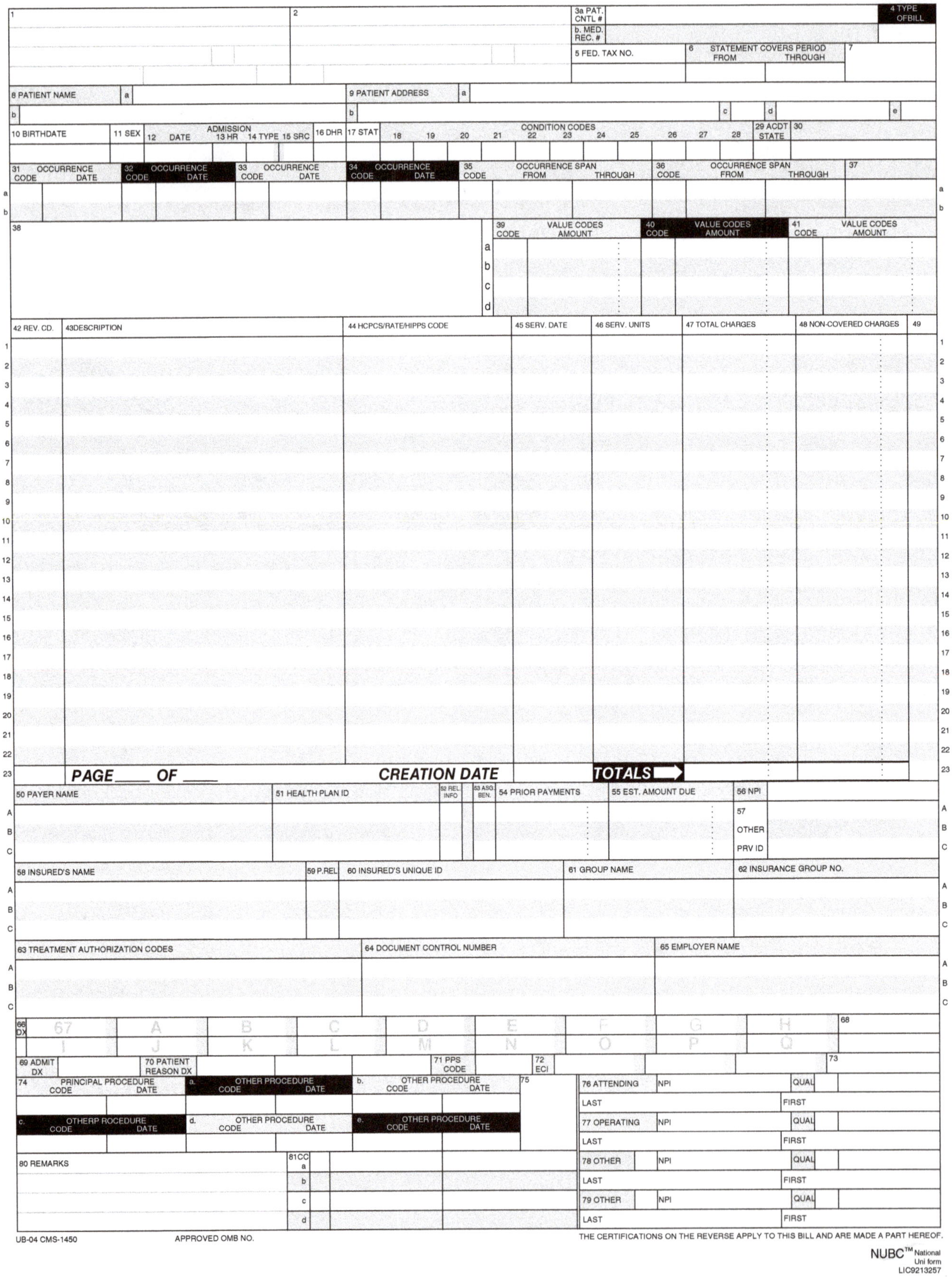

1 | 2 | 3a PAT. CNTL # | b. MED. REC. # | 4 TYPE OF BILL

5 FED. TAX NO. | 6 STATEMENT COVERS PERIOD FROM THROUGH | 7

8 PATIENT NAME a b | 9 PATIENT ADDRESS a b c d e

10 BIRTHDATE | 11 SEX | ADMISSION 12 DATE 13 HR 14 TYPE 15 SRC | 16 DHR | 17 STAT | CONDITION CODES 18 19 20 21 22 23 24 25 26 27 28 | 29 ACDT STATE | 30

31 OCCURRENCE CODE DATE | 32 OCCURRENCE CODE DATE | 33 OCCURRENCE CODE DATE | 34 OCCURRENCE CODE DATE | 35 OCCURRENCE SPAN CODE FROM THROUGH | 36 OCCURRENCE SPAN CODE FROM THROUGH | 37

38 | 39 VALUE CODES CODE AMOUNT | 40 VALUE CODES CODE AMOUNT | 41 VALUE CODES CODE AMOUNT

42 REV. CD. | 43 DESCRIPTION | 44 HCPCS/RATE/HIPPS CODE | 45 SERV. DATE | 46 SERV. UNITS | 47 TOTAL CHARGES | 48 NON-COVERED CHARGES | 49

PAGE ___ OF ___ CREATION DATE TOTALS

50 PAYER NAME | 51 HEALTH PLAN ID | 52 REL. INFO | 53 ASG. BEN. | 54 PRIOR PAYMENTS | 55 EST. AMOUNT DUE | 56 NPI | 57 OTHER PRV ID

58 INSURED'S NAME | 59 P.REL | 60 INSURED'S UNIQUE ID | 61 GROUP NAME | 62 INSURANCE GROUP NO.

63 TREATMENT AUTHORIZATION CODES | 64 DOCUMENT CONTROL NUMBER | 65 EMPLOYER NAME

66 DX | 67 A B C D E F G H I J K L M N O P Q | 68

69 ADMIT DX | 70 PATIENT REASON DX | 71 PPS CODE | 72 ECI | 73

74 PRINCIPAL PROCEDURE CODE DATE | a. OTHER PROCEDURE CODE DATE | b. OTHER PROCEDURE CODE DATE | 75 | 76 ATTENDING NPI QUAL LAST FIRST

c. OTHER PROCEDURE CODE DATE | d. OTHER PROCEDURE CODE DATE | e. OTHER PROCEDURE CODE DATE | 77 OPERATING NPI QUAL LAST FIRST

80 REMARKS | 81CC a b c d | 78 OTHER NPI QUAL LAST FIRST | 79 OTHER NPI QUAL LAST FIRST

UB-04 CMS-1450 APPROVED OMB NO. THE CERTIFICATIONS ON THE REVERSE APPLY TO THIS BILL AND ARE MADE A PART HEREOF.

NUBC™ National Uniform Billing Committee LIC9213257

FIGURE 10-2 UB-04 or CMS-1450 Inpatient Medical Service Claim Form.[6]

TABLE 10-2 • CPT Codes for Pharmacist Services

Section	Description	Codes
Medicine	Medication Therapy Management Services (MTMS)	99605, 99606, 99607
E/M[a]	Office or Other Outpatient Services "Incident to"	99211, 99212, 99213, 99214, 99215
E/M	Transitional Care Management Services (TCMS)	99495, 99496
E/M	Chronic Care Management Services (CCMS)	99490
E/M	Complex Chronic Care Management Services (CCCMS)	99487, 99489

[a] Production: Evaluation and management.

third-party administrators and assist the PDPs with the identification of MTM-eligible patients based on specific selection criteria defined by CMS within Part D. The MTM third-party administrators provide patient and program outcomes data to the PDPs and to CMS as part of the PDPs' contract obligations. The positive impact of pharmacist services has been highlighted with the implementation of this organization and infrastructure to document MTM services and their impact on PDP performance.

Historically, CMS contracts a PDP to execute the Medicare Part D drug benefit delivery and infers that the PDP is contractually required to perform some degree of MTM oversight or intervention for patients who meet the Medicare Part D MTM demographic criteria. The payment to a PDP from CMS is not dependent on the type, nature, or volume of MTM initiatives performed by the PDP. The PDP contract does not assign a discreet value or rate for MTM interventions. The CMS does not reimburse PDPs or pharmacists for MTM services provided to Medicare beneficiaries. MTM participation is lower than predicted, and it is still not possible to evaluate whether Part D MTM programs are working as intended. This has frustrated Part D plan sponsors and the federal government, especially considering MTM's success in some Medicaid and private-sector programs. The MTM program expenses have been viewed by the market as an unfunded mandate or contract compliance requirement for Medicare Part D PDPs, even considering the significant positive impacts that pharmacist services have had on federal spending and patient outcomes (Figure 10-4). In order to promote participation in Part D MTM and decrease expenses, CMS has announced the Enhanced MTM Model which began in January 2017 across five Part D regions (see Chapter 2, "Medicare Part D's Medication Therapy Management and Other Related Services").

Medication Therapy Management Services

Codes: 99605, 99606, 99607. MTM is the global term denoting the clinical services that pharmacists provide to patients. MTM services are provided as a supportive and collaborative effort toward optimizing drug therapy in addition to the services provided by prescribers.[11] In 2006, the Pharmacist Services Technical Advisory Coalition (PSTAC), comprising several national pharmacy organizations, presented the application for pharmacists' patient care services specific codes to the AMA CPT editorial panel. These CPT MTMS codes (Table 10-3) are designed to describe the scope and diversity of services provided by pharmacists and are valued in 15-minute increments (eg, time-based billing).[12] The MTMS codes for pharmacists describe all nondispensing activities related to patient care services. These may be clinical, financial, communication, or administrative services related to the management of a patient's medications and medical conditions. The CPT MTMS codes are unique in the fact that the codes are intended for use by pharmacists.

Office or Other Outpatient Services ("Incident to")

Codes: 99211, 99212, 99213, 99214, 99215. When an allied healthcare professional, such as a pharmacist, provides patient care services in conjunction with a physician, the service may be billed using an "incident to" billing method. "Incident to" billing, is when a physician serves as the primary billing party to facilitate payment for patient care services provided by another healthcare professional or staff member (Figure 10-5). The definitions and guidelines for "incident to" billing vary among different types of payers (ie, insurance, health plans, and CMS).

The physician or other qualified healthcare provider will initially evaluate the patient and create a treatment or care plan. Following this, a secondary provider or support staff will perform a task or service in accordance with the established treatment or care plan. In each case, the primary provider must be directly accessible (although not necessarily physically present) to serve as a resource while the secondary provider performs the service. By definition, the service should be provided under the primary provider's direct supervision or the provider must be in the area where care is delivered and be immediately available to provide assistance or greater supervision. CMS has historically been the most restrictive regarding the definition of provider accessibility; however, its own criteria have become more flexible over time, as have those of other payers. The reimbursement for the respective CPT code is 100% of the primary provider's fee and is not reduced because the provider's participation and accountability is maintained throughout the course of care.

The baseline CPT codes utilized within the "incident-to" billing process are the "Office or Other Outpatient Services-Established Patient" codes (viz, 99211, 99212, 99213, 99214, 99215).[8] Originally 99211, the lowest level of intensity code, served as the primary billing code for "incident to" services. However, many healthcare settings that utilize the "incident to" billing method now bill at all levels of intensity including, 99212, 99213, 99214, and 99215[13] (Table 10-4). Clinical documentation for the service provided must support the code level selected. Under the "incident to" reimbursement method, the payer tracks and processes payment to the primary provider, regardless of who the secondary provider is or what percentage of service that individual provides.

Care Management Services

The Care Management Services section of the AMA CPT codebook was added in 2015 to describe management and support services provided by a physician or other qualified healthcare

Date of service:	Account #:	Previous balance:
Patient name:	Insurance:	Today's charges:
		Today's payment:
Address:	Physician name:	Balance due:
Phone:	NPI#	
DOB: Age: Sex:	Tax ID#	

RANK	Office visit	New	Est
	Minimal		99211
	Problem focused	99201	99212
	Exp problem focused	99202	99213
	Detailed	99203	99214
	Comp (established pt)	99204	99215
	Comp (new pt)	99205	
	Significant, sep serv	−25	−25
	Well visit	**New**	**Est**
	< 1 y	99381	99391
	1-4 y	99382	99392
	5-11 y	99383	99393
	12-17 y	99384	99394
	18-39 y	99385	99395
	40-64 y	99386	99396
	65 y +	99387	99397
	Medicare preventive services		
	Annual wellness visit, initial		G0438
	Annual wellness visit, subsequentlvic		G0439
	Pap		Q0091
	Pelvic & breast		G0101
	Prostate/PSA		G0103
	Tobacco counseling/3-10 min		G0436
	Tobacco counseling/>10 min		G0437
	Welcome to Medicare exam		G0402
	ECG w/Welcome to Medicare		G0403
	Flexible sigmoidoscopy		G0104
	Hemoccult, immunoassay		G0328
	Flu shot		G0008
	Hep B shot		G0010
	Pneumonia shot		G0009
	Consultation/preop clearance		
	Expanded problem focused		99242
	Detailed		99243
	Comprehensive/mod complex		99244
	Comprehensive/high complexity		99245
	Other services		
	After posted hours		99050
	Evening/weekend appointment		99051
	Home health certification		G0180
	Home health recertification		G0179
	Post-op follow-up		99024
	Prolonged/30-74 min		99354
	Special reports/forms		99080
	Disability/Workers comp		99455
	Trans care mgmt/mod complex		99495
	Trans care mgmt/high complex		99496
	Radiology		
Diagnoses			
1			
2			
3			
4			
Next office visit			
Recheck · Prev · PRN	_______DWMY		
Instructions:			
Referral			
To:			
Instructions:			
Physician signature			
X______________________________			

RANK	Office procedures		
	Anoscopy		46600
	Audiometry		92551
	Cerumen removal per ear		69210
	Colposcopy		57452
	Colposcopy w/biopsy		57455
	ECG, w/interpretation		93000
	ECG, rhythm strip		93040
	Endometrial biopsy		58100
	Flexible sigmoidoscopy		45330
	Flexible sigmoidoscopy w/biopsy		45331
	Fracture care, cast/splint Site: ____________		29____
	Nebulizer		94640
	Nebulizer demo		94664
	Spirometry		94010
	Spirometry, pre and post		94060
	Tympanometry		92567
	Vasectomy		55250
	Skin procedures		**Units**
	Burn care, initial	16000	
	Foreign body, skin, simple	10120	
	Foreign body, skin, complex	10121	
	I&D, abscess	10060	
	I&D, hematoma/seroma	10140	
	Laceration repair, simple Site: ________ Size: _____	120___	
	Laceration repair, layered Site: ________Size: _____	120___	
	Lesion, biopsy, one	11100	
	Lesion, biopsy, each add'l	11101	
	Lesion, destruct., benign, 1-14	17110	
	Lesion, destruct., premal., single	17000	
	Lesion, destruct., premal., ea. add	17003	
	Lesion, excision, benign Site: ________Size: _____	114___	
	Lesion, excision, malignant Site: ________Size: _____	116___	
	Lesion, paring/cutting, one	11055	
	Lesion, paring/cutting, 2-4	11056	
	Lesion, shave Site: ________ Size: _____	113___	
	Nail removal, partial	11730	
	Nail removal, w/matrix	11750	
	Skin tag, 1-15	11200	
	Medications		**Units**
	Ampicillin, up to 500 mg	J0290	
	B-12, up to 1,000 mcg	J3420	
	Adrenalin epinephrine inj. 0.1 mg	J0171	
	Kenalog, 10 mg	J3301	
	Lidocaine, IV, 10 mg	J2001	
	Methylprednisolone	J1030	
	Methylprednisolone sodium	J2930	
	Normal saline, 1000 cc	J7030	
	Phenergan, up to 50 mg	J2550	
	Progesterone, 1 mg	J1050	
	Rocephin, 250 mg	J0696	
	Testosterone, 200 mg	J1080	
	Tigan, up to 200 mg	J3250	
	Toradol, 15 mg	J1885	
	Flu vaccine		
	Afluria	Q2035	
	FluLaval	Q2036	
	Fluvirin	Q2037	
	Fluzone	Q2038	

RANK	Laboratory		
	Venipuncture		36415
	Blood glucose, monitoring device		82962
	Blood glucose, visual dipstick		82948
	CBC, w/auto differential		85025
	CBC, w/o auto		85027
	Cholesterol		82465
	Hemoccult, guaiac		82270
	Hemoccult, immunoassay, non-Medicare		82274
	Hemoglobin A1C		83036
	Lipid panel		80061
	Liver panel		80076
	KOH prep (skin, hair, nails)		87220
	Metabolic panel, basic		80048
	Metabolic panel, comprehensive		80053
	Mononucleosis		86308
	Pregnancy, blood		84703
	Pregnancy, urine		81025
	Renal panel		80069
	Sedimentation rate		85651
	Strep, rapid, antibody		86403
	Strep culture		87081
	Strep A, rapid, direct, observatiion		87880
	TB		86580
	UA, complete, non-automated		81000
	UA, w/o micro, non-automated		81002
	UA, w/ micro, non-automated		81003
	Urine colony count		87086
	Urine culture, presumptive		87088
	Wet mount/KOH		87210
	Vaccines		
	DT, <7 y		90702
	DtaP, <7 y		90700
	Flu, preservative-free, 6-35 months		90655
	Flu, preservative-free, 3 y +		90656
	Flu, quadrivalent, live, intranasal		90672
	Flu, inectivated, subunit, adjuvanted, IM		90653
	Hep A, adult		90632
	Hep A, ped/adol, 2 dose		90633
	Hep B, adult		90746
	Hep B, adult, 2 dose		90739
	Hep B, ped/adol 3 dose		90744
	Hep B-Hib		90748
	Hib, 4 dose		90645
	HPV, bivalent		90650
	HPV, quadrivalent		90649
	IPV		90713
	MMR		90707
	Pneumonia		90732
	Pneumonia conjugate, <5 y		90669
	Tdap, >7 y+		90715
	Varicella		90716
	Immunizations & Injections		**Units**
	Allergen, one	95115	
	Allergen, multiple	95117	
	Imm admin, one	90471	
	Imm admin, each add'l	90472	
	Imm admin, intranasal, one	90473	
	Imm admin, intranasal, each add'l	90474	
	Imm admin, <19 y, face-to-face couns	90460	
	Imm admin, <19 y, face-to-face couns, each additional	90461	
	Injection, joint, small	20600	
	Injection, joint, intermediate	20605	
	Injection, joint, major	20610	
	Injection, ther/proph/diag	90772	
	Injection, trigger point	20552	

FIGURE 10-3 An example of a superbill.[9]

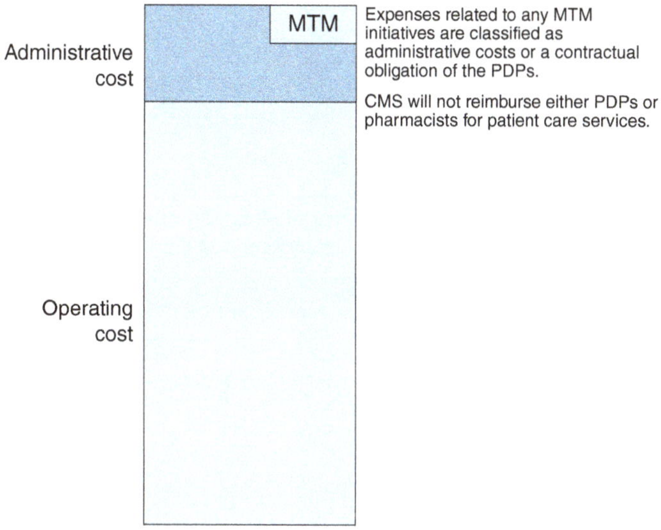

FIGURE 10-4 CMS payments to prescription drug plans.

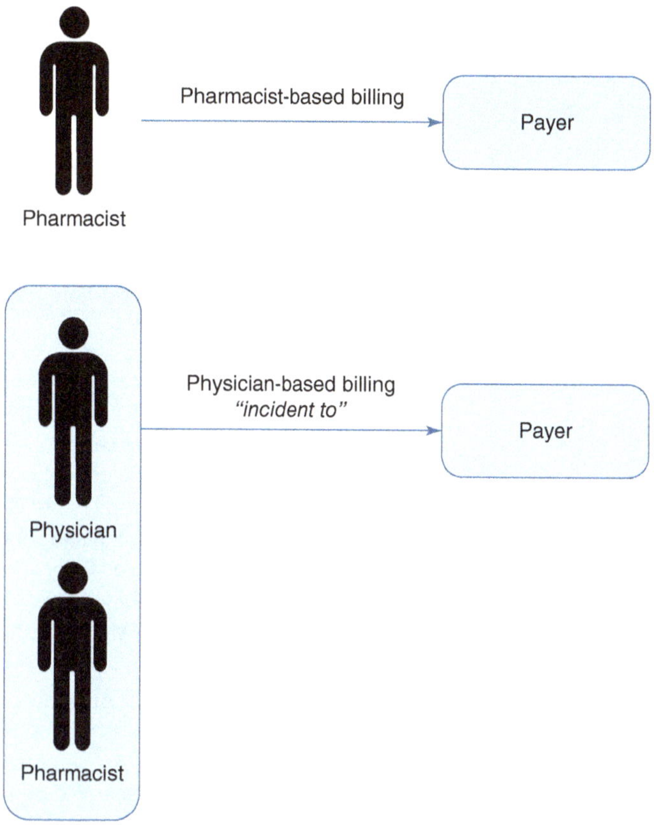

FIGURE 10-5 Pharmacist- and physician-based billing models.

professional to a patient, whether at home or in a healthcare facility, and includes the provision, management, and/or coordination of services as needed for all medical conditions, psychosocial needs, and activities of daily living. Pharmacists are included within the definition of "other qualified healthcare provider" as defined by the AMA CPT Professional Edition codebook. The Care Management Service codes support the multidisciplinary approach that is consistent with healthcare reform payment modeling. These services described within this section include Transitional Care Management Services, Chronic Care Management Services, Complex Chronic Care Management Services, and Advanced Care Planning.

Facilitating all these care management services is a documented plan of care that is shared with the patient and/or caregiver. It is a comprehensive plan for all the health problems based on a physical, mental, cognitive, social, functional and environmental assessment.

The care management office/practice must have the following capabilities:

- Provide to patients and/or caregivers 24/7 access to physicians or other qualified healthcare professionals or clinical support staff
- Provide continuity of care with a designated member of the care team

TABLE 10-3 • CPT MTMS Codes

CPT code type:	Category I
CPT chapter:	Medicine Chapter
Code title:	Medication Therapy Management Services (MTMS)
Code background	Medication Therapy Management Services describe face-to-face patient assessment and intervention as appropriate, by a pharmacist, on request; MTMS is provided to optimize the response to medications or to manage treatment-related medication interactions or complications MTMS includes the following documented elements: review of the pertinent patient history, medication profile (prescription and nonprescription), and recommendations for improving health outcomes and treatment compliance; these codes are not to be used to describe the provision of product-specific information at the point of dispensing or any other routine dispensing-related activities
Codes:	99605 Medication therapy management services provided by a pharmacist, individual, face-to-face with patient, with assessment and intervention if provided; initial 15 minutes, new patient 99606 Initial 15 minutes, established patient 99607 Each additional 15 minutes (list separately in addition to the code for primary service)
The caveats for these codes include the following: 1. A patient is considered new if it is the first encounter or if it has been more than 3 years since the last encounter. 2. Payers may authorize MTMS reimbursement for both face-to-face and remote encounters. 3. Time-based billing codes are used in block increments, not the exact length of the encounter in minutes (eg, a 25-minute encounter with a new patient would be submitted as 1 × 99605 and 1 × 99607).	

TABLE 10-4 • CPT "Incident to" Codes

CPT code type:	Category I	
CPT chapter:	Evaluation & Management	
Code title:	Office or Other Outpatient Services	
Code description:	Established patient	
Codes:	99211	Office or other outpatient visit for the evaluation and management of an established patient, which may not require the presence of a physician or other qualified healthcare professional Usually, the presenting problems are minimal; typically, 5 minutes are spent performing these services
	99212	Office or other outpatient visit for the evaluation and management of an established patient, which requires at least 2 of 3 key components: • A problem-focused history • A problem-focused examination • Straightforward medical decision-making Counseling and coordination of care with other physicians, other qualified healthcare professionals, or agencies are provided consistent with the nature of the problems and the patient's or family's needs Usually the presenting problems are self-limited or minor; typically, 10 minutes are spent face-to-face with the patient or family
	99213	Office or other outpatient visit for the evaluation and management of an established patient, which requires at least 2 of 3 key components: • An expanded problem-focused history • An expanded problem-focused examination • Medical decision-making of low complexity Counseling and coordination of care with other physicians, other qualified healthcare professionals, or agencies are provided consistent with the nature of the problems and the patient's or family's needs. Usually the presenting problems are self-limited or minor; typically, 15 minutes are spent face-to-face with the patient or family
	99214	Office or other outpatient visit for the evaluation and management of an established patient, which requires at least 2 of 3 key components: • A detailed focused history • A detailed focused examination • Medical decision-making of moderate complexity Counseling and coordination of care with other physicians, other qualified healthcare professionals, or agencies are provided consistent with the nature of the problems and the patient's or family's needs Usually the presenting problems are self-limited or minor; typically, 25 minutes are spent face-to-face with the patient or family
	99215	Office or other outpatient visit for the evaluation and management of an established patient, which requires at least 2 of 3 key components: • A comprehensive focused history • A comprehensive focused examination • Medical decision-making of high complexity Counseling and coordination of care with other physicians, other qualified healthcare professionals, or agencies are provided consistent with the nature of the problems and the patient's or family's needs Usually the presenting problems are self-limited or minor; typically, 40 minutes are spent face-to-face with the patient or family

- Provide timely access and management for follow-up after emergency department visit
- Utilize electronic health record (EHR)
- Use standardized methodology to identify patients who require care management services
- Employ an internal care management process to ensure identified patients start receiving care management services in a timely manner
- Use a standardized form and format within the medical record
- Engage and educate patients and caregivers
- Coordinate care among all service professionals for each patient

TABLE 10-5 • CPT TCMS Codes

CPT code type:	Category I	
CPT chapter:	Evaluation & Management	
Code title:	Transitional Care Management Services (TCMS)	
Codes:	99495	Transitional Care Management Services with the following required elements: • Communication (direct contact, telephone, electronic) with the patient or caregiver within 2 business days of discharge • Medical decision-making of at least moderate complexity during the service period • Face-to-face visit, within 14 calendar days of discharge
	99496	Transitional Care Management Services with the following required elements: • Communication (direct contact, telephone, electronic) with the patient or caregiver within 2 business days of discharge • Medical decision-making of high complexity during the service period • Face-to-face visit, within 7 calendar days of discharge
The caveats for these codes include the following: 1. Only 1 provider is supposed to report these codes during the 30-day period following the patient's transition. 2. The TCMS billing provider may not submit MTM codes (99605, 99606, and 99607) during the same period.		

Transitional Care Management Services

Codes: 99495, 99496. The TCMS codes were added to the AMA CPT codebook in 2013 (Table 10-5). These codes were developed in response to the increased focus on improving the coordination and management of patient care services during the transition from hospital or inpatient setting to a community setting, such as a patient's home or assisted-living facility. These codes focus on patients whose medical and/or psychosocial problems require either moderate or high-complexity medical decision-making during transitions from an inpatient setting (eg, acute hospital, rehabilitation facility, long-term acute-care or skilled nursing facility) to the patient's community setting. TCMS codes may be used by a physician or other qualified healthcare professionals from the date of discharge throughout the next 29 days.[8]

The TCMS involve one face-to-face visit in combination with remote services. An initial face-to-face visit must occur within designated timeframes and additional remote services are provided by the physician, other qualified healthcare provider, or clinical support staff. Services provided by the physician or other qualified healthcare providers include the following

- Collection and review of discharge information
- Determination of need for follow-up activities
- Interaction with other healthcare providers
- Education (patient or caregivers)
- Coordination of referrals
- Coordination with follow-up activities with other providers and services

Remote services provided by clinical support staff under the direction of the physician or other qualified healthcare provider include the following:

- Communications regarding aspects of care (patient or caregivers)
- Communications with other care providers or services
- Patient and/or family/caregiver education
- Assessment for treatment regimens
- Identification of community and health resources
- Facilitating access to care and services

Chronic Care Management Services

Code: 99490. The CCMS codes (Table 10-6) were added in 2015 and describe patient-centered condition management and

TABLE 10-6 • CPT CCMS Codes

CPT code type:	Category I	
CPT chapter:	Evaluation & Management	
Code title:	Chronic Care Management Services (CCMS)	
Codes:	99490	Chronic Care Management Services, at least 20 minutes of clinical staff time directed by a physician or other qualified health care professional, per calendar month with the following required elements: 1. Multiple (≥2) chronic conditions expected to last at least 12 months or until the death of the patient. 2. Chronic conditions place the patient at significant risk of death, acute exacerbation/decompensation, or functional decline. 3. Comprehensive care plan established, implemented, revised, or monitored.
The caveats for these codes include the following: 1. Chronic care management services of less than 20 minutes duration, in a calendar month, are not reported separately.		

clinical support services provided by clinical staff when the medical and/or psychosocial needs of the patient require establishing, implementing, revising, or monitoring of the care plan.[8] Chronic Care Management Services patients have two or more chronic health or episodic health conditions that are expected to last at least 12 months, or until death of the patient, and that place the patient as significant risk of death, acute exacerbation/decompensation, or functional decline. This code is used when at least 20 minutes of clinical staff time is spent on care management activities during a month.

Care management services performed by support staff typically include the following:

- Communication and engagement with patient, family members, guardian, caregivers, surrogate decision-makers and/or other professionals
- Communication with home health agencies and other community services utilized by the patient
- Collection of health outcomes data and registry documentation
- Patient and/or family/caregiver education to support self-management, independent living, and activities of daily living
- Assessment and support for treatment regimen adherence and medication management
- Identification of available community and health resources
- Facilitating access to care and services
- Management of care transitions not reported as part of Transitional Care Management
- Ongoing review of patient status, including review of laboratory and other studies not reported as part of an E/M service
- Development, communication, and maintenance of a comprehensive care plan

Complex Chronic Care Management Services

Codes: 99487, 99489. The CCCMS codes (Table 10-7) describe the following services offered during a given month that includes criteria for CCMS as well as establishment or substantial revision of a comprehensive care plan; medical, functional, and/or psychosocial problems requiring moderate or high-complexity medical decision-making; and clinical staff care management for at least 60 minutes under the direction of a physician or other healthcare professional. Medical decision making is determined by the problems addressed by the reporting individual as defined by the evaluation and management (E/M) guidelines.

Patients who require CCCMS may be identified by practice-specific or other published algorithms that recognize multiple illnesses, multiple medication use, inability to perform functions of daily living, requirement for a caregiver, and/or repeat admissions or visits to the emergency department. All patients must have two or more chronic continuous or episodic conditions expected to last more than 12 months or until death of the patient and that place the patient at significant risk of death, acute exacerbation/decompensation, or functional decline. Typical patients have complex conditions and morbidities and may demonstrate one or more of the following conditions:

- Need for the coordination of a number of specialties and services
- Inability to perform activities of daily living and/or cognitive impairment resulting in poor adherence to the treatment plan without substantial assistance from a caregiver
- Psychiatric and other medical comorbidities (eg, dementia and chronic obstructive pulmonary disease or substance abuse and diabetes) that complicate their care
- Social support requirements or difficulty with access to care

In general, typical adult patients requiring CCCMS have three or more prescription medications and may be receiving other types of therapeutic interventions (eg, physical therapy, occupational therapy), and typical pediatric patients require three or more therapeutic interventions (medications, nutritional support, respiratory support).

Pharmacists play a critical role in the medical decision-making and ongoing complex chronic-care coordination process.

TABLE 10-7 • CPT CCCMS Codes

CPT code type:	Category I	
CPT chapter:	Evaluation & Management	
Code title:	Complex Chronic Care Management Services	
Codes:	99487	Complex Chronic Care Coordination Services (60-89 minutes) with the following elements: 1. Multiple (≥2) chronic conditions expected to last at least 12 months or until the death of the patient 2. Chronic conditions place the patient at significant risk of death, acute exacerbation/ decompensation, or functional decline 3. Establishment or substantial revision of a comprehensive care plan 4. Moderate or high-complexity decision-making 5. 60 minutes of clinical staff time directed by a physician or other qualified health care professional, per calendar month
	99489	Each additional 30 minutes of clinical staff time directed by a physician or other qualified healthcare professional, per calendar month (list separately in addition to code for primary procedure)
The caveats for these codes include the following: 1. Only 1 provider is supposed to report these codes during a calendar month. 2. Physicians or other healthcare providers may not report CCCMS if the care plan is unchanged or requires minimal change (eg, only a medication is changed or an adjustment in a treatment modality is ordered). 3. Do not bill CCCMS for duration of services less than 60 minutes or for care management services of <30 minutes additional to the first 60 minutes of CCCMS during a calendar month. 4. The CCCMS billing provider may not submit MTM codes (99605, 99606, and 99607) during the same month.		

According to their level of professional training, scope of practice, and established patient care services, pharmacists meet the definition of "other qualified healthcare provider" as defined within the AMA CPT codebook.

Current Procedural Terminology Code Valuation

There are multiple methods for determining the value or value range for medical billing codes. Following the development and approval of medical billing codes within the AMA's CPT editorial panel process, the codes are typically submitted to the AMA/Specialty Society RVS Update Committee (RUC). The RUC is a multispecialty and multidisciplinary committee that is sanctioned by CMS to perform a standardized financial survey that determines a value range for the codes.[14]

The *resource-based relative value scale* (RBRVS) is a schema used to determine the code values and ranges of payments to healthcare providers. The RBRVS then provides for variations or adjustments in payment ranges based on the US geographic regions. Each code is composed of three primary elements: (1) the work, (2) the practice expense, and (3) the liability (medical malpractice expense) relevant to the code.

To ensure practical and functional results, the RUC engages providers and specialty organizations affected by the codes as participants and resources to determine realistic estimates of professional time, support staff time, overhead, liability, and resources involved with performing the specific codes.

It should be noted that the RUC, by design, is charged with and restricted to performing the valuation process on codes that are applicable to Medicare Part B providers. If codes are used primarily by providers who do not deliver Part B services, then they are not valued by the AMA's RUC. Codes that are not valued by the RUC are referred to as *market value*, which implies that there is no RUC-derived value range for the codes. Payers may conduct their own calculations and surveys to determine the rate schedule for market-value codes.

From a provider's perspective, determining a medical service code rate should include the following: professional time, support staff time, resources, liability, overhead, and profit margin. Attempting to base medical service rates solely on the provider's time and professional service rate is a common mistake that does not provide for sufficient revenue to support the delivery of the service and related expenses. There are numerous algorithms and methods that perform service rate estimates, and the approach will vary relative to the service type (ie, diagnostic, procedural, or cognitive).

As the demand for and reliance on clinical interventions from pharmacists have increased, both practitioners and payers have begun to analyze the costs associated with MTM in various practice settings. Practitioner surveys, practice management data, and cost analysis software all provide the information that will ultimately determine accurate fee schedules for the diversity of services provided by pharmacists. A thorough cost analysis should include assessments of the direct cost, indirect costs, breakeven analysis, and cost margin—all prior to applying a desired profit margin. Failing to evaluate these key components could negatively affect the sustainability of the pharmacist's practice model.[15]

In an effort to emulate the tiered-intensity model of the AMA CPT E/M coding, pharmacists in Minnesota have developed a rate schedule based on tiered criteria.[16] The E/M codes for a new office or other outpatient service involve five tiers (99201, 99202, 99203, 99204, and 99205); 99201 is the lowest-intensity code, and 99205 is the highest-intensity code. Providers are responsible for selecting, based on a combination of criteria (ie, level of history, level of examination, and level of medical decision-making), which code and corresponding payment level transpired during the patient encounter. The Minnesota MTM pricing model utilized a more pharmacist-centric set of criteria (ie, number of medical indications, number of medications, and number of drug therapy problems) as a foundation for articulating the level of intensity of a pharmacist's patient care encounter. However, attempting to apply an RBRVS method similar to the Minnesota model may cause documentation confusion if it is applied as a standardized algorithm. Patient risks for complications and negative outcomes are not directly correlated with these types of criteria. For example, a patient with a single serious medical condition who may be taking only one or two high-risk medications would score low on this scale, but the impact and value of the MTM encounter would be of high significance. RBRVS intensity criteria should always ensure that the provider has the ability to interpret the intensity on the basis of the patient's risk factors and supportive services provided and not be constricted by pure numerical calculations. Minnesota's efforts to develop an RBRVS-like scoring system have been productive and improved payer implementation of payment systems to pharmacists for both commercial and Medicaid patient populations.

Healthcare providers should be actively involved in the determination and maintenance of CPT code value ranges to ensure that payers are using rational methods and appropriate value ranges that ensure the delivery of quality healthcare services.

Preservice Payment Determination

Prior to providing a clinical service, providers should assess a patient's healthcare coverage and scope of benefits. This is to ensure that both the patient and the provider have complied with the payer's guidelines and policies. If the patient does not have healthcare coverage or if the payer does not cover the provider, specialty type, or the specific service, then the reimbursement method is private pay. If the patient has healthcare coverage, then it is important to determine whether the scope of benefits includes pharmacists and their patient care services.

Insurance companies and health plans are accustomed to giving providers rapid access to descriptions of patients' scopes of benefits or patient eligibility for specific services and procedures. Pharmacists should contact a payer's provider services department as a primary point of contact for this information. In many cases, on obtaining the patient's healthcare coverage details (ie, patient ID, date of birth, group number, and policy number), this information may even be accessible online from the payer's website.

It is imperative to identify and confirm in advance whether the payer is able to pay for the services or procedures. Payers typically have prior authorization systems to confirm or deny payment for noncovered services, procedures, and healthcare products. MTMS providers frequently receive prior authorization approvals, even on a case-by-case basis, to provide direct patient care services.

It is important to track and record the details of this process as well as to use a payer's forms and processes to optimize payment potential. Historical information concerning prior authorization and payment is also critical. This can ensure future efficiencies in case the patient needs to be seen for subsequent services.

CASE STUDIES

Case Study 1

Setting	Outpatient clinic
Practice model	Pharmacist practice
Payment	Health plan, included in scope of benefits (no prior authorization required)
Service description	MTMS: comprehensive medication review (face-to-face), new patient
Service time	45 minutes
Codes	CPT: MTMS 1 × 99605 (initial 15 minutes) 2 × 99607 (each additional 15 minutes)
Form	CMS-1500

Case Study 2

Setting	Outpatient clinic
Practice model	Physician practice (pharmacist service is provided "Incident to" physician)
Payment	Health plan, included in scope of benefits (no prior authorization required)
Service description	Anticoagulation services visit, face-to-face, laboratory monitoring, medication dosage adjustment, and patient as well as caregiver education; includes the following criteria: (1) expanded problem-focused history, (2) expanded problem-focused examination, and (3) medical decision making of low complexity
Service Time	20 minutes
Codes	CPT: "Incident to" 1 × 99213
Form	CMS-1500

Case Study 3

Setting	Outpatient clinic
Practice model	Pharmacy
Payment	Private pay
Service description	MTMS: medication review and pharmacogenetic analysis (face-to-face), established patient
Service time	30 minutes
Codes	CPT: MTMS 1 × 99606 (initial 15 minutes) 1 × 99607 (each additional 15 minutes)
Form	Patient invoice + CMS-1500 (if requested by patient to submit to payer)

Case Study 4

Setting	Outpatient clinic
Practice model	Pharmacist practice with physician team member
Payment	Health plan
Service description	Transitional Care Management Service (TCMS), face-to-face visit within 2 days of discharge from hospital to home, face-to-face visit within 7 days of discharge, patient was of high complexity
Service time	2.0 hours
Codes	CPT: TCMS 1 × 99496 TCMS with face-to-face visit, high-complexity patient, and follow-up within 7 days of discharge
Form	CMS-1500

Case Study 5

Setting	Outpatient clinic
Practice model	Pharmacist practice with physician team member
Payment	Accountable-care organization
Service description	Complex Chronic Care Management Services (CCCMS)
Service time	3.5 hours
Codes	CPT-CCCMS 1 × 99487 first hour 5 × 99489 each additional half hour
Form	CMS-1500

CONCLUSION

Pharmacists provide essential healthcare services that include the coordination, preparation, and delivery of medication therapy as well as direct patient care services focused on proper treatment, optimizing health outcomes, improving patient safety, and preserving medication access for patients both with and without healthcare coverage. With the development of CPT codes for MTM, payers have the mechanical and logistical tools to include pharmacists and MTM services within the standard scope of healthcare benefits. While many commercial health plans, state Medicaid programs, and Medicare Part D vendors (ie, prescription drug plans) have included varying degrees of access and payment for pharmacist services, MTM is not universally included in the standard scope of health benefits. CMS does not currently pay for pharmacist services based on an administrative clause within the Medicare law. The Medicare law includes a section referred to as "Medicare Part B Eligible Provider Status." This paragraph within the law presents a list of healthcare professionals who are eligible to receive payment for patient care services with Medicare funding. Currently, pharmacists are not included in this list and are precluded from receiving reimbursement from Medicare for services provided to Medicare beneficiaries. With CMS representing the largest of payers on a national level, it is imperative for Medicare beneficiaries, physicians, and pharmacists that the definition be expanded to include pharmacists.

Even though CMS represents a logical challenge for providing MTM services for Medicare patients, there is nothing restricting pharmacists from developing functional reimbursement models for services from direct pay patients and other health plans.

REFERENCES

1. AMA. *CPT® Process: How a Code Becomes a Code*; American Medical Association. Available at https://www.ama-assn.org/practice-management/cpt®-process-how-code-becomes-code. Accessed February 6, 2017.
2. AMA. *Current Procedural Terminology (CPT) 2015, Introduction*. Chicago, IL: American Medical Association; 2014.
3. Buffington DE. Pharmacist current procedural terminology codes and medication therapy management. *Am J Health Syst Pharm*. 2006;63(11):1008-1010.
4. Medication Therapy Management Service Codes. *PSTAC Pharmacist Services Technical Advisory Coalition*; 2010. Available at http://www.pstac.org/services/mtms-codes.html. Accessed February 6, 2017.
5. CMS. *Medicare Billing: 837P and Form CMS-1500*. Available at https://www.cms.gov/Outreach-and-Education/Medicare-Learning-Network-MLN/MLNProducts/Downloads/837P-CMS-1500.pdf. Accessed February 6, 2017.
6. Blue Cross Blue Shield. *Guide for Completing the CMS-1450 (Institutional Claims) Form*. Available at https://www.bcbsil.com/pdf/education/tutorials_user_guides/ub_user_guide.pdf. Accessed February 6, 2017.
7. National Provider Identifier. *NPPES*. Available at https://nppes.cms.hhs.gov/NPPES/StaticForward.do?forward=static.npistart. Accessed January 25, 2013.
8. AMA. *Current Procedural Terminology (CPT) 2015, Evaluation & Management*. Chicago, IL: American Medical Association; 2014.
9. AAFP. *Superbill*. American Academy of Family Physicians. Available at http://www.aafp.org/fpm/icd9/fpmsuperbill.pdf. Accessed January 5, 2013.
10. *Superbills: ICD-9 vs. ICD-10*. Available at https://www.aapc.com/ICD-10/superbills.aspx. Accessed September 29, 2014.
11. American Pharmacists Association (APA), National Association of Chain Drug Stores Foundation. *Medication Therapy Management in Community Pharmacy Practice: Core Elements of an MTM Service*, version 2.0. Available at http://www.pharmacist.com/sites/default/files/files/core_elements_of_an_mtm_practice.pdf. Accessed March 19, 2012.
12. AMA. *Current Procedural Terminology (CPT) 2015, Evaluation & Management*. Chicago, IL: American Medical Association; 2014.
13. Nicoletti B. *Billing Incident to Services*. *Physicians Practice*, April 29, 2010. Available at http://www.physicianspractice.com/pearls/billing-incident-services. Accessed February 6, 2013.
14. AMA. *RBRVS Overview*; 2013. Available at https://www.ama-assn.org/rbrvs-overview. Accessed January 15, 2013.
15. Rupp MT. Analyzing the costs to deliver medication therapy management services. *J Am Pharm Assoc*. 2011;51(3):19-27.
16. Isetts BJ. *Evaluating Effectiveness of the Minnesota Medication Therapy Management Care Program*. Available at http://archive.leg.state.mn.us/docs/2008/mandated/080113.pdf. Accessed January 23, 2013.

Review Questions

1. Payment to the pharmacist for MTM services may come from all of the following EXCEPT
   a. private payment (patient, family, caregivers)
   b. health insurance
   c. Medicare
   d. MA-PD plans
   e. PDPs

2. The CPT payment code for MTM-only services is
   a. 99605
   b. 99495
   c. 99487
   d. 99211
   e. 99215

3. A superbill is
   a. the same as 99606.
   b. required by CMS for MTM billing.
   c. required by PDPs for MTM payment.
   d. useful for services beyond MTM.
   e. required in transition care management

4. A requirement for CPT 99605 is
   a. face-to-face interaction with the patient.
   b. the patient's goals for therapy.
   c. a completed care plan.
   d. a reduction in polypharmacy
   e. improvement in patient outcomes

5. A requirement of incident to billing is
   a. creation of the first care plan.
   b. an extra payment for the primary provider.
   c. done in the area where the care was delivered.
   d. that the physician be physically present.
   e. that adverse drug events must be reduced.

6. Transitional care management services that may be delegated include
   a. collection and review of discharge information.
   b. determination of need for follow-up activities.
   c. interaction with other healthcare providers.
   d. coordination of follow-up activities with other providers and services.
   e. all of the above.

7. Care coordination services may include all of the following EXCEPT
   a. communications with the patient or caregiver
   b. communications with supportive-care agencies and service providers
   c. guaranteed health outcomes
   d. self-management education (patient or caregiver)
   e. assessment of treatment adherence and medication management

8. RBRVS calculation includes all of the following EXCEPT
   a. pharmacy fees
   b. geographic variation
   c. expertise
   d. practice expense
   e. malpractice cost

9. All of the following is true about the RUC EXCEPT
   a. AMA committee
   b. sets charges for Part B physician services
   c. involves physician specialty societies
   d. sets market-value prices
   e. does not include profit margin in charges

10. MTM payment determination by a commercial insurance plan
    a. uses the RUC market value payments amounts.
    b. will match the Minnesota Medicaid payment model.
    c. factors in if the pharmacist is APhA MTM certified.
    d. will require discussion with the plan's chief medical officer.
    e. depends on the scope of the patient's benefit.

ANSWERS

1. c	2. a	3. d
4. a	5. c	6. e
7. c	8. a	9. d
10. e		

11

The Complicated Patient

Kelechi C. Ogbonna, PharmD, MSHA, BCGP, Krista L. Donohoe, PharmD, BCPS, BCGP, Jenna S. Clemons, PharmD, and Jeffrey C. Delafuente, MS, FCCP, FASCP

KEY POINTS

- Multiple chronic conditions (MCCs) present challenges to older adults and their healthcare providers.
- Geriatric syndromes are not specific diseases but a constellation of symptoms common in older adults.
- The extensive use of medications by the geriatric population increases the risk of adverse drug events (ADEs), drug-drug interactions, disease-drug interactions, and food-drug interactions, and often contributes to medication nonadherence among patients.
- Poor care coordination and insufficient communication among providers caring for a patient is a cause of ADEs in older adults.
- The prescribing cascade commonly contributes to what is referred to as *polymedicine* or *polypharmacy*.
- Healthcare delivery for people with MCCs is often fragmented, less effective, complex as well as confusing, and more expensive.
- As older adults move from one healthcare setting to another, they are vulnerable to consequences of poor communication between settings and between providers.
- Many of the existing clinical practice guidelines do not take into consideration populations with physical disability, multiple medications, and multiple comorbidities, all of which are commonly seen in older adults.
- Providing care to older adults with complex conditions requires a specific skill set and knowledge about geriatric pharmacotherapy.
- The Beers criteria, The Screening Tool of Older Person's Prescriptions (STOPP) / Screening Tool to Alert Doctors to Right Treatment (START), and the Medication Appropriateness Index (MAI) provide a variety of methods to assess medication appropriateness.
- Little research exists to help identify the most effective means to improve health outcomes in patients with MCCs.
- Patients with complex multiple conditions need a team approach to improve and coordinate care.
- *Caregiver burden* describes the toll on people providing care and has been defined as "a multidimensional response to physical, psychological, emotional, social, and financial stressors associated with the caregiving experience."

CHARACTERISTICS OF THE AGING POPULATION

Older adults—those aged ≥65 years—numbered 46.2 million, or 14.5% of the entire population, in the United States in 2014. In the 10 years between 2000 and 2010 the older adult population increased by 5.4 million or 15.3%, almost twice the rate of those aged <65 years, and is expected to increase by 36% in the next decade (Figure 11-1).[1,2] By 2030 the number of older people is expected to be at 72.1 million—more than twice that of 2000. The 2010 US census identified 53,365 individuals aged ≥100 years, a 53% rate of increase from 20 years earlier, and this trend is expected to continue. Among older adults, women outnumber men by a ratio of 1.32 to 1; for those aged ≥85 years, the female-to-male ratio increases to 2.06 to 1.[2]

On average, a 65-year-old woman can expect to live an additional 20.5 years and her male counterpart, another 18 years. Since the mid-1990s, life expectancy for older adults in the United States has increased by more than 4 years because of improvements in healthcare. However, this increased longevity is less than that of other high-income countries, mainly because of heavy smoking among older adults when they were younger.[2] Other factors, such as obesity, diet, exercise, and economic inequality, also contribute to the divergence in life expectancy between the United States and other high-income countries.

Chronic Conditions of Older Adults

Chronic medical conditions are common among older adults. The most common chronic conditions in the Medicare population are

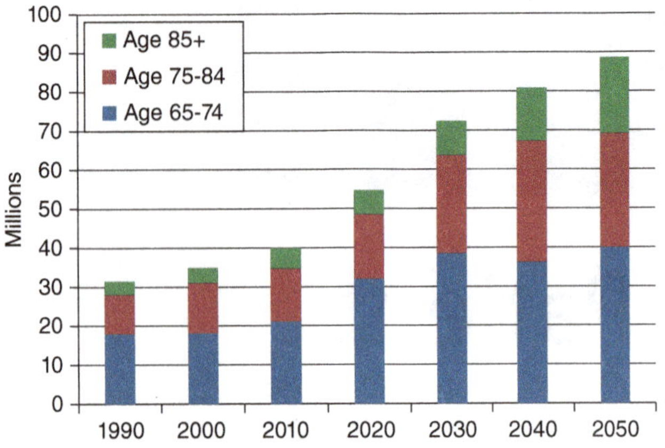

FIGURE 11-1 There will be a steep rate of increase in the older adult population over the next 25 years.

Source: Administration for Community Living, U.S. Department of Health and Human Services. *Aging. Projected Future Growth of the Older Population*. Available at http://aoa.gov/AoARoot/Aging_Statistics/future_growth/future_growth.aspx. Accessed May 23, 2014.

shown in Table 11-1. Hypertension, hyperlipidemia, and arthritis are more common in women, while ischemic heart disease is more common in men. Two-thirds of the Medicare population have MCCs, defined as two or more chronic conditions, and having three or more chronic conditions is common (Figure 11-2). For example, about 50% of Medicare beneficiaries with heart failure or stroke also have five or more additional diseases.[3] Overall, 33% of older adults have two to three chronic conditions, and 21% have five or more. The number of multiple chronic diseases increases with age; in the oldest group, those aged ≥85 years, more than 50% have four or more chronic conditions (Table 11-2). Among Medicare beneficiaries with three chronic conditions, hypertension, and hyperlipidemia are the most commonly found conditions in combination with other ailments such as diabetes mellitus, ischemic heart disease, and arthritis (Table 11-3). MCCs in older adults vary little by race or ethnicity.[3] As baby boomers age, the prevalence of chronic conditions will grow significantly.

MCCs lead to poorer health outcomes and functional limitations among patients, along with higher hospitalization rates and costs.[3] Hospitalization rates, readmission rates, emergency department visits, and use of home healthcare services rise as the

TABLE 11-1 • Prevalence of Common Chronic Diseases in Medicare Beneficiaries Aged ≥65 Years

Chronic Condition	Prevalence (%)
Hypertension	58
Hyperlipidemia	48
Arthritis	31
Ischemic heart disease	29
Diabetes	27
Chronic kidney disease	17
Heart Failure	15
Depression	14

Source: Centers for Medicare and Medicaid Services (CMS). *Chronic Conditions Among Medicare Beneficiaries*; Chart Book, 2014 ed. Baltimore, MD.

number of chronic conditions increases.[4] Activities of daily living (ADLs) include bathing, dressing, feeding, getting in or out of a bed or chair, walking, and toileting. Instrumental activities of daily living (IADLs) include high levels of function, such as cooking, managing money, using a telephone, and taking medications correctly. Impairment in carrying out ADLs and IADLs increases within the aging population (Figure 11-3). Over 27% of community-dwelling residents older than 65 had difficulties with one or more ADLs, and almost 13% needed help with IADLs.[2] Other types of disabilities, such as those affecting vision, hearing, cognition, ambulation, or self-care, may occur in approximately 37% of older adults.[2] People with limited abilities to take care of themselves require caregiving to maintain adequate function. A small percentage of the older Medicare population (11%) require personal care from a caregiver, either paid or unpaid.

Challenges Associated With Services for Older Adults With Complex Conditions

Comprehensive assessments of complex older adults requires expertise and time. In addition to a physical exam, functional, psychological, and social assessments also need to be made. Obtaining a past medical history may be difficult if a patient has cognitive, visual, or hearing impairments or is unable to communicate. Older adults may underreport symptoms because they are afraid of being diagnosed with a catastrophic illness (dementia, cancer), or institutionalization, or because they consider their symptoms to be part of normal aging. Asking questions about functional abilities is critical to uncovering underlying illness. For example, asking an older person to describe what she/he did yesterday may indicate a sedentary lifestyle. However, further questioning might reveal that pain is causing limitations in mobility.

Obtaining a comprehensive and accurate medication list for a patient with MCCs can also be difficult. Insurance claim data do not include nonprescription drugs and medications for which the patient paid out of pocket, and patients may use multiple pharmacies. Patients with multiple conditions usually consult multiple physicians, and one physician might not know that another is caring and prescribing for the patient as well.

Time must be spent understanding a senior's social situation. The patient's living situation must be identified. Does she/he live alone? Can she/he care for her/himself? Caregivers and guardians need to be identified and included in the coordination of care decisions. It is also important to understand the patient's financial status to ensure adequate resources for medications, food, and healthcare are available. If not, the patient may need to be connected with local social services.

It is common for older adults to have atypical presentations of disease, requiring a greater degree of sophistication in diagnosis. Physiologic reserves are diminished, and homeostasis is easily disrupted. Disease in one system may present with symptoms in another. Delirium and cognitive impairment are often seen because of the weakened physiologic reserve of older brains, even when the causative illness is centered on another organ system. The stress of an infection or anemia may present as heart failure in an older person with preexisting risk factors. This might lead to treatment for heart failure when the appropriate therapy should be directed elsewhere. A myocardial infarction might present as weakness or confusion rather than the classic chest pain. Pain may be absent with peptic

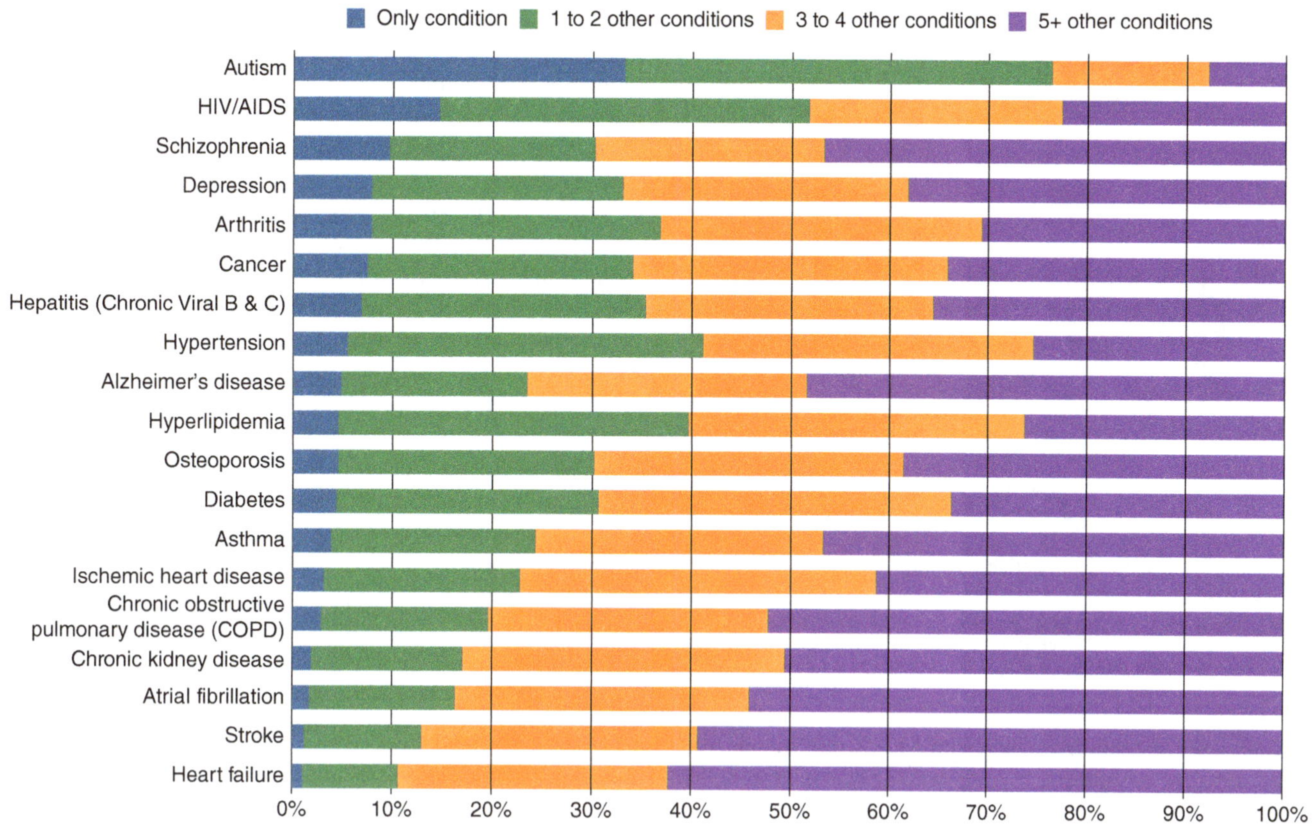

FIGURE 11-2 Comorbidity with three or more chronic conditions is common among Medicare beneficiaries.
Source: *Chronic Conditions among Medicare Beneficiaries*, Chart Book, 2014 ed. Baltimore, MD: Centers for Medicare & Medicaid Services.

ulcer disease. Misdiagnosis may occur because it can be difficult to diagnosis new symptoms in patients with multiple chronic diseases, as some coexisting diseases have similar symptoms. In addition, it is important to differentiate symptoms of an existing chronic condition from those of a new condition; this, too, can be challenging.

Geriatric syndromes are not specific diseases, but a constellation of symptoms common in older adults. Geriatric syndromes have various definitions but commonly include symptoms such as falling, acute confusion, syncope, weight loss, urinary incontinence, and dizziness. Geriatric syndromes are associated with increased morbidity, functional decline, and mortality. Underlying diseases as well as medications must be considered as potential causes of these syndromes. Adverse drug effects can cause geriatric syndromes and impair a person's ability to accomplish ADLs and IADLs.

Frailty is often defined as a constellation of symptoms, including unintentional weight loss of >10 pounds in 12 months, physical exhaustion, weakness as measured by grip strength, a decline in walking speed, and low physical activity.[5] People with three or more of these symptoms are considered to be frail. The term *prefrail* is used to describe people with one or two of these symptoms.[6] Because of varying definitions of frailty there is a wide range of prevalence estimations, from 4% to 59% among community-dwelling older adults. On average, approximately 42% of community-dwelling older adults are prefrail and about 11% are frail. Frailty increases with age; there is a 15.7% prevalence among 80- to 84-year-olds and a 26.1% prevalence in those aged ≥85 years.[7] Frailty contributes to

TABLE 11-2 • Percentage of Medicare Fee-for-Service (FFS) Beneficiaries by Number of Chronic Conditions and Age in 2010

Number of Chronic Conditions	65-74 Years (%)	75-84 Years (%)	≥85 Years (%)
2-3	34	33	29
4-5	20	27	29
≥6	9	18	25

Source: Centers for Medicare and Medicaid Services (CMS). *Chronic Conditions Among Medicare Beneficiaries*; *Chart Book*, 2012 ed. Baltimore, MD.

TABLE 11-3 • Chronic Condition Combinations in Medicare FFS Beneficiaries

Chronic Condition Combinations	Prevalence (%)
Hyperlipidemia, hypertension, ischemic heart disease	33.7
Hyperlipidemia, hypertension, diabetes mellitus	29.9
Hyperlipidemia, hypertension, arthritis	25.7
Hyperlipidemia, diabetes mellitus, ischemic heart disease	21.5
Hyperlipidemia, ischemic heart disease, arthritis	19.3

Source: Centers for Medicare and Medicaid Services (CMS). *Chronic Conditions Among Medicare Beneficiaries*; Chart Book, 2012 ed. Baltimore, MD.

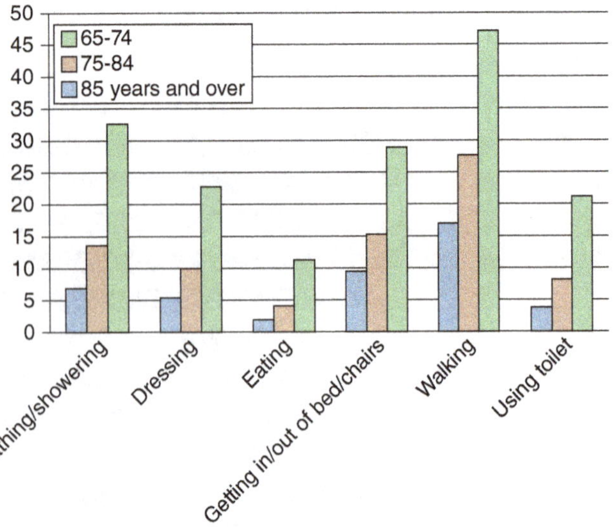

FIGURE 11-3 Impairment in activities of daily living increases with increasing age.

Source: Administration on Aging, US Department of Health and Human Resources. *A Profile of Older Americans;* 2011. Available at http://www.aarp.org/content/dam/aarp/livable-communities/learn/demographics/a-profile-of-older-americans-2011-aarp.pdf

the complexity of treating patients with MCCs. A comprehensive medication review is imperative in identifying whether frailty may be at least partially attributable to medication therapy. However, medications can also have a role in improving frailty, such as in improving grip strength or walking speed with better arthritis therapy or treating previously unrecognized depression.

Treating patients with MCCs present difficult challenges. Since the percentage of older adults with MCCs is high (see Figure 11-2), the number of medications they take also tends to be high. In older adults the incidence of ADEs increases with the number of medications taken. Polypharmacy also contributes to medication adherence problems and increased costs. Symptoms from ADEs are often misdiagnosed as a worsening of an existing condition or as a new condition.

Many older adults' chronic illnesses began when they were younger, but manifest as end-stage disease as they age. For example, a patient with long-standing diabetes may present with neuropathy, which increases falling risk, retinopathy, and peripheral vascular disease among other chronic conditions requiring specific treatment. Or a senior patient may have had rheumatoid arthritis for decades, but now her/his hands are so crippled that she/he may no longer be able to self-administer medications. Other challenges include deciding on drug therapy when two or more chronic conditions have contraindications for drug therapy, for example, using an anticholinergic medication for overactive bladder in a patient with dementia who is using an acetylcholinesterase inhibitor. The anticholinergic medication may worsen the dementia and lessen the effects of the acetylcholinesterase inhibitor.

PRESCRIBING IATROGENESIS

The Growing Problem

In the United States, older adults account for over 33% of outpatient spending on prescription medications.[2,8] This figure excludes herbals, supplements, and over-the-counter (OTC) medications, which would further increase the disproportionality between population size and medication usage. The extensive use of medications by the geriatric population increases the risk of ADEs, drug-drug interactions, disease-drug interactions, food-drug interactions, and often contributes to medication nonadherence among patients.[9,10]

Why is this population different, and how do we create such complex regimens? These questions are important, but are often multifactorial and not easily answered. Aging is associated with physiologic decline as well as increased prevalence of disease, and the increased lifespan of older adults has led to more individuals living with chronic conditions.[11] To combat many of these ailments, medications are prescribed either to sustain life or to improve quality of life. However, finding the line between benefit and harm, particularly when treating older adults, can be difficult. As patients age, the rate of medication addition is greater than the rate of medication reassessment and withdrawal.[12] This unbalanced approach not only increases the number of prescribed medications, but also can lead to unintended consequences.

Inappropriate Prescribing

Prescribing iatrogenesis, also known as the *prescribing cascade*, has been described extensively.[13-16] The most widely accepted definition was proposed in the 1990s by Rochon et al, who suggested that the prescribing cascade occurs when a drug side effect is mistaken for a new medical condition, which results in initiation of a second drug.[16] All too often in older adults, the initiation of an additional agent to treat what is believed to be a new condition results in the 14th, 15th, or even 19th medication prescribed.

Practitioner and patient characteristics play a substantial role in prescribing complexity, with no one factor identified as the primary cause.[17] A clinician's failure to recognize and act on an ADE may be due to the older adult's inability to associate the appearance of new symptoms with a medication or the healthcare provider attributing the patient's new physical or psychological complaints to aging rather than an ADE.[18] Regardless of the cause, an unidentified ADE can have severe consequences.

Figure 11-4 illustrates potential unintended consequences of the prescribing cascade. A patient may treat joint pain with OTC ibuprofen, which, in turn, may adversely affect her/his blood pressure (BP). During the patient's next primary-care appointment, a diuretic is prescribed to treat the elevated BP. The patient now presents to the urologist with urinary frequency and is prescribed oxybutynin. This inadvertent prescribing of medications for drug side effects appears obvious on paper, but is often difficult for practitioners to identify in practice. As stated previously, lack of awareness by either the patient or healthcare provider can contribute to prescribing iatrogenesis. In addition, poor care coordination can hinder identification of medication-related adverse effects.

Poor care coordination, in this case illustrated by insufficient communication among several providers caring for an individual patient, has been cited as a potential cause of drug-drug interactions and ADEs in older adults.[19-21] Green et al evaluated the correlation between the number of physicians prescribing medications to an older adult patient and the likelihood of that patient self-reporting an ADE. A telephone survey regarding the number of prescribing physicians, chronic conditions, medications, ADEs, and general health status was given to 405 Medicare managed care

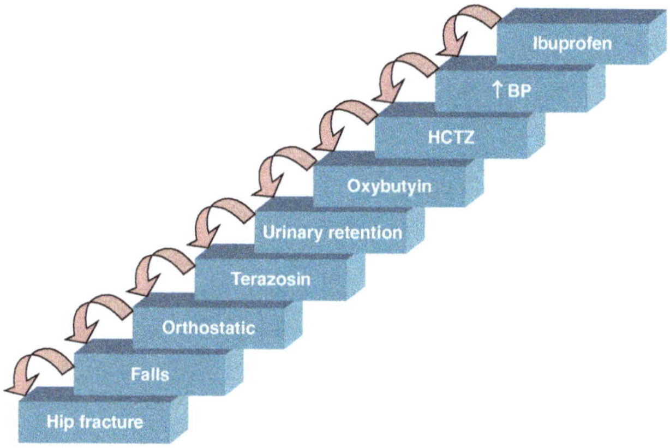

FIGURE 11-4 The prescribing cascade occurs when an adverse drug event is treated with another medication, which, in turn, causes another medication-related problem, which then gets treated with another medication. In this illustration, ibuprofen increases blood pressure; then a diuretic is added to treat the hypertension but causes urinary frequency that is misdiagnosed and the patient receives oxybutynin, which causes urinary retention treated with terazosin. The terazosin causes orthostatic hypotension, leading to a fall that results in a fracture.
Abbreviation: HCTZ = Hydrochlorothiazide.

enrollees aged ≥65 years. The researchers found that the number of prescribing physicians was an independent risk factor for patients self-reporting an ADE. In fact, each additional provider prescribing medications to a particular patient in this study increased the odds of reporting an ADE by approximately 29%.[22]

As one might expect, making a comprehensive assessment of an older adult is essential for providing that person with appropriate care. Providers must carefully investigate the etiology of a new condition and repeatedly reassess the need for each medication taken by their patients. As stated by Gurwitz, "Any symptom in an elderly patient should be considered a drug side effect until proven otherwise."[23] Following this advice can help identify medication-related adverse effects rather than perpetuating the prescribing cascade.

Polypharmacy

As a result of successful disease-focused research, many new drugs that are effective in treating acute and chronic conditions have come to market. However, much of the research substantiating a new drug is directed at proving its efficacy and safety for a single condition. In addition, complex patients are usually excluded from premarketing clinical trials. Very little has been done to evaluate the concomitant use of multiple agents to treat multiple conditions in older adults.[24] Because of the lack of data on treating older patients with MCCs, many providers prescribe a medication for each disease rather than prioritizing treatment. As a result, the complex older adult is more likely to have poor adherence, higher healthcare costs, and more adverse events attributed to excessive medication use.[25]

The prescribing cascade frequently contributes to what is referred to as *polymedicine* or *polypharmacy*. The term *polymedicine* is used to describe the escalation of medication usage as it relates to an increase in the number of associated medical problems, while *polypharmacy* denotes the unnecessary administration of more medications than clinically indicated.[26] The definition of *polypharmacy* can be further refined to describe the number of medications needed to deem the regimen excessive. This number varies depending on the patient and setting; however, it is most commonly understood as five or more medications.[27,28] As demonstrated by the prescribing cascade, understanding and identifying polypharmacy can help a clinician to decrease a patient's medication burden and regimen complexity.

The increasing use of medications among patients of increasing age provides an opportunity for providers to evaluate and reassess medication usage. Strategies to reduce polypharmacy should include comprehensive medication reviews, patient-provider communication, care coordination, and, most importantly, goals of care that are identified by the patient.

BARRIERS TO APPROPRIATE CARE

People with MCCs have healthcare needs and desires that differ from those of individuals with fewer medical issues. As people progress from a single chronic condition to MCCs, their needs change. Healthcare providers must focus on multiple complaints, but population-based approaches for caring for single complaints may impair this process. Time limits in the physician's office hinder proper attention to older adults with complex conditions, when these patients require extra time. Lack of time leads to additional visits, which may be difficult for people with transportation issues, limited funds for copayments, and mobility problems that make getting to an office visit difficult and unpleasant. Obtaining adequate care affects not only the patient, but also the family or caregiver. Lack of adequate social systems may contribute to poor health outcomes.

Convenient access to healthcare providers is important to older adults. These people also want clearly communicated care plans that are individualized for them, one person to coordinate their care as well as prioritize competing demands from their multiple conditions, and a permanent relationship with caring providers, including medical specialists and physician extenders.[29] Lack of coordination and continuity of care creates a barrier to optimal care.[30] Patients also want their providers to listen to them and understand their needs. Patient priorities may be different from that of their providers, and this conflict may create another barrier.

Care Coordination

Healthcare delivery systems for people with MCCs are often fragmented, less effective, complex as well as confusing, and expensive.[31] Table 11-4 identifies patient and caregiver perceptions of barriers to quality care that lead to poor health outcomes.[32] Patients and their caregivers identify poor care coordination, poor communication among providers, and lack of confidence in the healthcare system among the top reasons contributing to poor health outcomes. An American Association of Retired Persons (AARP) survey found that some caregivers report lacking the necessary skills to provide care.[32] The survey also found that most people with MCCs have many medical specialist visits, with almost 30% of patients visiting a specialist ≥13 times and 46% of patients visiting a specialist 5 to 12 times in a 3-year period. Patients and caregivers also reported receiving conflicting information from multiple providers, and 20% of survey respondents believe that their health had worsened because of poor communication among providers.

TABLE 11-4 • Quality-of-Care Issues Reported by Patients with Chronic Conditions and Their Caregivers

Perceived Issue	Reported by Patient (%)	Reported by Caregiver (%)
No follow-up visit after contact with healthcare facility	5.5	14.9
Patient did not receive care although it was needed	8.7	16.8
Poor transition of care coordination	18.2	25.2
Poor communication among providers	19.7	30.9
Lack of confidence in healthcare system	24.9	34.9

Source: AARP Public Policy Institute. *Beyond 50.09 Chronic Care: A Call to Action for Health Reform*; 2009. Available at https://www.giaging.org/documents/beyond_50_hcr.pdf (page 59).

Transitional Care

As older adults move from one healthcare setting to another, they become more vulnerable to the consequences of poor communication between settings and providers. Transitional care comprises a broad range of services designed to provide continuity of care to prevent poor outcomes, especially as high-risk chronically ill people move from one level of care to another. There are no set standards for transitional care, as the practice is still evolving.[33] Patients are often at risk as they transition from an acute-care setting to their homes, rehabilitation facilities, or long-term-care facilities. One problem is that acute-care providers are seldom not involved in post-acute care and post-acute-care providers receive little or no communication from the hospital on discharge.[34] The trend of hospitalists further adds to the problem. Data from Medicare beneficiaries indicate that >30% of patients discharged from a hospital had two or more care setting transitions in a 30-day period following discharge, with medication management and continuity of the care plan as major causes for transitions of care.[34] As more transitions in care settings occur, the risk of medication errors and poor communication increases.[35]

Rehospitalization within 30 days of discharge is common among Medicare recipients.[33] Transfer documents are often inadequate and lack specific details about the hospital course and patient care plan; in addition, documentation may be brief, handwritten, and difficult to read.[34] Approximately 20% of Medicare beneficiaries are rehospitalized within 30 days, 34% within 90 days, and >50% within 1 year.[36] The cause of rehospitalization is often different from the original admitting diagnosis. For example, patients hospitalized for heart failure are often readmitted within 30 days because of pneumonia, renal failure, and nutrition-related or metabolic problems.[36] Older adults are vulnerable to poor outcomes from hospitalization, which can lead to further decline and frailty. Hospitalization frequently leads to sleep deprivation, emotional and physical stress, deconditioned muscles due to bed rest, and poor nutrition because of missed meals owing to diagnostic testing. Hospitalized older adults often have delirium, which is a risk factor of extended hospital stays and postdischarge problems. These types of iatrogenic hospital-related events put older adults at risk for post-discharge adverse health outcomes, termed *posthospital syndrome*.[37] This syndrome is an acquired, transient condition that occurs while patients recover from acute illness. Older adults are particularly vulnerable to posthospitalization syndrome because of reduced physiologic reserves. To prevent posthospitalization syndrome, clinicians should pay more attention to avoiding its causes—sleep deprivation, malnutrition, and poor pain control, among others—both during hospitalization and after discharge.[37] Providing attention to the patient as a whole and not just the immediate cause of a hospitalization may decrease rehospitalization rates.

Inadequate medication reconciliation strongly contributes to poor transitional care. Obtaining an inaccurate list of medications at the time of hospital admission adds to the problem, particularly when there is no single database of information that all providers can review. Incomplete medication histories at the time of hospital admission account for >25% of all hospital prescribing errors. Discrepancies in prescription and nonprescription medication histories at hospital admission ranged from 27% to 48% of patients using at least one medication.[38]

Comprehensive Medication Review in Long-Term-Care Facilities

Medicare Part D beneficiaries residing in long-term-care facilities (LTCFs) must be offered a comprehensive medication review (CMR) if they meet eligibility criteria. The CMR must be conducted face to face or via telehealth. This creates several difficulties. First, many LTCF residents have severe dementia, which is the reason why they no longer live in the community. Having a face-to-face interaction will likely be unproductive. Second, many facilities neither provide telephones to residents nor have videotechnology for conducting CMRs with residents who are not cognitively impaired. The pharmacist conducting the CMR may also become yet another provider in the mix, contributing conflicting information for the patient or recommendations that are contrary to the facility's consultant pharmacist. In an ideal situation, the consultant pharmacist who reviews all residents' medication regimens monthly for appropriateness and monitors for adverse events would also provide the CMR. However, it is the responsibility of the prescription drug plan (PDP) to arrange for CMR services, and the PDP may not be able to contract with the consultant pharmacist or may provide her/his own CMR pharmacist. Coordinating the CMR pharmacist's recommendations with the consultant pharmacist and the LTCF staff may be a daunting task.

The CMR pharmacist must overcome other barriers in order to be effective. Providing a CMR annually without knowing a complex patient's history is difficult. To review multiple years' worth of data in order to make rational medication recommendations is time consuming, and it is unlikely that such detailed investigations would be reimbursable. Centers for Medicare and Medicaid Services (CMS) estimates the time needed to conduct an annual CMR is 40 minutes. Although this may be reasonable for community-dwelling older adults without significant medical complications, it may be an underestimation for residents of LTCFs with complex conditions.

Most consultant pharmacists know their residents well because they visit the facility monthly and may have served a particular facility for years. Families or powers of attorney of cognitively impaired residents may have made treatment decisions that may not be known to the CMR pharmacist, adding to the layers of conflicting or contradictory recommendations. As the CMR requirement for LTCF residents is new, many of these issues will need to be dealt with and solutions will need to be created.

GUIDING PRINCIPLES FOR APPROPRIATE CARE

Guideline-Based Practice: Quality Over Quantity

Most older adults have at least three chronic conditions.[39] Decisions on how and when to treat a patient with chronic diseases is often based on clinical practice guidelines (CPGs). These guidelines provide a summary of clinical evidence, expert consensus, and best practices to improve overall care. The utilization of CPGs for older adults with multiple conditions is limited because of the focus on only a single disease.[39] For instance, the available CPGs for diabetes do not take into account every drug-disease or drug-drug interaction that might occur in relation to a patient's comorbidities as a result of enacting recommendations. Furthermore, many of the available guidelines were not created on the basis of populations with physical disabilities, multiple medications, and multiple comorbidities, all of which are common among older adults.[40, 41]

To further complicate matters, pay-for-performance models and quality- of-care standards established using CPGs may not reflect the patient's goals of care or accurately portray the provider's care for a geriatric patient.[39,41,42] For example, a primary-care provider has a quality-of-care indicator that is dependent on achieving a hemoglobin A1c goal of <7% for all patients with diabetes. A 95-year-old patient with diabetes comes in for a follow-up appointment with a healthcare provider, and laboratory tests reveal an A1c of 8%. The provider decides not to push the patient or prescribe an additional medication to achieve the goal of <7%, given the potential risk for hypoglycemia and falls.[43] Yet, if the quality-of-care indicator has been set at an A1c of <7% and is the only determining factor for appropriate care, then this provider may be seen as an outlier.

Newer guidelines, such as HEDIS 2016 and the ADA Standards of Medical Care in Diabetes, offer less stringent A1c goals for special populations including older adults.[44,45] The Eighth Joint National Committee (JNC8) published evidence-based guidelines for treating hypertension in adults in 2014. JNC8 recommends a relaxed BP goal for adults aged ≥60 years with a systolic BP goal of <150 mmHg and diastolic blood pressure goal of <90 mmHg.[46]

The recognition that older adults require a different approach is important and a step in the right direction. Unfortunately, in some disease states such as hyperlipidemia, there may not be a sufficient number of older adults (those aged >75 years old) enrolled in randomized controlled trials to make an evidence-based recommendation on deciding when and if to initiate, continue, or discontinue statin therapy in these individuals.[47] The complexity of older adults requires more deliberation, patient perspective, and consideration of quality of life prior to recommending therapeutic interventions. More guidelines with geriatric focus and randomized controlled trials in this population are needed to ensure appropriate evidence-based care for older adults.

Boyd et al[39] evaluated the applicability of CPGs in a hypothetical 79-year-old woman with five chronic conditions (hypertension, diabetes mellitus, osteoarthritis, chronic obstructive pulmonary disease, and osteoporosis). From each available guideline, the authors extracted type of medication, tests, diet, exercise, self-monitoring, environmental changes, involvement of specialists and other clinicians, and frequency of follow-up with the goal of creating a comprehensive care plan for this patient.

If each disease-specific guideline were applied, the patient's regimen would include 12 medications costing over $406/month and 14 nonpharmacologic recommendations and activities. This regimen would require 19 medication doses per day taken at five separate intervals. The study's most alarming finding was the potential for drug-drug and drug-disease interactions accompanied by the lack of patient input. None of the CPGs evaluated considered the burden of the comprehensive treatment plan on the patient or caregivers.[39]

This study emphasizes the limitations of using CPGs as the sole source of information when treating older adults. To optimize the care of a senior patient, the provider should use CGPs as a reference point but consider each disease as it relates to the patient's comorbidities and goals of care. Successful management of a complex patient is not determined by the number of medications used for a specific disease. Only when a regimen provides more benefit than harm without significant impact on quality of life, as defined by the patient, can therapy be deemed a success.

Patient Considerations

The concept of including patient preference in decision-making is not uncommon or new; however, the assumption that the correct treatment choice is based on science alone remains heavily embedded in clinical practice.[48] The Institute of Medicine's (IOM) 2001 report, *Crossing the Quality Chasm*, introduced the idea of patient-centered care in which patients are involved in clinical decision-making. The report went on to say that clinicians should ensure "that patient values guide all clinical decisions."[49] Providers often select treatment options for their patients with the intention of improving health but without fully disclosing alternatives or risks associated with the selected treatment. This type of treatment decision is usually based on the provider's beliefs, preferences, and aversions rather than those of the patient.[50]

Shared decision-making is defined as a process of communication in which the physician and patient review the benefits and risks associated with all available treatment options in an unbiased fashion while incorporating patient-specific personal factors to decide which option is preferable.[50] Some patients may find solace in the notion that "doctor knows best" but forget that the clinician has very little insight into what they value or consider to be a good quality of life. Promoting shared decision-making is particularly important in a population where medical decisions to treat or not to treat can substantially impact quality of life and have a higher probability of causing treatment-related complications or even death.[51]

Provider Considerations

Providing care to older adults with MCCs requires a specific skill set and knowledge about geriatric pharmacotherapy. Caring providers can cause unintentional harm when they believe that they are treating the patient properly, but lack appropriate geriatric-focused knowledge. A prime example is the recurring prescribing cascade.

Understanding age-related changes in pharmacokinetics and pharmacodynamics is essential, as is recognizing unusual presentations of symptoms related to diseases and medication adverse effects. Being able to assess functional, psychological, and economic status in older adults is equally important as assessing physical status. Interviewing older adults also may require a special skill, as many older adults have cognitive, hearing, and vision impairments that complicate communication and increase the duration of the medication therapy management (MTM) encounter. Pharmacists, like other healthcare providers, may harm older adults by not applying geriatric principles of care.

Pharmacists providing MTM to older adults should have geriatric pharmacotherapy knowledge. Resources that can help establish essential baseline knowledge include the American Geriatrics Society website, available at http://www.americangeriatrics.org. The organization publishes a handbook (available in print, web-based, and mobile versions), *Geriatrics at Your Fingertips*, which provides geriatric medication use and dosing guidelines, clinical guidelines, calculators, assessment instruments, and more. The American Society of Consultant Pharmacists (available at http://www.ascp.com) is another useful resource. This organization's website contains useful clinical information for pharmacists providing care to older adults, including online continuing education on geriatric pharmacotherapy. This organization also provides live continuing education specific to geriatric pharmacy practice.

MEDICATION ASSESSMENT

There are multiple aspects of drug prescribing that affect both the quality and appropriateness of treatment. Avoiding inappropriate medications, identifying medication-related adverse events and drug interactions, and encouraging patient participation can have favorable effects on patient outcomes.[52] Screening tools that identify appropriate and inappropriate medications is one approach for assessing and improving the quality of prescribing.

Beers Criteria

The *Beers Criteria*, initially developed by expert consensus in 1991, is the most widely used tool to assess inappropriate prescribing.[53] The original criteria were an explicit list of 30 medications that should generally not be prescribed to elderly nursing home residents regardless of diagnosis. The *Beers Criteria* has since been updated 4 times (1997, 2003, 2012, and 2015) to make the list more current and applicable to the wider elderly population.[54-56] The most recent revision by the American Geriatrics Society includes the previously noted list of potentially inappropriate medications in older adults. New to the latest update are a list of drugs that require dose adjustments based on an individual's renal function and an overview of drug-drug interactions that may pose particular harm when combined for use in an older adult.

The first section of the criteria provides recommendations on medications to avoid independent of diagnosis or condition. This means that, regardless of a patient's comorbidities, any drug identified in this section should raise a red flag to the provider. As an example, the criteria recommend avoiding doxazosin in favor of an alternative with a superior risk-benefit profile. The rationale for the inclusion of doxazosin in this section is its high risk of orthostatic hypotension and the availability of alternative agents. This section provides a fairly consistent method for screening a patient for potentially inappropriate medications.

The second section discusses medications to avoid because of drug-disease or drug-syndrome interactions. Medications are identified that may exacerbate or worsen a condition or syndrome. For example, antipsychotics are presented in this section as a class of medications that should be avoided in patients with dementia. Antipsychotics have been associated with an increased risk of stroke and mortality in dementia patients. The *Beers Criteria* recommends judicious use of antipsychotics in this population unless nonpharmacologic options have failed and patients are a threat to themselves or others. This section highlights the effect of prescribing for one ailment in relation to other conditions.

The third section of the revised criteria provides general guidance on medications that should be used with caution in older adults. This section takes into account age-related decline in physiological reserves. For example, dabigatran is listed as a medication to be used with caution because of a greater risk of bleeding in older adults. In addition, use of dabigatran in renal impairment has not been thoroughly evaluated in clinical trials. Caution is emphasized in this section, because the medications presented may have severe consequences in older adults but the evidence surrounding the avoidance of use is not well defined.

The fourth section of *Beers Criteria*, a recent addition, focuses on drug-drug interactions that have shown to cause harm when prescribed concomitantly. This section highlights non-anti-infective drugs and describes the additive effect that can occur when certain agents are prescribed together. For instance, the criteria recommend avoiding the combination of corticosteroids with nonsteroidal anti-inflammatory drugs (NSAIDs) due to increased risk for peptic ulcer disease and gastrointestinal bleed. Moreover, this section provides guidance in case the combination cannot be avoided such as considering gastrointestinal protection in the previous scenario.

The fifth section provides a list of drugs that should be either dose-adjusted or completely avoided on the basis an individual's kidney function. These recommendations are evidence-based and also consider the degree of renal impairment (eg, mild, moderate, or severe). The *Beers Criteria* concludes by listing drugs that are known to be highly anticholinergic. A list of alternative medications is now available in a companion paper-making avoidance of the aforementioned drugs more feasible.

The *Beers Criteria* is advantageous because it allows broad application to all types of geriatric patients in multiple settings. On the other hand, it does not consider patient-specific characteristics or special circumstances that would make prescribing of one of the identified medications appropriate. It is important to keep in mind that this list was originally designed as a research tool and identifies only potentially inappropriate medications. Users should use the *Beers Criteria* only as an identification tool. Once a potentially inappropriate medication is identified, consider the context in which the medication is prescribed and then make a clinical decision regarding its appropriateness. Generally, there are better alternatives to the medications listed on the *Beers Criteria*. However, there are instances when a *Beers Criteria* drug is appropriate. Patients using a Beers drug should be monitored carefully for ADEs and efficacy.

Screening Tool of Older Person's Prescriptions/ Screening Tool to Alert Physicians to Right Treatment

The Screening Tool of Older Person's Prescriptions (STOPP) and Screening Tool to Alert physicians to Right Treatment (START) are additional sets of tools developed to improve prescribing in the geriatric population. Both were updated in 2015 to include drugs that are affected by renal function.[57]

The STOPP toolset identifies 80 clinically significant criteria for potentially inappropriate prescribing, with emphasis on eliminating acts of commission (prescribing of drugs that are potentially unsuitable). For example, if oxybutynin were to be prescribed to an older adult, STOPP would flag this drug as inappropriate if the patient has dementia, glaucoma, chronic constipation, or benign prostatic hyperplasia (BPH). STOPP also provides the clinical concern associated with the use of each agent. In this case, the tool identifies confusion (dementia), condition exacerbation (glaucoma and constipation), and urinary retention (BPH) as potential concerns for the use of oxybutynin in older adults. Similar to the updated *Beers Criteria*, STOPP also provides a therapeutic alternative for the inappropriate therapy. Instead of oxybutynin, STOPP recommends behavioral therapy for urge incontinence and diet therapy for constipation.

The START toolset consists of 34 prescribing indicators for common conditions observed in the geriatric population. It was developed to identify acts of underprescribing or omission (failure to prescribe an appropriate drug deemed beneficial in older adults). START provides common conditions encountered in older adults and recommends medications that should be considered if contraindications do not exist. For instance, calcium and vitamin D are recommended for patients with osteoporosis. The tool helps providers ensure patients are receiving complete and appropriate therapy for each condition. It is important, however, to ensure that patients will derive benefit from the proposed therapy, as outlined by START, and that the therapy aligns with the patient's goals of care.

The ability of the STOPP and START toolsets to consider patient characteristics and identify underprescribing provides an advantage over the *Beers Criteria*. However, neither STOPP nor START provides an exhaustive list of scenarios to cover the entirety of geriatric practice. Clinicians can use these tools to identify potential medication-related problems and errors of omission to optimize the care of their patients, keeping in mind that the proposed recommendations will not apply to all patients.

Medication Appropriateness Index

The *Medication Appropriateness Index* (MAI) is a list of 10 questions that clinicians should ask themselves about each individual medication:[58]

1. Is there an indication for the medication?
2. Is the medication effective for the condition?
3. Is the dosage correct?
4. Are the directions correct?
5. Are the directions practical?
6. Are there clinically significant drug-drug interactions?
7. Are there clinically significant drug-disease/condition interactions?
8. Is there unnecessary duplication with other medications?
9. Is the duration of therapy acceptable?
10. Is this medication the least expensive alternative compared with others of equal utility?

The questionnaire provides the clinician with a streamlined approach for assessing each medication in an organized and systematic fashion. Unlike traditional screening tools, the MAI can and should be used at each patient encounter.

The MAI focuses on indication, effectiveness, dose, correct directions, practical directions, drug-drug interactions, drug-disease interactions, duplications, duration, and cost. For example, if a patient has to take a medication 8 times over the course of a day, but does not receive relief from the ailment and cannot afford the medication, then the prescription is likely inappropriate. In this case, the directions are not practical, the drug is ineffective, and cost was not considered. All of these parameters impact adherence, tolerability, and patient outcomes.[58] The MAI should become a mental checklist for providers detailing the parameters that should be addressed for all medications at each visit.

Beyond Claims Data

The *Beers Criteria*, STOPP/START, and the MAI are tools for assessing medication appropriateness. However, they are not sufficiently comprehensive to be considered exhaustive for all patients. Prescription claims data should also be used with caution. When performing MTM reviews, the provider should not use claims data as the sole source of information. Prescription claims data can be used as a guide to better understand which medications the patient is receiving, but these data fail to capture the context surrounding medication use. Obtaining enough information to make evidence-based recommendations can be difficult for providers lacking access to a patient's medical records. Under these circumstances, the patient interview becomes increasingly important. Patients may be taking medications not included in claims data, they may be taking prescription medication for which they paid cash because their cost is less than deductibles and copays through their prescription drug plan, or they may be taking nonprescription medications and medications prescribed to others. The patient or caregiver can provide essential insight into how, when, and why a particular medication is being taken. The MTM provider should expect the patient to produce documents or provide information necessary to make an informed decision. To rely on claims data alone in the absence of a thorough interview can result in misinformation and patient harm.

INTERVENTIONS TO IMPROVE HEALTH OUTCOMES

Establishing Patient-Pharmacist Relationships

Effective MTM requires a trusting patient-pharmacist relationship. Patients may be reluctant to engage in an open and honest dialog with a pharmacist whom they do not know, especially when the MTM pharmacist initiates the process via a telephone conversation. A patient-pharmacist relationship must be established in situations where the pharmacist is a stranger to the patient. This can be accomplished by introducing yourself and including a brief background of your professional experience. As MTM services are relatively new, many patients will feel suspicious of a stranger who asks personal information and offers to provide a service that they may not know exists. They may feel that their physicians provide medication management and that pharmacist-provided MTM is unnecessary. It is more difficult to get the patient to agree to an

MTM encounter if that patient has no prior interaction with the pharmacist. The patient must understand the purpose of the MTM encounter and know what the pharmacist will do with the information gleaned from the MTM service. Allow the patient to ask questions and provide straight, unambiguous answers before delving into the MTM process. To help establish a trusting relationship, patients must feel that their interests are central to the pharmacist and the MTM encounter. Rushing through an interview and not addressing the patient's concerns will impede a quality patient-pharmacist relationship. Patients must feel comfortable with the pharmacist before they are likely to discuss medication issues, such as poor adherence, affordability of medications, and potential ADEs.

Patient Empowerment

Ensuring implementation of recommendations after the MTM review can be challenging because MTM pharmacists are not the primary care providers. Collaboration between the MTM pharmacist and the prescriber can be essential to enhancing care coordination, medication management, as well as patient outcomes. That being said, the pharmacist-provider relationship is not the only impetus for positive change. The patient is the key constituent in the MTM process. When collaboration between the pharmacist and provider has not been established, patients should be given the necessary information to understand and champion for all aspects of their healthcare. This empowers the patient to ask questions and expect results. Appropriate follow-up and action always start with the patient.

Recognizing the Decline

The Health Foundation of Western and Central New York and the Syracuse University Aging Studies Institute developed a model for identifying potential events or changes that can trigger a decline into frailty in vulnerable community-dwelling older adults.[59] These triggers can result from an individual (eg, financial challenges, mental and behavioral health conditions, acute illnesses, chronic conditions, access to food/nutrition), family/community (eg, care coordination confusion, elder abuse, caregiver issues), and/or society/system level (eg, medication management, transportation challenges, care transitions/system navigation, resource disparities).[60] While scientific evidence on interventions to help reduce the risk of frailty for all triggers is lacking, there are tools that can be useful.[59] Implementing screening procedures to identify older adults at risk of frailty with the Program of Research to Integrate Services for the Maintenance of Autonomy (PRISMA-7)[61,62] and following up with the Comprehensive Frailty Assessment Index[63] are two such tools. Once identified, older adults should be referred to multidimensional patient-centered care programs and to chronic disease management specialists in geriatrics, depending on their needs.[60] Recognizing triggers of decline and helping intervene when possible may help to keep older adults living independently in the community longer.

Effects of Interventions

Little research exists to help identify the most effective means to improve health outcomes in patients with MCCs.[64,65] A Cochrane Database review identified that interventions targeted at managing specific risk factors or in areas where patients have difficulty in performing specific tasks—such as medication management or functional abilities—are more likely to be effective.[64] Other data corroborate that patients with MCCs have problems with polypharmacy and managing complex medication regimens, and targeting these problems may be more effective than other strategies.[66] Broader approaches, such as case management or modifications in care delivery, are less effective than targeted interventions. Outpatient case management for adults with chronic diseases and complex care needs does not reduce overall mortality, improve functional status, reduce expenditures, or reduce hospitalization.[67]

Care Coordination

Care coordination must be enhanced to improve the quality of care for patients with MCCs. Dr. Gerard Anderson, a health policy expert, at a hearing before the US Senate Special Committee on Aging, stated: "Improved care coordination is critical if the Medicare program is going to lower spending and simultaneously improve outcomes. The need for better care coordination in the Medicare program is quite compelling. Care coordination is especially important for the 23 percent of Medicare beneficiaries with 5+ chronic conditions and for beneficiaries with dementia who may have difficulty coordinating their own care."[68]

Unfortunately, the US healthcare system is mostly uncoordinated, with hospitals, LTCFs, and ambulatory care as well as homecare providers working in silos.[69] There is some evidence that interprofessional primary care teams, consisting of a primary physician and other healthcare providers, produce better outcomes than usual care, reduced healthcare utilization, and lower costs.[69] Pharmacists as team members have been shown to improve medication adherence, prescribing, as well as disease-specific patient outcomes and reduce hospitalizations.[69]

New models of care delivery are being tested in order to improve care coordination and health outcomes. Patient-centered medical homes (PCMHs) and accountable-care organizations (ACOs) have been designed to solve some of the problems, particularly for complex patients. Coordination of care is a core function of primary care, but this is difficult to manage in a fragmented system. PCMHs and ACOs should help improve care coordination, which has two fundamental goals:

1. "To transfer information, such as medical history, medication lists, test results, and patient preferences, appropriately from one participant in a patient's care to another. This includes transferring information to or from the patient."
2. "To establish accountability by clarifying who is responsible for each aspect of a patient's overall care. This includes specifying who is primarily responsible for key care delivery activities, the extent of that responsibility, and when that responsibility will be transferred to other care participants. The accountable entity (whether a healthcare professional, care team, or healthcare organization) accepts responsibility for failures in the aspect(s) of care for which it is accountable. The patient or family also at times may be the accountable entity."[70]

Patients with MCCs need a team approach to improve and coordinate care. Selected members of a team might have a specific responsibility to ensure coordination of care, improve functional status, and reduce hospitalization risk.[70] Care coordination has six specific activities:

1. Determine and update care coordination needs.
2. Create and update a proactive plan of care.
3. Communicate among healthcare providers and patients as well as their families, within teams of healthcare providers, and across care teams along with settings.
4. Facilitate transitions.
5. Connect with community resources.
6. Align resources with population needs.

A person's coordination should be based on her/his physical, social, and psychological needs. The patient's preferences for care and health-related goals also must be determined. An established care plan must be periodically reviewed to determine whether the goals are being achieved and if gaps in care or outcomes exist as well as updated as needed. Communication among providers, with patients along with caregivers, and between healthcare settings is critical for good care coordination. Patients are vulnerable when transitions between healthcare settings occur. To minimize potential risks, there must be transfer of accountability and information between care settings. Community resources may be required to meet the care needs of older adults. Local Area Agency on Aging organizations can help connect people to needed resources. Search for community resources and help by zip code or city at www.eldercare.gov.

The Therapeutic Plan

Managing complex conditions of older adults does not stop at problem identification. It is up to the clinician and patient to develop a therapeutic plan to resolve each issue. A successful therapeutic plan for an older adult takes into account life expectancy, time until benefit, treatment target, and goals of care.[71] Once the therapeutic plan has addressed each of these factors, the provider and patient can determine whether certain medications should be initiated, continued, or discontinued.

Both quality and quantity of life must also be considered when setting therapeutic goals. Particularly among the oldest old (aged ≥85 years), quality of life is usually more important to patients than quantity of life. In terms of patient or caregiver preferences, not treating may be an appropriate option if the therapeutic intervention may reduce the quality of remaining life. Because complex patients have MCCs and likely multiple medications, additional drug therapy to treat a new problem may cause more harm. Part of therapeutic decision-making includes the complexity of the plan. Will the patient be able to adhere to it? Can the patient afford the medications, come in for therapeutic monitoring, or comprehend the instructions? A patient with cognitive impairment may have a higher risk of adverse events from medications with narrow therapeutic indices, such as warfarin. Is the risk of harm greater than the potential benefit if the patient is likely to take too much or too little?

Problem Prioritization

Complex patients often present with multiple problems, and setting therapeutic goals as well as priorities can be difficult. The acuteness and severity of a problem will usually dictate the therapeutic priority. Problems identified and deemed important by a clinician may not be perceived as important by the patient or caregiver. This situation dictates a candid discussion with the patient or caregiver. It is fruitless to put together a therapeutic plan if the patient will not adhere to it. The patient's therapeutic goals should also be considered when prioritizing problems. If the patient has diabetes and an A1c of 10.5% but also has osteoarthritic knee pain, the patient may be unwilling to tackle lifestyle modifications and work on their diabetes control until the knee pain is addressed.

During the CMR, focus on problems that have the biggest impact on the patient's day-to-day life, giving those problems the highest prioritization. Maybe cost is an issue for the patient, so switching to cheaper generic alternatives may be useful. Maybe the patient's regimen is too complicated, leading to poor adherence, so simplifying the regimen and number of medications and/or doses would be the highest priority for this patient.

When the situation allows, it is best to tackle one problem at a time. If two or more interventions are started at the same time, and the patient's condition changes, there may be no way to tell which intervention caused the change. In addition, implementing too many therapeutic approaches simultaneously may be confusing to the patient or caregiver.

CAREGIVER BURDEN

The term *caregiver burden* denotes the toll on people providing care and has been described as "a multidimensional response to physical, psychological, emotional, social, and financial stressors associated with the caregiving experience."[72] Caregivers may show symptoms of depression, anxiety, or stress, and report other physical and psychological symptoms.[73,74] Caregivers tend to neglect their own health, and caregiver burden is a risk factor for a higher mortality rate compared to noncaregivers.[73,74] Older caregivers are particularly vulnerable to adverse health outcomes from caring for a spouse.[75,76] The more help a person needs with ADLs and IADLs, the greater the caregiver burden. The number of hours required for caregiving also correlates with caregiver burden.[73]

Women, often a daughter or daughter-in-law, make up the majority of caregivers. Caregiving can interfere with a job, adding increased stress to the caregiver. Caregiving may require working less, which can decrease income, affect promotion and advancement, and add additional hours to a workweek. Job loss may also be a consequence of taking time to provide care. Leisure time, vacations, and quality time with family diminish as caregiver time commitments increase. Spouses have a higher level of burden than do children, due to the constant physical and emotional closeness of the couple.[74] Caregivers who live with the person receiving care also have a higher level of burden because of daily interactions and greater commitment to keeping the person at home.[74]

Dementia is common in older adults, with nearly 50% of the oldest elderly having symptoms of dementia.[77] Caregivers of older adults with dementia are more likely to be spouses than caregivers of people without dementia. The number of hours of care is greater for people with dementia, further adding to the caregiver burden.[78] Since dementia is a progressive disease, the patient's needs continue to expand as the patient's ability to carry out ADLs and IADLs diminishes.

Helping Caregivers

It is important to always ask caregivers how they are coping and identify their healthcare as well as resource needs. Screening tools can help assess caregiver burden, which will help a clinician to identify specific areas in which to provide help.[79] Local Area Agency on Aging organizations are a good resource for caregivers to help lessen their burden. Help with care, such as a nursing aide, food delivery, and respite care, may be available for free or at a nominal cost.

The AARP recommends 10 ways to help caregivers deal with stress:[80]

1. *Put your physical needs first.* Proper diet, exercise, and sleep are essential. Seek professional help for physical or mental ailments.
2. *Connect with friends.* Isolation increases stress; caregivers should spend time with friends and family.
3. *Ask for help.* Recruit others to help with caregiving or help the caregiver.
4. *Call on community resources.* Contact community resource agencies or faith-based organizations for help.
5. *Take a break.* Get help from friends or family, or find community respite care facilities to care for the patient while away for part of a day, a whole day, or a vacation.
6. *Deal with your feelings.* Share your feelings with friends or family members. Bottling up emotions can affect mental and physical health.
7. *Find time to relax.* Find something enjoyable and take time to do it. Relaxation is imperative.
8. *Get organized.* Prioritize responsibilities. Tackle the most important tasks first and don't feel that you must manage everything.
9. *Just say no.* Don't feel guilty by saying no when others ask for your help.
10. *Stay positive.* Don't dwell on what you can't do well, but on what you have done well.

CONCLUSION

As older adults age, the number and severity of their chronic conditions increases, as does the number of their prescribed medications. Differentiating between new or worsening disease and a medication-induced adverse event can be challenging, and often medication is not considered as a potential cause of clinical problems, leading to the prescribing cascade. Tools have been developed to help clinicians identify medications to avoid in older patients.

Improved care coordination and transitional care is needed to ensure that therapeutic plans are effective and improve health outcomes. With patients being treated by many providers there is often poor communication or miscommunication among providers and between healthcare settings. Lack of care coordination is a risk factor for poor outcomes.

Clinicians treating older adults must remember their caregivers, whose own health is paramount to caring for the patient. Caregiver burden is a risk factor for poor health, and caregivers may be reluctant to find help. Taking time to empathize with caregivers and asking them how they are doing may uncover problems that may be mitigated with available community resources. Although there are many barriers and challenges associated with caring for complex older adults, there are a variety of ways the patient, caregiver, and provider can have positive impacts on health outcomes.

REFERENCES

1. Administration on Aging, US Department of Health and Human Services. *Projected Future Growth of the Older Population.* Available at https://aoa.acl.gov/Aging_Statistics/future_growth/future_growth.aspx#age. Accessed December 29, 2016.
2. Administration on Aging. *A Profile of Older Americans: 2015.* Available at https://aoa.acl.gov/Aging_Statistics/Profile/2015/docs/2015-Profile.pdf. Accessed December 29, 2016.
3. CMS. *Chronic Conditions Among Medicare Beneficiaries.* Chart Book, 2011 ed., Baltimore, MD. Available at http://www.cms.gov/Research-Statistics-Data-and-Systems/Statistics-Trends-and-Reports/Chronic-Conditions/Downloads/2011Chartbook.pdf. Accessed December, 2012.
4. CMS. *Chronic Conditions among Medicare Beneficiaries,* Chart Book, 2012 ed., Baltimore, MD. Available at http://www.cms.gov/Research-Statistics-Data-and-Systems/Statistics-Trends-and-Reports/Chronic-Conditions/Downloads/2012Chartbook.pdf. Accessed December, 2012.
5. Morley JE, Haren MT, Rolland Y, Kim MJ. Frailty. *Med Clin North Am.* 2006;90:837-847.
6. Lacas A, Rockwood K. Frailty in primary care: A review of its conceptualization and implications for practice. *BMC Med.* 2012;10:4.
7. Collard RM, Boter H, Schoevers RA, Oude Voshaar RC. Prevalence of frailty in community-dwelling older persons: a systematic review. *J Am Geriatr Soc.* 2012;60:1487-1492.
8. National Institute on Drug Abuse. *Prescription Drugs: Abuse and Addiction.* Washington, DC: Nida Nih Dhhs; 2011;8.
9. Hepler C, Strand LM. Opportunities and responsibilities in pharmaceutical care. *Am J Hosp Pharm.* March 1990;47(3):533-543.
10. Salazar JA, Poon I, Nair M. Clinical consequences of polypharmacy in elderly: Expect the unexpected, think the unthinkable. *Expert Opin Drug Safety.* 2007;6:695-704.
11. Hanlon J, Artz MB. Drug-related problems and pharmaceutical care: what are they, do they matter, and what's next? *Med Care.* 2001;39(2):113-122.
12. Knight E, Avorn J. Quality indicators for appropriate medication use in vulnerable elders. *Ann Intern Med.* 2001;135(8 Pt 2):703-710.
13. Burkhardt H, Gladisch R. Pharmacotherapy of elderly patients from the clinical viewpoint. *Internist* (Berlin). 2003;44:959-967.
14. Gill SS, Mamdani M, Naglie G, et al. A prescribing cascade involving cholinesterase inhibitors and anticholinergic drugs. *Arch Intern Med.* 2005;165:808-813.
15. Rochon PA, Gurwitz JH. Optimising drug treatment for elderly people: The prescribing cascade. *Br Med J.* 1997;315:1096-1099.
16. Rochon PA, Gurwitz JH. Drug therapy. *Lancet.* 1995;346:32-36.
17. Simonson W, Fau-Feinberg, Janice L, Feinberg JL. Medication-related problems in the elderly: Defining the issues and identifying solutions. *Drugs Aging.* 2005;22(7):559-569.
18. Bates DW. Frequency, consequences and prevention of adverse drug events. *J Qual Clin Pract.* 1999;19(1):13-17.
19. Tierney WM. Adverse outpatient drug events: a problem and an opportunity. *N Engl J Med.* 2003;348:1587-1589.
20. Hajjar ER, Hanlon JT, Artz MB, et al. Adverse drug reaction risk factors in older outpatients. *Am J Geriatr Pharmacother.* 2003;1:82-89.
21. Zhan C, Correa-de-Araujo R, Bierman AS, et al. Suboptimal prescribing in elderly outpatients: Potentially harmful drug-drug and drug-disease combinations. *J Am Geriatr Soc.* 2005;53:262-267.
22. Green JL, Hawley JN, Rask KJ. Is the number of prescribing physicians an independent risk factor for adverse drug events in an elderly outpatient population? *Am J Geriatr Pharmacother.* 2007;5:31-39.
23. Gurwitz J, Monane M, Monane S, Avorn J. Polypharmacy. In: Morris JN, Lipsitz LA, Murphy K, Bellville-Taylor P, eds. *Quality Care in the Nursing Home.* St. Louis, MO: Mosby-Year Book; 1997;13-25.
24. Stewart RB, Cooper JW. Polypharmacy in the aged. Practical solutions. *Drugs Aging.* 1994;4:449-461.

25. Mansur N, Weiss A, Beloosesky Y. Looking beyond polypharmacy: Quantification of medication regimen complexity in the elderly. *Am J Geriatr Pharmacother*. 2012;10:223-229.

26. Hajjar ER, Cafiero AC, Hanlon JT. Polypharmacy in elderly patients. *Am J Geriatr Pharmacother*. 2007;5:345-351.

27. Rollason V, Vogt N. Reduction of polypharmacy in the elderly: A systematic review of the role of the pharmacist. *Drugs Aging*. 2003;20:817-832.

28. Fulton MM, Allen ER. Polypharmacy in the elderly: A literature review. *J Am Acad Nurse Pract*. 2005;17:123-132.

29. Bayliss EA, Edwards AE, Steiner JF, Main DS. Processes of care desired by elderly patients with multimorbidities. *Fam Pract*. 2008;25:287-293.

30. Bower P, Macdonald W, Harkness E, et al. Multimorbidity, service organization and clinical decision making in primary care: A qualitative study. *Fam Pract*. 2011;28:579-587.

31. Mollica RL, Gillespie P. *Care Coordination for People With Chronic Conditions*. Baltimore, MD: Partnership for Solutions, Johns Hopkins University; 2003. Available at http://www.partnershipforsolutions.org/DMS/files/Care_coordination.pdf. Accessed May 23, 2014.

32. AARP Public Policy Institute. *Beyond 50.09 Chronic Care: A Call to Action for Health Reform*. Available at http://www.aarp.org/health/medicare-insurance/info-03-2009/beyond_50_hcr.html. Accessed December 2012.

33. Naylor MD, Aiken LH, Kurtzman ET, Olds DM, Hirschman KB. The care span: The importance of transitional care in achieving health reform. *Health Aff* (Millwood, VA). 2011;30:746-754.

34. Boling PA. Care transitions and home health care. *Clin Geriatr Med*. 2009;25:135-148, viii.

35. Kane RL. Finding the right level of posthospital care: We didn't realize there was any other option for him. *JAMA*. 2011;305:284-293.

36. Jencks SF, Williams MV, Coleman EA. Rehospitalizations among patients in the Medicare fee-for-service program. *N Engl J Med*. 2009;360:1418-1428.

37. Krumholz HM. Post-hospital syndrome: An acquired, transient condition of generalized risk. *N Engl J Med*. 2013;368:100-102.

38. Tam VC, Knowles SR, Cornish PL, et al. Frequency, type and clinical importance of medication history errors at admission to hospital: a systematic review. *Can Med Assoc J*. 2005;173:510-515.

39. Boyd CM, Darer J, Boult C, et al. Clinical practice guidelines and quality of care for older patients with multiple comorbid diseases: implications for pay for performance. *JAMA*. 2005;294:716-724.

40. Tinetti ME, Fried T. The end of the disease era. *Am J Med*. 2004;116: 179-185.

41. Tinetti ME, Bogardus ST Jr, Agostini JV. Potential pitfalls of disease-specific guidelines for patients with multiple conditions. *N Engl J Med*. 2004;351:2870-2874.

42. Mangin D, Sweeney K, Heath I. Preventive health care in elderly people needs rethinking. *Br Med J*. 2007;335:285-287.

43. Hornick T, Aron DC. Managing diabetes in the elderly: Go easy, individualize. *Cleve Clin J Med*. 2008;75:70-78.

44. Anonymous. Standards of medical care in diabetes–2016. *Diabetes Care*. 2016;39(Suppl 1):S1-S112.

45. National Committee for Quality Assurance. *The Healthcare Effectiveness Data and Information Set (HEDIS) & Quality Management*. Available at http://www.ncqa.org/tabid/59/default.aspx. Accessed December 5, 2016.

46. James PA, Oparil S, Carter BL, et al. Evidence-based guideline for the management of high blood pressure in adults report from the panel members appointed to the eighth joint national committee (JNC 8). *JAMA*. 2014;311(5):507-520.

47. Stone NJ, Robinson JG, Lichtenstein AH. 2013 ACC/AHA guideline on the treatment of blood cholesterol to reduce atherosclerotic cardiovascular risk in adults: A report of the American College of Cardiology/American Heart Association Task Force on Practice Guidelines. *Circulation*. 2014; 129(25 Suppl 2):S1-S45 (Epub Nov. 12, 2013).

48. Mulley AG, Trimble C, Elwyn G. Stop the silent misdiagnosis: Patients' preferences matter. *Br Med J*. 2012;345:e6572.

49. National Research Council. *Crossing the Quality Chasm: A New Health System for the 21st Century*. Washington, DC: National Academies Press; 2001.

50. Moulton B, King JS. Aligning ethics with medical decision-making: The quest for informed patient choice. *J Law Med Ethics*. 2010;38:85-97.

51. Welch HG, Albertsen PC, Nease RF, Bubolz TA, Wasson JH. Estimating treatment benefits for the elderly: The effect of competing risks. *Ann Intern Med*. 1996;124:577-584.

52. Spinewine A, Schmader KE, Barber N, et al. Appropriate prescribing in elderly people: How well can it be measured and optimised? *Lancet*. 2007;370:173-184.

53. Beers MH, Ouslander JG, Rollingher I, et al. Explicit criteria for determining inappropriate medication use in nursing home residents. UCLA Division of Geriatric Medicine. *Arch Intern Med*. 1991;151:1825-1832.

54. Beers MH. Explicit criteria for determining potentially inappropriate medication use by the elderly. An update. *Arch Intern Med*. 1997;157:1531-1536.

55. Fick DM, Cooper JW, Wade WE, et al. Updating the Beers criteria for potentially inappropriate medication use in older adults: results of a US consensus panel of experts. *Arch Intern Med*. 2003;163:2716-2724.

56. American Geriatrics Society 2015 Beers Criteria Update Expert Panel. American Geriatrics Society 2015 updated Beers Criteria for potentially inappropriate medication use in older adults. *J Am Geriatr Soc*. 2015;63:2227-2246.

57. O'Mahony D, O'Sullivan D, Byrne S, O'Connor MN, Ryan C, Gallagher P. STOPP/START criteria for potentially inappropriate prescribing in older people: Version 2. *Age Aging*. 2015;44:213-218

58. Hanlon JT, Schmader KE, Samsa GP, et al. A method for assessing drug therapy appropriateness. *J Clin Epidemiol*. 1992;45:1045-1051.

59. Brown MT, Williams K. *White Paper: Identifying Interventions to Address Triggers of Decline in Vulnerable Older Adults*, 2016. Available at http://asi.syr.edu/wp-content/uploads/2016/03/Policy-Brief-WHITE-PAPER-1.pdf. Accessed December 5, 2016.

60. Health Foundation of Western and Central New York. *Triggers of Decline*. Available at https://hfwcny.org/resource/the-triggers-of-decline/. Accessed December 5, 2016.

61. Clegg A, Rogers L, Young J. Diagnostic test accuracy of simple instruments for identifying frailty in community-dwelling older people: A systematic review. *Age Aging*. 2015;44(1):148-152.

62. Hoogendijk EO, Van Hout HPJ. The identification of frail older adults in primary care: Comparing the accuracy of five simple instruments. *Age Aging*. 2013;42(2):262-265.

63. De Witte N, Verte D. The comprehensive frailty assessment instrument: Development, validity and reliability. *Geriatr Nurs*. 2013;34(4):274-281.

64. Smith SM, Soubhi H, Fortin M, Hudon C, O'Dowd T. Interventions for improving outcomes in patients with multimorbidity in primary care and community settings. *Cochrane Database Syst Rev*. 2012;4:CD006560.

65. Smith SM, Soubhi H, Fortin M, Hudon C, O'Dowd T. Managing patients with multimorbidity: Systematic review of interventions in primary care and community settings. *Br Med J*. 2012;345:e5205.

66. Haynes RB, Ackloo E, Sahota N, McDonald HP, Yao X. Interventions for enhancing medication adherence. *Cochrane Database Syst Rev*. 2008;(2): CD000011. doi:CD000011.

67. Hickam DH, Weiss JW, Guise J-M, et al. *Outpatient Case Management for Adults With Medical Illness and Complex Care Needs*, Comparative Effectiveness Review 99 (prepared by the Oregon Evidence based Practice Center under Contract 290-2007-10057-I.); AHRQ Publication 13-EHC031-EF. Rockville, MD: Agency for Healthcare Research and Quality; January 2013. Available at http://effectivehealthcare.ahrq.gov/ehc/products/240/733/CER99_OutpatientCaseManagement_FinalReport_20130102.pdf. Accessed May 23, 2014.

68. Anderson G. The future of Medicare: Recognizing the need for chronic care coordination. Hearing before the Special Committee on Aging. United State Senate 110th Session, Washington, DC, May 9 2007. Available at http://aging.senate.gov/publications/592007.pdf.

69. Boult C, Green AF Boult LB, et al. Successful models of comprehensive care for older adults with chronic conditions: Evidence for the Institute of Medicine's retooling for an aging America report. *J Am Geriatr Soc*. 2009;57:2328-2337.

70. Meyers D, Peikes D, Genevro J, et al. *The Roles of Patient-Centered Medical Homes and Accountable Care Organizations in Coordinating Patient Care*. AHRQ Publication 11-M005-EF. Rockville, MD: Agency for Healthcare Research and Quality. December 2010. Available at https://pcmh.ahrq.gov/sites/default/files/attachments/Roles%20of%20PCMHs%20And%20ACOs%20in%20Coordinating%20Patient%20Care.pdf. Accessed January 14, 2017.
71. Holmes HM, Hayley DC, Alexander GC, Sachs GA. Reconsidering medication appropriateness for patients late in life. *Arch Intern Med*. 2006;166:605-609.
72. Etters L, Goodall D, Harrison BE. Caregiver burden among dementia patient caregivers: A review of the literature. *J Am Acad Nurse Pract*. 2008;20:423-428.
73. Kim H, Chang M, Rose K, Kim S. Predictors of caregiver burden in caregivers of individuals with dementia. *J Adv Nurs*. 2012;68:846-855.
74. Carretero S, Garces J, Rodenas F, Sanjose V. The informal caregiver's burden of dependent people: Theory and empirical review. *Arch Gerontol Geriatr*. 2009;49:74-79.
75. von Kanel R, Mausbach BT, Dimsdale JE, et al. Cardiometabolic effects in caregivers of nursing home placement and death of their spouse with Alzheimer's disease. *J Am Geriatr Soc*. 2011;59:2037-2044.
76. Capistrant BD, Moon JR, Berkman LF, Glymour MM. Current and long-term spousal caregiving and onset of cardiovascular disease. *J Epidemiol Community Health*. 2012;66:951-956.
77. Alzheimer's Association. 2012 Alzheimer's disease facts and figures. *Alzheimer Dement*. 2012;8:131-168.
78. Ory MG, Hoffman RR, 3rd, Yee JL, Tennstedt S, Schulz R. Prevalence and impact of caregiving: A detailed comparison between dementia and nondementia caregivers. *Gerontologist*. 1999;39:177-185.
79. Parks SM, Novielli KD. A practical guide to caring for caregivers. *Am Fam Physician*. 2000;62:2613-2622.
80. AARP. *10 Ways to Deal With Caregiver Stress*. Available at http://www.aarp.org/relationships/caregiving/info-06-2010/crc-10-caregiver-stress-managment-tips.html. Accessed December, 2012.

Review Questions

1. Which of the following is NOT listed as one of the top 10 chronic conditions in the elderly?
   a. Insomnia
   b. Diabetes
   c. Hypertension
   d. Heart failure
   e. Ischemic heart disease

2. Geriatric syndromes are best characterized as
   a. specific disease states.
   b. not caused by drug therapy.
   c. found only in dementia-related patients.
   d. associated with increased mortality.
   e. characterized by chronic pain.

3. Which of the following is a characteristic of frailty?
   a. Unintentional weight loss of >10 lb in 12 months
   b. Decline in walking speed
   c. Weak grip strength
   d. Having a prevalence of >25% in those aged >85 years
   e. All of the above

4. Common chronic condition constellations in older adults include
   a. hyperlipidemia, hypertension, ischemic heart disease, and dementia.
   b. hyperlipidemia, hypertension, diabetes, and stroke.
   c. hyperlipidemia, diabetes mellitus, and ischemic heart disease.
   d. hyperlipidemia, ischemic heart disease, and sleep apnea.
   e. hyperlipidemia, arthritis, depression, and dementia.

5. Barriers to appropriate care for patients with multiple chronic conditions include
   a. lack of communication.
   b. lack of research in this area.
   c. involvement of multiple healthcare providers.
   d. caregiver burden.
   e. all of the above.

6. Which of the following contribute to rehospitalization in the older adults?
   a. Inadequate discharge documentation
   b. Lack of a detailed care plan
   c. Delirium while hospitalized
   d. Sleep deprivation while hospitalized
   e. All of the above

7. Current consensus regarding therapeutic guidelines are not as useful in older adults with MCCs, because of all of the following EXCEPT
   a. lack of strong evidence for combinations of chronic diseases.
   b. lack of strong evidence for the elderly.
   c. no allowance for differing life expectancies.
   d. promoting use of expensive brand-name drugs.
   e. exclusion of the patient's goals for treatment.

8. Which of the following statements about medication assessment in the elderly with MCCs is true?
   a. The *Beers Criteria* identifies medications that are ineffective.
   b. STOPP is hospital-specific.
   c. START focuses on common omissions in therapy.
   d. The combination of STOPP and START includes the patient's goals for therapy.
   e. The MAI measures therapeutic outcomes.

9. Which of the following statements about care coordination of the MCC patient is true?
   a. Patient-centered medical home and Accountable Care Organizations were created to improve coordination.
   b. Connection with community resources is essential.
   c. Every patient handoff has the potential to disrupt coordination.
   d. A comprehensive care plan is essential.
   e. All of the above

10. Caregivers can address stress by
    a. putting their physical needs first. Proper diet, exercise, and sleep are essential, and caregivers should seek professional help for physical or mental ailments.
    b. connecting with friends or family, as isolation increases stress; caregivers should spend time with friends and family.
    c. asking for help; others should be recruited to help with caregiving or help the caregiver.
    d. taking a break; getting friends, family, or find community-respite care facilities to care for the patient while away for part of a day, a whole day, or a vacation.
    e. all of the above.

ANSWERS

1. a	2. d	3. e
4. c	5. e	6. e
7. d	8. c	9. e
10. e		

12

Overview of Medication Therapy Management Data Sets

Karen Whalen, PharmD, BCPS, CDE, and Heather C. Hardin, PharmD, BCACP

KEY POINTS

- The medication therapy management (MTM) data set is a concise disease-based guide to providing a medication therapy review.
- The sections of the MTM data set include Introduction, Core Element 1 - Comprehensive Medication Review, Core Element 2 - Personal Medication List, Core Element 3 - Medication Action Plan, Core Element 4 - Intervention and Referral, and Core Element 5 - Documentation, and Follow-Up.
- The compendium of data sets is beneficial for those who work with student pharmacists or MTM provider trainees. The collection of MTM data sets is a valuable complement to MTM software and drug database programs.
- Limitations of the MTM data sets include an abbreviated listing of adverse drug reactions and limited information on drug interactions.
- With appropriate use, MTM data sets may facilitate better communication and collaboration between healthcare professionals, promote safe and effective medication use, and maximize therapeutic outcomes.

INTRODUCTION TO MEDICATION THERAPY MANAGEMENT (MTM) DATA SETS

To provide a little background on the rationale for creation of the MTM data sets, review the following scenario:

> Imagine that you have an excellent opportunity to start a new MTM business where you will provide MTM services to hundreds of patients per week via telephone or face-to-face interviews. To accomplish this mission, you will employ several pharmacists (MTM providers) and pharmacy technicians, and you will have the assistance of pharmacy interns and senior pharmacy students completing advanced pharmacy practice experiences (APPEs). All of this sounds wonderful until you realize that you need to have everyone trained, and the service up and running within a matter of a few months. To make matters more interesting, new pharmacy students will rotate into the practice site every month, necessitating the need for training of students on an ongoing basis. You quickly discover that you need an expeditious way to train all of these new employees and students. In addition, it would be handy to have a quick reference guide to prepare them for an MTM interview and to consult during MTM sessions in case they find themselves stumped or in unfamiliar territory.

The hypothetical scenario above is very similar to the experience at the University of Florida College of Pharmacy, as the faculty there established the MTM Communication and Care Center (now the Center for Quality Medication Management [CQM]).[1] When faced with the challenge of having to prepare multiple pharmacists and trainees to perform MTM services, the faculty rapidly gravitated toward the idea of creating data sets that would provide baseline information needed to conduct a successful medication therapy review. In short, trainees needed a resource that could provide answers to the following questions in the context of MTM:

- How do I interview the patient?
- What types of information do I need to gather?
- How do I explain complex health concepts or medical terminology to the patient?

- What medication-related problems (MRPs) might I commonly identify in patients with a given disease state?
- What types of interventions are routinely recommended for patients with a given disease state?
- How do I document interventions and follow-up with the patient?

Practitioners with hands-on MTM and clinical experience developed each of the MTM data sets. Since the data sets were originally designed as a resource to be utilized by both practitioners and students in a clinical setting, the writing style is simple and succinct, not highly technical. Each data set is a stand-alone disease-based guide to conducting a medication therapy review, and each incorporates practical aspects for performing the core elements of MTM:[2]

- Comprehensive medication review
- Personal medication list (PML)
- Medication action plan
- Intervention and/or referral
- Documentation

What is an MTM data set? It is a stand-alone disease-based guide to conducting a medication therapy review. Each data set incorporates practical aspects of performing the core elements of MTM for a given disease state.

In addition to knowing how to perform and document the core elements, practitioners also need to have an understanding of disease processes to conduct an optimal medication therapy review. Therefore, the introduction section of each MTM data set contains a basic overview of the disease state and current therapeutic goals. Since the objective of the MTM data sets is to be concise and functional, rather than comprehensive in nature, readers are often referred to tables, figures, and algorithms that summarize the necessary information in an efficient manner.

Whereas the MTM data sets are certainly useful in a busy MTM practice with multiple trainees such as the Center for Quality Medication Management at the University of Florida,[1] they have significant value in other settings, as well. Lack of communication skills, interview techniques, or outdated therapeutic knowledge are often listed as barriers for pharmacists in the provision of MTM.[3] In these areas, the disease-state-specific MTM data sets can offer guidance for professionals seeking to enhance their communication and clinical skills before getting started in the provision of MTM services. The MTM data sets serve as guides to performing high-quality comprehensive medication reviews, and developing personal medication lists, patient-specific medication action plans, and provider communications with recommendations to address MRPs. For healthcare professionals who are new to the MTM arena, MTM data sets may function as a resource for refining clinical expertise and keeping up-to-date with current clinical practice. Additionally, the MTM data sets may assist pharmacists in learning how to efficiently collaborate with other healthcare professionals, optimize medication use to positively impact clinical and economic outcomes, and reduce medication-related adverse events.

In summary, the MTM data set is a concise disease-based guide to providing MTM services. Each data set includes an overview of a disease state and information needed to conduct the core elements of MTM for that specific disease state. The overall collection of MTM data sets encompasses the top 10 targeted disease states for MTM programs,[4] along with several other disorders commonly encountered by MTM providers. The compendium is intended to be a companion text to the online version of *Pharmacotherapy: A Pathophysiologic Approach*, 10th edition.[5] As such, many of the tables and figures in the data sets are extracted from or linked to tables and figures in the corresponding chapter of *Pharmacotherapy*.

SECTIONS OF THE MTM DATA SET

All MTM data sets follow a similar format, which consists of an introduction to the disorder followed by five sections, one for each of the MTM core elements. When applicable, the chapter includes an additional section on key quality measures pertinent to the disorder. Table 12-1 outlines the contents for the various sections of the MTM data set. Following the table are detailed discussions on each section of the data set, which provide insight to optimize use of this helpful tool when conducting medication therapy reviews. The MTM data set for hypertension serves as an example for illustrative purposes.

Introduction

The first section of the MTM data set introduces the disease state. It defines the disorder and outlines any staging or classification system. For example, hypertension may be classified according to the systolic and diastolic blood pressure levels as prehypertension, stage 1 hypertension, or stage 2 hypertension.[6] Other definitions related to the disorder may be included in this section (eg, hypertensive crisis, isolated systolic hypertension, orthostatic hypertension, pseudohypertension) to give the MTM provider a broader perspective on the disorder and associated conditions.

The introduction also lists secondary causes of the disease, such as other medical conditions, medications, or situations that contribute to, or worsen the primary disease. For instance, secondary causes of hypertension include, but are not limited to, chronic kidney disease, obesity, obstructive sleep apnea, prescription medications, street drugs, over-the-counter (OTC) drugs, natural products, and food substances.[6,7] It is important for the MTM provider to be aware of secondary causes of the disease so that they may be discussed or ruled out during the medication review. Successful treatment of secondary causes of a disorder can substantially affect the need for treatment of the primary disease and alter the medication management plan. Complications of the disease state are also included in the introductory section. The MTM provider should familiarize themselves with possible complications of the disease state and be prepared to recommend pharmacotherapy to prevent or manage complications.

Finally, the introduction covers therapeutic goals for the disease state. For example, the goal blood pressure for most patients with hypertension is less than 140/90 mmHg. However, in certain circumstances, the goal may vary to less than 150/90 or 130/80.[6,8,9] The MTM data set assists providers in determining an appropriate goal for each patient. Setting therapeutic goals provides a means to assess therapeutic success or failure, and facilitates appropriate

TABLE 12-1 • Sections of the MTM Data Set

Section	Contents
Introduction	Definition of primary disease state Secondary causes/contributing factors Complications Therapeutic goals Therapeutic success defined Therapeutic failure defined
Core Element 1—Comprehensive Medication Review	Questions to ask to assess disease state and medication use Questions to ask for prevention/assessment of medical emergencies Questions to anticipate from patients Living room language
Core Element 2—Personal Medication List	Sample personal medication list in CMS-standardized format
Core Element 3—Medication Action Plan	Sample medication action plan in CMS-standardized format
Core Element 4—Intervention and/or Referral	Nonpharmacologic treatment Diet/lifestyle Devices or procedures Supportive therapies Complementary and alternative medicine Cognitive behavioral therapy Medications Prescription and OTC medications Herbals Common/serious side effects Blackbox warnings Current treatment algorithm Referral (emergent or other)
Core Element 5—Documentation and Follow-up	Sample pharmacist documentation of medication-related problems Sample provider communications Suggested intervals for follow-up (if applicable)

monitoring of the patient. Regarding hypertension, it is helpful to note that not all methods of blood pressure monitoring are equally precise. The MTM data set enlightens MTM providers on nuances of blood pressure monitoring, such as differences between in-clinic and out-of-office (ambulatory, self) blood pressure monitoring, and possible reasons for inaccurate readings.[10,11] Disease-specific therapeutic failures are outlined in each data set to help MTM providers recognize situations in which patients do not achieve their therapeutic goals, ascertain factors that put patients at higher risk for treatment failures (eg, nonadherence), and target interventions that aid in reducing complications and hospitalizations.

CORE ELEMENT 1—COMPREHENSIVE MEDICATION REVIEW

Conducting an effective patient interview and gathering key pieces of information are essential components of the comprehensive medication review (CMR), and are vitally important in identifying MRPs. Preparation and planning prior to the interview is critical, especially for the new or inexperienced MTM provider. This section of the MTM data set provides a convenient set of disease-related questions to ask patients during the CMR. For example, general questions that can be asked for hypertension are as follows:

1. How long have you had high blood pressure? When were you diagnosed as being hypertensive?
2. What do you know about the risks of uncontrolled blood pressure?
3. How often do you check your blood pressure at home?

One of the key components of the MTM interview is to ask direct questions that help patients prevent or plan for emergencies related to current disorder(s). For hypertension, questions might include the following:

1. What are the warning signs of a heart attack or stroke, and what is your action plan?
2. Have you fallen, felt dizzy, or had blurred vision or racing heart when getting up from sitting or lying down?
3. Have you ever been hospitalized for high blood pressure?

Many MTM providers are very comfortable following the example interview questions. However, they may feel uneasy because they are uncertain of questions that patients might ask in return. Just like preparing for a job interview, part of CMR preparation involves anticipating questions that are likely to arise. MTM providers should prepare by reviewing questions commonly asked by patients and the corresponding answers contained within this section of the MTM data set. Example questions to anticipate for hypertension include the following:

1. What is high blood pressure?
2. What causes high blood pressure?
3. What health problems are associated with high blood pressure?
4. Why are blood pressure medications so important?
5. I can't tell when my blood pressure is high. Can I just stop my medications if I feel okay?

During the MTM encounter, the MTM provider should encourage patients to play an active role in understanding and controlling their medication therapy and overall heath. However, it is often difficult for patients to understand and act on health information due to the use of complicated or confusing medical jargon by healthcare professionals. Many patients have low health literacy and, as such, have trouble processing and understanding basic medical information related to anatomy, physiology, diagnosis, prognosis, medications, other treatments, and therapeutic goals. According to the Institute of Medicine, nearly half of all American adults have difficulty understanding and appropriately using health information, which leads to increased hospitalizations, use of emergency services, and healthcare costs.[12] The use of "living room language," or lay terminology, may assist patients in overcoming barriers to medical understanding and interpretation. To help patients stay well informed and allow MTM providers to better communicate and collaborate with patients regarding healthcare decisions, pertinent living room language is included in each MTM data set. For instance, when asking a patient about a diuretic for hypertension, the MTM provider should inquire about the "water pill" used for blood pressure.

CORE ELEMENT 2—PERSONAL MEDICATION LIST

This section of the MTM data set contains a sample PML in CMS-standardized format.[13] The sample is representative only of medications used to treat the specific disease and/or its complications covered in the data set. Providers should create a comprehensive medication list by including additional medications for all other disease states in the medical history. MTM providers should remember to use plain language when creating the PML. Figure 12-1 provides a sample PML for a patient with hypertension. The example is representative only of antihypertensive medications.

CORE ELEMENT 3—MEDICATION ACTION PLAN

This section of the MTM data set contains a sample medication action plan (MAP) in CMS-standardized format.[13] The sample is representative only of action steps for the patient with the specific disease covered in the data set. MAPs for other disease states or other MRPs should be added and listed separately. In general, only a few of the most important action steps should be listed, so as not to overwhelm the patient. Providers can address other areas for patient self-management at later visits. MTM providers should remember to use plain language when creating the MAP. Figure 12-2 provides a sample MAP for a patient with hypertension. This example is representative only of action steps for a patient with hypertension.

CORE ELEMENT 4—INTERVENTION AND/OR REFERRAL

This section of the MTM data set covers both nonpharmacologic and pharmacologic treatment modalities. Nonpharmacologic

PERSONAL MEDICATION LIST FOR *(Insert patient's name, DOB: mm/dd/yyyy)*	
Medication: Hydrochlorothiazide 25 mg tablet	
How I use it: Take one pill (25 mg) every morning	
Why I use it: Blood pressure (water pill)	**Prescriber:** Jones
Date I started using it: 1/6/2016	**Date I stopped using it:** *(Leave blank for patient's notes)*
Why I stopped using it: *(Leave blank for patient's notes)*	
Medication: Ramipril 2.5 mg capsule	
How I use it: Take one capsule (2.5 mg) every night at bedtime	
Why I use it: Blood pressure	**Prescriber:** Jones
Date I started using it: 10/9/11	**Date I stopped using it:** *(Leave blank for patient's notes)*
Why I stopped using it: *(Leave blank for patient's notes)*	

FIGURE 12-1 Example of a personal medication list for hypertension medications.

	Date prepared: *(Insert date)*
What we talked about: Need to see how well new medicine is working for blood pressure	
What I need to do: 1. Check blood pressure at home at least 3 times weekly. 2. Write down my blood pressure in the logbook. Notify the clinic if my blood pressure is higher than 180/120 mmHg or lower than 110/60 mmHg. 3. Bring logbook and my blood pressure machine the next time I come to clinic.	**What I did and when I did it:** *(Leave blank for patient's notes)*

FIGURE 12-2 Sample medication action plan for a hypertensive patient.

interventions such as lifestyle modifications, surgery, and supportive therapy, are critical components of management and control of any disease. The MTM provider should be familiar with these modalities, as their use may have implications for drug therapy, such as recommending that prescription medications be stopped, started, changed, or closely monitored. Lifestyle modifications include diet, exercise, weight reduction, smoking cessation, and moderation in alcohol consumption, among others. Surgical procedures involve device placement (eg, pacemaker, stents), coronary artery bypass grafting (CABG), and other procedures. Finally, supportive therapy may consist of physical, occupational, cognitive behavioral, and/or speech therapy.

Each MTM data set outlines pharmacologic options for a given disease state. When available, a current treatment algorithm is included. MTM providers can utilize this information when making patient-specific recommendations for prescription or OTC medications. In this section, medications are organized by therapeutic class (eg, for hypertension—thiazide diuretics, β-blockers, calcium channel blockers). Unfortunately, medications may cause unwanted adverse effects when a patient begins taking the medication, when doses are altered, or when medications are stopped abruptly. Some adverse effects may be severe, significantly affect patient compliance, or necessitate drug discontinuation or dosage adjustment. The MTM data set lists several of the most common and serious adverse effects. MTM providers are encouraged to use this tool to acquaint patients with frequent or significant adverse effects of medications, and to screen for potential adverse effects that may affect medication adherence. Additionally, it will assist MTM providers in making treatment decisions, monitoring and advising patients, and identifying root causes of particular adverse effects.

Because MTM data sets are succinct and deliver only the most clinically relevant information to MTM providers, the list of medication adverse effects is not all-inclusive and does not cover adverse effects that are infrequent and minor in nature. For providers needing comprehensive information, complete adverse effect profiles can be found in the adverse reactions section of the prescription labeling for individual drug products. Blackbox warnings, contraindications, and FDA pregnancy categories are also provided for each medication class in the MTM data set. MTM providers must use this critical information to help prevent or reduce the frequency and severity of adverse drug events. For example, the hypertension data set advises against the use of angiotensin-converting enzyme (ACE) inhibitors, angiotensin receptor blockers, or direct renin inhibitors for the management of hypertension in pregnancy.

In addition to prescription and OTC medications used to treat primary disease states, it is important for MTM providers to ask patients about the use of herbal supplements. Many patients take herbal or natural remedies, and although some natural products may be beneficial, others may be potentially harmful or prone to interactions with more proven therapies. The herbal supplement data provided in the MTM data sets is derived from Natural Medicines, which was founded by healthcare providers and researchers to provide evidence-based information about complementary and alternative therapies.[14] The MTM data set outlines products with strong or fair evidence of benefit, along with the typical dosage, cost, and grade of supportive scientific evidence for each supplement. For hypertension, garlic and coenzyme Q10 are two of the listed products.

For MTM providers, a concise and thorough understanding of various health conditions is crucial, but not enough. They should also prepare for medical emergencies, be able to recognize an emergent or urgent medical situation, and know actions to take in the event of a medical emergency. Thus, for each disease state this section of the MTM data set delineates circumstances that are appropriate for instructing patients to call 9-1-1, go to the emergency room, or, for more routine problems, inform the physician at the next appointment. Since MTM interactions may occur over the telephone, the data set assists MTM providers with assessment of potential crises via this communication route as well. Finally, it is essential that MTM providers work closely with their patients to develop a crisis action plan, so that patients are best prepared for emergencies.

Core Element 5—Documentation and Follow-up

The final section of the MTM data set contains information related to documentation and follow-up. Clear and succinct documentation of MRPs and recommendations is a key component of the MTM consultation.

Documentation must be sufficient to detail patient problems, recommendations, and progress, and to serve as a record for reimbursement purposes, if necessary. To support MTM providers, examples of disease-specific MRPs and sample communications are included in each data set. Table 12-2 outlines examples of potential MRPs in patients with hypertension.

TABLE 12-2 • Medication-Related Problems (MRPs) in Patients with Hypertension

Category of MRP	Example Medication-Related Problem
Nonadherence	Suboptimal control of blood pressure due to patient missing doses of antihypertensive medication Patient not taking antihypertensive medication due to cost
Unnecessary medication	Duplicate therapy (eg, two calcium channel blockers)

Scenario: Patient given samples of valsartan, but cannot afford Rx once samples are finished.
Medication-related problem: Nonadherence

Assessment: Patient with uncontrolled blood pressure on valsartan 80 mg. Lack of BP control likely secondary to nonadherence with valsartan. Patient nonadherent with valsartan because of cost issues. Switching valsartan to an ACE inhibitor would provide for more affordable BP control and renal protection in this patient with type 2 diabetes mellitus.
Plan: Consider discontinuation of valsartan and addition of lisinopril 10 mg daily with titration to blood pressure goal < 140/90 mm Hg.
Source: ADA. Standards of medical care in diabetes—2017. *Diabetes Care.* 2017;40(Suppl 1):575-587.

FIGURE 12-3 Sample prescriber communication for hypertension.

Sample communications and recommendations to providers to address medication-related issues are found in Figure 12-3. The physician communications allow for simple substitution of medications and/or alert physicians to important MRPs and patient-related concerns. By having these statements scripted in advance, MTM providers are able to easily document and relay interventions to prescribers in an expedited manner. Fax, phone, or other means of written or secure electronic communication are appropriate methods to transmit recommendations. Examples provided below are for illustrative purposes only. MTM providers should individualize actual communications to prescribers based on the type of recommendation, patient specific characteristics, and the nature of the relationship with the prescriber.

To determine achievement of therapeutic goals and to ensure safety and efficacy of the care plan, close patient monitoring and follow-up must take place. The interval for follow-up will depend on a number of factors, including severity of the disease state, type of intervention, and patient-specific factors such as age, comorbid conditions, and ability to return for follow-up.

Each MTM data set outlines appropriate monitoring parameters and suggested intervals for follow-up to minimize the occurrence of MRPs. In patients with hypertension, blood pressure response is a marker for therapeutic success. Other monitoring parameters may include potassium, blood urea nitrogen (BUN), serum creatinine, and heart rate, depending on the antihypertensive regimen.

QUALITY MEASURES

Many payers of MTM services are accountable for providing high-quality care to their beneficiaries, the patients. These payers, usually healthcare plans, are "graded" on a 5-star rating system, where 1 reflects low quality and 5 reflects the highest quality standard. Plans are assessed across multiple categories, ranging from specific disease state measures to customer service measures. Providers of MTM services have an opportunity to assure the safe and effective use of medications and to improve the management of many health conditions. Therefore, payers view MTM as a valuable service for addressing medication usage and disease management, thus improving star ratings. The MTM data sets include, where appropriate, the identification of specific quality measures affected by MTM services. Table 12-3 displays an example of a quality measure impacted by MTM providers conducting medication reviews in patients with hypertension.

TABLE 12-3 • Medicare Star Ratings Measures Related to Hypertension

Measure (Part D Measure)	Measure Target
Medication Adherence for Hypertension (RAS antagonists)	Percent of plan members with a prescription for a blood pressure medication who fill their prescription often enough to cover ≥80% of the time they are supposed to be taking the medication. ("Blood pressure medication" means an ACE [angiotensin-converting enzyme] inhibitor, an ARB [angiotensin receptor blocker], or a direct renin inhibitor drug.) • For a 5-star rating ≥ 83% • For a 4-star rating ≥ 79% through <83%

Source: Reference 15.

POTENTIAL USES OF THE MTM DATA SET

As mentioned previously, the collection of MTM data sets definitely has practicality in a large MTM practice with multiple practitioners and trainees. However, the compendium could be of benefit to anyone who works with student pharmacists or MTM provider trainees. It has many conceivable applications, including the didactic classroom environment, professional practice laboratories, and the experiential setting. The MTM data sets are also a helpful resource for independent practitioners looking to build a new MTM practice. Additionally, some MTM software packages incorporate several pieces of the MTM data sets, as well as clinical decision support tools. However, current MTM software and drug databases do not contain the unique combination of items found in the data sets, such as living room language, OTC medications, herbal products and sample documentation. Therefore, the collection of MTM data sets is a valuable complement to MTM software and drug database programs.

LIMITATIONS

It is important to understand the limitations of using the MTM data sets. On average, providers may have 45 minutes or less for each initial CMR. This is usually not enough time to fully dissect each health condition and the entire medication therapy regimen. Because of time constraints, MTM providers must use clinical judgment to prioritize MRPs based on severity and patient concerns. For information on how to prioritize MRPs in a complex patient, refer to Chapter 11, "The Complicated Patient." MTM data sets can aid providers with the prioritization process by condensing each disease state into a concise, easy-to-read format.

As mentioned earlier, the list of medication adverse effects provided in the intervention section of the MTM data set is not all-inclusive. Comprehensive information on adverse effects can be found in the prescription labeling information or through consultation with patient safety organizations for the most up-to-date information. In addition, the data sets do not cover information on drug interactions. Due to the extensive list of potential interactions with many medications, MTM providers should consult a comprehensive drug interaction database before performing a CMR or making medication therapy recommendations.

Finally, it is important to remember that each patient is a unique individual. While guidelines and treatment algorithms outline suggested therapies, treatment plans must be customized to meet patient-specific characteristics, wants, needs, and cost considerations. The MTM provider must rely on clinical judgment in the design of patient-centered medication management plans.

CONCLUSION

In conclusion, MTM affords an exceptional opportunity for pharmacists, pharmacy interns, and pharmacy technicians to become involved in patient care, improve patient health, and reduce overall healthcare costs. The MTM data sets are a unique and comprehensive collection of information that serves as a useful tool for pharmacists, student pharmacists, and others practicing MTM. The MTM data sets provide a disease-state based practical guide to conducting a comprehensive medication therapy review. The data sets encompass the top ten targeted diseases and many more, including clinical pearls, living room language, and question sets. With appropriate use, MTM data sets may facilitate better communication and collaboration between healthcare professionals, promote safe and effective medication use, and maximize therapeutic outcomes.

REFERENCES

1. Center for Quality Medication Management. Report available at http://cqm.pharmacy.ufl.edu/. Accessed May 11, 2017.
2. APhA (American Pharmacists Association). Medication therapy management in pharmacy practice: Core elements of an MTM service model (version 2.0). *J Am Pharm Assoc.* 2008;48(3):341-353.
3. APhA. *Medication Therapy Management Digest 2011.* Available at http://www.pharmacist.com/sites/default/files/files/mtm_2011_digest.pdf. Accessed May 11, 2017.
4. CMS. *2016 Medicare Part D Medication Therapy Management (MTM) Programs Fact Sheet.* Available at https://www.cms.gov/Medicare/Prescription-Drug-Coverage/PrescriptionDrugCovContra/Downloads/CY2016-MTM-Fact-Sheet.pdf. Accessed May 11, 2017.
5. DiPiro JT, Talbert RL, Yee GC, Matzke GR, Wells BG, Posey LM, eds. *Pharmacotherapy: A Pathophysiologic Approach,* 10th ed. New York, NY: McGraw-Hill Education; 2017. Available at http://accesspharmacy.mhmedical.com.lp.hscl.ufl.edu/book.aspx?bookID=1861. Accessed May 11, 2017.
6. Chobanian AV, Bakris GL, Black HR, et al. Seventh Report of the Joint National Committee on Prevention, Detection, Evaluation, and Treatment of High Blood Pressure. *Hypertension.* 2003;42:1206-1252.
7. Saseen JJ, MacLaughlin EJ. Hypertension. In: DiPiro JT, Talbert RL, Yee GC, Matzke GR, Wells BG, Posey LM, eds. *Pharmacotherapy: A Pathophysiologic Approach,* 10th ed., Chapter 13. Available at http://accesspharmacy.mhmedical.com.lp.hscl.ufl.edu/content.aspx?bookid=1861&sectionid=146233698. Accessed May 11, 2017.
8. James PA, Oparil S, Carter BL, et al. 2014 evidence-based guideline for the management of high blood pressure in adults. Report from the panel members appointed to the Eighth Joint National Committee (JNC8). *JAMA.* 2014;311(5):507-520.
9. Anonymous: Blood pressure management in CKD ND patients without diabetes mellitus. In: *Kidney Disease Improving Global Outcomes,* Chapter 3; *Kidney Int Suppl.* 2012;2:357-362.

10. Pickering TG, White WB. ASH position paper: Home and ambulatory blood pressure monitoring. When and how to use self (home) and ambulatory blood pressure monitoring. *J Clin Hypertens*. 2008;10:850-855.

11. Hodgkinson J et al. Relative effectiveness of clinic and home blood pressure monitoring compared with ambulatory blood pressure monitoring in diagnosis of hypertension: Systematic review. *Br Med J*. 2011;342:d3621.

12. Institute of Medicine. *Health Literacy: A Prescription to End Confusion*. Washington, DC: National Academy Press; 2004:81-103.

13. CMS. *Medicare Part D Medication Therapy Management Program Standardized Format*. Available at https://www.cms.gov/Medicare/Prescription-Drug-Coverage/PrescriptionDrugCovContra/Downloads/MTM-Program-Standardized-Format-English-and-Spanish-Instructions-Samples-v032712.pdf. Accessed May 11, 2017.

14. Natural Medicines [database online]. Somerville, MA: Therapeutic Research Center; 2017. Report available from: https://naturalmedicines.therapeuticresearch.com/.

15. Centers for Medicare and Medicaid Services (CMS). *Medicare 2017 Part C & D Star Rating Technical Notes*. Available at https://www.cms.gov/medicare/prescription-drug-coverage/prescriptiondrugcovgenin/performancedata.html. Accessed May 13, 2017.

Review Questions

1. Which of the following best describes the rationale for creation of the MTM data sets?
   a. The need to train multiple MTM providers on an ongoing basis
   b. The need for a comprehensive drug information resource
   c. The need for a clinical decision support tool for MTM
   d. The need to define the core elements of MTM

2. All of the following are potential uses of the compendium of MTM data sets EXCEPT:
   a. A tool for educating trainees in an MTM practice setting
   b. A resource to supplement MTM software programs
   c. A resource for an MTM practitioner starting a new MTM program
   d. A tool to use in screening for drug interactions in MTM patients

3. Which of the following is a limitation of the MTM data sets?
   a. Lack of a treatment algorithm
   b. Lack of a complete listing of adverse effects
   c. Lack of suggested MTM interview questions
   d. Lack of sample medication action plans

4. Which of the following best describes the basic organizational structure for each MTM data set?
   a. Organized by type of medication-related problem
   b. Organized by core elements of MTM
   c. Organized by level of reimbursement for MTM services
   d. Organized by complexity of patient problems

5. An MTM provider is scheduled to see a patient with low health literacy and multiple medical conditions. Which section of the MTM data set provides guidance on how to communicate complex medical concepts to this patient?
   a. Living room language
   b. Questions to anticipate from the patient
   c. Sample provider communications
   d. Supportive therapies

6. Which of the following is a unique component of the MTM data sets, as compared to traditional drug databases?
   a. Categorization of prescription medications by drug therapy class
   b. Provision of common or serious adverse effects of medications
   c. Notation of black box warnings for medications
   d. Inclusion of referral strategies for treatment-emergent adverse events

7. All of the following items are located in the "Introduction" section of the MTM data set EXCEPT:
   a. Overview of the disease state
   b. Secondary causes or contributing factors
   c. Complications of the disease state
   d. Common therapeutic interventions

8. A first-time MTM provider is anxious about an upcoming MTM session with a new patient. Which of the following sections of the MTM data set contains a set of guided questions for the provider to ask during the patient interview?
   a. Comprehensive medication review
   b. Medication action plan
   c. Intervention
   d. Introduction

9. Which of the following sections of the MTM data set contains an outline of therapeutic goals for a given disease state?
   a. Comprehensive medication review
   b. Documentation
   c. Intervention
   d. Introduction

10. A student pharmacist wants to review some examples of medication-related problems that she should be screening for during an upcoming MTM encounter. Which of the following sections of the MTM data set is most likely to provide her with the needed information?
    a. Personal medication list
    b. Medication action plan
    c. Documentation
    d. Intervention

ANSWERS

1. a	2. d	3. b
4. b	5. a	6. d
7. d	8. a	9. d
10. c		

13

Asthma MTM Data Set

Maria Maniscalco-Feichtl, PharmD, and Kyle Melin, PharmD, BCPS, AE-C

KEY POINTS

- Asthma is a condition that may go into remission or present differently throughout the stages of life. The presence of airway inflammation remains a consistent feature.
- Symptoms of asthma are preventable and manageable with lifestyle modification and, when needed, pharmacotherapy.
- To achieve optimal outcomes, the medication therapy management (MTM) consult process must include patient education on trigger avoidance and self-management techniques.
- MTM providers should assess inhaler and/or device technique at each visit to help ensure maximal efficacy of asthma pharmacotherapy.

INTRODUCTION TO ASTHMA

Asthma is a disease that is characterized by airway inflammation and airway obstruction. In individuals with a genetic predisposition, the airways become inflamed and hyperresponsive when exposed to various environmental triggers, resulting in bronchoconstriction, formation of mucus plugs, and airway obstruction. Common symptoms of asthma are cough, dyspnea, wheeze, and/or chest tightness. Asthma is a serious lung condition affecting all age groups in many countries.[1,2] Although a common health condition, the clinical presentation is highly variable because of the intrinsic nature of the disease. Thus, global measures were created to assist clinicians in disease state management (Table 13-1).

Severity of asthma symptoms in patients who are not currently taking a long-term controller medication (also known as *maintenance medication*) is assessed using the impairment and risk domains illustrated in Table 13-2. To determine whether a patient is presenting with intermittent, mild, moderate, or severe asthma impairment, the following symptoms are assessed: nighttime awakenings, use of short-acting bronchodilator for quick relief of acute symptoms, workdays missed, patient ability to engage in normal daily activities, and quality of life. In general, patients are considered at higher risk for uncontrolled asthma if they have a history of two or more asthma exacerbations requiring treatment with oral corticosteroids. Table 13-3 outlines symptom criteria and corresponding pharmacotherapy for patients with persistent asthma symptoms in need of starting a controller therapy. In addition to methods for assessing asthma symptoms, there are several validated patient self-assessment instruments that may be useful in assessing level of control, including the Asthma Therapy Assessment Questionnaire© (ATAQ) and Asthma Control Test™ (ACT)".[1]

Spirometric data is another tool used in the assessment of asthma. The forced expiratory volume (measured during the first second of forced breath)/forced vital capacity (FEV_1/FVC) ratio is a more sensitive measure of severity in the impairment domain, as compared to FEV_1, which appears to be a useful measure in indicating risk for exacerbations.[1] Spirometry is generally used at diagnosis and may be used every 1 to 2 years for monitoring.

Other terms associated with asthma are as follows:

- *Acute exacerbations* (also called "flare-up")—transient worsening of asthma resulting from exposure to risk factors or triggers such as air pollutants, exercise, viral infection, allergen exposure, and/or change in weather conditions.[2]
- *Difficult-to-treat asthma*—patients with asthma in whom ongoing factors such as comorbidities, poor adherence to treatment and/or allergen exposure result in poor control of symptoms. Genetic predisposition may also be a factor.[2]
- *Exercise-induced bronchospasm* (EIB)—exacerbation that occurs during or within minutes after vigorous activity. Defined as a drop in FEV_1 by ≥10% from preexercise baseline value. Late-phase reaction may occur hours after exercise.[1,3]

TABLE 13-1 • Overview of Global Measures of Asthma Assessment

Assessment and monitoring are linked to the concepts of severity, control, and responsiveness to treatment
Severity[a] refers to the individual's intrinsic intensity of the disease process
Control refers to symptom control and the future risk of an adverse outcome
Responsiveness indicates the ease with which asthma symptoms are controlled by pharmacologic therapy
Both severity and control include the domains of "impairment" and "risk"[b]
Impairment describes the frequency of symptoms and subsequent functional limitations that the patient is experiencing or has recently experienced
Risk describes the likelihood of asthma exacerbations, progressive decline in lung function, or risk of an adverse effect from medication

[a] Severity is measured most easily in a patient who is not receiving long-term controller therapy.

[b] Impairment is assessed by interviewing the patient and/or caregiver recall of events during the previous 2-4 weeks; risk is based on symptoms and lung function reported over the last year.[1]

Source: References 1 and 2.

- *Nocturnal asthma*—symptoms worsening during sleep. Usually a sign of inadequately treated persistent asthma.[3]
- *Severe asthma*—patients who develop progressive airflow limitation that is not fully reversible with available therapies (refractory).[2]

The condition of asthma is associated with worsening symptoms when a patient is exposed to certain triggers. A *trigger* is an event (eg, respiratory infection) or exposure to a substance (eg, mold) that causes uncomfortable symptoms of shortness of breath, chest tightness, or cough. Symptoms may resolve when the trigger is removed. Patients should be encouraged to keep a trigger diary to determine factors that may worsen asthma symptoms. The diary should include triggers from the environment (eg, allergens), foods, psychosocial reactions, and seasonal changes. Table 13-4 lists common triggers of asthma symptoms. In addition, host factors such as allergic rhinitis, menstruation, gastroesophageal reflux disease (GERD), or obesity may cause or worsen symptoms.

Complications of Asthma

Complications of asthma vary depending on patient factors such as age, duration of uncontrolled symptoms, severity of hyperresponsiveness to triggers, airway physiology, comorbid conditions (eg, chronic obstructive pulmonary disease, heart failure). Table 13-5 provides examples of asthma complications.

Therapeutic Goals for Asthma

The therapeutic goal for patients with asthma is to attain adequate control of asthma, maintain or improve quality of life, reduce risk for exacerbations, and prevent airway remodeling. Figure 13-1 outlines recommended goals for asthma. Control is assessed by looking at the asthma impairment and risk. Impairment measures symptoms, nighttime awakening, ability to perform daily activities, use of a short-acting bronchodilator, FEV_1/peak flow, and completion of a validated

TABLE 13-2 • Classification of Asthma Severity for Patients Who Are Not Currently Taking Long-Term-Control Medications

		Children 0-4 and 5-11 Years of Age			
			Persistent		
	Components	**Intermittent**	**Mild**	**Moderate**	**Severe**
Impairment	Symptoms	≤2 days/wk	>2 days/wk but not daily	Daily	Throughout the day
	Nighttime awakenings (0-4 years)	0	1-2 x month	3-4 x month	>1 x week
	5-11 years	≤2 x month	3-4 x month	>1 x week, but not nightly	Often 7 x week
	SABA use for Sx control	≤2 days/wk	>2 days/wk but not daily	Daily	Several times per day
	Interference with normal activity	None	Minor limitation	Some limitation	Extremely limited
	Lung function	FEV_1 > 80%	FEV_1 > 80%	FEV_1 60%-80%	FEV_1 < 60%
	5-11 years	FEV_1/FVC >85% (>0.85)	FEV_1/FVC >80% (>0.80)	FEV_1/FVC 75%-80% (0.75-0.80)	FEV_1/FVC <75% (0.75)
	Exacerbations	**Intermittent**	**Persistent**		
Risk	0-4 years	0-1/y	≥2 in 6 months or ≥4 wheezing episodes/1 year lasting >1 day		
	5-11 years	0-2/y	>2 in 1 year →		
	Recommended step for initiating treatment	Step 1	Step 2	Step 3 and consider short course of oral corticosteroids	

(Continued)

TABLE 13-2 • Classification of Asthma Severity for Patients Who Are Not Currently Taking Long-Term-Control Medications (*Continued*)

		Youths ≥12 Years of Age and Adults			
			Persistent		
	Components	Intermittent	Mild	Moderate	Severe
Impairment	Symptoms	≤2 days/wk	>2 days/wk but not daily	Daily	Throughout the day
	Nighttime awakenings	≤2 x month	3-4 x month	>1 x week, but not nightly	Often 7 x week
	SABA use for Sx control	≤2 days/wk	>2 days/wk, but not >1 x day	Daily	Several times per day
	Interference with normal activity	None	Minor limitation	Some limitation	Extremely limited
	Lung function[a]	FEV_1 > 80%	FEV_1 > 80%	FEV_1 60%-80%	FEV_1 < 60%
		FEV_1/FVC normal	FEV_1/FVC normal	FEV_1/FVC reduced 5% (0.05)	FEV_1/FVC reduced >5% (> 0.05)
	Exacerbations	**Intermittent**	**Persistent**		
Risk		0-2/y	>2 in 1 year →		
	Recommended step for initiating treatment	Step 1	Step 2	Step 3 and consider short course of oral corticosteroids	Step 4 or 5 and consider course of oral corticosteroid

[a] Normal FEV_1/FVC: 8-19 years 85% (0.85); 20-39 years 80% (0.80); 40-59 years 75% (0.75); 60-80 years 70% (0.70).

Abbreviations: FEV_1 = forced expiratory volume in 1 second; FVC = forced vital capacity; SABA = short-acting β_2-agonist.

Source: Reproduced, with permission, from DiPiro, JT, Talbert RL, Yee GC, Matzke GR, Wells BG, Posey LM, eds. *Pharmacotherapy: A Pathophysiologic Approach*. 10th ed. New York, NY: McGraw-Hill; 2017.

TABLE 13-3 • GINA Recommendations for Initial Controller Treatment in Adults and Adolescents

Symptom Presentation	Preferred Treatment
Symptoms of asthma or need for SABA < 2×/month; no waking due to asthma in last month; and no risk factors for exacerbations, including in prior year	No controller
Infrequent symptoms, but patient has risk factors for exacerbation, eg, low lung function, use of OCS for asthma in prior year, intensive-care treatment for asthma	Low-dose ICS
Symptoms of asthma or need for SABA between 2×/month and 2×/week, or patient wakes because of asthma ≥ once per month	Low-dose ICS
Symptoms or need for SABA > 2×/week	Low-dose ICS[a]
Troublesome symptoms most days or waking ≥ 1×/week, especially if any risk factors exist	Medium/high-dose ICS(A) or low-dose ICS/LABA[b]
Symptoms consistent with severely uncontrolled asthma, or with an acute exacerbation	OCS short course *and* start of high-dose ICS (A) or moderate-dose ICS/LABA[b]

[a] Less effective options are LTRA or theophylline.

[b] Not recommended for initial controller treatment in children 6-11 years.

Abbreviations: GINA = Global Initiative for Asthma; ICS = inhaled corticosteroids; LABA = long-acting β_2-agonist; LTRA = leukotriene receptor antagonist; OCS = oral corticosteroids; SABA = short-acting β_2-agonist.

Source: Reference 2.

patient self-assessment questionnaire. Risk focuses on exacerbations, and monitoring for loss of lung function or treatment-related side effects. Controlled asthma symptoms deemed stable over 3 consecutive months is a prompt for clinical assessment to step down in use of pharmacologic treatment (eg, go from step 3 down to step 2 therapy), as illustrated in Table 13-6. Table 13-7 outlines activities to be completed when conducting an asthma consultation.

TABLE 13-4 • Agents and Events Triggering Asthma

Respiratory infection: respiratory syncytial virus (RSV), rhinovirus, influenza, parainfluenza, *Mycoplasma pneumonia, Chlamydia*
Allergens: airborne pollens (grass, trees, weeds), house-dust mites, animal danders, cockroaches, fungal spores
Environment: cold air, fog, ozone, sulfur dioxide, nitrogen dioxide, tobacco smoke, wood smoke, air pollution
Emotions: anxiety, stress, laughter
Exercise: particularly in cold, dry climate
Drugs/food preservatives: aspirin, NSAIDs (cyclooxygenase inhibitors), sulfites, benzalkonium chloride, nonselective β-blockers
Occupational stimuli: bakers (flour dust); farmers (hay mold); spice and enzyme workers; printers (arabic gum); chemical workers (azo dyes, anthraquinone, ethylenediamine, toluene diisocyanates, polyvinyl chloride); plastics, rubber, and wood workers (formaldehyde, western cedar, dimethylethanolamine, anhydrides)
Host factors: obesity, African-American race, Hispanic ethnicity, low socioeconomic status

TABLE 13-5 • Complications of Asthma

Type of Complication	Examples
Acute exacerbations	Difficulty breathing Difficulty performing normal activities Loss of sleep Possible need for mechanical ventilation
Chronic complications	Persistent cough Permanent decrease in lung function Adverse effects of medication, eg corticosteroids
During and after surgery	Asthma increases the risk for the following conditions: Acute bronchoconstriction triggered by intubation Hypoxemia Hypercapnia Impaired effectiveness of cough Atelectasis Respiratory infection Latex exposure, which may trigger exacerbation Prior use of some anesthetic agents may trigger exacerbation on reexposure to agent
Pregnancy[a]	Asthma increases risk for the following conditions: Preeclampsia Preterm birth Low-birth-weight infant Perinatal mortality

[a] Adequate asthma control is essential for health of mother and baby.

Source: References 1 and 2.

Pulmonary function

- Maintain baseline FEV_1
- Prevent airway remodeling
- Reduce complications secondary to infection, e.g., influenza, viral upper respiratory infection

Medication

- Achieve optimal symptom control with lowest dose of medication
- Require infrequent use (≤2 days a week) of short-acting inhaled β_2-agonist for quick relief of symptoms (not including prevention of EIB)
- Minimize adverse effects of asthma medications

Quality of life

- Be able to participate fully in any activity of choice
- Avoid missed work/school because of asthma symptoms
- Prevent recurrent exacerbations of asthma and minimize the need for emergency department visits or hospitalization
- Minimize daytime airway symptoms and sleep through the night

FIGURE 13-1 Therapeutic goals for asthma.
Source: References 1, 2, and 3.

TABLE 13-6 • GINA Stepwise Approach to Control Symptoms and Minimize Future Risk[2,3-4]

Step	Preferred Option (Evidence Level)	Other Recommended Options (Evidence Level)
1	As-needed SABA (A)	Consider low-dose ICS, in addition to as-needed SABA, for patients at risk for exacerbations (B)
2	Low dose ICS, plus as-needed SABA (A)	LTRA (A) Low-dose ICS/LABA (A) ICS started with symptoms of allergic asthma, for seasonal treatment only (D)
3	Low dose ICS/LABA, plus as-needed SABA for adults/adolescents (A) *Or* low-dose ICS/formoterol as both maintenance and reliever (A) For children aged 6-11 years, medium-dose ICS, plus as-needed SABA	Medium-dose ICS, for adults/adolescents (A) Low-dose ICS plus either LTRA (A) or low-dose, sustained-release theophylline (B)
4	Medium-dose ICS/LABA, plus as-needed SABA for adults/adolescents (B) *Or* medium-dose ICS/formoterol as both maintenance and reliever (A) For children aged 6-11 years, refer child to asthma specialist	Add-on therapy with tiotropium for adults or adolescents with exacerbation history (B) High-dose ICS/LABA Medium-dose ICS/LABA plus either LTRA or low-dose sustained-release theophylline
5	Referral to specialist and consideration of add-on treatment	Tiotropium for ages 12 and older (B) Omalizumab for moderate-severe allergic asthma (A) Mepolizumab or reslizumab for ages 12 and over with severe eosinophilic asthma (B) Sputum-guided treatment adjusted by eosinophilia >3% (A) Bronchial thermoplasty in some adults with severe asthma (B) Add-on low dose OCS (≤7.5 mg/day prednisone equivalent) (D)

Abbreviations: GINA = Global Initiative for Asthma; ICS = inhaled corticosteroids; LABA = long-acting β_2-agonist; LTRA = leukotriene receptor antagonist; OCS = oral corticosteroids; SABA = short-acting β_2-agonist.

Source: References 2, 3, and 4.

TABLE 13-7 • Recommendations for Initial Visit for Asthma

Framework	Information	Skills
Expectations of visit Assess Asthma control Patient's goals for therapy Medications Quality of life	Review definition of asthma using living room language Review definition of asthma control: Few daytime symptoms No nighttime awakenings secondary to asthma Engaging in normal daily activities Normal lung function	Teach/review or demonstrate the following: Inhaler technique Spacer or valved holding chamber technique Peak flow meter monitoring Review patient self-monitoring skills: Recognizing changes from baseline in intensity or frequency of symptoms Monitoring asthma-induced night awakenings Use of quick-relief inhaler and/or medication use Recognizing reduced exercise tolerance Create/review written asthma action plan Provide/educate on recommended vaccinations: Influenza "flu vaccine" yearly Pneumococcal "pneumonia vaccine" between ages 2 and 64 years and one time booster at age >65 • For adults aged ≥60 years, the zoster "shingles vaccine" • Tdap "prevent whooping cough and tetanus vaccine"

Source: References 1, 3, 4, 5, and 6.

TABLE 13-8 • Characteristics of Various Inhalation Devices

Device	Drugs	Breath-Activated	Dose Counter	Other Excipients	Disadvantages
MDI	All classes	No	No/yes	Propellants, surfactants, cosolvents	Requires coordination of actuation and inhalation; large pharyngeal deposition; difficult to teach
Pressair	Aclidinium	Yes	Yes	Lactose filler	Requires rapid inhalation to activate
Respiclick	Albuterol	Yes	Yes	Lactose filler	Requires rapid inhalation to activate
MDI plus valved holding chamber	All classes	No	No		More expensive than MDI alone; less portable; inconsistent effect on delivery; nonstatic preferred
Jet nebulizers	All classes	No	—	Preservatives in some solutions	Significant interbrand variability; expensive and time consuming; less efficient than MDIs; contamination possible; preparations may be light- and temperature-sensitive (short shelf life)
Ultrasonic nebulizer	Cromolyn solution, short-acting β_2-agonist solutions	No	—	Preservatives in some solutions	Same as for jet nebulizers plus cannot be used for suspensions; battery-operated models are portable
Flexhaler	Budesonide	Yes	Yes	Lactose filler	Requires high inspiratory flow (60 L/min); pharyngeal deposition Not approved for patients <6 years of age
Diskus	Fluticasone; salmeterol; fluticasone/salmeterol	Yes	Yes	Lactose filler	Not approved for patients <4 years of age Requires inspiratory flow of 30-60 L/min
Ellipta	Fluticasone furoate Fluticasone/vilanterol	Yes	Yes	Lactose filler	Not approved for patients <12 years of age (18 years for fluticasone/vilanterol) Requires inspiratory flow of 60 L/min
Aerolizer	Formoterol	Yes	—	Lactose filler	Single-dose capsules; not approved for patients <5 years of age Requires flow of 30-60 L/min
Neohaler	Indacaterol	Yes	—	Lactose filler	Single-dose capsules; not approved for children; requires flow of 60 L/min
Handihaler	Tiotropium	Yes	—	Lactose filler	Single-dose capsule; not approved for children; requires flow of 20 L/min
Twisthaler	Mometasone	Yes	Yes	Lactose filler	Not approved for children <4 years of age
Respimat	Tiotropium Albuterol/ipratropium Olodaterol	No	Yes	Preservative	Requires slow deep breath; not approved for children aged <12 years

Source: Reproduced, with permission, from DiPiro, JT, Talbert RL, Yee GC, Matzke GR, Wells BG, Posey LM, eds. *Pharmacotherapy: A Pathophysiologic Approach*. 10th ed. New York, NY: McGraw-Hill; 2017.

The inhaler technique is an essential skill for each person with asthma to master. Technique is dependent on the type of device. Multiple types of devices exist as shown in Table 13-8, and new devices are currently being created by drug manufacturers. To assist the patient in learning proper technique, MTM providers should use resources such as instructions in the drug package insert, manufacturer website and online tutorials.

The *peak flow meter* (PFM) is a tool for persons with asthma to use on a daily basis to monitor their airway symptoms. The tool assists in predicting when an exacerbation may occur, as a drop in the normal peak expiratory flow (PEF) reading occurs. This drop is a signal to patients to ensure that they have a quick-relief inhaler with them at all times throughout the day, and may signify a need for a temporary increase in asthma medications. Peak flow meters may be purchased in a pharmacy or durable medical equipment store, or may be provided by staff from the local chapter of the American Lung Association.

Therapeutic Failure

Drug treatment for asthma is deemed a *therapeutic failure* if a patient currently on a controller medication does not achieve adequate control of asthma symptoms. For example, asthma is considered to be uncontrolled when a patient reports use of a SABA on >2 days per week, one to three awakenings from sleep at night per week, or scores of 16 to 19 on the ACT. Very poorly controlled asthma is characterized by use of a SABA several times per day, four or more night awakenings from sleep per week, and/or a score on the ACT score of ≤15.

CORE ELEMENT 1—COMPREHENSIVE MEDICATION REVIEW FOR PATIENTS WITH ASTHMA

Following is a list of suggested questions to use when conducting a medication therapy review in a patient with asthma (Table 13-9). Table 13-10 summarizes questions for a follow-up consultation. During the follow-up the MTM provider should gather information to determine appropriate management for current asthma symptoms while aiming to reduce overall asthma risk and impairment. The number and types of questions will depend on several factors, including the amount of time for the interview, number of concurrent MRPs, urgency of MRPs, and the reliability of the patient in providing accurate information, among others. In time-limited interactions or in complex cases with multiple medical issues, the MTM provider may choose to target questions that help to identify or rule out issues of an urgent nature (see list of questions to ask for prevention/assessment of medical emergencies in Table 13-11). MTM providers should remember to use living room language during the interview (Figure 13-2), and to be prepared for questions that patients might ask regarding asthma (Table 13-12).

In addition to the suggested questions, validated instruments such as the ATAQ, the Asthma Control Questionnaire (ACQ), and the ACT are available via the NHLBI guidelines and may be utilized for conducting a complete or targeted medication review.[1]

TABLE 13-9 • Suggested Questions for the Asthma Patient

Initial Assessment of Asthma[1,3]
In the past 12 months…
Have you had a sudden severe episode or recurrent episodes of: coughing, wheezing, chest tightness, or shortness of breath? (*Note*: Initially ask about each symptom separately. Asking as a whole sentence is a cognitive burden for the patient to process.)
Have you had colds that "go to the chest" or take more than 10 days to recover from?
Have you experienced coughing, wheezing, or shortness of breath during a particular season?
Have you experienced coughing, wheezing, or shortness of breath in certain places or when exposed to certain things such as pets/animals, tobacco smoke, or perfumes?
Have you used any medication that helped you breath better? How often?
Are your symptoms relieved when you take those medications?
In the past 4 weeks, have you experienced coughing, wheezing, or shortness of breath:
At night that has awakened you?
On waking up?
After running, moderate exercise or other physical activity?
How do you use your inhalers? (Ask the patient to demonstrate the procedure.)
Assessing and Monitoring Asthma Control[1]
To assess and monitor asthma control, you would ask the patient the following questions:
Has your asthma awakened you at night or early in the morning?
Have you needed more quick-relief bronchodilator medication than usual?
Have you needed any urgent medical care for your asthma, such as an unscheduled visit to a physician or urgent care/emergency department?
Are you participating in your usual and desired activities?
If you are measuring your peak flow, has it been below your personal best?
How do you feel about taking medication?
Have you missed or stopped taking any regular doses of your medications? In the last week?
Have you had trouble filling your prescriptions (eg, is cost a burden?)?
How many puffs of your inhaled quick-relief medicine do you use per day?
How many inhalers have you been through in the past month?
Have you tried any other medicines or remedies?
Has your asthma medicine caused you any problems such as shakiness, nervousness, bad taste, sore throat, cough, upset stomach, hoarseness, or bruising?

Source: References 1 and 3.

TABLE 13-10 • Questions to Ask When Conducting a Follow-up Visit with an Asthma Patient

Monitoring Signs and Symptoms of Asthma
The following questions would be appropriate: Has your asthma been better or worse since the last visit? Have you noticed your asthma getting worse during a specific season? Event? In the past 2 weeks, how many days have you: Experienced coughing, wheezing, shortness of breath, or chest tightening during the day? Awakened at night from sleep due to coughing or other asthma symptoms? Awakened in the morning with asthma symptoms that didn't improve within 15 minutes of using a quick-relief inhaler? Experienced symptoms while exercising or playing? Been unable to perform a usual activity, such as walking up a flight of stairs, because of asthma?
Monitoring Pulmonary Function
The following questions would be appropriate: Do you have a peak flow meter? What have been the highest and lowest values since the last visit? Has it dropped below 80% of your personal best since last visit? If yes, what did you do to manage your asthma? How do you measure your peak flow? (Ask the patient to demonstrate this.) At what time of day do you usually measure your peak flow?
Measuring Quality of Life
Since your last visit, how many days have your asthma symptoms caused you to: Miss work or school? Reduce your ability to engage in activities? (For caregivers: Have you changed your schedule because of your child's asthma?) Have you had any unscheduled visits to emergency department or hospital?
Monitoring Exacerbation History
Since the last visit, have you experienced asthma episodes that were a lot worse than usual? If yes, then: Describe what you thought was the trigger for the worsening symptoms. Describe what you did to control the symptoms. Have there been changes in your work or home environment eg, adopting a pet or cigarette smoker moved into apartment next door?
Monitoring Pharmacotherapy
The following request and question would be appropriate: Please list all medications that you are currently taking. How do you feel about taking medication? Review each medication for the following criteria: Do you know what this medication is for? Describe how you take this medication. How often do you forget to take it? What do you do you when you realize that you forgot to take your prescribed dose? Do you find using the device (eg, MDI or nebulizer) easy to operate? Show me how you use it. Is it difficult for you to get this medication? (For instance, is cost a burden? Not on formulary?) What side effects do you have with this medication? When taking this medication, do you experience shakiness? Nervousness? Bad taste? Sore throat? Cough? Upset stomach? Hoarseness? Which inhaler is used for quick relief? For maintaining/controlling symptoms? Please demonstrate how you use this inhaler. Have you received your influenza vaccination this year? Have you received a pneumonia vaccine?

Source: Reference 1.

TABLE 13-11 • Questions to Ask for Prevention/Assessment of Medical Emergencies

Crisis planning:
Have you ever gone to the hospital to treat an asthma attack?
Describe the signs of an asthma attack. What is your action plan when you experience these symptoms?
Let's review important information: Tell me the asthma symptoms that make you think you should take more asthma medication. Which medication(s) would you use more if you have symptoms?
Describe symptoms that would prompt you to call me or your provider.
If you cannot reach anyone, which emergency department would you go to?
Show me the breathing techniques you use to handle acute shortness of breath (that sudden feeling when you cannot catch your breath).
Review the "belly breathing" (also known as the *abdominal breathing*) exercise.
You can lie down or sit.
Focus on breathing slowly through your nose.
When you inhale, you should feel your abdomen expand (not your chest).
Exhale slowly while pulling your abdomen inward.
(Ideally, exhalation should be twice as long as inhalation.)

Source: References 1, 2, 3, and 5

ACE inhibitor—a medicine used to help lower blood pressure; may also help prevent changes or damage to the heart and kidney. Most common side effect of ACEI is a cough.

Adverse event—an uncomfortable or bad reaction and/or unexplained or unwanted effects.

AHRQ—Agency for Healthcare Research and Quality.

Airways—tube-like structures in the lungs that allows air to enter and leave the body.

Allergens (see *Triggers*)—substance that you are exposed to such as dust, pets, smoke, perfume, or change in weather that make your asthma symptoms worse.

AQLQ—Asthma-related Quality of Life Questionnaire- a form you fill out to help you make the best choice in changing your lifestyle or medication for asthma.

Arrhythmia—irregular heartbeat, skipped heartbeat, heart problem; this might be a side effect of some asthma medications.

Arterial blood gas—the amount of oxygen in the blood.

Asthma—a condition of the lungs that will make it difficult to breathe.

Asthma action plan—a written plan that helps you recognize symptoms and what to do about them, including which medicine to take and when to take it.

Asthma Control Test—a form that you fill out to help you make the best choice in changing your lifestyle or medication for asthma.

Asthma flare-up (also known as *exacerbation* or *attack*)—when you suddenly find it difficult to breathe, and experience chest tightness, coughing, or wheezing.

ATAQ—Asthma Therapy Assessment Questionnaire; a form you fill out to help you make the best choice in changing your lifestyle or medication for asthma.

Beta-blocker (usually written with the Greek symbol, β-blocker)—some asthmatic patients experience worsening of their asthma symptoms when they begin taking this type of blood pressure or heart medication.

BMI—body mass index. A measure of weight in relation to height. Higher BMI indicates obesity, and obesity puts one at higher risk for worsening asthma symptoms.

CBC—complete blood count, a blood test that looks at different types of blood cells and measures how many you have.

Chronic—constant, never-ending, does not go away.

Controller (maintenance) medicine—medicine that you take daily to manage asthma and reduce or not feel symptoms.

Cough—the most common asthma symptom. Exposure to substances that irritate the air passages causes your body to take action to get rid of the substance (eg, mucus). A dry cough may occur when the substance gets into your blood and you cannot spit it out.

CPAP—continuous positive airway pressure provided by a device to help maintain oxygen while you sleep.

Diskus—a type of inhaler device that delivers a powder that you inhale directly into your lungs.

Dose counter—a window on a device that you look at to find out how many doses you have left in that inhaler.

EIB—exercise-induced bronchospasm; a condition that is asthma-like. This is prevented with use of quick-relief medication prior to any exercise or activity.

EKG—a test that looks for any damage to or problems with your heart.

Electrolytes—a type of necessary salt found in blood, such as salt, potassium, and calcium.

Elevate—raise, make higher.

eNO—exhaled nitric oxide; a chemical the body produces that is currently being studied as a marker of how well your body is managing asthma symptoms. May also be measured to help you with quitting cigarette smoking.

Exacerbation (also known as "asthma flare-up" or "attack")—when you suddenly find it difficult to breathe, have chest tightness, or experience coughing or wheezing.

FEF—forced expiratory flow, which measures your ability to force air out of your lungs.

FEV_1—forced expiratory volume (amount of air that you forcefully breathe out) in 1 second.

FEV_6—forced expiratory volume (amount of air that you forcefully breathe out) in 6 seconds.

FIGURE 13-2 Living room language for asthma.

FVC—forced vital capacity; the total amount of air that you can push out of your lungs.

GERD—gastroesophageal reflux disease; sometimes GERD can trigger asthma symptoms.

GINA—Global Initiative for Asthma. This is a document that a clinician can use to help you determine the best steps to take to relieve and /or prevent your asthma from getting worse.

Heart rate—how many times your heart beats each minute.

Hematocrit—a blood test that measures the number of red blood cells that you have. A very low number could be a sign of anemia.

HEPA—high-efficiency particulate air; the recommended type of filter used in air conditioners, vacuums, and air purifiers to remove allergens (also known as "triggers") from the air that you breathe.

HFA—hydrofluoroalkane; an inhaler propellant that causes the drug to spray out of a canister.

Hyperkalemia—a high amount of potassium found in the blood. Very high potassium is a medical emergency and may change the way your heart beats.

Hypokalemia—low potassium, which may cause muscle weakness and cramping.

ICS—inhaled corticosteroid(s); medications used as a "controller medicine." When taken as directed, they can prevent worsening of asthma symptoms. ICS are not used when you need to open the airway quickly (see *Quick-relief medication*).

ICU—intensive-care unit. The department in the hospital where they treat you when your asthma is completely uncontrolled and your body cannot provide oxygen to its own organs.

Inhaler—a device that you use to inject medication directly into your lungs (eg, Diskus, Turbohaler, Aerolizer, Handihaler, or metered-dose inhaler [MDI]).

IVIG—intravenous immunoglobulin, a medication given directly into the vein and used in patients who have severe uncontrolled asthma and allergies.

LABA—long-acting β_2-agonist(s); a controller (maintenance) inhaled medicine.

Lifestyle changes—changes that you make in your lifestyle to help you prevent worsening asthma symptoms. Includes maintaining a healthy weight, avoiding certain foods, and avoiding cigarette smoke/smoking.

LTRA—leukotriene receptor antagonist; a medication you take by mouth that stops the release of a certain chemical when you are exposed to a trigger. By blocking this chemical, your body will suffer fewer and less severe asthma symptoms. This medication also helps you manage allergy symptoms.

Lungs—the organ in your body used for breathing.

MDI—metered-dose inhaler; a device that delivers a specific amount of medicine per dose.

Mucus—the thick, sticky substance produced in your lungs in response to inflammation in your airway.

NAEPP—National Asthma Education and Prevention Program; a document that a clinician might use to help you determine the best course of action to relieve and/or prevent your asthma from getting worse.

Nebulizer—a device that delivers asthma medicine through a pump and mask/mouthpiece.

NHLBI—National Heart, Lung, and Blood Institute. This is the organization that coordinates all the health professionals who write the NAEPP.

NO or NO_2—nitric oxide, a chemical that the body produces and a marker of how well your body is managing asthma symptoms.

NSAID—nonsteroidal anti-inflammatory drug; a medicine such as aspirin or ibuprofen that provides pain relief. Many people with asthma experience worsening of asthma symptoms after taking a NSAID.

Obese—having a body mass index (BMI) of >30. This increases your risk of having high blood pressure, diabetes, cardiovascular disease, and asthma symptoms.

Overweight—having a BMI of >25. This increases your risk of experiencing asthma symptoms.

PCP—primary-care provider (or physician).

Peak expiratory flow (PEF)—the amount of air in liters/ per minute (L/min) that you can breathe out; measured with a peak flow meter.

Peak flow meter (PFM)—a handheld device that measures how well you are able to force air out of your lungs.

Quick-relief medications—inhaled medicine that you take when you are coughing/wheezing or feeling chest discomfort. It works rapidly to help you breathe better. Make sure that your physician knows if you use this more than twice a week.

SABA—short-acting β_2-agonist(s) (inhaled); also known as *quick-relief inhalers*, to be used when your asthma symptoms make you feel uncomfortable (chest tightness or coughing, etc).

SaO_2—oxygen saturation; the amount of oxygen in your blood circulating throughout your body.

Serum potassium—a test checking the amount of potassium in your blood (see *Hyperkalemia* and *Hypokalemia*).

Side effect—an unintended effect of taking a medication. For example, taking Benadryl might make you secrete mucus that you would have to spit out.

Sleep apnea—a sleep disorder that often involves pauses in breathing during the night; this may cause worsening of asthma since it reduces the amount of oxygen that you get into your lungs while you sleep.

Smoking cessation—a process to help you quit smoking. Avoiding cigarette smoke reduces the risk of having an asthma flare-up or exacerbation and reduces direct damage to the lungs.

Spacer device—a tube-like device that you use with your inhaler to help you get the full amount of medication directly into your lungs.

Spirometry—tests that your physician will ask you to perform where you breathe in and breathe out as fully and as rapidly as possible. These tests measure how well your lungs are working and, if you are given medication to use (eg, albuterol), how well your lungs respond to that medication.

Symptoms of asthma—physical changes in your body that you feel when you have asthma, such as coughing, wheezing, or chest discomfort/tightness.

Tachycardia—a rapid heartbeat, >100 times per minute; a possible adverse effect of some asthma medications.

Triggers (see *Allergens*)—substances or conditions such as dust, pet dander, smoke, perfume, or changes in weather that make your asthma symptoms worse. Triggers vary from patient to patient.

Wheeze—a whistling noise that occurs in your lungs when you are experiencing difficulty breathing.

FIGURE 13-2 *(Continued)*

It is important to discuss the unpredictable nature of asthma and assess how well the patient is prepared to handle sudden onset of symptoms, especially acute intense shortness of breath. Table 13-9 consists of questions to assess the ability of the asthma patient to provide quality self-care, with a focus on reducing impairment and risk by engaging in early intervention.

CORE ELEMENT 2—PERSONAL MEDICATION LIST[7]

Figure 13-3 presents a sample PML for a patient with asthma. This example is representative only of medications administered for asthma. Additional medications for other disease states should be

TABLE 13-12 • Questions to Anticipate Regarding Asthma

Asthma patients commonly ask the following questions:
What is asthma? Asthma is a condition of the airways that sometimes makes it difficult to breathe. People with asthma have airways that are very sensitive to certain triggers, resulting in feeling short of breath, coughing or gasping for air.
What causes asthma? Many factors known as 'triggers' cause asthma. Triggers can be related to the environment, such as exposure to pollen, pet dander, rapid change in temperature, allergies to grass or trees, or work-related exposure to dust or chemical fumes. Other triggers include exposure to cigarette smoke (passive or active) or odors like car fumes or potent perfume. Your body's response to a head cold/infection or stress can also trigger asthma. For some people, laughing so hard that they cannot catch their breath may trigger asthma.
What is uncontrolled asthma? Feeling short of breath or coughing or wheezing for >2 days per week and/or feeling like you need to use your quick-relief inhaler ≥2 days per week (not including use preexercise).
What health problems are associated with uncontrolled asthma? Quality of life is directly impacted. Fear and anxiety of not being able to breathe from initiating an activity becomes an unfortunate priority. Use and subsequent cost of going to the emergency department is an issue. Inability to do daily chores and calling out sick because of lack of energy are common. Children avoid exercise or activities requiring heavy breathing out of fear of passing out while playing. Long-term uncontrolled asthma can cause the structure of the airway to change permanently, resulting in a constant feeling of not being able to catch your breath that is not relieved by using medication.
How do I know if I have asthma? If you feel short of breath or have chest tightness or coughing often, write down each day you have these symptoms. Think about what you ate or inhaled or changes in weather that day and write it down. If you have a family history of asthma, write that down. Show your provider and ask about tests to see if you have asthma.
Why are asthma medications so important? When you cannot breathe, nothing else matters. Asthma medications help your lungs respond normally to everyday events and conditions (triggers) that bother you but do not bother other people. Asthma medications keep your airway open to help you feel better. Children are able to run and play because the medicine helps air get in and out of their lungs easily. People who need medicine and don't take it can develop uncontrolled asthma symptoms, which may lead to hospitalization, missed work/school, and cause anxiety about performing routine daily activities such as climbing stairs.
I can't tell when my asthma is uncontrolled. Can I just stop my medications if I feel okay? Asthma medicines do not cure your symptoms. Taking medicine to treat asthma is intended to help your body manage the triggers that you encounter daily. The goal of medicine is to prevent shortness of breath, chest tightness, and cough. Asthma gets worse for some people during certain seasons (eg, spring or fall). They may use more medication during the season and less when the season is over. It is important to create a plan with your physician regarding when you can stop taking medication. Avoid stopping on your own. Review your Asthma Action Plan with your physician, as well. Everyone who has a history of asthma should always have access to a quick-relief inhaler for emergency use.
What can happen if I stop taking my asthma medications? Stopping asthma medicine without a working plan or consent from your physician can lead to an asthma attack and possibly hospitalization. The effect can also be more subtle—not feeling well on a daily basis while performing routine tasks such as trying to do laundry or climb the stairs, which may lead to anxiety or fear of not being able to breathe.
When should I call my physician about my asthma? Call your physician if you are not responding to the prescribed treatment (you are feeling short of breath walking or climbing stairs or waking from sleep with chest discomfort or coughing), or if you are having side effects. Call if you experience the following symptoms of asthma: coughing, chest tightness, shortness of breath not relieved by use of quick-relief inhaler, *or* when you need your quick-relief inhaler for >2 days per week (not including use preexercise).
What should I do if I do not know how to use the inhaler? Inhaled medications are delivered in many different devices. Each device should come with directions for use in the drug leaflet you receive from the pharmacy. If you did not receive the leaflet, call the pharmacy where you obtained the inhaler and ask them for the copy. Even better, ask the pharmacist to show you how to use the device itself. Double-check by bringing the device to your physician and ask the physician or nurse to watch you give yourself a dose of inhaled medicine. If you are looking for other visual instruction, the internet site YouTube offers short videos on how to use inhalers.

added and listed separately. MTM providers should remember to use living room language when creating the PML.

CORE ELEMENT 3—MEDICATION ACTION PLAN[7]

Figure 13-4 provides sample medication action plans (MAPs) for a patient with asthma. These examples are representative only of action steps for the patient with asthma. MAPs for other disease states or other MRPs should be added and listed separately. In general, only a few of the most important action steps should be listed, so as not to overwhelm the patient. Other areas for patient self-management can be addressed at later visits. MTM providers should remember to use plain language when creating the MAP. In addition to the MAP, a Personal Written Asthma Action Plan as recommended by the NHLBI is available via the Regional Asthma Management and Prevention site.[5] Asthma action plans are available in different languages and include provider instructions, a plan guide to be completed by the practitioner/patient, review of triggers form, and school authorization form.

PERSONAL MEDICATION LIST FOR (*Insert patient's name, DOB: mm/dd/yyyy*)	
Medication: ProAir HFA (albuterol) inhaler	
How I use it: Inhale 1-2 puffs every 4 hours as needed for shortness of breath	
Why I use it: Asthma, shortness of breath	**Prescriber:** Ruggieri
Date I started using it: On/off since toddler	**Date I stopped using it:** (*Leave blank for patient's notes*)
Why I stopped using it: (*Leave blank for patient's notes*)	
Medication: Advair (fluticasone and salmeterol) Diskus 100/50	
How I use it: Use 1 inhalation twice daily	
Why I use it: Asthma symptom prevention	**Prescriber:** Ruggieri
Date I started using it: 3/1/2013	**Date I stopped using it:** (*Leave blank for patient's notes*)
Why I stopped using it: (*Leave blank for patient's notes*)	

FIGURE 13-3 Sample personal medication list for asthma control.

	DATE PREPARED: (*Insert date*)
What we talked about: Need to restart Advair to help with asthma symptoms due to seasonal pollen	
What I need to do: 1. Review how to use my inhaler 2. Start using Advair in morning and evening before I brush my teeth 3. Rinse my mouth out after inhaling Advair 4. Make sure that I refill my inhaler when the counter on the device tells me I have 14 doses (approximately 1 week of medication) left	**What I did and when I did it:** (*Leave blank for patient's notes*)
What we talked about: What to do when I have asthma symptoms—coughing, chest tightness, or wheezes	
What I need to do: 1. Breathe in and out slowly 2. Remind myself to employ the belly breathing technique, which will help me breathe better and feel less anxiety 3. Use 2-6 puffs of ProAir (albuterol) HFA "quick-relief inhaler." Breathe in and out slowly through pursed lips (like giving a kiss). If symptoms continue after 20 minutes, repeat inhaling 2-6 puffs of ProAir (albuterol) HFA. If still in discomfort 20 minutes after that, go to urgent-care clinic or hospital emergency department. 4. Write down in my airway diary when this occurs and bring to my next visit	**What I did and when I did it:** (*Leave blank for patient's notes*)

FIGURE 13-4 Sample medication action plan for an asthma patient.

CORE ELEMENT 4—INTERVENTION AND/OR REFERRAL

Interventions for management of asthma may include lifestyle modifications and/or drug therapy. Patients not adequately controlled with lifestyle modifications should be started on drug therapy. Lifestyle modifications, trigger avoidance, and medication management are all included in standards of asthma care. Table 13-13 outlines nonpharmacologic management of asthma. Table 13-14 highlights medications used for the management of asthma, but does not include therapies recommended for comorbid conditions (eg, allergic rhinitis, GERD).

In addition to prescription medication, patients may show interest in taking herbal therapy (Table 13-15). To date, there are limited data for most herbal products in asthma, and risks are largely unknown.[9] Green or black tea contains caffeine, which is assumed to cause bronchodilation since the chemical structure is similar to that of methylxanthines.[8-10] Inhaled L-arginine should be avoided, as it can exacerbate asthma symptoms.

Severity of asthma is utilized as a guide for clinical decision-making and treatment recommendations. The severity of asthma is determined by assessing the level of asthma impairment and risk (see Tables 13-1 and 13-2). The severity may be classified as intermittent, mild-persistent, moderate-persistent, or severe-persistent. For the intermittent group and/or patients with a history of exercise-induced bronchospasms, the use of a short-acting β-agonist (SABA) as needed prior to exercise is considered standard of care. Patients with persistent asthma are candidates for inhaled corticosteroids and/or other agents (eg, LABA or leukotriene antagonist) in addition to the SABA.

Preferred and alternative treatment recommendations for asthma for different age groups are displayed in Table 13-6. Pharmacotherapy always includes a short-acting bronchodilator as needed, regardless of severity or level of current control. With worsening asthma symptoms, adding medication or increasing the dose of therapy is considered to be a "step up" to gain airway control. Guidelines recommend that patients step up in therapy every 2 to 4 weeks until symptoms are stable. Following that, symptoms should be reevaluated every 3 months for patients with a mild-, moderate-, or severe-persistent classification. If a patient has well-controlled asthma for 3 consecutive months, a reduction in the current dose and/or elimination of one controller therapy may be considered. This is known as "step-down" therapy. The goal for all persons with asthma is to control or prevent asthma symptoms with the minimal amount of medication. Therefore, evaluating when to step down is a lifelong process. MTM providers should review the trigger diary to recognize any patterns that may exist (eg, the change of season worsens symptoms) and plan accordingly.

Once medication therapy is initiated, the clinical perspective focuses on assessing control (see Table 13-6) to adjust therapy using the stepwise approach. A patient currently on long-term controller therapy may experience worsening of asthma symptoms, for example, shifting from a well-controlled classification to a non-well-controlled classification secondary to exposure to a trigger. MTM providers should review the severity of symptoms over the past 2 to 4 weeks and the use of quick-relief medication, and assess triggers to determine appropriate changes, if needed, for the current medication regimen.

TABLE 13-13 • Nonpharmacologic Management of Asthma[a]

Intervention	Recommendation	Goal
Manage weight	Maintain normal body weight (body mass index: 18.5-24.9 kg/m^2)	Healthy weight reduces risk for asthma exacerbations
Avoid triggers	Allergens: indoor/outdoor air pollution, certain foods, noxious fumes, seasonal changes, weather, etc; keep a diary of what caused asthma symptoms (season of the year, foods, stress level, exercise without prior inhaler treatment are all examples) and consciously avoid triggers	Prevent hospitalization Prevent using sick days Feel in top shape
Increase physical activity	Engage in regular aerobic physical activity (brisk walking) at least 30 minutes per day most days of the week	Maintain and improve lung function
Stop smoking	For overall asthma symptom risk reduction, smoking is the number one lifestyle change	Preserve/improve lung function Reduce episodes of cough and shortness of breath
Carry quick-relief inhaler	Have a short-acting bronchodilator easily accessible; it is unpredictable when patients will encounter a trigger; therefore, a good rule of thumb is to carry one at all times	Prevent hospitalization Prevent using sick days Feel in top shape
Review inhaler technique	Correct inhaler technique will increase potency and efficacy of the medications.	Prevent asthma symptoms Maintain quality of life
Monitor peak flow	Perform peak expiratory flow monitoring (PEF) at the same time every day; record personal best; maintain diary of PEF readings	Utilizing PEF reading and asthma action plan, determine when to seek medical attention Prevent hospitalization

[a] Results will vary per patient depending on adherence to lifestyle modification and duration of implementation.

Source: References 1, 2, and 5.

TABLE 13-14 • Medications for Management of Asthma

Medication Class and Example Drugs	Common/Serious Side Effects[a]	Blackbox Warnings / Contraindications	Pregnancy Category[b]
Bronchodilators: β_2-agonists Short-acting β_2-agonists (SABA) Albuterol Levalbuterol Long-acting β_2-agonists (LABA) Arformoterol Formoterol Indacaterol Salmeterol	QT prolongation Tachycardia Hypokalemia Nervousness Tremor	Long-acting β_2-agonists may increase risk of death in asthma patients when used without inhaled corticosteroid	C
Bronchodilators: anticholinergics Ipratropium Tiotropium	Bronchospasm Pharyngitis Xerostomia Constipation Sinusitis	Hypersensitivity to atropine	B (ipratropium) C (tiotropium)
Bronchodilators: inhaled mast-cell stabilizers Cromolyn	Sore throat Bad taste in mouth	Hypersensitivity to cromolyn	B
Bronchodilators: methylxanthines Theophylline	Tachyarrhythmia Atrial fibrillation Nausea/vomiting Insomnia Tremor Irritability	Hypersensitivity to theophylline	C

(Continued)

TABLE 13-14 • Medications for Management of Asthma (*Continued*)

Medication Class and Example Drugs	Common/Serious Side Effects[a]	Blackbox Warnings / Contraindications	Pregnancy Category[b]
Inhaled corticosteroids (ICS) Beclomethasone Budesonide Ciclesonide Fluticasone Mometasone	Secondary hypocortisolism when used at high doses Pharyngitis Upper respiratory infection	Hypersensitivity to milk proteins	B (budesonide), C (all others)
Leukotriene modifiers Leukotriene receptor antagonist (LTRA) Montelukast Zafirlukast 5-Lipoxygenase inhibitor Zileuton[c]	Upper respiratory infection Fever Headache Neuropsychiatric changes in behavior/mood Hepatic dysfunction with zafirlukast Elevated liver function tests (LFTs)	Avoid chewable tablet in patient with phenylketonuria	B
Monoclonal antibody Mepolizumab Omalizumab Reslizumab (administered at provider's office)	Urticaria and anaphylactic reactions in 0.2% of users; may occur within hours to days, and may happen after several injections Injection-site pain and bruising up to 20% of patients Viral infection Upper respiratory infection	Pregnancy and omalizumab[d] Hypersensitivity to drug	Refer to product insert

[a] This is a general list and does not include all side effects that can occur from these drugs. Consult a drug reference source for a more inclusive list before making any recommendations. MTM providers should also consult a comprehensive drug interaction database before making pharmacotherapy recommendations.

[b] Product labeling for all prescription drugs is being updated to reflect the new FDA Pregnancy Labeling and Lactation Rule. Please check individual product labeling for the most accurate and updated pregnancy information.

[c] Zileuton is least desirable because of the paucity of efficacy data and need for liver function monitoring.

[d] Women exposed to omalizumab within 8 weeks prior to conception or any time during pregnancy should enroll in Pregnancy Exposure Registry by calling 866-496-5247.

Source: References 1, 2, and 8.

Since ICS are the preferred therapy for any patient presenting with either persistent asthma symptoms or non-well-controlled to very poorly controlled asthma symptoms, Table 13-16 provides an overview of ICS products and doses. Although low to medium doses of inhaled corticosteroid therapy do not result in the same intensity of adverse effects as does the oral formulation, prolonged use of high-dose ICS is more likely to result in effects on the immune system and other adverse effects. Table 13-17 highlights the potential adverse effects of ICS. It is essential to assess all patients taking the maximum dose of ICS to determine whether symptoms have been stable for 3 consecutive months. If so, the MTM provider should work with patient/provider to initiate a "step-down" by recommending a decrease in the ICS dose.

TABLE 13-15 • Herbal Supplements for Asthma

Herbal Product	Recommended Dosage	Effectiveness[a]	Cost[b]
Black tea/green tea	none	Insufficient evidence	$
Boswellia	300 mg 3× daily has been used	Insufficient evidence	$
Butterbur	none	Insufficient evidence	NA
Choline	500-1000 mg of choline 3× daily	Possibly effective	$$
Coleus	10 mg of forskolin powder, using a Spinhaler inhalator has been used	Insufficient evidence	NA

[a] Level of evidence: Likely effective. This product has a very high level of reliable clinical evidence supporting its use for a specific indication. Products rated "likely effective" are generally considered appropriate to recommend; "possibly effective"—This product has some clinical evidence supporting its use for a specific indication; however, the evidence is limited by quantity, quality, or contradictory findings. Products rated "possibly effective" might be beneficial, but do not have enough high-quality evidence to be recommended for most people; "insufficient evidence"—there is not enough reliable scientific evidence to provide an effectiveness rating.

[b] Cost: $ = ≥$10/month supply in recommended dosage; $$ = $11-$20/month.

Source: References 9 and 10.

TABLE 13-16 • Available Inhaled Corticosteroid Products, Lung Delivery, and Comparative Dosage

ICS	Product	Lung Delivery[a]
Beclomethasone dipropionate (BDP)	40 and 80 µg/actuation HFA MDI	50%-60%
Budesonide (BUD)	90 or 180 µg/dose DPI, Flexhaler	15%-30%
	200- and 500-µg ampules, 1 mg	5%-8%
Ciclesonide (CIC)	80 or 160 µg/actuation HFA MDI	50%
Flunisolide (FLU)	80 µg/actuation HFA MDI	68%
Fluticasone furoate (FF)	100, 200 µg/actuation DPI, Ellipta	80%-85%
Fluticasone propionate (FP)	44, 110, and 220 µg/actuation HFA MDI	20%
	50, 100, and 250 µg/dose DPI, Diskus	15%
Mometasone furoate (MF)	110 and 220 µg/dose DPI, Twisthaler; 100 and 200 µg/actuation HFA MDI	11%

	Comparative Daily Dosages (g) of Inhaled Corticosteroids		
	Low Daily Dose Child[a]/Adult	**Medium Daily Dose Child[a]/Adult**	**High Daily Dose Child[a]/Adult**
BDP			
HFA MDI	80-160/80-240	>160-320/>240-480	>320/>480
BUD			
DPI	180-360/180-540	>360-720/>540-1,080	>720/>1,080
Nebules	500/UK	1,000/UK	2,000/UK
CIC HFA MDI	80-160/160-320	>160-320/>320-640	>320/>640
FLU			
HFA MDI	160/320	320/320-640	≥640/>640
FFDPI		UK/100	UK/200
FP			
HFA MDI	88-176/88-264	176-352/264-440	>352/>440
DPIs	100-200/100-300	200-400/300-500	>400/>500
MF, DPI	110/110-220	220-440/>220-440	>440/>440

[a] Age range is 5-11 years, except for BUD Nebules, which is 2-11 years.

Abbreviations: DPI = dry powder inhaler; HFA = hydrofluoroalkane propellant; MDI = metered-dose inhaler; UK = unknown.

Source: References 2 and 11.

All MTM providers should keep in mind that treatment of other diseases may influence asthma treatment and control. In persons with asthma who continue to have poor symptom control even with optimal medication management, comorbid conditions such as gastroesophageal reflux disease, obstructive sleep apnea, allergic rhinitis, and obesity should be evaluated. For instance, adequate treatment of GERD symptoms with a proton pump inhibitor or H2-blocker may decrease nighttime reflux and associated asthma symptoms. Conversely, patients who initiate β-blocker therapy (eg, for atrial fibrillation) may experience a worsening of asthma control. Alternative medications should be considered when possible. If β-blocker therapy is necessary, cardioselective β-blockers such as metoprolol or atenolol should be used preferentially, starting with a low dose and titrating relative to patient tolerability. In pregnancy, asthma symptoms may improve, stay the same, or worsen. A patient who is well controlled on current therapy and becomes pregnant should continue therapy. Use of most asthma medications is justified in pregnancy, since maintaining oxygenation is essential to prevent preterm labor and low birth weight. When initiating inhaled corticosteroid therapy, budesonide should be considered first-line for use in pregnancy.

Recommendations for managing an acute exacerbation or asthma flare-up at home are illustrated in Figure 13-5. Strategies that are *not* effective and should be avoided when managing an exacerbation at home include drinking large volumes of liquids, breathing warm, moist air (eg, mist from a hot shower), or purchasing over-the-counter (OTC) bronchodilators such as Asthmanefrin (racepinephrine). Racepinephrine may provide transient bronchodilation, but is not a recommended treatment and should never cause a delay in seeking medical care.

Figure 13-6 is an overview of symptoms and/or criteria that must be vigilantly assessed when performing an MTM consultation for a patient with asthma. Observation of labored breathing and inability to speak a full sentence warrant immediate referral to the emergency department. Table 13-18 highlights key educational messages that should be reviewed with asthma patients.

TABLE 13-17 • Effects of Inhaled Corticosteroids

Beneficial Effects	Potential Adverse Effects
Decrease eosinophil numbers	Hoarseness, dysphonia, thrush
Decrease mast-cell numbers	Growth retardation, skeletal muscle myopathy
Decrease T-lymphocyte cytokine production	Osteoporosis, fractures and aseptic necrosis of hip
Inhibit transcription of inflammatory genes in airway epithelium	Posterior subcapsular cataract formation and glaucoma
Reduce endothelial cell leak	Adrenal axis suppression, immunosuppression
Upregulate β_2-receptor production	Impaired wound healing, easy bruising, skin striae
Reduce airway epithelial subbasement membrane thickening	Hyperglycemia/hypokalemia, hypertension
	Psychiatric disturbances

Source: References 1 and 11.

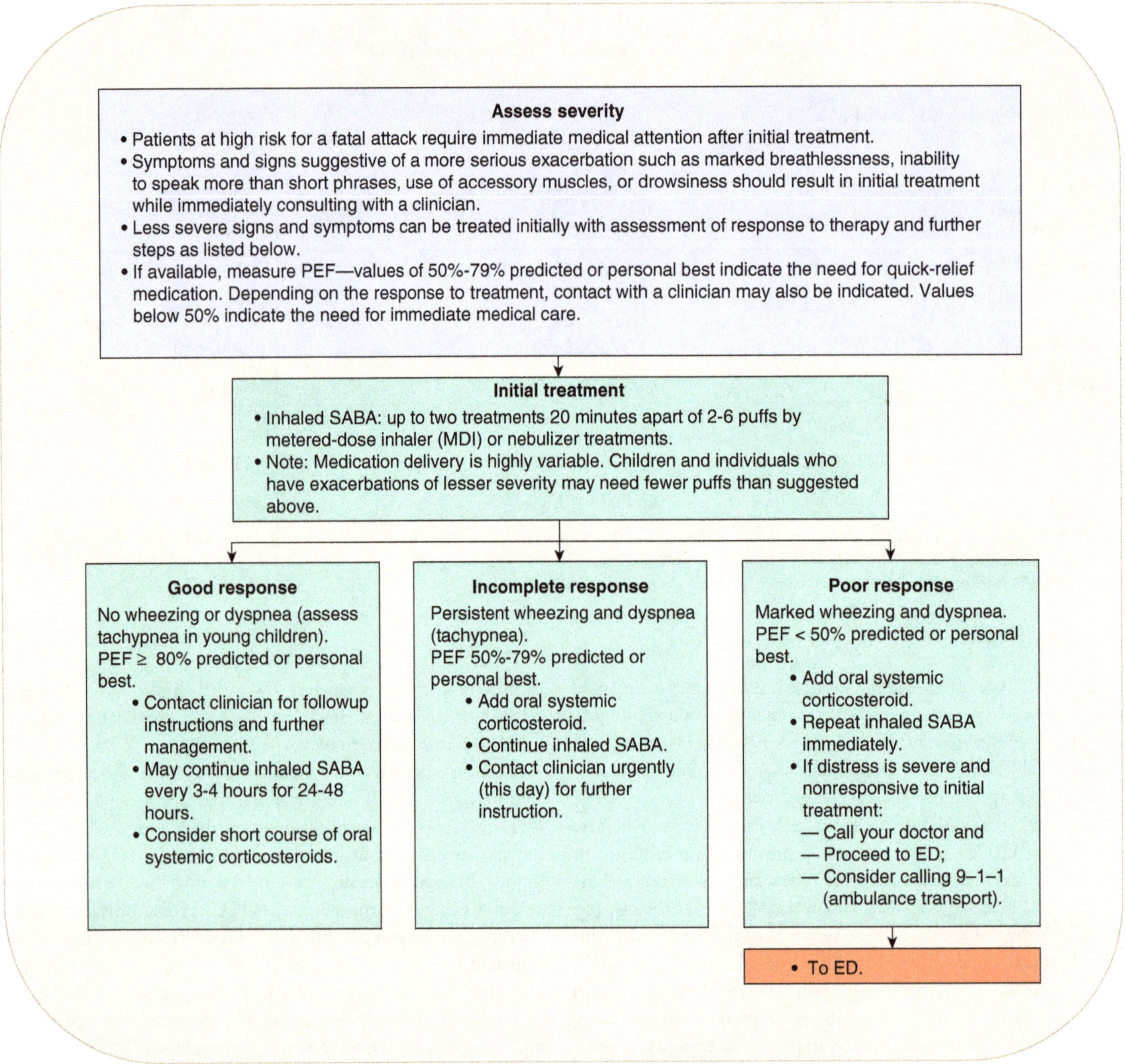

FIGURE 13-5 Self-management of worsening asthma in adults and adolescents with a written asthma action plan.

Abbreviations: ED = emergency department; MDI = metered-dose inhaler; PEF = peak expiratory flow; SABA = short-acting β-agonist [quick-relief inhaler].

Source: Reproduced with permission from Global Initiative for Asthma. Global strategy for asthma management and prevention, 2015. Available from www.ginasthma.org. See also Reference 2, this chapter.

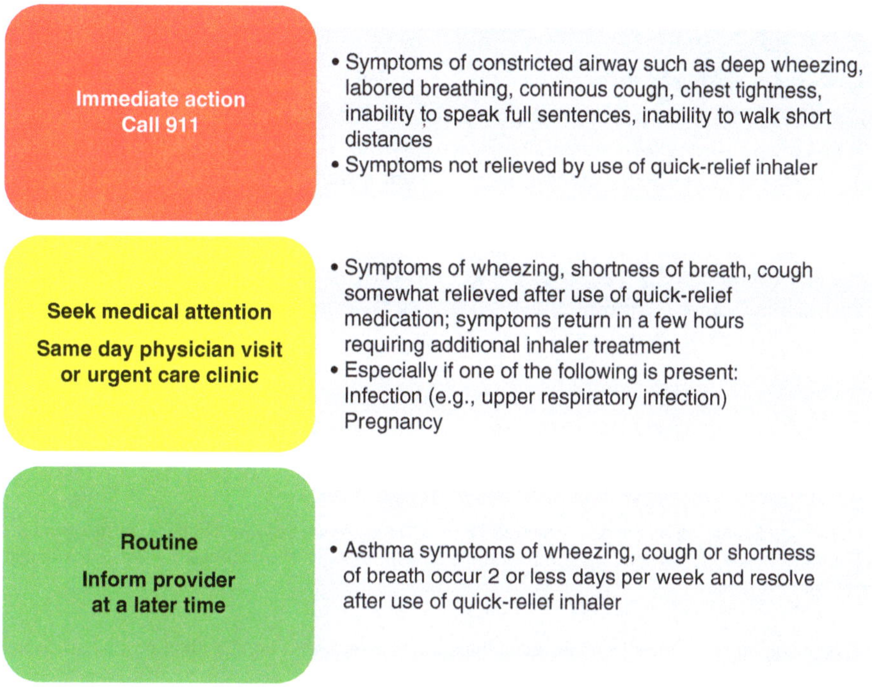

FIGURE 13-6 Referral for management of asthma.
Source: References 1 and 2.

TABLE 13-18 • Key Educational Messages for Patients

Key Educational Messages for Patients
Basic facts about asthma
Explain the difference between asthmatic and normal airways
Describe what happens to the airways in an asthma attack
Role of medications
Educate the patient how medications work
Explain difference between a controller (maintenance) medication and a quick-relief medication
Stress importance of using a quick-relief inhaler for sudden onset of symptoms; ask patient to show you which inhaler is the quick-relief device to confirm understanding via teach-back
Skills
Ask patient to demonstrate use of inhalers and, if applicable, use with the spacer or holding chamber
Review use of the nebulizer
Assess patient's ability to recognize and monitor symptoms; review peak flow monitoring, and recognition of early signs of worsening symptoms
Discuss the goal for using medication and how to monitor for symptom control
Environmental control measures
Educate on how to identify and avoid environmental triggers such as tobacco smoke
When and how to adjust treatment
Use written action plan
Respond appropriately to changes in asthma control

CORE ELEMENT 5—DOCUMENTATION AND FOLLOW-UP

Clear and succinct documentation of MRPs and recommendations is a key component of the MTM consult. Examples of potential MRPs in patients with asthma are provided in Table 13-19. Sample communications and recommendations to providers to address medication-related issues are found in Figure 13-7. Recommendations may be communicated via fax, phone, or other means of written or secure electronic communication. Actual communications to providers should be individualized according to the type of recommendation, patient-specific characteristics, and the nature of the relationship with the provider.

Follow-up to assess asthma triggers, effects of medications since last visit, and potential adverse effects is essential in patients with asthma. The interval for follow-up will depend on a number of factors, including severity of asthma, type of intervention, and patient-specific factors such as age, comorbid conditions, and ability to return for follow-up. Depending on the control of the patient's asthma, regular follow-up contact is recommended at 1- to 6-month intervals.[1] Suggested intervals for follow-up are provided in Table 13-20.

Scenario: Patient given samples of Flovent (fluticasone propionate), but cannot afford Rx once samples are finished

MRP: Nonadherence

Assessment:

Patient with uncontrolled asthma on Flovent (fluticasone propionate) HFA 110 mcg twice daily and Foradil (formoterol fumarate) 12 µg daily. Patient reports nonadherence to Flovent therapy because cost of both inhalers simultaneously is a financial burden. Lack of symptom improvement likely secondary to nonadherence with Flovent.

Plan:

Provider: Please consider replacing current Flovent and Foradil inhaled therapies with a combination product such as <(insert formulary agent here)> to reduce out-of-pocket copay.

Follow-up MTM appointment in 2 to 4 weeks to assess need for changes to medication regimen, assess patient inhaler technique, and evaluate symptoms/signs of airway stabilization.

Scenario: Opportunity to reduce asthma symptoms by technique assessment

MRP: Ineffective medication

Assessment:

Based on pharmacy claims and/or patient report, your patient is currently receiving:

- Advair (fluticasone and salmeterol), Diskus
- ProAir (albuterol) HFA

Please note: Cough has not resolved since taking Advair for past month. Requesting early refills for ProAir HFA due to increased use. Assessed inhaler technique and patient not inhaling Diskus device properly—finds it too difficult to inhale.

Plan:

Provider: Please consider switching patient to the Advair (fluticasone and salmeterol) HFA formulation to assist with maximizing therapy, as patient is having difficulty operating Diskus device.

Follow-up MTM appointment in 1 to 2 weeks to assess inhaler technique and symptoms.

Scenario: Asthma patient with allergy-induced asthma symptoms not on antihistamine therapy

MRP: Need for additional therapy

Assessment:

Patient currently using Symbicort (budesonide and formoterol HFA) twice daily as directed and albuterol HFA approximately 1 to 2 inhalations per day. Reports daily symptoms of runny nose, itchy eyes, and occasional cough.

Plan:

Provider: Please consider initiation of second-generation antihistamine such as fexofenadine, cetirizine, or loratadine daily.

Follow-up MTM appointment in 2 to 4 weeks. Patient to keep a symptom diary including use of SABA. Pt to report SABA use and symptoms at follow up visit. If antihistamine is insufficient, would consider contacting provider for addition of an intranasal inhaled steroid for additional treatment of allergic rhinitis.

Scenario: Asthma patient ran out of refills for albuterol HFA, so decided to purchase an Asthmanefrin (racepinephrine) inhaler. Has been using twice a day with inadequate relief.

MRP: Ineffective medication

Assessment:

Asthma symptoms are uncontrolled as determined by use of Asthmanefrin (racepinephrine) inhaler for airway distress. Reviewed triggers with patient and determined change of weather (cold spell) causing current symptoms. Prior to past 2 days, patient has not needed his albuterol for past few months. Educated patient that OTC Asthmanefrin is an inappropriate therapy for asthma symptoms.

Plan:

Patient to be seen at local walk-in clinic or PCP as soon as possible or if symptoms dramatically worsen, report to ED immediately.

Patient to obtain new prescription for SABA.

Patient to take SABA as prescribed and maintain a trigger diary.

Follow-up MTM appointment in 2 weeks.

FIGURE 13-7 Sample provider communications for asthma.

TABLE 13-19 • Medication-Related Problems (MRPs) in Patients with Asthma

Category of MRP	Example of a Medication-Related Problem
Nonadherence	Suboptimal control of asthma symptoms due to nonadherence with lifestyle modifications (eg, smoking cessation) Suboptimal control of asthma due to patient missing doses of asthma medication Patient not taking asthma medication due to cost
Unnecessary medication	Duplicate therapy (eg, two ICS therapies)
Need for additional medication	Active asthma symptoms for >2 days/week or sleep interruption due to asthma symptoms Patient with history of well-controlled asthma symptoms in past year, but recently started using SABA >2 days/week for symptoms (not related to preventing EIB) New onset of and/or comorbid condition that is not well controlled, resulting in worsening asthma symptoms (eg, allergic rhinitis, GERD) Patient experiencing active respiratory infection
Ineffective medication	Adequate trial of new asthma medication without significant clinical response Incorrect inhaler technique
Dosage too low	Asthma symptoms uncontrolled, risk for hospitalization, inability to perform daily activities without discomfort or fear of not catching breath
Dosage too high	Patient taking high or maximum doses of ICS for >3 months consecutively without trial of stepdown Overuse of β-agonist causing hypokalemia, hyperglycemia, tachycardia, or tremors
Adverse drug event	Dysphonia/thrush from inhaled steroid

Abbreviations: EIB = exercise-induced bronchospasm; GERD = gastroesophageal reflux disease; ICS = inhaled corticosteroid; SABA = short-acting β-agonist.

TABLE 13-20 • Suggested Intervals for Follow-up and Monitoring in Patients with Asthma

Have patient bring in all medications and peak flow meter (if using one)
Review
Patient self-assessment of asthma symptoms and trigger diary
Inhaler and/or spacer or valved holding chamber technique
Peak flow meter technique and results
Asthma action plan; update if appropriate
Need for vaccinations
Hospitalizations or emergency room visits
Airway response[1,2]
2-4 weeks after initiating or making changes in therapy.
Every 2-6 weeks while gaining control.
Every 1-6 months to monitor control.
Every 3 months if step-down in therapy is anticipated.
On determining whether asthma symptoms are stable, including use of quick-relief inhaler for ≤2 days per week, patients should be monitored every 3-6 months.
Patients with ≥2 hospitalizations within the past 12 months, comorbid conditions, history of poor control, nonadherence, or symptoms of adverse drug effects should be followed more frequently.
Toxicity[1,2]
Monitor for adverse drug effects 2-4 weeks after starting a new agent to assess tolerance
Once airway symptoms are stable, monitor every 1-6 months to assess need for step-down therapy
Serum potassium and blood glucose should be monitored at least yearly and monitored closely during flare-ups that require hospitalization

Source: References 1, 2, and 5.

REFERENCES

1. NHLBI. *NHLBI Guidelines for the Diagnosis and Treatment of Asthma*. Available at http://www.nhlbi.nih.gov/guidelines/asthma/. Accessed May 6, 2017.
2. Global Initiative for Asthma (GINA). *Global Strategy for Asthma Management and Prevention*. Updated 2017. Available at http://www.ginasthma.org/. Accessed May 6, 2017.
3. Sorkness CA, Blake, Kathryn V. Asthma. In: DiPiro JT, Talbert RL, Yee GC, Matzke GR, Wells BG, Posey LM, eds. *Pharmacotherapy: A Pathophysiologic Approach*. 10th ed. New York, NY: McGraw-Hill; 2017, Chapter 26. Available at http://accesspharmacy.mhmedical.com/content.aspx?bookid=1861&sectionid=146058008 Accessed May 6, 2017.
4. Gelfand EW. Pediatric asthma: A different disease. *Proc Am Thorac Soc*. 2009; 6:278-282.
5. Regional Asthma Management and Prevention. *Asthma Actions Plans*. Available at http://www.rampasthma.org/info-resources/asthma-action-plans. Accessed May 6, 2017.
6. HHS. *Vaccines*. US Department of Health and Human Services Center for Disease Control and Prevention. Available at https://www.cdc.gov/vaccines/ed/patient-ed.html. Accessed May 6, 2017.
7. CMS. *Medicare Part D Medication Therapy Management Program Standardized Format*. Available at https://www.cms.gov/Medicare/Prescription-Drug-Coverage/PrescriptionDrugCovContra/Downloads/MTM-Program-Standardized-Format-English-and-Spanish-Instructions-Samples-v032712.pdf. Accessed May 6, 2017.
8. Barnes PJ. Pulmonary pharmacology. Methylxanthines. In: Brunton LL, Chabner BA, Knollmann BC, eds. *Goodman & Gilman's The Pharmacological Basis of Therapeutics*, 12th ed. New York, NY: McGraw-Hill; 2011, Chapter 36. Available at http://www.accesspharmacy.com/content.aspx?aID=16671685. Accessed May 6, 2017.
9. Natural Medicines [database online]. Somerville, MA: Therapeutic Research Center; 2017. Available at https://naturalmedicines.therapeuticresearch.com/. Access May 6, 2017.
10. *Herbal Medications Cost Estimated*. Available from Drugstore.com. Accessed on May 6, 2017.
11. Raissy HH, Kelly HW, Harkins M, et al. Inhaled corticosteroids in lung diseases. *Am J Respir Crit Care Med*. 2013;187(8):798-803.

Review Questions

1. Assessment and monitoring of asthma are linked to which of the following?
   a. Severity, control, and responsiveness to treatment
   b. Severity, control, and responsiveness to triggers
   c. Severity, control, and responsiveness to inhaler technique
   d. Severity and control

   Please use the following case to answer the next three questions.

   A 45-year-old female requests a refill of her albuterol inhaler. Her last refill was 2 weeks ago, and you ask her why she is getting it refilled so soon. She replies that she is having some discomfort in her chest, so she is using the inhaler a few times every day to prevent an asthma attack. In addition, she reports that she has awakened from coughing every night this week. She does not use a peak flow meter and reports that her last asthma attack was "years ago." She does not take a controller medication.

2. Which of the following best classifies the severity of her asthma?
   a. Mild intermittent
   b. Mild persistent
   c. Severe persistent
   d. Nocturnal symptoms

3. Which of the following is the most important goal in managing her asthma?
   a. Initiation of a peak flow meter
   b. Completion of the Asthma Control Test and ATAQ
   c. Prevention of thrush by using proper inhaler technique
   d. Lessening of symptoms—few daytime symptoms and no nighttime awakenings

4. On the basis of the case described above, which of the following best summarizes actions to document on the medication action plan for that patient?
   a. Maintain symptom diary; document use of albuterol.
   b. Document the use of albuterol and the start date of controller therapy.
   c. Maintain symptom diary and document use of albuterol and instructions for when to go to the emergency department.
   d. Document the use of albuterol, the start date of controller therapy, and instructions for when to go to the emergency department.

5. Using living room language, which of the following best describes an asthma action plan?
   a. A written plan that helps a person recognize asthma symptoms and how to take care of them.
   b. A written prescription for oral corticosteroids to take for emergency purposes.
   c. A tool to document peak flow meter results.
   d. A tool to document the number of albuterol inhalations used.

6. A patient comes to clinic complaining of shortness of breath and inability to complete normal activities due to difficulty breathing for the last 3 days. He is unable to speak a full sentence and wheezes audibly. He currently uses budesonide/formoterol inhaler one inhalation in the morning, and albuterol inhaler two to four puffs as needed (at least 3 times daily for the past few days). He is worried because the elevator in his building is broken and he lives on the fourth floor. Which of the following is the best recommendation to address his current asthma symptoms?
   a. See a physician within the next week.
   b. Go to the emergency room or seek urgent care today.
   c. Repeat spirometric testing.
   d. Stay with a friend who lives on the first floor.

   Please use the following case to answer the next two questions.

   A 68-year-old asthmatic female reports episodes of shortness of breath when spending time outside. This has occurred a few times over the past 2 weeks. She describes her symptoms as a "tickle and itching in the back of my throat that makes me cough at times." She has history of seasonal allergies. Current medications include albuterol inhaler as needed and trospium 60 mg in the morning.

7. Which of the following best describes her medication-related problem?
   a. Nonadherence
   b. Unnecessary medication
   c. Need for additional medication
   d. Dose too low

8. Which of the following is the most appropriate recommendation to send to this patient's physician?
   a. Recommend scheduled use of albuterol two puffs before going outdoors.
   b. Recommend diphenhydramine at bedtime.
   c. Consider addition of an oral steroid.
   d. Consider addition of an intranasal steroid.

9. The patient has a history of asthma, environmental allergies, and hypertension. His asthma symptoms have been controlled for 2 months on a regimen of fluticasone/salmeterol inhaler twice daily, montelukast daily, and albuterol inhaler as needed. He started lisinopril for hypertension about one month ago. His chief complaint is a "dry annoying cough" that occurs intermittently throughout the day for the last few weeks. He thinks that he needs to adjust his asthma medications. Which of the following is the most appropriate recommendation to make to his provider?
   a. Step up dose of fluticasone/salmeterol.
   b. Discontinue lisinopril for a few days to see if cough resolves.
   c. Discontinue albuterol and start levalbuterol.
   d. Step up allergy prevention by adding cetirizine 5 mg one tablet daily.

10. The patient has been using high-dose fluticasone/salmeterol inhaler twice daily for the past 6 months to control asthma symptoms. She also uses albuterol inhaler as needed (less than once per week) and fexofenadine daily when her allergies bother her. She started the high-dose fluticasone/salmeterol inhaler when she suffered an upper-respiratory infection that required two courses of antibiotics and a methylprednisolone dose pack. She has not seen her physician since she recovered from the infection. She is picking up the last refill of fluticasone/salmeterol today. Which of the following is the most appropriate education to provide to the patient at this time?
    a. Remember to rinse your mouth after inhaling fluticasone/salmeterol to prevent thrush.
    b. Your voice may have changed secondary to using a high dose of an inhaled steroid.
    c. Consider discussing a step down in the dose of fluticasone/salmeterol with your physician.
    d. Go to the urgent-care clinic today if you cannot see your physician.

ANSWERS

1. a	2. c	3. d
4. c	5. a	6. b
7. c	8. d	9. b
10. c		

14

Atrial Fibrillation MTM Data Set

Katherine Vogel Anderson, PharmD, BCACP, and Sarah E. Honaker, PharmD

KEY POINTS

- Atrial fibrillation (AF) is a common supraventricular tachycardia.
- The management of AF centers on rate and/or rhythm control and prevention of stroke.
- Risk of thromboembolic stroke must be assessed in every patient with AF so that appropriate preventive measures can be implemented. Medication therapy management (MTM) providers should be familiar with risk assessment tools and strategies for stroke prevention.
- Medications used for stroke prevention, rate control, and rhythm control in AF have many important drug interactions (eg, warfarin, amiodarone). MTM providers should be vigilant for drug interactions in patients with AF and, when possible, recommend alternative therapies for other disorders that minimize the risk of significant interactions.

INTRODUCTION TO ATRIAL FIBRILLATION

Atrial fibrillation (AF) is the most common supraventricular tachycardia seen in clinical practice.[1] It is estimated that 6 million Americans were diagnosed with AF in 2010; this number is projected to double by the year 2030.[2] Atrial flutter is less common than AF, yet the management is essentially the same. In general, the management of AF centers on rate and/or rhythm control and prevention of stroke. Table 14-1 lists risk factors for developing AF.

AF Definitions

- *AF*—irregularly, irregular heart rate, which may present as tachycardia (atrial rate of 400 to 600 beats per minute [bpm]; ventricular rate of 120 to 180 bpm); characterized by disorganized atrial activation
- *Acute AF*—onset of AF within the last 48 hours
- *Nonvalvular AF*—AF in the absence of rheumatic mitral stenosis, a mechanical or bioprosthetic heart valve, or mitral valve repair
- *Paroxysmal AF*—AF that terminates spontaneously within 7 days
- *Permanent AF*—AF that does not terminate, despite therapy with drugs or electrical cardioversion
- *Persistent AF*—AF that lasts longer than 7 days and does not terminate spontaneously
- *Postoperative AF*—AF that occurs 3 to 5 days after surgery; usually self-terminating
- *Recurrent AF*—two or more AF episodes

> The management of AF is the same, irrespective of the type of AF - except for postoperative AF, which typically is treated for only one month.

Complications of AF

Data suggest that Medicare patients with AF are more likely to be hospitalized than are their age- and sex-matched counterparts who do not have AF.[1,3] However, perhaps the most important complication of AF is stroke.[3] The use of anticoagulant therapy has decreased ischemic stroke significantly since the mid-1990s, but the

TABLE 14-1 • Risk Factors for AF

Standard risk factors	Family history	Genetics
Increasing age Hypertension Diabetes Myocardial infarction Valvular heart disease Heart failure Obesity Obstructive sleep apnea Cardiothoracic surgery Smoking Exercise Alcohol Hyperthyroidism European ancestry	Early-onset familial lone AF Having one parent with AF A first-degree relative with AF at age <65 years **ECG/echocardiographic** Left ventricular hypertrophy Left atrial enlargement Increased left ventricular wall thickness Decreased left ventricular fractional shortening	Mutations in genes coding for sodium and potassium channels, gap junction protein Single-nucleotide polymorphism (SNP) in chromosomes 4q25, 16q22, 1q21 **Biomarkers** Increased C-reactive protein (CRP) Increased B-type natriuretic peptide (BNP)

Source: References 1 and 3.

rate of hemorrhagic stroke has remained fairly steady.[1] The complications of stroke are listed in Table 14-2. AF and chronic heart failure (CHF) share many of the same risk factors. For example, 40% of patients with AF will develop CHF, and 40% of patients with CHF will develop AF, substantiating the common phrase "AF begets CHF and CHF begets AF."[4]

Therapeutic Goals for AF

It is important to determine whether the patient with AF requires rate or rhythm control. Generally speaking, patients with mild AF symptoms (or, no symptoms at all) should receive rate control with a β-blocker or nondihydropyridine calcium channel blocker. Guidelines for the management of AF recommend a resting heart rate of <80 bpm.[3] Patients with AF who have symptoms despite rate control, are hemodynamically unstable, or who have CHF should receive rhythm control with a Class Ic or Class III antiarrhythmic.[3] Prevention of strokes is an important therapeutic goal for AF. As such, stroke prophylaxis must be considered for all patients with AF.[3] Finally, it should be noted that the newer oral anticoagulant drugs (apixaban, dabigatran, edoxaban, and rivaroxaban) should not be used for stroke prevention in patients with valvular AF.[3] Patients with valvular AF are at a higher risk of stroke; to date, the evidence suggests that anticoagulation with warfarin is the best option for patients with valvular AF.[3]

TABLE 14-2 • Complications of AF versus Stroke Complications

AF Complications	Stroke Complications
Cardioembolic stroke (see next column) CHF Rapid ventricular response → can induce CHF, or cause cardiomyopathy	Hemiparesis Inability to walk without assistance Cognitive deficit Depression Aphasia Dependence on others for activities of daily living Death

Abbreviations: AF = atrial fibrillation; CHF = congestive heart failure.

Source: References 5 and 6.

Therapeutic Failures

Patients who continue to have symptoms of AF despite adequate rate control may be considered for rhythm control. This may be accomplished with antiarrhythmic drugs or electrical cardioversion.[1,3] Embolic stroke, as a result of inadequate anticoagulation therapy, would be considered a treatment failure, as would a life-threatening bleed that results from excessive anticoagulation. Patients who have an uncontrolled heart rate with hypotension are particularly complicated since treatment options are limited.

CORE ELEMENT 1—COMPREHENSIVE MEDICATION REVIEW FOR PATIENTS WITH AF

Following is a list of suggested questions to use when conducting a medication therapy review in a patient with AF (Table 14-3). The number and types of questions will depend on several factors, including the amount of time for the interview, number of concurrent medication-related problems (MRPs), urgency of MRPs, and the reliability of the patient in providing accurate information, among others. In time-limited interactions or in complex cases with multiple medical issues, the MTM provider may choose to target questions that help to identify or rule out issues of an urgent nature (see questions to ask for prevention/assessment of medical emergencies). MTM providers should remember to use living room language during the interview (Figure 14-1), and to be prepared for questions that patients may ask regarding AF (Table 14-4).

CORE ELEMENT 2—PERSONAL MEDICATION LIST[7]

Figure 14-2 presents a sample personal medication list (PML) for a patient with AF. Additional medications for other disease states should be added and listed separately. MTM providers should remember to use plain language when creating the PML.

CORE ELEMENT 3—MEDICATION ACTION PLAN[7]

Figure 14-3 provides a sample medication action plan (MAP) for a patient with AF. These examples are representative only of action steps for a patient with AF. MAPs for other disease states or other MRPs should be added and listed separately. In general, only a few of the most important action steps should be listed, so as not to overwhelm the patient. Other areas for patient self-management

TABLE 14-3 • Questions to Ask When Conducting a Comprehensive Medication Review in a Patient with AF

Suggested Questions for the Patient with Atrial Fibrillation
How long have you had atrial fibrillation? When were you diagnosed?
Who else in your family has atrial fibrillation?
What do you know about the health risks associated with atrial fibrillation?
Have you ever experienced the following signs/symptoms of atrial fibrillation:
Heart palpitations (feeling your heart beat hard and fast)
Shortness of breath
Dizziness or lightheadedness
Chest pain or pressure
Fatigue (feeling tired)
Weakness, inability to perform exercises?
What medications do you take for your atrial fibrillation? How do you take them?
Has your physician placed you on an anticoagulant (blood thinner) after diagnosing you with atrial fibrillation?
If yes, what is the dose/schedule of your anticoagulant?
How often and for what reasons do you miss a dose of your anticoagulant?
Have you experienced any abnormal bleeding or bruising which may be associated with your anticoagulant?
As foods containing vitamin K may interact with your anticoagulant, what does your diet typically consist of?
How often do you miss a dose of your atrial fibrillation medication?
What other medications have you taken in the past for your atrial fibrillation?
Have you ever stopped taking any of your prescribed atrial fibrillation medications without telling your physician? If so, why?
What over-the-counter (OTC) medications or herbals do you use for your atrial fibrillation?
What has your physician discussed with you regarding OTC medications that you should avoid because they can worsen your atrial fibrillation and/or risk of stroke?
Questions to Ask for Prevention/Assessment of Medical Emergencies
Crisis planning: What are the warning signs of a heart attack and stroke, and what is your action plan?
Have you fallen, felt dizzy, or had blurred vision or racing heart when performing activities or at rest?
Have you ever been hospitalized for your atrial fibrillation?
(If on anticoagulant) Have you experienced dark or red urine, black or red stool, coughing or vomiting blood or coffee ground-like material? These are all signs of internal bleeding and should be reported immediately if experienced.

can be addressed at later visits. MTM providers should remember to use plain language when creating the MAP.

CORE ELEMENT 4—INTERVENTION AND/OR REFERRAL

Interventions for AF management include lifestyle modifications and drug therapy. Medications should be selected on the basis of evidence and patient characteristics, such as renal function, other comorbidities (eg, diabetes, cardiovascular disease), bleeding risk, and cost. Table 14-5 summarizes lifestyle modifications that may help reduce the risk of stroke in AF. Table 14-6 provides an overview of drug categories for management of AF. A treatment algorithm for AF is presented in Figure 14-4, and Tables 14-7 and 14-8 include treatment recommendations for managing rate and rhythm.

Figure 14-5 outlines the selection of therapy for prevention of thromboembolism. When assessing thromboembolic risk, it is prudent to calculate a patient's CHA_2DS_2-VASc score, where points are assigned as follows:[3]

- C = chronic heart failure, 1 point
- H = hypertension, 1 point
- A_2 = age ≥75 years, 2 points
- D = diabetes, 1 point
- S_2= stroke, transient ischemic attack, thromboembolism, 2 points
- V = vascular disease (myocardial infarction, peripheral arterial disease, aortic plaque), 1 point
- Sc= sex category (eg, female sex), 1 point

Patients with a CHA_2DS_2-VASc equal to 0 are considered low-risk and do not require anticoagulation therapy. Patients with a CHA_2DS_2-VASc equal to 1 may receive treatment with aspirin (325 mg) or anticoagulation therapy, or no therapy at all. A CHA_2DS_2-VASc score of ≥2 indicates the need for anticoagulation therapy with warfarin or a direct oral anticoagulant.[3]

Table 14-9 reviews nonpharmacologic therapies for AF, while Table 14-10 provides information about herbal supplements that might be useful. Figure 14-6 highlights situations where emergency referral for evaluation of stroke may be needed.

CORE ELEMENT 5—DOCUMENTATION AND FOLLOW-UP

Clear and succinct documentation of medication-related problems and recommendations is a key component of the MTM consult. Examples of potential MRPs in patients with AF are provided

Ablation—a technique using a catheter to burn away and block the source of rhythm abnormality in patients with atrial fibrillation or flutter.

Acute coronary syndrome—term used to cover any symptoms caused by decreased blood flow to the heart, such as a heart attack or chest pain.

Adverse event—something bad that happens, bad reaction, unexplained or unwanted effects.

Angina—chest pain or discomfort caused by decreased blood flow through the heart, which could be a sign of heart attack.

Angioedema—a rare side effect of angiotensin-converting enzyme (ACE) inhibitors and some antiarrhythmics; a medical emergency involving rapid swelling of the lips, tongue, and throat that may affect breathing.

Antiarrhythmic—a medication used to control the beating of the heart in patients with an abnormal heartbeat such as atrial fibrillation.

Anticoagulant—a medication used to prevent blood clots from forming in the body as a result of atrial fibrillation; blood clots may lead to stroke.

Antithrombotic—see *Anticoagulant.*

Arrhythmia—irregular heartbeat, skipped heartbeat, heart problem; an example is atrial fibrillation.

Arteries—blood vessels that carry blood away from the heart.

Atrial fibrillation (A fib)—an irregular and often rapid heart rate that commonly causes poor blood flow to the body.

Atrial flutter—an abnormal heart rhythm similar to atrial fibrillation with similar complications.

Atrium—the top chamber on each side of the heart, where heart rhythm originates and where abnormalities develop in atrial fibrillation.

β-blocker—a medicine used to help lower blood pressure and control how rapidly the heart beats; works by decreasing the body's reaction to stress.

BMI—body mass index; a measure of weight in relation to height that assigns people to a weight class of underweight, normal weight, overweight, or obese on the basis of their amount of excess weight.

Bradycardia—low pace for the heart to beat, <60 times in a minute.

Calcium channel blocker—a medicine used in atrial fibrillation to control heart rate.

Cardiac—related to the heart.

Cardiologist—physician specialized in treating heart disease and disorders.

Cardioversion—restoring a patient experiencing atrial fibrillation to a normal heart rhythm using either surgery or medication.

Chronic—constant, never-ending, not going away.

Diastolic—the bottom blood pressure number, smaller number; the pressure in the arteries when the heart relaxes.

Diuretic—water pill.

Edema—swelling because of the buildup of excessive fluid.

ECG—a test that looks for any damage to or problems with your heart.

Electrolytes—a type of necessary salt found in blood, such as salt, potassium, and calcium.

Elevate—raise, make higher.

Embolus—a mass, such as an air bubble, detached blood clot, or other material, that travels in the bloodstream and lodges in a blood vessel, blocking the flow of blood through that vessel.

Gingival hyperplasia—excessive growth of gum tissue in your mouth, which could be caused by calcium channel blockers.

Heart failure—a condition in which the heart can no longer pump enough blood to meet the needs of your body; can often develop as a result of high blood pressure and atrial fibrillation.

Heart rate—how many times your heart beats each minute.

Hematocrit—a blood test looking at the amount of red blood cells you have, a very low amount could be a sign of anemia.

Hemorrhage—bleed.

Hemorrhagic stroke—a stroke due to decreased blood flow to brain tissue caused by bleeding from an artery.

Hyperkalemia—high potassium; very high potassium is a medical emergency and could cause a deadly change in the way your heart beats.

Hypertension—high blood pressure that increases the chance of heart attack, stroke, and kidney disease.

Hypotension—low blood pressure.

Ischemia—insufficient blood supply and oxygen to an organ or tissue due to blockage of an artery.

Ischemic stroke—a stroke due to decreased blood flow to brain tissue caused by blockage of an artery.

Left ventricular hypertrophy—when the left side of the heart becomes large, which may change the way the heart beats and could lead to heart failure.

Lifestyle changes—your physician may have recommended changes in lifestyle to help control blood pressure and heart problems, which for some patients include reaching a goal weight, decreasing the amount of alcohol you consume, exercising, or quitting smoking.

Low-sodium diet—a diet with <2 g (2000 mg) of salt each day, which may lower blood pressure and may be beneficial to people with heart problems or kidney disease.

Myocardial Infarction—heart attack, damage to the heart.

Obese—having a body mass index (BMI) of >30, which increases your risk of having high blood pressure, diabetes, and cardiovascular disease.

Oral contraceptives—birth control medicine, may be a cause of high blood pressure and increase risk of stroke and heart attack.

Orthostatic hypotension—dizziness or lightheadedness on standing because of low blood pressure.

Overweight—having a body mass index (BMI) of >25, which increases your risk of having high blood pressure, diabetes, and heart disease.

Peripheral edema—swelling, usually of the legs, that may be a side effect of calcium channel blockers.

Serum potassium—a test to check the amount of potassium in your blood (see *Hyperkalemia*).

Smoking cessation—quitting smoking, which can lower your chance of heart disease.

Sodium—salt, which can increase blood pressure if consumed.

Stroke—a condition caused by bleeding or lack of blood in the brain, which may cause a loss of speech, memory, or other abilities.

Systolic—the top blood pressure number, the larger number; the pressure in the arteries when the heart contracts.

Tachycardia—a rapid heart beat, >100 times in a minute.

Thromboembolism—formation in a blood vessel of a clot (thrombus) that breaks loose and is carried by the bloodstream to plug another vessel.

Unstable angina—pain or a feeling of pressure on the chest, which is a medical emergency and may lead to a heart attack.

Veins—blood vessels that carry blood toward the heart.

FIGURE 14-1 Living room language for AF patients.

TABLE 14-4 • Questions to Anticipate from Patients Regarding Atrial Fibrillation

What is atrial fibrillation? Atrial fibrillation is an irregular and often rapid heart rate that commonly causes poor blood flow to the body. This rapid heart rate is due to dysfunction of the upper chambers of the heart (atria) causing abnormal signals and beating of the heart. The heart rate in atrial fibrillation may range from 100 to 175 bpm. The normal range for a heart rate is 60 to 100 bpm. **What causes atrial fibrillation?** Atrial fibrillation is usually caused by long-term damage and changes to the heart's structure. Health conditions that may contribute to the development of atrial fibrillation include high blood pressure, heart attacks, previous heart surgery, congenital heart defects, viral infections, overactive thyroid gland, sick sinus syndrome, abnormal heart valves, emphysema and other lung diseases, stress due to pneumonia, surgery or other illnesses, and sleep apnea. Exposure to stimulants, such as medications, caffeine or tobacco, or to alcohol may also contribute to developing atrial fibrillation. **What health problems are associated with atrial fibrillation?** Because of the abnormal rhythm created by atrial fibrillation, blood has a chance to sit and pool within the upper chambers (atria) and form clots. These clots may break away from the heart and block off blood flow to the brain, causing a stroke. Atrial fibrillation may also lead to heart failure if left uncontrolled, as the increased work load on the heart weakens the heart's ability to pump blood effectively. **Why are atrial fibrillation medications so important?** Medications that you may be taking for atrial fibrillation control heart rate and/or rhythm to return the heart to a normal state of function. You may also need a blood-thinning agent to reduce the risk of a stroke due to atrial fibrillation.
Can I just stop my medications if I feel okay? Some medications may relieve your symptoms of atrial fibrillation and make you feel better. It is important to continue taking these medications to consistently keep your heart rate under control and prevent possible complications associated with atrial fibrillation. Medications used to reduce risk of stroke (blood-thinning agents) will not cause any noticeable difference in how you feel, but are very important to take as directed to achieve the greatest benefit. **When should I call my physician?** Contact your physician if you experience new symptoms while performing normal activities. If you experience signs or symptoms of atrial fibrillation, call your physician or seek immediate medical attention elsewhere. If you allow your atrial fibrillation to go untreated, your risk of having a stroke is greatly increased. **What should I do if I have a problem with my medications?** Never stop taking your atrial fibrillation medications without first talking to your physician. Speak with your physician and/or pharmacist to let them know about any problems or side effects that you are having, and together you can make sure your medications are the right ones for you.

PERSONAL MEDICATION LIST FOR *(Insert patient's name, DOB: mm/dd/yyyy)*	
Medication: Eliquis (apixaban) 5 mg	
How I use it: One tablet (5 mg) every morning and every evening	
Why I use it: To prevent stroke (blood thinner)	**Prescriber:** Jones
Date I started using it: 10/27/2016	**Date I stopped using it:** (*Leave blank for patient's notes*)
Why I stopped using it: (*Leave blank for patient's notes*)	
Medication: Cardizem CD (diltiazem) 120 mg	
How I use it: One capsule (120 mg) every morning	
Why I use it: Heart rate	**Prescriber:** Jones
Date I started using it: 10/27/2016	**Date I stopped using it:** (*Leave blank for patient's notes*)
Why I stopped using it: (*Leave blank for patient's notes*)	

FIGURE 14-2 Sample personal medication list of atrial fibrillation medications.

<table>
<tr><td colspan="2" align="right">DATE PREPARED: (Insert date)</td></tr>
<tr><td colspan="2">What we talked about:
Importance of taking blood thinner (warfarin) to reduce my risk of stroke caused by my irregular heart beat (atrial fibrillation)</td></tr>
<tr><td>What I need to do:
Take my warfarin therapy every day as directed.
Keep my scheduled appointments to check my blood.
Report any unusual bruising or bleeding to my provider.
Ask my physician or pharmacist which medications or herbal supplements I should avoid, as they may cause your blood thinner to be more or less effective.</td><td>What I did and when I did it: (Leave blank for patient's notes)</td></tr>
<tr><td colspan="2">What we talked about:
You reported having a history of atrial fibrillation, which can increase your risk for having a stroke. It is important to speak with your physician about your stroke risk and prevention options.</td></tr>
<tr><td>What I need to do:
1. Ask my healthcare provider about my risk of stroke and if I should be taking medication to prevent it.
2. Learn to identify signs and symptoms of stroke, as well as inform my friends and family of what to watch for.
3. Seek medical attention if I experience any of the following signs and symptoms:
Paralysis and/or numbness of face, arm, or leg on one side of body
Trouble walking
Dizziness
Severe, sudden headache
Trouble speaking, slurring words
Vision problems, blackened vision, seeing double</td><td>What I did and when I did it: (Leave blank for patient's notes)</td></tr>
</table>

FIGURE 14-3 Sample medication action plan for a patient with AF.

TABLE 14-5 • Lifestyle Modifications for Prevention of Stroke in Patients with AF

Modification	Recommendation
Cigarette smoking	Cigarette smoking *and* exposure to secondhand smoke can increase stroke risk. Patients should be encouraged to quit smoking through use of counseling, nicotine replacement products, or prescription medications.
Nutrition	Consume a diet rich in fruits, vegetables, and low-fat dairy products with a reduction in dietary cholesterol, saturated fat, and total fat content. Dietary sodium should be reduced to ≤100 mmol per day (2.4 g sodium). Ideally, patients should consume <1.5 g of salt per day. Routine supplementation with vitamins is not recommended.
Increase physical activity	Engage in regular aerobic physical activity (brisk walking) at least 30 minutes per day most days of the week. If there is disability present secondary to stroke, then supervised physical therapy or cardiac rehabilitation is recommended.
Decrease alcohol consumption	Heavy drinking/alcoholism increases stroke risk. Limiting alcohol as follows is reasonable: men—≤2 drinks/day; women and lighter persons—≤1 drink/day. Of note, 1 drink equals 12 oz beer, 5 oz wine, or 1.5 oz of 80-proof whiskey.

Source: Reference 8.

TABLE 14-6 • Medications for Management of AF

Medication Class Drug Examples	Common/Serious Side Effects[a]	Blackbox Warnings/Contraindications	Pregnancy Category[b]
Class IA antiarrhythmics Disopyramide Procainamide Quinidine	Constipation, diarrhea, headache, nausea, rash, vomiting, xerostomia, muscle weakness, blurred vision, delay when starting to pass urine, urinary retention, generalized aches and pains, congestive heart failure, heart block, hypotension, prolonged QT interval, torsade de pointes, hypoglycemia, agranulocytosis, thrombocytopenia, hepatotoxicity, hypotension, ventricular arrhythmia, anemia, systemic lupus erythematosus, angioedema	Disopyramide QT prolongation Cardiac arrhythmias Myocardial infarction Torsade des pointes Atrioventricular (AV) block Cardiogenic shock Procainamide Cardiac arrhythmias Bone marrow suppression Systemic lupus erythematosus AV block Ester local anesthetic hypersensitivity QT prolongation Torsade des pointes Quinidine Cardiac arrhythmias AV block Bundle-branch block Myasthenia gravis Quinidine hypersensitivity	C
Class IC antiarrhythmics Flecainide Propafenone	Chest pain, palpitations, nausea, dizziness, edema, anxiety, headache, blurred vision, photopsia, dyspnea, fatigue, bundle-branch block, cardiac arrest, cardiac dysrhythmia, cardiogenic shock, abnormal electrocardiogram, heart block, heart failure, prolonged QT interval, syncope, torsade des pointes, agranulocytosis, systemic lupus erythematosus, renal failure, respiratory failure	Flecainide Chronic atrial fibrillation Cardiac arrhythmias Cardiogenic shock Propafenone Cardiac arrhythmias History of myocardial infarction (MI) Acute bronchospasm Asthma AV block Bradycardia Brugada syndrome Cardiogenic shock Electrolyte imbalance Heart failure Hypotension Sick sinus syndrome	C
β-Blockers (Class II antiarrhythmics) Metoprolol (M) Nadolol (N) Propranolol (P)	Bradyarrhythmia, heart failure, hypotension, constipation, diarrhea, nausea, dizziness, fatigue, headache, depression, dyspnea, pruritus, rash, heart block, cardiac dysrhythmia (N), anaphylaxis, seizure, bronchospasm, asthma (P), pulmonary edema, Stevens-Johnson syndrome (P)	Metoprolol Abrupt discontinuation Acute heart failure AV block β-Blocker hypersensitivity Bradycardia Cardiogenic shock Hypotension Pheochromocytoma Sick sinus syndrome	C

(Continued)

TABLE 14-6 • Medications for Management of AF (*Continued*)

Medication Class Drug Examples	Common/Serious Side Effects[a]	Blackbox Warnings/Contraindications	Pregnancy Category[b]
		Nadolol Abrupt discontinuation Asthma AV block Bradycardia Cardiogenic shock Acute heart failure Propranolol Abrupt discontinuation Asthma AV block Bradycardia Cardiogenic shock Sick sinus syndrome	
Class III antiarrhythmics Amiodarone (A) Dofetilide (DO) Dronedarone (DR) Ibutilide (I) Sotalol (S)	Abdominal pain, bradyarrhythmia, chest pain, diarrhea, dizziness, dyspnea, fatigue, headache, nausea, palpitations, vomiting, raised serum creatinine (DR), heart block, heart failure, QT prolongation, torsade de pointes, cerebrovascular accident, liver failure (A, DR), Stevens-Johnson syndrome (A), rhabdomyolysis (A), acute respiratory distress syndrome (A), pulmonary fibrosis and toxicity (A), hyperthyroidism (A), hypothyroidism (A), systemic lupus erythematosus (A)	Amiodarone Cardiac arrhythmias Hepatic disease Pneumonitis Pulmonary fibrosis Requires an experienced clinician AV block Benzyl alcohol hypersensitivity Bradycardia Cardiogenic shock Iodine hypersensitivity Sick sinus syndrome Dofetilide QT prolongation Renal failure Torsade des pointes Cardiac arrhythmias Renal disease Renal impairment Ventricular arrhythmias Ventricular tachycardia Dronedarone Heart failure Permanent atrial fibrillation AV block Bradycardia Breastfeeding Pregnancy QT prolongation Sick sinus syndrome	D (A) C (DO) X (DR) C (I) B (S)

(*Continued*)

TABLE 14-6 • Medications for Management of AF (*Continued*)

Medication Class Drug Examples	Common/Serious Side Effects[a]	Blackbox Warnings/Contraindications	Pregnancy Category[b]
		Ibutilide Cardiac arrhythmias QT prolongation Requires a specialized care setting Requires an experienced clinician Torsade des pointes Ventricular arrhythmias Ventricular tachycardia Sotalol QT prolongation Cardiac arrhythmias Requires specialized care setting Ventricular arrhythmias Asthma AV block Bradycardia Heart failure Hypokalemia Pulmonary edema Renal failure Renal impairment	
Calcium channel blockers (Class IV antiarrhythmics) Diltiazem (D) Verapamil (V)	Bradycardia, headache (D), nausea (D), constipation (V)	Acute MI AV block Cardiogenic shock Hypotension Heart failure/left ventricular systolic dysfunction Sick sinus syndrome Ventricular tachycardia Wolff-Parkinson-White syndrome	C
Cardiac glycoside Digoxin	Headache, blurred or yellow vision, rash, gynecomastia, nausea, vomiting, diarrhea, AV block, cardiac arrest, cardiac dysrhythmia, hypokalemia, hyperkalemia, thrombocytopenia, ventricular tachycardia, supraventricular tachycardia	Ventricular fibrillation	C
Antiplatelet salicylate Aspirin	Gastrointestinal ulcer, bleeding, age-related macular degeneration, tinnitus, bronchospasm, angioedema, Reye syndrome	Salicylate hypersensitivity	D

(*Continued*)

TABLE 14-6 • Medications for Management of AF (*Continued*)

Medication Class Drug Examples	Common/Serious Side Effects[a]	Blackbox Warnings/Contraindications	Pregnancy Category[b]
ADP receptor antagonist Clopidogrel	Bleeding, fixed-drug eruption, Stevens-Johnson syndrome, colitis, gastrointestinal (GI) hemorrhage, agranulocytosis, pancytopenia, thrombotic thrombocytopenic purpura, hepatitis, hepatotoxicity, liver failure, epidural hematoma, intracranial hemorrhage, intraocular hemorrhage, interstitial pneumonia, pulmonary edema, respiratory tract hemorrhage, drug withdrawal, rebound effect	Poor metabolizers Bleeding GI bleeding Intracranial bleeding	B
Vitamin K antagonist Warfarin	Alopecia, cholesterol embolus syndrome, gangrenous disorder, tissue necrosis, hemorrhage, hypersensitivity reaction, compartment syndrome, intracranial hemorrhage, intraocular hemorrhage	Bleeding Alcoholism Aneurysm Aortic dissection Dementia Eclampsia Endocarditis Epidural anesthesia GI bleeding Head trauma Hematological disease Intracranial bleeding Lumbar puncture Pericardial effusion Pericarditis Preeclampsia Pregnancy Psychosis Retinal bleeding Spinal anesthesia Stroke Surgery	X
Oral thrombin inhibitor Dabigatran	Esophagitis, gastritis, gastroesophageal reflux disease, GI hemorrhage, GI ulcer, indigestion, bleeding, MI, anaphylaxis, intracranial hemorrhage	Bleeding Mechanical heart valves	C
Oral factor Xa inhibitors Apixaban (A) Edoxaban (E) Rivaroxaban (R)	Anemia, bleeding (GI, vaginal, bruising), hypersensitivity reaction, intracranial hemorrhage, intraocular hemorrhage, epidural hematoma	Apixaban Abrupt discontinuation Bleeding Epidural anesthesia Lumbar puncture Spinal anesthesia Mechanical heart valves	B (A) C (E) C (R)

(*Continued*)

TABLE 14-6 • Medications for Management of AF (*Continued*)

Medication Class Drug Examples	Common/Serious Side Effects[a]	Blackbox Warnings/Contraindications	Pregnancy Category[b]
		Edoxaban Abrupt discontinuation Bleeding Epidural anesthesia Lumbar puncture Creatinine clearance (CrCl) > 95 mL/min or < 15 mL/min Spinal anesthesia Mechanical heart valves Rivaroxaban Bleeding Abrupt discontinuation Epidural anesthesia Spinal anesthesia Mechanical heart valves	
Low-molecular-weight heparin Dalteparin Enoxaparin Tinzaparin	Diarrhea, hematoma, nausea, anemia, bleeding, thrombocytopenia, increased liver function tests, fever, atrial fibrillation, heart failure, eczematous drug eruption, skin necrosis, hemorrhage, intracranial hemorrhage, paraplegia, pneumonia	All Epidural anesthesia Lumbar puncture Spinal anesthesia Bleeding Heparin hypersensitivity Porcine protein hypersensitivity Enoxaparin Heparin-induced thrombocytopenia Thrombocytopenia Dalteparin Thrombocytopenia Tinzaparin Benzyl alcohol hypersensitivity Renal impairment Sulfite hypersensitivity	B
Factor Xa inhibitor Fondaparinux	Injection-site reaction, rash, fever, anemia, bleeding	Epidural anesthesia Lumbar puncture Spinal anesthesia Bleeding Endocarditis Renal failure Thrombocytopenia	B

[a] This is a general list and does not include all side effects that can occur from these drugs. This list also includes a class of medications; the side effects and their degree of effect may vary from drug to drug in each drug class. Consult a drug reference source for a more inclusive list before making any recommendations. MTM providers should also consult a comprehensive drug interaction database before making pharmacotherapy recommendations.

[b] Product labeling for all prescription drugs is being updated to reflect the new FDA Pregnancy Labeling and Lactation Rule. Please check individual product labeling for the most accurate and updated pregnancy information.

Source: Reference 9.

in Table 14-11. Sample communications and recommendations to providers to address medication-related issues are found in Figure 14-7. Recommendations may be communicated via fax, phone, or other means of written or secure electronic communication. The examples below are for illustrative purposes. Actual communications to providers should be individualized according to the type of recommendation, patient-specific characteristics, and the nature of the relationship with the healthcare provider.

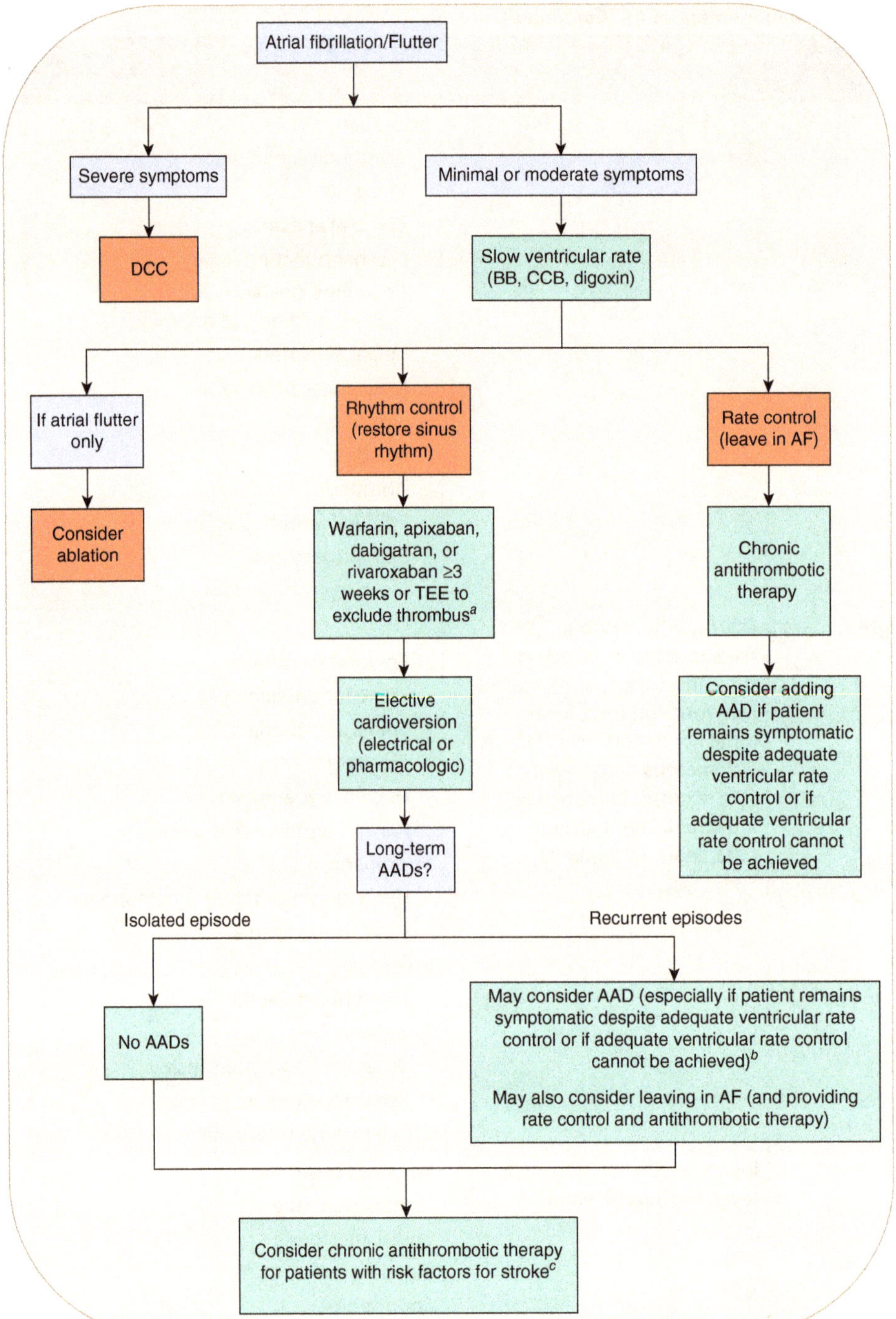

FIGURE 14-4 Algorithm for the treatment of AF and atrial flutter. [a]If AF is < 48 hours in duration, anticoagulation prior to cardioversion is unnecessary; initiate anticoagulation with unfractionated heparin, a low-molecular-weight heparin, apixaban, dabigatran, or rivaroxaban as soon as possible either before or after cardioversion for patients at high risk for stroke (this anticoagulant regimen or no antithrombotic therapy may be considered in low-risk patients). [b]Ablation may be considered for patients who fail or do not tolerate at least 1 AAD or as first-line therapy (before AAD therapy) for select patients with recurrent symptomatic paroxysmal AF. [c]Chronic antithrombotic therapy should be considered in all patients with AF and risk factors for stroke regardless of whether or not they remain in sinus rhythm.

Abbreviations: AAD = antiarrhythmic drug; AF = atrial fibrillation; BB, β-blocker; CCB = calcium channel blocker [ie, verapamil or diltiazem]; DCC = direct-current cardioversion; TEE = transesophageal echocardiogram.

Source: Reproduced, with permission, from DiPiro, JT, Talbert RL, Yee GC, Matzke GR, Wells BG, Posey LM, eds. *Pharmacotherapy: A Pathophysiologic Approach*. 10th ed. New York, NY: McGraw-Hill; 2017.

Follow-up to assess heart rate, symptoms, and other risk factors for stroke such as blood pressure, lipid panel, and blood glucose is essential in patients with AF. The interval for follow-up will depend on a number of factors, including antithrombotic regimen, severity of AF, type of intervention, and patient-specific factors such as age, comorbid conditions, and ability to return for follow-up. Suggested intervals for follow-up are provided in Table 14-12.

TABLE 14-7 • Evidence-Based Pharmacologic Treatment Recommendations for Controlling Ventricular Rate, Restoring Sinus Rhythm, and Maintaining Sinus Rhythm in Patients with Atrial Fibrillation

Treatment Recommendations	ACC/AHA/ESC Guideline Recommendation
Ventricular rate control (acute setting)	
In the absence of an accessory pathway, IV β-blockers or IV non-DHP CCBs are recommended for patients without hypotension or HF.	Class I
In the absence of an accessory pathway, IV digoxin or IV amiodarone is recommended for patients with HF.	Class I
IV amiodarone can be used to control the ventricular rate in patients who are refractory to or have contraindications to IV β-blockers, non-DHP CCBs, or digoxin.	Class IIa
IV procainamide or ibutilide is a reasonable alternative in patients with an accessory pathway when DCC is not necessary.	Class IIa
IV procainamide, ibutilide, or amiodarone may be considered for hemodynamically stable patients with an accessory pathway.	Class IIb
IV non-DHP CCBs are not recommended in patients with decompensated HF.	Class III
Ventricular rate control (chronic setting)	
Oral digoxin is effective for controlling the ventricular rate at rest in patients with HF or LV dysfunction, and in those who are sedentary.	Class I
Combination therapy with oral digoxin and either an oral β-blocker or non-DHP CCB is reasonable to control the ventricular rate both at rest and during exercise.	Class IIa
Oral amiodarone can be used when the ventricular rate cannot be adequately controlled at rest and during exercise with an oral β-blocker, non-DHP CCB, and/or digoxin.	Class IIb
Digoxin should not be used as the only agent for controlling the ventricular rate in patients with paroxysmal AF.	Class III
Restoration of sinus rhythm	
Flecainide, dofetilide, propafenone, or ibutilide is recommended for pharmacologic cardioversion of AF.	Class I
Amiodarone is a reasonable option for pharmacologic cardioversion of AF.	Class IIa
The "pill-in-the-pocket" approach (see text) can be used to terminate persistent AF on an outpatient basis once the treatment has been used safely in the hospital, in patients without sinus or AV node dysfunction, bundle-branch block, QT interval prolongation, Brugada syndrome, or SHD. (*Note*: AV node must be adequately blocked before initiating this therapy.)	Class IIa
Amiodarone can be used on an outpatient basis in patients with paroxysmal or persistent AF when rapid restoration of sinus rhythm is not necessary.	Class IIa
Quinidine or procainamide might be considered for pharmacologic cardioversion of AF, but their efficacy is not well established.	Class IIb
Digoxin and sotalol should not be used for pharmacologic cardioversion of AF (may be harmful).	Class III
Quinidine, procainamide, disopyramide, and dofetilide should not be initiated on an outpatient basis.	Class III
Maintenance of sinus rhythm	
Antiarrhythmic therapy can be useful for maintaining sinus rhythm and preventing tachycardia-induced cardiomyopathy.	Class IIa
Outpatient initiation of antiarrhythmic therapy is reasonable in patients without SHD.	Class IIa
Propafenone or flecainide may be initiated on an outpatient basis in patients with paroxysmal AF who have no SHD and are in sinus rhythm at the time therapy is initiated.	Class IIa
Sotalol may be initiated on an outpatient basis in patients without SHD, QT interval prolongation, electrolyte abnormalities, or other risk factors for proarrhythmia.	Class IIa
An antiarrhythmic drug should not be used when patients have risk factors for proarrhythmia with that particular agent.	Class III
Antiarrhythmic therapy is not recommended in patients with sinus or AV node dysfunction unless a pacemaker is present.	Class III

Abbreviations: ACC = American College of Cardiology; AF = atrial fibrillation; AHA = American Heart Association; AV = atrioventricular; CCB = calcium channel blocker; DCC = direct-current cardioversion; DHP = dihydropyridine; ESC = European Society of Cardiology; HF = heart failure; IV = intravenous; LV = left ventricular; SHD = structural heart disease.

Source: Adapted from References 6 and 10.

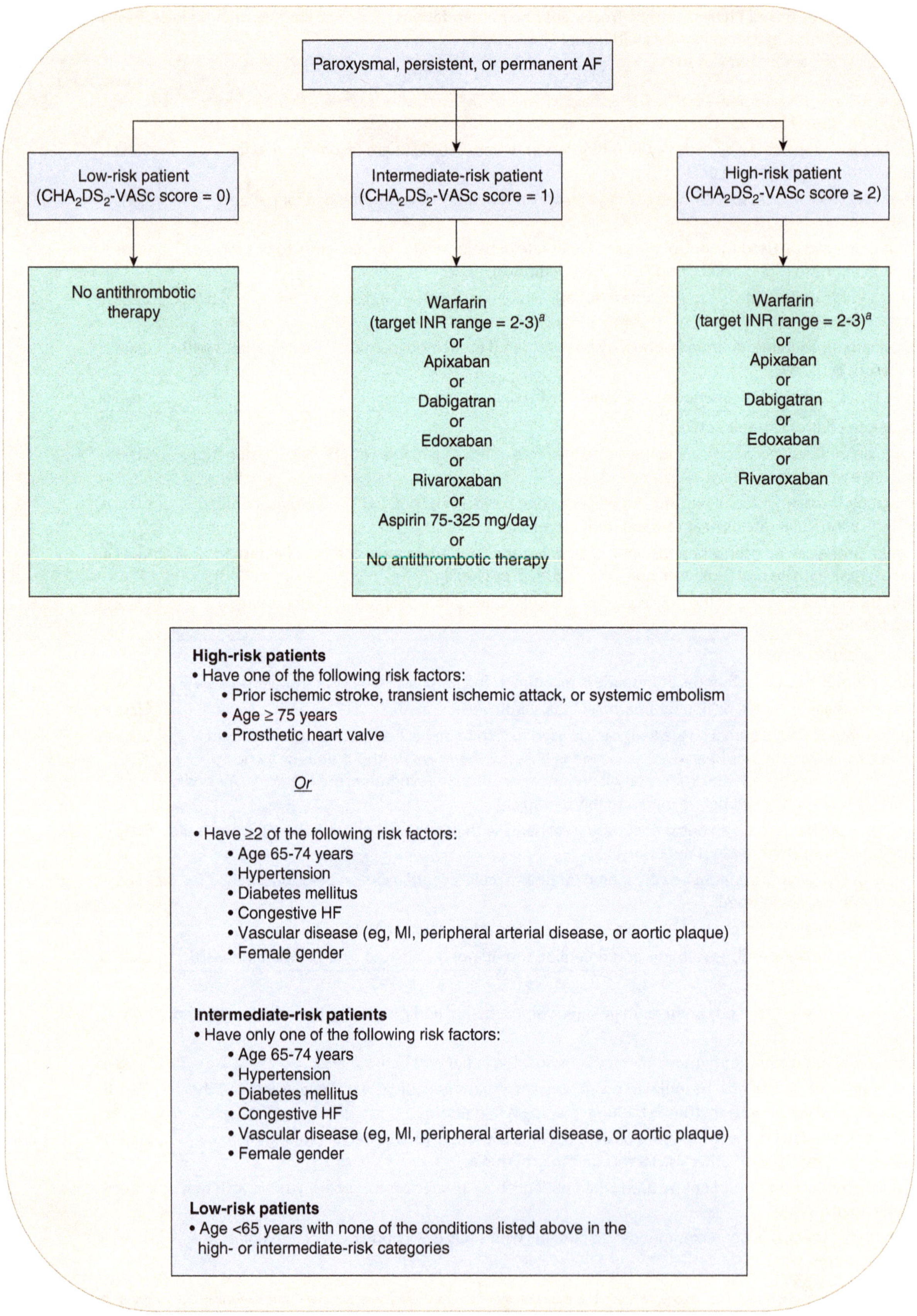

FIGURE 14-5 Algorithm for prevention of thromboembolism in paroxysmal, persistent, or permanent AF.

[a] Note: The target INR for patients with prosthetic heart valves should be based on the type of valve that is present.

Abbreviations: AF = atrial fibrillation; HF = heart failure; INR = international normalized ratio; MI = myocardial infarction.

Source: Reproduced, with permission, from DiPiro, JT, Talbert RL, Yee GC, Matzke GR, Wells BG, Posey LM, eds. *Pharmacotherapy: A Pathophysiologic Approach*. 10th ed. New York, NY: McGraw-Hill; 2017.

TABLE 14-8 • Guidelines for Selecting Antiarrhythmic Drug Therapy for Maintenance of Sinus Rhythm in Patients with Recurrent Paroxysmal or Recurrent Persistent Atrial Fibrillation

No structural heart disease[a] (absence of heart failure, coronary artery disease, signifi cant LVH, and valvular disease) First line:[b] dofetilide, dronedarone, flecainide, propafenone, or sotalol Second line:[c] amiodarone
Heart failure[a] First line[b]: amiodarone or dofetilide Second line: catheter ablation
Coronary artery disease[a] First line:[b] dofetilide, dronedarone,[d] or sotalol[d] Second line:[c] amiodarone
Hypertension[a] Presence of signifi cant LVH: First line:[b] amiodarone or dronedarone Second line: catheter ablation Absence of signifi cant LVH: First line:[b] dofetilide, dronedarone, flecainide, propafenone, or sotalol Second line:[c] amiodarone

LVH, left ventricular hypertrophy.

[a] Drugs are listed alphabetically and not in order of suggested use.

[b] Catheter ablation may also be considered first-line therapy in select patients with paroxysmal atrial fibrillation.

[c] Catheter ablation may also be considered when patients are refractory or intolerant to at least 1 antiarrhythmic drug.

[d] Should only be used in this situation if the patient has normal left ventricular systolic function.

TABLE 14-9 • Nonpharmacologic Considerations for AF

Direct-current cardioversion (DCC)	When rapid ventricular response does not respond to drug therapy, if the patient is hemodynamically unstable, or when patient is unable to tolerate AF symptoms, cardioversion may be considered.
Surgery	Ablation—radiofrequency ablation, or catheter ablation, to shut down signaling MAZE procedure—small incisions made in the heart to create scar tissue, which is not able to conduct electric signals
Holding anticoagulants for surgical procedures	Warfarin *High-risk patients* are those who have had a TIA or stroke within the last 3 months, have a CHA_2DS_2-VASc score of 5 or 6, or have a mechanical heart valve. For these patients, interruption of warfarin therapy could increase risk of stroke, so bridging with a low-molecular-weight heparin is recommended while off warfarin. *Moderate-risk patients* are those with a CHA_2DS_2-VASc score of 3 or 4. The benefits of bridging should be weighed against the risk of bleeding for each individual patient. *Low-risk patients* are those who have never had a TIA or stroke, and have a CHA_2DS_2-VASc score of 0 to 2. Most clinicians would recommend holding warfarin 5-7 days prior to a procedure without bridging.

Source: Reference 3.

TABLE 14-10 • Herbal Supplements for AF

Supplement	Typical Dose	Effectiveness[a]	Cost[b]
Magnesium	Dietary allowances: Men aged 19-30 years: 400 mg Women aged 19-30 years: 310 mg Males aged >30 years: 420 mg Women aged 30 years: 320 mg	Possibly effective	$$
L-Carnitine	2 g used daily, in divided doses, to prevent cardiovascular disease	Insufficient evidence	$$$$

[a] Level of evidence: "likely effective"—this product has a very high level of reliable clinical evidence supporting its use for a specific indication. Products rated "likely effective" are generally considered appropriate to recommend. Products rated "possibly effective" have some clinical evidence supporting their use for a specific indication; however, the evidence is limited by quantity, quality, or contradictory findings. Products rated "possibly effective" might be beneficial, but do not have enough high-quality evidence to recommend use for most people. The rating "insufficient evidence" indicates that there is insufficient reliable scientific evidence to provide an effectiveness rating.

[b] Cost: $ = ≤$10/month supply in recommended dosage; $$$$ = >$50/month.

Source: Reference 10.

Stroke Warning Signs: F.A.S.T.[11]

Face – Ask the person to smile. Does the face look uneven?

Arms – Ask the person to raise both arms. Does one arm drift down or is unable to move?

Speech – Ask the person to repeat a simple phrase. Does their speech sound strange? Speech may be slurred, the wrong words may come out, or the person may be unable to speak.

Time – to call 9-1-1.

Immediate action Call 911	• Chest pain • Symptoms of heart attack or angina • Symptoms of stroke
Seek medical attention Emergency room	• Symptoms of AF including: Palpitations, faintness, dizziness, weakness, or shortness of breath
Routine Inform provider at a later time	• Medication side effects or problems obtaining medications • New medications, especially antibiotics, which may interfere with warfarin

FIGURE 14-6 Referral for management of AF. Stroke warning signs: **FAST**.
Source: Reference 11.

TABLE 14-11 • **Medication-Related Problems (MRPs) in Patients with AF**

Category of MRP	Examples of Medication-Related Problems
Nonadherence	Suboptimal control of AF symptoms due to patient missing doses of rate-controlling medication Patient not taking anticoagulant medication due to cost
Unnecessary medication	Duplicate therapy (eg, aspirin and clopidogrel without an approved indication for both)
Need for additional medication	Patient with risk for stroke not on antithrombotic therapy (ie, CHA_2DS_2-VASc ≥2)
Ineffective medication	Adequate trial of new rhythm control medication without significant clinical response Use of an herbal supplement instead of an FDA-approved therapy
Dosage too low	Palpitations on a starting dose of metoprolol Low INR while on warfarin (without a modifiable reason)
Dosage too high	Elevated INR on warfarin (without a modifiable reason) Addition of enzyme-inhibiting medication resulting in elevated INR in patient on warfarin Heart rate too low on diltiazem for rate control strategy Dose of apixaban too high if patient has two of the following criteria: age ≥80 years, serum creatinine ≥1.5 mg/dL, weight ≤60 kg
Adverse drug event	Nosebleed from warfarin Patient not taking diltiazem because of headaches and/or constipation Gastroesophageal reflux symptoms while on dabigatran

Scenario: Patient has atrial fibrillation with a CHA_2DS_2-VASc score of 3 without anticoagulation **MRP:** Need for additional therapy
Assessment: Per pharmacy claims and patient report, patient has atrial fibrillation with a CHA_2DS_2-VASc score of 3 with no stroke prevention medication. Addition of Pradaxa (dabigatran) would reduce risk of stroke in this patient. **Plan:** If appropriate, please consider addition of Pradaxa 150 mg twice daily to reduce risk of stroke.
Scenario: Patient experiencing severe headaches associated with diltiazem **MRP:** Adverse drug event
Assessment: Patient experiencing severe headaches associated with initiation of diltiazem 60 mg 3 times daily for atrial fibrillation rate control. Headaches are a documented adverse effect associated with diltiazem. Adverse effects may impact patient compliance with medication. **Plan:** Address reported adverse effect at next appointment. If appropriate, please consider switching to another rate control agent such as metoprolol tartrate 25 mg twice daily, titrating to effect.
Scenario: Patient receiving amiodarone and warfarin therapy **MRP:** Dosage too high (drug-drug interaction)
Assessment: Per patient report and pharmacy claims, patient is receiving o Amiodarone 400 mg daily o Warfarin 5 mg daily Amiodarone may result in a significant rise in INR when initiated in a patient taking warfarin. **Plan:** Consider increasing frequency of INR monitoring and reduction in dose of warfarin by 30%-50% when adding amiodarone therapy.
Scenario: Patient with history of atrial fibrillation and CHA_2DS_2-VASc score of 0 receiving warfarin **MRP:** Unnecessary medication
Assessment: Per pharmacy claims and patient report, patient has atrial fibrillation and a CHA_2DS_2-VASc score of 0 and is receiving warfarin 5 mg daily for stroke prophylaxis. Use of warfarin in patients with a CHA_2DS_2-VASc of score 0 is not recommended because of risk of bleed outweighing the benefit of stroke prevention in a patient at low risk for stroke. **Plan:** If there is no other indication for anticoagulation in this patient, please consider discontinuing warfarin therapy.

FIGURE 14-7 Sample provider communications for AF.

TABLE 14-12 • Suggested Intervals for Follow-up and Monitoring in Patients with AF

Atrial fibrillation management
Clinical symptoms such as palpitations or dyspnea should trigger ECG monitoring to demonstrate AF, or to correlate symptoms with the underlying rhythm. In patients receiving antiarrhythmic medications, ECG should be monitored regularly to detect possible QT interval prolongation. Following ablation procedures, patients should initially follow-up after 3 months, then every 6 months for 2 years to identify recurrence of atrial fibrillation. During follow-up visits, provider should assess: • Changes in risk profile (need for anticoagulation therapy) • Improvement of symptoms • Signs or risk of proarrhythmia • Progression of paroxysmal AF to persistent/permanent AF • 12-lead ECG to document rate, rhythm, and disease progression
Anticoagulant monitoring
Patients taking warfarin should have INR monitored every 1 to 2 weeks until within therapeutic range consistently. Follow-up time may be lengthened in well-controlled patients. No routine anticoagulation monitoring is necessary for the direct oral anticoagulants, although there should be follow-up with providers at regular intervals for assessment of bleeding and compliance. Checking renal function and a complete blood count at least twice per year is reasonable.
Toxicity
Monitor for adverse drug effects 2-4 weeks after starting a new agent or dose increase. Monitor adverse bleeding events due to anticoagulants at each visit.

REFERENCES

1. Sanoski CA, Bauman JL. The arrhythmias. In: DiPiro JT, Talbert RL, Yee GC, Matzke GR, Wells BG, Posey L. eds. *Pharmacotherapy: A Pathophysiologic Approach*, 10th ed. New York, NY: McGraw-Hill. Available at http://accesspharmacy.mhmedical.com/content.aspx?bookid=1861&sectionid=146057036. Accessed May 8, 2017.
2. Benjamin EJ, Blaha MJ, Chiuve SE, et al. Heart disease and stroke statistics 2017 update: A report from the American Heart Association. *Circulation.* 2017;135:e229-e268.
3. January CT, Wann LS, Alpert JS, et al. 2014 AHA/ACC/HRS guideline for the management of patients with atrial fibrillation: A report of the American College of Cardiology/American Heart Association Task Force on Practice Guidelines and the Heart Rhythm Society. *Circulation.* 2014;130(23):e199-e267.
4. Wang TJ, Larson MG, Levy D, et al. Temporal relations of atrial fibrillation and congestive heart failure and their joint influence on mortality; the Framingham Heart Study. *Circulation.* 2003;107:2920-2925.
5. Kelly-Hayes M, Beiser A, Kase CS, et al. The influence of gender and age on disability following ischemic stroke: The Framingham Study. *J Stroke Cerebrovasc Dis.* 2003;12:119-126.
6. Fagan SC and Hess DC. Stroke. In: DiPiro JT, Talbert RL, Yee GC, Matzke GR, Wells BG, Posey L. eds. *Pharmacotherapy: A Pathophysiologic Approach*, 10th ed. New York, NY: McGraw-Hill. Available at http://accesspharmacy.mhmedical.com/content.aspx?bookid=1861&sectionid=132515962. Accessed May 8, 2017.
7. *Medicare Part D Medication Therapy Management Program Standardized Format.* Available at http://www.cms.gov/Medicare/Prescription-Drug-Coverage/PrescriptionDrugCovContra/Downloads/MTM-Program-Standardized-Format-Revisions-v071514-[ZIP-2MB].zip. Accessed May 7, 2017.
8. Walter NK, Ovbiagele BO, Black HR, et al. Guidelines for the prevention of stroke in patients with stroke and transient ischemic attack: A guideline for healthcare professionals from the American Heart Association/American Stroke Association. *Stroke.* 2014;45:2160-2236.
9. Clinical Pharmacology [database online]. Tampa, FL: Gold Standard, Inc.; 2017. Report available at http://www.clinicalpharmacology.com. Accessed May 7, 2017.
10. Natural Medicines [database online]. Somerville, MA: Therapeutic Research Center; 2017. Report available at https://naturalmedicines.therapeuticresearch.com/. Accessed May 7, 2017
11. American Heart Association. *Heart Attack or Stroke? Call 911 First and Fast.* Available at http://www.heart.org/HEARTORG/Affiliate/Heart-Attack-or-Stroke-Call-911-First-And-Fast_UCM_435652_Article.jsp. Accessed May 7, 2017.

Review Questions

1. Risk factors for atrial fibrillation include all of the following EXCEPT:
   a. Increased age
   b. Diabetes
   c. Genetics
   d. Low body mass index

2. A 65-year-old female was just diagnosed with atrial fibrillation. She has no symptoms, and states that she's "never been sick a day in my life." Her past medical history is significant for seasonal allergies, for which she uses loratadine as needed. She takes no other medications, and has no drug allergies. Which of the following is the BEST choice for initial management of her atrial fibrillation?
   a. Amlodipine 5 mg once daily
   b. Amiodarone 400 mg three times daily
   c. Metoprolol 12.5 mg twice daily
   d. Sotalol 80 mg twice daily

3. When counseling a patient about treatment goals in the management of atrial fibrillation, a reasonable target heart rate would be:
   a. 100-115 beats per minute (bpm) at rest or during exercise.
   b. a 30% decrease from baseline.
   c. 75 bpm during exercise.
   d. <80 bpm at rest.

4. Which of the following is the most appropriate definition of atrial fibrillation using living room language?
   a. An irregular and often rapid heart rate that commonly causes poor blood flow to the body.
   b. An arrhythmia that may be the result of long-standing hypertension, heart failure, or other cardiac issues.
   c. A condition that will give you a stroke.
   d. A rapid heart rate originating in the atria resulting in a lack of sufficient blood circulation within the periphery.

5. A 75-year-old male with a history of heart failure with reduced ejection fraction and atrial fibrillation has a resting heart rate of 61 bpm. He was admitted to the hospital 4 weeks ago for acute heart failure. Today, in clinic, his provider determines that he still has symptoms related to atrial fibrillation. Which of the following would be the BEST medication to add?
   a. Dronedarone 400 mg twice daily
   b. Metoprolol 50 mg twice daily
   c. Verapamil 180 mg once daily
   d. Amiodarone 200 mg once daily

6. Which of the following is correct regarding a patient with newly diagnosed atrial fibrillation who has a CHA_2DS_2-VASc score of 0 and is hemodynamically stable?
   a. This patient does not require antithrombotic therapy.
   b. This patient should be treated with aspirin, 325 mg daily.
   c. This patient should be treated with warfarin.
   d. This patient should be cardioverted as soon as possible.

7. All of the following statements are appropriate for inclusion in the "What I need to do" section of the MAP for a patient regarding usage of warfarin EXCEPT:
   a. Take my warfarin therapy every day as directed.
   b. Keep track of my scheduled appointments to check my blood.
   c. Don't eat any foods high in vitamin K.
   d. Report any unusual bruising or bleeding to my healthcare provider.

8. Regarding the warning signs of a stroke, what does the acronym FAST represent?
   a. Face, Arms, Speech, Time
   b. Feet, Arms, Speech, Time
   c. Face, Arms, Speech, Tongue
   d. Fall, Ache, Speech, Tongue

9. Which of the following medication-related problems is matched with the correct category of MRP?
   a. Dosage too low—high INR while on warfarin
   b. Dosage too high—low INR while on warfarin
   c. Nonadherence—suboptimal control of atrial fibrillation symptoms due to patient missing doses of rate-controlling medication
   d. Unnecessary medication—patient with risk for stroke not on antithrombotic therapy (ie, aspirin, clopidogrel, or warfarin)

10. Which is correct regarding usage and monitoring of rivaroxaban?
   a. INR monitoring is required.
   b. Renal function should be checked twice per year.
   c. There is no risk of gastrointestinal bleeding.
   d. Rivaroxaban should not be used when creatinine clearance is less than 95 mL/min.

ANSWERS

1. d 2. c 3. d
4. a 5. d 6. a
7. c 8. a 9. c
10. b

15

Bipolar Disorder MTM Data Set

Megan J. Ehret, PharmD, MS, BCPP

KEY POINTS

- Bipolar disorder is a lifelong illness, which requires adherence to medications to prevent repeated episodes.
- Polypharmacy is the rule in the treatment of bipolar disorder, rather than the exception.
- Adverse effects, drug interactions, and cost of medications can lead to nonadherence. Medication therapy management (MTM) providers should be watchful of nonadherence and work with the patient to create a regimen that is both tolerable and affordable.
- Inclusion of the patient in a therapeutic alliance can increase adherence to treatment and medications.

INTRODUCTION TO BIPOLAR DISORDER

Bipolar disorder (previously known as *manic-depressive disorder*) is a cyclic mood disorder characterized by recurrent fluctuations in mood, energy, and behavior.[1,2] Bipolar disorder is a lifelong illness with a variable course, which requires both nonpharmacologic and pharmacologic treatment.[1,2] Episodes of bipolar disorder include not only major depression but also hypomania, mania, and mixed (Table 15-1).

Types and Causes of Bipolar Disorder

There are two major types of bipolar disorder:

- *Bipolar disorder type I* —involves periods of severe mood episodes ranging from mania to depression
- *Bipolar disorder type II*—milder form of mood elevation, involving milder episodes of hypomania that alternate with periods of severe depression

Some medical conditions and medications can induce mania or depressive symptoms. Secondary causes of mania (Table 15-2) or depression (Table 15-3) should be ruled out before a diagnosis of bipolar disorder is confirmed. In addition, treatment of secondary causes of mania or depression may affect the need for drug therapy for the management of bipolar disorder.

Complications of Bipolar Disorder[1,2,15-17]

Stopping medication(s) or treatment can worsen symptoms of bipolar disorder. It can lead to alcohol and/or drug abuse; problems with relationships, work, and finances; and suicidal thoughts or behaviors. Bipolar disorder is difficult to treat. Patients, their families, friends, and caregivers must know the risks of not treating bipolar disorder. Table 15-4 provides an overview of the complications of bipolar disorder.

Therapeutic Goals for Bipolar Disorder

Adequate control of bipolar disorder can be challenging, as mood variations are not predictable. It can be difficult to determine whether a patient with bipolar disorder is responding to treatment or is emerging from an episode naturally. The main goal of treatment is to treat and reduce the severity of acute episodes when they occur, while also reducing the frequency of new episodes. An additional goal of importance is to help the patient maintain a high quality of life between episodes. Table 15-5 outlines therapeutic goals for the treatment of bipolar disorder. The assessment of a patient with bipolar disorder is detailed in Table 15-6, and rating scales used during the assessment are described in Table 15-7.

Treatment resistance or treatment failure in bipolar disorder can be difficult to define. In the literature it has been defined

TABLE 15-1 • Evaluation and Diagnosis of Mood Episodes

Diagnosis Episode	Impairment of Functioning or Need for Hospitalization[a]	DSM-5 Criteria[b]
Major depressive	Yes	At least 2-week period of either depressed mood or loss of interest or pleasure in normal activities, associated with at least five of the following symptoms: Depressed, sad mood (adults); can be irritable mood in children Decreased interest and pleasure in normal activities Decreased or increased appetite, weight loss or weight gain Insomnia or hypersomnia Psychomotor retardation or agitation Decreased energy or fatigue Feelings of excessive guilt or worthlessness Impaired concentration or indecisiveness Recurrent thoughts of death, suicidal thoughts or attempts
Manic	Yes	At least 1-week period of abnormally and persistently elevated mood (expansive or irritable) and energy, associated with at least three of the following symptoms (four if the mood is only irritable): Inflated self-esteem (grandiosity) Decreased need for sleep Increased talking (pressure of speech) Racing thoughts (flight of ideas) Distractibility (poor attention) Increased goal-directed activity (socially, at work, or sexually) or psychomotor agitation Excessive involvement in activities that are pleasurable but have a high risk for serious consequences (buying sprees, sexual indiscretions, poor judgment in business ventures)
Hypomanic	No	At least 4 days of abnormally and persistently elevated mood (expansive or irritable) and energy, associated with at least three of the following symptoms (four if the mood is only irritable): Inflated self-esteem (grandiosity) Decreased need for sleep Increased talking (pressure of speech) Racing thoughts (flight of ideas) Distractibility (poor attention) Increased goal-directed activity (socially, at work, or sexually) or psychomotor agitation Excessive involvement in activities that are pleasurable but have a high risk for serious consequences (buying sprees, sexual indiscretions, poor judgment in business ventures)

[a] Impairment in social or occupational functioning; may include need for hospitalization because of potential self-harm, harm to others, or psychotic symptoms.

[b] The disorder is not caused by a medical condition (eg, hypothyroidism) or substance-induced disorder (eg, antidepressant treatment, medications, drugs of abuse). Numerous specifiers are available to further characterize episodes (eg, with mixed features, with anxious distress, with rapid cycling, with melancholic features).

Source: Compiled from reference 1.

as nonresponse to a combination of two standard medications in a specific period, such as 6 weeks for mania, and 6 months or 3-cycle lengths for maintenance.[20] The reemergence of symptoms or treatment-resistant symptoms can lead a clinician to consider increasing a dose, changing a medication, or admitting the patient to a hospital. Almost half of patients with bipolar disorder with symptom remission will have a recurrence in 2 years under standard care, so clinicians need to constantly review symptoms with each patient.

CORE ELEMENT 1—COMPREHENSIVE MEDICATION REVIEW FOR PATIENTS WITH BIPOLAR DISORDER

Table 15-8 contains a list of questions to use when conducting a medication therapy review in a patient with bipolar disorder. The number and types of questions will vary from patient to patient depending on the type of episodes, the time for the interview, the number of medication-related problems (MRPs), and the urgency of the MRPs. If time is limited or in the case of a highly complex patient, the MTM provider should choose target questions that will help to identify or rule out issues of an urgent nature (see questions to ask for prevention/assessment of medical emergencies). MTM providers should remember to use living room language during the interview (Table 15-9), and to be prepared to answer questions that patients may ask regarding bipolar disorder (Table 15-10).

CORE ELEMENT 2—PERSONAL MEDICATION LIST[24]

Figure 15-1 is a sample personal medication list (PML) for a patient with bipolar disorder. This example is representative of typical medications used for bipolar disorder and is not encompassing of all

TABLE 15-2 • Secondary Causes of Mania

Medical conditions that induce mania
CNS disorders (brain tumor, strokes, head injuries, subdural hematoma, multiple sclerosis, systemic lupus erythematosus, temporal lobe seizures, Huntington disease)
Infections (encephalitis, neurosyphilis, sepsis, human immunodeficiency virus)
Electrolyte or metabolic abnormalities (calcium or sodium fluctuations, hyperglycemia or hypoglycemia)
Endocrine or hormonal dysregulation (Addison disease, Cushing disease, hyperthyroidism or hypothyroidism, menstrual-related or pregnancy-related or perimenopausal mood disorders)
Medications or drugs that induce mania
Alcohol intoxication
Drug withdrawal states (alcohol, α_2-adrenergic agonists, antidepressants, barbiturates, benzodiazepines, opiates)
Antidepressants (MAOIs, TCAs, 5-HT and/or NE and/or DA reuptake inhibitors, 5-HT antagonists)
DA-augmenting agents (CNS stimulants: amphetamines, cocaine, sympathomimetics; DA agonists, releasers, and reuptake inhibitors)
Hallucinogens (LSD, PCP)
Marijuana intoxication precipitates psychosis, paranoid thoughts, anxiety, and restlessness
NE-augmenting agents (α_2-adrenergic antagonists, β-agonists, NE reuptake inhibitors)
Steroids (anabolic, adrenocorticotropic hormone, corticosteroids)
Thyroid preparations
Xanthines (caffeine, theophylline)
Nonprescription weight loss agents and decongestants (ephedra, pseudoephedrine)
Herbal products (St. John's wort)
Somatic therapies that induce mania
Bright-light therapy
Deep-brain stimulation
Sleep deprivation

Abbreviations: CNS = central nervous system; DA = dopamine; 5-HT = serotonin; LSD = lysergic acid diethylamide; MAOI = monoamine oxidase inhibitor; NE = norepinephrine; PCP = phencyclidine; TCA = tricyclic antidepressant.

Source: Data from references 1, 3-12.

TABLE 15-3 • Common Medical Conditions, Substance Use Disorders, and Medications Associated with Depressive Symptoms

General Medical Conditions		**Substance Use Disorders (Including *Intoxication* and *Withdrawal*)**
Endocrine diseases	Metabolic disorders	Alcoholism
Hypothyroidism	Electrolyte imbalance	Marijuana abuse and dependence
Addison or Cushing disease	Hypokalemia	Nicotine dependence
Deficiency states	Hyponatremia	Opiate abuse and dependence (eg, heroin)
Pernicious anemia	Hepatic encephalopathy	Psychostimulant abuse and dependence (eg, cocaine)
Wernicke encephalopathy	Cardiovascular disease	**Drug therapy**
Severe anemia	Coronary artery disease	Antihypertensives
Infections	Congestive heart failure	Clonidine
AIDS	Myocardial infarction	Diuretics
Encephalitis	Neurologic disorders	Guanethidine sulfate
Human immunodeficiency virus	Alzheimer disease	Hydralazine hydrochloride
Mononucleosis	Epilepsy	Methyldopa
Sexually transmitted diseases	Huntington disease	Propranolol
Tuberculosis	Multiple sclerosis	Reserpine
Collagen disorder	Pain	Hormonal therapy
Systemic lupus erythematosus	Parkinson disease	Oral contraceptives
	Post-stroke	Steroids/adrenocorticotropic hormone
	Malignant disease	Acne therapy
		Isotretinoin
		Other
		Interferon-β_{1a}

Source: Data from references 2, 3, and 14.

TABLE 15-4 • Complications of Bipolar Disorder

Alcohol and substance abuse	Drugs of abuse have significant impact on the age of onset, course of illness, and response to treatment: Earlier onset of illness Mixed states Higher rates of relapse Poorer response to treatment Comorbid personality disorders Increased suicide risk More psychiatric hospitalizations
Functional disability	More than half of patients have some degree of disability, including psychosocial and occupational functioning: Legal problems Financial problems Relationship problems
Mortality rate	Higher mortality rate; up to 50% of patients will have at least one suicide attempt, with approximately 10%-19% with bipolar I disorder committing suicide. Accidental deaths are more frequent in those with mania, due to grandiosity, hallucinations, or delusions that result in risk-taking behaviors. Higher mortality rates also result from endocrine, respiratory, and cardiovascular disease, which result from higher rates of obesity, smoking, alcohol, substance abuse, infections, and lack of medical care.

TABLE 15-5 • Therapeutic Goals for the Treatment of Bipolar Disorder

Eliminate mood episode with complete remission of symptoms
Prevent recurrences or relapses of mood episodes
Return to complete psychosocial functioning
Maximize adherence with therapy
Minimize adverse effects
Use medications with the best tolerability and fewest drug interactions
Treat comorbid substance use and abuse

Source: Data from references 2, 18, and 19.

TABLE 15-6 • General Principles of Management for Bipolar Disorder

- Perform a diagnostic evaluation
  - Assess for presence of an alcohol or substance abuse use disorder or any other factors that may contribute to the disease
  - Inquire about a history of time with mood dysregulation or ability accompanied by associated manic symptoms
- Ensure the safety of the patient and others and determine a treatment setting
  - Consider hospitalization in those who:
    - Pose a serious threat of harm to themselves or others
    - Are severely ill and lack adequate social support outside a hospital setting or demonstrate significant impaired judgment
    - Have a complicating psychiatric or general medical condition
    - Have not responded adequately to outpatient treatment
- Establish and maintain a therapeutic alliance with the patient
- Monitor the patient's psychiatric status
- Educate the patient and her/his family regarding bipolar disorder
- Enhance treatment adherence
- Promote awareness of stressors and regular patterns of activity and sleep
- Work with the patient to anticipate and address early signs of relapse
- Evaluate and manage functional impairments

Source: Data from reference 2.

TABLE 15-7 • Rating Scales for the Assessment of Bipolar Disorder

Mood Disorder Questionnaire[21]	Developed by a team of psychiatrists, researchers, and consumer advocates to address the need for timely and accurate evaluation of bipolar disorder. Designed for screening purposes; available at http://www.dbsalliance.org/pdfs/MDQ.pdf
Brief Bipolar Disorder Symptom Scale[22]	10-item measure of symptom severity for bipolar disorder, which is derived from the Brief Psychiatric Rating Scale; available at http://www.argos2001.org/TIMABipolar.pdf
Young Mania Rating Scale[23]	11-item scale for assessing the severity of manic symptoms over the previous 48 hours; available at http://dcf.psychiatry.ufl.edu/files/2011/05/Young-Mania-Rating-Scale-Measure-with-background.pdf

Source: Data from references 21, 22, and 23.

medications that a patient may take. Additional medications, over-the-counter (OTC) products, and herbal supplements should be added to the list for each patient. MTM providers should remember to use plain language when creating the PML for the patient.

CORE ELEMENT 3—MEDICATION ACTION PLAN[24]

Figure 15-2 provides a sample medication action plan (MAP) for patients with bipolar disorder. This example is representative only of action steps for the patient with bipolar disorder, and does not include plans for other disease states or other MRPs. These should be listed and addressed separately. Typically, only a few of the most important action steps should be listed, so as not to overwhelm the patient. Additional areas for patient self-management can be addressed at later visits. MTM providers should remember to use plain language when creating medication action plans.

CORE ELEMENT 4—INTERVENTION AND/OR REFERRAL

Interventions for bipolar disorder management include many lifestyle modifications and medication therapy. Patients will need both in order to prevent future episodes of bipolar disorder. Mood stabilizers should be chosen on the basis of patient-specific characteristics including the current episode, chronicity of illness, cost of medication, potential or actual adverse effects, drug-drug interactions, family history of response, and patient preference. Patients should be encouraged to monitor their own illness at home through mood logs. Polypharmacy is typically the rule with bipolar disorder, rather than the exception. Table 15-11

TABLE 15-8 • Questions to Ask When Conducting a Medication Therapy Review in a Patient with Bipolar Disorder

Suggested Questions for the Patient with Bipolar Disorder
When were you diagnosed with bipolar disorder? What types of symptoms were you experiencing then? How often did you experience these symptoms prior to the diagnosis of bipolar disorder?
How many episodes of depression have you had? How long did each episode typically last?
How many episodes of mania/hypomania have you had? How long did each episode typically last?
How many episodes per year do you typically experience? What is the maximum number of episodes per year you have experienced?
Does anyone else in your family have a mental illness? If so, who and which illness?
What do you know about the risks of untreated bipolar disorder?
How often do you see your clinician regarding the treatment of bipolar disorder?
How do you monitor your symptoms of bipolar disorder?
What triggers do you have for the development of a new episode of bipolar disorder?
What medications do you take for the treatment of bipolar disorder? How do you take them?
What medications have you tried in the past to treat bipolar disorder? Why did you stop taking them? How long did you try each medication?
How often do you miss a dose of your medications? What do you do when you realize you have missed a dose?
Have you ever stopped taking any of your prescribed medications without telling your clinician? If so, why? What happened?
What over-the-counter (OTC) medications or herbals do you use for the treatment of bipolar disorder?
Other than medications, what else have you tried to treat bipolar disorder? Exercise? Yoga?
Do you ever have thoughts of hurting yourself? If so, can you describe these thoughts?
What do you do when you have these thoughts? Do you want to hurt yourself now?
Questions to Ask for Prevention/Assessment of Medical Emergencies
Crisis planning: What are your triggers for a manic or depressive episode?
Have you experienced these recently?
What is your typical mood? How do you feel now?
Are you suicidal? Do you have a plan?
Can you tell someone if you don't feel safe?
Have you ever been hospitalized for bipolar disorder?

TABLE 15-9 • Living Room Language for Bipolar Disorder

Adverse event—something bad that happens, bad reaction, unexplained or unwanted effects.
Alopecia—loss of hair; baldness; potential adverse effect from valproic acid.
Ammonia—forms when bacteria in the gut break down protein. The liver normally changes ammonia into urea, which is then eliminated in the urine. Ammonia may rise when the liver is not able to change ammonia to urea. May be caused by liver diseases (cirrhosis or severe hepatitis).
Antianxiety medication—medications used for the treatment of anxiety.
Antidepressant—medications used for the treatment of depression.
Antimanic medication—medication that is effective in the treatment of mania or hypomania.
Antipsychotic—tranquilizer used to treat psychotic conditions when a calming effect is desired.
Basic metabolic panel—blood test that measures your sugar (glucose) level, electrolyte and fluid balance, and kidney function.
Bipolar disorder—mood disorder with recurrent ups and downs in mood, energy, and behavior.
Bipolar disorder due to a general medical condition—disorder characterized by symptoms of bipolar disorder which are caused by another medical condition.
Bipolar disorder not otherwise specified (NOS)—a disorder that is diagnosed when a person has symptoms of the illness that do not meet criteria for either bipolar disorder type I or II. The symptoms may not last long enough, or the person may have too few symptoms, to be diagnosed with type I or II. However, the symptoms are clearly out of the person's normal range of behavior.
Bipolar disorder type I— defined mainly by manic or mixed episodes that last at least 7 days, or by manic symptoms that are so severe that the person needs immediate hospital care. Usually, the person also has periods of depression episodes, typically lasting at least 2 weeks. The symptoms of mania or depression must be a major change from the person's normal behavior.
Bipolar disorder type II—defined by a pattern of depressive episodes shifting back and forth with hypomanic episodes, but no full-blown manic or mixed episodes.
BMI—body mass index; a measure of weight in relation to height that assigns people to a weight class of underweight, normal weight, overweight, or obese on the basis of their amount of excess weight.
Chronic—constant, never-ending, does not go away.
Complete blood count—test that measures the following factors:
  The number of red blood cells (RBC count)
  The number of white blood cells (WBC count)
  The total amount of hemoglobin in the blood
  The fraction of the blood composed of red blood cells (hematocrit)
  The platelet count, which is also usually included in the CBC.
Creatinine test—a test that checks how well the kidneys are working; an increase means that the kidneys are not working well.
Cyclothymic disorder—a mild form of bipolar disorder. People who have cyclothymia have episodes of hypomania that shift back and forth with mild depression for at least 2 years. However, the symptoms do not meet the diagnostic requirements for any other type of bipolar disorder.
Depression—medical illness that causes a persistent feeling of sadness and loss of interest.
ECT—electroconvulsive therapy; procedure in which electric currents are passed through the brain, causing a seizure.
Elevate—raise, make higher.
Episode—one of a series of related events in the course of a continuous account.
Euphoric—feeling of great happiness or well-being.
Euthymia—periods of time when people are in a normal mood.
Fasting lipid panel—a test of the fats in your blood taken after 8-12 hours without eating any food, because the test results can change depending on what you eat.
Gastrointestinal—of or relating to the stomach and intestines.
Genetics—a branch of biology that deals with how disease susceptibilities and traits are passed down through families in different generations.
Gingival hyperplasia—excessive growth of gum tissue in your mouth, which could be caused by phenytoin.
Glucose test—a blood glucose test that measures the amount of a type of sugar, called *glucose*, in your blood. Glucose comes from carbohydrate foods. It is the main source of energy used by the body. Increased glucose can be a side effect from antipsychotic medications.
Too much glucose can result in diabetes.
Hyperthyroidism—a condition in which your thyroid gland produces too much of the hormone thyroxine. Hyperthyroidism can speed up your body's metabolism significantly, causing sudden weight loss, a rapid or irregular heartbeat, sweating, and nervousness or irritability; can mimic mania.
Hypomania—a mild degree of mania characterized by optimism; excitability; energetic, productive behavior; marked hyperactivity and talkativeness; heightened sexual interest; quick anger and irritability; and a decreased need for sleep. It may be observed before a full-blown manic episode.
Hypothyroidism—a condition in which your thyroid gland does not produce enough of certain important hormones. Can mimic depression, can be an adverse effect from lithium?
Insomnia—difficulty sleeping, despite good conditions and sufficient time for sleep, which affects your ability to function during the day; possible side effect of many psychotropic medications.
Lithium level—level taken of the amount of lithium in the blood; normal range is 0.6-1.2 mEq/L.

(*Continued*)

TABLE 15-9 • Living Room Language for Bipolar Disorder (*Continued*)

Liver function tests—common tests that are used to see how well the liver is working. This is called *liver function*.
Mania—abnormally elevated mental status, characterized by feelings of euphoria, lack of inhibitions, racing thoughts, diminished need for sleep, excessive talkativeness, risk taking, and irritability.
Metabolic syndrome—a syndrome marked by the presence of usually three or more of a group of factors (eg, high blood pressure, abdominal obesity, high triglyceride levels, low levels of good cholesterol, and high fasting levels of blood sugar) that are linked to an increased risk of heart disease and type 2 diabetes.
Mixed features—a period during which the symptoms of both a major depressive episode and of a manic episode occur nearly every day, with rapidly changing moods.
MRI—magnetic resonance imaging; uses a large circular magnet and radiowaves to generate signals from atoms in the body. The signals are used to construct images of structures inside the body.
NAMI—the National Alliance on Mental Illness, the nation's largest grassroots mental health organization dedicated to building better lives for the millions of Americans affected by mental illness. NAMI supports access to services, treatment, and funds research. NAMI is also committed to raising awareness and building a community for hope for all of those in need.
Neuron—a cell with specialized processes that is the core functional unit of nervous tissue.
Neurotransmitter—a substance that transmits nerve signals across a synapse in the brain.
NMS—neuroleptic malignant syndrome; a life-threatening disorder most often caused by a reaction to neuroleptic or antipsychotic drugs. Symptoms include high fever, sweating, unstable blood pressure, lack of mental function, and rigid muscle.
Pharmacogenomics—the study of how genes affect a person's response to medications.
Psychiatrist—a medical physician with an MD degree who specializes in preventing, diagnosing, and treating mental illness.
Psychologist—a mental health specialist with a doctoral degree (PhD, PsyD, or EdD) or master's degree in psychology, which is the study of the mind and behaviors. Graduate school provides a psychologist an education in evaluating and treating mental and emotional disorders.
Psychotherapy—a general term for treating mental health problems by talking with a psychiatrist, psychologist, or other mental health provider.
Psychotropic medication—a term for psychiatric medicines that alter chemical levels in the brain which impact mood and behavior.
Rapid cycling—a pattern of symptoms in bipolar disorder where a person with bipolar disorder experiences four or more episodes of mania or depression in one year.
Receptor—part of a cell that binds and responds to a specific substance; receptors are potential targets for medications used to treat mood disorders.
Sedative—an agent or drug having a soothing, calming, or tranquilizing effect.
Serotonin syndrome—a potentially life-threatening drug reaction that causes the body to contain too much serotonin.
SIADH—syndrome of inappropriate diuretic hormone; excessive levels of antidiuretic hormones (hormones that help the kidneys and body conserve the correct amount of water) are produced. This syndrome causes the body to retain water and certain levels of electrolytes in the blood to fall (such as sodium); can be a side effect of antidepressants, especially in the elderly.
Social worker—a professional who seeks to improve the quality of life and well-being of an individual, group, or community.
Sodium—an essential element. Enables the neurons to fire signals in the brain.
Substance abuse—harmful use of psychoactive substances, including alcohol and illicit drugs, such as cocaine, heroin, or crack.
Substance-induced bipolar disorder—disorder characterized by symptoms of bipolar disorder that are induced by a substance, either of abuse or another medication or treatment such as antidepressants or ECT.
Suicide—the action of killing oneself on purpose.
Synapse—the point at which a nerve signal passes from one neuron to another in the brain.
Therapeutic drug level—blood tests designed to look for the presence and the amount of specific drugs in the blood.
Thyroid—a gland that secretes and stores hormones that help regulate the heart rate, blood pressure, body temperature, and the rate at which food is converted into energy.
TMS—transcranial magnetic stimulation, procedure that uses magnetic fields to excite nerve cells in the brain to improve symptoms of depression.
Tremor—a trembling or shaking usually from physical weakness, emotional stress, or disease.
Unipolar depression—a major depressive episode without a manic phase that occurs in the classic form of bipolar disorder.
Valproic acid level—level of valproic acid in the blood; normal range 50-100 μg/mL.

summarizes lifestyle modifications that are beneficial for patients diagnosed with bipolar disorder. Table 15-12 provides an overview of the different classes of medications used in the treatment of bipolar disorder. Additionally, Table 15-13 outlines hepatic enzymes affected by carbamazepine and other anticonvulsants that may be used for mood stabilization. Table 15-14 describes the use of herbal supplements for the treatment of bipolar disorder.

Guidelines for the treatment of bipolar disorder can be complex and change frequently as new medications and indications are introduced. Table 15-15 outlines the current treatment guidelines for the treatment of bipolar disorder. Figure 15-3 details scenarios in which the MTM provider may need to seek emergency treatment for those with bipolar disorder.

TABLE 15-10 • Questions to Anticipate from Patients Regarding Bipolar Disorder

What is bipolar disorder?

A condition in which people go back and forth between periods of a very good or irritable mood and depression. The "mood swings" between mania and depression can be very quick.

How often can I switch from mania to depression?

Everyone with bipolar disorder is different. Some people may experience only a couple of episodes in their entire life, while others may experience a couple of episodes every year.

What is manic-depressive disorder?

The term previously used to define bipolar disorder.

What causes bipolar disorder?

The exact cause of bipolar disorder is unknown, but it occurs more often in relatives of people with bipolar disorder. In most people, there is no clear cause for the manic or depressive episodes. However, the following events or conditions may trigger a manic episode in people with bipolar disorder: life changes such as childbirth, medications such as antidepressants or steroids, periods of sleeplessness, recreational drug use.

What health problems are associated with bipolar disorder?

Without prior treatment, complications from bipolar disorder can develop, such as alcohol and/or drug abuse; problems with relationships, work, and finances; and suicidal thoughts and behaviors.

How do I know if I have bipolar disorder?

Many factors are involved in diagnosing bipolar disorder. Your healthcare provider may perform some or all of the following procedures to determine the appropriate diagnosis: (1) ask about your family medical history, such as whether anyone has bipolar disorder; (2) ask you about your mood swings and for how long you have had them; (3) perform an examination to look for other illnesses or medications that may be causing your symptoms; (4) order laboratory tests to check for thyroid problems or drug levels; (5) discuss your behavior with your family members; (6) obtain a medical history, including any medical problems you have and any medications you take; and/or (7) monitor your behavior and mood.

What medications can be used to treat bipolar disorder?

Your healthcare provider may first try to determine what might have triggered the mood episode and whether you need to be hospitalized for treatment. Typically, a mood stabilizer such as carbamazepine, lamotrigine, lithium, or valproic acid are used first line for the treatment of bipolar disorder. Other anticonvulsants may be tried according to your response and adverse effects experienced. Depending on the type of episode and severity, antipsychotic, antianxiety, or antidepressant medications may be added to control additional symptoms.

Can I stop my medications if I feel better?

This is not recommended. Most people who stop taking their medication because they feel better will end up having another episode. Continuing to take your medication will prevent future episodes. If you don't experience any episodes for a length of time, your provider may be able to decrease the dose of your medication or eliminate extra medications and maintain you on one medication.

What if I become pregnant while taking medications, should I stop taking them?

No, you should never stop taking medications without your clinician's instructions. Your physician may change your medications due to potentially negative effects from the medications on your baby. You should take a multivitamin supplement with folic acid, even if you aren't pregnant but could become pregnant, to help prevent any negative effects from your antiepileptic mood stabilizer medication.

When should I call my physician about my bipolar disorder?

You should call your physician if you are having any thoughts of death or suicide, experiencing severe symptoms of depression or mania, or if you have been diagnosed with bipolar disorder and your symptoms have returned or you are having any new symptoms.

What should I do if I experience an adverse reaction or have a question about my medications?

If you experience an adverse effect or have a question about your medications, continue your medications and call your physician or pharmacist, who will be able to evaluate the problem and make an alternate plan for you.

Whom can I contact to find out more about bipolar disorder?

Several organizations are available to provide you with more information on bipolar disorder:

Depression and Bipolar Support Alliance (DBSA)

www.dbsalliance.org

National Alliance on Mental Illness (NAMI)

www.nami.org

The Center for Patient Partnerships

www.patientpartnerships.org

Substance Abuse and Mental Health Services Administration (SAMHSA)

www.samhsa.gov

Why do I have to have my blood drawn while taking these medications?

Many of the medications used for the treatment of bipolar disorder may affect different chemicals in your blood or organs within your body, such as the kidney or liver. The blood levels are used to determine whether the medication is changing these chemicals or organs too much. Additionally, some of the medications have levels at which they work best. The blood is drawn to check the levels of medications in your blood.

Are there any medications that I don't have to take them every day?

Some of the antipsychotic medications are available in an injectable formulation, which allows for twice- or once-monthly injections of a medication instead of daily oral medications. Some of these medications are approved for the use of bipolar disorder, and your physician can decide with you whether one of these medications would be appropriate for you.

PERSONAL MEDICATION LIST FOR *(Insert patient's name, DOB: mm/dd/yyyy)*	
Medication: Lithium 300 mg	
How I use it: Take one capsule (300 mg) 3 times daily	
Why I use it: Controls mood	**Prescriber:** Smith
Date I started using it: 1/12/2013	**Date I stopped using it:** (*Leave blank for patient's notes*)
Why I stopped using it: (*Leave blank for patient's notes*)	
Medication: Risperdal (risperidone) 2 mg	
How I use it: Take one pill (2 mg) every morning and every evening	
Why I use it: Controls mood	**Prescriber:** Smith
Date I started using it: 12/4/2011	**Date I stopped using it:** (*Leave blank for patient's notes*)
Why I stopped using it: (*Leave blank for patient's notes*)	

FIGURE 15-1 Example personal medication list for bipolar disorder medications.

	DATE PREPARED: (*Insert date*)
What we talked about: You reported having some stomach upset following your dose of lithium. This is a very common side effect of lithium. There are several different options to help treat this, without changing the medication, since you state that you are feeling better.	
What I need to do: Here are some of the things you can do to help lessen the amount of stomach upset that you experience: • Take each dose of lithium with food. • If you still have stomach upset, take your entire dose of lithium at bedtime to prevent the stomach upset from occurring during the day. If you still have stomach upset, we can discuss switching your medication to an long-acting product.	**What I did and when I did it:** (*Leave blank for patient's notes*)
What we talked about: Need to remember to take my medications on time each day	
What I need to do: Here are some things that you can do to help yourself remember to take your medications: • Use a pillbox with multiple daily dosing holders. • Fill the box on a weekly basis. • Set an alarm on my watch, phone, or in the house to buzz when I should take my medication. • Tell a family member to remind me when to take my medications.	**What I did and when I did it:** (*Leave blank for patient's notes*)

FIGURE 15-2 Sample medication action plan for a patient with bipolar disorder.

TABLE 15-11 • Lifestyle Modifications for Management of Bipolar Disorder

Get adequate nutrition, sleep, and exercise, and practice stress reduction.
Obtain supportive counseling: individual or group, couples or family therapy, medication adherence counseling.
Generate coping skills for triggers for future manic or depressive episodes.
Eliminate alcohol and substances of abuse.
Minimize nicotine use and stop caffeine intake at least 8 hours prior to bedtime.
Avoid stressors or substances that precipitate an acute episode.

TABLE 15-12 • Medications for Management of Bipolar Disorder

Medication	Common/Serious Side Effects[a]	Blackbox Warnings/Contraindications	Pregnancy Category[b]
Lithium	Gastrointestinal distress, diarrhea, muscle weakness, lethargy, polydipsia with polyuria and nocturia, headache, memory impairment, confusion, poor concentration, fine hand tremor, nephrogenic diabetes insipidus, hypothyroidism, T-wave flattening or inversion, atrioventricular block, bradycardia, benign reversible leukocytosis, dermatologic effects, weight gain, sexual dysfunction, morphologic renal changes Toxicity—worsening in several key symptoms: Gastrointestinal, coordination, and cognition. Seizures, cardiac dysrhythmia, permanent neurologic impairments with ataxia and deficits in memory, and kidney damage can also occur	Toxicity is closely related to serum Li levels and can occur at doses close to therapeutic levels. Contraindications: Cardiovascular disease Concomitant use of diuretics Debilitation Dehydration Renal disease Sodium depletion	D

(*Continued*)

TABLE 15-12 • Medications for Management of Bipolar Disorder (*Continued*)

Medication	Common/Serious Side Effects[a]	Blackbox Warnings/Contraindications	Pregnancy Category[b]
Valproic acid, divalproex sodium	GI upset, sedation, unsteadiness, tremor, thrombocytopenia, alopecia, polycystic ovary-like syndrome, weight gain, menstrual cycle irregularities Acute hepatic failure, acute pancreatitis, hyperammonemia are rarer side effects	Hepatic failure Contraindications: Hepatic disease or significant hepatic dysfunction, hypersensitivity to valproic acid, urea cycle disorders	D
Carbamazepine	Diplopia, dizziness, drowsiness, nausea, unsteadiness, blood dyscrasias, rash, hyponatremia	Fatal dermatologic reactions- HLA-B*1502 genetic polymorphism especially in those of Asian descent Aplastic anemia Agranulocytosis Contraindications: Bone marrow depression, concomitant use of MAOI or within 14 days of discontinuing an MAOI, concomitant use of nefazodone, delavirdine, or other nonnucleoside reverse transcriptase inhibitors, hypersensitivity to carbamazepine or to any of the tricyclic compounds	D
Oxcarbazepine	Sedation, dizziness, ataxia, nausea, rash, hyponatremia	Contraindications: Hypersensitivity to any component	C
Lamotrigine	Diplopia, dizziness unsteadiness, headache, rash	Warning: Serious, life-threatening rash Contraindications: Hypersensitivity to lamotrigine	C
Second-generation antipsychotics Aripiprazole Asenapine Brexpiprazole Cariprazine Iloperidone Lurasidone Olanzapine Olanzapine/fluoxetine Paliperidone Quetiapine Risperidone Ziprasidone	Dose-related extrapyramidal symptoms, increased prolactin, tardive dyskinesia, anticholinergic, lowering of seizure threshold, orthostatic hypotension, increased LFTs, sedation, weight gain, NMS, agranulocytosis, lipid abnormalities, glucose intolerance, QTc prolongation, myocarditis, sudden cardiac death	All second-generation antipsychotics: Elderly people with dementia-related psychosis treated with antipsychotic drugs are at an increased risk of death compared to placebo Quetiapine/aripiprazole/brexpiprazole: Can increase the risk of suicidal thinking and behavior in children, adolescents, and young adults Contraindications: *Ziprasidone*: Concomitant administration with QTc prolonging medications, heart failure, uncompensated hypersensitivity to ziprasidone, MI, acute and recent QT prolongation, including congenital long QT syndrome *Lurasidone*: Coadministration with strong CYP3A4 inducers and coadministration with strong CYP3A4 inhibitors	All are category C, except lurasidone and clozapine which are B
Selective serotonin reuptake inhibitors (SSRIs) Citalopram Escitalopram Fluoxetine Fluvoxamine Paroxetine Sertraline	Gastrointestinal, sexual dysfunction, headache, insomnia, discontinuation syndrome, serotonin syndrome, SIADH	Increased risk of suicidal thinking and behavior in children, adolescents, and young adults Contraindications: *All SSRIs*: Concomitant use with an MAOI, including linezolid or IV methylene blue, or use within 14 days of discontinuation of an MAOI, concomitant use with pimozide *Fluoxetine/paroxetine*: Concomitant use with thioridazine *Sertraline*: Concomitant use with disulfiram	All are category C except paroxetine, which is category D

(*Continued*)

TABLE 15-12 • Medications for Management of Bipolar Disorder (*Continued*)

Medication	Common/Serious Side Effects[a]	Blackbox Warnings/Contraindications	Pregnancy Category[b]
Serotonin norepinephrine reuptake inhibitors (SNRIs) Desvenlafaxine Duloxetine Levomilnacipran Venlafaxine	Nausea, sexual dysfunction, activation, dose-related increase in blood pressure, decreased appetite, increased sweating, serotonin syndrome, SIADH	Increased risk of suicidal thinking and behavior in children, adolescents, and young adults Contraindications: *All SNRIs*: Concomitant use with an MAOI, including linezolid or IV methylene blue, or use within 14 days of discontinuation of an MAOI *Duloxetine*: narrow-angle glaucoma, uncontrolled	All are category C
Tricyclic antidepressants Amitriptyline Clomipramine Doxepin Imipramine Desipramine Nortriptyline	Anticholinergic effects, orthostatic hypotension, cardiac conduction delays, serotonin syndrome	Increased risk of suicidal thinking and behavior in children, adolescents, and young adults Contraindications: *All*: Concomitant use with an MAOI, including linezolid or IV methylene blue, or use within 14 days of discontinuation of an MAOI MI, during the acute recovery period *Doxepin*: untreated narrow angle glaucoma, urinary retention, tendency toward urinary retention	All are category C
Others Bupropion Nefazodone Trazodone Mirtazapine Vilazodone Vortioxetine	*Bupropion*: Nausea, vomiting, tremor, insomnia, dry mouth, skin reactions, dose-related seizures, activation, agitation *Nefazodone/trazodone*: Orthostatic hypotension, sedation, cognitive slowing, dizziness, priapism, serotonin syndrome	Increased risk of suicidal thinking and behavior in children, adolescents, and young adults Contraindications: *All*: Concomitant use with an MAOI, including linezolid or IV methylene blue, or use within 14 days of discontinuation of an MAOI *Bupropion*: Abrupt discontinuation of alcohol or sedative Bulimia or anorexia, prior or current diagnosis Concomitant use of MAOI Seizure disorder *Nefazodone*: Treatment should not be initiated in individuals with active liver disease or with elevated baseline serum transaminases. Contraindications: Previous withdrawal of nefazodone due to evidence of liver injury, coadministration of carbamazepine, or coadministration with full doses of triazolam	All are category C

[a] This is a general list and does not include all side effects that can occur from these drugs. Consult a drug reference source for a more inclusive list before making any recommendations. MTM providers should also consult a comprehensive drug interaction database before making pharmacotherapy recommendations.

[b] Product labeling for all prescription drugs is being updated to reflect the new FDA Pregnancy Labeling and Lactation Rule. Please check individual product labeling for the most accurate and updated pregnancy information.

Abbreviations: GI = gastrointestinal; IV = intravenous(ly); LFT = liver function test; Li = lithium; MAOI = monoamine oxidase inhibitor; MI = myocardial infarction; NMS = neuroleptic malignant syndrome; SIADH = syndrome of inappropriate antidiuretic hormone.

TABLE 15-13 • Carbamazepine and Other Antiepilepsy Drug Elimination Pathways and Major Effects on Hepatic Enzymes

Antiepilepsy Drugs	Major Hepatic Enzymes	Renal Elimination (%)	Induced	Inhibited
Carbamazepine	CYP3A4; CYP1A2; CYP2C8	<1	CYP1A2; CYP2C; CYP3A; GT	None
Clobazam	CYP3A4; CYP2C19; CYP2B6	0	CYP3A4 (weak)	CYP2D6
Eslicarbazepine	Undergoes hydrolysis	<90% parent drug, >60% active metabolite	GT (mild)	CYP2C19
Ethosuximide	CYP3A4	12-20	None	None
Ezogabine	GT; acetylation	85	None	None
Felbamate	CYP3A4; CYP2E1; other	50	CYP3A4	CYP2C19; β-oxidation
Gabapentin	None	Almost completely	None	None
Lacosamide	CYP2C19	70	None	None
Lamotrigine	GT	10	GT	None
Levetiracetam	None (undergoes nonhepatic hydrolysis)	66	None	None
Oxcarbazepine (MHD is active oxcarbazepine metabolite)	Cytosolic system	1	CYP3A4; CYP3A5; GT	CYP2C19
		(27 as MHD)		
Perampanel	CYP3A4/5; CYP1A2; CYP2B6	Undefined	CYP3A4/5;GT	CYPA3A4/5
Phenobarbital	CYP2C9; other	25	CYP3A; CYP2C; GT	None
Phenytoin	CYP2C9; CYP2C19	5	CYP3A; CYP2C; GT	
Pregabalin	None	100	None	None
Rufinamide	Hydrolysis	2	CYP3A4 (weak)	CYP2E1 (weak)
Tiagabine	CYP3A4	2	None	None
Topiramate	Not known	70	CYP3A (dose dependent)	CYP2C19
Valproate	GT; β-oxidation	2	None	CYP2C9; GT epoxide hydrolase
Vigabatrin	None	Almost completely	CYP2C9	None
Zonisamide	CYP3A4	35	None	None

Abbreviations: CYP = cytochrome P450 isoenzyme system; GT = glucuronyl transferase.

Source: Data from references 25, 26, 27, 28, 29, 30, 31, 32, 33, and 34.

TABLE 15-14 • Herbal Supplements for Bipolar Disorder

Supplement	Use in Bipolar Disorder	Typical Dose	Effectiveness[a]	Cost[b]
St. John's wort	Depressive episodes	Starting dose of 300 mg 3 times daily and a maintenance dose of 300-600 mg daily	Likely Effective	$
Omega-3 fatty acids, fish oil, α-linolenic acid	Depressive episodes	Seven capsules twice daily (total daily dose of 6.2 g of eicosapentaenoic acid and 3.4 g of docosahexanoic acid) for 4 months with conventional therapy	Possibly Effective	$$
Folate	Depressive episodes	500 μg of folic acid or 15-50 mg of methylenetetrahydrofolate daily for 8 weeks to 6 months	Possibly effective	$
SAMe (S-adenosyl-L-methionine)	Depressive episodes	800-1600 mg daily for 6 weeks	Likely effective	$$$$

[a] Level of evidence: "likely effective"—this product has a very high level of reliable clinical evidence supporting its use for a specific indication. Products rated "likely effective" are generally considered appropriate to recommend; "possibly effective"—this product has some clinical evidence supporting its use for a specific indication; however, the evidence is limited by quantity, quality, or contradictory findings. Products rated "possibly effective" might be beneficial, but do not have enough high-quality evidence to be recommended for most people; "insufficient evidence" indicates that there is insufficient reliable scientific evidence to provide an effectiveness rating.

[b] Cost: $ = ≤$10/month supply in recommended dosage; $$ = $11-$20/month; $$$$ = >$50/month.

Source: References 35, 36, and 37.

TABLE 15-15 • Current Treatment Algorithm for Bipolar Disorder

<table>
<tr><th colspan="2">Acute Manic or Mixed Episode: General Guidelines</th><th colspan="2">Acute Depressive Episode</th></tr>
<tr><td colspan="2">Assess for secondary causes of mania or mixed states (eg, alcohol or drug use)
Discontinue antidepressants
Taper off stimulants and caffeine if possible
Treat substance abuse
Encourage good nutrition (with regular protein and essential fatty-acid intake), exercise, adequate sleep, stress reduction, and psychosocial therapy</td><td colspan="2">Assess for secondary causes of depression (eg, alcohol or drug use)
Taper off antipsychotics, benzodiazepines, or sedative-hypnotic agents if possible
Treat substance abuse
Encourage good nutrition (with regular protein and essential fatty-acid intake), exercise, adequate sleep, stress reduction, and psychosocial therapy</td></tr>
<tr><th>Hypomania</th><th>Mania</th><th>Mild to Moderate Depressive Episode</th><th>Severe Depressive Episode</th></tr>
<tr><td>First, optimize current mood stabilizer or initiate mood-stabilizing medication: lithium,[a] valproate,[a] carbamazepine,[a] or SGAs
Consider adding a benzodiazepine (lorazepam or clonazepam) for short-term adjunctive treatment of agitation or insomnia if needed
Alternative medication treatment options: oxcarbazepine
Second, if response is inadequate, consider a two-drug combination:
Lithium[a] plus an anticonvulsant or an SGA
Anticonvulsant plus an anticonvulsant or SGA</td><td>First, two- or three-drug combinations (lithium,[a] valproate,[a] or SGA) plus a benzodiazepine (lorazepam or clonazepam) and/or antipsychotic for short-term adjunctive treatment of agitation or insomnia; lorazepam is recommended for catatonia
Do not combine antipsychotics
Alternative medication treatment options: carbamazepine;[a] if patient does not respond or tolerate, consider oxcarbazepine
Second, if response is inadequate, consider a three-drug combination:
Lithium[a] plus an anticonvulsant plus an antipsychotic
Anticonvulsant plus an anticonvulsant plus an antipsychotic
Third, if response is inadequate, consider ECT for mania with psychosis or catatonia,[d] or add clozapine for treatment-refractory illness</td><td>First, initiate and/or optimize mood-stabilizing medication: lithium,[a] quetiapine, lurasidone
Alternative anticonvulsants: lamotrigine,[b] valproate;[a] antipsychotics: fluoxetine/olanzapine combination</td><td>First, optimize current mood stabilizer or initiate mood-stabilizing medication: lithium[a] or quetiapine or lurasidone
Alternative fluoxetine/olanzapine combination
If psychosis is present, initiate an antipsychotic in combination with above
Do not combine antipsychotics
Alternative anticonvulsants: lamotrigine,[b] valproate[a]
Second, if response is inadequate, consider carbamazepine[a] or adding antidepressant
Third, if response is inadequate, consider a three-drug combination:
Lithium plus lamotrigine[b] plus an antidepressant
Lithium plus quetiapine plus antidepressant[c]
Fourth, if response is inadequate, consider ECT for treatment-refractory illness and depression with psychosis or catatonia[d]</td></tr>
</table>

[a] Use standard therapeutic serum concentration ranges if clinically indicated; if partial response or breakthrough episode, adjust dose to achieve higher serum concentrations without causing intolerable adverse effects; valproate is preferred over lithium for mixed episodes and rapid cycling; lithium and/or lamotrigine is preferred over valproate for bipolar depression.

[b] Lamotrigine is not approved for the acute treatment of depression, and the dose must be started low and slowly titrated up to decrease adverse effects if used for maintenance therapy of bipolar I disorder. Lamotrigine may be initiated during acute treatment with plans to transition to this medication for long-term maintenance. A drug interaction and a severe dermatologic rash can occur when lamotrigine is combined with valproate (ie, lamotrigine doses must be halved from standard dosing titration).

[c] Controversy exists concerning the use of antidepressants, and they are often considered third-line in treating acute bipolar depression, except in patients with no recent history of severe acute mania or potentially in bipolar II patients.

[d] ECT is used for severe mania or depression during pregnancy and for mixed episodes; prior to treatment, anticonvulsants, lithium, and benzodiazepines should be tapered off to maximize therapy and minimize adverse effects.

Abbreviations: ECT = electroconvulsive therapy; SGA = second-generation antipsychotic.

Source: Data from references 2, 38, and 39.

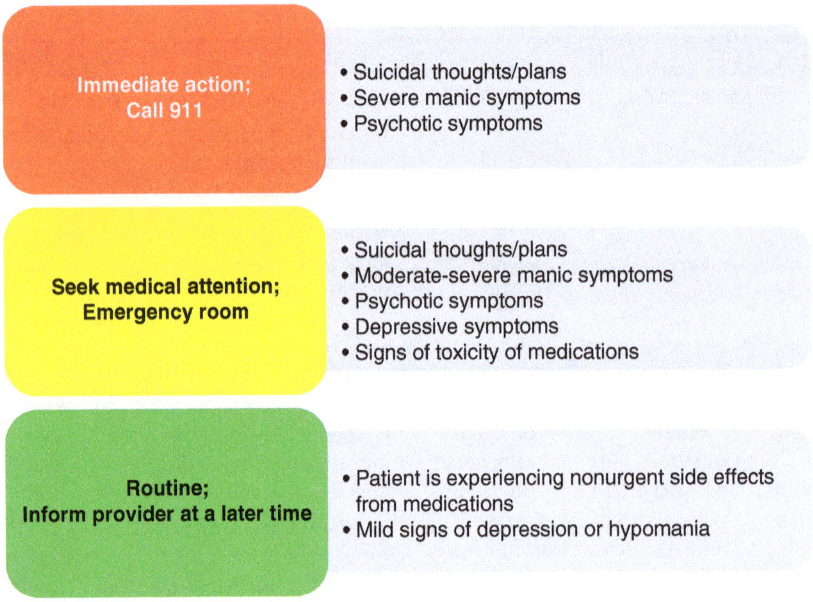

FIGURE 15-3 Referral for management of bipolar disorder.

CORE ELEMENT 5—DOCUMENTATION AND FOLLOW-UP

Clear and concise documentation of MRPs and recommendations by the MTM provider is a key component of the MTM consult. Examples of potential MRPs in patients with bipolar disorder are provided in Table 15-16. Sample communications and recommendations to clinicians to address MRPs are found in Figure 15-4. Recommendations should be communicated to the provider via fax, telephone, email, or notes written into the medical chart. Each of these methods should be a secure method to protect the private health information that it contains. Actual communications and recommendations to providers should be individualized according to the type of recommendation, the specific characteristics of the patient's case, and the nature of the relationship with the provider.

The development of a therapeutic alliance is key in monitoring the symptoms of bipolar disorder, promoting adherence, and minimizing adverse reactions and drug interactions. The evaluation of outcomes (ie, therapeutic drug monitoring, symptom management, and side effect minimization) requires regular monitoring. More frequent visits (eg, weekly during a drug titration or taper period, or every 3 to 6 months during maintenance phases), telephone calls, and intensive outpatient programs may be needed to prevent rehospitalization. Patients and family members should be actively involved with the treatment and should be educated to monitor symptoms, treatment adherence, and adverse effects.[2]

TABLE 15-16 • Medication-Related Problems (MRPs) in Patients with Bipolar Disorder

MRP Category	Example of MRP
Nonadherence	Suboptimal control of depressive symptoms because of nonadherence with medication and psychotherapy Patient not taking medication because of adverse effects of nausea/vomiting
Unnecessary medication	Patient experienced a manic episode and was placed on an antipsychotic medication along with a mood stabilizer; after recovering from the episode, the medication regimen was not reevaluated and the patient is still receiving the antipsychotic medication
Need for additional medication	Patient still experiencing depressive symptoms after starting a mood stabilizer Patient still experiencing symptoms of insomnia after starting a mood stabilizer
Ineffective medication	Adequate trial of a new mood stabilizer without significant clinical response Monotherapy with an antidepressant without a mood stabilizer for depressive symptoms
Dosage too low	Suboptimal mood stabilization because of a low dose of a mood stabilizer (eg, lithium level of 0.2 mEq/L)
Dosage too high	Patient experiences signs of toxicity of lithium (eg, nausea/vomiting, coarse tremor, lithium level 1.2 mEq/L)
Adverse drug reaction	Rash from lamotrigine Patient not taking valproic acid because of nausea/vomiting (could also be classified under nonadherence)

Scenario: Patient prescribed valproic acid capsules, experiencing nausea/vomiting **MRP:** Nonadherence
Assessment: Patient with hypomanic symptoms started on valproic acid 500 mg twice daily. Patient experiencing upset stomach and nausea at each dosing interval. Switching patient from valproic acid capsules to divalproex sodium would provide a delayed-release product, which is associated with less nausea/vomiting. **Plan:** Consider discontinuation of valproic acid capsules and addition of divalproex sodium 500 mg twice daily with titration to a therapeutic dose.
Scenario: Patient prescribed lithium 3 months ago, has not had any follow-up blood monitoring **MRP:** Potential adverse event (need for monitoring)
Assessment: Patient currently on lithium 450 mg twice daily without follow-up laboratory monitoring. Patient would benefit from continued follow-up monitoring to verify whether appropriate blood levels of lithium have been obtained and adverse effects from lithium are not occurring. **Plan:** Recommend ordering a trough lithium level, basic metabolic panel, and a thyroid panel for the patient at this time. Every 6 months the patient should have a thyroid panel and basic metabolic panel. Lithium levels should be obtained as needed.
Scenario: Depressed patient currently taking lithium 900 mg twice daily, with a blood level of 0.8 mEq/L. **MRP:** Need for additional therapy
Assessment: Patient is still experiencing depressive symptoms, even with a therapeutic dose of lithium. An additional medication may help alleviate the residual depressive symptoms. **Plan:** Consider initiation of lamotrigine 25 mg daily or an antidepressant such as citalopram 20 mg daily for this patient. If symptoms worsen, consider hospitalization for change in therapy.
Scenario: Patient on lamotrigine 25 mg daily for 3 weeks, with residual depressive symptoms **MRP:** Ineffective medication
Assessment: Patient has been taking lamotrigine 25 mg daily for 3 weeks and is still experiencing depressive symptoms. Patient would benefit from an increase in dosage. **Plan:** Recommend increasing the dose of lamotrigine to 50 mg daily for 2 weeks, then to 100 mg daily for one week, then to 200 mg daily. Patient to monitor depressive symptoms and follow-up in 1 week.

FIGURE 15-4 Sample provider communications for bipolar disorder.

REFERENCES

1. American Psychiatric Association. *Diagnostic and Statistical Manual of Mental Disorders*, 5th ed. Arlington VA: American Psychiatric Association; 2013; 123-169.
2. American Psychiatric Association. Practice guideline for the treatment of patients with bipolar disorder (revision). *Am J Psychiatry*. 2002;159:1-50.
3. Ceide MF, Rosenberg PB. Brief manic episode after rituximab treatment of limbic encephalitis. *J Neuropsychiatry Clin Neurosci*. 2011;23(4):E8.
4. Chopra A, Tye SJ, Lee KH, et al. Underlying neurobiology and clinical correlates of mania status after subthalamic nucleus deep brain stimulation in Parkinson's disease: A review of the literature. *J Neuropsychiatry Clin Neurosci*. 2012;24(1):102-110.
5. Dias RS, Lafer B, Russo C, et al. Longitudinal follow-up of bipolar disorder in women with premenstrual exacerbation: Findings from STEP-BD. *Am J Psychiatry* 2011;168(4):386-394.
6. Goldsmith M, Singh M, Chang K. Antidepressants and psychostimulants in pediatric populations: Is there an association with mania? *Pediatr Drugs*. 2011;13(4):225-243.
7. Habek M, Brian M, Brian VV, et al. Psychiatric manifestations of multiple sclerosis and acute disseminated encephalomyelitis. *Clin Neurol Neurosurg*. 2006;108(3):290-294.
8. Navines R, Castellvi P, Sola R, Martin-Santos R. Peginterferon-and-ribavirin-induced bipolar episode successfully treated with lamotrigine without discontinuation of antiviral therapy. *Gen Hosp Psychiatry*. 2008;30(4):387-389.
9. Plante DT, Winkelman JW. Sleep disturbance in bipolar disorder: Therapeutic implications. *Am J Psychiatry*. 2008;165(7):830-843.
10. Santos CO, Caeiro L, Ferro JM, Figueira ML. Mania and stroke: A systematic review. *Cerebrovasc Dis*. 2011;32(1):11-21.
11. Spiegel DS, Weller AL, Pennell K, et al. The successful treatment of mania due to acquired immunodeficiency syndrome using ziprasidone: A case series. *J Neuropsychiatry Clin Neurosci*. 2010;22(1):111-114.
12. Valenti M, Pacciarotti I, Bonnin CM, et al. Risk factors for antidepressant-related switch to mania. *J Clin Psychiatry*. 2012;73(2):e271-e276.
13. Patten SB, Barbui C. Drug-induced depression: A systematic review to inform clinical practice. *Psychother Psychosom*. 2004;73(4):207-215.
14. Botts S, Ryan M. Depression. *Drug-Induced Diseases: Prevention, Detection, and Management*, 2nd ed. Bethesda, MD: American Society of Health-System Pharmacists; 2010.
15. Goldberg JF, Harrow M, eds. *Bipolar Disorders: Clinical Course and Outcome*. Washington, DC: American Psychiatric Press; 1999.
16. Post RM, Denicoff KD, Leverich GS, et al. Morbidity in 258 bipolar outpatients followed for 1 year with daily prospective ratings on the NIMH life chart method. *J Clin Psychiatry*. 2003;64:680-690.
17. Abreu LN, Lafer B, Baca-Garcia E, Oquendo MA. Suicidal ideation and suicide attempts in bipolar disorder type I: An update for the clinician. *Rev Bras Psiquiatr*. 2009;31:271-280.
18. Goodnick PJ, ed. *Mania: Clinical and Research Perspectives*. Washington, DC: American Psychiatric Press; 1998.

19. Suppes T, Dennehy EB, Hirschfeld RM, et al. The Texas implementation of medication algorithms: Update to the algorithms for treatment of bipolar I disorder. *J Clin Psychiatry*. 2005;66:870-886.
20. Sachs GS. Treatment-resistant bipolar depression. *Psychiatr Clin North Am.* 1996;19:215-224.
21. Hirschfeld RMA. The mood disorder questionnaire: A simple patient-rated screening instrument for bipolar disorder. *J Clin Psychiatry Primary Care Compan.* 2002;4:9-11.
22. Dennehy EB, Suppes T, Crismon ML, et al. Development of the brief bipolar disorder symptom scale for patients with bipolar disorder. *Psychiatry Res.* 2004;127:137-145.
23. Young RC, Biggs JT, Ziegler VE, et al. Young mania rating scale. In: *Handbook of Psychiatric Measures*. Washington, DC: American Psychiatric Association; 2000:540-542.
24. *Medicare Part D Medication Therapy Management Program Standardized Format.* Available at https://www.cms.gov/Medicare/Prescription-Drug-Coverage/PrescriptionDrugCovContra/Downloads/MTM-Program-Standardized-Format-English-and-Spanish-Instructions-Samples-v032712.pdf. Accessed May 5, 2017.
25. Engel J. Antiseizure drugs. In: *Seizures and Epilepsy*, 2nd ed. New York, NY: Oxford University Press; 2013:541-602.
26. Onfi [package insert]. Deerfield, IL: Lundbeck Inc.; October 2011.
27. Garnett WR, Bainbridge JL, Johnson SL. Ethosuximide. In: Murphy J, ed. *Clinical Pharmacokinetics*. Bethesda, MD: American Society of Health-System Pharmacists; 2008:153-159.
28. Felbatol [package insert]. Somerset, NJ: Meda Pharmaceuticals; July 2011.
29. Vimpat [package insert]. Smyrna, GA: UCB, Inc.; August 2014.
30. Lamictal [package insert]. Research Triangle Park, NC: GlaxoSmithKline; May 2015.
31. Keppra [package insert]. Smyrna, GA: UCB, Inc.; September 2013.
32. Trileptal [package insert]. East Hanover, NJ. Novartis Pharmaceuticals; July 2014.
33. Fycompa [package insert]. Woodcliff Lake, NJ: Eisai Inc.; June 2015.
34. Dilantin [package insert]. New York, NY: Pfizer; April 2009.
35. Chiappedi M, Bejor M. Herbals and natural dietary supplements in psychiatric patients. *Recent Patents on CNS Drug Discovery* 2010;5:164-171.
36. Chiappedi M, de Vincenzi S, Bejor M. Nutraceuticals in psychiatric practice. *Recent Patents on CNS Drug Discovery* 2012;7:163-172.
37. Natural Medicines [database online]. Somerville, MA: Therapeutic Research Center; 2017. Report available at https://naturalmedicines.therapeuticresearch.com/. Accessed May 11, 2017.
38. Miklowitz DJ, Otto MW, Frank E, et al. Psychosocial treatments for bipolar depression: A 1- year randomized trial from the Systematic Treatment Enhancement Program. *Arch Gen Psychiatry*. 2007;64:419-427.
39. Yatham LN, Kennedy SH, Parkh SV, et al. Canadian Network for Mood and Anxiety Treatments (CANMAT) and International Society for Bipolar Disorders (ISBD) Collaboration update of CANMAT guidelines for the management of patients with bipolar disorder: Update 2013. *Bipolar Disord.* 2013;15:1-44.

Review Questions

1. A patient experiencing five episodes of bipolar disorder in one year should be classified by which of the following diagnostic criteria?
   a. Bipolar disorder type I
   b. Bipolar disorder type II
   c. A mixed specifier
   d. Rapid cycling

2. Which of the following rating scales would be useful as a screening tool to detect symptoms of bipolar disorder?
   a. Mood Disorder Questionnaire
   b. Brief Bipolar Disorder Symptom Scale
   c. Young Mania Rating Scale
   d. Hamilton Rating Scale for Depression

3. Which of the following is the primary goal for the treatment of bipolar disorder?
   a. Reduce the severity of acute attacks.
   b. Minimize adverse effects.
   c. Maximize adherence with therapy.
   d. Treat comorbid substance abuse.

4. Which of the following terms could be described as a mild degree of mania?
   a. Depression
   b. Euthymia
   c. Hypomania
   d. Cyclothymia

5. When developing a medication action plan for a patient to remember to take medications, which of the following techniques would be useful to include in the patient's "What I need to do" section?
   a. Decrease the number of medications that the patient takes to one per day.
   b. Use and fill a pillbox on a weekly basis to track missed doses.
   c. Carry all medications in one pill vial for less confusion.
   d. Increase the number of times per day that the patient takes a medication.

6. A patient is experiencing gastrointestinal upset following an increase in dosage of valproic acid over the past week. Which of the following is the most appropriate course of action?
   a. Refer the patient to the emergency room because of potential dehydration.
   b. Discontinue the use of valproic acid.
   c. Consider a switch from valproic acid to divalproex sodium.
   d. Provide the patient with a prescription for ondansetron.

7. A euthymic patient with bipolar disorder type I is receiving citalopram and lithium after a depressive episode 8 months ago. The use of citalopram in this patient would be classified in which of the following medication-related problem types?
   a. Nonadherence
   b. Need for additional medication
   c. Unnecessary medication
   d. Need for additional monitoring

For questions 8-10 please use the following case:

A 34-year-old white female has a 10-year history of bipolar disorder, type I. She currently takes the following medications:

Divalproex sodium 750 mg twice daily
Lurasidone 40 mg daily
Escitalopram 20 mg daily
Trazodone 50 mg daily as needed for sleep

Labs:

VPA level: 65 μg/L
LFTs: within normal limits (WNL)
CBC: WNL
Thyroid: WNL

Current mood: some depression, no energy, inability to concentrate

8. The patient presents with a prescription today for lamotrigine 25 mg daily. Which of the following is the most appropriate recommendation prior to dispensing the lamotrigine to this patient?
   a. No changes are needed. Fill the prescription as written.
   b. Increase the lamotrigine from 25 mg daily to 50 mg daily.
   c. Decrease the lamotrigine from 25 mg daily to 25 mg every other day.
   d. Decrease the divalproex sodium from 750 mg twice daily to once daily.

9. You have identified that this patient is missing another medication. Which of the following medications would be the most appropriate to recommend for this patient?
   a. Lithium 450 mg twice daily
   b. Zolpidem 10 mg at bedtime
   c. Levothyroxine 25 mcg daily
   d. Folic acid 1 mg daily

10. This patient is experiencing symptoms of increased energy and quick speech. She is not sleeping at night and is spending time surfing the internet to buy all new things for her house. Which of the following medications is most likely contributing to these symptoms?
   a. Divalproex sodium
   b. Lamotrigine
   c. Escitalopram
   d. Lurasidone

ANSWERS

1. d	2. a	3. a
4. c	5. b	6. c
7. c	8. c	9. d
10. c		

16

Chronic Kidney Disease MTM Data Set

Katie E. Cardone, PharmD, BCACP, FNKF, FASN

KEY POINTS

- Estimating kidney function is essential for drug dosing, staging kidney disease, and screening for complications. Creatinine-based estimation equations are commonly used for these purposes.
- Slowing progression of chronic kidney disease (CKD) is important to reduce risk of end-stage kidney disease, dialysis, cardiovascular complications, and other CKD-related conditions.
- Patients with CKD tend to have numerous medications prescribed by multiple practitioners. Medication reconciliation is therefore an essential Medicare Therapy Management (MTM) service component for patients with CKD.
- Hospital admissions and readmissions are frequent for patients with CKD. Discharge counseling and educational interventions are important strategies for improving medication use in patients with kidney disease.

INTRODUCTION TO CHRONIC KIDNEY DISEASE

Chronic kidney disease (CKD) is a significant public health concern, affecting nearly 15% of the U.S. population.[1] It is progressive and may ultimately lead to end-stage renal disease (ESRD) requiring dialysis or transplantation. The Kidney Disease Outcomes Quality Initiative clinical practice guideline defined CKD in 5 stages, spanning from normal glomerular filtration rate with structural damage (stage 1) to end-stage kidney disease (stage 5).[2] The staging was modified by the Kidney Disease Improving Global Outcomes (KDIGO) group to include a notation of cause of CKD, glomerular filtration rate (GFR), and amount of albuminuria.[3] Table 16-1 describes the staging further. For example, a patient who has diabetic kidney disease with a GFR 35 mL/min/1.73m^2 and a urinary albumin to creatinine ratio of 400 mg/g would be staged as follows: diabetic kidney disease, G3b, A3.

CKD is often the result of another underlying condition. Diabetes mellitus is the leading cause of CKD, and hypertension is the second most common cause. Therefore, management of CKD involves treatment of the underlying condition.[1] Efforts should be taken to prevent progression of CKD and identify and treat complications of kidney disease. As CKD progresses, complications such as anemia, mineral and bone disorders, hypertension, hyperkalemia, edema, and acid-base disorders may develop.[4] Cardiovascular disease is also highly prevalent and is the leading cause of death in CKD.[1] A high medication burden is typically required to treat the multiple conditions and complications in these patients.[5] Once a patient is on dialysis, the average patient takes 12 home medications, putting him/her at especially high risk for medication-related problems (MRPs).[5] Therefore, medication management and education are of utmost importance in the management of CKD and ESRD.

Because of the high frequency of MRPs, patients with CKD are an ideal population for MTM services. Additionally, patients with ESRD qualify for Medicare benefits regardless of age.[6] Therefore, a large proportion of them will receive benefits from a Medicare part D plan.[1] In 2013, the Centers for Medicare & Medicaid Services (CMS) added ESRD as one of core chronic conditions that Part D plans may use to target beneficiaries for MTM services.[7] Currently, ESRD is a targeted condition by over 15% of Medicare-sponsored MTM programs.[8] Because patients with CKD, particularly those with ESRD, are frequently hospitalized, preventing readmissions becomes an important target for the MTM provider.[1] In addition, since the End-Stage Renal

TABLE 16-1 • Staging of Chronic Kidney Disease

GFR Category[b]	
G1[a]	≥90
G2[a]	60-89
G3a	45-59
G3b	30-44
G4	15-29
G5	<15
Albuminuria Category[c]	
A1	<30
A2	30-300
A3	>300

[a] Kidney damage must be present to have CKD stage G1 or G2.

[b] mL/min/1.73m².

[c] Albumin excretion rate in mg urinary albumin/24 hours or albumin to creatinine ratio in mg urinary albumin per g urinary creatinine.

TABLE 16-2 • Equations for the Estimation of Creatinine Clearance and GFR in Adults with Stable Renal Function

Cockroft and Gault[13]	Men: $CL_{cr} = (140 - age)\ ABW/(S_{cr} \times 72)$ Women: $CL_{cr} \times 0.85$
Jelliffe[14]	Men: $CL_{cr} = (100/S_{cr}) - 12$ Women: $CL_{cr} = (80/S_{cr}) - 7$
Jelliffe[15]	Men: $CL_{cr} = 98 - [0.8\ (age - 20)]/S_{cr}$ Women: $CL_{cr} \times 0.9$
Mawer et al[16]	Men: IBW $[29.3 - (0.203 \times age)]$ $[1 - (0.03 \times S_{cr})]/(14.4 \times S_{cr})$ Women: IBW $[25.3 - (0.175 \times age)]$ $[1 - (0.03 \times S_{cr})]/(14.4 \times S_{cr})$
Hull et al[17]	Men: $CL_{cr} = [(145 - age)/S_{cr}] - 3$ Women: $Cl_{cr} \times 0.85$
Levey et al (MDRD6)[18]	$GFR = 170 \times (S_{cr})^{-0.999} \times [age]^{-0.176} \times$ [0.762 if patient is female] × [1.180 if patient is Black] × $[SUN]^{-0.170} \times [Alb]^{0.318}$
Levey et al (MDRD4)[18]	$GFR = 186 \times (S_{cr})^{-1.154} \times [age]^{-0.203} \times$ [0.742 if patient is female] × [1.210 if patient is Black]
Levey et al (MDRD4-IDMS)[18]	$GFR = 175 \times (S_{cr})^{-1.154} \times [age]^{-0.203} \times$ [0.742 if patient is female] × [1.210 if patient is Black]
Levey et al (CKD-EPI)[19]	$GFR = 141 \times \min(S_{cr}/\kappa, 1)^{\alpha} \times \max(S_{cr}/\kappa, 1)^{-1.209} \times 0.993^{Age} \times 1.018$ [if patient is female] × 1.159 [if patient is Black]
Rule et al (MCQ)[20]	$GFR = \exp[1.911 + (5249/S_{cr}) - (2.114/S_{cr}{}^{2}) - 0.00686 \times Age - 0.205$ (if female)]

κ is 0.7 for women and 0.9 for men, α is –0.329 for women and –0.411 for men; min indicates the minimum of S_{cr}/κ or 1, and max indicates the maximum of S_{cr}/κ or 1. (If S_{cr} <0.8 mg/dL, use 0.8 for S_{cr}.)

Abbreviations: ABW = actual body weight; Alb = serum albumin concentration (g/dL); CL_{cr} = creatinine clearance in mL/min; GFR = glomerular filtration rate; IBW = ideal body weight (kg); S_{cr} = serum or plasma creatinine (mg/dL); SUN = serum urea nitrogen concentration (mg/dL).

Source: From Table 50-5 in DiPiro JT, Talbert RL, Yee GC, Matzke GR, Wells BG, Posey LM, Schwinghammer T, eds. *Pharmacotherapy: A Pathophysiological Approach.* 8th ed. New York: McGraw-Hill; 2011.

Disease Prospective Payment System (PPS, aka "the Bundle") was implemented in dialysis units in 2011, medication use patterns have changed in recent years, and adherence and quality of care have become even more important.[9] The "Bundle" pays a composite rate for dialysis services, with no additional payment for injectable ESRD-related medications and their oral equivalents. This has thus contributed to increased vigilance and a reduction in the use of expensive ESRD medication such as erythropoiesis stimulating agents. Additional oral medications are slated to be added to the "Bundle" in 2024.[10] It is expected that this change will further affect prescribing patterns and will further warrant MTM services. In addition to the ESRD PPS, a value-based purchasing program was implemented in dialysis facilities, which also affects medication management and MTM services in this population. The ESRD Quality Incentive Program (QIP) is the first federally funded pay-for-performance program, with quality measures that change annually.[11] The MTM provider should be familiar with these measures, as they may be logical targets for the MTM provider. For example, one current measure is hypercalcemia, where more cases lead to a lower quality score. The MTM provider might therefore include an evaluation of the patient's serum calcium and medications that might contribute to hypercalcemia (eg, calcium-based phosphate binders or vitamin D).

Assessing Kidney Function

As an MTM provider, assessment of kidney function is necessary to evaluate drug dosing, identify rate of GFR decline, and assess risk for CKD complications (ie, anemia, mineral and bone disorders (MBD), etc). Creatinine alone should not be used to evaluate kidney function; however, trends in creatinine or acute rises in serum creatinine may be useful in the clinical evaluation of the patient and may assist in recognizing acute kidney injury. Measuring GFR is rarely done in practice. Measuring creatinine clearance with a timed urine collection is occasionally used in the outpatient setting; however, use of estimation equations is much more common. Many equations have been used to estimate kidney function, as described in Table 16-2.

For staging, the Modification of Diet in Renal Disease (MDRD) or the Chronic Kidney Disease Epidemiology Collaboration (CKD-EPI) equations that estimate glomerular filtration rate (eGFR) are recommended.[3] The Cockroft-Gault equation, used to calculate estimated creatinine clearance, is used principally for drug dosing, although other equations may be used.[21,22] Most package inserts of currently approved medications include dosing adjustment recommendations based on the Cockroft-Gault equation, and dosing adjustments based on eGFR estimates are beginning to appear within prescribing information.

While some aspects surrounding use of these equations is controversial within the nephrology community, it is important to remember that they all have limitations and represent only *estimates* of kidney function. Accuracy should be questioned in cases where a patient has an abnormal amount of muscle mass, either more or less than average. In patients who weigh less than ideal body weight, actual body weight should be used in the Cockroft-Gault equation. For patients who are morbidly obese, an alternative body weight descriptor should be used in the equation, for example, lean body weight.[23]

Risk Factors for CKD

The MTM pharmacist should be familiar with risk factors for CKD. Table 16-3 includes susceptibility and initiation factors for CKD. Many of these risk factors are nonmodifiable; however, patients at high risk may be undiagnosed and screening for CKD may be warranted. Medication use may be affected by CKD stage.

Preventing Progression of CKD

Once a patient has been diagnosed with CKD, delaying progression of the disease is important to limit complications of CKD, prevent cardiovascular events, and avoid dialysis. Progression factors are generally modifiable and become important targets for therapy in patients with CKD.[2] Blood pressure control is paramount for any patient with CKD to prevent both the progression of CKD and cardiovascular events.[24] Clinical practice guidelines are available for the management of blood pressure in CKD, most recently from the KDIGO group.[24] The KDIGO recommendations are summarized in Table 16-4. In addition to blood pressure reduction, ACE inhibitors and ARBs reduce proteinuria. For patients with proteinuria and hypertension, blood pressure should be the primary target, and ACEi and angiotensin receptor blocker (ARBs) are first-line agents in this case. ACEi or ARBs may also be used to treat proteinuria in patients without hypertension. In the treatment of proteinuria, doses toward the higher end of the dosing range may be required, but the patient should be maintained on the lowest effective dose to prevent both hypotension and hyperkalemia.

TABLE 16-3 • Risk Factors for Susceptibility to and Initiation of Chronic Kidney Disease

Clinical Factors
Diabetes
Hypertension
Obesity
Autoimmune diseases
Systemic infections
Urinary tract infections
Urinary stones
Lower urinary tract obstruction
Neoplasia
Family history of CKD
Recovery from acute kidney injury
Reduction in kidney mass
Exposure to certain drugs
Low birth weight
Sociodemographic Factors
Older age
US ethnic minority status: African American, American Indian, Hispanic, Asian, or Pacific Islander
Exposure to certain chemical and environmental conditions
Low income/education

Used with permission from Inker LA, Astor BC, Fox CH, et al. KDOQI US commentary on the 2012 KDIGO clinical practice guideline for the evaluation and management of CKD. *Am J Kidney Dis.* 2014;63:713-735.

TABLE 16-4 • KDIGO Recommendations for Blood Pressure Management in Patients with CKD (Nondialysis Dependent)

Diabetes Status	Albuminuria Status	BP Goal	First Line Medication
With or without diabetes	A1	≤140/90 mm Hg	No preferred agent
With or without diabetes	A2 or A3	≤130/80 mm Hg	ACE inhibitor or ARB

Source: Reference 24.

For people with diabetes, intensive blood glucose control is an important intervention to prevent progression of CKD.[25,26] The American Diabetes Association recommends an A1c target of below 7% in most people.[25] Maintaining A1c below 6.5% has been shown to prevent albuminuria in patients with diabetes and is therefore recommended in patients at low risk for hypoglycemia. The National Kidney Foundation's Kidney Disease Outcomes Quality Initiative (KDOQI) also recommends A1c maintenance around 7% to prevent microvascular complications, including diabetic kidney disease.[26]

Other Interventions

Smoking cessation, controlling lipids, and maintaining a healthy weight should also be stressed in patients with CKD.[4] Although the impact of these interventions on preventing progression is not as clear as blood pressure and glucose control, they are important for overall cardiovascular health. Protein restriction in predialysis stages of CKD is generally recommended to delay progression of CKD, although data for this intervention are also relatively weak.[21]

Nephrotoxins should be avoided in patients with preexisting CKD whenever possible. Patients should be counseled on avoiding nonsteroidal anti-inflammatory drugs (NSAIDs), especially those available over-the-counter. A list of common nephrotoxins can be found in Table 16-5.

The overall therapeutic goals of treating the patient with CKD are to prevent progression of CKD, and prevent or treat CKD-related complications, including cardiovascular disease. Additionally, the pharmacist should assist with dosage selection for medications used for any indication based on kidney function. Despite aggressive intervention, some patients' kidney function will decline, and dialysis may be necessary to extend life.

TABLE 16-5 • Drug-Induced Kidney Structural—Functional Alterations

Tubular Epithelial Cell Damage	**Glomerular Disease (*Cont.*)**
Acute tubular necrosis	Membranous disease
• Aminoglycoside antibiotics	• NSAIDs
• Radiographic contrast media	• Penicillamine
• Cisplatin, carboplatin	• Captopril
• Amphotericin B	Focal segmental glomerulosclerosis
• Cyclosporine, tacrolimus	• Pamidronate
• Adefovir, cidofovir, tenofovir	• Interferon-α and -β
• Pentamidine	• Lithium
• Foscarnet	• Sirolimus
• Zoledronate	• Anabolic steroids
Osmotic nephrosis	**Tubulointerstitial Disease**
• Mannitol	Acute allergic interstitial nephritis
• Dextran	• Penicillins
• IV immunoglobulin	• Ciprofloxacin
Hemodynamically Mediated Kidney Injury	• NSAIDs, cyclooxygenase-2 inhibitors
• Angiotensin-converting enzyme inhibitors	• Proton pump inhibitors
• Angiotensin II receptor blockers	• Loop diuretics
• Nonsteroidal anti-inflammatory drugs (NSAIDs)	Chronic interstitial nephritis
• Cyclosporine, tacrolimus	• Cyclosporine
• OKT3	• Lithium
Obstructive Nephropathy	• Aristolochic acid
Crystal nephropathy	Papillary necrosis
• Acyclovir	• NSAIDs, combined phenacetin, aspirin, and caffeine analgesics
• Sulfonamides	**Renal Vasculitis, Thrombosis, and Cholesterol Emboli**
• Indinavir	Vasculitis and thrombosis
• Foscarnet	• Hydralazine
• Methotrexate	• Propylthiouracil
Nephrolithiasis	• Allopurinol
• Sulfonamides	• Penicillamine
• Triamterene	• Gemcitabine
• Indinavir	• Mitomycin C
Nephrocalcinosis	Methamphetamines
• Oral sodium phosphate solution	• Cyclosporine, tacrolimus
Glomerular Disease	• Adalimumab
Minimal change disease	• Bevacizumab
• NSAIDs, COX-2 inhibitors	Cholesterol emboli
• Lithium	• Warfarin
• Pamidronate	• Thrombolytic agents
• Interferon-α and -β	

Source: From Table 46-1 in DiPiro JT, Talbert RL, Yee GC, Matzke GR, Wells BG, Posey L, eds. *Pharmacotherapy: A Pathophysiological Approach*. 10th ed. New York, NY: McGraw-Hill; 2017.

CORE ELEMENT 1—COMPREHENSIVE MEDICATION REVIEW FOR PATIENTS WITH CKD

The following section contains a list of suggested questions that might be used during a medication therapy review (Table 16-6). Plain language or "living room language" should generally be used during the medication review (Figure 16-1). However, health literacy levels vary, and there is a significant amount of training and education that patients receive once they are on dialysis. In many cases, patients know dialysis vernacular well. In addition, it is important to be prepared for questions from patients during the medication review (Figure 16-2).

CORE ELEMENT 2—PERSONAL MEDICATION LIST

Many patients with CKD have extensive medication lists including drugs from many prescribers. Medications may be administered in the physician's office or infusion clinic (ie, intravenous iron

TABLE 16-6 • Questions to Ask When Conducting a Medication Review in a Patient with Chronic Kidney Disease

Suggested Questions for Patients with CKD	
Medication Reconciliation • What medications do you take (prescription or over-the-counter)? • Do you use any herbals or supplements? • Do you ever take medication for pain, either prescription or over-the-counter? (To determine if NSAIDs are being used) • How often do you miss a dose of medication? • What physicians do you see? • What pharmacy or pharmacies do you use? • Do you have any allergies, or have you had bad reactions to any medications? **CKD History** • How long have you had kidney disease? • What caused your kidney disease? • Do any of your family members have kidney disease? • Have you ever had protein or blood in your urine? • Do you have a copy of your recent laboratory values? • Do you know what stage kidney disease you have? • Do you currently see a nephrologist/kidney physician? • Do you ever have edema/swelling in your legs, ankles or feet? • Do you ever have shortness of breath? • Have you ever been told your potassium is too high or too low? • Have you been hospitalized recently? If so, why? **Hypertension/CVD** (see also questions from Chapter 27, "Hypertension MTM Data Set") • What does your blood pressure typically run? Do you check your blood pressure at home? • How often does your blood pressure get too low? • What medications do you currently take for blood pressure? • (If not on an ACEi or ARB): Were you ever on a medication called an ACE inhibitor? Do you recall ever being on a blood pressure medication that caused a cough or swelling in your face? **Diabetes** (see also questions from Chapter 21, "Diabetes Mellitus MTM Data Set") • What medications do you use for diabetes? • Do you know your current A1c value?	• Do you check your blood sugar at home? • What is your blood sugar when you get up in the morning? • What is your blood sugar throughout the day or after you eat? • What do you do when your blood sugar is too low? **Lipids** (see also questions from Chapter 22, "Dyslipidemia MTM Data Set") • Do you take any medications for your cholesterol? **Vaccines** • Have you had your flu shot this year? • Have you ever had the pneumonia vaccine? • Have you had the hepatitis vaccine? • Have you had the shingles vaccine? **Anemia** • Do you take over-the-counter iron? • Do you get any medications for anemia? Some you might use at home as an injection, or you might go to the physician's office to get it there. • Have you ever been told you have anemia? • Have you ever had a blood transfusion? **CKD Mineral and Bone Disorder** • Do you take a phosphate binder? Which one? • How often do you miss a dose of phosphate binder? • Are you taking vitamin D? (either over-the-counter or prescription) **Additional Questions for Patients on Hemodialysis** • How much weight do you usually gain between dialysis sessions? • Do you still urinate? • How do you take your medications on nondialysis days? Is it different on dialysis days? • Do you get dialysis through a fistula, graft, or catheter? • Does your blood pressure ever get too low during dialysis? • Do you work? **Additional Questions for Patients on Peritoneal Dialysis** • What dialysate do you use? • What is your dialysis regimen like? Do you use a cycler at night? • Have you ever had an infection of your peritoneal membrane (peritonitis)?
Questions to Ask for Prevention/Assessment of Medical Emergencies	
Crisis planning • Have you ever been hospitalized for your kidney disease or complications of kidney disease? • Have you ever been treated for high potassium? • Have you ever needed a blood transfusion to treat anemia? • What do you do if you experience increasing shortness of breath?	**For patients on dialysis** • How often do you miss dialysis days? What is your plan if you are unable to make it to dialysis? • Have you ever had an infection following dialysis? How do you know if you have an infection?

or erythropoiesis stimulating agent), or may be received at dialysis. These medications should be reconciled and included in the medication list.

The following is an example personal medication list for a patient on dialysis in the Centers for Medicare & Medicaid Services' (CMS) standardized format (Figure 16-3).[28] Note that the list contains medications for the underlying cause of CKD, for complications of CKD, and other medications for comorbid diseases. Some patients may prefer a separate, single-page medication list in addition to this version that outlines which medications are to be dosed in the morning, afternoon, or evening, which are to be taken with meals, and which should be held prior to dialysis.

CORE ELEMENT 3—MEDICATION ACTION PLAN

The following are example medication action plans for patients with CKD (Figure 16-4) using the CMS standardized format.[28]

Acidosis—a build-up of acids in the body.

Anemia—low red blood cell count.

Anuria—no longer urinates (pees).

Arteriovenous fistula—a surgical connection between an artery and a vein that hemodialysis needles can be inserted into.

Arteriovenous graft—a connection between an artery and a vein that hemodialysis needles can be inserted into, made of a synthetic material.

Central venous catheter—a thin tube that is inserted into your body to help access the blood. The dialysis tubing would be attached to this tube when you get dialysis.

Dry weight—the goal weight after dialysis; the weight when there is not extra fluid in the body, nor too little fluid in the body.

Edema—swelling due to too much fluid.

End-stage renal disease—when the kidneys work very little and either dialysis or kidney transplant is required to live.

Erythropoiesis stimulating agent—a medication that tells the body to make more red blood cells.

Ferritin—a measure of how much iron is stored in the body.

Hematuria—blood in the urine.

Hemodialysis—procedure to remove extra fluid and toxins when the kidneys do not work; involves running the blood through tubing, through a filter, and then pumping the cleaned blood back to the body.

Hemoglobin—a molecule that carries oxygen in your blood. The concentration can be measured to see if you have anemia.

Hyperkalemia—high potassium.

Hyperparathyroidism—high parathyroid hormone (PTH); an indicator of bone health.

Hyperphosphatemia—high phosphorus.

Hypertension—high blood pressure.

Nephrologist—kidney physician.

Peritoneal dialysis—procedure to remove extra fluid and toxins when the kidneys do not work; involves putting dialysis fluid in the abdomen, keeping it there for some time, the replacing it.

Proteinuria—protein in the urine.

Renal—having to do with the kidney.

Transferrin saturation (TSAT)—a measure of iron in the body.

Ultrafiltration—the removal of fluid.

Vascular access—the way hemodialysis is connected to the body; could be AV fistula, graft or catheter.

FIGURE 16-1 Living Room language for CKD.

What health problems are associated with CKD?

CKD is usually caused by one of many different health conditions, most commonly from diabetes or high blood pressure. As kidney function worsens, patients are prone to certain complications such as high blood pressure that is difficult to control, anemia, and bone changes. If you have diabetes, you might notice that your blood sugars are lower. CKD also contributes to heart disease.

Why is it important to take my medications regularly?

Your regimen contains medications that are used to prevent worsening of your kidney function, some to treat complications of CKD and others to treat conditions not related to CKD. It is important to take your medications regularly to prevent worsening of kidney function and to treat any kidney-related complications. For example, if your blood pressure is not well controlled, then your kidney function might be lost faster than if it was kept controlled. Once your kidney function is very low, you may need dialysis to live.

What can happen if I stop taking my medications?

You take medications for several different conditions. If you stop taking your medications for the condition that caused your CKD, your kidney function would likely worsen faster than it would otherwise. You might also put yourself at risk for a serious medical problem. For example, if you stopped taking your diabetes medication, you could have become ill or need to be hospitalized for treatment of high blood sugar.

What should I do if I have a problem with my medications?

You should call your physician's office or pharmacist about specific problems with your medications. Some issues require changing medications and others do not. Some side effects from medications only last a short time while your body adjusts, while others may not go away.

Why do some of my medication doses need to be changed?

Your kidneys are responsible for removing some medications from your body. When your kidney function declines, some medications can build up. In that case, you would have more medication in your body than we would like. Sometimes this can lead to more side effects or can be dangerous. To prevent this, some medications require lower doses in patients with CKD.

How will my medications change as my kidneys get worse?

As your kidney function declines, you may notice that some of your medication doses change. You may need lower doses of some, and higher doses of others. You will probably see more medications added to your regimen. Blood pressure is sometimes more difficult to control and might require multiple medications. You might need a high dose water pill (diuretic) for fluid. You might also need new medications for anemia or bone health.

When should I dose my medications around dialysis?

That depends on the medication. Some medications are removed by dialysis and others are not. We can review each medication separately to see if it will be affected by the dialysis procedure. Sometimes people will need to adjust when they take their medications around dialysis. If your blood pressure tends to run low during dialysis, for example, your physician's might have you not take your blood pressure medication in the morning before dialysis treatment.

Why do I have to take phosphate binders?

Phosphorus is in many foods we eat. As your kidney function declines, your body is less able to remove that phosphorus. Extra phosphorus can combine with calcium and deposit in your arteries and veins where it can affect blood pressure control and heart disease risk.

If I miss a dose of phosphate binder, should I take it when I remember?

You should take your phosphate binders at mealtimes only. If you forget at mealtime, skip that dose, and resume at your next meal.

What medications can I take for pain?

Over-the-counter acetaminophen is usually best for occasional pain. You should avoid taking ibuprofen or naproxen. These can raise your blood pressure and could affect your kidney function.

FIGURE 16-2 Questions commonly asked by patients with chronic kidney disease.

PERSONAL MEDICATION LIST FOR *<Insert Member's name*, DOB: *mm/dd/yyyy>*

This medication list was made for you after we talked. We also used information from *<insert sources of information>*.

- Use blank rows to add new medications. Then fill in the dates you started using them.
- Cross out medications when you no longer use them. Then write the date and why you stopped using them.
- Ask your physicians, pharmacists, and other healthcare providers in your care team to update this list at every visit.

Keep this list up-to-date with:

- ☐ prescription medications
- ☐ over the counter drugs
- ☐ herbals
- ☐ vitamins
- ☐ minerals

If you go to the hospital or emergency department, take this list with you. Share this with your family or caregivers too.

DATE PREPARED: Month day, 20XX

Allergies or side effects: None reported

Medication: Prilosec 40 mg (omeprazole 40 mg capsule)	
How I use it: Take 1 capsule (40 mg) by mouth every day morning.	
Why I use it: Acid reflux	**Prescriber:** Dr. Mantey (primary physician)
Date I started using it:	**Date I stopped using it:**
Why I stopped using it:	

Medication: Toprol XL 50 mg (metoprolol succinate ER 50 mg tablet)	
How I use it: Take 1 tablet (50 mg) by mouth every day at bedtime.	
Why I use it: Blood pressure, heart failure and atrial fibrillation	**Prescriber:** Dr. Jones (cardiologist)
Date I started using it:	**Date I stopped using it:**
Why I stopped using it:	

Medication: Lipitor 20 mg (atorvastatin 20 mg tablet)	
How I use it: Take 1 tablet (20 mg) by mouth every evening.	
Why I use it: High cholesterol	**Prescriber:** Dr. Jones (cardiologist)
Date I started using it:	**Date I stopped using it:**
Why I stopped using it:	

Medication: Coumadin 5 mg (warfarin 5 mg tablet)	
How I use it: Take 1 tablet by mouth daily.	
Why I use it: Blood thinner (for atrial fibrillation)	**Prescriber:** Dr. Jones (cardiologist)
Date I started using it:	**Date I stopped using it:**
Why I stopped using it:	

Medication: Lantus Solostar Pen 100 units/mL (insulin glargine)	
How I use it: Inject 22 units subcutaneously at bedtime.	
Why I use it: Long-acting insulin for diabetes	**Prescriber:** Dr. Ramirez (endocrinologist)
Date I started using it:	**Date I stopped using it:**
Why I stopped using it:	

Medication: Novolog FlexPen 100 units/mL (insulin aspart)	
How I use it: Inject 8 units subcutaneously at mealtimes.	
Why I use it: Mealtime insulin for diabetes	**Prescriber:** Dr. Ramirez (endocrinologist)
Date I started using it:	**Date I stopped using it:**
Why I stopped using it:	

Medication: Renvela 800 mg tablet (sevelamer carbonate 800 mg)	
How I use it: Take 3 tablets (2400 mg) 3 times a day with meals.	
Why I use it: Phosphate binder to lower phosphorus	**Prescriber:** Dr. Dan (nephrologist)
Date I started using it:	**Date I stopped using it:**
Why I stopped using it:	

FIGURE 16-3 Example personal medication list for a patient with chronic kidney disease.

Medication: Lasix 80 mg (furosemide 80 mg tablet)	
How I use it: Take 1 tablet by mouth in the morning of nondialysis days.	
Why I use it: Water pill to remove extra fluid	**Prescriber:** Dr. Dan (nephrologist)
Date I started using it:	**Date I stopped using it:**
Why I stopped using it:	
Medication: Nephro-Vite tablet	
How I use it: Take 1 tablet by mouth daily.	
Why I use it: daily vitamin	**Prescriber:** Dr. Dan (nephrologist)
Date I started using it:	**Date I stopped using it:**
Why I stopped using it:	
Medication: Hectorol Injection (doxercalciferol injection)	
How I use it: This medicine is given to you at dialysis. Your dose changes are made based on a protocol.	
Why I use it: Vitamin D supplement	**Prescriber:** Dr. Dan (nephrologist)
Date I started using it:	**Date I stopped using it:**
Why I stopped using it:	
Medication: Venofer Injection (iron sucrose injection)	
How I use it: This medicine is given to you at dialysis. Your dose changes are made based on a protocol. Your current dose is 100 mg IV once a week.	
Why I use it: Iron supplement for anemia	**Prescriber:** Dr. Dan (nephrologist)
Date I started using it:	**Date I stopped using it:**
Why I stopped using it:	
Medication: Epogen injection (epoetin alfa injection)	
How I use it: This medicine is given to you at dialysis. Your dose changes are made based on a protocol. Your current dose is 6000 units IV three times a week.	
Why I use it: Anemia	**Prescriber:** Dr. Dan (nephrologist)
Date I started using it:	**Date I stopped using it:**
Why I stopped using it:	
Other Information: Primary care physician: Dr. Mantey Nephrologist (kidney physician): Dr. Dan Endocrinologist (physician you see for diabetes): Dr. Ramirez Cardiologist (heart physician): Dr. Jones	
If you have any questions about your medication list, call Katie Cardone, PharmD at 555-5555, M-F 8:30-5 pm.	

FIGURE 16-3 (*Continued*)

	DATE PREPARED: *<Insert date>*
What we talked about: Low blood sugar: When your blood sugar is too low, you are currently using orange juice to bring your sugar up. We talked about avoiding orange juice because it has a lot of potassium.	
What I need to do: Instead of drinking orange juice when my sugar is low, take 4 glucose tablets.	**What I did and when I did it:**
What we talked about: Pain reliever: You mentioned that you take naproxen over-the-counter when you have body aches or headaches. We discussed that naproxen may be bad for your heart and could harm your remaining kidney function.	
What I need to do: Use acetaminophen 500 mg 1 to 2 tablets every 4-6 hours if needed. Avoid over-the-counter products like ibuprofen and naproxen sodium.	**What I did and when I did it:**
What we talked about: Phosphate binder: You mentioned that you often forget to take your phosphate binder when you go out to eat.	
What I need to do: Ask my pharmacist for an extra, labeled prescription vial in a small size that I can put a few doses in and carry in my purse for when I am out. This way I will not need to carry the large bottle with you.	**What I did and when I did it:**
What we talked about: Blood pressure: You mentioned that you have a blood pressure kit at home, but do not use it on a regular basis.	
What I need to do: Try to check my blood pressure at home on your nondialysis days. Share this number with my physician. The blood pressures I take at home are important in helping the physician adjust my medications.	**What I did and when I did it:**

FIGURE 16-4 Example medication action plan for a patient with chronic kidney disease.

CORE ELEMENT 4—INTERVENTION AND/ OR REFERRAL

Nonpharmacologic Interventions

Interventions that are necessary in CKD include many nonpharmacologic recommendations. Among the most important are dietary changes.

Potassium. Hyperkalemia is an important complication for patients with CKD and contributes to high rates of sudden cardiac death. Avoidance of excess potassium should be stressed. Many foods contain a high concentration of potassium. Some common ones are listed in Table 16-7.

Phosphorus. Limiting phosphorus intake is generally recommended in patients with advanced kidney disease either as monotherapy or in combination with phosphate binder medications. Phosphorus is found in many foods, especially in those high in protein. Thus, phosphorus restriction may be difficult for patients who are instructed to increase protein intake while limiting phosphorus, which is common for patients on dialysis. Working closely with a dietitian may be helpful in this case. Common foods high in phosphorus include beans, peas, nuts, cola, dairy products, and whole grain breads.[30] Additionally, phosphate-containing solutions are often used in processed meats. The packages of these products typically say "moist and tender," "tender and juicy," or "extra tender."

TABLE 16-7 • Foods That Are High in Potassium

High Content (>250 mg)	Very High Content (>500 mg)
Kidney beans, cooked	Potato, baked, flesh, and skin
Lentils, cooked	Sweet potato, baked in skin
Soybeans, green, cooked	Juice, canned
Lima beans, cooked	Prunes
Soybeans, mature, cooked	Carrot
Pinto beans, cooked	Tomato
Lentils, cooked	Tomato paste
Halibut, cooked	Tomato puree
Rockfish, Pacific, cooked	Beet greens, cooked
Cod, Pacific, cooked	White beans, canned
Tuna, yellowfin, cooked	Plain yogurt, nonfat or low-fat
Rainbow trout, cooked	Clams, canned
Evaporated milk, nonfat	
Low-fat (1%) or reduced fat (2%) chocolate milk	
Skim milk (nonfat)	
Low-fat milk or buttermilk (1%)	
Orange juice, fresh	
Bananas	
Peaches, dried, uncooked	
Prunes, stewed	
Apricots, dried, uncooked	
Plantains, cooked	
Tomato sauce	
Pork loin, center rib, lean, roasted	
Spinach, cooked	

Source: Reproduced, with permission, from DiPiro, JT, Talbert RL, Yee GC, Matzke GR, Wells BG, Posey LM, eds. *Pharmacotherapy: A Pathophysiologic Approach*. 10th ed. New York, NY: McGraw-Hill; 2017.

Fluid. Fluid restriction is often recommended in conjunction with sodium restriction for most patients with late stages of CKD, especially once dialysis has begun. Fluid overload may precipitate heart failure exacerbations, contribute to resistant hypertension, and increase risk of death. For patients with anuria, fluid restrictions can be especially difficult to follow. Sodium restriction is important to manage thirst.

Sodium. In addition to managing the amount of table salt that is used, patients should avoid other foods high in sodium. Common items include processed foods, breads and rolls, cheese, chips, cold cuts, pizza, popcorn, pretzels, soups, and soy sauce.

Protein. At GFR <30 mL/min, limiting daily protein intake to 0.8 g/kg is commonly recommended.[3] However, once a patient is on dialysis, prevention of malnutrition is important, and protein intake is usually not restricted. Many patients on dialysis are prescribed protein supplements.

Depending on each patient's comorbid conditions, there may be additional dietary restrictions or recommendations, including glucose and cholesterol. Because of the large number of dietary restrictions, working with a dietitian is advised for many patients. Dialysis facilities in the United States are required to have a registered dietitian on staff.[31]

Dialysis. Patients may choose one of several dialysis modalities, if needed, in stage 5 CKD. Hemodialysis is the most common selection in the United States.[1] Patients on hemodialysis typically go to a dialysis center three times weekly to receive a 3- to 4-hour treatment, although some receive different schedules or home hemodialysis.[32] Blood is pumped through a dialysis filter, where solutes and excess fluid are removed. Common complications include intradialytic hypotension, vascular access thrombosis, infection, and uremic pruritus. The pharmacist should be familiar with these conditions if providing MTM to a patient on hemodialysis, since the medication regimen may be affected. For example, blood pressure medications may be withheld on dialysis days if hypotension is an issue. Midodrine is a commonly prescribed medication for intradialytic hypotension.

Peritoneal dialysis is another common dialysis modality where the patient is able to dialyze at home. Dialysate is pumped into the peritoneal cavity in the abdomen, allowed to "dwell" for a specified amount of time, and then drained.[32] The dialysate usually contains glucose, which can affect blood glucose control. In some cases, patients may add insulin to the dialysate to control blood glucose. Intraperitoneal insulin should be included in the medication list. Additionally, if the patient is infected (particularly peritonitis), antibiotics may be administered intraperitoneally.[32,33]

With any dialysis modality, medication scheduling is particularly important, especially if a medication is likely to be removed by dialysis. A common resource to determine dialyzability of a medication is the *Dialysis of Drugs* handbook, which is available electronically online (http://renalpharmacyconsultants.com/publications and as an app on iTunes).[34]

Multidisciplinary Team. Patients with CKD often have multiple prescribers, so it is important to share the reconciled medication list and recommendations with the entire care team. This might include, for example, the primary care physician, nephrologist, endocrinologist, and cardiologist. For patients on dialysis, a multidisciplinary team is available through the dialysis center. Facilities are required to have a medical director, nursing staff, dietitian, and social worker on staff.[31] These professionals can assist in the coordination of care of these patients.

Pharmacologic Therapy

Preventing Progression of CKD. All classes of blood pressure agents are used to treat hypertension in CKD, which is often difficult to control (see Chapter 27, "Hypertension MTM Data Set"). Sodium restriction and fluid management are paramount to managing hypertension in CKD. ACE inhibitors or ARBs are used as well. In treating proteinuria, high doses of ACE inhibitors or ARBs are generally required. Potassium accumulation is problematic in CKD, and potassium should generally be checked within a week of adding or increasing an ACE inhibitor. In cases of mild hyperkalemia, thiazide or loop diuretics may be used in conjunction with dietary interventions to manage serum potassium. A recently approved option is patiromer, a potassium binder for the treatment of nonemergent hyperkalemia.[35] This medication is administered once a day and may allow for continuation of an ACEi, for example, which would have otherwise been stopped with increasing serum potassium.

Antidiabetic agents are used to control blood glucose in patients with diabetes. Insulin is commonly used, especially in late stages of CKD (see Chapter 21, "Diabetes Mellitus MTM Data Set"), but there are now many other options with data in the CKD population. It is important to remember that many medications for diabetes will require dose adjustment in CKD based on kidney function and frequency and severity of hypoglycemia.

Addressing Common Complications of CKD

Anemia. Screening for anemia should occur at least annually in stage 3 CKD, twice a year in stages 4 or 5 (nondialysis dependent), and every 3 months in patients on dialysis.[36] Monitoring generally consists of serum hemoglobin, transferrin saturation, and ferritin. The first step to therapy is usually repletion of iron stores. Oral iron may be trialed in patients for up to 3 months, although gastrointestinal side effects may limit utility. However, oral iron is inexpensive and convenient, and many insurance companies require a trial of oral iron before IV iron will be covered. If oral iron is used, 200 mg of elemental iron should be given in divided doses, for example, ferrous sulfate 325 mg TID. Oral iron preparations are reviewed in Table 16-8.

For many patients, including almost all on hemodialysis, intravenous iron will be required to maintain adequate iron stores. Intravenous iron preparations are listed in Table 16-9.

An important serious side effect of intravenous iron products is anaphylactic-type reactions. Only iron dextran and ferumoxytol products have blackbox warnings for anaphylaxis; however, all IV iron agents have the potential to cause hypersensitivity reactions. Free iron reactions are also an important effect, more likely to occur with smaller molecular weight products (eg, iron sucrose or sodium

TABLE 16-8 • Oral Iron Preparations

Iron Product	Common Agents and Available Units	Amount of Elemental Iron Per Unit	Number of Units Per Day[a]
Ferrous sulfate	Fer-In-Sol (75 mg/0.6 mL)	75 mg	2-3
	Feosol (200 mg)	65 mg	3-4
	Ferrous sulfate, various preparations (325 mg)	65 mg	3-4
	Slow FE (160 mg)	50 mg	4
Ferrous fumarate	Ferrous fumarate, various preparations (300 mg)	99 mg	2
	Femiron (63 mg)	20 mg	10
	Nephro-Fer (350 mg)	115 mg	2
	Vitron-C (65-125 mg)	65 mg	3
Ferrous gluconate	Ferrous gluconate, various (325 mg)	36 mg	5
	Fergon (240 mg)	27 mg	6
Polysaccharide iron	Niferex (50 mg)	50 mg	4
	Hytinic (150 mg)	150 mg	1-2
Heme iron polypeptide	Proferrin-ES (12 mg)	12 mg	17

[a] Number of units per day depends on the amount of elemental iron per unit; 200 mg elemental iron per day is recommended.

Source: From Table 53-6 in DiPiro JT, Talbert RL, Yee GC, Matzke GR, Wells BG, Posey L, eds. *Pharmacotherapy: A Pathophysiological Approach*. 8th ed. New York, NY: McGraw-Hill; 2011.

TABLE 16-9 • IV Iron Preparations

IV Iron Preparations						
Iron Compounds	**Brand Name(s)**	**Half-life (Hours)**	**Molecular Weight (Daltons)**	**FDA-Approved Indications**	**FDA-Approved Dosing[a]**	**Dose Ranges (mg)[b]**
Ferric carboxymaltose	Injectafer	7-12	150 000	Adult patients with intolerance to oral iron or who have had an unsatisfactory response to oral iron and in adult patients with CKD not on dialysis	Give 2 doses separated by at least 7 days of 750 mg per dose (if body weight is ≥50 kg) or 15 mg/kg per dose (if body weight is <50 kg) not to exceed 1500 mg per course. Give either IV push (100 mg per min) or diluted in not more than 250 mL of 0.9 NaCl as an infusion over at least 15 minutes	750
Ferumoxytol	Feraheme	15	750 000	Adult patients with iron-deficiency anemia associated with chronic kidney disease	510 mg (17 mL) as a single dose, followed by a second 510 mg dose 3-8 days after the initial dose. Dilute in 50-200 mL of 0.9% NaCl or 5% dextrose and administer as an IV infusion over 15 minutes	510
Iron dextran	INFeD Dexferrum	40-60	96 000 265 000	Patients with iron deficiency in whom oral iron is unsatisfactory or impossible	100 mg over 2 minutes (25-mg test dose required) Note: Equation provided by manufacturer to calculate dose based on desired Hb	25-1000
Iron sucrose	Venofer	6	43 000	Adult and pediatric CKD 5HD patients aged 2 years and older	Adult: 100 mg over 2-5 minutes or 100 mg in maximum of 100 mL of 0.9% NaCl over 15 minutes per consecutive HD session Pediatric: 0.5 mg/kg not to exceed 100 mg per dose over 5 minutes or diluted in 25 mL of 0.9% NaCl administered over 5-60 minutes (give dose every 2 weeks for 12 weeks)	25-1000
				Adult and pediatric ND-CKD patients aged 2 years and older	Adult: 200 mg over 2-5 minutes on 5 different occasions within 14-day period. There is limited experience with administration of 500 mg diluted in a maximum of 250 mL of 0.9% NaCl over 3.5 to 4 hours on day 1 and day 14 Pediatric: see pediatric dosing for CKD 5HD (give dose every 4 weeks for 12 weeks)	
				Adult and pediatric CKD 5PD patients aged 2 years and older	Adult: Give 3 divided doses within 28 days as 2 infusions of 300 mg over 1.5 hours 14 days apart followed by one 400 mg infusion over 2.5 hours 14 days later. Dilute in a maximum of 250 mL of 0.9% NaCl Pediatric: see pediatric dosing for CKD 5HD (give dose every 4 weeks for 12 weeks)	

(*Continued*)

TABLE 16-9 • IV Iron Preparations (*Continued*)

IV Iron Preparations						
Iron Compounds	Brand Name(s)	Half-life (Hours)	Molecular Weight (Daltons)	FDA-Approved Indications	FDA-Approved Dosing[a]	Dose Ranges (mg)[b]
Sodium ferric gluconate	Ferrlecit	1	350 000	Adult and pediatric CKD 5HD patients aged 6 years and older receiving ESA therapy	Adult: 125 mg over 10 minutes or 125 mg in 100 mL of 0.9% NaCl over 60 minutes Pediatric: 1.5 mg/kg in 25 mL of 0.9% NaCl over 60 minutes; maximum dose 125 mg per dose	62.5-1000

[a] Monitor for 30 minutes following an infusion; KDIGO guidelines recommend monitoring for 60 minutes (1B recommendation for iron dextran, 2C recommendation for nondextran products).

[b] With the exception of ferric carboxymaltose and ferumoxytol, small doses (eg, 25-150 mg/wk) are generally used for maintenance regimens. Larger doses (eg, 1 g) should be administered in divided doses.

Abbreviations: CKD = chronic kidney disease; ESA = erythropoiesis stimulating agent; ND-CKD = nondialysis CKD patients.

Source: Reproduced, with permission, from DiPiro JT, Talbert RL, Yee GC, Matzke GR, Wells BG, Posey L, eds. *Pharmacotherapy: A Pathophysiological Approach*. 10th ed. New York, NY: McGraw-Hill; 2017.

ferric gluconate). This can result in hypotension after administering the iron too rapidly or at too high a dose.

Erythropoiesis stimulating agents (ESAs) are also generally required in the treatment of anemia as CKD progresses.[36] Four ESAs are currently available in the United States: Procrit (epoetin alfa), Epogen (epoetin alfa), Aranesp (darbepoetin alfa), and Mircera (methoxy PEG-epoetin beta) (Table 16-10). ESAs should be avoided if possible, and if used, should be at the lowest possible dose to prevent blood transfusions.[4,36] If iron stores are replete and hemoglobin remains low, or a patient still exhibits signs or symptoms of anemia, an ESA should be considered (usually at hemoglobin concentrations <10 g/dL).[34] In certain circumstances, more drug will be used to maintain a higher hemoglobin for improvements in quality of life or prevention of symptoms of anemia. For patients with CKD on ESA therapy, hemoglobin concentrations are generally maintained below 11.5 g/dL.[36] Dose increases should occur no more frequently than every 4 weeks at 25% increases.[37] There are several blackbox warnings on ESA products relating to patients with CKD and patients with cancer. The warning for CKD states:

> In controlled trials, patients experienced greater risks for death, serious adverse cardiovascular reactions, and stroke when administered erythropoiesis-stimulating agents (ESAs) to target a hemoglobin level of greater than 11 g/dL. No trial has identified a hemoglobin target level, ESA dose, or dosing strategy that does not increase these risks. Use the lowest Epogen dose sufficient to reduce the need for red blood cell (RBC) transfusions.[37]

Common adverse events related to ESAs include hypertension and hemodialysis vascular access thrombosis.[37]

TABLE 16-10 • Erythropoiesis-Stimulating Agents in Chronic Kidney Disease

Drug Name	Brand Name(s)	Starting Dose	Route of Administration	Half-life (Hours)
Epoetin alfa	Epogen, Procrit	Adults: 50-100 units/kg 3 times per week Pediatrics: 50 units/kg 3 times per week	IV or SubQ	8.5 (IV) 24 (SubQ)
Darbepoetin alfa	Aranesp	Adults: ND-CKD: 0.45 µg/kg once every 4 weeks CKD 5HD or CKD 5PD: 0.45 µg/kg once per week or 0.75 µg/kg every 2 weeks Pediatrics: 0.45 µg/kg once weekly; may give 0.75 µg/kg once every 2 weeks in ND-CKD patients	IV or SubQ	25 (IV) 48 (SubQ)
Methoxy PEG-epoetin beta	Mircera	All adult CKD patients: 0.6 µg/kg every 2 weeks; after Hb stabilizes, double the dose and administer monthly (eg, if administering 0.6 µg/kg every 2 weeks, give 1.2 µg/kg every month)	IV or SubQ	134 (IV) 139 (SubQ)

Abbreviations: CKD = chronic kidney disease; ND-CKD = nondialysis CKD patients; PEG = polyethylene glycol; SubQ = subcutaneous.

Source: Reproduced, with permission, from DiPiro JT, Talbert RL, Yee GC, Matzke GR, Wells BG, Posey L, eds. *Pharmacotherapy: A Pathophysiological Approach*. 10th ed. New York, NY: McGraw-Hill; 2017.

Anemia medications (ESAs and IV iron) may be covered by Medicare Part B (as opposed to Part D) in certain cases. Therefore, these medications may be missing from Part D claims data or from the pharmacy medication list. The MTM pharmacist should be on the outlook for these treatments.

Mineral and Bone Disorders (CKD-MBD). As CKD progresses, CKD-MBD is very common. CKD leads to changes in the bone, as well as calcification in the vasculature. It is monitored mainly with serum parathyroid hormone, phosphorus, and calcium concentrations.[38]

Phosphate binders are used to control hyperphosphatemia, a very common complication in advanced CKD. These medications are taken in conjunction with dietary restriction of phosphorus. They should be taken at mealtimes throughout the day. Phosphate binders are listed in Table 16-11.

Calcium citrate should not be used as a phosphate binder because of increased absorption of aluminum. Adherence to phosphate binders is notoriously low, and counseling is usually warranted to verify adherence. Because there are numerous phosphate binder dosage forms available, the pharmacist should work to assist with selecting an agent acceptable to the patient. Another consideration when selecting an agent is calcium content, particularly if the patient has hypercalcemia, since patients with CKD are prone to vascular calcification. Calcium should be maintained in the normal range.[38] Phosphorus should be maintained in the normal range for patients not on dialysis, and "toward the normal range" in patients on dialysis.[38]

In a patient with osteoporosis and CKD-MBD, calcium supplements are generally not used except in the case of hypocalcemia or as calcium-based phosphate binders. In this case, the primary bone disease target becomes secondary hyperparathyroidism, managed with vitamin D products, phosphate binders, and potentially a calcimimetic agent.

Secondary hyperparathyroidism is primarily treated with vitamin D therapy.[37] In early stages of kidney disease, replenishing 25-hydroxyvitamin D stores with ergocalciferol or cholecalciferol may be effective in reducing parathyroid hormone (PTH) since the kidney has some ability to convert inactive vitamin D to 1,25 dihydroxyvitamin D. A new FDA-approved option for predialysis CKD patients is extended release calcifediol.[39] This medication is used in patients with CKD stages 3 and 4 who have vitamin D levels <30 ng/mL.[39] If 25-OH vitamin D stores are replenished and PTH remains elevated, activated vitamin D should be considered.[37] This includes calcitriol (oral or IV) or a vitamin D analog (ie, doxercalciferol or paricalcitol). Vitamin D products are listed in Table 16-12. For patients on dialysis, activated vitamin D products are administered within dialysis clinics, so may not appear on the Part D medication claims information.

Recent studies suggest benefits of replenishing 25-OH vitamin D with ergocalciferol or cholecalciferol for reasons other than PTH reduction in CKD, such as cardiovascular benefits, reduced ESA use, and improved mortality risk.[40] Therefore, it is not uncommon to see a patient with stage 4 or 5 CKD receiving both ergocalciferol and an active vitamin D analog.

Calcimimetic agents (cinacalcet and etelcalcetide) are additional options to lower parathyroid hormone in patients on dialysis by lowering the parathyroid gland's sensitivity to calcium.[41,42] These medications are usually used in conjunction with vitamin D analogs. Cinacalcet is available as an oral tablet under the brand name Sensipar, and dosing ranges from 30 mg to 180 mg daily.[41] The main side effects are gastrointestinal, including nausea and vomiting. Hypocalcemia is also common and may be serious, occurring in approximately two-thirds of patients who take it. Therefore, cinacalcet should be used very cautiously in patients with history of seizure.[41] Cinacalcet has not been shown to improve mortality risk or cardiovascular outcomes in patients on dialysis.[43] Etelcalcetide is a new IV calcimimetic, given at dialysis, which may be advantageous from an adherence standpoint. Like cinacalcet, hypocalcemia is a significant adverse event with etelcalcetide. Both medications will be billed by the ESRD PPS under Medicare Part B, so they may not appear on Part D medication claims data.

Other Interventions

Lipids. HMG-CoA reductase inhibitors may be used in patients with CKD. They have been shown to reduce the incidence of atherosclerotic events in this population.[44] Patients on dialysis who are stable on statin therapy may be continued on it, if warranted. However, statin therapy should generally not be initiated in patients on dialysis.[26,45,46] This recommendation is based on several prospective clinical trials that have failed to show a benefit in this patient population.[45,46] When choosing a statin, several factors should be considered including potential for drug interactions, lipid lowering effect, and rapidity of change in kidney function. The dose of rosuvastatin should be decreased in patients with stages 4 or 5 CKD.[26] Other statins may require lower initial dosing, and some sources suggest limiting the maximum dose, as well.[26]

Tobacco Cessation. Smoking cessation should be encouraged in patients with CKD. Of note, chewing tobacco is high in potassium and should be avoided to prevent hyperkalemia. In addition to the many health benefits of quitting, smoking cessation may be necessary to qualify for organ transplantation. Nicotine replacement products may be used. Other options may be used, as well. Depending on kidney function, medication doses may require adjustment.

Vaccines. Vaccines that are recommended in this population include hepatitis B, influenza, Tdap, pneumococcal (both 23 valent and 13 valent), and, if indicated, human papilloma virus (HPV) and Zoster. Particularly for patients awaiting transplant, HPV and Zoster should be considered.[46]

Herbal Supplements. Several herbal supplements have been used in kidney disease with varying efficacy. Table 16-13 lists some common ones.

Referral for Management of CKD

Figure 16-5 lists some examples of conditions that would indicate emergent referral of a patient with CKD. Circumstances can involve acute or chronic changes in kidney function or CKD-associated complications (ie, hypertension, cardiovascular disease, anemia, edema, etc). Abnormal laboratory results may trigger a healthcare provider to send a patient to seek

TABLE 16-11 • Phosphate-Binding Agents Used for the Treatment of Hyperphosphatemia in CKD Patients

Category	Drug	Brand Name(s)	Compound Content	Starting Doses	Dose Titration[a]	Comments[b]
Calcium-based binders	Calcium acetate (25% elemental calcium)	PhosLo	25% elemental calcium (169 mg elemental calcium per 667 mg capsule)	1334 mg 3 times a day with meals	Increase or decrease by 667 mg per meal (169 mg elemental calcium)	Comparable efficacy to calcium carbonate with lower dose of elemental calcium Approximately 45 mg phosphorus bound per 1 g calcium acetate Evaluate for drug interactions with calcium
		Phoslyra	667 mg calcium acetate per 5 mL			
	Calcium carbonate[c]	Tums, Os-Cal, Caltrate	40% elemental calcium	0.5-1 g (elemental calcium) 3 times a day with meals	Increase or decrease by 500 mg per meal (200 mg elemental calcium)	Dissolution characteristics and phosphate binding may vary from product to product Approximately 39 mg phosphorus bound per 1 g calcium carbonate Evaluate for drug interactions with calcium
Iron-based binders	Ferric citrate	Auryxia	210 mg tablets (= 1 g ferric citrate)	420 mg ferric iron 3 times daily with meals	Increase or decrease dose by 1 or 2 tablets per meal	May increase serum iron, ferritin, and TSat May cause discolored (dark) stools Evaluate for drug interactions with iron
	Sucroferric oxyhydroxide	Velphoro	500 mg chewable tablets	500 mg 3 times daily with meals	Increase or decrease by 500 mg per day	May cause discolored (dark) stools Evaluate for drug interactions with iron
Resin binders	Sevelamer carbonate	Renvela	800 mg tablet 0.8 and 2.4 g powder for oral suspension	800-1600 mg 3 times a day with meals (once-daily dosing also effective)	Increase or decrease by 800 mg per meal	Also lowers low-density lipoprotein cholesterol Consider in patients at risk for extraskeletal calcification Risk of metabolic acidosis with sevelamer hydrochloride (less risk with carbonate formulation) May interact with 36 ipro and mycophenolate mofetil
	Sevelamer hydrochloride	Renagel	400 and 800 mg caplets	800-1600 mg 3 times a day with meals	Increase or decrease by 800 mg per meal	
Other elemental binders	Lanthanum carbonate	Fosrenol	500, 750, and 1000 mg chewable tablets 750 and 1000 mg oral powder	1500 mg daily in divided doses with meals	Increase or decrease by 750 mg/day	Potential for accumulation of lanthanum because of GI absorption (long-term consequences unknown) Evaluate for drug interactions (eg, cationic antacids, quinolone antibiotics)
	Aluminum hydroxide	AlternaGel	Content varies (range 100-600 mg/unit)	300-600 mg 3 times a day with meals	Not for long-term use requiring titration	Not a first-line agent; risk of aluminum toxicity; do not use concurrently with citrate-containing products Reserve for short-term use (4 weeks) in patients with hyperphosphatemia not responding to other binders Evaluate for drug interactions

[a] Based on phosphorus levels, titrate every 2 to 3 weeks until phosphorus goal reached.

[b] GI side effects are possible with all agents (eg, nausea, vomiting, abdominal pain, diarrhea, or constipation).

[c] Multiple preparations available that are not listed.

Abbreviation: Tsat = transferrin saturation.

Source: Reproduced, with permission, from DiPiro JT, Talbert RL, Yee GC, Matzke GR, Wells BG, Posey L, eds. *Pharmacotherapy: A Pathophysiological Approach*. 10th ed. New York, NY: McGraw-Hill; 2017.

TABLE 16-12 • Vitamin D Agents

Nutritional Vitamin D						
Generic Name	**Brand Name**	**Form of Vitamin D**	**Dosage Forms**	**Initial Dose[a]**	**Dosage Range**	**Frequency of Dosing**
Ergocalciferol	Drisdol	D_2	po	Varies based on 25(OH) D levels	400-50 000 international units	Daily (doses of 400-2000 international units)
Cholecalciferol[b]	Generic	D_3	po			Weekly or monthly for higher doses (50 000 international units)
Vitamin D and Analogs						
Generic Name	**Brand Name**	**Form of Vitamin D**	**Dosage Forms**	**Initial Dose[a,c]**	**Dosage Range**	**Dose Titration[d]**
Calcitriol	Rocaltrol	D_3	po	0.25 μg daily	0.25-5 μg	Increase by 0.25 μg/day at 4-8 week intervals
	Calcijex		IV	1-2 μg 3 times per week	0.5-5 μg	Increase by 0.5-1 μg at 2- to 4-week intervals
Doxercalciferol[e]	Hectorol	D_2	po	ND-CKD: 1 μg daily ESRD: 10 μg 3 times per week	5-20 μg	Increase by 0.5 μg at 2-week intervals for daily dosing or by 2.5 μg at 8-week intervals for 3 times per week dosing
			IV	ESRD: 4 μg 3 times per week	2-8 μg	Increase by 1-2 μg at 8-week intervals
Paricalcitol	Zemplar	D_2	po	ND-CKD: 1 μg daily or 2 μg 3 times per week if PTH ≤500 pg/mL (ng/L; ≤54 pmol/L); 2 μg daily or 4 μg 3 times per week if PTH >500 pg/mL (ng/L; >54 pmol/L)	1-4 μg	Increase by 1 μg (for daily dosing) or 2 μg (for 3 times per week dosing) at 2-4 week intervals
			IV	ESRD: 0.04-1 μg 3 times per week	2.5-15 μg	Increase by 2-4 μg at 2-4 week intervals

[a] Dose ratios are as follows: 1:1 for IV paricalcitol to oral doxercalciferol; 1.5:1 for IV paricalcitol to IV doxercalciferol; and 1:1 for IV to oral calcitriol.

[b] Multiple preparations are available that are not listed.

[c] Daily orally dosing most common for nonhemodialysis CKD patients, IV dosing 3 times per week more often used in the hemodialysis population.

[d] Based on PTH, calcium, and phosphorus levels. Decreases in dose are necessary if PTH is oversuppressed and/or if calcium and phosphorus are elevated.

[e] Prodrug that requires activation by the liver.

Abbreviations: ESRD = end-stage renal disease; ND-CKD = nondialysis chronic kidney disease; PTH = parathyroid hormone.

Source: Reproduced, with permission, from DiPiro JT, Talbert RL, Yee GC, Matzke GR, Wells BG, Posey L, eds. *Pharmacotherapy: A Pathophysiological Approach*. 10th ed. New York, NY: McGraw-Hill; 2017.

urgent or emergent care, but many times there are no specific symptoms to warn the MTM pharmacist. Clinical judgment must be used when deciding whether to refer for immediate or urgent care.

CORE ELEMENT 5—DOCUMENTATION AND FOLLOW-UP

Clear recommendations should be made when conducting an MTM consultation. It is important to remember the large number of providers that are often involved in the care of the CKD patient. Therefore, it may be necessary to reach out to multiple providers to solve an MRP. If the patient is on dialysis, be sure to send a copy of the updated medication list there as well as to the nephrologist's office. The dialysis center is often where changes are made for these patients. Table 16-14 lists common MRPs with examples. Table 16-15 provides example assessments and plans for patients with CKD.

Patients with CKD often require frequent follow-up to assess achievement of therapeutic goals, rate of CKD progression, and severity of CKD-related complications. Recommendations for follow-up are listed in Table 16-16.

TABLE 16-13 • Herbal Supplements for Chronic Kidney Disease

Herbal Product	Specific Uses	Recommended Dosage	Level of Evidence[a]	Cost[b]
Vitamin D	Vitamin D deficiency; hypocalcemia; hypophosphatemia; hyperparathyroidism	1000 international units or more daily	A	\$-\$\$
Omega-3 fatty acids (fish oil)	Cyclosporine-induced hypertension and nephropathy, IgA nephropathy; prevention of hemodialysis graft thrombosis, uremic pruritus, hypertension	• Hypertension: 4 g daily • Cyclosporine-induced nephrotoxicity: 12 g daily • Prevent graft thrombosis: 4-6 g daily • Uremic pruritus: 6 g daily	A (hyperlipidemia, hypertension) C (dialysis, IgA nephropathy, inflammation, nephrotic syndrome)	\$\$-\$\$\$
Astragalus (huangqi)[c]	Nephrotic syndrome; proteinuria; diabetic nephropathy; promotes diuresis; antioxidant and anti-inflammatory properties	Varies greatly. • 20-500 mg extract 3-4 times a day • 1-60 g dried root daily; • 500-1000 mg root capsules 3 times daily • May be added to food or drink. • Often used with angelica	C	\$
Angelica (dong quai)[c]	Glomerulonephritis	Varies greatly • Weight based dosing: <100 lb: 520 mg TID; • 100-175 lb: 1040 mg TID; >175 lb 1560 mg TID • 1-15 g whole root once daily (boiled or soaked in wine) • Often used with astragalus	C	\$
Rhubarb (dahuang)[c]	Prevention of CKD progression	• 1 g once daily, then titrated to 6-9 g once daily for up to 22 weeks • 0.5 g once daily titrated to 3 g daily for 4 weeks • Retention enema dosing: 10 g rhubarb powder in 0.5 L water once daily for 2 weeks or 30 g raw rhubarb in 200 mL water BID for 1 week	B	\$

[a] Evidence-based grading: A = strong; B = good; C = conflicting evidence.

[b] Cost: \$ = \$10/month supply in the recommended dosage; \$\$ = \$11-\$20/month; \$\$\$ = >\$50/month.

[c] Traditional Chinese herb.

Source: References 48, 49, and 50.

TABLE 16-14 • Medication-Related Problems in Chronic Kidney Disease

Category of MRP	Sample Medication-Related Problem
Nonadherence	Suboptimal control of blood pressure because of nonadherence with fluid restriction Suboptimal control of phosphorus because of patient missing phosphate binder doses Patient not taking calcimimetic medication because of cost
Unnecessary medication	Diuretic prescribed in an anuric patient
Need for additional medication	Iron stores are replete, other contributing causes of anemia ruled out, yet hemoglobin is low. Erythropoiesis stimulating agent may be needed Patient with diabetes not on ACE inhibitor or ARB for hypertension with proteinuria
Ineffective medication	Probenecid prescribed for gout in a patient with creatinine clearance 30 mL/min Nitrofurantoin is prescribed for UTI in a patient with creatinine clearance 15 mL/min Hydrochlorothiazide prescribed for a patient with creatinine clearance 15 mL/min
Dosage too low	Medication significantly removed by dialysis without appropriate adjustment Suboptimal blood pressure control on low dose of antihypertensive agent Patient on ESA therapy with hemoglobin maintained at 9.5 g/dL, yet requires frequent transfusions
Dosage too high	Patient on ESA with hemoglobin maintained at 13 g/dL Patient on insulin and now reports frequent hypoglycemia
Adverse drug event	Patient develops cough from ACE inhibitor Patient has constipation from calcium acetate

Abbreviations: ACE = angiotensin converting enzyme; ARB = angiotensin receptor blocker; ESA = erythropoiesis stimulating agent; UTI = urinary tract infection.

Immediate action

- Symptoms of uremia: mental status change, shortness of breath, nausea and vomiting, weakness, bleeding, uremic fetor, uremic frost
- Emergent blood pressure: >180/120 mm Hg with evidence of target organ damage
- Severe edema, shortness of breath
- Urgent side effects from angiotensin converting enzyme inhibitor (angioedema)
- Fistula rupture

Seek medical attention

- Symptoms of acute kidney injury - acute changes in urine (color or decreased quantity)
- Urgent blood pressure without target organ damage
- Changes in fluid status (fluid overload - edema, weight gain, shortness of breath; fluid depletion - new onset orthostatic hypotension, tenting of the skin)
- Heart failure exacerbation: rales, edema
- Shortness of breath
- Prolonged severe vomiting, diarrhea, or constipation

Routine
Inform provider at a later time

- Blood pressure routinely above goal, not emergent or urgent
- Patient is experiencing nonurgent side effects from angiotensin converting enzyme inhibitor (dry cough)
- Increased frequency of hypoglycemia
- Mild edema
- Mild symptoms of anemia: cold, tired, easily fatigued

FIGURE 16-5 Referral for selected chronic kidney disease-related issues.

TABLE 16-15 • **Sample Provider Communications for the Patient with CKD**

	Assessment	Plan
1	The patient was prescribed lanthanum carbonate 1000 mg TID with meals 3 months ago and reports nonadherence because of taste. Patient has consistent hyperphosphatemia.	Consider switching phosphate binder to sevelamer carbonate 800 mg tablets, 2 TID with meals.
2	The patient was prescribed sitagliptin 100 mg daily. Current creatinine clearance is approximately 25 mL/min.	Suggest reducing the sitagliptin dose to 25 mg daily.
3	The patient has been taking furosemide 80 mg daily on nondialysis days. However, she is now anuric.	Consider discontinuing furosemide.
4	The patient's hemoglobin has risen to 12 g/dL. She is currently treated with epoetin alfa 8000 units 3 times a week.	Suggest reducing the dose by 25% to 6000 units 3 times weekly.
5	The patient has a urinary albumin to creatinine ratio of 200 mg/g). His blood pressure is 140/90 mm Hg; potassium is 4.2 mEq/L.	Consider initiating lisinopril 10 mg daily.

TABLE 16-16 • Follow-up Assessment in Patients with Chronic Kidney Disease

Measurement	Follow-up Recommendations
Glomerular filtration rate	• Check at least annually • Check more frequently in patients at risk for CKD progression
Albuminuria	• Measure at least annually • Assess more frequently in patients at risk for CKD progression
Serum creatinine	• Use to calculate GFR as previously recommended • Check 2 and 4 weeks following initiation of ACE inhibitor/angiotensin receptor blocker (ARB) • Check when acute kidney injury (AKI) is suspected; frequency of monitoring should be individualized based on severity of AKI
Blood pressure	• Assess at each clinic visit • Consider use of home blood pressure monitors and/or ambulatory blood pressure monitoring • Check at every hemodialysis session (pre- and post-HD)
Potassium	• Check within 1 week of ACE inhibitor/ARB initiation or adjustment, then monthly after dose stabilization • Assess frequently in patients with CKD and heart failure requiring adjustment of diuretics and/or ACE inhibitors • Assess monthly in patients on dialysis
Hemoglobin	• Assess when anemia is suspected • In patients without anemia diagnosis, check at least once a year in patients with stage 3, every 6 months in patients with stages 4 or 5 (nondialysis dependent), and every 3 months in people on dialysis • In patients with an anemia diagnosis not using an ESA, check at least every 3 months in CKD patients not on hemodialysis and monthly in patients on hemodialysis • In patients on an ESA, assess at least monthly until dose stabilization. For patients not on dialysis on a stable ESA dose, assess at least every 3 months. For patients on dialysis on a stable ESA dose, assess at least monthly
Iron indices	• For patients on an ESA, assess transferrin saturation (TSAT) and ferritin at least every 3 months • Assess when clinically indicated (eg, following blood loss or when ESA dose is increased)

Parathyroid hormone	• Assess 1 to 2 times per year in stages 3-4 CKD and every 3 to 6 months in stage 5 CKD
	• For patients on dialysis receiving vitamin D:
	  • Predialysis: levels should be checked at least every 3 months
	  • Dialysis: assess monthly for 3 months following dose change then every 3 months once stable
	• Following calcimimetic initiation or adjustment: assess within one to 4 weeks, then every 1 to 3 months after dose stabilization (Sample should be taken at least 12 hours after the last dose)

Phosphorus	• Assess 1 to 2 times per year in stage 3 CKD, every 3 to 6 months in stage 4 CKD, and every 1 to 3 months in stage 5 CKD • Phosphorus should be assessed during phosphate binder use

Calcium	• Assess 1 to 2 times per year in stage 3 CKD, every 3 to 6 months in stage 4 CKD and every 1 to 3 months in stage 5 CKD
	• For patients on vitamin D therapy:
	  • Stages 3-4: assess at least monthly after initiation of therapy for 3 months, then at least every 3 months thereafter
	  • Dialysis: Check every 2 weeks for the first month after dose change, then assess monthly thereafter
	  • During initiation or dose adjustment of intravenous active vitamin D analog, may check up to twice weekly, then at least monthly once stable
	• Following cinacalcet initiation or adjustment: assess within a week, then monthly after dose stabilization
	• During initiation or dose adjustment of a calcium-based phosphate binder, assess up to twice a week

Source: References 3, 23, 24, 36, 38, 41, 42, and 51.

REFERENCES

1. United States Renal Data Systems (USRDS). *2016 Annual Data Report.* Bethesda, MD: National Institutes of Health, National Institute of Diabetes, Digestive, and Kidney Diseases; 2016.
2. National Kidney Foundation. K/DOQI clinical practice guidelines for chronic kidney disease: evaluation, classification, and stratification. *Am J Kidney Dis.* 2002;39(2 suppl 1):S1-266.
3. Kidney Disease: Improving Global Outcomes (KDIGO) CKD Work Group. KDIGO 2012 clinical practice guideline for the evaluation and management of chronic kidney disease. *Kidney Int.* 2013;3(suppl):1-150.
4. Hudson JQ, Wazny LD. Chronic kidney disease. In: DiPiro JT, Talbert RL, Yee GC, Matzke GR, Wells BG, Posey L, eds. *Pharmacotherapy: A Pathophysiological Approach.* 10th ed. New York, NY: McGraw-Hill; 2017.
5. Cardone KE, Bacchus S, Assimon MM, Pai AB, Manley HJ. Medication-related problems in CKD. *Advances in Chronic Kidney Dis.* 2010;17(5):404-412.
6. CMS. Medicare coverage of kidney dialysis and kidney transplant services. May 2016. Available at https://www.medicare.gov/Pubs/pdf/10128-Medicare-Coverage-ESRD.pdf.
7. CMS. Contract Year 2013 Medication Therapy Management Program guidance and submission instructions. April 10, 2012. Available at http://www.cms.gov/Medicare/Prescription-Drug-Coverage/PrescriptionDrugCovGenIn/Downloads/Memo-Contract-Year-2013-Medication-Therapy-Management-MTM-Program-Submission-v041012.pdf.
8. CMS. 2016 Medicare Part D Medication Therapy Management (MTM) programs, fact sheet, summary of 2016 MTM Programs. May 4, 2016. Available at https://www.cms.gov/Medicare/Prescription-Drug-Coverage/PrescriptionDrugCovContra/Downloads/CY2016-MTM-Fact-Sheet.pdf.
9. CMS. CMS-1418-F—Medicare programs; end-stage renal disease prospective payment system. August 12, 2010. Available at http://edocket.access.gpo.gov/2010/pdf/2010-18466.pdf.
10. CMS. Part D payment for drugs for beneficiaries receiving renal dialysis services. November 14, 2014. Available at https://www.cms.gov/Medicare/Medicare-Fee-for-Service-Payment/ESRDpayment/Downloads/Memo-PartD-ESRD-Guidance.pdf.
11. CMS. ESRD quality incentive program. Available at https://www.cms.gov/Medicare/Quality-Initiatives-patient-Assessment-Instruments/ESRDQIP/.
12. Dowling TC. Clinical assessment of kidney function. In: DiPiro JT, Talbert RL, Yee GC, Matzke GR, Wells BG, Posey LM, Schwinghammer T, eds. *Pharmacotherapy: A Pathophysiological Approach.* 8th ed. New York: McGraw-Hill; 2011.
13. Cockroft DW, Gault MH. Prediction of creatinine clearance from serum creatinine. *Nephron.* 1976;16:31-41.
14. Jelliffe RW. Creatinine clearance: bedside estimate. *Ann Intern Med.* 1973; 79: 604-605.
15. Mawer CE, Knowles BR, Lucas SB, et al. Computer-assisted prescribing of kanamycin for patients with renal insufficiency. *Lancet.* 1972;1:12-15.
16. Hull JH, Hak LJ, Koch GC, et al. Influence of range of renal function and liver disease on predictability of creatinine clearance. *Clin Pharmacol Ther.* 1981; 29: 516-521.
17. Levey AS, Bosch JP, Lewis JB, et al. A more accurate method to estimate glomerular filtration rate from serum creatinine: a new prediction equation. *Ann Intern Med.* 1999;130:461-470.
18. Levey AS, Greene T, Kusek J, Beck G. A simplified equation to predict glomerular filtration rate from serum creatinine. *J Am Soc Nephrol.* 2000;11:155A.
19. Levey AS, Stevens LA, Schmid CH, et al. A new equation to estimate glomerular filtration rate. *Ann Intern Med.* 2009;150:604-612.
20. Rule AD, Larson TS, Bergstralh EJ, et al. Using serum creatinine to estimate glomerular filtration rate: Accuracy in good health and in chronic kidney disease. *Ann Intern Med.* 2004;141:929-937.
21. Nyman HA, Dowling TC, Hudson JQ, Peter WL, Joy MS, Nolin TD. Comparative evaluation of the Cockcroft-Gault Equation and the Modification of Diet in Renal Disease (MDRD) study equation for drug dosing: an opinion of the Nephrology Practice and Research Network of the American College of Clinical Pharmacy. *Pharmacotherapy.* 2011;31:1130-1144.
22. Matzke GR, Aronoff GR, Atkinson AJ Jr, et al. Drug dosing consideration in patients with acute and chronic kidney disease-a clinical update from Kidney Disease: Improving Global Outcomes (KDIGO). Kidney Int. 2011;80:1122-1137.
23. Dowling TC. Evaluation of kidney function. In: DiPiro JT, Talbert RL, Yee GC, Matzke GR, Wells BG, Posey L, eds. *Pharmacotherapy: A Pathophysiologic Approach.* 10th ed. New York, NY: McGraw-Hill; 2017.
24. Kidney Disease: Improving Global Outcomes (KDIGO) CKD Work Group. KDIGO Clinical practice guideline for the management of blood pressure in chronic kidney disease. *Kidney Int.* 2012;2(suppl):337-414.
25. American Diabetes Association. Standards of medical care in diabetes—2017. *Diab Care.* 2017;40:S1-134.
26. National Kidney Foundation. KDOQI clinical practice guideline for diabetes and CKD: 2012 Update. Am J Kidney Dis. 2012;60(5):850-886.
27. Nolin TD. Drug-induced kidney disease. In: DiPiro JT, Talbert RL, Yee GC, Matzke GR, Wells BG, Posey L, eds. *Pharmacotherapy: A Pathophysiologic Approach.* 10th ed. New York, NY: McGraw-Hill; 2017.
28. CMS. MTM Program standardized format revisions (v07.15.14). Available at https://www.cms.gov/Medicare/Prescription-Drug-Coverage/PrescriptionDrugCovContra/Downloads/MTM-Program-Standardized-Format-Revisions-v071514-[ZIP-2MB].zip.
29. Flurie RW, Brophy DF. Disorders of potassium and magnesium homeostasis. In: DiPiro JT, Talbert RL, Yee GC, Matzke GR, Wells BG, Posey L, eds. *Pharmacotherapy: A Pathophysiologic Approach.* 10th ed. New York, NY: McGraw-Hill; 2017.
30. Kalantar-Zadeh K, Gutekunst L, Mehrotra R, et al. Understanding sources of dietary phosphorus in the treatment of patients with chronic kidney disease. *Clin J Am Soc Nephrol.* 2010;5:519-530.
31. CMS. Medicare and Medicaid programs; conditions for coverage for end-stage renal disease facilities, final rule. 42 CFR Parts 405, 410, 413, 414, 488, and 494. Available at https://www.cms.gov/CFCsAndCoPs/downloads/ESRDfinalrule0415.pdf.
32. Sowinski KM, Churchwell MD, Decker BS. Hemodialysis and peritoneal dialysis. In: DiPiro JT, Talbert RL, Yee GC, Matzke GR, Wells BG, Posey L, eds. *Pharmacotherapy: A Pathophysiologic Approach.* 10th ed. New York, NY: McGraw-Hill; 2017.
33. Li PK, Szeto CC, Piraino B, et al. Peritoneal dialysis-related infections recommendations: 2010 update. *Perit Dial Int.* 2010;30:393-423.
34. Bailie GR, Mason NA. 2016 dialysis of drugs. Saline, MI: Renal Pharmacy Consultants; 2016.
35. Veltassa (patiromer) [package insert]. Relypsa; Redwood City, CA: 2016.
36. Kidney Disease: Improving Global Outcomes (KDIGO) CKD Work Group. KDIGO clinical practice guideline for anemia in chronic kidney disease. *Kidney Int.* 2012;2(suppl):279-335.
37. Epogen (epoetin alfa) [package insert]. Amgen; Thousand Oaks, CA: 2017.
38. Kidney Disease: Improving Global Outcomes (KDIGO) CKD-MBD Work Group. KDIGO clinical practice guideline for the diagnosis, evaluation, prevention, and treatment of chronic kidney disease-mineral and bone disorder (CKD-MBD). *Kidney Int.* 2009;113(suppl):S1-130.
39. Rayaldee (calcifediol) [package insert]. Miami, FL, Opko: 2016.
40. Nigwekar SU, Bhan I, Thadhani R. Ergocalciferol and cholecalciferol in CKD. *Am J Kidney Dis.* 2012;60:139-156.
41. Sensipar (cinacalcet) [package insert]. Amgen; Thousand Oaks, CA: 2017.
42. Parsabiv (etelcalcetide) [package insert]. Amgen; Thousand Oaks, CA: 2017.
43. Chertow GM, Block GA, Correa-Rotter R, et al. Effect of cinacalcet on cardiovascular disease in patients undergoing dialysis. *N Engl J Med.* 2012;367:2482-2494.
44. Baigent C, Landray MJ, Reith C, et al. The effects of lowering LDL cholesterol with simvastatin plus ezetimibe in patients with chronic kidney disease (Study of Heart and Renal Protection): a randomised placebo-controlled trial. *Lancet.* 2011;377:2181-2192.
45. Wanner C, Krane V, Marz W, et al, for the German Diabetes and Dialysis Study Group. Atorvastatin in patients with type 2 diabetes mellitus undergoing hemodialysis. *N Engl J Med.* 2005;353:238-248.

46. Fellström BC, Jardine AG, Schmieder RE, et al. Rosuvastatin and cardiovascular events in patients undergoing hemodialysis. *N Engl J Med*. 2009; 360:1395-1407.

47. ACIP Adult Immunization Work Group. Recommended immunization schedule for adults aged 19 years or older by medical conditions and other indications, United States, 2017. Available at https://www.cdc.gov/vaccines/schedules/hcp/imz/adult-conditions.html.

48. Natural Medicines [database online]. Somerville, MA: Therapeutic Research Center; 2017. Available at https://naturalmedicines.therapeuticresearch.com/.

49. Li X, Wang H. Chinese herbal medicine in the treatment of chronic kidney disease. *Adv Chron Kid Dis*. 2005;12:276-281.

50. Lok CE, Moist L, Hemmelgarn BR, et al. Effect of fish oil supplementation on graft patency and cardiovascular events among patients with new synthetic arteriovenous hemodialysis grafts: a randomized controlled trial. *JAMA*. 2012;307:1809-1816.

51. Kidney Disease: Improving Global Outcomes (KDIGO) Acute Kidney Injury Workgroup. KDIGO clinical practice guideline for acute kidney injury. *Kidney Int*. 2012;2(suppl):1-138.

Review Questions

1. Which is the most common cause of chronic kidney disease?
   a. Hypertension
   b. Diabetes mellitus
   c. Glomerulonephritis
   d. Drug-induced kidney injury

2. A patient with a glomerular filtration rate of 12 ml/min/1.73m^2 and a spot albumin to creatinine ratio of 20 mg/g has which stage of CKD?
   a. G4, A2
   b. G4, A1
   c. G5, A2
   d. G5, A1

3. Which is an appropriate blood pressure target for a 49-year-old patient with type 2 diabetes and an albumin to creatinine ratio of 300 mg/g?
   a. <150/100 mm Hg
   b. <140/90 mm Hg
   c. <130/80 mm Hg
   d. <120/80 mm Hg

4. A patient was told by his prescriber that he is not reaching his dry weight and should double his furosemide dose on nondialysis days. Which is the best interpretation of this statement in plain language?
   a. When you leave dialysis, there is extra fluid left in your body, which can strain your heart. You should now take more of your water pills, two tablets of furosemide instead of one tablet, on your nondialysis days (Tuesdays, Thursdays, Saturdays, and Sundays).
   b. Your physician changed your furosemide dose. You should now take 80 mg on nondialysis days.
   c. Your weight after dialysis is far from your dry weight. Your physician wants you to double your dose of furosemide.
   d. Dialysis is a procedure that removes extra fluid from your body. You should take more tablets of furosemide on your nondialysis days (Tuesdays, Thursdays, Saturdays, and Sundays).

5. All of the following are appropriate self-management recommendations for inclusion on the MAP of a patient with late stage CKD **EXCEPT**:
   a. Orange juice should be avoided due to potassium content.
   b. Ibuprofen should be used in preference to acetaminophen for mild pain.
   c. If you forget a dose of phosphate binder at lunch, skip that dose and resume taking your medication at your next meal.
   d. You should check your blood pressure at home, in addition to having it checked at your physician's office.

6. All of the following would necessitate urgent or emergent evaluation and treatment **EXCEPT**:
   a. Blood pressure 200/110 mm Hg.
   b. Serum potassium concentration of 7.5 mEq/L.
   c. Serum phosphorus concentration of 7.5 mg/dL.
   d. Severe edema and shortness of breath.

7. A pharmacist identified four medication-related problems for a patient with chronic kidney disease. Which should take priority over the others?
   a. The patient has stage 5 CKD and has mildly elevated LDL.
   b. The patient frequently forgets to take his phosphate binder, and phosphorus is 6.5 mg/dL.
   c. The patient is on hemodialysis and has a predialysis blood pressure of 157/87 mm Hg.
   d. The patient had a recent dose increase in his epoetin alfa, and hemoglobin has risen 2 g/dL in the past month to 12.5 g/dL.

8. Which agent is most appropriate to treat anemia in a patient with stage 5 CKD on hemodialysis, with declining hemoglobin (currently 9.8 g/dL) and low TSAT (10%) and ferritin (85 ng/mL)?
   a. Epoetin alfa
   b. Darbepoetin alfa
   c. Iron dextran
   d. Iron sucrose

9. Which agent should be used to treat a low 25-OH vitamin D level in a patient with stage 5 CKD?
   a. Calcitriol
   b. Paricalcitol
   c. Ergocalciferol
   d. Doxercalciferol

10. A patient is prescribed epoetin alfa to treat anemia of CKD. Which is correct regarding selection of a hemoglobin target for this patient?
    a. All patients prescribed erythropoiesis-stimulating agents should have hemoglobin maintained at or below 10 g/dL.
    b. Hemoglobin should be maintained at 15 g/dL for men and 13 g/dL for women.
    c. Hemoglobin target should be individualized, usually at a hemoglobin less than 11.5 g/dL.
    d. The hemoglobin target is between 11 and 12 g/dL for all patients.

ANSWERS

1. b	2. d	3. c
4. a	5. b	6. c
7. d	8. d	9. c
10. c		

17

Chronic Obstructive Pulmonary Disease MTM Data Set

Kyle Melin, PharmD, BCPS, AE-C, and Maria Maniscalco-Feichtl, PharmD

KEY POINTS

- Unlike asthma, the airflow limitation caused by chronic obstructive pulmonary disease is not fully reversible.
- The single most important intervention for prevention and treatment of chronic obstructive pulmonary disease is smoking cessation. Medication therapy management (MTM) providers should work with patients to incorporate a strategy for smoking cessation into the medication action plan.
- Adherence to pharmacotherapy is key in reaching treatment goals, and guidelines for chronic obstructive pulmonary disease emphasize the importance of routine assessment and discussion of the therapeutic regimen with patients. Through provision of MTM, MTM providers can assist patients and other providers in improving treatment and achieving therapeutic goals.

INTRODUCTION TO CHRONIC OBSTRUCTIVE PULMONARY DISEASE

Chronic obstructive pulmonary disease (COPD) is a preventable and treatable disease characterized by persistent airflow limitation that is usually progressive.[1] The airflow limitation is most often caused by a mixture of small airway disease and parenchymal destruction (Figure 17-1).

The underlying etiology of COPD is due to an enhanced chronic inflammatory response of the airways and lungs to noxious particles or gases. The most common exposure leading to chronic inflammation in COPD is tobacco smoke, accounting for 85% to 90% of cases of COPD. Other environmental risk factors include occupational dusts, chemicals, and air pollution (Table 17-1). A variety of host factors also influence the risk of developing COPD following exposure to these environmental risk factors.

Patients with COPD may experience symptoms that include cough, excess mucus production, chest tightness, breathlessness, difficulty sleeping, and fatigue. The term *COPD* is often used interchangeably with the terms chronic bronchitis and emphysema. However, the terms are not synonymous. Chronic bronchitis is defined as the presence of cough and sputum production for at least 3 months in each of 2 consecutive years, whereas emphysema is an increase in the size of the air spaces caused by irreversible expansion of the alveoli and/or destruction of alveolar walls. It is important to note that most COPD patients have some combination of both emphysema and chronic bronchitis. Clinical diagnosis of COPD requires persistent airflow limitation that is not fully reversible, as defined by a forced expiratory volume in one second to forced vital capacity ($FEV_{1/FVC}$) ratio of less than 0.70 post bronchodilator. Beyond this, COPD is further classified by risk of exacerbations and level of symptoms.

The 2017 report of the Global Initiative for Chronic Obstructive Lung Disease (GOLD) guidelines uses a system of grades based upon FEV_1 measurement from spirometric testing to define the level of airflow limitation. The grading system starts with grade 1 as the lowest amount of airflow limitation and goes up to grade 4 for patients with the most severe airflow limitation (Table 17-2).

Patients with COPD are also classified according to level of symptoms. The GOLD guidelines recommend using one of two validated questionnaires to assess symptoms in patients with COPD. The first is the *Breathlessness Measurement Using the*

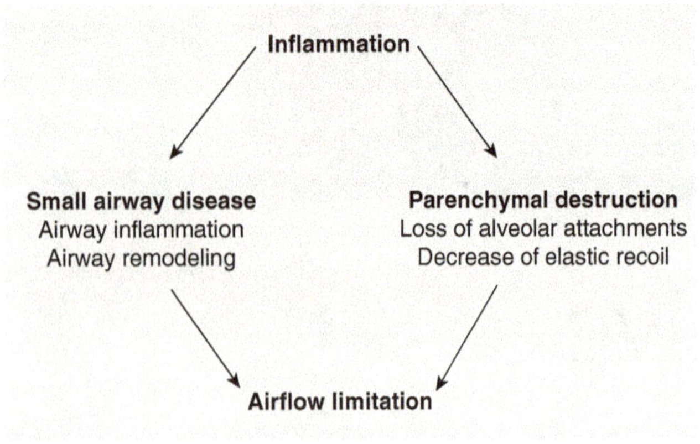

FIGURE 17-1 Mechanisms for developing chronic airflow limitation in COPD.[1]

TABLE 17-1 • Risk Factors for Development of Chronic Obstructive Pulmonary Disease (COPD)

Exposures	Host Factors
Environmental tobacco smoke	Genetic predisposition (Alpha-1-antitrypsin deficiency)
Occupational dusts and chemicals	Airway hyperresponsiveness
Air pollution	Impaired lung growth

TABLE 17-2 • Classification of Severity of Airflow Limitation in COPD (Based on Post Bronchodilator FEV_1)

In Patients with FEV_1/FVC <0.70		
GOLD 1	Mild	FEV_1 ≥80% predicted
GOLD 2	Moderate	50% ≤ FEV_1 <80% predicted
GOLD 3	Severe	30% ≤ FEV_1 <50% predicted
GOLD 4	Very severe	FEV_1 <30% predicted

Source: Reproduced, with permission, from Global Initiative for Chronic Obstructive Lung Disease (GOLD). Global strategy for the diagnosis, management and prevention of COPD; 2017.

Modified British Medical Research Council (mMRC) Questionnaire, and the second is the *COPD Assessment Test (CAT)*. The CAT questionnaire is preferred by the guidelines, as it provides a more comprehensive assessment of symptomatic impact of the disease. A CAT score ≥10 or an mMRC grade of ≥2 is indicative of a high level of symptoms. CAT can be accessed online in a variety of languages at the following URL: http://www.catestonline.org/. Once risk of exacerbation and level of symptoms have been determined, a patient can then be placed in a combined COPD assessment group (Table 17-3).

An exacerbation that leads to a hospitalization automatically places a patient in patient group C or D. It is important to assess exacerbation history thoroughly, as risk directly impacts which group and treatment the patient receives. Recommended treatment regimens for each COPD combined assessment group are outlined later in the chapter.

Complications of COPD

Unfortunately, many patients will experience declining lung function over time, even with the best available care. Therefore, symptoms and objective measures of airflow limitation should be monitored routinely to identify need for modification of treatment and development of complications.[1] As the disease progresses, patients may subjectively report an increase of symptoms including cough and sputum, breathlessness, fatigue, activity limitation, and sleep disturbances. Objectively, these may be manifested as an increase in grade on the mMRC or increasing CAT score. A decrease in FEV_1 marks worsening of airflow limitation. Disease progression may also lead to more unscheduled visits to providers, telephone calls for assistance, and use of urgent or emergency care facilities. Additionally, COPD patients requiring surgery for any indication may commonly develop postoperative pulmonary complications. The severity of COPD may be one factor in the determination of whether a patient is a surgery candidate.

Therapeutic Goals for COPD

The therapeutic goals for stable COPD involve reducing both current symptoms and future risks. Goals for symptom relief include a decrease in dyspnea, cough and sputum production, and improvement in exercise tolerance and health status. Risk reduction goals involve the prevention of disease progression, prevention and treatment of exacerbations, and reduction in mortality (Figure 17-2).

TABLE 17-3 • Combined Assessment of COPD

Assess Exacerbation Risk and Symptoms		
Exacerbation history		
≥2 or ≥1 leading to hospital admission	**C**	**D**
0 or 1 (did not result in a hospital admission)	**A**	**B**
	mMRC 0-1 CAT <10	*mMRC ≥2 CAT ≥10*
	Symptoms	

Characteristics by patient grouping	
A	Low Risk Less Symptoms
B	Low Risk More symptoms
C	High risk Fewer symptoms
D	High risk More symptoms

Source: Reference 1.

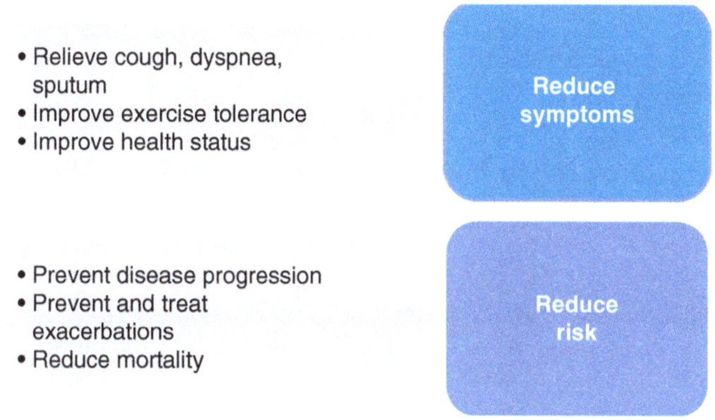

FIGURE 17-2 Treatment goals for stable COPD patients.
Source: Reproduced, with permission, from Global Initiative for Chronic Obstructive Lung Disease (GOLD). Global strategy for the diagnosis, management and prevention of COPD; 2017.

The combined COPD assessment group directs treatment for COPD. Due to the progressive nature of COPD, therapeutic success is not clearly defined by the GOLD guidelines and is determined at the individual patient level. For most patients, at a minimum, success means stabilization in symptoms, if not improvement. Experiencing COPD exacerbations may be indicative of therapeutic failure and is therefore incorporated into the guidelines by placing all patients with 2 or more exacerbations (or 1 or more exacerbations requiring hospitalization) in the past year in the high-risk COPD combined assessment groups C and D.

Currently, COPD is estimated to be the fourth leading cause of death in the United States.[2] Healthy People 2020 has set ambitious goals to decrease the number of hospitalizations and emergency department visits for patients with COPD.[3] Adherence to pharmacotherapy is key in reaching this goal, and treatment guidelines emphasize the importance of routine assessment and discussion of therapeutic regimen. Through MTM and the techniques discussed in this chapter, MTM providers can assist patients and other providers in improving COPD treatment and achieving therapeutic goals.

CORE ELEMENT 1—COMPREHENSIVE MEDICATION REVIEW FOR PATIENTS WITH COPD

Following is a list of suggested questions to use when conducting a medication therapy review in a patient with COPD (Table 17-4). As with most medication reviews, the specific questions used and depth of COPD assessment performed by the MTM provider will vary depending on a variety of factors, including the amount of time for the interview, number of concurrent medication-related problems (MRPs), urgency of MRPs, and the reliability of the patient in providing accurate information, among others. In time-limited interactions or in complex cases with multiple medical issues, the MTM provider may choose to target questions which help to identify or rule out issues of an urgent nature (see questions to ask for prevention/assessment of medical emergencies). One particular point to discuss with all patients is the use of long-acting bronchodilators and/or inhaled corticosteroids. As many patients are more familiar with "as needed" use of inhalers or breathing treatments, it is important to assess if controller medications are being used inconsistently due to misunderstanding of the intended use.

TABLE 17-4 • Questions to Ask When Conducting a Medication Review in a Patient with COPD

Suggested Questions for the Patient with COPD

- How long have you had COPD? When were you diagnosed?
- How does having COPD affect your life today? In 10 years?
- Which of these symptoms do you experience from COPD?
  - Cough
  - Extra phlegm/mucus in your chest
  - Chest tightness
  - Breathlessness or shortness of breath
  - Difficulty doing activities around your house
  - Difficulty walking outside of your home
  - Difficulty sleeping
  - Tiredness or fatigue
- What inhalers do you take for your COPD?
  - Do you use them regularly or as needed if you are having trouble breathing?
- What breathing treatments do you take for your COPD? How do you take them?
  - Which treatment do you use every day? Which do you use when you have trouble breathing?
- Do you know what a controller inhaler is/which of your inhalers is a controller?
- Do you know what a quick-relief inhaler is/which of your inhalers is fast-acting?
- What oral medications (tablets/capsules/liquids) do you take for your COPD?
- How often do you miss a dose of your COPD medication?
- What other medications have you taken in the past for your COPD?
- Have you ever stopped taking any of your prescribed COPD medications? If so, why? Does your physician know that you stopped taking them?
- What over-the-counter medications or herbals do you use for your COPD?
- Other than medicines, what have you tried for your COPD (eg, pulmonary rehab)?
- What exercise regimen do you follow?
- Have you had your "flu shot" (influenza vaccination) this year?
- Have you ever had a "pneumonia" (pneumococcal) vaccination?
- Do you smoke any tobacco products?
  - If so, have you ever tried to quit?
  - What strategies have you tried to quit in the past? Have any of them worked?
- Do you smoke any other substances (eg, marijuana)?

Questions to Ask for Prevention/Assessment of Medical Emergencies

- Crisis planning: What are the warning signs that your COPD is getting worse?
- Have you had to go to the hospital or urgent care for your COPD in the last year? How many times?
- When you get short of breath, does your medication give you relief?
- Have you had any situations recently where you got short of breath and your inhaler did not help?
- Have you gotten short of breath and gotten dizzy/light headed, had a fall, or passed out?

TABLE 17-5 • Living Room Language for COPD

Adverse event—something bad that happens, bad reaction, unexplained or unwanted effects.
Airways—tube-like structures in your lungs that permit air to enter and exit the body.
Chronic—constant, never ending, does not go away.
Chronic obstructive pulmonary disease (COPD)—a long-term disease that causes blockage in the lungs. Symptoms include shortness of breath, cough, chest tightness, and excess sputum/mucus production in the chest.
Controller inhaler—a medicine for COPD or asthma that works for a long time (12 to 24 hours) and helps PREVENT someone from having symptoms like shortness of breath or cough.
Cushing's syndrome—a group of symptoms and changes in normal body processes that may result if a class of drugs known as steroids are taken over a long period of time; this may be a cause of high blood pressure, weight gain, changes in mood and other symptoms.
Exacerbation—a sudden worsening of COPD symptoms. You will likely need to use your inhaled medication to catch your breath. Sometimes requires a visit to urgent care or emergency room for relief.
FEV_1 (forced expiratory volume)—the total amount of air you can breathe out in 1 second.
FVC (forced vital capacity)—the total amount of air you can breathe out of your lungs after taking a full breath.
Heart rate—how many times your heart beats each minute.
Lifestyle changes—your physician may have recommended changes in lifestyle to help improve your COPD symptoms, which for some patients include reaching a goal weight, exercising, or quitting smoking.
Lungs—the organ in your body that is used for breathing.
Metered dose inhaler (MDI)—a type of inhaler that delivers the same amount of medicine in each puff.
Mucus—thick, sticky stuff made by your lungs in response to inflammation.
Obese—having a body mass index (BMI) over 30. Being obese and having excess belly fat may worsen your ability to breathe.
Overweight—having a body mass index (BMI) over 25, which increases your risk of having high blood pressure, diabetes, and cardiovascular disease.
Pulmonologist—a physician that specializes in lung disease.
Quick-relief medication—a medicine for COPD or asthma that works very quickly (within minutes) to help treat shortness of breath or breathlessness.
Sleep apnea—a sleep condition that often involves pauses in breathing during the night. May occur in patients who have COPD.
Smoking cessation—quitting smoking, which can lower your chance of COPD getting worse and improve how you breathe.
Spirometry—sometimes referred to as pulmonary function testing; this is a measure of how well your lungs can move air in and out.
Tachycardia—a fast pace for the heart to beat, more than 100 times in a minute.

MTM providers should remember to use living room language during the interview (Table 17-5) and to be prepared for questions that patients may ask regarding COPD (Table 17-6).

CORE ELEMENT 2—PERSONAL MEDICATION LIST

The following is a sample personal medication list[4] (PML) for a patient with COPD (Figure 17-3). This example is representative only of respiratory medications. Additional medications for other disease states should be added and listed separately. MTM providers should remember to use living room language when creating the PML.

CORE ELEMENT 3—MEDICATION ACTION PLAN

Figure 17-4 contains a sample medication action plan[4] [MAPs] for a patient with COPD. The examples provided only include action steps related to COPD. MAPs for other disease states or other MRPs should be added and listed separately. In general, it is best to limit your action items to only a few points that are of the highest priority to avoid overwhelming the patient. Other areas for patient self-management can be addressed at later visits. MTM providers should remember to use living room language when creating the MAP.

CORE ELEMENT 4—INTERVENTION AND/OR REFERRAL

Smoking Cessation

The single most important intervention for prevention and treatment of COPD is smoking cessation.[1] Additionally, removal of any other contributing environmental factors that are modifiable (see Table 17-1) is imperative. However, of all interventions, including both lifestyle modifications and pharmacologic treatments, smoking cessation has the greatest capacity to affect the progression of COPD. For this reason, health care providers should encourage all patients who smoke to quit. The tobacco cessation guidelines from the U.S. Public Health Service are summarized in Table 17-7. First-line pharmacotherapy treatment options for tobacco cessation are outlined in Table 17-8.

TABLE 17-6 • Questions Commonly Asked by COPD Patients

- **What is COPD?**
  COPD stands for chronic obstructive pulmonary disease. COPD means that the air does not move in and out of your lungs as well as it should. This can cause shortness of breath, cough, chest tightness, and extra mucus or sputum in your chest.
- **What causes COPD?**
  COPD is usually caused by breathing in some dangerous chemicals. The most common of these is tobacco smoke. It accounts for 85% to 90% of cases of COPD. Other risk factors include occupational dusts, chemicals, and air pollution.
- **How do I know if I have COPD?**
  Symptoms of COPD include shortness of breath, cough, chest tightness, and extra mucus or sputum in your chest. However, your physician will have to do special testing to confirm if you have COPD. This testing is called spirometry. A spirometer tests how difficult it is for the lungs to move air in and out of the body. Poor airflow in and out of the body means a diagnosis of COPD.
- **Why is it important to take my controller medications on days when I feel fine?**
  Controller medications are very important to prevent and/or manage the symptoms of COPD. They must be used every day as prescribed to get the full benefit of the medicine. This means that even if you are feeling fine or not having any symptoms, it is still important to take your controller medication to prevent your symptoms from returning.
- **Can I just stop my COPD medications if I feel okay?**
  No. When you feel ok and think about stopping your COPD medications, call your physician. Do not stop taking medicine until you have talked about it with your physician. Most people with COPD need to take medication every day to prevent symptoms from returning.
- **What can happen if I stop taking my COPD medications?**
  If you stop taking your COPD medicine without talking to your physician first, your symptoms may return. In some cases, your breathing may get worse very quickly, and you may need to go to the urgent care or hospital to get help.
- **When should I call my physician about my COPD?**
  Many COPD patients will notice that their symptoms may be worse on some days than others. However, you should call your physician if you experience any of the following:
  - Coughing more deeply or more often than normal
  - Increase in mucus (sputum) or a change in the color of the mucus you cough up
  - Shortness of breath or symptoms that do not go away after taking your medication and resting for 15 to 30 minutes
  - Fever over 101°F or flu-like symptoms
- **What should I do if I have a problem with my COPD medications?**
  If you are having a problem with any of your COPD medications, it is very important to let your physician or pharmacist know. Together, you and your healthcare provider can make sure you are on the right medications or, if needed, change them to the best treatment for you.

Nonpharmacologic Treatment

Nonpharmacologic treatment of COPD includes pulmonary rehabilitation and regular physical exercise. Physical activity can increase exercise tolerance and even reduce symptoms of dyspnea and fatigue in COPD patients. All patients with COPD should be provided rehabilitation and encouraged to maintain physical activity.[1] Even when no changes in spirometry are seen, pulmonary rehabilitation can produce long-term improvement in activities of daily living, quality of life, exercise tolerance, and dyspnea for patients with moderate to severe COPD.[6]

PERSONAL MEDICATION LIST FOR *<Insert Patient's name*, **DOB:** *mm/dd/yyyy>*	
Medication: Spiriva (tiotropium) 18 mcg capsule with handihaler	
How I use it: Inhale contents of one capsule (18 mcg) with handihaler every morning with 2 breaths	
Why I use it: COPD (breathing)	**Prescriber:** Dr. Warner
Date I started using it: 5/17/2017	**Date I stopped using it:** *(Leave blank for patient's notes)*
Why I stopped using it: *(Leave blank for patient's notes)*	
Medication: ProAir HFA (albuterol) inhaler	
How I use it: Take 1 to 2 puffs (separated by at least 1 minute) every 4 to 6 hours as needed for shortness of breath.	
Why I use it: COPD (breathing)	**Prescriber:** Dr. Warner
Date I started using it: 11/1/2016	**Date I stopped using it:** *(Leave blank for patient's notes)*
Why I stopped using it: *(Leave blank for patient's notes)*	

FIGURE 17-3 Example personal medication list for respiratory medications.

	DATE PREPARED: *<Insert date>*
What we talked about: Importance of using Spiriva regularly for control of COPD symptoms	
What I need to do: • Spiriva is a controller inhaler that must be used every day to PREVENT shortness of breath. It does not work well to quickly relieve symptoms that have already started. • Use the Spiriva inhaler once every morning as prescribed (even on the days I wake up feeling well). • Inhale slowly and deeply two times to get the full dose of medicine. • If I experience shortness of breath during the day, use the Proair inhaler as prescribed for quick relief of symptoms.	**What I did and when I did it:** *(Leave blank for patient's notes)*
	DATE PREPARED: *<Insert date>*
What we talked about: How to gain control of increasing COPD symptoms	
What I need to do: • Continue to use fluticasone/salmeterol inhaler twice daily. • Use albuterol inhaler as prescribed for quick relief of shortness of breath throughout the day. • Use albuterol inhaler 4 to 6 times a day if needed. • Talk to the physician about my shortness of breath at the next office visit. An adjustment in treatment may help control symptoms. • Keep this medication with me at all times – "quick relief inhaler."	**What I did and when I did it:** *(Leave blank for patient's notes)*

FIGURE 17-4 Example medication action plan for a patient with COPD.

Immunizations

Both the influenza and pneumococcal vaccinations are recommended for all patients with COPD, regardless of age. The influenza vaccination should be provided to all COPD patients annually and has the potential to reduce serious illness and death by 50%.[7,8] Current guidelines recommend the vaccination for all patients, unless they have a history of life-threatening or anaphylactic reaction to the vaccine in the past. A history of egg allergy is no longer considered a justifiable reason to withhold vaccination for influenza. While the evidence of benefit for the pneumococcal vaccine is not as robust as that of influenza, it should be administered to all COPD patients, as well. Current vaccination guidelines call for

TABLE 17-7 • Key Guideline Recommendations Regarding Tobacco Use and Dependence

Tobacco dependence is a chronic disease that often requires repeated intervention and multiple attempts to quit. Effective treatments are available that can significantly improve rates of long-term abstinence.
Clinicians and healthcare delivery systems should consistently identify and document tobacco use status and treat every tobacco user.
Tobacco-dependence treatments are effective over a broad range of populations. Clinicians should encourage every patient willing to make a quit attempt to use counseling treatments and medications recommended in the guideline.
Brief tobacco-dependence treatments are effective. Clinicians should offer every patient who uses tobacco at least these brief treatments.
Individual, group, and telephone counseling are effective, and their effectiveness increases with treatment intensity. Practical counseling (problem-solving and/or skills training) and social support are especially effective and should be employed as a part of treatment.
There are numerous effective medications for tobacco dependence, and clinicians should encourage their use by patients during a quit attempt, except when medically contraindicated or with populations in which the evidence of effectiveness is insufficient (pregnancy, smokeless tobacco users, light smokers, and adolescents). Seven first-line medications (5 nicotine and 2 nonnicotine) consistently increase long-term abstinence rates. Clinicians should also consider the use of combinations as identified in the guideline.
Counseling and medication are effective when used by themselves for treating tobacco dependence. The combination of the two is more effective than either alone. Patients should be encouraged to use both counseling and medication.
Telephone quitline counseling is effective for diverse populations and offers the advantage of broad reach. Clinicians should ensure patient access to quitlines and promote quitline use.
For a tobacco user who is currently unwilling to make a quit attempt, clinicians should use motivational treatments that have been shown to be effective in increasing future quit attempts.
Tobacco-dependence treatments are both clinically effective and highly cost-effective relative to interventions for other clinical disorders. Providing coverage for these treatments increases quit rates. Insurers and purchasers should ensure that all insurance plans include the counseling and medications identified as effective in the guideline as covered benefits.

Source: Reference 5.

TABLE 17-8 • First-Line Pharmacotherapies for Smoking Cessation

Agent	Usual Dose	Duration	Common Complaints
Bupropion SR	150 mg orally daily for 3 days, then twice daily	12 weeks, up to 6 months	Insomnia, dry mouth
Nicotine gum	2-4 mg gum prn, up to 24 pieces daily	12 weeks	Sore mouth, dyspepsia
Nicotine inhaler	6-16 cartridges daily	Up to 6 months	Sore mouth and throat
Nicotine nasal spray	8-40 doses daily	3-6 months	Nasal irritation
Nicotine patches	Various, 7-21 mg every 24 hours	Up to 8 weeks	Skin reaction, insomnia
Varenicline	0.5 mg daily for 3 days, then 0.5 mg twice daily for 4 days, then 1 mg twice daily	12 weeks	Nausea, sleep disturbances

a one-time administration of the 23-valent pneumococcal polysaccharide (PPSV23) vaccine for all COPD patients under the age of 65. For all patients 65 years of age or older, a single administration of 13-valent pneumococcal conjugate vaccine (PCV13) is indicated, followed by a one-time booster of PPSV23 at least one year later (if the first PPSV23 vaccination was administered more than five years prior). Table 17-9 details the Advisory Committee on Immunization Practices (ACIP) recommendations for use of PCV13 and PPSV23.

Pharmacologic Treatment of COPD

Pharmacologic treatment of COPD is used to reduce symptoms, reduce frequency and severity of exacerbations, and improve health status and exercise tolerance.[1] As mentioned previously, treatment for COPD is directed by the combined COPD assessment group (Table 17-10). However, due to great interpatient variability, treatment should be individualized as much as possible based upon individual response. A notable difference from the treatment of asthma is the limited use of short-acting bronchodilators for as-needed use. Table 17-11 provides an overview of the different medications used for COPD.

Figure 17-5 provides criteria for referral in the management of COPD. It is important for the MTM provider to make appropriate referrals to different levels of care based upon disease state assessment. It may also be necessary to educate patients about when medical attention should be sought for changes in symptoms (Table 17-6).

TABLE 17-9 • ACIP Recommendations for the Use of PCV13 and PPSV23

Vaccine Naïve Adults • PCV13 first with PPSV23 administered at least 8 weeks later • Second dose of PPSV23 at 5-year interval and PPSV23 at age 65 years and at least 5 years after last dose
PPSV23-immunized Adults • PCV13 at least 1 year after last dose of PPSV23 • Second dose of PPSV23 at 5-year interval and PPSV23 at age 65 years and at least 5 years after last dose

Indications for PCV13 for Adults 19 Years and Older
• Functional or anatomic asplenia
• Immunocompromising conditions
  • Congenital or acquired immunodeficiencies
  • HIV infection
  • Chronic renal failure or nephrotic syndrome
  • Leukemias, lymphomas, Hodgkin's lymphoma
  • Generalized malignancy
  • Diseases requiring treatment with immunosuppressive drugs, including long-term systemic corticosteroids or radiation therapy
  • Solid organ transplantation
  • Multiple myeloma
• Cerebral spinal fluid leaks or cochlear implants

Abbreviations: PCV13 = 13-valent pneumococcal conjugate vaccine; PPSV23 = 23-valent pneumococcal polysaccharide vaccine.

Source: Reference 9.

Other Treatments

The GOLD guidelines also address the use of several other pharmacologic and nonpharmacologic treatments for stable COPD. Mucolytic agents (eg, carbocysteine), antitussives, and vasodilators are all specifically discussed. However, as data is limited and sometimes contradictory, treatment with any of these agents is not routinely recommended. Additionally, the GOLD guidelines do not recommend the use of any herbal medicines for the treatment of COPD due to inadequate evidence. Still, many patients will use herbal products in place of or in addition to their prescribed treatments (Table 17-12). Other alternatives, including acupuncture and homeopathy have not been adequately tested and are not recommended as treatment options. Long-term oxygen administration (greater than 15 hours per day) may be beneficial in patients with severe resting hypoxemia. Leukotriene modifiers and mast cell stabilizers have not been adequately tested in COPD patients and are not currently recommended.

CORE ELEMENT 5—DOCUMENTATION AND FOLLOW-UP

Clear and succinct documentation of MRPs and recommendations is a key component of the MTM consult. Examples of potential MRPs in patients with COPD are provided in Table 17-13. Sample communications and recommendations to providers to address medication-related issues are found in Figure 17-6. Recommendations may be communicated via fax, telephone, or other means of written or secure electronic communication. The examples that follow are for illustrative purposes. Actual communications to providers should be individualized based on the type of recommendation, patient specific characteristics, and the nature of the relationship with the provider.

TABLE 17-10 • Initial Pharmacologic Treatment Based on Combined COPD Assessment Group

Patient Group	Recommended First Choice	Recommended Escalation if Symptoms Persist	Notes
A Low risk Fewer symptoms	Bronchodilator (May be either short-acting or long-acting)	Continue, stop, or try alternative class of bronchodilator	
B Low risk More symptoms	Long-acting bronchodilator (LABA or LAMA)	Add a second long-acting bronchodilator from another class to regimen	Address comorbidities that may add to airway symptoms
C High risk Fewer symptoms	LAMA	**Preferred**: Add a second long-acting bronchodilator (LABA) Nonpreferred: Switch to LABA+ICS	ICS increases risk for pneumonia in some patients
D High risk More symptoms	LAMA + LABA	**Preferred**: Escalation to LABA+LAMA+ICS Nonpreferred: Switch to LABA+ICS	If exacerbations persist with LABA+LAMA+ICS: • Add PDE-4 if FEV_1 <50% predicted and chronic bronchitis • Add macrolide in previous smokers If symptoms well controlled with LABA+LAMA+ICS, consider discontinue ICS

Abbreviations: LABA = long-acting β_2-agonist; LAMA = long-acting antimuscarinic antagonist; ICS = inhaled corticosteroid; PDE-4 = phosphodiesterase-4.

Source: Reference 1.

TABLE 17-11 • Common Medications for the Management of Stable COPD

Medication Class and Example Drugs	Common/Serious Side Effects[a]	Blackbox Warnings/ Contraindications	Pregnancy Category[b]
Bronchodilators—anticholinergics Aclidinium bromide Ipratropium Tiotropium Umeclidinium	Bronchospasm Pharyngitis Xerostomia Constipation Sinusitis	Hypersensitivity to atropine	B (ipratropium) C (tiotropium)
Bronchodilators—β_2-agonists Albuterol Arformoterol Formoterol Indacaterol Levalbuterol Olodaterol Salmeterol	QT prolongation Tachycardia Hypokalemia Nervousness Tremor	Long-acting β_2-agonist may increase risk of death in asthma patients when used without inhaled corticosteroid	C
Bronchodilators—methylxanthines Theophylline	Tachyarrhythmia Atrial fibrillation Nausea/vomiting Insomnia Tremor Irritability	Hypersensitivity to theophylline	C
Inhaled corticosteroids (ICS) Beclamethasone Budesonide Ciclesonide Fluticasone Mometasone	Secondary hypocortisolism when used at high doses Pharyngitis Upper respiratory infection	Hypersensitivity to milk proteins	B (budesonide) C (all others)
Phosphodiesterase-4 inhibitors Roflumilast	Weight loss Nausea/diarrhea	Moderate to severe liver impairment	C

[a] This is a general list and does not include all side effects that can occur from these drugs. Consult a drug reference source for a more inclusive list before making any recommendations. MTM providers should also consult a comprehensive drug interaction database before making pharmacotherapy recommendations.

[b] Product labeling for all prescription drugs is being updated to reflect the new FDA Pregnancy Labeling and Lactation Rule. Please check individual product labeling for the most accurate and updated pregnancy information.

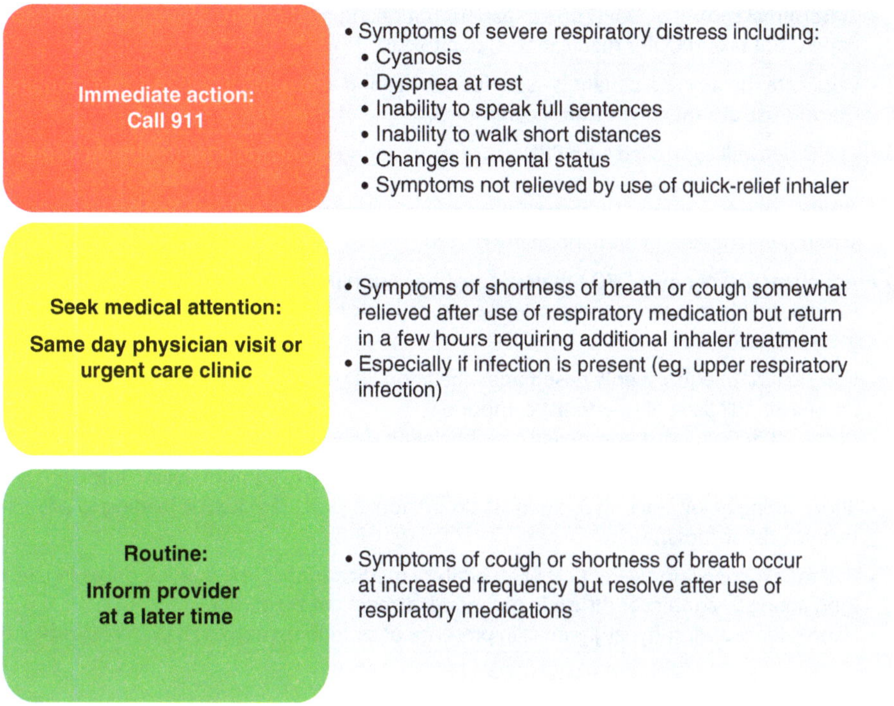

FIGURE 17-5 Referral for management of COPD.

TABLE 17-12 • Herbal Supplements for COPD

Herbal Product	Recommended Dosage	Level of Evidence	Cost[a]
Choline	1.5 g to 3 g daily	Possibly effective when taken orally for asthma. No data for COPD.	$$
Ephedra	N/A	Contains the chemicals ephedrine and pseudoephedrine. There is insufficient reliable information available about the effectiveness of ephedra for its use in COPD, and it is NOT recommended due to serious health risks including MI, CVA, and HF.	Not available
Beta-carotene	The Institute of Medicine has reviewed beta-carotene, but did not make recommendations for daily intake, citing lack of sufficient evidence.	The prevalence of bronchitis and dyspnea in male smokers with chronic obstructive pulmonary disorder (COPD) seems to be lower in those patients who consume a diet containing high amounts of beta-carotene. However, taking beta-carotene supplements does not seem to help.	$
Panax ginseng	100 mg to 6 g 3 times daily for up to 3 months has been used	A meta-analysis of clinical trials evaluating the use of panax ginseng orally in patients with stable COPD shows that panax ginseng significantly improves pulmonary function tests and quality of life compared to placebo after 3-6 months of treatment. However, panax ginseng only modestly improved FEV_1. Panax ginseng improved COPD symptoms by approximately 53% compared to placebo.	$ to $$$$
N-acetyl cysteine	600-1200 mg daily	In patients with moderate-to-severe COPD, taking N-acetyl cysteine orally can decrease the number of acute exacerbations by about 40% when used in addition to standard therapy.	$

[a] Cost: $ = $10/month supply in the recommended dosage; $$ = $11-$20/month, and $$$$ = >$50/month.

Abbreviations: COPD = chronic obstructive pulmonary disease; CVA = cerebrovascular accident; HF = heart failure; MI = myocardial infarction.

Sources: References 1 and 10.

TABLE 17-13 • Medication-Related Problems (MRPs) in Patients with COPD

Category of MRP	Example Medication-Related Problem
Nonadherence	• Suboptimal control of COPD due to patient not taking medications regularly or as prescribed • Patient not taking COPD medication(s) due to cost
Unnecessary medication	• Duplicate therapy (eg, patient is using ICS inhaler and also using ICS/ β_2-agonist combination inhaler) • Chronic use of a mucolytic (not recommended)
Need for additional medication	• COPD not well controlled with PRN use of short acting bronchodilator (requiring addition of scheduled long-acting bronchodilator) • COPD not well controlled with scheduled use of a single long-acting bronchodilator (requiring additional scheduled long-acting bronchodilator or ICS)
Ineffective medication	• Adequate trial of new COPD medication without significant clinical response • Patient unable to operate inhaler device (eg, arthritic hands find it difficult to grasp Spiriva handihaler) • Incorrect technique
Dosage too low	• Combo ICS/ β_2-agonist only dosed one inhalation BID for an inhaler that requires two inhalations BID to administer full dose of β_2-agonist component • Combo ICS/ β_2-agonist only dosed one inhalation daily for an inhaler that is indicated for BID dosing
Dosage too high	• Short-acting or long-acting bronchodilators dosed above maximum dosing intervals • Short-acting or long-acting β_2-agonists dosed above indicated dosage leading to adverse effects (eg, tachycardia, restlessness)
Adverse drug event	• Patient experiencing side effects of respiratory medications at appropriate doses (eg, tachycardia after taking long acting β_2-agonist or thrush in the mouth after initiation of ICS) • Hypokalemia and/or hyperglycemia in presence of continuous administration of short- or long-acting β_2-agonists

Abbreviations: BID = twice daily; COPD = chronic obstructive pulmonary disease; ICS = inhaled corticosteroid; PRN = as needed.

Scenario: Patient given samples of indacaterol but cannot afford Rx once samples are finished
MRP: Nonadherence

- Assessment:
  Patient unable to afford full cost of Arcapta (indacaterol) and prescription formulary does not cover. Currently uses sample only on days when she is having difficulty breathing instead of every day as prescribed. Switching to formulary long-acting beta agonist would provide for more affordable COPD treatment and allow patient to use daily as prescribed.
- Plan:
  Consider discontinuation of indacaterol daily and addition of twice-daily salmeterol or formoterol for daily control of COPD symptoms.

Scenario: Opportunity to reduce COPD inhaler burden
MRP: Nonadherence (or the potential to minimize nonadherence by simplifying regimen)

- Assessment:
  Based on pharmacy claims and/or patient report, your patient is currently receiving:
  - ProAir HFA (albuterol) inhaler, 2 puffs every 6 hours scheduled
  - Pulmicort (budesonide) 90mcg Flexhaler, 2 puffs twice daily

  Please note: Utilizing a combination long-acting beta agonist and inhaled corticosteroid inhaler dosed twice daily would provide similar control of COPD symptoms and simplify the inhaler burden.
- Plan:
  If appropriate, please consider switching your patient to a combination long-acting beta agonist/inhaled corticosteroid medication (Advair or Symbicort) to help reduce medication burden and optimize current therapy.

Scenario: COPD with reported poorly controlled symptoms and only one bronchodilator
MRP: Need for additional therapy

- Assessment:
  COPD symptoms reportedly not well controlled over the last few months with limitations in ability to clean house and work in garden noted several times per week. Patient reports currently taking tiotropium daily and denies any missed doses in the last 2 weeks.
- Plan:
  Consider addition of BID long acting beta agonist to improve symptoms or an ICS if airflow limitation is severe or very severe. Patient to keep log of COPD symptoms and report if improvement in symptoms to provider after 2 weeks of regular usage.

Scenario: COPD with poorly controlled symptoms and incorrect dose of long-acting beta agonist
MRP: Dosage too low

- Assessment:
  COPD symptoms reportedly not well controlled over the last few months. Patient currently prescribed Advair HFA 45/21 (fluticasone/salmeterol), 1 inhalation twice daily, which only provides half of the indicated salmeterol dose. Increase in dose to 2 inhalations twice daily may improve symptoms by providing adequate dose of long-acting beta agonist component.
- Plan:
  Recommend increase Advair dose to 2 inhalations twice daily.
  Patient to keep log of COPD symptoms and report if improvement in symptoms to provider after 2 weeks of regular usage.

FIGURE 17-6 Sample provider communications for COPD.

Regular follow-up is essential in COPD, as some patients may have worsening lung function over time despite the best available care. Symptoms should be discussed at every visit, as well as the current therapeutic regimen. The optimal interval for follow-up has not been clearly defined and depends on several factors, including severity of disease, type of intervention, and patient-specific factors such as age, comorbid conditions, and ability to return for follow-up. However, at a minimum, it is prudent to perform spirometry testing annually.[1] Additionally, questionnaires such as the CAT may be performed every 2 to 3 months.

REFERENCES

1. Global Initiative for Chronic Obstructive Lung Disease (GOLD). Global strategy for the diagnosis, management and prevention of COPD, 2017. Available at http://goldcopd.org. Accessed May 14, 2017.
2. Centers for Disease Control and Prevention (CDC), National Center for Health Statistics. Compressed mortality file 1999-2006. CDC WONDER on-line database, compiled from compressed mortality file 1999-2006 Series 20 No. 2L. Atlanta: CDC; 2009. Available at http://wonder.cdc.gov/cmf-icd10.html. Accessed May 14, 2017.
3. U.S. Department of Health and Human Services, Healthy People 2020. (2011, June 29). Respiratory diseases: objectives. Available at http://www.healthypeople.gov/2020/topicsobjectives2020/objectiveslist.aspx?topicId=36. Accessed July 31, 2017.
4. CMS. Medicare Part D medication therapy management program standardized format. Available at https://www.cms.gov/Medicare/Prescription-Drug-Coverage/PrescriptionDrugCovContra/Downloads/MTM-Program-Standardized-Format-English-and-Spanish-Instructions-Samples-v032712.pdf. Accessed May 14, 2017.
5. Fiore MC, Jaén CR, Baker TB, et al. *Treating Tobacco Use and Dependence: 2008 Update. Clinical Practice Guideline.* Rockville, MD: U.S. Department of Health and Human Services; May 2008.
6. American Thoracic Society. Pulmonary rehabilitation—1999: official statement of the American Thoracic Society. *Am J Respir Crit Care Med.* 1999;159:1666-1682.
7. Kim DK, Riley LE, Harriman KH, Hunter P, Bridges CB. Advisory Committee on Immunization Practices recommended immunization schedule for adults aged 19 years or older—United States, 2017. *MMWR Morb Mortal Wkly Rep.* 2017;66:136-138.
8. Nichol KL, Margolis KL, Wourenma J, Von Sternberg T. The efficacy and cost effectiveness of vaccination against influenza among elderly persons living in the community. *New Engl J Med.* 1994;331:778-784.
9. Centers for Disease Control and Prevention. Use of 13-valent pneumococcal conjugate vaccine and 23-valent pneumococcal polysaccharide vaccine among adults aged ≥65 years: recommendations of the Advisory Committee on Immunization Practices (ACIP). *MMWR Morb Mortal Wkly Rep.* 2014;63:822-825.
10. Natural Medicines [database online]. Somerville, MA: Therapeutic Research Center; 2017. Available at https://naturalmedicines.therapeuticresearch.com/. Accessed May 11, 2017.

Review Questions

1. Which host factor can influence the risk of developing COPD following exposure to environmental risk factors?
   a. Tobacco smoke
   b. Air pollution
   c. Occupational dusts and chemicals
   d. Airway hyperresponsiveness

2. Which factor is indicative of a patient who is "high risk" for future COPD exacerbations?
   a. Daily use of both long-acting beta2-agonist and anticholinergic bronchodilator.
   b. COPD Assessment Test (CAT) score of 12.
   c. Grade 3 airflow limitation.
   d. A history of 2 COPD exacerbations in the previous 12 months.

3. Which directive is a component of the goal of risk reduction for COPD patients?
   a. Prevent and treat exacerbations.
   b. Improve exercise tolerance.
   c. Use quick-relief medication per schedule.
   d. Reduce quick-relief medication use.

4. Which term can be defined, in living-room language, as the "total amount of air you can breathe out in 1 second?"
   a. FVC
   b. FEV1
   c. FEV1/FVC
   d. FEV6

5. Which information would be appropriate to include in the MAP for a COPD patient?
   a. Tiotropium is a controller inhaler that may be used as needed to treat shortness of breath.
   b. Use your tiotropium inhaler once every morning as prescribed (even on the days you wake up feeling well).
   c. Fluticasone/salmeterol is a quick-relief inhaler that may be used as needed to treat shortness of breath.
   d. If you experience shortness of breath during the day, use your fluticasone/salmeterol inhaler as prescribed for quick relief of your symptoms.

6. Which symptom requires IMMEDIATE referral to a physician?
   a. Shortness of breath after climbing several flights of stairs that is relieved upon rest.
   b. New onset of shortness of breath not relieved by use of quick-relief inhaler.
   c. COPD symptoms of cough or shortness of breath that occur at increased frequency but resolve after use of respiratory medications.
   d. Fever of 99°F (37°C) without flu-like symptoms for a duration of 2 days.

7. In which situation should the MTM provider assess for the medication-related problem "need for additional medication"?
   a. Chronic use of a mucolytic to treat a cough after inhalation of tobacco smoke
   b. Suboptimal control of COPD because of patient not taking medications as prescribed
   c. COPD not well controlled with as-needed use of short-acting bronchodilator
   d. Combination inhaled corticosteroid /beta2-agonist dosed 1 inhalation daily

8. Which statement is correct regarding immunizations for a COPD patient?
   a. Patients with COPD should receive the 23-valent pneumococcal polysaccharide (PPSV23) vaccine every 5 years.
   b. Patients with a history of serious allergy to egg should not receive the influenza vaccine.
   c. Influenza vaccination has the potential to reduce serious illness and death by 50%.
   d. Patients with COPD should receive the 13-valent pneumococcal conjugate vaccine (PCV13) vaccine every 3 years.

9. Based on the 2017 GOLD guidelines, what is a recommended first-line monotherapy for a patient in group C?
   a. Long-acting anticholinergic
   b. Long-acting beta2-agonist
   c. Inhaled corticosteroid
   d. PDE-4 inhibitor

10. Which supplement is not recommended for COPD patients due to serious risks including myocardial infarction, cerebrovascular accident, and heart failure?
    a. Beta-carotene
    b. Choline
    c. Ephedra
    d. Boswellia

ANSWERS

1. d	2. d	3. a
4. b	5. b	6. b
7. c	8. c	9. a
10. c		

18

Chronic Stable Angina MTM Data Set

Shawn D. Anderson, PharmD, BCACP, and Kristyn M. Pardo, PharmD, BCPS, CACP

KEY POINTS

- Stable ischemic heart disease (SIHD) is caused by atherosclerotic plaque buildup in the coronary arteries.
- Angina results when the heart's demand for oxygen exceeds the available supply.
- Stable angina is reproducible and relieved by rest or nitroglycerin. An increase in angina frequency, severity, or duration characterizes it as "unstable." A patient with unstable angina should be referred for medical evaluation.
- Acute angina attacks that do not resolve with rest may require the use of nitroglycerin. Medication therapy management (MTM) providers should counsel on proper use of nitroglycerin, including when to call 911.
- Management of chronic stable angina aims to reduce the frequency of angina attacks. β-Blockers, calcium channel blockers, and long-acting nitrates are common treatments.
- MTM providers should stress the importance of adherence to medications for chronic stable angina, and counsel on appropriate use of medications to maximize the therapeutic effect, eg, the importance of a nitrate-free interval for patients on long-acting nitrates.

INTRODUCTION

Chronic stable angina (CSA) describes a syndrome in which the cardiac demand for oxygen exceeds the available supply in patients with stable ischemic heart disease (SIHD). Over time, atherosclerotic plaques build up in the coronary arteries. The plaques narrow the diameter of the arteries that supply blood to the heart. When oxygen demand increases (for example, during exercise or stress), the healthy heart compensates by increasing blood flow and consequently increasing oxygen supply. This compensatory increase in blood flow is not always achieved in patients with chronic stable angina.[1,2] When myocardial demand exceeds the supply from the coronary arteries, the patient may feel chest pain, pressure, or tightness (angina). Pain may radiate to the jaw, shoulder, back, or arm. Table 18-1 reviews typical angina symptoms. It is important to note that not all patients will present with these classic symptoms; in fact, some patients may have no symptoms at all. This is called silent ischemia.[1] Women are also more likely to present with atypical symptoms such as nausea, vomiting, or sharp chest pain.[2]

Noncardiac chest pain or discomfort can mimic angina pain (Table 18-2).[1,2] Careful questioning can help to determine whether a patient's chest pain may be related to a noncardiac cause. However, the MTM provider should err on the side of caution and refer patients to their healthcare provider or emergency department if they report worsening symptoms.

Distinguishing Chronic Stable Angina from Acute Coronary Syndromes

CSA is reproducible with a specific amount of exertion and is relieved either with rest or with the use of vasodilators such as nitroglycerin.[4] The reproducibility and reversibility of angina pain separates chronic stable angina from the acute coronary syndromes (unstable angina, non-ST elevation myocardial infarction, and ST-elevation myocardial infarction), although they all are indicative of SIHD. An increase in the frequency, severity, or duration of angina pain may suggest that the angina is "unstable," rather than stable. Further workup may be needed to determine

TABLE 18-1 • Typical Anginal Symptoms

Description	Character	Radiation of Pain	Provoking Factors	Associated Symptoms
Discomfort Squeezing Tightness Pressure	Gradual in onset and offset Not localized to one specific area	Upper abdomen Shoulders Arms Lower jaw/teeth	Physical activity Emotional stress Sexual intercourse Cold weather	Shortness of breath Sweating Dizziness or lightheadedness

Source: Compiled from reference 3.

whether additional pharmacological or procedural interventions are necessary.[1,2]

Classification of Severity of Angina

Various criteria have been developed to classify stages and severity of angina (Table 18-3 and 18-4). More severe degrees of coronary artery blockage may result in more severe symptoms, but this is not always the case. Coronary angiography can be used to determine the extent of atherosclerotic disease in the coronary arteries. Coronary angioplasty or revascularization with stents or bypass surgery may be appropriate if there are severe or multiple blocked arteries.[1]

Many factors influence outcomes in chronic stable angina patients (Table 18-5). Efforts should focus on cardiovascular disease management and control of modifiable risk factors.[1,2]

Therapeutic Goals for Chronic Stable Angina

The immediate goal of therapy for CSA is to maximize functional status and improve quality of life. Specific goals may include reducing chest pain frequency or allowing the patient to perform specific activities without chest pain. A well-conducted patient interview will help the MTM provider determine whether the CSA regimen is meeting this goal (Table 18-6). Adjustments to antianginal medications may be warranted if quality of life or ability to carry out activities is significantly affected by chest pain. Any increase in the frequency, severity, or duration of chest pain may constitute unstable angina, which could warrant immediate referral for work-up. MTM providers must also assess whether the patient is receiving appropriate medications that aim to reduce long-term morbidity and mortality.[2] For this reason, the MTM provider should carefully review the medication list and identify any potential gaps in therapy.

TABLE 18-2 • Differential Diagnosis of Episodic Chest Pain Resembling Angina Pectoris

	Duration	Quality	Provocation	Relief	Location	Comment
Effort angina	5-15 minutes	Visceral (pressure)	During effort or emotion	Rest, NTG	Substernal, radiates	First episode vivid
Rest angina	5-15 minutes	Visceral (pressure)	Spontaneous (with exercise?)	NTG	Substernal, radiates	Often nocturnal
Mitral prolapse	Minutes to hours	Superficial (rarely visceral)	Spontaneous (no pattern)	Time	Left anterior	No pattern, variable
Esophageal reflux	10 minutes to 1 hour	Visceral	Spontaneous, cold liquids, exercise, lying down	Foods, antacids, H_2 blockers, proton pump inhibitors, NTG	Substernal, radiates	Mimics angina
Peptic ulcer	Hours	Visceral, burning	Lack of food, "acid" foods	Foods, antacids, H_2 blockers, proton pump inhibitors	Epigastric, substernal	
Biliary disease	Hours	Visceral (wax and wane)	Spontaneous, food	Time, analgesia	Epigastric, radiates	Colic
Cervical disk	Variable (gradually subsides)	Superficial	Spontaneous, food	Time, analgesia	Arm, neck	Not relieved by rest
Hyperventilation	2-3 minutes	Visceral	Emotion, tachypnea	Stimulus removed	Substernal	Facial paraesthesia
Musculoskeletal	Variable	Superficial	Movement, palpation	Time, analgesia	Multiple	Tenderness
Pulmonary	30 minutes	Visceral (pressure)	Often spontaneous	Rest, time bronchodilator	Substernal	Dyspneic

Abbreviation: NTG = nitroglycerin.

Source: Reproduced, with permission, from DiPiro JT, Talbert RL, Yee GC, Matzke GR, Wells BG, Posey L, eds. *Pharmacotherapy: A Pathophysiologic Approach.* 10th ed. New York, NY: McGraw-Hill; 2017.

TABLE 18-3 • Criteria for Determination of the Specific Activity Scale Functional Class

	Any Yes	No
1. Can you walk down a flight of steps without stopping (4.5-5.2 MET)?	Go to 2	Go to 4
2. Can you carry anything up a flight of 8 steps without stopping (5-5.5 MET)? Or can you a. Have sexual intercourse without stopping (5-5.2 MET) b. Garden, rake, weed (5.6 MET) c. Roller skate, dance foxtrot (5-6 MET) d. Walk at a 4 miles/h rate on level ground (5-6 MET)	Go to 3	Class III
3. Can you carry at least 24 lb up 8 steps (10 MET)? Or can you a. Carry objects that weigh at least 80 lb (18 MET) b. Do outdoor work, shovel snow, spade soil (7 MET) c. Do recreational activities such as skiing, basketball, touch football, squash, handball (7-10 MET) d. Jog/walk 5 miles/h (9 MET)	Class I	Class II
4. Can you shower without stopping (3.6-4.2 MET)? Or can you a. Strip and make bed (3.9-5 MET) b. Mop floors (4.2 MET) c. Hang washed clothes (4.4 MET) d. Clean windows (3.7 MET) e. Walk 2.5 miles/h (3-3.5 MET) f. Bowl (3-4.4 MET) g. Play golf, walk, and carry clubs (4.5 MET) h. Push a power lawnmower (4 MET)	Class III	Go to 5
5. Can you dress without stopping because of symptoms (2-2.3 MET)?	Class III	Class IV

Abbreviation: MET = metabolic equivalents of activity.

Source: Reproduced, with permission, from Goldman L, Hashimoto B, Cook EF, Loscalzo A. Comparative reproducibility and validity of systems for assessing cardiovascular functional class: advantages of a new specific activity scale. *Circulation.* 1981;64:1227-1234.

TABLE 18-4 • Grading of Angina Pectoris by the Canadian Cardiovascular Society Classification System

Class	Description of Stage
Class I	Ordinary physical activity does not cause angina such as walking and climbing stairs. Angina occurs with strenuous, rapid, or prolonged exertion at work or recreation.
Class II	Slight limitation or ordinary activity. Angina occurs on walking or climbing stairs rapidly, on walking uphill, on walking or stair climbing after meals, in cold, in wind, under emotional stress, or only during the few hours after wakening. Walking more than two blocks on the level and climbing more than one flight of ordinary stairs at a normal pace and in normal condition.
Class III	Marked limitations of ordinary physical activity. Angina occurs on walking one to two blocks on the level and climbing one flight of stairs in normal conditions and at a normal pace.
Class IV	Inability to carry on any physical activity without discomfort—anginal symptoms may be present at rest.

Source: Reproduced, with permission, from Campeau L. Grading of angina [letter]. *Circulation.* 1976;54:522-523.

TABLE 18-5 • Factors that May Aggravate Chronic Stable Angina

Medical Conditions	Patient Factors
Hypertension, hypotension	Smoking/tobacco use
Anemia	Stress, anxiety, depression
Tachycardia	Exercise
Hyperthyroidism	Cocaine abuse
Pulmonary disease	Methamphetamine abuse
Obstructive sleep apnea	

Source: References 2 and 3.

TABLE 18-6 • Suggested Questions to Ask When Conducting a Medication Therapy Review in a Patient with Chronic Stable Angina

Questions Assessing Identification and Control of Chronic Stable Angina

• Describe your angina or "chest pain" symptoms.
  • What brings it on?
  • What makes it better?
  • What makes it worse?
  • How long does it typically last?
• How often does it occur? How does chest pain limit you from doing activities?
• How long have you had problems with angina?
• Have you ever been hospitalized for chest pain? Have you had a heart attack? Open heart surgery? Stents placed in your heart? When?

Questions Assessing General Medication Use and Adherence
• What medications do you take to treat or prevent angina? How do you take them? • How do you use nitroglycerin? How often do you need to use it? • How often do you replace your bottle of nitroglycerin? • How often do you miss a dose of your medications? • Have you ever stopped taking any of your prescribed medications without telling your physician? If so, why? • What over-the-counter medications or herbals do you use?
Questions Assessing Additional Risk Factors

• What tobacco products do you use?
• How is your blood pressure?
  • How often do you check your blood pressure?
  • What is a "typical" blood pressure for you?
• How is your cholesterol? What "statin" medicine do you take?
• How is your blood sugar?
• What kinds of physical activity do you do on a regular basis?
• What is your weight? What is your height? How do you feel about your weight? What did your physician tell you about your weight?

Questions to Ask for Prevention/Assessment of Medical Emergencies
• Crisis planning: What are the warning signs of a heart attack and stroke, and what is your action plan? • What would you do if your nitroglycerin does not relieve your chest pain?

CORE ELEMENT 1—COMPREHENSIVE MEDICATION REVIEW FOR PATIENTS WITH CHRONIC STABLE ANGINA

Table 18-6 contains a list of suggested questions to use when conducting a medication therapy review in a patient with CSA. The number and types of questions will depend upon several factors, including the amount of time for the interview, number of concurrent medication-related problems, urgency of MRPs, and the reliability of the patient in providing accurate information, among others. In time-limited interactions or in complex cases with multiple medical issues, the MTM provider may choose to target questions that help to identify or rule out issues of an urgent nature (see questions to ask for prevention/assessment of medical emergencies). MTM providers should remember to use living room language during the interview (Figure 18-1) and be prepared for questions that patients may ask regarding their condition (Table 18-7).

CORE ELEMENT 2—PERSONAL MEDICATION LIST

The following is a sample personal medication list[8] (PML) for a patient with CSA (Figure 18-2). This example is representative only of CSA medications. Additional medications for other disease states should be added and listed separately. MTM providers should remember to use plain language when creating the PML.

CORE ELEMENT 3—MEDICATION ACTION PLAN

Figure 18-3 contains a sample medication action plan[8] (MAP) for a patient with CSA. This example is representative only of action steps for a patient with CSA. MAPs for other disease states or other MRPs should be added and listed separately. In most cases, only a few of the most important action steps should be listed, so as not

ACE inhibitor—a medicine used to help lower blood pressure, may also help prevent changes or damage to the heart and kidney.

Acute coronary syndrome—decreased blood flow to the heart which may lead to a heart attack.

Adverse event—something bad that happens, bad reaction, unexplained or unwanted effects.

Angina—chest pain or discomfort caused by decreased blood flow to the heart muscle.

Antihypertensive medication—a medicine that lowers blood pressure.

Antiplatelet—a medicine that prevents blood from forming clots.

Arteries—blood vessels that carry blood away from the heart.

Atherosclerosis—hardening or clogging of the arteries due to a buildup of fatty material, may lead to decreased blood flow to the heart.

β-blocker—a medicine used to help lower blood pressure and control heart rate; can be used to prevent chest pain.

Calcium channel blocker—a medicine used to lower blood pressure. Some of these medicines also control heart rate. Can be used to prevent chest pain.

Cardiac—related to the heart.

Cardiac catheterization—procedure that allows a physician to examine the heart and heart vessels.

Cardiologist—heart physician.

Chronic—constant, long-lasting, persistent.

Coronary angiography—procedure that allows a physician to see blockages in the heart vessels.

Coronary artery disease—narrowing and hardening of the small blood vessels that supply blood and oxygen to the heart.

Coronary artery bypass surgery—open-heart surgery that helps restore good blood flow to the heart.

Crescendo angina—chest pain attack that happens with increasing frequency, intensity or duration.

Direct vasodilator—a medicine used to treat or prevent chest pain or lower blood pressure; it works by relaxing blood vessels.

ECG—a test that looks for any damage to or problems with your heart.

Fasting lipid panel—a test of the fats in your blood taken after 8-12 hours without eating any food (fasting).

Heart rate—how many times your heart beats each minute.

Hypertension—high blood pressure.

Hypotension—low blood pressure.

Lifestyle changes—your Physician may have recommended changes in lifestyle to lower your blood pressure, which for some patients include reaching a goal weight, decreasing the amount of alcohol you consume, exercising, or quitting smoking.

Myocardial infarction—heart attack, damage to the heart.

Nitrate—a medicine used to relieve chest pain.

Obese—having a body mass index (BMI) over 30; increases your risk of having high blood pressure, diabetes, and heart disease.

Obstructive sleep apnea—a sleep disorder that often involves pauses in breathing during the night.

Orthostatic hypotension—dizziness or lightheadedness upon standing because of low blood pressure.

Overweight—having a body mass index (BMI) over 25; increases your risk of having high blood pressure, diabetes, and heart disease.

Presyncope—almost fainting, "blacking out" or "passing out."

Revascularization—a procedure that restores good blood flow to the heart.

Smoking cessation—quitting smoking.

Stable ischemic heart disease—heart problems caused by a lack of blood flow to the heart.

Statin—a medicine used to lower the risk of heart disease; can also lower cholesterol.

Stent—a tube-like device that is used to open up a clogged blood vessel in the heart.

Stroke—a condition that can cause a loss of speech, memory, or physical abilities due to damage to the brain.

Syncope—fainting, "blacking out" or "passing out."

Tachycardia—a fast heartbeat, more than 100 times in a minute.

Unstable angina—an increase in the frequency, intensity or duration of chest pain, which should be evaluated by a physician.

Veins—blood vessels that carry blood toward the heart.

FIGURE 18-1 Living room language for chronic stable angina.

TABLE 18-7 • Questions to Anticipate Regarding Chronic Stable Angina

- **What is angina?**
  Angina is a feeling that people with heart disease get when their heart muscle is not getting enough oxygen from blood flow. It may feel like pressure or tightness. It usually comes on with physical activity or stress and gets better with rest or quick-acting medicines like nitroglycerin.
- **What is chronic stable angina?**
  Chronic means constant. Stable means that the condition is not getting worse. Angina is what happens when the heart is not getting enough blood flow (see "What is angina?" section). A person with chronic stable angina can generally manage their condition with simple things such as rest or medicine. If the condition is getting worse, it is no longer "stable" and should be assessed by a physician.

(*Continued*)

TABLE 18-7 • Questions to Anticipate Regarding Chronic Stable Angina (*Continued*)

- **What causes chronic stable angina?**
  Over your lifetime, cholesterol builds up in the blood vessels that bring oxygen to the heart. This is called atherosclerosis. When the blockages get very thick, they can block blood flow going to the heart muscle. The heart has to pump more blood during physical activity or stress than it does when you are resting. To do that, the heart muscle needs more blood (and oxygen) for itself. Usually the blood vessels in the heart can supply extra blood when it is needed, but if there are large blockages this may not happen. A person may feel "angina" or chest pain/pressure when the heart's demand for blood is not met by an increase in blood supply. Medicines such as nitroglycerin widen the heart vessels to increase blood supply. Resting will decrease the heart's demand for blood.
- **What health problems are associated with chronic stable angina?**
  Cardiovascular disease is an umbrella term for many health problems affecting the heart and blood vessels in the body, including chronic stable angina. High blood pressure, high cholesterol, and diabetes are examples of cardiovascular diseases. Heart attack, stroke, and death are possible results of long-term cardiovascular disease.
- **Why are medications so important?**
  Medications used to treat chronic stable angina can improve symptoms and quality of life. Some medications help to prevent other problems such as heart attack and stroke. Taking medications as prescribed is one of the best things you can do to prevent further health problems and early death.
- **What can happen if I stop taking my medications?**
  If you stop taking your medicines suddenly, your angina symptoms may get worse. You may have a life-threatening heart attack or stroke.
- **When should I seek medical attention for my angina?**
  Call 911 if your angina or chest pain is does not get better after your first dose of nitroglycerin or if it is not completely relieved after three doses. Waiting to call 911 may cause a delay in getting the appropriate emergency treatment. Call your physician or seek emergency medical attention if your symptoms happen more frequently, last longer than usual, or are more severe. You may need to have tests to evaluate your heart condition. Your physician may also adjust your medicines.
- **How should I store my nitroglycerin tablets?**
  Be sure to have your nitroglycerin tablets available to you at all times so that you always have them when you need them. Store your tablets in the original bottle, and make sure you keep the top tightly closed to protect the tablets from moisture. Keep at room temperature, and avoid exposing the tablets to very hot or very cold environments. The tablets are good until the expiration date on the bottle if they are stored properly. If your tablets appear powdery, you should order a new bottle. Some providers may suggest replacing the bottle every six months.
- **Can I take nitroglycerin before I exercise to prevent chest pain?**
  Yes, as long as your physician has told you that it is safe for you to exercise. You can take nitroglycerin just before you begin, and the effects should last.
- **What should I do if I have a problem with my medications?**
  Never stop taking your medications without first talking to your physician. Speak with your physician and/or pharmacist to let them know about any problems you are having, and together you can make sure your medications are the right ones for you.

PERSONAL MEDICATION LIST FOR *<Insert Patient's name*, DOB: *mm/dd/yyyy>*	
Medication: Metoprolol tartrate 25 mg tablet	
How I use it: Take one pill (25 mg) every 12 hours	
Why I use it: Blood pressure and heart	**Prescriber:** Smith
Date I started using it: 1/6/2015	**Date I stopped using it:** *(Leave blank for patient's notes)*
Why I stopped using it: *(Leave blank for patient's notes)*	
Medication: Nitroglycerin 0.4 mg sublingual tablet	
How I use it: Place one pill (0.4 mg) under the tongue for relief of chest pain. May repeat dose every 5 minutes for a total of 3 doses. Call 911 if chest pain is not better after first dose or completely gone after 3 doses.	
Why I use it: Chest pain (angina)	**Prescriber:** Smith
Date I started using it: 1/6/2015	**Date I stopped using it:** *(Leave blank for patient's notes)*
Why I stopped using it: *(Leave blank for patient's notes)*	

FIGURE 18-2 Example personal medication list for chronic stable angina.

	DATE PREPARED: *<Insert date>*
What we talked about: Importance of taking nitroglycerin correctly when I have chest pain	
What I need to do: • Place one pill under the tongue for relief of chest pain. • May repeat dose every 5 minutes for a total of 3 doses. • Call 911 if chest pain is not better after first dose or completely gone after 3 doses.	**What I did and when I did it:** *(Leave blank for patient's notes)*
What we talked about: • Need to see how well new medicine is working to reduce angina episodes and severity	
What I need to do: 1. Write down the number and severity of angina episodes. Severity can be graded on a scale of 0 to 10 with 10 being the most severe. Notify clinic if episodes are more frequent or more severe. Always seek immediate medical attention for chest pain at rest not relieved with nitroglycerin. 2. Check and record blood pressure at home. Notify the clinic if my blood pressure is higher than 180/120 mm Hg or lower than 100/60 mm Hg. 3. Check and record heart rate at home. Notify the clinic if my heart rate is higher than 100 bpm or lower than 60 bpm. 4. Bring log book every time I come to clinic.	**What I did and when I did it:** *(Leave blank for patient's notes)*

FIGURE 18-3 Example medication action plan for a patient with chronic stable angina.

to overwhelm the patient. Other areas for patient self-management can be addressed at later visits. MTM providers should remember to use plain language when creating the MAP.

CORE ELEMENT 4—INTERVENTION AND/OR REFERRAL

Interventions for the management of CSA because of SIHD can be separated into short- and long-term strategies. Short-term interventions prevent or limit symptoms of angina to maximize quality of life and exercise capacity.[1,2] Long-term strategies attempt to limit the progression of atherosclerosis and ultimately prevent cardiovascular events (eg, acute coronary syndromes).[1,9] Both strategies include lifestyle modifications and/or drug therapy. Patients not adequately controlled with lifestyle modifications should be started on drug therapy. In addition, patients likely will have to take cardioprotective medications, regardless of adherence to and success of lifestyle modifications. Fortunately, some cardioprotective medications are also effective at reducing anginal symptoms.

Many patient factors should be considered when selecting an antianginal medication. These factors include, but are not limited to: compelling indications, comorbid disease states, concomitant medications, cost, and adherence. Patients should be encouraged to monitor vital signs (blood pressure, heart rate, weight) at home and to follow up at regular intervals so that progression to treatment goals can be assessed. Table 18-8 summarizes modifiable risk factors that contribute to progression of SIHD and worsening angina.

TABLE 18-8 • Modifiable Risk Factors in Stable Ischemic Heart Disease and Chronic Stable Angina

Risk Factor	Treatment Consideration
Smoking cessation	Encourage smoking cessation and avoidance of second hand smoke. Utilize a stepwise strategy (Ask, Advise, Assess, Assist, Arrange, Avoid) for smoking cessation.
Hypertension	Refer to Chapter 27 and follow most recent guidelines.
Dyslipidemia	Refer to Chapter 22 and follow most recent guidelines.
Diabetes	Refer to Chapter 21 and follow most recent guidelines.
Obesity	Initial weight loss of 5% to 10% from baseline through physical activity and reduced caloric intake. Goal is to maintain or achieve a BMI between 18.5 and 24.9 kg/m^2.
Alcohol consumption	Men: ≤2 drinks/day Women and lighter persons: ≤1 drink/day 1 drink equals 12 oz beer, 5 oz wine, or 1.5 oz of 80-proof whiskey
Sedentary lifestyle	Most patients should participate in 30 to 60 minutes of moderate-intensity aerobic activity at least 5 days per week. High-risk patients should participate in a medically supervised cardiac rehabilitation program.
Psychological (stress, anxiety, depression)	Refer to Chapter 20. It is reasonable to screen for mental illness and refer to mental health provider, if indicated.

Abbreviations: BMI = body mass index; oz = ounces.

Source: References 1, 2, and 9.

Table 18-9 provides an overview of antianginal drug therapy. Key concepts for nitrate therapy can be found in Table 18-10. Considerations for antianginal drug therapy such as compelling indications and individualization of drug therapy are found in Tables 18-11 and 18-12, respectively. In addition, Table 18-13 outlines herbal remedies that may be useful in the management of angina. A CSA treatment algorithm and criteria for referral for management of unstable and stable angina are found in Figures 18-4 and 18-5, respectively. In addition to antianginal therapy, patients with SIHD may also benefit from the addition of other medications for secondary coronary artery disease prevention (briefly outlined in Table 18-14).

TABLE 18-9 • Medications for Management of Angina

Medication Class and Example Drugs	Common/Serious Side Effects[a]	Blackbox Warnings/Contraindications	Pregnancy Category[b]
β-Blockers Atenolol Bisoprolol Metoprolol Propranolol	Mask hypoglycemia in diabetics; Worsen insulin sensitivity, breathing disorders, and PVD; Bradycardia, Dizziness, Exercise intolerance, Fatigue, Orthostatic hypotension (especially mixed α- and β-blockers)	• Abrupt discontinuation • Asthma (avoid nonselective BB or high-dose selective BB) • AV block • Bradycardia • Cardiogenic shock • Heart failure (except bisoprolol, carvedilol, metoprolol succinate) • Hypotension • Pheochromocytoma (if not on α-blocker) • Sick sinus syndrome	C D (atenolol)
Calcium channel blockers dihydropyridines Amlodipine Felodipine Nifedipine	Dizziness, Flushing, Gingival hyperplasia, Headache, Nausea, Peripheral edema, Postural hypotension, IR preparations: reflex tachycardia	• Avoid short-acting dihydropyridines that may worsen angina (ie, immediate-release nifedipine or nicardipine)	C
Calcium channel blockers nondihydropyridines Diltiazem Verapamil	Bradycardia, Hypotension, Peripheral edema Diltiazem: headache, nausea Verapamil: constipation	• Acute MI • AV block • Cardiogenic shock • Hypotension • Heart failure with reduced EF • Sick sinus syndrome • Ventricular tachycardia • Wolff-Parkinson-White syndrome	C
Nitrates Nitroglycerin (SL, spray, patch, ointment), Isosorbide dinitrate, Isosorbide mononitrate	Headache, Dizziness, Hypotension, Flushing, Nausea	• Concomitant use with PDE inhibitors • Constrictive pericarditis • Restrictive cardiomyopathy • Tolerance may occur at high doses or with administration without a nitrate-free interval	C
Antianginal (other) Ranolazine	Dizziness, Headache, QT prolongation	• Potent CYP3A4 inhibitors and inducers • QT interval prolongation at baseline (>500 ms) • Hepatic cirrhosis	C

[a] This is a general list and does not include all side effects that can occur from these drugs. Consult a drug reference source for a more inclusive list before making any recommendations. MTM providers should also consult a comprehensive drug interaction database before making pharmacotherapy recommendations.

[b] Product labeling for all prescription drugs is being updated to reflect the new FDA Pregnancy Labeling and Lactation Rule. Please check individual product labeling for the most accurate and updated pregnancy information.

Abbreviations: AV = atrioventricular; BB = β-blocker; CYP3A4 = cytochrome P450 3A4; EF = ejection fraction; IR = immediate-release; MI = myocardial infarction; ms = milliseconds; PVD = peripheral vascular disease; SL = sublingual; PDE = phosphodiesterase.

Source: References 1, 2, and 10.

TABLE 18-10 • Key Concepts for Nitrate Use in Chronic Stable Angina

Sublingual Nitroglycerin	Long-acting Nitrates
Available as tablet or spray.	Available as tablet or transdermal patch.
For treatment of acute attacks: place 1 tablet (or spray) under the tongue every 5 minutes for a total of 3 doses. Call 911 if pain is not improved after the first dose or if pain is not completely resolved after the third dose.	Consider as add-on therapy after optimizing β-blocker and/or calcium channel blocker.
Prophylaxis of symptoms when engaging in activities known to precipitate angina: Place 1 tablet (or spray) under the tongue approximately 5 minutes prior to initiation of activity. Antianginal effects should last approximately 30 minutes.	A nitrate-free period of at least 8 to 12 hours per day can prevent tolerance.

TABLE 18-11 • Compelling Indications in Chronic Stable Angina

Compelling Indication	Preferred Drug Options
Heart failure with reduced ejection fraction (EF ≤40%)	β-Blocker (bisoprolol, carvedilol, or metoprolol succinate) at very low doses and titrate slowly based on tolerability Caution: Ranolazine may induce negative inotropy Avoid: CCB (except amlodipine and felodipine)
Post-myocardial infarction	β-Blocker without intrinsic sympathomimetic (ISA) activity Avoid: IR dihydropyridine CCBs, β-blockers with ISA activity (acebutolol, penbutolol, pindolol)
Vasospastic or Prinzmetal's angina	Non-DHP or DHP CCB as monotherapy preferred May combine a non-DHP CCB and DHP CCB if angina persists on optimal monotherapy dose and nitrates Avoid: β-blockers may worsen angina because of vasoconstriction (may consider using a β-blocker with α-blocking activity as last-line [eg, carvedilol])
Atrial arrhythmias	β-Blocker without ISA activity or non-DHP CCBs Avoid: IR dihydropyridine CCBs (reflex tachycardia)
Ventricular arrhythmias	β-Blocker without ISA activity Verapamil is a first-line option for rare idiopathic ventricular tachycardias

Abbreviations: CCB = calcium channel blocker; DHP = dihydropyridine; IR = immediate-release; ISA = intrinsic sympathomimetic activity.

Source: References 1, 2, and 9.

TABLE 18-12 • Considerations in Individualizing Therapy for Chronic Stable Angina

Condition	Drug Options
Hypertension	All drug therapy options will lower blood pressure, except for ranolazine. Recommend optimizing blood pressure prior to adding ranolazine.
Low blood pressure or hypotension	There are some data to suggest that a diastolic blood pressure <60 mm Hg may worsen angina and is associated with poor prognosis. Most patients can tolerate a low dose of antianginal drugs. If symptomatic hypotension is problematic, ranolazine is a reasonable option.
Bradycardia	Use DHP CCBs, nitrates, and/or ranolazine.
Aortic stenosis	Patients with moderate-to-severe AS may not be able to tolerate arterial vasodilators such as non-DHP CCBs and DHP CCBs. May consider utilizing β-blockers without α activity, nitrates, and/or ranolazine. Avoid: non-DHP and DHP CCBs.
Erectile dysfunction	Nitrates are contraindicated with concomitant phosphodiesterase (PDE) inhibitors (sildenafil, tadalafil, vardenafil). Most clinicians will not prescribe an IR nitrate and PDE inhibitor together. If a nitrate must be used, an alternate treatment option for ED may be explored. If a nitrate and a PDE inhibitor are prescribed together, the patient must wait at least 24 hours after sildenafil and vardenafil and 48 hours after tadalafil before taking a nitrate. Use β-blockers, CCBs, and/or ranolazine per CSA algorithm (Figure 18-4).

Abbreviations: AS = aortic stenosis; CCB = calcium channel blocker; CSA = chronic stable angina; DHP = dihydropyridine; ED = erectile dysfunction; IR = immediate-release; PDE = phosphodiesterase.

Source: References 1,2,9, and 11.

TABLE 18-13 • Herbal Supplements for Chronic Stable Angina

Supplement	Typical Dose	Effectiveness[a]	Cost[b]
Coenzyme Q10	60 mg daily	Insufficient evidence	$
Hawthorn	100 mg TID	Possibly effective	$$
L-Carnitine	1.5-2 g daily	Possibly effective	$$$
N-Acetyl Cysteine	400-600 mg TID	Possibly effective	$$

[a] Level of evidence: Likely effective. This product has a very high level of reliable clinical evidence supporting its use for a specific indication. Products rated "likely effective" are generally considered appropriate to recommend. Possibly effective: This product has some clinical evidence supporting its use for a specific indication; however, the evidence is limited by quantity, quality, or contradictory findings. Products rated "possibly effective" might be beneficial, but do not have enough high-quality evidence to recommend for most people; "insufficient evidence"—there is not enough reliable scientific evidence to provide an effectiveness rating.

[b] Cost: $ = $10/month supply in the recommended dosage; $$ = $11-$20/month; $$$ = $21-$50/month.

Source: Data compiled from reference 2.

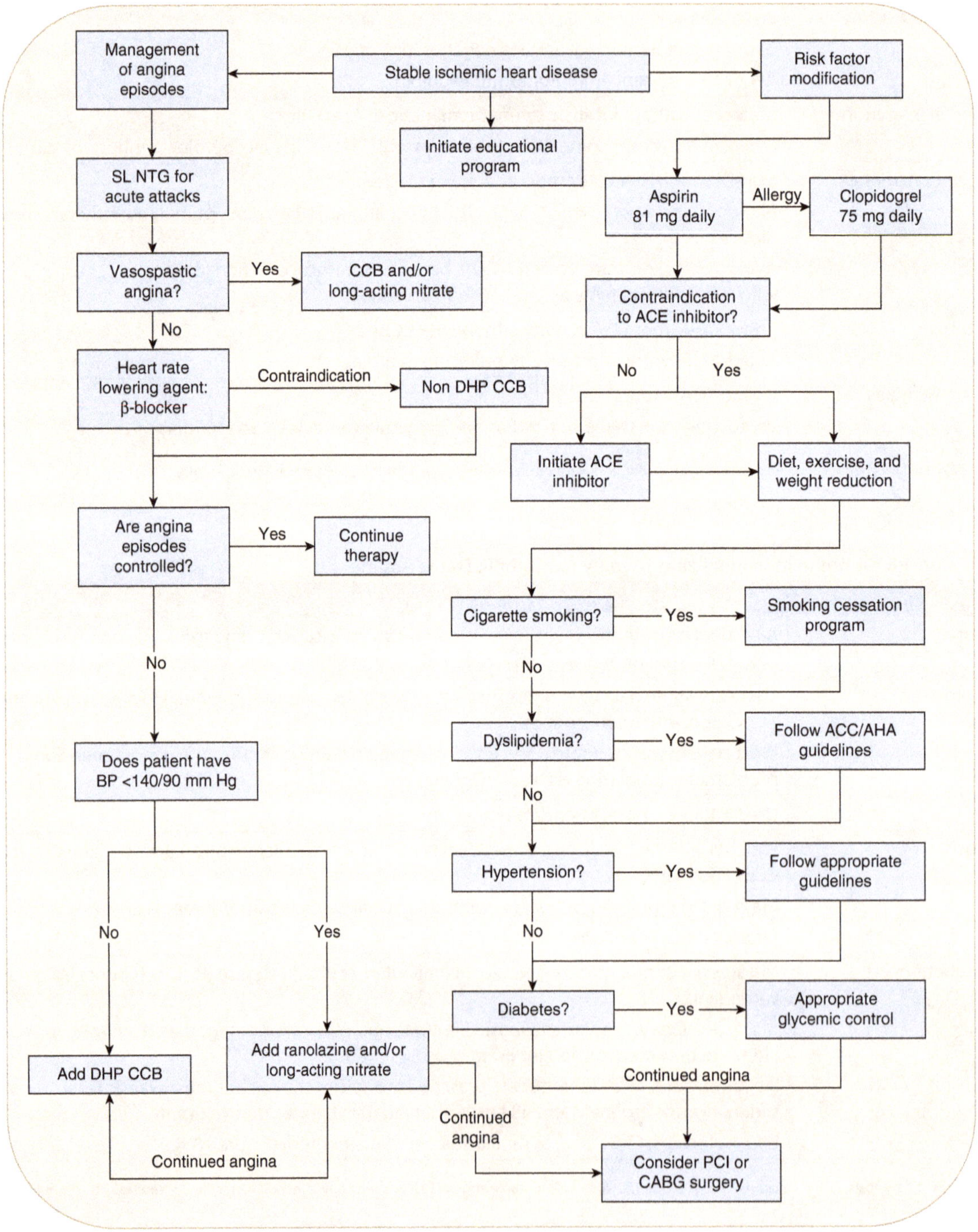

FIGURE 18-4 Current treatment algorithm for stable ischemic heart disease.[2]

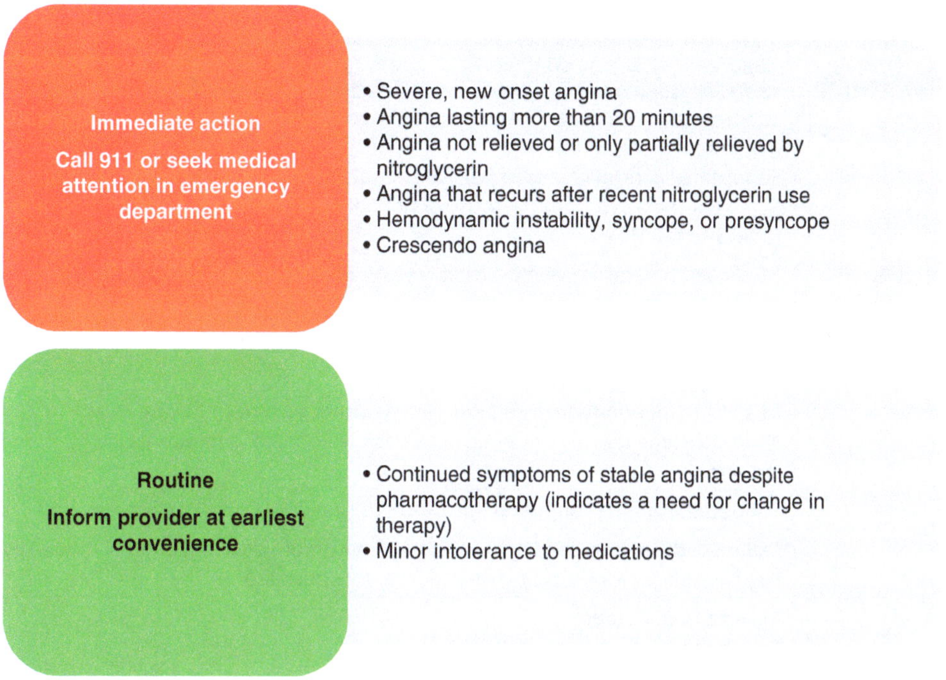

FIGURE 18-5 Referral for management of angina.[2]

TABLE 18-14 • Medications for Management of Stable Ischemic Heart Disease

Medication Class and Example Drugs	Recommendations
Antiplatelets Aspirin Clopidogrel	Aspirin 75 to 162 mg daily should be continued indefinitely in the absence of contraindications. Clopidogrel 75 mg daily may be used in those with an aspirin allergy. Treatment with both aspirin (75 to 162 mg daily) and clopidogrel 75 mg daily might be reasonable in certain high-risk SIHD patients.
β-Blockers Metoprolol Atenolol	Initiate a β-blocker after an MI or ACS once stable and continue for at least 3 years. May consider indefinite therapy if patient is tolerating therapy well. Carvedilol, metoprolol succinate, or bisoprolol should be used in all patients with HFrEF (EF ≤40%) unless contraindicated.
ACE inhibitors Lisinopril Perindopril	ACE inhibitors should be prescribed in all patients with concomitant hypertension, diabetes, HFrEF or CKD, unless contraindicated. It is reasonable to treat patients with an ACE inhibitor who have both SIHD and other vascular disease.
Angiotensin receptor blocker Valsartan Losartan	ARBs are recommended in patients who are ACE inhibitor intolerant.
Lipid-lowering drugs Atorvastatin Simvastatin	A moderate or high intensity statin regimen should be used unless contraindicated or patient is intolerant. Niacin, bile acid sequestrant, gemfibrozil, or a PCSK-9 inhibitor can be utilized in those not able to tolerate statins.
Vaccines Influenza	All patients should receive an annual influenza vaccine unless contraindicated.

Abbreviations: ACE = angiotensin converting enzyme; ACS = acute coronary syndrome; ARB = angiotensin receptor blocker; CKD = chronic kidney disease; EF = ejection fraction; HFrEF = heart failure with reduced ejection fraction; MI = myocardial infarction; PCSK-9 = proprotein convertase subtilisin kexin type 9; SIHD = stable ischemic heart disease.

Source: References 1, 2, and 9.

TABLE 18-15 • Medication-Related Problems (MRPs) in Patients with Chronic Stable Angina

Category of MRP	Example Medication-Related Problem
Nonadherence	• Suboptimal control of angina because of nonadherence with lifestyle modifications (eg, smoking cessation) • Suboptimal control of angina because of patient missing doses of antianginal medications • Acute coronary syndrome because of nonadherence with cardioprotective medications (eg, ASA, statin)
Unnecessary medication	• Duplicate therapy (eg, two β-blockers or ACE inhibitor with ARB)
Need for additional medication	• Patient taking an optimal regimen for CSA, but not taking ASA for SIHD • Suboptimal angina control in a patient with low blood pressure (systolic 100 mm Hg); patient not prescribed ranolazine
Ineffective medication	• Isosorbide mononitrate dosed twice daily without a nitrate-free interval • No improvement in angina symptoms despite adherence to maximum recommended daily dose of ranolazine
Dosage too low	• Suboptimal angina control on low dose of a non-DHP CCB and HR is elevated
Dosage too high	• Patient with symptomatic hypotension on maximum dose antianginal medication • Headache from a long-acting nitrate recently uptitrated
Adverse drug event	• Myalgia from a statin • Peripheral edema from a DHP CCB

Abbreviations: ACE = angiotensin converting enzyme; ASA = aspirin; CCB = calcium channel blocker; CSA = chronic stable angina; DHP = dihydropyridine; HTN = hypertension; HR = heart rate; SIHD = stable ischemic heart disease.

Scenario: Patient was given samples of ranolazine but could not afford prescription.
MRP: Nonadherence.

- Assessment:
  Patient with stable angina still having symptoms on a maximum β-blocker dose and ranolazine 500 mg bid. No improvement in anginal symptoms is likely secondary to nonadherence with ranolazine. Patient is nonadherent with ranolazine due to cost. BP slightly elevated and HR low. Switching to a DHP CCB may provide for more affordable angina and BP control.
- Plan:
  Consider discontinuation of ranolazine and addition of amlodipine 5 mg daily with titration to 10 mg daily based on anginal symptoms and blood pressure. Reassess tolerability in 2 weeks.

Scenario: Patient with chronic stable angina on a low-dose β-blocker with heart rate of 60 beats per minute. This medication has decreased the frequency of his anginal symptoms; however, angina still limits his ability to perform household chores.
MRP: Need for additional medication.

- Assessment:
  β-blockers are first-line for management of chronic stable angina. The HR does not allow for further titration. An additional agent should be considered for management of anginal symptoms.
- Plan:
  Please consider adding an additional medication to help control CSA symptoms, such as a DHP CCB.

Scenario: Patient given a β-blocker for vasospastic angina, which has not reduced frequency or severity of angina symptoms.
MRP: Ineffective medication.

- Assessment:
  Symptoms of vasospastic angina not relieved with β-blocker. Patient may obtain more benefit from first-line drugs for vasospastic angina such as non-DHP or DHP CCBs.
- Plan:
  Consider stopping metoprolol 25 mg bid and starting diltiazem 120 mg qam with close monitoring of BP, HR, and angina symptom burden.

Scenario: Patient recently increased amlodipine from 5 mg to 10 mg daily with improvement in anginal symptoms, but worsening peripheral edema. Patient is taking isosorbide mononitrate 30 mg every morning and no β-blocker (HR 55 beats per minute).
MRP: Adverse effect.

- Assessment:
  Peripheral edema is a common adverse effect from a CCB. The adverse effect is dose-dependent and reversible with downtitration or discontinuation.
- Plan:
  Reduce amlodipine to 5 mg daily, and increase isosorbide mononitrate to 60 mg every morning. Reassess tolerability in 2 weeks.

FIGURE 18-6 Sample provider communications for chronic stable angina.

CORE ELEMENT 5—DOCUMENTATION AND FOLLOW-UP

Clear, concise, and evidence-based documentation of MRPs and recommendations is a key component of the MTM consult. Examples of potential MRPs in patients with CSA are provided in Table 18-15. Sample communications and recommendations to providers to address medication-related issues are found in Figure 18-6. Recommendations may be communicated via fax, telephone, or other means of written or secure electronic communication. The examples are for illustrative purposes. Actual communications to providers should be individualized based on the type of recommendation, patient specific characteristics, and the nature of the relationship with the provider.

The exact follow-up interval in patients with CSA is not well defined. However, follow-up to assess symptom progression, adherence, effectiveness of interventions, and potential adverse effects is essential. The time frame for follow-up will depend on several factors, including severity of ischemic heart disease and symptoms and comorbidities. Patients with worsening angina symptoms or reduced exercise tolerance should be seen promptly in clinic. Those with unstable symptoms should seek immediate medical attention. Suggested intervals for follow-up are provided in Table 18-16. Since ranolazine has multiple drug interactions and can prolong the QT interval, monitoring to ensure safety is also provided in Table 18-16.

TABLE 18-16 • Suggested Intervals for Follow-up in Patients with Chronic Stable Angina

Follow-up and Monitoring in Patients with Chronic Stable Angina
Antianginal response • Reassess 2 to 4 weeks after initiating or making changes in therapy • Newly diagnosed patients should be reassessed at least every 4 to 6 months for the first year • After angina symptoms are minimized and patient is stable, monitor every 6 to 12 months • Patients with more severe symptoms, multiple comorbidities, history of nonadherence, or symptoms of adverse drug effects should be followed more frequently
Toxicity • Monitor for adverse drug effects 2 to 4 weeks after starting a new agent or dose increase • Monitor for adverse effects every 6 to 12 months in stable patients • Since ranolazine can prolong QTc interval, an ECG and serum potassium and magnesium should be obtained at baseline and within 6 weeks of starting therapy or increasing dose.[a] Reassess QTc interval and electrolytes periodically and if drug interactions occur.

[a] Clinical trials of ranolazine reassessed QTc interval at 1 to 2 weeks and 6 weeks after initiating therapy.

Source: References 1, 2, 13, 14, and 15.

REFERENCES

1. Dobesh PP. Stable ischemic heart disease. In: DiPiro JT, Talbert RL, Yee GC, Matzke GR, Wells BG, Posey L, eds. *Pharmacotherapy: A Pathophysiologic Approach*. 10th ed. New York, NY: McGraw-Hill; 2017. Available at http://accesspharmacy.mhmedical.com.lp.hscl.ufl.edu/content.aspx?bookid=1861&sectionid=146056655. Accessed May 07, 2017.
2. Fihn SD, Gardin JM, Abrams J, et al. 2012 ACCF/AHA/ACP/AATS/PCNA/SCAI/STS guideline for the diagnosis and management of patients with stable ischemic heart disease: a report of the American College of Cardiology Foundation/American Heart Association task force on practice guidelines, and the American College of Physicians, American Association for Thoracic Surgery, Preventive Cardiovascular Nurses Association, Society for Cardiovascular Angiography and Interventions, and Society of Thoracic Surgeons. *Circulation*. 2012;126:e354-e471.
3. Morrow DA. Chest discomfort. In: Kasper D, Fauci A, Hauser S, Longo D, Jameson J, Loscalzo J, eds. *Harrison's Principles of Internal Medicine*. 19th ed. New York, NY: McGraw-Hill; 2014. Available at http://accesspharmacy.mhmedical.com.lp.hscl.ufl.edu/content.aspx?bookid=1130&sectionid=79724231. Accessed May 07, 2017.
4. Antman EM, Loscalzo J. Ischemic heart disease. In: Kasper D, Fauci A, Hauser S, Longo D, Jameson J, Loscalzo J, eds. *Harrison's Principles of Internal Medicine*. 19th ed. New York, NY: McGraw-Hill; 2014. Available at http://accesspharmacy.mhmedical.com.lp.hscl.ufl.edu/content.aspx?bookid=1130&sectionid=79743463. Accessed May 07, 2017.
5. Talbert RL. Ischemic heart disease. In: DiPiro JT, Talbert RL, Yee GC, Matzke GR, Wells BG, Posey L, eds. *Pharmacotherapy: A Pathophysiologic Approach*. 9th ed. New York, NY: McGraw-Hill; 2014. Available at http://accesspharmacy.mhmedical.com.lp.hscl.ufl.edu/content.aspx?bookid=689&sectionid=48811455. Accessed May 07, 2017.
6. Goldman L, Hashimoto B, Cook EF, Loscalzo A. Comparative reproducibility and validity of systems for assessing cardiovascular functional class: advantages of a new specific activity scale. *Circulation*. 1981;64:1227-1234.
7. Campeau L. Grading of angina [letter]. *Circulation*. 1976;54:522-523.
8. CMS. *Medicare Part D Medication Therapy Management Program Standardized Format*. Available at https://www.cms.gov/Medicare/Prescription-Drug-Coverage/PrescriptionDrugCovContra/Downloads/MTM-Program-Standardized-Format-English-and-Spanish-Instructions-Samples-v032712.pdf. Accessed May 7, 2017.
9. Smith SS, Benjamin EJ, Bonow RO, et al. AHA/ACCF secondary prevention and risk reduction therapy for patients with coronary and other atherosclerotic vascular disease: 2011 Update: A guideline From the American Heart Association and American College of Cardiology Foundation. *Circulation*. 2011;124:2458-2473.
10. Clinical Pharmacology [database online]. Tampa, FL: Gold Standard, Inc.; 2017. Available at http://clinicalpharmacology.com.
11. Rosendorff C, Black HR, Cannon CP, et al. Treatment of hypertension in the prevention and management of ischemic heart disease: a scientific statement. *Circulation*. 2007;115(21):2761-2788.
12. Natural Medicines [database online]. Somerville, MA: Therapeutic Research Center; 2017. Available at https://naturalmedicines.therapeuticresearch.com/. Accessed May 7, 2017.
13. Chaitman BR, Pepine CJ, Parker JO, et al. Effects of ranolazine with atenolol, amlodipine, or diltiazem on exercise tolerance and angina frequency in patients with severe chronic angina: a randomized controlled trial. *JAMA*. 2004;291(3):309-316.
14. Chaitman BR, Skettino SL, Parker JO, et al. Anti-ischemic effects and long-term survival during ranolazine monotherapy in patients with chronic severe angina. *J Am Coll Cardiol*. 2004;43(8):1375-1382.
15. Stone PH, Gratsiansky NA, Blokhin A, et al. Antianginal efficacy of ranolazine when added to treatment with amlodipine: the ERICA (Efficacy of Ranolazine in Chronic Angina) trial. *J Am Coll Cardiol*. 2006;48(3):566-575.

Review Questions

1. All of the following actions may induce an angina attack **EXCEPT:**
   a. walking up a flight of stairs.
   b. participating in a heated argument.
   c. engaging in sexual intercourse.
   d. eating a spicy meal.

2. What question is most helpful for the MTM provider to determine whether the patient's chronic stable angina is controlled on the current medication regimen?
   a. "How many times have you had to call 911 for chest pain?"
   b. "What is your usual blood pressure and heart rate?"
   c. "How does chest pain limit you from doing the activities you enjoy?"
   d. "What actions do you take when you get chest pain?"

3. What is an "immediate" goal of chronic stable angina therapy?
   a. Reduce the frequency of angina attacks.
   b. Control blood pressure and blood sugar.
   c. Prevent a second heart attack.
   d. Avoid activities that induce angina.

4. Which statement regarding angina is appropriate for patient education?
   a. "Angina may be caused by atherosclerotic buildup or vasospasm."
   b. "Angina or chest pain happens when the heart muscle does not get enough blood."
   c. "Angina occurs when there is an imbalance of myocardial oxygen demand and supply."
   d. "Hypertension, tachycardia, and anemia can induce angina in patients with ischemic heart disease."

5. Which information should be included in the medication action plan regarding appropriate nitroglycerin use?
   a. Chew nitroglycerin for faster onset of action.
   b. If pain is not improved after the third dose, call 911.
   c. Repeated dosing is not recommended.
   d. Nitroglycerin should be stored in the original container and sealed tightly.

6. All of the following cases require referral for further evaluation **EXCEPT:**
   a. Patient reports chest pain used to occur only with exertion but is now happening at rest.
   b. Patient manages exertional angina by taking sublingual nitroglycerin 5 minutes prior to walking up the stairs to his apartment.
   c. Patient admits that he/she is having active chest pain during the MTM interview.
   d. Patient tells you that his/her most recent episodes of angina pain was rated 7/10 in intensity; prior to last week, the worst angina pain he/she ever experienced was rated 4/10.

7. A patient admits that she does not take her metoprolol consistently because she feels that her blood pressure is well controlled without it. She had a heart attack 6 months ago. What is the correct category for this medication-related problem?
   a. Dosage too high
   b. Unneccesary medication
   c. Adverse drug event
   d. Nonadherence

8. A patient experiences angina attacks about 5 to 6 times per week, limiting his ability to do household chores. His blood pressure is 171/85 mm Hg, which is consistent with readings from the home blood pressure log. He is adherent to a maximized dose of a β-blocker, with a heart rate in the 55 to 60 bpm range. His provider has tried to increase his dose of isosorbide mononitrate in the past, but he could not tolerate it due to headache. Which medication would be the most appropriate addition to his anti-anginal therapy?
   a. Verapamil
   b. Ranolazine
   c. Amlodipine
   d. Aspirin

9. A patient experiences angina symptoms that are rare and always relieved after the first dose of nitroglycerin. The patient had a heart attack last year and is compliant with metoprolol tartrate therapy. All of the following medications would be an appropriate recommendation for add-on therapy for secondary coronary artery disease prevention **EXCEPT:**
   a. aliskiren.
   b. lisinopril.
   c. atorvastatin.
   d. valsartan.

10. Which counseling point is especially important for patients with diabetes and chronic stable angina who are taking β-blockers?
   a. β-Blockers increase insulin sensitivity.
   b. Diabetics should not take β-blockers unless their blood sugar is well-controlled.
   c. Diabetes is a compelling indication for β-blocker therapy.
   d. β-Blockers can cause hypoglycemic unawareness.

ANSWERS

1. d	2. c	3. a
4. b	5. d	6. b
7. d	8. c	9. a
10. d		

19

Dementia-Related Disorders MTM Data Set

Joshua Caballero, PharmD, BCPP, FCCP, and Jordan Sedlacek, PharmD, BCACP

KEY POINTS

- When working with patients with dementia and related disorders, it is important to gain an understanding of the support system surrounding the patient and the primary caregiver.
- Before recommending therapy for dementia-related disorders, Medication therapy management (MTM) providers should make sure to review the entire medication profile (including neutraceuticals and over-the-counter products) to assess for items that may be contributing to or causing cognitive impairment.
- The MTM provider should remember to address other comorbid conditions that may manifest because of dementia (eg, depression, anxiety, insomnia).
- The use of scales and inventories is valuable to track cognitive status and functioning in activities of daily life.

INTRODUCTION

Dementia causes significant cognitive decline that occurs over time, resulting in poor self-care and death. There are different types of dementia (Table 19-1); however, Alzheimer disease is the most common. While most think of dementia as occurring in old age, some patients may develop early-onset dementia in their 40s or 50s.[1] Dementia can be devastating not only to the patient, but also to caregivers and families. Although medications may offer some relief and comfort, they basically delay the inevitable . . . death. The provision of medication therapy management (MTM) can play a vital role in making the journey and its transitions as painless and meaningful as possible.

Before interviewing the patient and/or caregiver, the MTM provider needs to place himself/herself in their situation. For those who have never had a personal experience working with a patient with Alzheimer disease, it may be a good idea to reflect.

Reflection: *Imagine, you have been told you have an illness that will in time erase your memories. It will start with recent things: what you had for breakfast, what sitcom you watched last night, if you spoke with your son, daughter, brother, or spouse. In time, you will lose your ability to work, the ability to care for your loved ones. Eventually, you will lose the ability to take care of yourself. You will be dependent on those around you, which, sadly, is not always a thing of comfort. You will begin to misplace things, perhaps blaming others for stealing them. With every hour and day that inevitably passes, you take a step closer to forgetting the names, faces, and voices of those you love, eventually sitting in a place where no one is recognizable or understandable. In time, you will not be able to communicate with them as the loss of language will occur. Imagine, you will forget the name of a "mortar and pestle," a laptop, an iPad. You will forget how to eat, or that you are hungry or thirsty. Eventually, you will forget who you are, your accomplishments, your desires and passions, until you end up in an empty vacuum, void of any communication, contact, or love. Now think of this person as your loved one, the one you have spent 40 years with, the one who has helped you become the person who you are today—the person sitting across from you.*

Before the Interview

The most important aspect to consider when talking to a patient and/or caregiver with Alzheimer disease is *time*. It is important to make sure that enough time is blocked off to adequately allow for all concerns to be addressed, especially for the first encounter. While there may be several issues to address, taking the time to listen and address concerns with empathy will be appreciated, and may be more valuable than any recommendations for adjustment to medications.

TABLE 19-1 • Common Types of Dementia in Late Life

Alzheimer disease
Vascular dementia
Dementia with Lewy bodies
Mixed dementia
Other (eg, Parkinson disease dementia, Frontotemporal dementia, Huntington disease, Creutzfeldt-Jakob disease)
Potentially reversible causes of cognitive dysfunction (eg, normal pressure hydrocephalus, thyroid dysfunction, vitamin B_{12} deficiency, delirium, depression, Wernicke–Korsakoff syndrome)

Source: Reproduced, with permission, from DiPiro JT, Tolbert RL, Yee GC, Matzke GR, Wells BG, Posey LM, eds. *Pharmacotherapy: A Pathophysiologic Approach*. 10th ed. New York: McGraw-Hill; 2017.

The MTM provider should make sure to face the patient, speak slowly, use layperson terminology, sit in a private area to ensure patient confidentiality, and explain the purpose of MTM services and its components. Patients should be asked about their living arrangements, thoughts or feelings about their condition, and medication use. In addition, the MTM provider should obtain immunization history, assess cultural issues, educational level, language barriers, health literacy level, and other characteristics of the patient's communication abilities that could affect outcomes.

The MTM provider should assess the patient's understanding of his/her condition and the purpose of the patient's current medication(s) if already on therapy. During this process, the MTM provider can elaborate or correct those answers, use patient information pamphlets or diagrams, and ask the patient or caregiver to repeat back what was explained, if possible. Instead of asking "*Do* you have questions or concerns?" MTM providers may prefer to ask, "*What* questions and concerns do you have?" This will allow for more open communication away from a simple "yes/no" answer. It is also important to ask the patient what he or she feels is the most significant or burdensome issue of the disease and explain to the patient what specific therapeutic responses he or she may expect to achieve with treatment. In other words, the MTM provider should be realistic, but encouraging and empathic. Finally, it is important to communicate some tips to the caregiver who will be managing the patient (Table 19-2).

TABLE 19-2 • Basic Principles of Care for the Alzheimer Patient

- Consider vision, hearing, or other sensory impairments.
- Find optimal level of autonomy and adjust expectations for patient performance over time.
- Avoid confrontation. Remain calm, firm, and supportive if the patient becomes upset.
- Maintain a consistent, structured environment with stimulation level appropriate to the individual patient.
- Provide frequent reminders, explanations, and orientation cues. Employ guiding, demonstration, and reinforcement.
- Reduce choices, keep requests and demands of the patient simple, and avoid complex tasks that lead to frustration.
- Bring sudden declines in function and the emergence of new symptoms to professional attention.

Source: Reproduced, with permission, from DiPiro JT, Tolbert RL, Yee GC, Matzke GR, Wells BG, Posey LM, eds. *Pharmacotherapy: A Pathophysiologic Approach*. 10th ed. New York: McGraw-Hill; 2017.

Secondary Causes of Dementia or Changes in Mental Status

Medications. Before initiating a medication for dementia, cognitive impairment related to medications should be ruled out. Reviewing the current medication regimen may identify medications that are causing cognitive impairment and, therefore, avoid unnecessary therapeutic regimens. This will avoid a potential prescribing cascade that could place a heavier burden on the patient and caregiver. Several classes of medications may cause cognitive impairment, including anticholinergics, sedative hypnotics (eg, diazepam, alprazolam), opioid analgesics (eg, morphine, meperidine), and psychiatric medications such as anticonvulsants (eg, topiramate) and antipsychotics (eg, quetiapine).[7,8] In the elderly, high doses of histamine H_2-receptor antagonists (eg, ranitidine), digoxin, amiodarone, antihypertensives, nonsteroidal anti-inflammatory drugs, and corticosteroids have also been reported to cause cognitive impairment.[7] Therefore, it is imperative to address these medications and adjust doses, if possible, before considering the initiation of cognitive agents.

Disease States. Additionally, disease states such as hypothyroidism, dehydration, constipation, vitamin deficiencies (eg, thiamine, vitamin B_{12}), and pain can contribute to cognitive impairment. Infectious diseases such as urinary tract infections, human immunodeficiency virus, or syphilis should also be ruled out.[9] Identifying and managing these illnesses appropriately may negate the need for initiation of cognitive medications.

Assessment of the Patient with Dementia

Several tests can be used to stage cognitive status. However, the mini-mental state examination (MMSE – available at http://www.heartinstitutehd.com/Misc/Forms/MMSE.1276128605.pdf) is traditionally used (Table 19-3). The MMSE is scored on a scale of

TABLE 19-3 • Stages of Alzheimer Disease

Mild (MMSE score 26-21)	Patient has difficulty remembering recent events. Ability to manage finances, prepare food, and carry out other household activities declines. May get lost while driving. Begins to withdraw from difficult tasks and give up hobbies. May deny memory problems.
Moderate (MMSE score 20-10)	Patient requires assistance with activities of daily living. Frequently disoriented with regard to time (date, year, season). Recall for recent events is severely impaired. May forget some details of past life and names of family and friends. Functioning may fluctuate from day to day. Patient generally denies problems. May become suspicious or tearful. Loses ability to drive safely. Agitation, paranoia, and delusions are common.
Severe (MMSE score 9-0)	Patient loses ability to speak, walk, and feed self. Incontinent of urine and feces. Requires care 24 hours a day, 7 days a week.

Abbreviation: MMSE = Mini-Mental Status Examination.

Source: Reproduced, with permission, from DiPiro JT, Tolbert RL, Yee GC, Matzke GR, Wells BG, Posey LM, eds. *Pharmacotherapy: A Pathophysiologic Approach*. 10th ed. New York: McGraw-Hill; 2017.

0 to 30, with lower scores indicating a greater degree of cognitive impairment. While the MMSE has limitations, especially in being able to identify clinically significant cognitive decline in the early stages, it is the test most commonly used in general practice.

Therapeutic Goals for Dementia

The therapeutic goals for treating dementia are to slow the progression of cognitive decline and maintain quality of life and functional status for as long as possible. Without treatment, the MMSE typically declines by 2 to 4 points per year.[1] While on treatment, a decline of <2 points per year is considered demonstration of efficacy. However, a rapid cognitive decline (eg, >3 to 4 points per year) while on medication signifies a therapeutic failure and the need for adjustment of the regimen. The following sections will provide insight and offer examples to assist in the development of MTM plans for patients with dementia.

CORE ELEMENT 1—COMPREHENSIVE MEDICATION REVIEW FOR DEMENTIA-RELATED DISORDERS

Following is a list of suggested questions to use when conducting a medication therapy review in a patient with dementia-related disorders (Table 19-4). The number and types of questions will depend upon several factors, including the amount of time for the interview, number of concurrent medication-related problems (MRPs), urgency of MRPs, and the reliability of the patient (or caregiver) in providing accurate information, among others. With dementia-related disorders, it is best to keep communication direct and to the point. The MTM provider should demonstrate empathy, but also state the facts and avoid "sugar coating" the information. Some conversations may be difficult, and patients/caregivers may become emotional and cry, but the vast majority will appreciate honesty and candor, especially when it comes to the efficacy of medications. The most important part is to show compassion and genuine concern in responses to the patient and caregiver. MTM providers should remember to use living room language during the interview (Table 19-5) and be prepared for questions patients may ask regarding their illness (Table 19-6).

TABLE 19-4 • Questions to Ask When Conducting a Medication Review in a Patient with Dementia-Related Disorders

Suggested Questions for the Patient with Dementia-Related Disorders

- How long since you were diagnosed with dementia?
- What do you know about your dementia (eg, what type, prognosis)?
- Do you use a diary or "to-do list" to remember things?
- What medications do you currently take for dementia?
- Since starting your medication, have you experienced any of the following:
  - Nausea or vomiting
  - Diarrhea
  - Sweating
- Do you feel the medications are helping? (if on current therapy)
- Overall, how is your memory?
- What over-the-counter pills or herbal medications do you take for dementia?
- What are your two greatest concerns?
- Do you have a living will?

Suggested Questions for the Caregiver

- Are relatives (eg, sons, daughters, brothers) or close friends aware of this condition?
- Over the last several weeks, has the patient experienced the following:
  - Bouts of crying
  - Disorientation
  - Aggressive behavior
  - Suspiciousness
  - Midnight awakenings
  - Shouting
  - Hallucinations or delusions
- Do you have any support to assist you with the care for your loved one?
- Do you or anyone else have power of attorney?
- Does your patient or loved one have a living will?

Questions to Ask for Prevention/Assessment of Medical Emergencies

- How often do you feel anxious, down, angry, guilty, agitated, like crying or actually cried, life is not worth living, or suicidal thoughts?
- If "yes," ask if the patient has a plan to end his/her life.
- What triggers these feelings? How often do they occur?
- If considering an agent for psychiatric complications, it is a good idea to ask:
  - What are your thoughts on using a medication for (depression, anxiety, aggressive behavior)?
  - Have you had any experiences with them?
  - Do you prefer any particular agent?

CORE ELEMENT 2—PERSONAL MEDICATION LIST

The following is a sample personal medication list[12] (PML) for a patient with dementia-related disorders (Figure 19-1). This example is representative only of medications for dementa-related disorders. Additional medications for other disease states should be added and listed separately. MTM providers should remember to use plain language when creating the PML.

CORE ELEMENT 3—MEDICATION ACTION PLAN

The following is a sample medication action plan[12] (MAPs) for a patient with dementia-related disorders (Figure 19-2). This example is representative only of action steps for a patient with dementia-related disorders. MAPs for other disease states or other MRPs should be added and listed separately. In general, only a few of the most important action steps should be listed, so as not to overwhelm the patient/caregiver. Other areas for patient self-management can be addressed at later visits. MTM providers should remember to use plain language when creating the MAP.

TABLE 19-5 • Living Room Language for Dementia-Related Disorders

Activities of daily living—sometimes are referred to as ADLs. These are the functions that we normally do during the day. They can include bathing, cooking, eating, grooming, managing your finances, using the restroom, and driving.
Alzheimer disease—it is the most common form of dementia. The disease causes a loss of memories, the ability to think, and a change in behaviors over time. As a result, this can affect daily tasks.
Amyloid plaques—sticky clumps of proteins that forms on nerve cells in the brain. This causes the nerve cells to not work efficiently and die over time.
Cholinesterase inhibitors—medications that slow down the progression of Alzheimer disease by increasing a chemical called acetylcholine.
Cognition—the ability to think.
Cognitive decline—a decrease in memory.
Delusion—thinking or beliefs that are not rational or real. For example, thinking that someone is stealing from you or moving objects around the house.
Dementia—it is not an actual disease. Overall, it is the word we use to describe the different types of symptoms associated with the loss of memory or ability to perform activities of daily living such as eating and bathing.
Hallucination—a false perception of an object or event that is not real or occurring. They usually include the senses. For example, seeing or hearing a person who is not living, such as a deceased relative.
Living will—a legal document that a person uses to let others know what their wishes are regarding medical treatments in case they are not able to do so.
NMDA receptor antagonist—a medication usually given with cholinesterase inhibitors that works on stabilizing a chemical in the brain called glutamate.
Power of attorney—a legal document that allows a person to make decisions on your behalf.

Source: Reference 4.

PERSONAL MEDICATION LIST FOR *<Insert Patient's name*, DOB: *mm/dd/yyyy>*	
Medication: Aricept (donepezil) 10 mg	
How I use it: Take 1 pill (10 mg) at bedtime	
Why I use it: For memory	**Prescriber:** Dr. Rockwell
Date I started using it: 11/18/15	**Date I stopped using it:** *(Leave blank for patient's notes)*
Why I stopped using it: *(Leave blank for patient's notes)*	
Medication: Zoloft (sertraline) 25 mg	
How I use it: Take 1 pill (25 mg) in the morning	
Why I use it: For depression	**Prescriber:** Dr. Hemingway
Date I started using it: 02/17/16	**Date I stopped using it:** *(Leave blank for patient's notes)*
Why I stopped using it: *(Leave blank for patient's notes)*	

FIGURE 19-1 Example personal medication list for dementia-related medications.

DATE PREPARED: *<Insert date>*	
What we talked about: You reported some stomach cramping and nausea with starting donepezil. This is one of the most common side effects of donepezil.	
What I need to do: Here are some things I can do to help lessen this effect: • Be patient: Sometimes the side effects decrease or go away after a few weeks • If the side effects do not get better, try taking it with a light snack like some soda crackers or slice of bread.	**What I did and when I did it:** *(Leave blank for patient's notes)*
What we talked about: You started sertraline 25 mg every morning for depression.	
What I need to do: Here are some things I need to be aware of: • Initially, the medication may cause nausea, diarrhea, or stomach pain. These side effects usually last two weeks and get better or disappear. However, if I cannot tolerate these side effects, I should stop the medication and call my provider. • During these two weeks, I can temporarily stop my laxative or stool softener and see if the diarrhea improves. • I might begin to feel an improvement in my mood after about two weeks, but the full effect may not be seen for at least 4-6 weeks—sometimes longer. I should be patient. • I should keep a daily log of my symptoms like side effects and overall how I am feeling. This helps my team make sure the medication is working and is the best one for me.	**What I did and when I did it:** *(Leave blank for patient's notes)*

FIGURE 19-2 Example medication action plan for a patient with dementia.

CORE ELEMENT 4—INTERVENTION AND/OR REFERRAL

Interventions for dementia-related disorders may include lifestyle modifications and pharmacotherapy. Medications primarily consist of cholinesterase inhibitors during mild to severe stages of Alzheimer disease. Memantine, an NMDA receptor antagonist, is used in moderate to severe stages. Table 19-7 summarizes lifestyle modifications that may be useful to minimize confusion, psychiatric complications (eg, agitation, anxiety), and sleep issues. Table 19-8 provides an overview of the available prescription agents used for dementia.

Initiation of Therapy

After staging the patient, recommendations are as follows:

1. Start a cholinesterase inhibitor in any patient who falls into the mild or moderate category.[1] While there is some disagreement on whether to start a cholinesterase inhibitor in someone who is classified as severe, general practice recommendations are to start an agent as well. It is acceptable to switch cholinesterase inhibitors if a lack of response is seen or intolerable adverse effects are noted.
2. The addition of an NMDA receptor antagonist (ie, memantine) to a cholinesterase inhibitor should be considered for any patient who falls into the moderate or severe stages of dementia.[1]

TABLE 19-6 • Questions to Anticipate Regarding Dementia-Related Disorders

Questions Commonly Asked by Patients
• **What is dementia?** Dementia is the progression of loss of memories over time. Loss of memory can occur fast or slow, depending on the person. There are several types of dementias, but Alzheimer disease is the most common. Alzheimer disease destroys neurons which are cells in the brain. With time, the more brain cells that are destroyed, the more your memory will decrease and the ability to learn becomes more difficult. This may be very difficult to accept. However, I am here to assist you in the best way I can and offer the support needed to make the necessary transitions. Are you familiar with support groups? Would you like me to call for you? (Have materials or websites handy where person can get support. In some cases, the MTM provider may make the initial call for them to an Alzheimer support group and communicate to them, "Here is the number. I called them as you requested, and they are expecting your call." This can go a long way in helping the caregiver and displaying empathy toward the disease.)
• **What should I expect from a therapeutic response?** Medication used to treat dementias only slows down the progression of the disease, but it does not cure it. Depending on the person, some medications in the same drug class work better than others. We do not know why, but believe it may be based on our genetics. We will start with one and see if you respond. If not, we can try a different one.
• **How long will I need to be on the medication?** You will probably be on the medication as long as it can slow down the progression of the disease. Typically, these medications usually work between 6 and 12 months for about 50% of the patients. For others, they can work longer or shorter.
• **What types of medications are there for dementia?** There are generally two types of medications. The first are called cholinesterase inhibitors. They work by increasing the amount of a chemical in the brain called acetylcholine. Examples of these medications include Aricept, Exelon, and Razadyne. Sometimes another class of drug is added when these other drugs are not working as well or the disease progresses to moderate or severe. This class of medications is called an NMDA (N-methyl-D-aspartate) receptor antagonist. There is only one medication in this class (Namenda). It works by balancing the amount of another chemical in the brain called glutamate which is also involved in memory and learning.
• **What side effects of the medications should I expect?** The most common side effects of cholinesterase inhibitors are: • Nausea or vomiting • Diarrhea • Indigestion or abdominal pain • Loss of appetite and weight loss The most common side effects of NMDA receptor antagonists are: • High blood pressure • Confusion • Constipation • Dizziness • Headaches • Cough
• **What happens if I have a problem with the medication?** If you have a problem with the medication, for example, you are having a side effect you cannot tolerate, there are several things we can do. We can decrease the dose of the current medication to see if you tolerate it better, change the time you take the medication, or change to a different medication, if needed. Each case will be different, but I will work with you to make sure we find the best therapy for you.
• **What happens if I stop taking my medications for dementia?** Usually, the progression of the disease may become worse. The medications work by increasing chemicals in the brain, such as acetylcholine, or regulating other chemicals in the brain such as glutamate.
• **What are some alternative medications or herbal products commonly used or tried for Alzheimer disease?** Herbal medications often used: • Acetyl-L-carnitine • Axona (caprylic triglyceride) • Bacopa (Brahmi) • Coenzyme Q10 • Ginkgo biloba (EGb 761) • Ginseng • Huperzine A • Lemon balm (Melissa officinalis) • Omega-3 fatty acids, Fish oil, fatty acid blends • Periwinkle (Vinpocetine) • Sage (Salvia officinalis) However, care must be used if trying these agents because they are not regulated and efficacy has not been determined. In some cases, they may worsen the condition.

TABLE 19-7 • Nonpharmacologic Management of Dementia and Psychiatric Symptoms

Targeted Behavior	Recommendation
Sundown syndrome (patient getting more anxious or confused as night approaches)	Have lights set on timers so that they turn on as evening approaches.
Patient wandering off by driving or walking	Place medical wristband with information (eg, name, emergency telephone, allergies). Try to limit driving. You may consider a GPS tracking device similar to what a child may use.
Sleep pattern off	Avoid daytime napping, schedule routine before bedtime.
Urinary incontinence	Schedule bathroom breaks.
Disorientation, especially when traveling	Bring familiar objects including a security object or photo album when traveling. Place familiar objects in new room or setting.

Herbal Medications

Table 19-9 provides a summary of herbals and OTC medications. While the use of herbals is usually discouraged, attempting to use an herbal may be recommended if it brings a therapeutic alliance (eg, caregiver does not want to use an antidepressant for depression, but wants to try an herbal). The MTM provider and patient may come to an understanding that the patient can try an herbal for 1 to 2 months, and if there is no improvement, an antidepressant can be prescribed. Additionally, if the patient has a cultural preference for herbal medicines, use may be warranted, provided that there are no drug-drug interactions, and the patient or caregiver is made aware of side effects that warrant discontinuation of therapy. Axona is a prescribed medical food. It is a medium chain triglyceride which may assist patients with mild to moderate Alzheimer disease, especially those that are Apo E4 negative.[13] It should be used concomitantly with FDA-approved medications for Alzheimer disease. Axona should be mixed with cool liquid or soft food and the dose titrated up over seven days. Gastrointestinal adverse events (eg, diarrhea, nausea, gas) are common and may be minimized by consuming 30 minutes after a full meal (best if meal has fat and protein), taking Axona slowly (sipping, adding ice), or using OTC medications (eg, simethicone, antacids).

Discontinuation of Therapy

Discontinuation of therapy may be considered in several instances. Examples include:

1. Discontinue cholinesterase inhibitors if the patient experiences a fast cognitive decline (eg, >3 to 4 points per year) despite switching and trying 2 to 3 different cholinesterase inhibitors. If discontinuing therapy, tapering is usually recommended.
2. Discontinue memantine if it has worsened cognitive or behavioral function.
3. Discontinue any agent that causes intolerable adverse effects.

TABLE 19-8 • Pharmacologic Agents Used in the Treatment of Dementia

Medication Class and Example Drugs	Approved Use	Common Side Effects[a]	Serious Side Effects
Cholinesterase inhibitors • Donepezil (Aricept®) • Galantamine (Razadyne®) • Rivastigmine (Exelon®)	 All stages Mild to moderate Mild to moderate	• Nausea or vomiting • Diarrhea • Indigestion or abdominal pain • Loss of appetite and weight loss (higher incidence of side effects with rivastigmine)	• Gastrointestinal bleed. Caution with NSAIDs or aspirin.
NMDA receptor antagonist • Memantine (Namenda®)	Moderate to severe	• High blood pressure • Confusion • Constipation • Dizziness • Headaches • Cough	• Significant increase in blood pressure (discontinue medication). • Interaction may occur if using amantadine or dextromethorphan (side effects may increase).
Cholinesterase inhibitor + NMDA receptor antagonist • Donepezil + Memantine (Namzaric®)	Moderate to severe	• Nausea/vomiting • Headache • Diarrhea • Dizziness • Loss of appetite and weight loss • Ecchymosis	• Gastrointestinal bleed. Caution with NSAIDs or aspirin. • Significant increase in blood pressure (discontinue medication). • Interaction may occur if using amantadine or dextromethorphan (side effects may increase).

[a] This is a general list and does not include all side effects that can occur from these drugs. Consult a drug reference source for a more inclusive list before making any recommendations. MTM providers should also consult a comprehensive drug interaction database before making pharmacotherapy recommendations.

Abbreviations: NSAIDS = nonsteroidal anti-inflammatory drugs; NMDA = N-methyl-D-aspartate.

TABLE 19-9 • Herbal Supplements for Dementia

Supplement	Recommended Daily Dose	Level of Evidence[a]	Cost[b]
Acetyl-L-carnitine	2-3 g	Possibly effective	$$$
Axona (caprylic triglyceride)	40 g	Insufficient evidence	$$$-$$$$
Bacopa (Brahmi)	100-450 mg	Possibly effective	$-$$
Coenzyme Q10	350 mg	Insufficient evidence	$$$
Ginkgo biloba (EGb 761)	120-240 mg	Possibly effective	$$
Ginseng	Varies on origin	Possibly effective	$-$$$
Huperzine A	300-800 mcg	Possibly effective	$$-$$$
Lemon balm (Melissa officinalis)	60 drops of extract	Possibly effective	$-$$
Omega-3 fatty acids, fish oil, fatty acid blends	Varies on formulation and proprietary blends	Insufficient evidence	$$-$$$
Periwinkle (Vinpocetine)	10-120 mg	Insufficient evidence	$-$$
Sage (Salvia officinalis)	60 drops of extract	Possibly effective	$$-$$$
Vitamin E	400-800 international units	Possibly effective	$$-$$$

[a] Level of evidence. Likely effective: This product has a very high level of reliable clinical evidence supporting its use for a specific indication. Products rated "likely effective" are generally considered appropriate to recommend. Possibly effective: This product has some clinical evidence supporting its use for a specific indication; however, the evidence is limited by quantity, quality, or contradictory findings. Products rated "possibly effective" might be beneficial, but do not have enough high-quality evidence to recommend for most people. Insufficient evidence: There is not enough reliable scientific evidence to provide an effectiveness rating.

[b] Cost: $ = $10 or less per month supply in the recommended dosage; $$ = $11-$20 per month; $$$ = $21-$50 per month; and $$$$ = more than $50.

Source: Compiled from reference 14.

4. Consider discontinuation of dementia medications if the patient is diagnosed with another terminal disease (eg, cancer).
5. Consider discontinuation of dementia medications if the patient is at a severe stage and palliative care is being considered.

Management of Common Comorbidities—Depression, Aggression, and Sleep Disorders

Depression. During the initial stages of Alzheimer disease, the patient may experience depressive symptoms. If depressive symptoms are suspected, antidepressant therapy should be offered.[15] Selective serotonin reuptake inhibitors (SRRIs) may be used with a preference toward those with less anticholinergic risk (eg, sertraline, citalopram).[16] Counseling points on antidepressants should include at a minimum:

1. The antidepressant will take 4 to 6 weeks before it starts to work.
2. Side effects include nausea, diarrhea, sweating, sleep disturbance (eg, insomnia or somnolence), or slight tremors. Adverse effects occur more commonly during the first 2 weeks, but then usually subside or go away. Therefore, if tolerated, have the patient try the medication for the first month and then reassess.

Aggressive Behavior. In the latter stages of dementia or Alzheimer disease, aggressive behaviors and hallucinations or delusions may become a concern. Medications to control aggressive or agitated behavior should be added when behavior modifications or treatment with dementia-related medications have failed. Second generation antipsychotics (SGAs) are first-line therapy for management of these behaviors.[15] Among the SGAs, risperidone, olanzapine, or aripiprazole are preferred, while quetiapine should be avoided.[15] Although SGAs carry a blackbox warning for increased mortality in the elderly, they still have a more favorable side effect profile than first generation antipsychotics (eg, haloperidol, fluphenazine). SGAs should be initiated at low doses and titrated carefully. Caution should be used with the long-acting injectable formulations of the SGAs. Patients with dementia sometimes have poor muscle mass, and this may cause erratic distribution or a dose-dumping effect which will place the patient at a high risk for adverse events. There is a fine balance between using *as needed* scheduling and having a patient on a *scheduled* regimen. Some clinicians advocate for *as needed* scheduling in patients who tend to have infrequent bouts or in which the caregiver can anticipate a trigger (eg, leaving the house to go shopping). However, *scheduled* administration is preferred with frequent behavioral disturbances or unpredictable behaviors. Counseling points on SGAs include at minimum:

1. Tremors may develop while taking these medications. If they occur, it may be okay, as long as they do not interfere with balance or place the patient at a risk for falls.
2. SGAs carry a blackbox warning for increased death. While the risk is small, it is possible. However, it is important to consider the quality of the remaining time over the quantity. Also, if the safety of the patient or the caregiver(s) is at risk (eg, patient wanders, takes the car for a drive, or becomes aggressive and pushes/strikes the caregiver causing an injury or fall), then SGAs should be used to prevent an injury that may lead to a higher mortality (eg, car accident, fall resulting in broken hip).

Issues with Sleep. Other issues that may occur are sleep complications, especially a shift in sleeping patterns. When this occurs, it is best to look at the current medications and determine if any medications may be causing excessive daytime drowsiness. Some medications may cause napping or sleeping during the day, which may result in the inability to sleep at nighttime. Conversely, cholinesterase inhibitors may cause insomnia, so administration of the medication in the morning may improve sleep at nighttime. Nonpharmacologic options for management of sleep are preferred and should be tried before initiating a medication for insomnia. Nonpharmacologic therapies may include exercise during the day, exposing the patient to direct sunlight (make sure they wear sunscreen), establishing a daily routine (eg, same time for meals, bathing), limiting alcohol and caffeine at night, emptying bladder before going to sleep, and offering security items in the evening (eg, blanket, photo album).[16,17] Pharmacologic agents used may include antidepressants (eg, SSRIs, trazodone, tricyclic antidepressants), benzodiazepines, or nonbenzodiazepines (eg, zolpidem, ramelteon).[16,18] However, data on the safety and efficacy of these agents are lacking in this population. Therefore, a risk-benefit assessment should be noted before initiating therapy. Finally, counseling and monitoring on adverse events, especially increased risk for cognitive impairment and falls, is crucial.

Referral (Emergent or Other)

The patient should call the provider or seek emergency treatment when the following occur: unexpected falls (eg, syncope), shortness of breath, or black tarry stools. The caregiver should call the provider or seek emergency treatment when the following occur in the patient: sudden, rapid cognitive decline, uncontrollable aggressive behavior which puts patient or others at risk for harm, unresponsiveness or excessive sedation, delusions (eg, paranoia), hallucinations, or suicidal thoughts or ideations.

TABLE 19-10 • Medication-Related Problems (MRPs) in Patients with Dementia

Category of MRP	Example of MRP
Nonadherence	• Patient not taking cholinesterase inhibitor because of perceived lack of efficacy
Unnecessary medication	• Memantine being used during mild stage of severity
Need for additional medication	• Patient now in moderate-severe stage of Alzheimer disease and currently only taking a cholinesterase inhibitor • Patient is depressed and needs an antidepressant • Patient displaying aggressive behavior not controlled by current medications or nonpharmacologic measures
Ineffective medication	• Current cholinesterase inhibitor is not effective (eg, decrease in MMSE of 4 points in 1 year)
Dosage too low	• Suboptimal control of depressive symptoms with antidepressant
Dosage too high	• Patient experiencing extrapyramidal symptoms causing imbalance with antipsychotic prescribed for hallucinations and aggressive behavior
Adverse drug event	• Significant nausea/upset stomach from current cholinesterase inhibitor • Significant increase in blood pressure from NMDA receptor antagonist

Abbreviations: MMSE = Mini-Mental State Examination; NMDA = N-methyl-D-aspartate.

CORE ELEMENT 5—DOCUMENTATION AND FOLLOW-UP

Clear and succinct documentation of MRPs and recommendations is a key component of the MTM consult. Examples of potential MRPs in patients with dementia are provided in Table 19-10. Recommendations must present a systematic reason for initiation/switch/discontinuation of pharmacologic agent(s). Sample communications and recommendations to providers to address medication-related issues are found in Figure 19-3. Recommendations may be communicated via fax, telephone, or other means of written or secure electronic communication. The following examples are for illustrative purposes. Actual communications to providers should be individualized based on the type of recommendation, patient specific characteristics, and the nature of the relationship with the provider. Documentation of therapeutic management must be dated (month/date/year) and signed.

Follow-up visits to monitor dementia-related medications (eg, donepezil, galantamine, memantine) should occur every 3 months with MMSE scores and overall assessment of behavior and function (eg, activities of daily life). During the assessment, it is important to gather as much information as possible from the caregiver. Sometimes a caregiver that is constantly with the patient has a harder time noticing changes in cognition or behavior, compared to a caregiver that sees the patient every couple of weeks. Therefore, it is vital that close attention is given to assessments from the caregiver about activities of daily life (eg, ability to use the television, making coffee, doing laundry, using the computer). While the Alzheimer's Disease Functional Assessment and Change Scale (ADFACS) is the one of the most common instruments for assessing this aspect, other tools are available that may be less time consuming or require less training (eg, https://www.alz.org/national/documents/brochure_toolsforidassesstreat.pdf, http://www.alz.org/careplanning/downloads/katz-adl-lawton-iadl.pdf). Also, some scales or inventories such as the Neuropsychiatric Inventory (http://npitest.net/) can be used to assess neuropsychiatric complications that may occur in patients with dementia. However, some of the scales are subject to copyright or are limited in the extent of activities of daily life that they assess. Overall, using an activity of daily living scale/inventory or formal assessment for psychiatric complications may help in staging and monitoring the patient more objectively.

Scenario: Patient has continued to suffer a decline in cognition on donepezil 10 mg per day.
MRP: Adverse drug event.

- Assessment:
  MMSE scores have declined by 5 points in 3 months on donepezil 10 mg daily. Patient currently taking Tylenol PM (which contains diphenhydramine). Patient also increased ranitidine to 150 mg bid to help with nausea/upset stomach when donepezil was started at 5 mg day (currently on 10 mg QAM). Both diphenhydramine and ranitidine in doses >150 mg/day can impair cognition.
- Plan:
  Recommend patient discontinue use of Tylenol PM.
  Recommend that patient reduce ranitidine to 150 mg day as currently prescribed.
  Educate that nausea/upset stomach is a common side effect with donepezil, but it usually diminishes over time.
  Recommend switching donepezil dose to evening to minimize nausea.
  Reassess patient in two weeks via phone call.

Scenario: Patient is not using Exelon patch 4.6 mg/day as prescribed.
MRP: Nonadherence.

- Assessment:
  Patient was prescribed Exelon Patch 4.6 mg/24 hours for moderate stage Alzheimer's disease (MMSE 16) but is unable to afford the medication. Donepezil is also effective in moderate stages of Alzheimer and is much more affordable.
- Plan:
  Recommend initiating donepezil 5 mg at bedtime with titration to 10 mg at bedtime after 4 weeks. (*Note: Reason for 4-week titration is based on patient and caregiver level of understanding and may be simpler to increase at next refill (1 month). Slower titration may also provide better tolerability of side effects.)*

Scenario: Patient with dementia experiencing hallucinations and aggressive behavior on quetiapine.
MRP: Dosage too low or need for additional medication.

- Assessment:
  Currently on quetiapine 150 mg at bedtime. Prior nonpharmacologic therapy has failed. Current MMSE is 9 (severe stage). Adjustment in antipsychotic therapy is warranted due to hallucinations and aggression.
- Plan:
  Consider one of the following antipsychotic regimens:
  1. Increase quetiapine to 200 mg at bedtime. However, doses over 150 mg/day may increase risk for extrapyramidal side effects. Additionally, quetiapine has a higher rate of anticholinergic activity compared to other antipsychotics and has lost favor in recent articles.
  2. Discontinue quetiapine and start low dose risperidone (0.25 mg - 0.5 mg per day). Low doses have good effectiveness with minimal extrapyramidal symptoms, and a lower anticholinergic profile compared to quetiapine. It is also available in generic. Dose may need to be titrated to 1-1.5 mg per day.

  Note: In psychiatry, there is typically more than one possibility. When initially developing trust with a physician (which the MTM provider has to earn), it is good practice to always provide the two best options. By providing two options:
  - *It demonstrates that the MTM provider looked at alternatives and did a comprehensive search assuming other possibilities.*
  - *The MTM provider is more likely to have one of the two choices/recommendations selected. With human nature, people do not like being cornered into a decision, especially with someone they do not know, so they may not pick the MTM provider's choice (i.e., accept the recommendation). That is why the best sales person will always narrow the choices to two (e.g., Car A or B, smartphone A or smartphone B). If given two choices, a person is more likely to "buy." On the other hand, more than two choices causes most of us confusion, so we don't buy anything (in this case choose a recommendation) and are more likely to have "buyer's remorse if we do choose. After developing trust, the physician will just ask the MTM provider which choice he/she prefers, and the MTM provider can discontinue offering two choices.*

FIGURE 19-3 Sample provider communications for dementia-related disorders.

REFERENCES

1. Peron EP, Slattum PW, Powers KE, Hobgood SE. Alzheimer disease. In: DiPiro JT, Tolbert RL, Yee GC, Matzke GR, Wells BG, Posey LM, eds. *Pharmacotherapy: A Pathophysiologic Approach*. 10th ed. New York: McGraw-Hill; 2017.
2. Reisberg B. Diagnostic criteria in dementia: a comparison of current criteria, research challenges, and implications for DSM-V. *J Geriatr Psychiatry Neurol.* 2006;19:137-146.
3. Rubin CD. The primary care of Alzheimer's disease. *Am J Med Sci.* 2006; 332:314-333.
4. Alzheimer's Association. 2016 Alzheimer's Disease Facts and Figures. Available at http://www.alz.org/documents_custom/2016-facts-and-figures.pdf. Accessed May 1, 2017.
5. Alzheimer's Association. http://www.alz.org. Accessed May 1, 2017.
6. Lyketsos CG, Colenda CC, Beck C, et al. Position statement of the American Association for Geriatric Psychiatry regarding principles of care for patients with dementia resulting from Alzheimer's disease. *Am J Geriatr Psychiatry.* 2006;14:561-573.
7. Moore AR, O'Keeffe ST. Drug-induced cognitive impairment in the elderly. *Drugs Aging.* 1999;15:15-28.
8. Boustani M, Campbell N, Munger S. Impact of anticholinergics on the aging brain: a review and practical application. *Aging Health.* 2008;4:311-320.
9. National Collaborating Centre for Mental Health (UK). Dementia: a NICE-SCIE guideline on supporting people with dementia and their careers in health and social care. Leicester (UK): British Psychological Society; 2007 (last update September 2016).
10. Robinson L, Tang E, Taylor JP. Dementia: timely diagnosis and early intervention. *BMJ.* 2015;350:h3029.
11. Folstein MF, Folstein SE, McHugh PR. Mini-mental state. A practical method for grading the cognitive state of patients for the clinician. *J Psychiatr Res.* 1975;12:189-198.
12. CMS. *Medicare Part D Medication Therapy Management Program Standardized Format.* Available at https://www.cms.gov/Medicare/Prescription-Drug-Coverage/PrescriptionDrugCovContra/Downloads/MTM-Program-Standardized-Format-English-and-Spanish-Instructions-Samples-v032712.pdf. Accessed May 1, 2017.

13. Axona. Fuel the brain. Available at http://www.about-axona.com/. Accessed May 1, 2017.

14. Natural Medicines [database online]. Somerville, MA: Therapeutic Research Center; 2017. Available at https://naturalmedicines.therapeuticresearch.com/. Accessed May 1, 2017.

15. Gauthier S, Patterson C, Chertkow H, et al. Recommendations of the 4th Canadian Consensus Conference on the Diagnosis and Treatment of Dementia (CCCDTD4). *Can Geriatr J*. 2012;15:120-126.

16. APA Work Group on Alzheimer's Disease and other Dementias; Rabins PV, Blacker D, Rovner BW, et al. American Psychiatric Association practice guideline for the treatment of patients with Alzheimer's disease and other dementias, second edition. *Am J Psychiatry*. 2007;164:5-56.

17. McCurry SM, Pike KC, Vitiello MV, Logsdon RG, Larson EB, Teri L. Increasing walking and bright light exposure to improve sleep in community-dwelling persons with Alzheimer's disease: results of a randomized, controlled trial. *J Am Geriatr Soc*. 2011;59:1393-1402.

18. Deschenes CL, McCurry SM. Current treatments for sleep disturbances in individuals with dementia. *Curr Psychiatry Rep*. 2009;11:20-26.

Review Questions

1. What is the most important component of an initial MTM interview with a patient or caregiver regarding dementia?
   a. Dedicate sufficient time for the visit.
   b. After the interview, ask the patient or caregiver, "Do you have any questions?"
   c. Avoid discussing any sensitive issues such as inevitable decline, psychiatric complications (eg, depression, anxiety), or family support.
   d. Do not focus on the patient's educational or health literacy status because the MTM form is going to the primary physician.

2. When performing a patient assessment in a patient with dementia it is crucial to:
   a. refer the patient to an assisted living facility.
   b. review the current medication profile and ask about over-the-counter products and neutraceuticals.
   c. avoid use of scales or inventories because their utility is limited in patients with dementia.
   d. stay emotionless and focus on obtaining a detailed patient history.

3. What is considered a therapeutic failure that may warrant a change in cognitive medications (eg, donepezil, galantamine)?
   a. No change from baseline in the MMSE scores
   b. A decrease from baseline in the MMSE by 1 to 2 points in a year
   c. A decrease from baseline in the MMSE by 5 points in a year
   d. Loose stools during the first 3 days of cholinesterase inhibitor therapy

4. Which statement demonstrates proper use of living room language?
   a. "You have Alzheimer disease. This is a neurocognitive disorder that will cause a deterioration of your cognitive abilities over time."
   b. "You have Alzheimer disease. This is a disease that affects your memory and the ability to take care of yourself over time."
   c. "You have Alzheimer disease. Pharmacologic treatment options include cholinesterase inhibitors and N-Methyl-D-aspartate inhibitors that work by regulating your neurotransmitters."
   d. "You have Alzheimer disease. This is a cognitive disease that can cause psychiatric conditions such as anhedonia, alogia, psychosis, and overall deterioration of your activities of daily life."

5. A 75-year-old patient was recently diagnosed with Alzheimer disease. His caregiver states he has become "depressed" and worried about the future. These feelings have caused a significant change in his daily life, including bouts of crying. After discussing these feelings with the patient, he is open to starting an agent. The patient takes approximately 10 medications but forgot his medication list at home. What is the most appropriate therapeutic option?
   a. Initiate citalopram 10 mg daily because drug–drug interactions with citalopram are minimal.
   b. Initiate paroxetine 20 mg daily because drug–drug interactions with paroxetine are minimal.
   c. Initiate quetiapine 100 mg at bedtime to minimize the symptoms of worrying.
   d. Avoid recommending an agent for depression.

6. An 81-year-old patient was diagnosed with Alzheimer disease 2 years ago and placed on donepezil. She was recently staged as moderate-severe Alzheimer disease and started on memantine 20 mg daily 3 days ago. She reports severe dizziness for the past 2 days. Assuming vital signs are normal, which therapeutic option is the best course of action?
   a. Discontinue memantine since it does not provide a favorable risk–benefit ratio.
   b. Reduce memantine to 5 mg daily, and monitor for improvement of dizziness.
   c. Recommend meclizine 25 mg daily for dizziness, and monitor for improvement.
   d. Encourage the patient to continue medication for 3 more weeks.

7. All of the following are indications for emergency or urgent referral in Alzheimer disease **EXCEPT:**
   a. a call from the caregiver reporting 2 syncopal episodes in 3 days.
   b. a call from the caregiver reporting the patient has black tarry stools.
   c. a call from the caregiver reporting patient is taking longer naps.
   d. a call from the caregiver reporting the patient has become hostile and aggressive and not responding to redirection.

8. A patient has had a significant decrease in cognitive function over the past 3 months. During the comprehensive medication review the patient reports taking Tylenol PM® to induce sleep for the last several weeks. Which medication-related problem would most appropriately describe this scenario?
   a. Nonadherence
   b. Dosage too high
   c. Adverse drug event
   d. Need for additional medication

9. Which scales and inventories can be appropriately used in staging cognitive function and activities of daily living, respectively, in patients with dementia?
   a. MMSE, ADFACS
   b. MMSE, PANSS
   c. ADFACS, PANSS
   d. NPI, ADFACS

10. What are the primary agents used to treat dementia-related disorders and obtain the intended goal of treatment?
   a. Cholinesterase inhibitors to reduce the decline of cognitive function
   b. N-Methyl-D-aspartate inhibitors to reduce the decline of cognitive function
   c. Cholinesterase inhibitors to improve cognitive function
   d. N-Methyl-D-aspartate inhibitors to improve cognitive function

ANSWERS

1. a	2. b	3. c
4. b	5. a	6. b
7. c	8. c	9. a
10. a		

20

Depression MTM Data Set

Stacey D. Curtis, PharmD, and Kristin W. Weitzel, PharmD, FAPhA

KEY POINTS

Depression is a common and chronic disease that can cause serious harm to patients and increases the risk of death.

- Treatment goals for depression include reduction or remission of current symptoms, return to a full level of functioning, and prevention of future depressive episodes and/or relapse.
- Medications commonly used to treat depression include selective serotonin reuptake inhibitors (eg, sertraline), serotonin-norepinephrine reuptake inhibitors (eg, venlafaxine), bupropion, and tricyclic antidepressants (eg, amitriptyline).
- MTM providers should educate patients and/or their support system (eg, family members) about the delay in onset of antidepressant effects.
- Medication therapy management (MTM) providers should explain the importance of adherence throughout the entire course of antidepressant treatment.
- MTM providers should advise care when patients are switching between antidepressants to avoid withdrawal symptoms and ensure a consistent therapeutic response.
- Patients with depression should be assessed for suicide risk, and MTM providers should be familiar with supportive resources for patients expressing suicidal ideation (eg, National Suicide Prevention Lifeline 1-800-273-8255).

INTRODUCTION TO MAJOR DEPRESSIVE DISORDER

Recognizing Depression

Major depressive disorder (MDD) is characterized by discrete episodes of at least 2 weeks' duration (although most episodes last considerably longer) involving clear-cut changes in affect, cognition, and neurovegetative functions, and interepisode remissions.[1] According to criteria listed in the *Diagnostic and Statistical Manual of Mental Disorders*, fifth edition, a major depressive episode is defined by the criteria listed in Table 20-1.[1]

Evidence demonstrates that depression is a common and chronic disease that can cause serious harm to patients and increases the risk of death. Table 20-2 reviews commonly encountered signs and symptoms of depression. These symptoms, especially physical symptoms, often cause patients to seek medical help from their physician.

All patients who are diagnosed with MDD should be assessed for suicidal thoughts. Factors associated with an increased risk for suicide include psychiatric and substance use disorders, adolescence and younger age adults, physical illness, recent stressful life event, childhood trauma, feelings of hopelessness, and male gender.[3]

Secondary Causes of Depression

Before a patient is diagnosed with depression, other contributing factors should be ruled out. These may include medications or other medical conditions, eg, patients with some neurological disorders may experience symptoms similar to depression.[1,4] Suspected drug- or disease-related factors that may contribute to depressive symptoms should be addressed before or along with treatment of depression to optimize response. Table 20-3 contains selected medications associated with drug-induced depressive symptoms, and Table 20-4 contains common medical conditions and substance use disorders that are associated with symptoms of depression.

TABLE 20-1 • DSM-5 Diagnostic Criteria for Major Depressive Disorder

A. Five (or more) of the following symptoms have been present during the same 2-week period and represent a change from previous functioning; at least one of the symptoms is either (1) depressed mood or (2) loss of interest or pleasure.
Note: Do not include symptoms that are clearly attributable to another medical condition.
1. Depressed mood most of the day, nearly every day, as indicated by either subjective report (eg, feels sad, empty, and hopeless) or observation made by others (eg, appears tearful). (Note: In children and adolescents, can be irritable mood.)
2. Markedly diminished interest or pleasure in all, or almost all, activities most of the day, nearly every day (as indicated by either subjective account or observation).
3. Significant weight loss when not dieting or weight gain (eg, a change of >5% of body weight in a month), or decrease or increase in appetite nearly every day. (Note: In children, consider failure to make expected weight gain.)
4. Insomnia or hypersomnia nearly every day.
5. Psychomotor agitation or retardation nearly every day (observable by others, not merely subjective feelings of restlessness or being slowed down).
6. Fatigue or loss of energy nearly every day.
7. Feelings of worthlessness or excessive or inappropriate guilt (which may be delusional) nearly every day (not merely self-reproach or guilt about being sick).
8. Diminished ability to think or concentrate, or indecisiveness, nearly every day (either by subjective account or as observed by others).
9. Recurrent thoughts of death (not just fear of dying), recurrent suicidal ideation without a specific plan, or a suicide attempt or a specific plan for committing suicide.

B. The symptoms cause clinically significant distress or impairment in social, occupational, or other important areas of functioning.

C. The episode is not attributable to the physiological effects of a substance or to another medical condition.
Note: Criteria A-C represent a major depressive episode.
Note: Responses to a significant loss (eg, bereavement, financial ruin, losses from a natural disaster, a serious medical illness or disability) may include the feelings of intense sadness, rumination about the loss, insomnia, poor appetite, and weight loss noted in Criterion A, which may resemble a depressive episode. Although such symptoms may be understandable or considered appropriate to the loss, the presence of a major depressive episode in addition to the normal response to a significant loss should also be carefully considered. This decision inevitably requires the exercise of clinical judgment based on the individual's history and the cultural norms for the expression of distress in the context of loss.
In distinguishing grief from a major depressive episode (MDE), it is useful to consider that in grief the predominant affect is feelings of emptiness and loss, while in MDE it is persistent depressed mood and the inability to anticipate happiness or pleasure. The dysphoria in grief is likely to decrease in intensity over days to weeks and occurs in waves, the so-called pangs of grief. These waves tend to be associated with thoughts or reminders of the deceased. The depressed mood of MDE is more persistent and not tied to specific thoughts or preoccupations. The pain of grief may be accompanied by positive emotions and humor that are uncharacteristic of the pervasive unhappiness and misery characteristic of MDE. The thought content associated with grief generally features a preoccupation with thoughts and memories of the deceased, rather than the self-critical or pessimistic ruminations seen in MDE. In grief, self-esteem is generally preserved, whereas in MDE feelings of worthlessness and self-loathing are common. If self-derogatory ideation is present in grief, it typically involves perceived failings vis-a-vis the deceased (eg, not visiting frequently enough, not telling the deceased how much he or she was loved). If a bereaved individual thinks about death and dying, such thoughts are generally focused on the deceased and possibly about "joining" the deceased, whereas in MDE such thoughts are focused on ending one's own life because of feeling worthless, undeserving of life, or unable to cope with the pain of depression.

D. The occurrence of the major depressive episode is not better explained by schizoaffective disorder, schizophrenia, schizophreniform disorder, delusional disorder, or other specified and unspecified schizophrenia spectrum and other psychotic disorders.

E. There has never been a manic episode or a hypomanic episode.
Note: This exclusion does not apply if all of the manic-like or hypomanic-like episodes are substance-induced or are attributable to the physiological effects of another medical condition.

Source: Reproduced, with permission, from *The Diagnostic and Statistical Manual of Mental Disorders*. 5th ed. American Psychiatric Association; 2013.

Depression Screening, Diagnosis, and Treatment

There is no blood test or physical examination finding that is diagnostic for depression. A diagnosis of depression is based on the patient's self-reported symptoms and the emotions that they have been experiencing. Ongoing monitoring of depressive symptoms and response to therapy may be challenging because many symptoms are general or subjective in nature and may be related to other conditions (eg, weight loss, insomnia). Several depression rating scales exist to help measure response to therapy. These scales help gauge the degree of depression a patient is experiencing and/or how the patient is responding to therapy.[9,10,11] Table 20-5 provides representative examples and comparisons of depression-rating instruments.

Treatment goals for depression include reducing symptoms acutely, achieving remission of symptoms, helping the patient return to a full level of functioning, and preventing a future episode or relapse. The primary goal of therapy is determined by the phase of treatment, although each patient's treatment will need to be individualized. Table 20-6 provides general guidance for treatment phases and corresponding goals.

TABLE 20-2 • Signs and Symptoms of Depression

Psychological
Sadness
Loss of interest
Pessimism
Guilt (increased risk of suicide)
Feelings of worthlessness (increased risk of suicide)
Anxiety (up to 90% of patients)
Decreased concentration
Poor memory
Auditory hallucinations
Physical
Fatigue
Pain
Headache
Sleep disturbances
Hypersomnia
Weight gain
Weight loss
Gastrointestinal complaints
Heart palpitations
Decreased libido

Source: Compiled from reference 2.

TABLE 20-3 • Selected Medications Associated with Drug-Induced Depressive Symptoms

Acne treatment
Isotretinoin
Anticonvulsants
Levetiracetam
Topiramate
Vigabatrin
Antimigraine agents
Triptans
Cardiovascular medications
β-blocker
Clonidine
Methyldopa
Reserpine
Hormonal therapy
Gonadotropin-releasing hormone
Oral contraceptives
Steroids (eg, prednisone)
Tamoxifen
Immunologic agents
Interferons
Smoking cessation medications
Varenicline

Source: Reproduced, with permission, from DiPiro JT, Talbert RL, Yee GC, Matzke GR, Wells BG, Posey L, eds. *Pharmacotherapy: A Pathophysiologic Approach*. 10th ed. New York, NY: McGraw-Hill; 2017.

TABLE 20-4 • Common Medical Conditions and Substance Use Disorders Associated with Depressive Symptoms

General Medical Conditions
Cardiovascular diseases
Coronary artery disease
Congestive heart failure
Myocardial infarction
Collagen disorder
Arthritis
Systemic lupus erythematosus
Deficiency states
Pernicious anemia
Severe anemia
Wernicke encephalopathy
Electrolyte imbalance
Hypokalemia
Hyponatremia
Endocrine diseases
Hypothyroidism
Addison or Cushing disease
Infections
AIDS
Encephalitis
Human immunodeficiency virus
Mononucleosis
Sexually transmitted diseases
Tuberculosis
Malignant disease
Any type
Metabolic disorders
Neurologic disorders
Alzheimer disease
Epilepsy
Hepatic encephalopathy
Huntington disease
Multiple sclerosis
Pain (chronic)
Parkinson disease
Post stroke
Renal diseases
Chronic kidney disease
End stage renal failure
Substance use disorders (including *intoxication* and *withdrawal*)
Alcoholism
Marijuana abuse and dependence
Nicotine dependence
Opiate abuse and dependence (eg, heroin)
Psychostimulant abuse and dependence (eg, cocaine)

Source: References 2, 7, and 8.

TABLE 20-5 • Depression and Bipolar Disorder Rating Scales

Rating Scale	Type	Scoring	Comments
Hamilton Depression Scale (HAMD or HDRS)	Clinician rated	17-item scale; <6 = normal mood; 17-25 = moderate depression; >25 = severe depression	Used to screen patients for drug studies and to determine severity of symptoms and treatment outcome. HDRS is the standard to compare other depression rating scales against.
Montgomery-Asberg Depression Rating Scale (MADRS)	Clinician rated	10-item, 7-point scale. For each item: 0 = no symptoms; 6 = severe symptoms	Differentiates between the intermediate grades of depression. Decreases bias in patients with other medical illnesses and increased somatization (varied unexplained physical symptoms).
Beck Depression Inventory (BDI)	Patient rated	21-item scale; 0-9 = normal; 10-15 = mild depression; 16-19 = mild-moderate; 20-29 = moderate-severe; 30-63 = severe depression	The standard for depression self-rating scales and an objective measure of change in symptoms as a result of treatment.
Zung Self-Rating Depression Scale (ZSDS)	Patient rated	20-item scale, 4-point severity; <50 = normal; 50-59 = minimal-mild; 60-69 = moderate-marked; ≥70 severe depression	Severity rated by frequency of occurrence of symptoms. May not be as sensitive in measuring changes in severity of symptoms.
Patient Health Questionnaire (PHQ-9)	Patient rated	9-item, 4-point scale. For each DSM-IV depression criteria item: 0 = not at all; 3 = nearly every day. Score <10 = minimal depression symptoms	Commonly used in primary care to establish a diagnosis of depression and assess severity of depressive symptoms.
Quick Inventory of Depressive Symptomatology (QIDS-C [Clinician] and QIDS-SR [Patient])	Clinician and patient rated	16-item scale; scores range from 0-27; 0-5 = none; 6-10 = mild; 11-15 = moderate; 16-20 = severe; 21-27 = very severe	Used to assess symptom severity and symptomatic change. QIDS-SR found to be as sensitive to symptom change as the HDRS. Has usefulness in both clinical and research settings.
Young Mania Rating Scale (YMRS)	Clinician rated	11-item scale; 5-point severity; 13 = minimal; 20 = mild; 26 = moderate; 38 = severe	Used to screen patients for drug studies and to determine severity of symptoms and treatment outcome. YMRS is the standard to compare other mania rating scales against.
Mood Disorder Questionnaire (MDQ)	Patient rated	15-item scale; score of ≥7 suggestive of bipolar spectrum disorder	Screens for a lifetime history of mania or hypomania. Does not assess severity of illness.

Source: Reproduced, with permission, from DiPiro JT, Talbert RL, Yee GC, Matzke GR, Wells BG, Posey L, eds. *Pharmacotherapy: A Pathophysiologic Approach*. 10th ed. New York, NY: McGraw-Hill; 2017.

The treatment phases described in Table 20-6 are general and do not apply to every patient. Treatment for depression should be individualized based on patient needs and response to treatment. Medications used for depression may take 2 to 4 weeks or longer to work completely. Response to therapy can be evaluated in 6 to 8 weeks using the same scale or measures used for baseline evaluation. Table 20-7 lists benchmarks to consider when monitoring response to therapy. Lifelong therapy may be indicated in patients at increased risk for experiencing another depressive episode (ie, patients younger than 40 years old who have had 2 or more depressive episodes, and patients of any age who have had 3 or more episodes).[4]

American Psychiatric Association practice guidelines for the treatment of depression recommend a therapy change in patients who only achieve a partial response to drug therapy. Potential drug therapy changes may include an increase in dosage, switch to an alternative antidepressant, or the addition of different antidepressant or nonpharmacologic therapy.[1,4] Definitive evidence does not support one option as being superior to another. The choice of treatment for partial responders is often based on patient considerations

TABLE 20-6 • Treatment Phases for Major Depression

Phase	Time Length	Goal
Acute	6-10 weeks	Achieve remission
Continuation	4-9 months	Prevent relapse
Maintenance	12-36 months	Prevent another depressive episode

Source: References 2, 4, and 12.

TABLE 20-7 • Monitoring Response to Depression Therapy

Response	Score Change from Baseline Symptoms
Nonresponse	<25% decrease
Partial Response	26-49% decrease
Partial Remission	>50% decrease
Remission	No symptoms present
Treatment Resistant	No remission after two adequate trials of antidepressant

Source: Reference 12.

TABLE 20-8 • Questions to Assess Patient Nonresponse to Treatment

Is the diagnosis of major depressive disorder correct?
Does the patient have symptoms of psychotic depression?
Has the patient received adequate dose and duration of treatment?
Do adverse effects preclude appropriate dosing?
Has the patient adhered to the prescribed regimen?
Has sexual dysfunction led to noncompliance?
Was a stepwise approach to treatment used?
Was treatment outcome adequately measured?
Is there a coexisting or preexisting medical or psychiatric disorder?
Are there other factors that interfere with treatment?

Source: References 2 and 4.

(eg, comorbid conditions) and/or preference, cost, insurance formulary, and prescriber preference. Table 20-8 lists questions to ask a patient who is not responding to therapy to help guide appropriate next steps.

CORE ELEMENT 1—COMPREHENSIVE MEDICATION REVIEW FOR PATIENTS WITH DEPRESSION

Interviewing the patient is an important step in the treatment and diagnosis of depression because the initial assessment and monitoring of response is largely based on the patient's description of symptoms. In the treatment of depression, it is especially important that the patient feels comfortable, secure, and open in discussing his/her symptoms with the health care provider. Following is a list of suggested questions to use when conducting a medication therapy review in a patient with depression (Table 20-9). MTM providers may need to establish rapport with patients and put patients at ease by talking through other conditions or medications first. Open-ended questions may be useful in allowing the patient freedom to bring up his/her own concerns about depression.

The number and types of questions will depend on multiple factors, including the stage of therapy, amount of time for the interview, and coexisting conditions or medication-related problems (MRPs). MTM providers should remain alert for patients expressing suicidal thoughts or behaviors. In addition, MTM providers should remember to use living room language for depression (Table 20-10) and be prepared for questions that patients may ask regarding depression or its treatment (Table 20-11).

TABLE 20-9 • Questions to Ask When Conducting a Medication Review in a Patient with Depression

Suggested Questions for the Patient with Depression

- How long have you had depression? When were you diagnosed?
- Who else in your family has depression?
- If someone else in your family is also taking medication, which one(s) have they taken and how did they work?
- Have you recently experienced any of the following signs/symptoms of depression?
  - Little interest or pleasure in doing things that you once found enjoyable
  - Feeling down, depressed, or hopeless
  - Changes in sleep patterns (trouble sleeping or sleeping too much)
  - Changes in appetite (eating more or less than usual)
  - Feeling bad about yourself
  - Difficulty concentrating or remembering things
  - Significant changes in your energy level (more or less energy)
  - Crying for no reason
  - Feelings of guilt or despair
  - Feeling like your life is not worth living
  - Thoughts of hurting yourself or suicide
- What medications do you take for your depression? How do you take them?
- How often do you miss a dose of your depression medication?
- What other medications have you taken in the past for your depression?
- Have you ever stopped taking any of your prescribed depression medications without telling your physician? If so, why?
- What over-the-counter medications or herbals do you use for your depression?
- Other than medicines, what have you tried for your depression (eg, counseling)?
- What has your physician discussed with you regarding over-the-counter medications that you should avoid because they can worsen your depression?

Questions to Ask for Prevention/Assessment of Suicide Risk

- Have you ever thought about death or dying?
- Have you ever thought that life was not worth living?
- Have you ever thought about ending your life?
- Have you ever attempted suicide?
- Are you currently thinking about ending your life?
- What are your reasons for wanting to die and your reasons for wanting to live?

Source: References 2, and 13.

Assessing Suicide Risk

Suicide is a leading cause of death among patients with depression.[2] All patients with depression should be assessed for suicidal thoughts or behavior. Patients at increased risk for committing suicide include those with a history of substance use disorders, adolescents and young adults, those with comorbid illnesses, a recent stressful event, presence of trauma from childhood, feelings of hopelessness, and male patients. The risk of suicide is highest at the beginning of treatment and increases as patients develop more specific plans for how and when they would commit suicide.[14]

Notably, the FDA added a blackbox warning to antidepressant medication labeling in 2004, stating that antidepressants may increase the risk of suicidal thoughts and behaviors in pediatric patients. This blackbox warning was expanded in 2007 to include young adults. MTM providers should be aware of this labeling and stay alert for patients who may express suicidal thoughts or behaviors. In addition, providers should counsel younger patients that antidepressants may increase agitation or anxiety at the start of therapy and should discuss suicide directly. Talking about suicide with a patient does not increase the patient's risk or chance of

TABLE 20-10 • Living Room Language for Depression

Aminoketone—a class of drugs used to treat depression; these work primarily by increasing dopamine in the brain. Bupropion is the only drug in this class.
Bipolar depression—a condition associated with periods of euphoria and happiness followed by periods of depression and sadness.
Chronic—constant, never ending, does not go away.
Dopamine—a neurotransmitter involved in mood and other bodily functions. Dopamine is increased by bupropion.
Electroconvulsive therapy (ECT)—electrical currents are passed through the brain to produce a seizure in order to treat some types of mood disorders.
Elevate—raise, make higher.
GI—gastrointestinal tract.
Heart palpitations—rapid heartbeat, feeling of one's heart pounding or racing.
Hypersomnia—excessive daytime sleepiness and/or excessive sleeping.
Insomnia—to have trouble falling or staying asleep; results in daytime drowsiness.
Libido—sexual drive.
Major depressive disorder—a condition associated with several periods of sadness, hopelessness, or feeling down consistently.
Mania—a condition where the patient has periods of euphoria and happiness.
Monoamine oxidase inhibitors (MAOIs)—a group of drugs used to treat depression, eg, phenelzine and tranylcypromine; these work by increasing norepinephrine and serotonin.
Neurotransmitter—chemicals in your brain that help different areas of your brain communicate with each other and function optimally.
Norepinephrine—a neurotransmitter involved in mood and other bodily functions. Norepinephrine is increased by SNRIs and TCAs.
Post-traumatic stress disorder (PTSD)—An anxiety disorder with onset after a person has experienced a traumatic event. May involve nightmares, sleep disturbances, and flashbacks of the event.
Selective serotonin reuptake inhibitors (SSRIs)—a group of medications used to treat depression; these work by increasing specific neurotransmitters in the brain (sertraline, fluoxetine, citalopram, escitalopram, paroxetine, and others).
Serotonin—a neurotransmitter involved in mood and other bodily functions. Serotonin levels are increased by SSRIs, SNRIs, and TCAs.
Serotonin-norepinephrine reuptake inhibitors (SNRIs)—a group of medications used to treat depression; these work by increasing serotonin and norepinephrine in the brain (desvenlafaxine, venlafaxine, and duloxetine).
St. John's wort—an herbal supplement sometimes used to treat depression.
Tetracyclic antidepressants—mirtazapine is the only drug in this class and is used to treat depression by increasing serotonin and norepinephrine.
Triazolopyridines—a class of drugs used to treat depression; these work by increasing serotonin levels in the brain and activating serotonin receptors (trazodone).
Tricyclic antidepressants (TCAs)—a class of drugs used to treat depression; these work by increasing norepinephrine and serotonin in the brain, but come with many undesirable side effects that sometimes limit their use (amitriptyline, nortriptyline, others).

TABLE 20-11 • Questions to Anticipate Regarding Depression

- **What causes depression?**
  Depression is not a simple disease to understand. There is not one thing that causes a person to feel depressed. A combination of genetics, environment, life events, and social surroundings are thought to all influence the likelihood of developing depression.
- **How is depression different than just feeling sad?**
  Depression is different from just feeling sad in that it lasts from weeks to month to years and interferes with a person's daily life. Depression is a medical illness that needs to be diagnosed and treated by a health care provider.
- **How do I know if I am depressed?**
  There are several symptoms of depression including fatigue, loss of interest in things you previously enjoyed, weight changes, feelings of guilt or worthlessness, anxiety, or others. A diagnosis of depression requires a complete workup by a health care provider. If you are feeling any of these symptoms, you should talk to your physician or other health care provider.
- **Is it my fault that I am depressed?**
  No. Depression is a medical condition just like high blood pressure or diabetes. It is a condition that affects the brain and impairs its ability to function properly.
- **Can children become depressed?**
  Children and adolescents can develop depression, just like adults, as they are also exposed to life changes that can affect their mood.
- **Why do women suffer from depression more than men do?**
  It is thought that women suffer from depression more than men do because of hormone changes that occur naturally or from pregnancy. This can lead to mood changes and could result in depression.
- **How long can depression last?**
  Depression, if left untreated, can last for years and result in severe life impairment. In Major Depressive Disorder, patients suffer from episodes of depression that last anywhere from 2 weeks to several months.
- **How long will it take for my depression medication to start working?**
  Medications used to treat depression can take 2 to 4 weeks or longer for effects to be seen.
- **Why does it take so long for the medications to help me feel better?**
  Researchers are not sure why it takes weeks for the medication's effect to been seen. This stems from the fact that we do not know what exactly causes depression.
- **How long will I have to stay on medication for depression?**
  There is no definite length of treatment, and each patient is different. How long you stay on depression medications will depend on how you react to the medication, how your mood improves while on it, how long you have been taking it, and whether you have had previous episodes of depression. Some individuals can taper off their antidepressants after 6 months or so, especially if it is their first episode of depression. Other patients may need longer or even lifelong therapy. When you and your provider feel it is right to get off the medication, your physician will instruct you on how to decrease the medication until you stop taking it altogether. Do not stop antidepressant medications abruptly, as this can cause nausea, anxiety, worsening depression, or other symptoms.

PERSONAL MEDICATION LIST FOR *<Insert patient's name*, DOB: *mm/dd/yyyy>*	
Medication: Sertraline 50 mg	
How I use it: Take one tablet (50 mg) by mouth every morning	
Why I use it: Depression	**Prescriber:** Smith
Date I started using it: 2/8/2017	**Date I stopped using it:** *(Leave blank for patient's notes)*
Why I stopped using it: *(Leave blank for patient's notes)*	

FIGURE 20-1 Example personal medication list for depression medications.

committing suicide. MTM providers who work with patients with depression should be aware of local and/or national resources for suicide prevention and counseling (eg, Suicide Prevention Lifeline) to refer patients if needed.[2,15] If a significant risk is observed, the patient must be referred immediately to an appropriate healthcare professional.

CORE ELEMENT 2—PERSONAL MEDICATION LIST[16]

Above is a sample personal medication list (PML) for a patient with depression (Figure 20-1). This is only an example for a person on antidepressants and does not include other classes of medications, which should be listed separately. MTM providers should remember to use plain language when creating the PML.

CORE ELEMENT 3—MEDICATION ACTION PLAN[16]

The following are sample medication action plans (MAPs) for patients with depression (Figure 20-2). These examples are representative only of patients with depression and do not represent other disease states that a patient may have in addition to his/her depression. MAPs for other disease states or other MRPs should be added and listed separately. MAPs should focus on the highest priority needs and instructions so as not to overwhelm the patient. MTM providers should remember to use plain language when creating the MAP.

CORE ELEMENT 4—INTERVENTION AND/OR REFERRAL

Treatment options for depression include nonpharmacologic and pharmacologic therapy. Appropriate treatment is chosen based on symptoms, severity, and other factors such as patient and prescriber preference, comorbid conditions, treatment cost, and concomitant medications. In some instances, pharmacologic and nonpharmacologic treatments are combined. Recommendations for nonpharmacologic therapy are summarized in Table 20-12 and an overview of pharmacotherapy options is provided in Table 20-13, with a treatment algorithm presented in Figure 20-3.

Many antidepressants can also inhibit enzymes that are responsible for the metabolism of other drugs that patients could be taking.[2,4] The following is a list of enzymes inhibited by antidepressants and the degree of inhibition (Table 20-15).

	DATE PREPARED: *<Insert date>*
What we talked about: You reported having some trouble sleeping since starting your medication for depression. You currently take your medicine at bedtime. This trouble sleeping may be caused by your depression medication, as some treatments can cause changes in sleep patterns.	
What I need to do: Here are some things I can do to help lessen this side effect: • Take my depression medication in the morning instead of just before bedtime to help prevent insomnia. • Try to take my medicine at the same time each day. • Practice good sleep habits, such as avoiding daytime naps or caffeine, vigorous exercise, or other stimulating activities in the evening.	**What I did and when I did it:** *(Leave blank for patient's notes)*
What we talked about: You reported that you do not see any difference yet with your depression medication. You do not feel any worse, but still not feeling better. You have been on the current dose of this medication for about 1 week. It is not uncommon for most depression medications to take 2 to 4 weeks or longer to see their full effects. You will likely continue to see improvement in symptoms over the next few weeks.	
What I need to do: Here are some things I can do until my medication starts to work fully: • Continue to take my medicine as prescribed every day. • Try to manage stress and promote wellbeing through regular physical activity, adequate sleep, balanced diet, etc. • Keep my follow-up appointment in 4 weeks so that we can see how the medication is working. • Contact my health care provider if my mood or depression worsens significantly or I have thoughts of harming myself or others.	**What I did and when I did it:** *(Leave blank for patient's notes)*

FIGURE 20-2 Example medication action plan for a patient with depression.

TABLE 20-12 • Nonpharmacologic Treatment Options for Depression

Nonpharmacologic Therapy	Recommendations	Adverse Events
Depression-focused psychotherapy	Not recommended to be used alone to treat severe MDD, with or without psychotic features. May be first-line if the depressive episode is mild to moderate in severity. Combination psychotherapy and pharmacotherapy may be useful initially, especially in patients with coexisting psychiatric or social disorders (psychosocial or interpersonal problems, etc). Psychotherapy may provide further symptom improvement in patients who have partial response to pharmacotherapy.	None
Electroconvulsive therapy (ECT)	Recommended primarily for severe depression or in certain patients with mild to moderate illness. In most cases, ECT candidates: Exhibit a need for rapid treatment response (ie, within 10-14 days). Have a favorable benefit/risk profile (ie, potential benefits outweigh the risk). Have a history of poor response to other depression treatments. Have had a good response to ECT in the past. Prefer ECT over other therapies.	Cognitive dysfunction (mostly transient) Cardiovascular dysfunction Prolonged apnea Treatment-emergent mania Headache Nausea Muscle aches Requires anesthesia
Bright light therapy	Effective in: Patients with seasonal affective disorder (SAD). Combination therapy to treat MDD in patients that present with seasonal exacerbations.	Minor visual discomfort (patients should receive baseline, then periodic eye exams as therapy continues)
Repetitive transcranial magnetic stimulation (rTMS)	Indicated for the treatment of MDD in adult patients who have failed to receive satisfactory improvement from prior antidepressant medication in the current episode. Requires written informed consent. Patient should wear earplugs.	Seizure Vasovagal syncope Scalp discomfort

Abbreviation: MDD = major depressive disorder.

Source: References 1, 2, 4, 17, 18, 19, and 20.

TABLE 20-13 • Medications Used to Treat Depression

Medication Class and Example Drugs	Common/Serious Side Effects[a]	Blackbox Warnings/ Contraindications	Pregnancy Category[b]
SSRIs Citalopram Escitalopram Fluoxetine Fluvoxamine Paroxetine Sertraline **Multi-modal** Vortioxetine	Headaches Nausea Insomnia Ejaculation dysfunction Drowsiness Asthenia Diarrhea Anxiety Anorexia Dizziness Tremor Libido decrease Inhibited orgasm Hyponatremia in elderly	Blackbox Warning: Increased risk of suicidal thoughts and behavior in children and young adults, particularly during the first few months of therapy. Not approved for use in children <6 years of age. Contraindications: MAOI therapy	Paroxetine: D Other SSRIs: C

(Continued)

TABLE 20-13 • Medications Used to Treat Depression (*Continued*)

Medication Class and Example Drugs	Common/Serious Side Effects[a]	Blackbox Warnings/ Contraindications	Pregnancy Category[b]
SNRIs Desvenlafaxine Duloxetine Levomilnacipran Venlafaxine	Nausea Withdrawal Dry mouth Drowsiness Insomnia Increased sweat Dizziness Ejaculation dysfunction Anorexia Constipation Hypertension (venlafaxine)	Blackbox Warning: Increased risk of suicidal thoughts and behavior in children and young adults, particularly during the first few months of therapy. Not approved for use in children. Contraindications: MAOI therapy Duloxetine is contraindicated for use in patients with uncontrolled closed-angle glaucoma.	C
NDRI Bupropion	Nausea Dry mouth Insomnia Dizziness Sore throat Stomach pain Agitation Anxiety Shakiness Seizures	Blackbox Warning: Increased risk of suicidal thoughts and behavior in children and young adults, particularly during the first few months of therapy. Not approved for use in children. Contraindications: Anorexia nervosa Bulimia nervosa Head trauma Intracranial mass MAOI therapy Seizure disorder Seizures Stroke	C
Triazolopyridines Nefazodone Trazodone	Serotonin syndrome Mania QT prolongation Hypotension Unusual bleeding Priapism Hyponatremia Sleepiness Dizziness Constipation Blurry vision	Blackbox Warning: Increased risk of suicidal thoughts and behavior in children and young adults, particularly during the first few months of therapy. Not approved for use in children. Treatment with nefazodone should not be initiated in individuals with active hepatic disease or with elevated baseline serum transaminases. Contraindications: Hepatic disease Hepatitis Jaundice MAOI therapy	C
SSRI and 5-HT$_{1A}$ Vilazodone	Headache Diarrhea Nausea Palpitations Dizziness Insomnia Drowsiness Fatigue	Blackbox Warning: Increased risk of suicidal thoughts and behavior in children and young adults, particularly during the first few months of therapy. Not approved for use in children. Contraindications: MAOI therapy	Not studied in pregnant women.

(*Continued*)

TABLE 20-13 • Medications Used to Treat Depression (*Continued*)

Medication Class and Example Drugs	Common/Serious Side Effects[a]	Blackbox Warnings/ Contraindications	Pregnancy Category[b]
SSRI and 5-HT$_{1A}$ Vilazodone (*Cont.*)	Abnormal dreams Restlessness Paresthesia Delayed ejaculation Migraine Sedation Panic attack		
Tetracyclic antidepressant Mirtazapine	Manic episodes Neutropenia Serotonin syndrome Seizures Hyponatremia Sleepiness Increased appetite Increased weight Increased cholesterol and triglycerides Dry mouth Constipation Dizziness Abnormal dreams	Blackbox Warning: Increased risk of suicidal thoughts and behavior in children and young adults, particularly during the first few months of therapy. Not approved for use in children. Contraindications: None	C
TCAs **Tertiary Amines:** Amitriptyline Clomipramine Doxepin Imipramine Trimipramine **Secondary Amines:** Amoxapine Desipramine Nortriptyline Protriptyline	Dry mouth Dizziness Drowsiness Tremor Headache Constipation Ejaculation dysfunction Fatigue Nausea Orthostatic hypotension	Blackbox Warning: Increased risk of suicidal thoughts and behavior in children and young adults, particularly during the first few months of therapy. Not approved for use in children. Contraindications: Acute myocardial infarction Carbamazepine hypersensitivity TCA hypersensitivity MAOI therapy Closed-angle glaucoma Glaucoma Urinary retention	C
MAOIs[c] Phenelzine Selegiline (transdermal) Tranylcypromine	Dizziness Headache Drowsiness Sleep disturbances (including insomnia and hypersomnia) Fatigue Weakness Tremors Twitching Myoclonic movements Hyperreflexia Constipation Dry mouth Gastrointestinal disturbances	Blackbox Warning: Increased risk of suicidal thoughts and behavior in children and young adults, particularly during the first few months of therapy. Not approved for use in children. Contraindications: Heart failure Hepatic disease Pheochromocytoma Renal disease Renal failure Renal impairment Surgery Cardiac disease	C

(*Continued*)

TABLE 20-13 • Medications Used to Treat Depression (*Continued*)

Medication Class and Example Drugs	Common/Serious Side Effects[a]	Blackbox Warnings/ Contraindications	Pregnancy Category[b]
MAOIs[c] Phenelzine Selegiline (transdermal) Tranylcypromine (*Cont.*)	Elevated serum transaminases Weight gain Orthostatic hypotension Edema Sexual disturbances	Cerebrovascular disease Headache Hypertension	

[a] This is a general list and does not include all side effects that can occur from these drugs. This list is also for a class of medications; the side effects and their degree of effect may vary from drug to drug in each drug class. Consult a drug reference source for a more inclusive list before making any recommendations. MTM providers should also consult a comprehensive drug interaction database before making pharmacotherapy recommendations.

[b] Product labeling for all prescription drugs is being updated to reflect the new FDA Pregnancy Labeling and Lactation Rule. Please check individual product labeling for the most accurate and updated pregnancy information.

[c] MAOIs also require food restriction in order to avoid adverse reactions. See Table 20-14 for a list of foods that should be avoided or consumed in limited amounts by patients currently taking MAOIs. Food interactions can occur for up to 2 weeks after stopping an MAOI.

Abbreviations: MAOIs = monoamine oxidase inhibitors; NDRI = norepinephrine dopamine reuptake inhibitor; SNRIs = serotonin norepinephrine reuptake inhibitors; SSRIs = selective serotonin reuptake inhibitors; TCAs = tricyclic antidepressants.

Source: References 2, 4, 21, 22, 23, and 24.

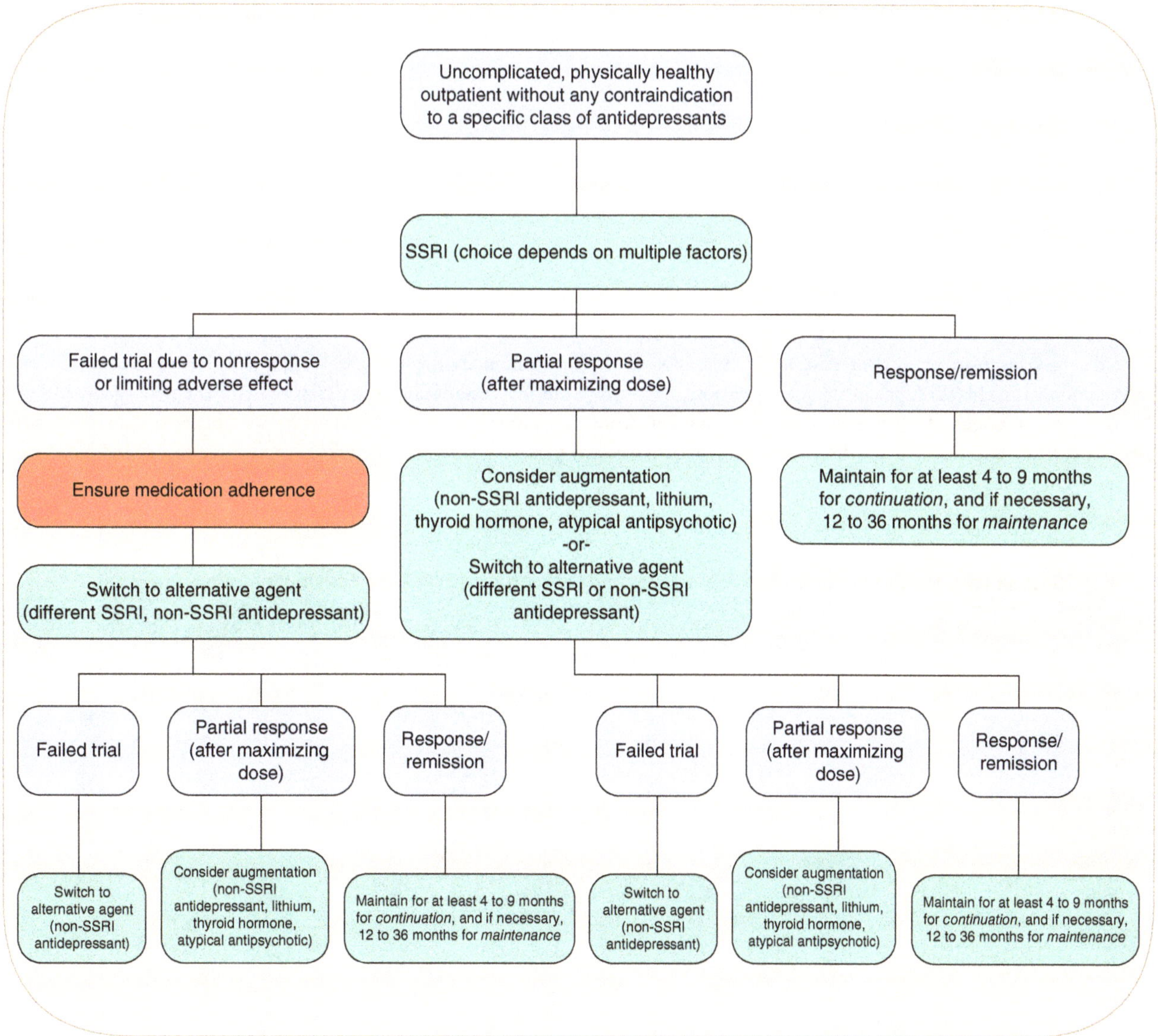

FIGURE 20-3 Algorithm for treatment of uncomplicated major depressive disorder.
(Reproduced, with permission, from DiPiro JT, Talbert RL, Yee GC, Matzke GR, Wells BG, Posey L, eds. *Pharmacotherapy: A Pathophysiologic Approach.* 10th ed. New York, NY: McGraw-Hill; 2017.)

TABLE 20-14 • Dietary and Medication Restrictions for Patients Taking Monoamine Oxidase Inhibitors

FOODS[a]	
Aged cheeses[b]	Monosodium glutamate
Sour cream[c]	Liver (chicken or beef, >2 days old)
Yogurt[c]	Raisins
Cottage cheese[c]	Pods of broad beans (fava beans)
American cheese[c]	Yeast extract and other yeast products
Mild Swiss cheese[c]	Soy sauce
Wine[d] (especially Chianti and sherry)	Chocolate[e]
Beer	Coffee[e]
Herring (pickled, salted, dry)	Ripe avocado
Sardines	Sauerkraut
Canned, aged, or processed meats	Licorice

MEDICATIONS	
Amphetamines	Levodopa
Appetite suppressants	Local anesthetics containing sympathomimetic/vasoconstrictors
Asthma inhalants	Meperidine
Buspirone	Methyldopa
Carbamazepine	Methylphenidate
Cocaine	Other antidepressants[f]
Cyclobenzaprine	Other MAOIs
Decongestants (topical and systemic)	Reserpine
Dextromethorphan	Rizatriptan
Dopamine	Stimulants
Ephedrine	Sumatriptan
Epinephrine	Sympathomimetics
Guanethidine	Tryptophan

[a] According to the FDA-approved prescribing information for the transdermal selegiline patch, patients receiving the 6-mg/24-hour dose are not required to modify their diet. However, patients receiving the 9- or 12-mg/24-hour dose are still required to follow the dietary restrictions similar to the other MAOIs.

[b] Clearly warrants absolute prohibition (eg, English Stilton, blue, Camembert, cheddar).

[c] Up to 2 oz (59 mL) daily is acceptable.

[d] 3 oz (89 mL) white wine or a single cocktail is acceptable.

[e] Up to 2 oz (59 mL) daily is acceptable; larger amounts of decaffeinated coffee are acceptable.

[f] Tricyclic antidepressants may be used with caution by experienced clinicians in treatment-resistant populations.

Source: Reproduced, with permission, from DiPiro JT, Talbert RL, Yee GC, Matzke GR, Wells BG, Posey L, eds. *Pharmacotherapy: A Pathophysiologic Approach*. 10th ed. New York, NY: McGraw-Hill; 2017.

Some herbal and/or dietary supplement products have also been investigated or used for treatment of depression symptoms. Table 20-16 reviews commonly used herbal supplements for depression.

MTM providers should advise care when switching patients from one antidepressant to another.[2] Abrupt discontinuation of antidepressant therapy can result in withdrawal symptoms, most commonly nausea, dizziness, fatigue, anxiety, or worsening depression symptoms. Additionally, there may be a lag time between discontinuation of one antidepressant and onset of efficacy of the new agent. Although the treatment approach should be individualized for each patient, it is generally recommended that a taper is not needed when switching from SSRI to SSRI, or from SSRI to SNRI (and vice versa), since

TABLE 20-15 • Second- and Third-Generation Antidepressants and Cytochrome (CYP) P450 Enzyme Inhibitory Potential

	CYP Enzyme			
Drug	*1A2*	*2C*	*2D6*	*3A4*
Buproprion	0	0	+	0
Citalopram	0	0	+	NA
Duloxetine	0	0	+++	0
Escitalopram	0	0	+	0
Fluoxetine	0	++	++++	++
Fluvoxamine	++++	++	0	+++
Mirtazapine	0	0	0	0
Nefazodone	0	0	0	++++
Paroxetine	0	0	++++	0
Sertraline	0	++	+	+
Desvenlafaxine	0	0	0/+	0

Abbreviations: ++++ = high; +++ = moderate; ++ = low; + = very low; 0 = absent.

Source: References 2, 21, 22, 26, 27, 28, and 29.

TABLE 20-16 • Herbal Supplements for Depression

Supplement	Recommended Dosage	Effectiveness[a]	Cost[b]
5-hydroxytryptophan	150-800 mg daily for 2 to 6 weeks	Possibly effective	$$
Deplin (L-methylfolate)	7.5 to 15 mg daily	Possibly effective	$$$$
DHEA (dehydroepiandrosterone)	30-450 mg daily for up to 6 weeks	Possibly effective	$
Fish oil, Omega-3 fatty acids	2-6.6 g daily for 8 to 10 weeks	Insufficient evidence	$
Folate; Folic Acid	200 mcg to 15 mg daily for up to 6 months	Possibly effective	$
Saffron	30 mg daily for 18 weeks	Possibly effective	$$
SAMe (S-Adenosyl methionine)	Up to 1600 mg daily in 2 divided doses for up to 8 weeks	Likely effective	$$$
St. John's wort	Starting dose of 300 mg TID Maintenance dose of 300-600 mg daily	Likely effective	$

[a] Level of Evidence. Likely effective: This product has a very high level of reliable clinical evidence supporting its use for a specific indication. Products rated "likely effective" are generally considered appropriate to recommend. Possibly effective: This product has some clinical evidence supporting its use for a specific indication; however, the evidence is limited by quantity, quality, or contradictory findings. Products rated "possibly effective" might be beneficial, but do not have enough high-quality evidence to recommend for most people. Insufficient evidence: There is not enough reliable scientific evidence to provide an effectiveness rating.

[b] Cost: $ = $10 or less per month supply in the recommended dosage; $$ = $11-$20 per month; $$$ = $21-$50 per month; and $$$$ = >$50.

Source: References 30 and 31.

both agents inhibit serotonin reuptake. In these cases, patients can stop one agent and begin the new agent the next day. When switching between agents with different mechanisms of action, a cross-taper is generally recommended. In these cases, the first agent is tapered over a few weeks while the dose of the second agent is slowly increased.[32] When discontinuing any antidepressant, it is recommended to taper therapy over a few weeks to avoid withdrawal symptoms. Fluoxetine is an exception to this rule because of its long half-life, which provides a prolonged self-taper with abrupt discontinuation.

CORE ELEMENT 5—DOCUMENTATION AND FOLLOW-UP

Communicating effectively with patients and prescribers is an important element of solving MRPs for patients with depression. Examples of potential MRPs in patients with depression are provided in Table 20-17. Once a medication-related problem is identified, it is important for the MTM provider to succinctly and accurately communicate recommendations to the patient's physician. Figure 20-4 provides examples of provider communications for depression. Recommendations may be communicated via fax, telephone, or other means of written or secure electronic communication. The examples that follow are for illustrative purposes. Actual communications to providers should be individualized based on the type of recommendation, patient specific characteristics, and the nature of the relationship with the provider.

Follow-up to assess antidepressant response and potential adverse effects is essential in patients with depression. Suggested intervals for follow-up are provided in Table 20-18.

TABLE 20-17 • Medication-Related Problems (MRPs) in Patients with Depression

Category of MRP	Sample Medication-Related Problem
Nonadherence	• Suboptimal control of depression because of patient missing doses of antidepressant therapy • Patient not taking antidepressant medication because of cost
Unnecessary medication	• Duplicate therapy (eg, two SSRIs)
Need for additional medication	• Monotherapy for treatment of depression in a patient with treatment-resistant depression that requires combination therapy with multiple agents
Ineffective medication	• Adequate trial of new antidepressant with no clinical response
Dosage too low	• Partial or no response on a low dose of an antidepressant • Patient's antidepressant dosage is not titrated appropriately
Dosage too high	• Patient with increased blood pressure from venlafaxine • Patient experiencing dose-related side effects (eg, nausea, diarrhea) from rapid dose titration of an SSRI
Adverse drug event	• Patient experiencing insomnia from bupropion • Patient experiencing nausea/diarrhea from an SSRI • Patient not taking antidepressant because of sexual dysfunction

Scenario: Patient given desvenlafaxine samples, but cannot afford to fill the Rx once samples are finished. **MRP:** Nonadherence
• Assessment: Patient with uncontrolled depression on desvenlafaxine 50 mg daily. Patient is not taking medication due to cost. Lack of medication is likely contributing to poor control of depression symptoms. Switching to a generic, low-cost antidepressant would provide an equally effective and affordable option for this patient. • Plan: Consider discontinuation of desvenlafaxine and addition of sertraline 50 mg daily with titration to response of depression symptoms.
Scenario: Patient taking amitriptyline for 4 weeks and has experienced dizziness and light-headedness when he stands up, accompanied by a drop in blood pressure, since starting amitriptyline. **MRP:** Adverse drug event
• Assessment: Patient is experiencing orthostatic hypotension, most likely related to amitriptyline therapy. Switching to an alternate agent that also affects serotonin and norepinephrine may help negate this side effect. • Plan: Consider discontinuation of amitriptyline and addition of venlafaxine extended-release at 75 mg daily with dose titration to response of depression symptoms.
Scenario: Patient currently taking sertraline 50 mg for 3 months with only a slight improvement in depressive symptoms. **MRP:** Dosage too low
• Assessment: Patient is partially responsive to sertraline therapy, so a dose increase is warranted. The usual dosage range of sertraline is 50 to 200 mg daily. Increasing dose as tolerated at not less than one-week intervals will increase likelihood of patient response to therapy. • Plan: Consider dose increase for sertraline to 100 mg daily, with reassessment at 4 weeks for further dose adjustment.

FIGURE 20-4 Sample provider communications for depression.

TABLE 20-18 • Suggested Intervals for Follow-Up in Patients with Depression

Follow-up and Monitoring in Patients with Depression
The American Psychiatric Association recommends the following follow-up intervals in patients treated for depression: • 4-8 weeks after initiation of a new antidepressant or dose change during the acute phase of treatment • Monitoring at regular intervals as determined by the prescriber for adverse events, adherence, and functional ability is recommended for patients in the continuation phase of treatment (may last for 4-9 months once patient shows antidepressant response in order to prevent return of depression symptoms) • Monitoring at less frequent intervals as determined by the prescriber to prevent patient from having another episode of depression for patients in the maintenance phase (may last for 12-36 months after the continuation phase) Additional considerations: • Lifelong treatment is recommended for patients who are younger than 40 years of age and have had 2 or more prior episodes of depression, or patients of any age who have had 3 or more prior episodes. • When a patient is discontinuing antidepressant medication, he or she should never abruptly stop the medication in order to avoid withdrawal symptoms. Rather, most antidepressant medications require a downward titration over a period of days to weeks.

Source: Compiled from reference 4.

REFERENCES

1. American Psychiatric Association. *Diagnostic and Statistical Manual of Mental Disorders*. 5th ed. Arlington, VA: American Psychiatric Publishing; 2013.
2. Teter CJ, Kando JC, Wells BG. Major depressive disorder. In: DiPiro JT, Talbert RL, Yee GC, Matzke GR, Wells BG, Posey L, eds. *Pharmacotherapy: A Pathophysiologic Approach*. 10th ed. New York, NY: McGraw-Hill; 2017. Available at http://accesspharmacy.mhmedical.com/content.aspx?bookid=1861&sectionid=146064868. Accessed May 08, 2017.
3. Jacobs D, Brewer M. APA practice guideline provides recommendations for assessing and treating patients with suicidal behaviors. *Psychiatric Annals*. 2004;34(5):373-380.
4. Gelenberg, AJ, Freeman, MP, Markowitz, JC, et al. Practice guidelines for the treatment of patients with major depressive disorder. 3rd ed. *Am J Psychiatry*. 2010;167(10):1-3,9-11,13-118.
5. American Psychiatric Association. *Practice Guideline for the Treatment of Patients with Major Depressive Disorder*. 3rd ed. Arlington, VA: American Psychiatric Association; 2010.
6. Patten SB, Barbui C. Drug-induced depression: a systematic review to inform clinical practice. *Psychother Psychosom*. 2004;73(4):207-215.
7. Botts S, Ryan M. Depression. In: *Drug-Induced Diseases: Prevention, Detection, and Management*. 2nd ed. Bethesda, MD: American Society of Health-System Pharmacists; 2010.
8. Sofuoglu M, Dudish-Poulsen S, Poling J, et al. The effect of individual cocaine withdrawal symptoms on outcomes in cocaine users. *Addict Behav*. 2005;30(6):1125-1134.
9. Leucht S, Kane JM, Kissling W, Hamann J, Etschel E, Engel R. Clinical implications of Brief Psychiatric Rating Scale scores. *Br J Psych*. 2005;187:366-371.
10. Fankhauser MP, German ML. Understanding the use of behavioral rating scales in studies evaluating the efficacy of antianxiety and antidepressant drugs. *Am J Hosp Pharm*. 1987;44:2087-2100.

11. Montgomery SA, Asberg M. A new depression scale designed to be sensitive to change. *Br J Psychiatry.* 1979;134:382-389.

12. Mann JJ. The medical management of depression. *N Engl J Med.* 2005;353(17):1819-1834.

13. Suicide Prevention Resource Center. Suicide risk: a guide for ED evaluation and triage. Suicide Prevention Resource Center website. Available at http://www.sprc.org/. Accessed May 22, 2017.

14. Jacobs DG, Baldessarini RJ, Fawcett JA, et al. Practice guidelines for the assessment and treatment of patients with suicidal behaviors. *Am J Psychiatry.* 2003;160(11 suppl):1-60.

15. Fawcett JA, Baldessarini RJ, Coryell WH. Defining and managing suicidal risk in patients taking psychotropic medications. *J Clin Psychiatry.* 2009;70(6):782-789.

16. CMS. Medicare Part D Medication Therapy Management Program standardized format. CMS website. Available at https://www.cms.gov/Medicare/Prescription-Drug-Coverage/PrescriptionDrugCovContra/Downloads/MTM-Program-Standardized-Format-English-and-Spanish-Instructions-Samples-v032712.pdf. Accessed May 22, 2017.

17. Marangell LB. Switching antidepressants for treatment-resistant major depression. *J Clin Psychiatry.* 2001;62(suppl 18):12-17.

18. George MS, Taylor JJ, Short EB. The expanding evidence base for rTMS treatment of depression. *Curr Opin Psychiatry.* 2013;26(1):13-18.

19. Perera T, George MS, Grammer G, Janicak PG, Pascual-Leone A, Wirecki TS. The Clinical TMS Society consensus review and treatment recommendations for TMS therapy for major depressive disorder. *Brain Stimul.* 2016;9(3):336-346.

20. Klapheke MM. Electroconvulsive therapy consultation: an update. *Convuls Ther.* 1997;13:227-241.

21. Medscape Reference. WebMD, LLC (Copyright 1994-2016). Available at reference.medscape.com. Accessed May 22, 2017.

22. Lexicomp Online. Lexi-Comp, Inc (Copyright 1978-2016). Available at http://online.lexi.com. Accessed May 22, 2017.

23. Clinical Pharmacology [database online]. Tampa, FL: Gold Standard, Inc; 2017. Available at http://clinicalpharmacology.com. Accessed June 1, 2017.

24. Lexi-comp online™ interaction analysis. Lexi-Comp Online, Lexi-Comp, Inc. http://online.lexi.com. Accessed June 1, 2017.

25. Anonymous. Drug interactions. Thomson MICROMEDEX Healthcare Series. Available at https://www.thomsonhc.com. Accessed June 1, 2017.

26. Hemeryck A, Belpaire FM. Selective serotonin reuptake inhibitors and cytochrome P-450 mediated drug-drug interactions: an update. *Curr Drug Metab.* 2002;3(1):13-37.

27. Kent JM. SNaRIs, NaSSAs, and NaRIs: new agents for the treatment of depression. *Lancet.* 2000;355(9207):911-918.

28. DeVane CL. Differential pharmacology of newer antidepressants. *J Clin Psychiatry.* 1998;59(suppl 20):S85-S93.

29. Preskorn SH. Clinically relevant pharmacology of selective serotonin reuptake inhibitors. An overview with emphasis on pharmacokinetics and effects on oxidative drug metabolism. *Clin Pharmacokinet.* 1997;32(suppl 1):S1-S21.

30. Natural Medicines [database online]. Somerville, MA: Therapeutic Research Center; 2017. Available at https://naturalmedicines.therapeuticresearch.com/. Accessed May 22, 2017.

31. Deplin. Available at http://www.deplin.com/. Accessed May 22, 2017.

32. Marangell LB. Switching antidepressants for treatment-resistant major depression. *J Clin Psychiatry.* 2001;62(suppl 18):12-17.

Review Questions

1. Which statement is correct regarding the symptoms included in the diagnostic criteria for major depressive episode?
   a. At least one symptom must be insomnia.
   b. Symptoms should be present for at least 6 months.
   c. Symptoms may include fatigue or loss of energy.
   d. Symptoms may be directly caused by a drug of abuse.

2. All of the following questions are appropriate when assessing the patient with depression **EXCEPT**:
   a. "Have you recently experienced changes in your sleep patterns?"
   b. "How often do you miss a dose of your blood pressure medication?"
   c. "How long have you had depression?"
   d. "Have you ever felt so depressed that you have had thoughts of harming yourself?"

3. What is the treatment goal for a patient in the "maintenance" phase of depression therapy?
   a. Reduce symptoms
   b. Induce remission
   c. Prevent relapse
   d. Prevent another depressive episode

4. Which statement is the most appropriate explanation of the term "neurotransmitter" using living room language?
   a. Neurotransmitters are chemicals that help different areas of your brain communicate with each other to carry out a function.
   b. Serotonin, norepinephrine, and dopamine are examples of neurotransmitters.
   c. Neurotransmitters are neurochemicals that transfer nerve impulses across a synapse.
   d. Neurotransmitters are chemicals that allow the transition of signals from one neuron to the next via a synapse.

Please use the following case to answer the next two questions.

A 48-year-old patient has been taking escitalopram for 4 weeks for a recent diagnosis of a major depressive episode. She reports that she has felt very drowsy since starting her medication. Her mood has improved, and she feels like she is responding, but she is very bothered by the constant fatigue. She is currently taking 10 mg daily at breakfast.

5. Which statement is correct regarding the medication action plan for this patient?
   a. The medication action plan should include a comprehensive list of all of her medications, including start and stop dates.
   b. The medication action plan should be written in healthcare professional language.
   c. The medication action plan should include a list and incidence of all side effects of escitalopram.
   d. The medication action plan should include a summary of what was discussed during the visit today.

6. Which statement is true regarding the categorization of this patient's medication-related problem?
   a. The patient is experiencing an adverse drug event from escitalopram.
   b. The patient's escitalopram dosage is too low.
   c. Escitalopram is an unnecessary medication for the patient.
   d. The patient is nonadherent to her escitalopram therapy.

7. A patient presents to the pharmacy for a follow-up medication therapy management visit for depression therapy. The patient appears tearful and very upset and states, "I just don't feel like I can handle it anymore." Which question would be most helpful in assessing the patient's suicide risk today?
   a. "What medication are you taking for depression?"
   b. "How is your depression medicine working for you?"
   c. "Have you ever had thoughts of hurting yourself or ending your life?"
   d. "What other medications have you taken in the past for your depression?"

8. Which antidepressant does not require an extended taper upon discontinuation because of its long half-life?
   a. Paroxetine
   b. Fluoxetine
   c. Venlafaxine
   d. Bupropion

9. A 32-year-old patient is being started on treatment for a first episode of major depression. The patient's past medical history is significant for epilepsy. All of the following antidepressants would be an appropriate choice for this patient **EXCEPT**:
   a. Desvenlafaxine
   b. Citalopram
   c. Sertraline
   d. Bupropion

10. A patient has been on sertraline 50 mg daily for 6 months for a first episode of major depression. He states today that he no longer has any symptoms of depression and his medication is working well. According to the patient's response to depression therapy, how would his status be categorized today?
    a. Nonresponse
    b. Partial response
    c. Partial remission
    d. Remission

ANSWERS

1. c	2. b	3. d
4. a	5. d	6. a
7. c	8. b	9. d
10. d		

21

Diabetes Mellitus MTM Data Set

Karen Whalen, PharmD, BCPS, CDE, and Karen R. Sando, PharmD, BCACP, BC-ADM

KEY POINTS

- Intensive glycemic control can reduce microvascular complications of diabetes.
- The hemoglobin A1c goal for most patients is <7%; however, goals for glycemic control should be individualized based on presence of concurrent illness or complications, risk of hypoglycemia, and life expectancy.
- To reduce macrovascular complications, management of cardiac risk factors such as hypertension and hyperlipidemia is necessary; reductions in glycemic control alone are unlikely to prevent significant cardiovascular morbidity and mortality.
- Medication therapy management (MTM) providers should work with the patient and members of the healthcare team to tailor medication regimens that achieve therapeutic goals, promote adherence, reduce the risk of complications, and maximize quality of life for patients with diabetes.

INTRODUCTION TO DIABETES

Diabetes mellitus (DM) is a group of disorders characterized by hyperglycemia because of insulin resistance, reduced insulin secretion, or both. Diabetes may result in chronic complications including microvascular, macrovascular, and neuropathic disorders.[1] Diabetes currently affects 29.1 million people in the United States, which represents approximately 9.3% of the population.[2] Prediabetes, defined as impaired fasting glucose or impaired glucose tolerance, affects about 37% of adults over the age of 20, or approximately 86 million people.[2] Diabetes also causes a large economic burden in the United States. Total costs are estimated at $245 billion, which includes $176 billion in direct medical costs and $69 billion in indirect medical costs because of reduced productivity.[3]

The most common forms of diabetes include type 1, type 2, and gestational diabetes. Type 2 diabetes mellitus (T2DM) is the most prevalent, accounting for 95% of cases of diabetes diagnosed in adults. Type 1 diabetes mellitus (T1DM) occurs in approximately 5% of those diagnosed with diabetes. It appears most often in children and young adults, although it may occur at any time. Table 21-1 provides an overview of the characteristics of T1DM and T2DM. Gestational diabetes mellitus (GDM) occurs in 2% to 10% of women during pregnancy, and most women will return to normoglycemia following pregnancy. However, women who have GDM during pregnancy have an increased likelihood of developing T2DM in the future.[4] Less common causes of diabetes include infections, genetic defects, pancreatic destruction, endocrinopathies, and certain medications (Table 21-2).

The diagnosis of diabetes is based on several glycemic cutpoints and recommendations from groups such as the American Diabetes Association.[5] Criteria for the diagnosis of diabetes are listed in Table 21-3.

Other Terms Associated with Diabetes

- **Adult onset diabetes** - an older term used to describe T2DM. Because T2DM can also occur in young adults and children, this term is no longer used to describe the disease.
- **Impaired fasting glucose (IFG)** - defined as a fasting plasma glucose of 100 to 125 mg/dL. Individuals with IFG can be diagnosed with prediabetes and are at increased risk for the development of T2DM.
- **Impaired glucose tolerance (IGT)** - defined as a plasma glucose of 140 to 199 mg/dL following a 2-hour oral glucose tolerance test (OGTT). Individuals with IGT can be diagnosed with prediabetes and are at increased risk for the development of T2DM.

TABLE 21-1 • Classical Clinical Presentation of Diabetes Mellitus[a]

Characteristic	Type 1 DM	Type 2 DM
Age	<30 years[b]	>30 years[b]
Onset	Abrupt	Gradual
Body habitus	Lean	Obese or history of obesity
Insulin resistance	Absent	Present
Autoantibodies	Often present	Rarely present
Symptoms	Symptomatic[c]	Often asymptomatic
Ketones at diagnosis	Present	Absent[d]
Need for insulin therapy	Immediate	Years after diagnosis
Acute complications	Diabetic ketoacidosis	Hyperosmolar hyperglycemic state
Microvascular complications at diagnosis	No	Common
Macrovascular complications at or before diagnosis	Rare	Common

[a] Clinical presentation can vary widely.

[b] Age of onset for type 1 DM is generally <20 years of age but can present at any age. The prevalence of type 2 DM in children, adolescents, and young adults is increasing. This is especially true in ethnic and minority children.

[c] Type 1 may present acutely with symptoms of polyuria, nocturia, polydipsia, polyphagia, and weight loss.

[d] Type 2 children and adolescents are more likely to present with ketones but after the acute phase may be treated with oral agents. Prolonged fasting can also produce ketones in individuals.

Source: Reproduced, with permission, from DiPiro JT, Talbert RL, Yee GC, Matzke GR, Wells BG, Posey L, eds. *Pharmacotherapy: A Pathophysiologic Approach*. 10th ed. New York, NY: McGraw-Hill; 2017.

TABLE 21-2 • Drug or Chemical-Induced Causes of Diabetes

Pyriminil
Pentamidine
Nicotinic acid
Glucocorticoids
Thyroid hormone
Diazoxide
β-Adrenergic agonists
Thiazides
Phenytoin
α-Interferon
Others

Note: Loop diuretics and protease inhibitors are other drug classes that may cause glucose intolerance or hyperglycemia.[6] Statins have also been linked to increased incidence of new onset diabetes.[8,9]

TABLE 21-3 • Criteria for the Diagnosis of Diabetes Mellitus[a]

1. HbA1c ≥6.5% (≥0.065; ≥48 mmol/mol Hb). The test should be performed in a laboratory using a method that is National Glycohemoglobin Standardization Program (NGSP) certified and standardized to the DCCT assay.[a]
2. Fasting plasma glucose ≥126 mg/dL (≥7.0 mmol/L). Fasting is defined as no caloric intake for at least 8 hours.[a]
3. Two-hour plasma glucose ≥200 mg/dL (≥11.1 mmol/L) during an OGTT. The test should be performed as described by the World Health Organization, using a glucose load containing the equivalent of 75 g anhydrous glucose dissolved in water.[a]
4. In a patient with classic symptoms of hyperglycemia or hyperglycemic crisis, a random plasma glucose concentration ≥200 mg/dL (≥11.1 mmol/L).

[a] In the absence of unequivocal hyperglycemia, criteria 1-3 should be confirmed by repeat testing.

Source: Reproduced, with permission, from DiPiro JT, Talbert RL, Yee GC, Matzke GR, Wells BG, Posey L, eds. *Pharmacotherapy: A Pathophysiologic Approach*. 10th ed. New York, NY: McGraw-Hill; 2017.

- **Juvenile diabetes** - an older term used to describe T1DM. Because T1DM can also occur in adults, this term is no longer used to describe the disease.
- **Latent autoimmune diabetes in adults (LADA)** - a disorder in which β-cell failure is slowed despite the presence of islet antibodies at time of diagnosis. LADA patients are therefore not insulin requiring, at least during the first 6 months after diagnosis of diabetes. This type of diabetes occurs in about 10% of individuals with phenotypic type 2 diabetes aged 40 to 75.
- **Maturity onset diabetes of youth (MODY)** - an inherited disorder characterized by impaired insulin secretion in response to a glucose stimulus. There is little or no insulin resistance in MODY. Six specific genetic defects are associated with MODY, which leads to mild hyperglycemia at an early age. Diagnosis is often delayed because of the mild presentation, but can vary based on patient severity.
- **Prediabetes** - presence of IFG, IGT, or hemoglobin A1c of 5.7% to 6.4%, making an individual high risk for the future development of diabetes. Prediabetes is commonly associated with obesity, hypertension, and dyslipidemia (high triglycerides and/or low HDL). Patients with prediabetes should be encouraged to increase physical activity to 150 minutes per week and achieve weight loss of at least 7%, as these interventions have been shown to reduce the risk of progression to T2DM.[7] In certain patients with prediabetes (eg, those with a BMI over 35 kg/m^2, age <60 years, or women with a history of GDM) metformin therapy may be considered for prevention of T2DM.

Complications of Diabetes

Diabetes can lead to both acute and chronic complications (Table 21-4). Poorly controlled diabetes increases the risk of development of chronic microvascular and macrovascular complications. Diabetes is the leading cause of end-stage renal disease, blindness, and nontraumatic lower limb amputations.[2] Additionally, patients with diabetes have a 2- to 4-fold increased risk of heart attack or stroke, and cardiovascular disease is the major cause of death in individuals with diabetes. The risk of death for a person with diabetes

TABLE 21-4 • Acute and Chronic Complications of Diabetes

Acute Complications	Chronic Complications
Hypoglycemia Diabetic ketoacidosis (DKA) Hyperosmolar hyperglycemic nonketotic syndrome (HHNS)	• Microvascular complications Retinopathy Neuropathy Nephropathy Albuminuria • Macrovascular complications Myocardial infarction Stroke or transient ischemic attack (TIA) Peripheral vascular disease Coronary artery disease

Sources: References 1 and 10.

TABLE 21-5 • Glycemic Goals of Therapy by Organization

Biochemical Index	ADA	ACE and AACE
Hemoglobin A1c	<7% (<0.07; <53 mmol/mol Hb)[a]	≤6.5% (≤0.065; ≤48 mmol/mol Hb)
Preprandial plasma glucose	80-130 mg/dL (4.4-7.2 mmol/L)	<110 mg/dL (<6.1 mmol/L)
Postprandial plasma glucose	<180 mg/dL[b] (<10 mmol/L)	<140 mg/dL (<7.8 mmol/L)

[a] Assay should be National Glycohemoglobin Standardization Program (NGSP) certified and DCCT standardized. More stringent glycemic control may be appropriate if accomplished without significant hypoglycemia or adverse effects. Less stringent HbA1c goals may be appropriate in patients with a history of severe hypoglycemia, limited life expectancy, advanced micro/macrovascular complications or comorbidities, at-risk elderly, dementia, or younger children.

[b] Postprandial glucose measurements should be made 1 to 2 hours after the beginning of the meal, generally the time of peak levels in patients with diabetes.

Abbreviations: AACE = American Association of Clinical Endocrinologists; ACE = American College of Endocrinology; ADA = American Diabetes Association; DCCT = Diabetes Control and Complications Trial.

Source: References 11 and 12.

is twice that of a person the same age without diabetes. Hyperglycemia also contributes to poor wound healing, impaired white blood cell function, and the appearance of classic symptoms of diabetes (eg, polyuria, polydipsia, polyphagia, and fatigue).[1] Intensive glycemic control has been shown to reduce the risk for development of microvascular complications of diabetes. Control of cardiovascular risk factors, such as dyslipidemia, hypertension, smoking cessation, and use of antiplatelet therapy is required to reduce the incidence of macrovascular disease.[1,10]

THERAPEUTIC GOALS FOR MANAGEMENT OF DIABETES

The goals of diabetes management are to reduce the risk of complications, improve symptoms, reduce mortality, and improve quality of life.[1] Appropriate care for the individual with diabetes requires goal setting for glycemia, management of common comorbidities (eg, hypertension and hyperlipidemia), regular monitoring for complications, lifestyle modifications, medications, and appropriate self-monitoring of blood glucose (SMBG).[1] Glycemic goals provided by the American Diabetes Association and the American Association of Clinical Endocrinologists are listed in Table 21-5.[1,11,12] Several large randomized controlled trials have demonstrated that tight glycemic control reduces the development of microvascular complications in T1DM and T2DM.[13-17] Intensive glycemic control alone is unlikely to reduce macrovascular complications. Management of traditional cardiovascular risk factors (eg, hypertension, hyperlipidemia, smoking cessation, use of antiplatelet therapy) is recommended to reduce cardiovascular morbidity and mortality.[10] Therapeutic failure should be considered when an individual does not meet glycemic goals after 3 months of therapy at adequate doses.[12,18]

CORE ELEMENT 1—COMPREHENSIVE MEDICATION REVIEW FOR PATIENTS WITH DIABETES

Following is a list of suggested questions to use when conducting a medication therapy review in a patient with diabetes (Table 21-6). The number and types of questions will depend upon several factors, including the amount of time for the interview, number of concurrent medication-related problems (MRPs), urgency of MRPs, and the reliability of the patient in providing accurate information, among others. In time-limited interactions or in complex cases with multiple medical issues, the MTM provider may choose to target questions that help identify or rule out issues of an urgent nature (see questions to ask for prevention/assessment of medical emergencies). MTM providers should remember to use living room language during the interview (Figure 21-1) and be prepared for questions that patients may ask regarding diabetes (Table 21-7).

CORE ELEMENT 2—PERSONAL MEDICATION LIST[19]

The following is a sample personal medication list (PML) for a patient with diabetes (Figure 21-2). This example is representative only of medications for diabetes or prevention of complications of diabetes. Additional medications for other disease states should be added and listed separately. MTM providers should remember to use plain language when creating the PML.

CORE ELEMENT 3—MEDICATION ACTION PLAN[19]

The following is a sample medication action plan (MAPs) for a patient with diabetes (Figure 21-3). This example representative only of action steps for a patient with diabetes. MAPs for other disease states or other MRPs should be added and listed separately. In general, only a few of the most important action steps should be listed, so as not to overwhelm the patient. Other areas for patient self-management can be addressed at later visits. MTM providers should remember to use plain language when creating the MAP.

TABLE 21-6 • Questions to Ask When Conducting a Medication Review in a Patient with Diabetes

Suggested Questions for the Patient with Diabetes

• How long have you had diabetes? When were you diagnosed?
• Who else in your family has diabetes?
• What do you know about the risks of uncontrolled diabetes?
• Do you monitor your blood sugar at home?
  • What meter do you use to check your blood sugar? How often do you check your blood sugar?
  • What is a "typical" blood sugar for you?
  • According to your physician, what should your blood sugar be (or what is a "good" blood sugar)?
  • Do you record your numbers in a diary or log book? If so, request to see.
  • If your blood sugar is high when you check it at home, what do you do? Has your physician given you any instructions to follow if your blood sugar is high?
  • If your blood sugar is low when you check at home, what do you do? Has your physician given you any instructions on how to manage a low blood sugar?
• Have you ever experienced the following signs/symptoms of low blood sugar (hypoglycemia):
  • Blurry vision
  • Confusion
  • Dizziness or light-headedness
  • Fatigue (feeling tired)
  • Weakness
  • Feeling nervous
  • Racing heartbeat
  • Sweating
  • Shaking
  • Irritability (feeling "on edge")
• Have you ever experienced the following signs/symptoms of high blood sugar (hyperglycemia):
  • Urinating frequently
  • Feeling very thirsty
  • Increase in appetite or hunger
  • Abdominal pain or nausea (feeling sick to your stomach)
  • Fatigue (feeling tired)
• What medications do you take for your diabetes? How do you take them?
• How often do you miss a dose of your diabetes medication?
• What other medications have you taken in the past for your diabetes?
• Have you ever stopped taking any of your prescribed diabetes medications without telling your physician? If so, why?
• What over-the-counter medications or herbals do you use for your diabetes?
• Other than medicines what have you tried for your diabetes (eg, lifestyle changes)?
• Has your physician recommended adjusting your carbohydrate intake? If so, what have you done?
• What exercise regimen do you follow?
• What has your physician discussed with you regarding over-the-counter medications that you should avoid because they can worsen your blood sugar control?

Questions to Ask for Prevention/Assessment of Medical Emergencies
Crisis planning: Has your physician discussed with you how to manage diabetes when you are sick?
Have you ever passed out from low blood sugar? Or received help from another person to treat a low blood sugar?
Have you ever experienced frequent urination, extreme thirst, nausea, or abdominal pain?
Have you ever tested positive for ketones? (urine test to measure for ketone bodies)
Have you ever been hospitalized for your diabetes?

A1c—also known as "hemoglobin A1c"; this is a blood test used to measure how well your diabetes has been controlled over the past 3 months.

ACE inhibitor—a medicine used to help lower blood pressure; may also help prevent changes or damage to the heart and kidney.

Acute—describes something that happens suddenly and for a short time. Opposite of chronic.

Albuminuria—a condition in which the urine has more than normal amounts of a protein called albumin. Albuminuria may be a sign of nephropathy (kidney disease).

Alpha cell—a type of cell in the pancreas. Alpha cells make and release a hormone called glucagon. The body sends a signal to the alpha cells to make glucagon when blood sugar falls too low. Then glucagon tells the liver to release sugar into the blood for energy.

Alpha-glucosidase inhibitor—a class of oral medicine for T2DM that blocks enzymes that digest starches in food.

Amylin—a hormone formed by beta cells in the pancreas. Amylin regulates the timing of glucose release into the bloodstream after eating by slowing emptying of the stomach.

Antibodies—proteins made by the body to protect itself from "foreign" substances such as bacteria or viruses. People get T1DM when their bodies make antibodies that destroy the body's own insulin-making beta cells.

ARB—an oral medicine that lowers blood pressure; ARB stands for angiotensin receptor blocker; may also help prevent changes or damage to the heart and kidney.

Aspartame—a dietary sweetener with almost no calories and no nutritional value (Brand names: Equal, NutraSweet).

Autoimmune disease—disorder of the body's immune system in which the immune system mistakenly attacks and destroys body tissue it believes to be foreign.

Autonomic neuropathy—a type of nerve damage affecting the lungs, heart, stomach, intestines, bladder or genitals.

Basal insulin—a long-acting type of insulin that may be delivered once or twice a day to help control blood sugar throughout the day and night (eg, insulin glargine, insulin detemir, insulin degludec, NPH insulin).

Beta cell—a cell that makes insulin. Beta cells are located in the pancreas.

Biguanides—a class of medication used to treat T2DM that lowers blood sugar by reducing the amount of sugar made by the liver and by helping the body respond better to insulin (generic name: metformin).

Blood glucose—the main sugar found in the blood and the body's main source of energy. Also called blood sugar.

Blood glucose level—the amount of sugar in a given amount of blood. It is noted in milligrams in a deciliter, or mg/dL.

BMI—body mass index; a measure of weight in relation to height that assigns people to a weight class of underweight, normal weight, overweight, or obese based on their amount of excess weight.

Bolus insulin—a fast-acting type of insulin that is typically given before a meal or to correct high blood sugar (eg, insulin lispro, insulin aspart, insulin glulisine).

C-peptide—"Connecting peptide." A substance the pancreas releases into the blood stream in equal amounts to insulin. A test of C-peptide levels shows how much insulin the body is making.

Calorie—a unit representing the energy provided by food. Carbohydrate, protein, fat, and alcohol provide calories in the diet. Carbohydrate and protein have 4 calories per gram, fat has 9 calories per gram, and alcohol has 7 calories per gram.

Carbohydrates—one of the main types of nutrients; can be simple or complex. Simple carbohydrates include sugars found naturally in foods such as fruits, vegetables, milk, and milk products. They also include sugars added during food processing and refining. Complex carbohydrates include whole grain breads and cereals, starchy vegetables and legumes.

Cardiovascular disease—a disease of the heart and blood vessels (arteries, veins, and capillaries).

Cerebrovascular disease—damage to blood vessels in the brain. Vessels can burst and bleed or become clogged with fatty deposits. When blood flow is interrupted, brain cells die or are damaged, resulting in a stroke.

Certified diabetes educator (CDE)—a health care professional with expertise in diabetes education who has met eligibility requirements and successfully completed a certification exam.

Cholesterol—a type of fat produced by the liver and found in the blood; it is also found in some foods. Cholesterol is used by the body to make hormones and build cell walls.

Chronic—describes something that is long-lasting; Opposite of acute.

Chronic kidney disease—When the kidneys are not able to work well, which may cause high blood pressure and other serious health problems.

Complications—harmful effects of diabetes such as damage to the eyes, heart, blood vessels, nervous system, teeth and gums, feet and skin or kidneys.

Dawn phenomenon—the early-morning (4 am to 8 am) rise in blood sugar.

Diabetic ketoacidosis (DKA)—an emergency condition in which extremely high blood sugar levels, along with a severe lack of insulin, result in the breakdown of body fat for energy and build-up of ketones in the blood and urine.

Diabetes mellitus—a condition characterized by high blood sugar resulting from the body's inability to use blood sugar for energy. In T1DM, the pancreas no longer makes insulin and, therefore, blood sugar cannot enter the cells to be used for energy. In T2DM, either the pancreas does not make enough insulin or the body is unable to use insulin correctly.

Diabetic retinopathy—diabetic eye disease; damage to the small blood vessels in the retina. Loss of vision may occur.

Dilated eye exam—a test done by an eye care specialist in which the pupil (the black center) of the eye is temporarily enlarged with eye drops to allow the specialist to see the inside of the eye more easily.

DPP-4 inhibitor—a class of oral medication to treat diabetes; examples include sitagliptin and saxagliptin.

Endocrinologist—a physician who treats people who have endocrine gland problems such as diabetes.

Exchange lists—one of several approaches for diabetes meal planning. Foods are categorized into three groups based on their nutritional content. Lists provide the serving sizes for carbohydrates, meat and meat alternatives, and fats.

Fasting blood glucose test—a check of a person's blood sugar level after the person has not eaten for 8 to 12 hours. This test is used to diagnose prediabetes and diabetes. It is also used to monitor people with diabetes.

Fructose—sugar that occurs naturally in fruits and honey.

Gastroparesis—a form of neuropathy that affects the stomach. Digestion of food can be incomplete or delayed, resulting in nausea, vomiting, or bloating, making blood sugar control difficult.

GLP-1 agonists—a class of medication to treat diabetes; examples include exenatide and liraglutide. These medicines must be injected.

Glucagon—a hormone produced by the alpha cells in the pancreas. It raises blood sugar. An injectable form of glucagon, available by prescription, may be used to treat severe low blood sugar.

Glycemic index—a ranking of carbohydrate-containing foods, based on the food's effect on blood sugar compared with a standard reference food.

FIGURE 21-1 Living room language for diabetes.

Hyperglycemia—high blood sugar, usually defined as a blood sugar greater than 200 mg/dL.

Hyperosmolar hyperglycemic nonketotic state (HHNS)—an emergency condition in which one's blood glucose level is very high and ketones are not present in the blood or urine. If untreated, can lead to coma or death.

Hypoglycemia—low blood sugar, usually defined as a blood sugar less than 70 mg/dL.

Hypoglycemia unawareness—a state in which a person does not feel or recognize the symptoms of low blood sugar.

Injection site rotation—changing the places on the body where insulin is injected.

Insulin—a hormone produced by cells in the pancreas that regulates blood sugar in the body. Insulin is like a "key" that unlocks our cells to allow sugar inside to give our body energy.

Insulin pen—a device for injecting insulin that looks like a fountain pen and holds insulin.

Insulin pump—an insulin-delivering device about the size of a deck of cards that can be worn on a belt or kept in a pocket. An insulin pump connects to a narrow, flexible plastic tubing that ends with a needle inserted just under the skin.

Insulin resistance—the body's inability to respond to and use the insulin it produces. Insulin resistance may be linked to obesity, high blood pressure, and high levels of fat in the blood.

Islets—group of cells located in the pancreas that make hormones that help the body break down and use food. Also called islets of Langerhans.

Ketones—a chemical produced when there is a shortage of insulin in the blood and the body breaks down body fat for energy. High levels of ketones can lead to diabetic ketoacidosis and coma. Sometimes referred to as ketone bodies.

Lipoatrophy—loss of fat under the skin resulting in small dents. Lipoatrophy may be caused by repeated injections of insulin in the same spot.

Lipohypertrophy—buildup of fat below the surface of the skin, causing lumps. Lipohypertrophy may be caused by repeated injections of insulin in the same spot.

Macrovascular disease—disease of the large blood vessels, such as those found in the heart. Lipids and blood clots build up in the large blood vessels and cause clogged arteries, heart disease, stroke, and peripheral vascular disease.

Meglitinide—a class of oral medicine for T2DM that lowers blood sugar by helping the pancreas make more insulin right after meals (generic name: repaglinide, nateglinide).

Microalbuminuria—the presence of small amounts of albumin, a protein, in the urine. Microalbuminuria is an early sign of kidney damage, or nephropathy, a common and serious complication of diabetes.

Microvascular disease—disease of the smallest blood vessels, such as those found in the eyes, nerves, and kidneys. The walls of the vessels become abnormally thick but weak. Then they bleed, leak protein, and slow the flow of blood to the cells.

Monofilament—a short piece of nylon, like a hairbrush bristle, mounted on a wand. To check the sensitivity of the nerves in the foot, the physician touches the filament to the bottom of the foot.

Nephropathy—disease of the kidneys. Uncontrolled high blood pressure and blood sugar can lead to damage of the kidneys and protein leaks out into the urine. Damaged kidneys can no longer remove waste and extra fluids from the bloodstream.

Obesity—a condition in which a greater than normal amount of fat is in the body; more severe than overweight; having a BMI of 30 or more.

Oral glucose tolerance test (OGTT)—a test to diagnose prediabetes and diabetes. The OGTT is given by a healthcare professional after an overnight fast. A blood sample is taken, then the patient drinks a high-sugar beverage. Blood samples are taken at intervals for 2 to 3 hours.

Overweight—having a body mass index (BMI) over 25, which increases your risk of having high blood pressure, diabetes, and cardiovascular disease.

Pancreas—the organ in the body that produces insulin, a key hormone that controls blood sugar. The pancreas is located behind the lower part of the stomach and is about the size of a hand.

Peripheral neuropathy—damaged nerves, which may be caused by high blood sugar and could lead to tingling or burning sensations in the hands or feet; could also lead to a reduced sensation to touch or pressure in the extremities.

Polydipsia—feeling very thirsty; a symptom of high blood sugar.

Polyphagia—extreme hunger; a symptom of high blood sugar.

Polyuria—frequent urination; a symptom of high blood sugar.

Postprandial blood glucose—the blood glucose level taken 1 to 2 hours after eating.

Preprandial blood glucose—the blood glucose level taken before eating.

Proteinuria—the presence of protein in the urine, indicating the kidneys are not working properly.

Retinopathy—damaged blood vessels in the eyes, which may be caused by high blood pressure and high blood sugar and could lead to loss of eyesight.

Risk factor—anything that raises the chances of a person developing a disease.

Self-monitoring blood glucose (SMBG)—checking your own blood sugar.

SGLT2 inhibitors—a class of oral medicine for T2DM that helps to reduce blood sugar by increasing sugar loss through the kidneys. (Generic names: canagliflozin, dapagliflozin, empagliflozin)

Sliding scale—a set of instructions for adjusting insulin on the basis of blood sugar results, meals, or activity levels.

Somogyi effect—when the blood glucose level swings high following a low blood sugar. The Somogyi effect may follow an untreated low blood sugar episode during the night and is caused by the release of stress hormones.

Sucralose—a sweetener made from sugar, but with no calories and no nutritional value.

Sugar alcohols—sweeteners that produce a smaller rise in blood glucose other than carbohydrates.

Sulfonylurea—a class of medication for diabetes treatment; they work by increasing the production of insulin from the pancreas; examples include glipizide, glimepiride, and glyburide.

Thiazolidinedione—a class of oral medicine for T2DM that helps insulin take sugar from the blood into cells for energy by making cells more sensitive to insulin. (Generic names: pioglitazone and rosiglitazone)

Type 1 diabetes (T1DM)—a condition characterized by high blood sugar levels caused by a total lack of insulin. Occurs when the body's immune system attacks the insulin-producing beta cells in the pancreas and destroys them. The pancreas produces little or no insulin. T1DM develops most often in young people, but can appear in adults.

Type 2 diabetes (T2DM)—a condition characterized by high blood sugar levels caused by either a lack of insulin or the body's inability to use insulin efficiently. Type 2 diabetes develops most often in middle-aged and older adults, but can appear in young people.

Unit of insulin—the basic measure of insulin. U-100 insulin means 100 units of insulin per milliliter (mL) or cubic centimeter (cc) of solution. Most insulin made today in the United States is U-100.

FIGURE 21-1 *(Continued)*

TABLE 21-7 • Questions to Anticipate Regarding Diabetes

Questions Commonly Asked by Patients with Diabetes
• **What causes diabetes?** Type 1 diabetes is triggered by genetics and possible environmental factors that lead to the immune system's destruction of the insulin producing cells in the pancreas (beta cells). The risk for type 2 diabetes can be increased by certain factors such as age, race, having a family history of diabetes, as well as obesity and physical inactivity. In type 2 diabetes, either the body does not produce enough insulin or the cells do not use insulin properly. Insulin is necessary for the body to be able to use glucose for energy. We do not know what causes gestational diabetes, but some research suggests it may be caused by hormones produced during pregnancy blocking the action of insulin in the mother's body.
• **Which type of diabetes is worse? Type 1 or type 2?** Neither type is worse than the other. The main difference between type 1 and type 2 diabetes is how the disease process starts and the age of onset. In individuals with type 1 diabetes, the body no longer produces insulin, so you must be on insulin from the time of diagnosis. Type 1 diabetes is usually diagnosed in children and adolescents. In type 2 diabetes, the body is resistant to insulin, and over time the body is unable to make enough insulin. Type 2 diabetes is usually diagnosed in adults, but may occur in children. Both type 1 and type 2 diabetes can lead to complications if poorly controlled.
• **What factors increase my risk for getting type 2 diabetes?** The following individuals may have increased risk of developing type 2 diabetes: people with impaired fasting glucose or impaired glucose tolerance, age >45, family history of diabetes, being overweight or obese, physical inactivity, people with low HDL-cholesterol (good cholesterol) or high triglycerides, certain racial and ethnic groups (eg, non-Hispanic Blacks, Hispanic/Latino Americans, Asian Americans, Pacific Islanders, and American Indians and Alaskan Natives), and women with a history of GDM.
• **What health problems are associated with diabetes?** Diabetes commonly occurs along with high blood pressure and high cholesterol. Poorly controlled diabetes can increase your risk of cardiovascular disease, heart attacks, strokes, kidney failure, blindness, and a condition called neuropathy (nerve damage) because of high levels of blood sugar.
• **How do I know if I have diabetes?** People with diabetes may experience symptoms of frequent urination, unusual thirst, extreme hunger, unusual weight loss, and extreme fatigue or irritability. People who have developed type 2 diabetes may also experience frequent infections, blurred vision, cuts or bruises that are slow to heal, tingling or numbness in the hands/feet, and recurring skin, gum, or bladder infections. If you have any of these symptoms, your physician will do certain blood tests and take a medical history to see if you have diabetes.
• **Why are diabetes medications so important?** It is important to keep your blood sugar within goal so that you can stay healthy. People with high blood sugars are more likely to develop complications of diabetes such as heart disease, kidney failure, blindness, and limb amputations, or other health issues.
• **Should I test my blood sugar? If so, how often should I test my blood sugar?** Testing blood sugar (also called self-monitoring of blood glucose) can provide valuable information on how well your medicines for diabetes are working, as well as how activity and food affect your blood sugar. If you are on insulin, testing blood sugar is important to make sure your insulin doses are correct and to detect low or high blood sugars. If you are on oral diabetes medicines, testing blood sugar may be useful. Your physician should tell you how often to test your blood sugar. It may helpful to keep a log or diary of your blood sugar so you can keep track and bring it to your physician.
• **What causes a low blood sugar?** A low blood sugar, usually defined as a blood glucose ≤70 mg/dL, can occur for several reasons such as decreased food intake, increase in physical activity, or too much insulin or certain diabetes medications (eg, sulfonylureas). Symptoms of a low blood sugar include dizziness, shaking, feeling nervous, sweating, confusion, and moodiness or behavior changes.
• **How should I treat a low blood sugar?** To treat a low blood sugar, consume 15 grams of fast-acting glucose (eg, 4 oz fruit juice, ½ can regular soda, 8 oz low fat milk, 8 to 10 hard candies). Once you have checked your blood glucose and treated your hypoglycemia, wait 15 or 20 minutes and check your blood again. If your blood glucose is still low and your symptoms of hypoglycemia do not go away, repeat the treatment. After you feel better, be sure to eat your regular meals and snacks as planned to keep your blood glucose level up.
• **When should I call my physician about high or low blood sugars?** Call your physician if you are not responding to the prescribed treatment (your blood sugar levels are not within goal), or if you are having side effects. Call your physician if you experience the following symptoms of high blood sugar: frequent urination, extreme thirst, extreme hunger, unusual fatigue, nausea/vomiting, or if you develop ketones, or have an infection or wound that will not heal. Call your physician if you experience frequent symptoms of low blood sugar such as: dizziness, shakiness, feeling nervous, sweating, confusion, moodiness, or behavior changes.
• **What can happen if I stop taking my diabetes medications?** You may experience symptoms of high blood sugar such as fatigue, frequent urination, unusual thirst, or extreme hunger. Over time serious health problems such as heart attack, stroke, kidney failure, blindness, or nerve damage can occur. Also, when you restart certain medicines, your dose may have to be lowered for a period of time to prevent side effects. Your prescriber will tell you how to slowly work your way back up to your usual dose.
• **What should I do if I have a problem with my diabetes medication(s)?** Never stop taking your diabetes medications without first talking to your physician. Speak with your physician and/or pharmacist to let them know about any problems you are having, and together you can make sure your diabetes medications are the right ones for you.

PERSONAL MEDICATION LIST FOR *<Insert Patient's name*, DOB: *mm/dd/yyyy>*	
Medication: Metformin 1000 mg	
How I use it: Take one pill (1000 mg) twice daily with food	
Why I use it: Diabetes	**Prescriber:** Jones
Date I started using it: 11/7/2010	**Date I stopped using it:** *(Leave blank for patient's notes)*
Why I stopped using it: *(Leave blank for patient's notes)*	
Medication: Januvia (sitagliptin) 100 mg	
How I use it: Take one pill (100 mg) daily	
Why I use it: Diabetes	**Prescriber:** Jones
Date I started using it: 10/9/12	**Date I stopped using it:** *(Leave blank for patient's notes)*
Why I stopped using it: *(Leave blank for patient's notes)*	
Medication: Lisinopril 20 mg	
How I use it: Take one pill daily (20 mg) at bedtime	
Why I use it: Blood pressure; protects kidneys from diabetes	**Prescriber:** Jones
Date I started using it: 10/9/12	**Date I stopped using it:** *(Leave blank for patient's notes)*
Why I stopped using it: *(Leave blank for patient's notes)*	
Medication: Pravastatin 40 mg	
How I use it: Take one pill daily (40 mg) at bedtime	
Why I use it: Cholesterol	**Prescriber:** Jones
Date I started using it: 1/6/13	**Date I stopped using it:** *(Leave blank for patient's notes)*
Why I stopped using it: *(Leave blank for patient's notes)*	
Medication: Enteric coated baby aspirin 81 mg	
How I use it: Take one pill (81 mg) daily	
Why I use it: To prevent heart disease	**Prescriber:** Jones
Date I started using it: 10/9/12	**Date I stopped using it:** *(Leave blank for patient's notes)*
Why I stopped using it: *(Leave blank for patient's notes)*	

FIGURE 21-2 Example personal medication list for diabetes medications.

	DATE PREPARED: *<Insert date>*
What we talked about: Importance of controlling blood sugar to prevent complications of diabetes	
What I need to do: 1. Take diabetes medication (metformin) as prescribed 2. Check blood sugar two times a day (first thing in the morning and two hours after a meal) and write down values 3. Notify provider if three sugar readings over 250 mg/dL or any one reading over 300 mg/dL 4. Notify provider if frequent low blood sugar readings (≤70 mg/dL) 5. Bring log book of my sugar readings and my meter to the next visit for review	**What I did and when I did it:** *(Leave blank for patient's notes)*
What we talked about: How to manage low blood sugar (hypoglycemia)	
What I need to do: 1. Check my blood sugar when I am having signs of low sugar (feeling shaky, sweaty, dizzy, moody, or hungry) 2. If my blood sugar is low (≤70), take at least 15 grams of carbohydrates (a source of sugar), eg, half a cup of regular soda or fruit juice, 4 teaspoons of table sugar, or 4 glucose tablets; avoid foods that are high in fat like candy bars and ice cream 3. Check my blood sugar again in 15 to 20 minutes to see if it has come up 4. Notify provider if frequent low blood sugar readings (≤70 mg/dL)	**What I did and when I did it:** *(Leave blank for patient's notes)*

FIGURE 21-3 Example medication action plan for a patient with diabetes.

CORE ELEMENT 4— INTERVENTION AND/OR REFERRAL

Interventions for diabetes management may include lifestyle modifications and/or drug therapy. Table 21-8 summarizes suggested lifestyle modifications for patients with diabetes.

Patients with T2DM who are not adequately controlled with lifestyle modifications should be started on drug therapy. Providers should select glucose-lowering agents based on the level of hyperglycemia, potential adverse effects, and other comorbid disease states. Many patients will require more than one medication to control their glucose, and some may require a combination of oral agents and insulin, or intensive insulin therapy. Table 21-9 provides an overview of oral antihyperglycemics for T2DM, Table 21-10 summarizes available insulin preparations, and Table 21-11 provides an overview of other injectable therapies. Considerations for individualizing antihyperglycemic therapy are found in Table 21-12. In addition, Table 21-13 outlines herbal remedies that may be useful in the management of diabetes. The treatment algorithm for type 2 diabetes is provided in Figure 21-4, and guidelines for the use of insulin therapy in type 2 diabetes are outlined in Figure 21-5. The management of type 1 diabetes consists mainly of insulin and sometimes pramlintide. For a review of the management of type 1 diabetes, the reader is referred to the *Medical Management of Type 1 Diabetes*, sixth edition.[21]

In addition to medications for glycemic control, some patients also need additional therapy to help prevent or reduce the risk of complications of diabetes. Table 21-14 provides an overview of medications used in the management of chronic complications of diabetes. The MTM provider should also ensure that recommended immunizations (ie, influenza, pneumococcal, and hepatitis B) are up to date in patients with diabetes.[5]

CORE ELEMENT 5—DOCUMENTATION AND FOLLOW-UP

Clear and succinct documentation of MRPs and recommendations is a key component of the MTM consult. Examples of potential MRPs in patients with diabetes are provided in Table 21-15. Sample communications and recommendations to providers to address medication-related issues are found in Figure 21-6. Recommendations may be communicated via fax, telephone, or other means of written or secure electronic communication. The examples that follow are for illustrative purposes. Actual communications to providers should be individualized based on the type of recommendation, patient specific characteristics, and the nature of the relationship with the provider.

Follow-up to assess glucose control, effects of interventions, and potential adverse effects is essential in patients with diabetes.

TABLE 21-8 • Lifestyle Modifications for Management of Diabetes

Modification	Recommendation
Weight loss	Weight loss is recommended for all insulin-resistant/overweight or obese individuals. Sustained weight loss of 5% of body weight is beneficial for glycemic control. Weight loss may be achieved with DASH, plant-based, or Mediterranean diets.
Medical nutrition therapy (MNT)	Monitoring carbohydrate intake is integral to glucose control. The relative mix of carbohydrate, protein, and fat in the diet should be individualized depending on the desired level of glycemic control. Intake of saturated fat intake should be <10% of total calories. The intake of trans fat should be minimized. Consultation with a registered dietitian is encouraged to help optimize MNT for patients with diabetes.
Physical activity	Patients with diabetes should have at least 150 minutes of moderate exercise per week (or 75 minutes of high intensity exercise). Exercise should occur on most days of the week. Patients should be encouraged to avoid going more than 2 days without exercise.
Alcohol consumption	Patients with diabetes should limit alcohol intake to the following: Men: ≤2 drinks/day Women and lighter persons: ≤1 drink/day. Patients should monitor for hypoglycemia if consuming alcohol.
Smoking cessation	For overall cardiovascular risk reduction, patients with diabetes should not smoke or use tobacco products or e-cigarettes. Patients should be strongly encouraged to quit smoking entirely.
Stress reduction	Stress may adversely affect glucose levels. Patients with diabetes are encouraged to reduce life stressors if possible and to practice stress management techniques.
Antioxidants	Regular supplementation with antioxidants (eg, beta carotene or vitamins C or E) is not recommended.

Source: Compiled from reference 20.

TABLE 21-9 • Oral Medications for Management of Diabetes

Medication Class and Example Drugs	Common/Serious Side Effects[a]	Blackbox Warnings/ Contraindications	Pregnancy Category[b]
Alpha-glucosidase inhibitors Acarbose Miglitol	Abdominal pain Flatulence Diarrhea	Diabetic ketoacidosis Gastrointestinal obstruction Ileus Inflammatory bowel disease	B
Biguanides Metformin[c]	Abdominal pain Diarrhea Dyspepsia Flatulence Lactic acidosis Vitamin B12 deficiency Weight loss	Lactic acidosis Diabetic ketoacidosis Metabolic acidosis Radiographic contrast administration Renal failure Type 1 diabetes	B
Bile acid sequestrants Colesevelam	Constipation Gastrointestinal obstruction Hypertriglyceridemia	Gastrointestinal obstruction Hypertriglyceridemia Pancreatitis	B
Dipeptidyl peptidase-4 (DPP-4) inhibitors Alogliptin[c,d] Linagliptin[d] Saxagliptin[d] Sitagliptin[d]	Angioedema Infection Lymphopenia (saxagliptin) Pancreatitis Urticaria	Angioedema Pancreatitis Type 1 diabetes	B
Dopamine-2 agonists Bromocriptine (quick release)	Anorexia Asthenia Constipation Dizziness Drowsiness Dyspepsia Fatigue Headache Nausea Orthostatic hypotension Xerostomia	Basilar/hemiplegic migraine Breastfeeding Eclampsia Ergot alkaloid hypersensitivity Hypertension Preeclampsia Type 1 diabetes History of heart disease (eg, coronary artery disease, MI, arrhythmias) History of mental health disorders (eg, depression, schizophrenia)	B However, use in pregnancy should be avoided if possible.
Glinides Nateglinide Repaglinide[d]	Arthralgia/arthropathy Dizziness Gastrointestinal upset Headache Hypoglycemia Secondary failure Upper respiratory infection Weight gain	Diabetic ketoacidosis Type 1 diabetes	C
Sodium glucose co-transporter 2 (SGLT2) inhibitor Canagliflozin[d] Dapagliflozin[d,e] Empagliflozin[d,f]	Dehydration Dizziness Hyperkalemia Hypoglycemia Hypotension Ketoacidosis Increases in LDL cholesterol Male and female genital fungal infections Syncope Urinary tract infections	Dialysis Renal failure Hypersensitivity Hypovolemia Renal impairment Type 1 diabetes	C

(Continued)

TABLE 21-9 • Oral Medications for Management of Diabetes (*Continued*)

Medication Class and Example Drugs	Common/Serious Side Effects[a]	Blackbox Warnings/ Contraindications	Pregnancy Category[b]
Sulfonylureas Glimepiride[c] Glipizide[d] Glyburide[d]	Hypoglycemia Rash/urticaria Secondary failure Weight gain	Diabetic ketoacidosis Sulfonamide hypersensitivity Sulfonylurea sensitivity Type 1 diabetes	B or C (glyburide[g]) C (others)
Thiazolidinediones Pioglitazone[d] Rosiglitazone[d]	Back pain Bone fractures Diarrhea Dizziness Edema/fluid retention Increased risk of bladder cancer Upper respiratory infection Weight gain	Acute heart failure Heart failure Bladder cancer Diabetic ketoacidosis Osteoporosis	C

[a] This is a general list and does not include all side effects that can occur from these drugs. Consult a drug reference source for a more inclusive list before making any recommendations. MTM providers should also consult a comprehensive drug interaction database before making pharmacotherapy recommendations.

[b] Product labeling for all prescription drugs is being updated to reflect the new FDA Pregnancy Labeling and Lactation Rule. Please check individual product labeling for the most accurate and updated pregnancy information.

[c] Available in combination with pioglitazone.

[d] Available in combination with metformin.

[e] Available in combination with sitagliptin.

[f] Available in combination with linagliptin.

[g] Pregnancy category varies for different manufacturers; glyburide is sometimes used for management of GDM.

Abbreviations: LDL = low-density lipoprotein; MI = myocardial infarction.

Source: References 6, 12, and 18.

TABLE 21-10 • Available Insulin Preparations

Generic Name	Manufacturer	Analog[a]	Administration Options	Room Temperature[b] Expiration
Rapid-acting insulins				
Humalog (insulin lispro)	Lilly	Yes	Insulin pen 3-mL, 3-mL and 10-mL vial, or 3-mL pen cartridge	28 days
NovoLog (insulin aspart)	Novo Nordisk	Yes	Insulin pen 3-mL, 10-mL vial, or 3-mL pen cartridge	28 days
Apidra (insulin glulisine)	Sanofi	Yes	Insulin pen 3-mL, 10-mL vial	28 days
Short-acting insulins				
Humulin R (regular) U-100	Lilly	No	10-mL vial, 3-mL vial	28 days
Novolin R (regular)	Novo Nordisk	No	10-mL vial	42 days
Intermediate-acting insulins				
NPH				
Humulin N	Lilly	No	3-mL and 10-mL vial, Insulin pen 3-mL	Vial: 31 days; pen: 14 days
Novolin N	Novo Nordisk	No	10-mL vial	42 days
Long-acting insulins				
Lantus (insulin glargine)	Sanofi	Yes	10-mL vial, Insulin pen 3-mL	28 days
Levemir (insulin detemir)	Novo Nordisk	Yes	10-mL vial, Insulin pen 3-mL	42 days
Tresiba (insulin degludec)	Novo Nordisk	Yes	Insulin pen 3-mL	56 days
Premixed insulins				
Premixed insulin analogs				
Humalog Mix 75/25 (75% neutral protamine lispro, 25% lispro)	Lilly	Yes	10-mL vial, Insulin pen 3-mL	Vial: 28 days; pen: 10 days

(*Continued*)

TABLE 21-10 • Available Insulin Preparations (*Continued*)

Generic Name	Manufacturer	Analog[a]	Administration Options	Room Temperature[b] Expiration
Novolog Mix 70/30 (70% aspart protamine suspension, 30% aspart)	Novo Nordisk	Yes	10-mL vial, Insulin pen 3-mL	Vial: 28 days; pen: 14 days
Humalog Mix 50/50 (50% neutral protamine lispro/50% lispro)	Lilly	Yes	10-mL vial, Insulin pen 3-mL	Vial: 28 days; pen:10 days
NPH-regular combinations				
Humulin 70/30	Lilly	No	3-mL and 10-mL vial, Insulin pen 3-mL	Vial: 31 days; pen: 10 days
Novolin 70/30	Novo Nordisk	No	10-mL vial	42 days
Concentrated insulins				
Regular insulin (U-500)	Lilly	No	20-mL vial, Insulin pen 3-mL	Vial: 40 days; pen: 28 days
Humalog (U-200 insulin lispro)	Lilly	Yes	Insulin pen 3-mL	28 days
Toujeo (U-300 insulin glargine)	Sanofi	Yes	Insulin pen 1.5-mL	42 days
Tresiba (U-200 insulin degludec)	Novo Nordisk	Yes	Insulin pen 3-mL	56 days
Inhaled insulin				
Afrezza (Technosphere insulin)	Mannkind	No	4 unit and 8 unit cartridges	Sealed-unopened blister card/strip 10 days; opened 3 days

[a] All diabetes injectables available in the United States are now made by human recombinant DNA technology. An insulin analog is a modified human insulin molecule that imparts particular pharmacokinetic advantages.

[b] Room temperature defined as 59°-86° F (15°-30° C). All products are good until expiration date on product if unopened and stored correctly.

Source: Reproduced, with permission, from DiPiro JT, Talbert RL, Yee GC, Matzke GR, Wells BG, Posey L, eds. *Pharmacotherapy: A Pathophysiologic Approach*. 10th ed. New York, NY: McGraw-Hill; 2017.

TABLE 21-11 • Available GLP-1 Receptor Agonists and Amylinomimetics

Generic Name	Administration Options	Room Temperature[b] Expiration	Pharmacokinetics/ Drug Interactions[a]	Major Adverse Events
Glucagon-like peptide-1 agonists				
Exenatide (Byetta)	5-mcg and 10-mcg pen, 60 doses/pen Dosed twice daily at or before meals	30 days (≤77°F [≤25°C])	Pharmacokinetics: 53% homology to GLP-1, t_{max} ~2 hours, and duration of action 4-6 hours Drug interactions: Caution with warfarin: May increase INR Delayed gastric emptying may delay absorption of medication. Move 1 hour before or at least 3 hours after injection.	Nausea >35% Vomiting/diarrhea 10%, respectively. Start with 5 mcg BID. Expect recurrence of GI with increase in dose to 10 mcg BID. Inject closer to meals to limit nausea, but maximal satiety may be achieved by injecting 1-2 hours prior to food intake. Drug class warning: Pancreatitis
Exenatide (Bydureon)	2-mg single use pen device, 2-mg vial with separate diluent, single-use system Dosed weekly	30 days (≤77°F [≤25°C])	Pharmacokinetics: Exenatide embedded in microspheres slowly release over 10 weeks upon injection. Levels gradually increase with each weekly injection; 6-8 weeks to steady-state. Attains therapeutic levels at week 2. Drug interactions: See exenatide.	Slightly less nausea and vomiting versus twice daily exenatide. Drug class warning: Pancreatitis Long-acting GLP-1 agonist—do not use in medullary thyroid CA, MEN2.

(*Continued*)

TABLE 21-11 • Available GLP-1 Receptor Agonists and Amylinomimetics (*Continued*)

Generic Name	Administration Options	Room Temperature[b] Expiration	Pharmacokinetics/ Drug Interactions[a]	Major Adverse Events
Liraglutide (Victoza)	3-mL pen, delivers 0.6 mg, 1.2 mg, or 1.8 mg dose. Dosed daily.	30-days	Pharmacokinetics: 97% homology to GLP-1 A C-16 fatty acid (palmitic acid) self-associates into heptamers, prolonging half-life to 13 hours. T_{max} is reached 8-12 hours after injection with steady state in 3 days. Drug interactions: Delay in gastric emptying may affect absorption of other medications.	Nausea: 1.2 mg—10%-30% Nausea: 1.8 mg—15%-40% Vomiting: 5% Diarrhea: 8%-15% Stay on titration dose of 0.6 mg (non-therapeutic dose) daily until GI side effects dissipate. Then increase dose to 1.2 mg daily. Drug class warning: Pancreatitis Long-acting GLP-1 agonist—do not use in medullary thyroid CA, MEN2.
Albiglutide (Tanzeum)	30-mg and 50-mg single use pen Dosed weekly	4 weeks (≤86°F [≤30°C])	Pharmacokinetics: Recombinant fusion protein consists of two copies of a 30-amino acid sequence of a modified human GLP-1 (fragment 7-36) that is fused to human albumin. Fragment 97% homology to GLP-1, half-life: 5 days. May not penetrate CNS. Drug interactions: Delay in gastric emptying may affect absorption of other medications.	Nausea 9%-15% Vomiting 5%-12% Diarrhea 12% Drug class warning: Pancreatitis Long-acting GLP-1 agonist—do not use in medullary thyroid CA, MEN2.
Dulaglutide (Trulicity)	0.75-mg and 1.5-mg single use pen (0.5 mL) 0.75-mg and 1.5-mg single use prefilled syringe (0.5 mL) Dosed weekly	14 days (≤86°F [≤30°C]))	Pharmacokinetics: Two identical disulfide-linked chains, each containing a modified human GLP-1 analog (90% homology to GLP-1) covalently linked to a modified human immunoglobulin G4 heavy chain fragment Half-life: 5 days Drug interactions: Delay in gastric emptying may affect absorption of other medications.	Nausea: 0.75 mg—8%-18% Nausea:1.5 mg—17%-28% Vomiting 3-5%, but as high as 17% with 1.5 mg dosing Diarrhea: 8%-17% Drug class warning: Pancreatitis Long-acting GLP-1 agonist—do not use in medullary thyroid CA, MEN2.
Amylinomimetic				
Pramlintide (Symlin)	1.5-mL pen: delivers 15-, 30-, 45-, or 60-mcg dose; 2.7-mL pen: delivers 60- or 120-mcg dose. Dosed with each meal.	30 days	Pharmacokinetics: The t_{max} is approximately 20 minutes. The $t_{1/2}$ is approximately 45 minutes. Metabolized by kidneys. One active metabolite (2-37 pramlintide) has a similar half-life as the parent compound. No accumulation seen in renal insufficiency. Injection into the arm—not recommended. Drug interactions: Pramlintide may delay gastric emptying.	Dosing: type 1 DM start at 15 mcg before meals, may increase as tolerated, most can advance dose to 30-45 mcg before meals. Type 2 DM—start with 60 mcg before meals, most advance to 120 mcg before meals Nausea: type 1 DM > type 2 DM Vomiting: type 1 DM > type 2 DM Severe hypoglycemia possible: decrease prandial insulin 30%-50% prior to initiation.

[a] All diabetes injectables available in the United States are now made by human recombinant DNA technology. An insulin analog is a modified human insulin molecule that imparts particular pharmacokinetic advantages.

[b] Room temperature defined as 59°-86° F (15°-30° C). All products are good until expiration date on product if unopened and stored correctly.

Abbreviations: CNS = central nervous system; GI = gastrointestinal; MEN2 = multiple endocrine neoplasia type 2; $t_{1/2}$ = half-life of medication; t_{max} = time at maximum concentration.

Source: Reproduced, with permission, from DiPiro JT, Talbert RL, Yee GC, Matzke GR, Wells BG, Posey L, eds. *Pharmacotherapy: A Pathophysiologic Approach*. 10th ed. New York, NY: McGraw-Hill; 2017.

TABLE 21-12 • Considerations in Individualizing Diabetes Therapy

Comorbid Condition	Drug Therapy Considerations
Bladder cancer	• Avoid pioglitazone
Chronic kidney disease	• Canagliflozin – dose adjustment required if eGFR < 60 mL/min/1.73 m^2; avoid if eGFR < 45 mL/min/1.73 m^2 • Dapagliflozin - do not initiate if eGFR < 60 mL/min/1.73 m^2; discontinue if eGFR falls below 60 mL/min/1.73 m^2 • Empagliflozin – do not initiate if eGFR < 45 mL/min/1.73 m^2; discontinue if eGFR falls below 45 mL/min/1.73 m^2 • DPP-4 inhibitors – all require renal dose adjustment except linagliptin • GLP-1 agonists – use of exenatide is not recommended with CrCl < 30 mL/min • Metformin – contraindicated in patients with severe renal dysfunction because of risk of lactic acidosis; reduce dose with eGFR < 45 mL/min/1.73 m^2; avoid use if eGFR < 30 mL/min/1.73 m^2 • Sulfonylureas – start at low dosages and titrate slowly; glyburide should not be used with CrCl < 50 mL/min
Diabetic gastroparesis	• Avoid GLP-1 agonists and pramlintide
Heart failure	• Avoid thiazolidinediones • Metformin may be used if heart failure is not severe and cardiac function is stable
Hepatic disease	• Pioglitazone may be beneficial for patients with fatty liver disease; avoid in patients with liver function tests > 2.5 times the upper limit of normal • Insulin is preferred in cases of severe hepatic dysfunction
Obesity	• Sulfonylureas, glinides, pioglitazone, and insulin may cause weight gain • DPP-4 inhibitors are weight neutral • Metformin, GLP-1 agonists, and SGLT2 inhibitors may be associated with weight loss
Osteoporosis	• Avoid pioglitazone
Pancreatitis	• Avoid DPP-4 inhibitors and GLP-1 agonists
Pregnancy	• Insulin is the preferred therapy • Glyburide and metformin may also be used
Thyroid cancer	• Avoid GLP-1 agonists

Abbreviations: CrCl = creatinine clearance; DPP-4 = dipeptidyl peptidase 4; eGFR = estimated glomerular filtration rate; GLP-1 = glucagon-like peptide-1; SGLT2 = Sodium glucose co-transporter 2.

Source: References 6, 12, and 18.

TABLE 21-13 • Herbal Supplements for Diabetes

Herbal	Typical Dose	Effectiveness[a]	Cost[b]
Alpha-lipoic acid	300 to 1800 mg daily in single or divided doses (type 2 diabetes and neuropathy)	Possibly effective	\$-\$\$
Berberine	500 mg twice daily	Possibly effective	\$\$-\$\$\$
Chromium	200 mcg chromium, 1-3 times a day; 1000 mcg chromium picolinate once daily	Possibly effective	\$
Cinnamon	120-6000 mg of cinnamon daily; 333 mg of cinnamon extract 3 times daily	Possibly effective	\$
Ginseng	3 g of American ginseng extract powder 100-200 mg of Panax ginseng (type 2 diabetes)	Possibly effective	\$
Milk thistle	200 mg 3 times daily of constituent silymarin	Possibly effective	\$\$-\$\$\$

[a] Level of evidence. Likely effective: This product has a very high level of reliable clinical evidence supporting its use for a specific indication. Products rated "likely effective" are generally considered appropriate to recommend. Possibly effective: This product has some clinical evidence supporting its use for a specific indication; however, the evidence is limited by quantity, quality, or contradictory findings. Products rated "possibly effective" might be beneficial but do not have enough high-quality evidence to recommend for most people. Insufficient evidence: There is not enough reliable scientific evidence to provide an effectiveness rating.

[b] Cost: \$ = \$10 or less per month supply in the recommended dosage; \$\$ = \$11-\$20 per month; \$\$\$ = \$21-\$50 per month; and \$\$\$\$ = more than \$50.

Source: Data compiled from reference 22.

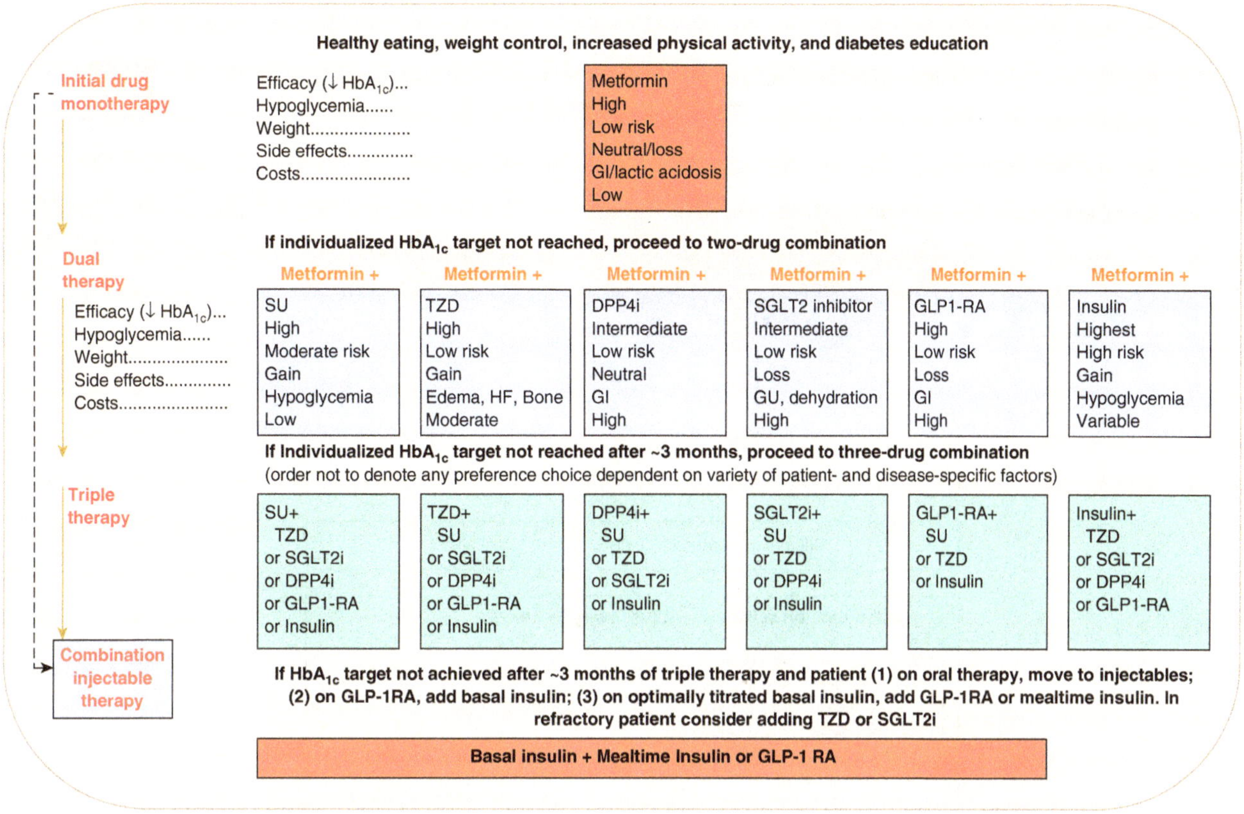

FIGURE 21-4 Current treatment algorithm for type 2 diabetes.

Source: Reproduced, with permission, from DiPiro JT, Talbert RL, Yee GC, Matzke GR, Wells BG, Posey L, eds. *Pharmacotherapy: A Pathophysiologic Approach*. 10th ed. New York, NY: McGraw-Hill; 2017.

TABLE 21-14 • Selected Evidence-Based Recommendations for Patients with Diabetes

Complication	Recommendations	Level of Evidence[a]
Cardiovascular disease–Blood pressure control	• Systolic blood pressure should be treated to <140 mm Hg	A
	• Consider systolic blood pressure target of <130 mm Hg for younger patients or those at high risk of cardiovascular disease, if it can be achieved without undue treatment burden	C
	• Diastolic blood pressure should be treated to <90 mm Hg	A
	• Initial drug therapy for hypertension in diabetes should include medications known to reduce cardiovascular events (ACE inhibitor, ARB, DHP CCB, or thiazides)	A
	• ACE inhibitors and ARBs are first-line therapy in diabetes with hypertension and albuminuria	A
Cardiovascular disease–Lipid management	• For patients 40-75 years without ASCVD risk factors, use a moderate-intensity statin and lifestyle modifications	A
	• For patients 40-75 years with ASCVD risk factors, use a high-intensity statin and lifestyle modifications	B
	• For patients over 75 without ASCVD risk factors use moderate-intensity statin and lifestyle modifications	B
	• For patients over 75 with ASCVD risk factors use high-intensity statin and lifestyle modifications	B
	• Addition of other lipid-lowering agents to statins does not improve ASCVD outcomes and is not recommended	A
	• A statin/fibrate combination may be considered for males with low HDL (≤34 mg/dL) and TG ≥ 204 mg/dL	B
Cardiovascular disease–Antiplatelet therapy	• Use aspirin (75-162 mg daily) for secondary prevention	A
	• Consider aspirin (75-162 mg daily) for primary prevention in patients with diabetes and increased CV risk	C
	• Clopidogrel (75 mg/day) is appropriate for patients with ASCVD and documented aspirin allergy	B
Nephropathy	• ACE inhibitors or ARBs are the preferred treatment for nonpregnant patients with albuminuria in the range of 30-299 mg/day	C
	• ACE inhibitors or ARBs are the preferred treatment for nonpregnant patients with urinary albumin excretion ≥300 mg/day	A

[a] Level of evidence: A = clear evidence from well-conducted, generalizable, randomized controlled trials that are adequately powered. B = supportive evidence from well-conducted cohort studies or well-conducted case-control study. C = supportive evidence from poorly controlled or uncontrolled studies or conflicting evidence with weight of evidence supporting the recommendation. E = expert consensus or clinical experience.

Abbreviations: ACE = angiotensin-converting enzyme; ARB = angiotensin receptor blocker; ASCVD = atherosclerotic cardiovascular disease; CV = cardiovascular; DHP CCB = dihydropyridine calcium channel blocker; HDL = high-density lipoprotein; TG = triglycerides.

Source: Data compiled from reference 10.

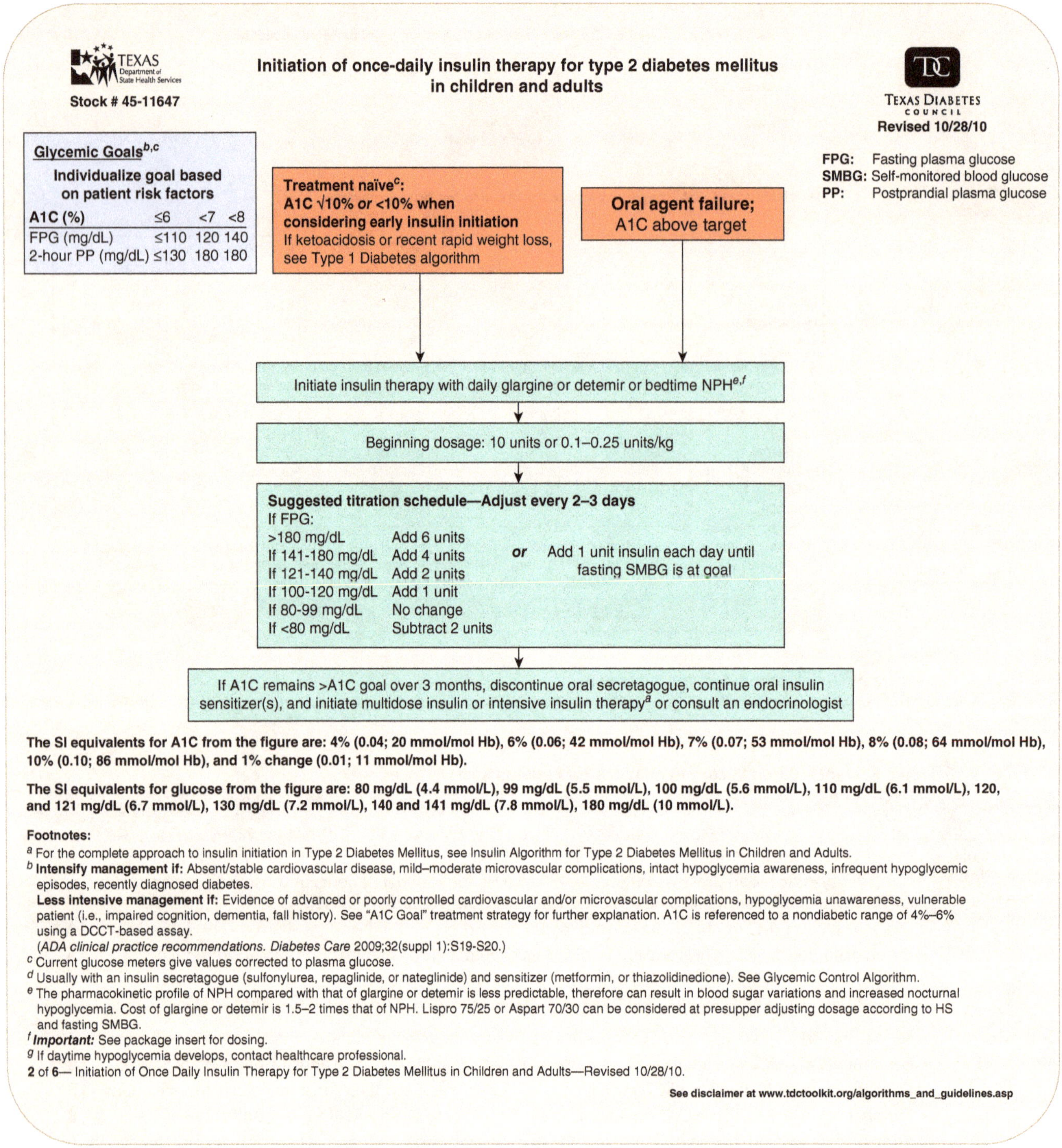

FIGURE 21-5 Algorithm for initiation of insulin therapy in type 2 diabetes.
Source: Texas Diabetes Council, Texas Department of State Health Services.

Patients should be encouraged to monitor blood glucose at home and to follow up at regular intervals so that glycemic control may be assessed. The interval for follow-up will depend on several factors, including severity of hyperglycemia, type of intervention, and patient-specific factors such as age, comorbid conditions, and ability to return for follow-up. Additionally, evidenced-based guidelines, such as those by the American Diabetes Association, provide recommendations on monitoring for diabetes complications. Suggested intervals for follow-up are provided in Table 21-16. Lastly, Figure 21-7 outlines criteria for referral for management of diabetes.

QUALITY MEASURES

Many payers of MTM services are accountable for providing high quality care to their beneficiaries, the patients. These payers, usually healthcare plans, are "graded" on a 5-star rating system (where 1 reflects low quality and 5 reflects the highest quality standard) by

TABLE 21-15 • Medication-Related Problems (MRPs) in Patients with Diabetes

Category of MRP	Example Medication-Related Problem
Nonadherence	• Suboptimal control of glucose because of nonadherence with lifestyle modifications (eg, carbohydrate intake) • Suboptimal control of glucose because of patient missing doses of insulin • Patient not taking medication (eg, DPP-4 inhibitor) because of cost
Unnecessary medication	• Duplicate therapy (eg, two sulfonylureas)
Need for additional medication	• Monotherapy with therapeutic doses of metformin with suboptimal glucose control • Patient with high postprandial glucose on basal insulin only (need for prandial insulin) • Patient with diabetes and microalbuminuria not on ACE or ARB inhibitor for renal protection
Ineffective medication	• Adequate trial of new antihyperglycemic without significant A1c lowering • Patient with increasing A1c despite increased dose of sulfonylurea
Dosage too low	• Suboptimal glucose control on low dose of metformin monotherapy
Dosage too high	• Patient with chronic kidney disease not receiving renally adjusted dose of DPP-4 inhibitor • Patient with frequent hypoglycemia from insulin
Adverse drug event	• Patient with pancreatitis from GLP-1 agonist • Patient with exacerbation of heart failure from thiazolidinedione

Scenario: Patient with type 2 diabetes given samples of Onglyza (saxagliptin) but cannot afford Rx once samples are finished

MRP: Nonadherence

• Assessment:

Patient with uncontrolled glucose on saxagliptin 5 mg daily. Lack of glucose control likely secondary to nonadherence with saxagliptin. Patient nonadherent with saxagliptin due to cost issues. Switching saxagliptin to metformin, the preferred therapy for T2DM would provide for more affordable glucose control. Serum creatinine is WNL for starting metformin therapy.

• Plan:

Consider discontinuation of saxagliptin and addition of metformin 500 mg po twice daily with food; titrate as needed based on glucose readings and patient tolerance.

Scenario: Patient with type 2 diabetes and renal dysfunction having hypoglycemia on glyburide

MRP: Adverse effect, dosage too high

• Assessment:

Patient with T2DM and chronic kidney disease (est CrCl 38 mL/min) experiencing frequent hypoglycemia on glyburide 5 mg twice daily. Current A1c 6.5%. Hypoglycemia likely secondary to glyburide accumulation related to decreased renal elimination. Changing to another sulfonylurea or another agent that does not increase insulin (eg, DPP-4 inhibitor) may lessen hypoglycemia.

• Plan:

Recommend discontinuation of glyburide.

Consider initiation of glipizide 2.5 mg twice daily with titration to desired level of glucose control OR initiation of a DPP-4 inhibitor such as Januvia (sitagliptin) 50 mg po daily (dose appropriate for renal function).

Scenario: Diabetes patient with elevated blood pressure not on antihypertensive

MRP: Need for additional medication

• Assessment:

Blood pressure above goal of <140/90 mm Hg in this patient with T2DM. Lifestyle modifications have not resulted in adequate response. ACE inhibitor may help achieve BP goals and provide renal protection.

• Plan:

Consider initiation of lisinopril 10 mg po daily.

Patient to check blood pressure at home three times weekly and bring log to next visit.

Scenario: Obese patient with type 2 diabetes on metformin with suboptimal glucose control

MRP: Need for additional medication

• Assessment:

Patient with A1c of 7.8% on metformin 1000 mg twice daily. Tolerating therapy well and reports adherence with medication and diet. Addition of a GLP-1 agonist may help achieve glycemic goals and contribute to weight loss. Goal A1c <7%.

• Plan:

Recommend continuation of metformin 1000 mg twice daily.

Consider initiation of Victoza (liraglutide) 0.6 mg SC once daily for one week, then increase to 1.2 mg daily.

FIGURE 21-6 Sample provider communications for diabetes.

TABLE 21-16 • Suggested Intervals for Follow-up in Patients with Diabetes

Monitoring Parameter	Recommendation
Glucose	• Home blood glucose monitoring is needed for patients on insulin therapy • Patients on other therapeutic interventions, including oral agents, may benefit from home blood glucose monitoring • When initiating or changing oral therapy, it is advisable to follow-up with patients by phone or in person in 2-4 weeks to assess glucose levels (note: therapeutic effects of thiazolidinediones may not be seen for several weeks) • More frequent follow-up may be needed for patients titrating insulin
A1c	• Perform quarterly in individuals not meeting glycemic goals • Perform twice yearly in individuals meeting glycemic goals
Toxicity	• Monitor for adverse drug effects 2-4 weeks after starting a new agent or increasing a dose (dependent on agent started) • Monitor every 6-12 months in stable patients
Routine screening/monitoring[a]	• Measure blood pressure at each visit • Obtain fasting lipid panel upon initiation of statin therapy and periodically thereafter • Assess urinary albumin at least annually in patients with type 2 diabetes and patients who have had type 1 diabetes for at least 5 years • Perform annual comprehensive foot exam • Screen patients for polyneuropathy within 5 years of diagnosis of T1DM and at diagnosis of T2DM; screen at least annually thereafter • Refer for a dilated eye exam within 5 years of diagnosis of T1DM, and shortly after diagnosis in T2DM, with follow-up every year 1 to 2 years as recommended by an eye specialist

[a] The MTM provider should recommend these screening and monitoring tests to the primary care provider if not routinely performed.

Sources: References 10, 11, and 18.

the Centers for Medicare & Medicaid Services. Plans are assessed across multiple categories, ranging from specific disease state measures to customer service measures. Providers of MTM services have an opportunity to assure the safe and effective use of medications and to improve the management of many health conditions. Therefore, payers view MTM as a valuable service for addressing medication usage and disease management, with a potential to improve star ratings. Table 21-17 displays examples of quality measures impacted by MTM providers conducting medication reviews in patients with diabetes.

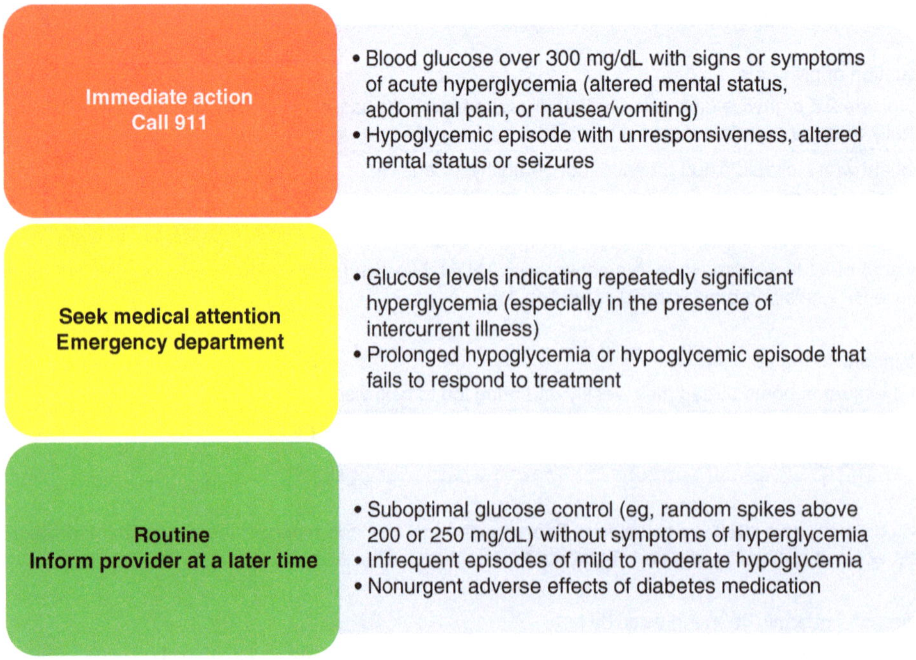

FIGURE 21-7 Referral for management of diabetes.

TABLE 21-17 • Medicare Star Ratings Measures Related to Diabetes

Measure	Measure Target
Part C Measures	
• Diabetes Care—Eye Exam	Dilated or retinal eye exam each year (or negative exam in year prior) • For 5-star rating ≥81% • For 4-star rating ≥73 to <81%
• Diabetes Care—Kidney Disease Monitoring	Nephropathy screening (eg, urinary albumin or protein) during the last year or evidence of ACE inhibitor or ARB therapy • For 5-star rating ≥98% • For 4-star rating ≥96% to <98%
• Diabetes Care—Blood Sugar Controlled	Percent of patients with hemoglobin A1c <9% • For 5-star rating ≥84% • For 4-star rating ≥76% to <84%
Part D Measures	
• Medication Adherence for Diabetes Medications	Percent of patients with a prescription for diabetes medications who fill their prescription often enough to cover 80% or more of the time they are supposed to be taking the medication (includes most oral diabetes drugs and GLP-1 agonists) • For 5-star rating ≥83% • For 4-star rating ≥79% to <83%

Source: Reference 24.

REFERENCES

1. Triplitt CL, Repas T, Alvarez C. Diabetes mellitus. In: DiPiro JT, Talbert RL, Yee GC, Matzke GR, Wells BG, Posey LM, eds. *Pharmacotherapy: A Pathophysiologic Approach*. 10th ed. New York: McGraw-Hill Education; 2017. Available at http://accesspharmacy.mhmedical.com.lp.hscl.ufl.edu/content.aspx?bookid=1861&sectionid=146065891. Accessed May 11, 2017.
2. Centers for Disease Control and Prevention. National diabetes statistics report, 2014. CDC website. Available at https://www.cdc.gov/diabetes/pubs/statsreport14/national-diabetes-report-web.pdf. Accessed May 12, 2017.
3. American Diabetes Association. Economic costs of diabetes in the U.S. in 2012. *Diabetes Care*. 2013;36(4):1033-1046.
4. American Diabetes Association. Management of diabetes in pregnancy. *Diabetes Care*. 2017;40(suppl 1):S114-S119.
5. American Diabetes Association. Classification and diagnosis of diabetes. 2017;40(suppl 1):S11-S24.
6. Clinical Pharmacology [database online]. Tampa, FL: Gold Standard, Inc.; 2017. Available at http://clinicalpharmacology.com.
7. American Diabetes Association. Prevention or delay of type 2 diabetes. *Diabetes Care*. 2017;40(suppl 1):S44-S47.
8. Sattar N, Preiss D, Murray HM, et al. Statins and risk of incident diabetes: a collaborative meta-analysis of randomised statin trials. *Lancet*. 2010;375(9716):735-742.
9. Ridker PM, Danielson D, Fonseca FAH, et al. Rosuvastatin to prevent vascular events in men and women with elevated C-reactive protein. *N Engl J Med*. 2008;359(21):2195-2207.
10. American Diabetes Association. Cardiovascular disease and risk management. *Diabetes Care*. 2017;40(suppl 1):S75-S87.
11. American Diabetes Association. Glycemic targets. *Diabetes Care*. 2017;40(suppl 1): S48-S56.
12. Garber AJ, Abrahamson MJ, Barzilay JI, et al. Consensus statement by the American Association of Clinical Endocrinologists and American College of Endocrinology on the Comprehensive Type 2 Diabetes Management Algorithm. *Endocr Pract*. 2017;23(2):207-238.
13. The Diabetes Control and Complications Trial Research Group. The effect of intensive treatment of diabetes on the development of long-term complications in insulin-dependent diabetes mellitus. *N Engl J Med*. 1993;329:977-986.
14. UK Prospective Diabetes Study (UKPDS) Group. Intensive blood-glucose control with sulphonylureas or insulin compared with conventional treatment and risk of complications in patients with type 2 diabetes (UKPDS 33). *Lancet*. 1998;352(9144):837-853.
15. The Diabetes Control and Complications Trial/Epidemiology of Diabetes Interventions and Complications (DCCT/EDIC) Study Research Group. Intensive diabetes treatment and cardiovascular disease in patients with type 1 diabetes. *N Engl J Med*. 2005;353(25):2643-2653.
16. Holman RP, Paul SK, Bethel MA, Matthews DR, and Neil HA. 10-year follow-up of intensive glucose control in type 2 diabetes. *N Engl J Med*. 2008;359:1577-1589.
17. UK Prospective Diabetes Study (UKPDS) Group. Effect of intensive blood-glucose control with metformin on complications in overweight patients with type 2 diabetes. *Lancet*. 1998;352:854-865.
18. American Diabetes Association. Pharmacologic approaches to glycemic treatment. *Diabetes Care*. 2017;40(suppl 1):S64-S74.
19. CMS. *Medicare Part D Medication Therapy Management Program Standardized Format*. Available at https://www.cms.gov/Medicare/Prescription-Drug-Coverage/PrescriptionDrugCovContra/Downloads/MTM-Program-Standardized-Format-English-and-Spanish-Instructions-Samples-v032712.pdf. Accessed May 11, 2017.
20. American Diabetes Association. Lifestyle management. *Diabetes Care*. 2017; 40(suppl 1):S33-S43.
21. Kaufman FR, ed. *Medical Management of Type 1 Diabetes*. 6th ed. Alexandria, VA: American Diabetes Association; 2012.
22. Natural Medicines [database online]. Somerville, MA: Therapeutic Research Center; 2017. Available at https://naturalmedicines.therapeuticresearch.com/. Accessed May 11, 2017.
23. Inzucchi SE, Bergenstal RM, Buse JB, et al. Management of hyperglycemia in type 2 diabetes, 2015: a patient-centered approach: update to a position statement of the American Diabetes Association and the European Association for the Study of Diabetes. *Diabetes Care*. 2015;38(1):140-149.
24. CMS. 2017 Part C & D Star Ratings Measures. CMS website. Available at https://www.cms.gov/Medicare/Prescription-Drug-Coverage/PrescriptionDrugCovGenIn/Downloads/2017-Measure-List.pdf. Accessed May 12, 2017.

Review Questions

1. Which finding is consistent with a diagnosis of diabetes?
   a. A1c of 6.0%
   b. Fasting plasma glucose of 137 mg/dL
   c. Two-hour plasma glucose of 186 mg/dL
   d. Random blood glucose of 179 mg/dL with polydipsia

2. According to the ADA, which clinical scenario would indicate a need for adjustment of pharmacotherapy in a patient with diabetes mellitus?
   a. A 65-year-old female with average fasting glucose of 127 mg/dL on metformin 1000 mg twice daily
   b. A 45-year-old male taking metformin 1000 mg twice daily and liraglutide 1.2 mg daily with postprandial glucose average of 167 mg/dL
   c. A 40-year-old male taking metformin 500 mg twice daily and home blood pressure values ranging 120-138/70-80 mm Hg
   d. A 50-year-old female taking metformin 1000 mg twice daily with a history of atherosclerotic cardiovascular disease not currently on statin therapy

3. A frail 81-year-old white male patient has a history of type 2 diabetes, hypertension, chronic kidney disease, and mild Alzheimer dementia. What is the most appropriate A1c goal for this patient?
   a. <6.5%
   b. <7%
   c. <8%
   d. <10%

4. Which description **best** explains the mechanism of metformin to a patient using living room language?
   a. A hypoglycemic medication that works by decreasing hepatic gluconeogenesis.
   b. A diabetes medicine that works by reducing the amount of sugar the liver makes.
   c. A diabetes medicine that works by reducing glucose synthesis and increasing peripheral insulin sensitivity.
   d. A diabetes medicine that does not cause hypoglycemia because it does not stimulate release of insulin.

5. All statements are appropriate for inclusion on the medication action plan of a patient with diabetes **EXCEPT**:
   a. Check blood sugar 2 times a day (first thing in the morning and 2 hours after a meal) and write down values.
   b. Notify the provider if 3 sugar readings are over 250 mg/dL or any reading is over 300 mg/dL.
   c. For low blood sugar (≤ 70 mg/dL), eat one-half a cup of ice cream, one-half of a candy bar, or drink one-half of a cup of fruit juice or soda
   d. Bring a log book of sugar readings and meter to the next visit for review.

6. Which finding would indicate the need for emergent referral of a patient with diabetes?
   a. Blood glucose of 300 mg/dL with nausea and vomiting
   b. Nausea after starting exenatide therapy
   c. Blood glucose of 250 mg/dL without symptoms of hyperglycemia
   d. Blood glucose of 50 mg/dL responsive to treatment with glucose tablets

7. A patient with type 2 diabetes and an A1c of 7.8% is started on metformin 500 mg daily and is increased to metformin 500 mg twice daily after 2 weeks. Four months later the A1c is 7.2%. What is the most appropriate categorization of the medication-related problem?
   a. Adverse effect
   b. Dosage too low
   c. Need for additional medication
   d. Ineffective medication

8. A 75-year-old female with type 2 diabetes is being treated with metformin 500 mg twice daily. At a recent visit her A1c was 7.5%. Other labs revealed a fasting glucose of 135 mg/dL and a serum creatinine of 1.7 mg/dL (estimated GFR 29 mL/min/1.73m^2). Which recommendation is **most** appropriate for her metformin therapy?
   a. Continue the current dose of metformin.
   b. Decrease the dose of metformin.
   c. Discontinue the metformin.
   d. Increase the dose of metformin.

9. A 70-year-old female has a history of type 2 diabetes, hypertension, depression, and gastroparesis. Her current A1c is 7.5%, and she is unable to tolerate metformin due to gastrointestinal side effects. Which agent should be avoided for management of this patient's diabetes?
   a. Exenatide
   b. Glipizide
   c. Pioglitazone
   d. Sitagliptin

10. During an MTM session, a patient is counseled about the importance of tight control of blood glucose to reduce the complications of diabetes. Specifically, the patient should be informed that controlling glucose is most likely to reduce which complication of diabetes?
    a. Hypoglycemia
    b. Myocardial infarction
    c. Neuropathy
    d. Stroke

ANSWERS

1. b	2. d	3. c
4. b	5. c	6. a
7. b	8. c	9. a
10. c		

22

Dyslipidemia MTM Data Set

Jason G. Powell, PharmD

KEY POINTS

- Lowering low-density cholesterol to target levels is no longer the primary goal of treatment.
- Patients with dyslipidemia as well as other diseases that put them at risk for atherosclerotic cardiovascular disease should be assessed for the need for treatment.
- Statins are the preferred medications for atherosclerotic cardiovascular disease risk reduction.
- Lifestyle modifications such as a low-fat diet and exercise should be instituted, along with medication for maximal treatment effect.
- Medication therapy management (MTM) providers should emphasize the importance of adherence to medications and the timing of administration to optimize efficacy.
- MTM providers should educate patients regarding the serious adverse effects of cholesterol medications and when to contact the prescriber or seek medical assistance.

INTRODUCTION TO DYSLIPIDEMIA

Cholesterol is a fat-like substance (lipid) that is present in cell membranes and is a precursor of bile acids and steroid hormones. Cholesterol travels in the blood in distinct particles containing both lipid and proteins (lipoproteins). The three major classes of lipoproteins are low-density lipoproteins (LDL), high-density lipoproteins (HDL), and very low-density lipoproteins (VLDL).[1] A major component of VLDL is triglycerides (TG), a storage form of fat. Dyslipidemia may be defined as an elevation in total cholesterol (TC), LDL cholesterol, or triglycerides, a low level of HDL cholesterol, or any combination of these abnormalities. Dyslipidemias, particularly those characterized by elevations in LDL cholesterol, are associated with an increased risk of coronary heart disease (CHD), cerebrovascular disease, and peripheral arterial disease.[1] Other studies have also suggested that low levels of HDL also correspond with an increased risk of cardiovascular disease.

Other Terms Associated with Dyslipidemia

- **Familial hypercholesterolemia**[1] - This term is used for individuals that meet the following three criteria:
  - High TC, TG usually normal
  - Deposition of LDL-derived cholesterol in tendons and arteries (xanthomas, atheromas)
  - Hypercholesterolemia caused by an inherited autosomal trait
- **Hyperlipidemia**[1] - Describes cholesterol abnormalities and simply refers to elevated lipid levels. Dyslipidemia and hyperlipidemia, along with hypercholesterolemia, are often used interchangeably to describe elevated cholesterol levels, even though they each have a unique meaning.
- **Hypertriglyceridemia**[1,2] - A state in which the TG levels are elevated. This can occur alone, or in conjunction with other lipid abnormalities.
- **Primary prevention**[2] - Treatment of dyslipidemia to prevent or delay the onset of atherosclerotic cardiovascular disease (ASCVD).
- **Secondary prevention**[2] - Treatment of dyslipidemia to prevent progression of ASCVD or recurrent ASCVD events.

Dyslipidemia is detected through a fasting lipoprotein profile including TC, LDL cholesterol, HDL cholesterol, and triglycerides. All adults aged ≥20 years should have a fasting lipoprotein profile measured at least every 4 to 6 years according to the American Heart Association (AHA).[2] Individuals should fast for at least 8 to 12 hours before getting blood drawn. If the lipid profile is obtained in the nonfasting state, only total cholesterol and HDL cholesterol will be valid. This is because TG are elevated in the nonfasting state, and the LDL cholesterol is usually a calculated value that will be inaccurate if the TG value is inflated. If the patient was nonfasting, non-HDL cholesterol is at or above 220 mg/dL, or if TG are greater than 500 mg/dL, a follow-up fasting lipoprotein panel should be obtained.[2] Classifications of lipid abnormalities are found in Table 22-1. A thorough review of patient history (Table 22-2)

TABLE 22-1 • Classification of Total-, LDL-, HDL-Cholesterol, and Triglycerides

Total Cholesterol	
<200 mg/dL (<5.17 mmol/L)	Desirable
200-239 mg/dL (5.17-6.20 mmol/L)	Borderline high
≥240 mg/dL (≥6.21 mmol/L)	High
LDL Cholesterol	
<100 mg/dL (<2.59 mmol/L)	Optimal
100-129 mg/dL (2.59-3.5 mmol/L)	Near or above optimal
130-159 mg/dL (3.36-4.13 mmol/L)	Borderline high
160-189 mg/dL (4.14-4.90 mmol/L)	High
≥190 mg/dL (≥4.91 mmol/L)	Very high
HDL Cholesterol	
<40 mg/dL (<1.03 mmol/L)	Low
≥60 mg/dL (≥1.55 mmol/L)	High
Triglycerides	
<150 mg/dL (<1.70 mmol/L)	Normal
150-199 mg/dL (1.70-2.25 mmol/L)	Borderline high
200-499 mg/dL (2.26-5.64 mmol/L)	High
≥500 mg/dL (≥5.65 mmol/L)	Very high

Abbreviations: HDL = high-density lipoprotein; LDL = low-density lipoprotein.

Source: Reproduced, with permission, from DiPiro JT, Talbert RL, Yee GC, Matzke GR, Wells BG, Posey L, eds. *Pharmacotherapy: A Pathophysiologic Approach*. 10th ed. New York, NY: McGraw-Hill; 2017.

TABLE 22-2 • Factors to Use in the Assessment of ASCVD Risk

Factors Used Directly to Calculate ASCVD Risk
Sex – Male or female
Age – 40 to 79 years
Race – African American, Caucasian, Other
Total Cholesterol level (mg/dL)
HDL level (mg/dL)
Systolic blood pressure (mm Hg)
Diastolic blood pressure (mm Hg)
Treatment for hypertension – Yes or No
Diabetes – Yes or No
Smoker – Yes or No
Factors to Consider When Evaluating Risk of ASCVD[a]
Family history of premature ASCVD with onset <55 years of age in a first-degree male relative or <65 years of age in a first-degree female relative
High-sensitivity C-reactive protein >2 mg/L
CAC score ≥300 Agatston units or ≥75 percentile for age, sex, and ethnicity
Ankle-brachial index <0.9

[a] These factors may indicate an increased risk for ASCVD but are not included in the risk calculator. These factors may be used in clinical decision-making when deciding to initiate statin therapy.

Source: References 1, 2, and 3.

should be performed to evaluate for the following: (1) disease states that increase risk of ASCVD, (2) tobacco use, (3) family history of premature cardiovascular disease, (4) secondary causes of lipid abnormalities (Table 22-3), and (4) presence of ASCVD (acute coronary syndromes, or a history of MI, stable or unstable angina, coronary or other arterial revascularization, stroke, Transient ischemic attack (TIA), or peripheral arterial disease presumed to be of atherosclerotic origin).[2] Treatment of secondary causes of dyslipidemia may reduce the need for antihyperlipidemic medications or necessitate a change in drug therapy.[1]

TABLE 22-3 • Secondary Causes of Lipoprotein Abnormalities

Hypercholesterolemia	Hypothyroidism
	Obstructive liver disease
	Nephrotic syndrome
	Anorexia nervosa
	Acute intermittent porphyria
	Drugs: progestins, thiazide diuretics, glucocorticoids, β-blockers, isotretinoin, protease inhibitors, cyclosporine, mirtazapine, sirolimus
Hypertriglyceridemia	Obesity
	Diabetes mellitus
	Lipodystrophy
	Glycogen storage disease
	Ileal bypass surgery
	Sepsis
	Pregnancy
	Acute hepatitis
	Systemic lupus erythematosus
	Monoclonal gammopathy: multiple myeloma, lymphoma
	Drugs: alcohol, estrogens, isotretinoin, β-blockers, glucocorticoids, bile-acid resins, thiazides, asparaginase, interferons, azole antifungals, mirtazapine, anabolic steroids, sirolimus, bexarotene
Hypocholesterolemia	Malnutrition
	Malabsorption
	Myeloproliferative diseases
	Chronic infectious diseases: AIDS, tuberculosis
	Monoclonal gammopathy
	Chronic liver disease
Low HDL	Malnutrition
	Obesity
	Drugs: non-ISA β-blockers, anabolic steroids, probucol, isotretinoin, progestins

Abbreviations: HDL = high-density lipoprotein; ISA = intrinsic sympathomimetic activity.

Source: Reproduced, with permission, from DiPiro JT, Talbert RL, Yee GC, Matzke GR, Wells BG, Posey L, eds. *Pharmacotherapy: A Pathophysiologic Approach*. 10th ed. New York, NY: McGraw-Hill; 2017.

COMPLICATIONS OF DYSLIPIDEMIA

Detection of dyslipidemia and increased risk of developing ASCVD may be delayed if patients fail to attend regular preventative health appointments. Individuals may develop lipid profile abnormalities before experiencing any vascular problems, which often makes this disease state difficult to detect. The development of atherosclerosis is a "silent" process until it reaches a severe level. Diseases such as peripheral vascular disease, cerebrovascular disease, CHD, ischemic heart disease (angina), myocardial infarction, stroke, and other ASCVD complications will develop and become hard to reverse without aggressive intervention, including lifestyle changes, medications, and surgery. Table 22-4 lists potential complications of dyslipidemia. Once medication therapy is initiated, the patient may not "feel" any different but may experience potential adverse effects from the medications, which can lead to adherence issues.

APPROACH TO TREATMENT OF DYSLIPIDEMIA[2]

In 2013, the American College of Cardiology and the American Heart Association (ACC/AHA) released a new clinical guideline on the approach to management of dyslipidemia and, more specifically, how to reduce the risk of ASCVD. This guideline completely changed the clinical approach to dyslipidemia. Rather than target specific LDL cholesterol goals, the primary target of therapy for management of dyslipidemia is prevention of ASCVD events. With this approach, treating to a specific targeted cholesterol level is not recommended. More precisely, the ACC/AHA guidelines focus on reducing the risk of ASCVD through identification of patients that fall into one of four main statin benefit groups. The benefit groups (Table 22-5) include patients with clinical ASCVD (secondary prevention) or patients at significant risk for ASCVD events (primary prevention). The ACC/AHA guidelines also suggest that treatment plans for all patients should include optimization of lifestyle modifications, such as improving diet and increasing exercise.

TABLE 22-4 • Complications of Dyslipidemia

Type of Complication	Examples
Cardiovascular disease	• Angina pectoris • Coronary artery disease • Coronary heart disease • Left ventricular hypertrophy • Heart failure • Myocardial infarction • Sudden death
Cerebrovascular disease	• Cognitive decline • Ischemic stroke • Transient ischemic attack (TIA) • Vascular dementia
Peripheral vascular disease	• Aneurysms (abdominal aortic, thoracic aortic) • Occlusive peripheral arterial disease
Other	• Pancreatitis may occur with very high (>500 mg/dL) triglyceride levels • Nonalcoholic steatohepatitis

Source: References 1 and 2.

Lifestyle Changes[4]

All patients, including those with ASCVD, risk of developing ASCVD, defined dyslipidemia, or even those without any overt risk factors for developing ASCVD should be counseled on appropriate lifestyle modifications to improve health. Recommended lifestyle modifications are provided in Table 22-6.

For patients that do not meet the criteria for defined ASCVD or have LDL cholesterol greater than 190 mg/dL, the risk of developing ASCVD must be estimated. To estimate ASCVD risk, the ACC/AHA guidelines recommend the Pooled Cohort Risk Equation[3,5] (http://tools.acc.org/ASCVD-Risk-Estimator/), which uses criteria similar to the Framingham risk assessment. Risk factors in the ASCVD risk estimator include gender, age, race, total cholesterol levels, HDL cholesterol, systolic blood pressure, treatment for hypertension, diabetes, and smoking status. The pooled cohort risk equation estimates the 10-year risk for developing ASCVD for patients aged 40 to 79, as well as the lifetime risk of developing ASCVD for patients aged 20 to 59. The risk assessment is then used to help determine need for and selection of therapy. Of note, the use of the risk calculator is limited to patients between the ages of 40 and 75 and those with a minimum TC level ≥130 mg/dL. The risk estimator assumes that patients are not currently taking lipid-lowering therapy, ie, lipid levels are baseline. For patients already on statins or other therapies that may alter cholesterol levels, the estimated 10-year risk may be underestimated when compared to those not on lipid-lowering therapies.

Making a Decision on the Statin Intensity[2]

As outlined in Table 22-5, statins are categorized by their ability to lower LDL levels (eg, high-intensity, moderate-intensity). High-intensity statin therapy lowers LDL by at least 50%, and moderate-intensity statin therapy lowers LDL cholesterol by 30% to 50%. The choice of therapy is simple for those in the statin benefit groups of clinical ASCVD or LDL cholesterol levels greater than 190 mg/dL. Both groups require high-intensity statin therapy, assuming they can tolerate such doses. Patients in other statin benefit groups may require either moderate-intensity or high-intensity statin therapy, depending on the 10-year risk for ASCVD. After distinguishing if the patient falls into one of the four statin benefit groups (and calculating the 10-year risk for ASCVD, if needed), the MTM provider needs to determine which statin therapy, if any, is required. In general, it is best to use the lowest dose of statin within the appropriate intensity category to help reduce possible risk of adverse effects. Table 22-7 outlines which statins fall into low-intensity, moderate-intensity, or high-intensity statin categories.

Alternative Goals for Dyslipidemia[2,7]

Patients should be treated with the appropriate intensity statin therapy as outlined in the ACC/AHA guidelines; however, some may be unable to tolerate maximal doses of statin therapy. In this case, the patient should be treated with the maximally tolerated intensity of statin. When treated with high-intensity statin therapy, the LDL cholesterol should drop by at least 50% from baseline. For those who cannot tolerate high-intensity statin therapy, an alternative goal of 30% to 40% reduction may be acceptable. This alternative

TABLE 22-5 • Key Recommendations to Reduce the Risk of ASCVD in Adults

Recommendations	ACC/AHA COR	ACC/AHA LOE
Heart healthy lifestyle for everyone		
Appropriate intensity of statin therapy should be initiated or continued		
1. Clinical ASCVD[a]		
a. Aged <75 years and no safety concerns: high-intensity statin therapy	I	A
b. Aged >75 years or safety concerns: moderate-intensity statin therapy	I	A
2. Primary prevention—Primary LDL ≥190 mg/dL		
a. Rule out secondary causes of dyslipidemia	I	B
b. Aged ≥21 years: high-intensity statin therapy	I	B
c. Achieve at least a 50% reduction in LDL	IIa	B
d. LDL-lowering nonstatin therapy may be considered to further reduce LDL	IIb	C
3. Primary prevention—diabetes 40-75 years of age and LDL 70-189 mg/dL		
a. Moderate-intensity statin therapy	I	A
b. Consider high-intensity statin when ≥7.5% 10-year ASCVD risk using the Pooled Cohort Equations	II	B
4. Primary prevention—no diabetes, 40-75 years of age and LDL 70-189 mg/dL		
a. Estimate 10-year ASCVD risk based on Pooled Cohort Equations in those not receiving a statin; estimate risk every 4-6 years	I	B
b. To determine if statin should be initiated, engage in a clinician-patient discussion concerning risk, adverse reactions, drug interactions, and patient preferences	IIa	C
c. Reemphasize heart-healthy lifestyle and address other risk factors	I	A
i. ≥7.5% 10-year ASCVD risk: moderate or high-intensity statin therapy	I	A
ii. 5%-7.5% 10-year ASCVD risk: consider moderate-intensity statin therapy	IIb	C
iii. Other risk factors may be considered: LDL ≥160 mg/dL, family history of premature ASCVD, hs-CRP ≥2 mg/dL, CAC score ≥300 Agaston units, ABI <0.9 or lifetime risk	IIb	C
5. Primary prevention when LDL <190 mg/dL and aged <40 or >75 years, or <5% 10-year ASCVD risk		
a. Statin therapy may be considered in selected individuals	IIb	C
6. Statin therapy is not routinely recommended for individuals with NYHA Class II-IV heart failure or who are receiving maintenance hemodialysis		

[a] Clinical ASCVD includes nonfatal MI, CHD death, and nonfatal and fatal stroke, TIA or peripheral arterial disease presumed to be of atherosclerotic origin.

Abbreviations: ABI = ankle-brachial index; ACC/AHA = American College of Cardiology/American Heart Association; ASCVD = atherosclerotic cardiovascular disease; CAC = coronary artery calcium; COR = class of recommendation; hsCRP = high-sensitivity C-reactive protein; LDL = low density lipoprotein; LOE = level of evidence; NYHA = New York Heart Association.

Source: Reproduced, with permission, from DiPiro JT, Talbert RL, Yee GC, Matzke GR, Wells BG, Posey L, eds. *Pharmacotherapy: A Pathophysiologic Approach*. 10th ed. New York, NY: McGraw-Hill; 2017.

TABLE 22-6 • Lifestyle Modifications

Recommendations
• Dietary intake should focus on whole grains (25%-35% of total calories), fresh fruits and vegetables, low-fat dairy products, fish, and lean proteins (15% of total calories). • Limit simple carbohydrates, sugary foods, trans fats, and red meats. • Target diet that has <7% of calories from saturated fats. • Consume 20-30 grams of dietary fiber daily and 2 grams of plant sterols. • Physical activity should include aerobic exercise for 30-40 minutes on 3-4 days per week for a total of 150 min/week of moderate exercise or 115 min/week of vigorous exercise.

Source: References 1, 2, and 4.

goal for LDL reduction correlates with LDL cholesterol reductions seen with moderate-intensity statin therapy. Some individuals may also present with extremely elevated TG (>500 mg/dL). For these patients, the focus should be on reduction of TG using both statin and nonstatin therapies to help reduce risk of pancreatitis. The goal is to reduce TG below 500 mg/dL, with the ideal goal of targeting TG below 150 mg/dL.[2,7-8]

CORE ELEMENT 1—COMPREHENSIVE MEDICATION REVIEW FOR PATIENTS WITH DYSLIPIDEMIA

Following is a list of suggested questions to use when conducting a medication therapy review in a patient with dyslipidemia (Table 22-8). The number and types of questions will depend upon

TABLE 22-7 • Intensity of Statin Therapy by Drug and Dose

High-Intensity Statin Therapy	Moderate-Intensity Statin Therapy	Low-Intensity Statin Therapy
Daily dose lowers LDL on average by ≥50% **Atorvastatin (40)-80 mg** **Rosuvstatin 20-**(40) **mg**	Daily dose lowers LDL on average by 30 to <50% **Atorvastatin 10** (20) **mg** **Rosuvastatin** (5)**-20 mg** **Simvastatin 20-40 mg**[a] **Pravastatin 40-**(80) **mg** **Lovastatin 40 mg** Fluvastatin XL 80 mg **Fluvastatin 40 mg BID** Pitavastatin 2-4 mg	Daily dose lowers LDL on average by <30% Simvastatin 10 mg **Pravastatin 10-20 mg** **Lovastatin 20 mg** Fluvastatin 20-40 mg Pitavastatin 1 mg

[a] Simvastatin is not recommended by the FDA to be started at 80 mg/day due to increased risk of myopathy and, rarely, rhabdomyolysis.

Note: Boldface type indicates specific statins that have been tested in RCT.

Abbreviations: FDA = Food and Drug Administration; RCT = randomized clinical trials.

Source: Reproduced, with permission, from DiPiro JT, Talbert RL, Yee GC, Matzke GR, Wells BG, Posey L, eds. *Pharmacotherapy: A Pathophysiologic Approach*. 10th ed. New York, NY: McGraw-Hill; 2017.

TABLE 22-8 • Questions to Ask When Conducting a Medication Review in a Patient with Dyslipidemia

Suggested Questions for the Patient with Dyslipidemia

- How long have you had high cholesterol? When were you diagnosed?
- Who else in your family has high cholesterol?
- What do you know about the risks of high cholesterol?
- When was the last time your physician talked to you about your cholesterol levels?
- Do you have any history of cardiovascular (heart) disease?
  - Have you ever suffered from a heart attack?
  - Have you been told by your physician you have angina or are you taking nitroglycerin for chest pain?
  - Has your physician told you that you have coronary artery disease or have you ever had a stent placed or bypass surgery?
  - Do you have peripheral artery disease or peripheral vascular disease?
- Have you ever suffered from a stroke/TIA?
- Have you been told you have a problem with your blood sugars or told you have diabetes?
  - Do you have a family history of diabetes?
- Are you currently or have you ever used tobacco products?
  - What risks are associated with using tobacco products and high cholesterol?
- Do you have a history of high blood pressure?
  - What medications are you taking to help control your blood pressure?
  - How often do you check your blood pressure?
  - What numbers do you see when you do check your blood pressure?
- Who in your family, if anyone, has had a history of heart disease?
  - How old was your family member when they were diagnosed or passed away from this?
- According to your physician, what is the goal for treating your cholesterol?
- Why is your physician treating your cholesterol?
  - Do you have a condition that makes your body produce more cholesterol?
  - Have you been told your triglycerides are elevated? How high were they?
- What medications do you take for your cholesterol? How do you take them? How long have you been on this/these medication(s)?
- What side effects, if any, are you experiencing from your cholesterol medication(s)?
- How often do you miss a dose of your cholesterol medication(s)?
- What other medications have you taken in the past for your cholesterol?
- Have you ever stopped taking any of your prescribed cholesterol medications without telling your physician? If so, why?
- What over-the-counter medications or herbals do you use for your cholesterol?
- Other than medicines, what have you tried to lower your cholesterol (eg, lifestyle changes)?
- Has your physician recommended making changes in your diet to help control your cholesterol? If so, what did they discuss with you? What changes have you made?
- What exercise regimen do you follow?
- What has your physician discussed with you regarding over-the-counter medications that you should avoid because they interact with your medications for cholesterol?
- When starting a new medication, herbal supplement or over-the-counter medication do you discuss it with your physician or pharmacist?

Questions to Ask for Prevention/Assessment of Medical Emergencies

- Crisis planning: What are the warning signs of a heart attack and stroke, and what is your action plan?
- Have you fallen, felt dizzy, had blurred vision, sudden memory lapses, or one-sided weakness?
- Have you had any sudden abdominal pain, muscle pain/weakness, or changes to your urine?
- Do you live by yourself? If not, does the person you live with know what the signs/symptoms of a heart attack or stroke are?

several factors, including the amount of time for the interview, number of concurrent MRPs, urgency of MRPs, and the reliability of the patient in providing accurate information, among others. In time-limited interactions or in complex cases with multiple medical issues, the MTM provider may choose to target questions that help to identify or rule out issues of an urgent nature (see questions to ask for prevention/assessment of medical emergencies). MTM providers should remember to use living room language during the interview (Figure 22-1) and be prepared for questions that patients may ask regarding dyslipidemia (Table 22-9).

Abdominal aortic aneurysm—widening or ballooning of the large blood vessel that supplies blood to the gut, hip area, and legs that happens because of weakness in the wall of the blood vessel. This may cause the blood vessel to burst and cut off blood flow to areas of the body.

Acute coronary syndrome—term used to cover any symptoms caused by decreased blood flow to the heart, such as a heart attack or chest pain.

Adverse event—something bad that happens, bad reaction, unexplained or unwanted effects.

ALT—alanine aminotransferase; enzyme found in liver; a blood test that can tell if there is liver damage.

Angina—chest pain or discomfort caused by decreased blood flow through the heart, which could be a sign of heart attack.

Arteries—blood vessels that carry blood away from the heart.

AST—aspartate aminotransferase; enzyme found in the liver; a blood test that can tell if there is liver damage.

Atherosclerosis—hardening or clogging of the arteries due to a buildup of fatty material; this could lead to decreased blood flow to important areas of the body and may cause a heart attack.

Atherosclerotic cardiovascular disease (ASCVD)—a disease that results from a hardening or clogging of your arteries/blood vessels due to cholesterol.

Blood glucose—blood sugar. If you have high blood cholesterol your physician will check your blood sugar to be sure you do not also have diabetes, as the two conditions are often seen together.

BMI—body mass index; a measure of weight in relation to height that assigns people to a weight class of underweight, normal weight, overweight, or obese based on their amount of excess weight.

Carbohydrates—one of the main types of nutrients, can be simple or complex. Simple carbohydrates include sugars found naturally in foods such as fruits, vegetables, milk, and milk products. They also include sugars added during food processing and refining. Complex carbohydrates include whole grain breads and cereals, starchy vegetables and beans.

Cardiac—related to the heart.

Cardiologist—heart physician.

Cholesterol—a naturally occurring substance made in the body and found in food which is used by body. Too much cholesterol can lead to health problems.

Chronic—constant, never ending, does not go away.

CK (creatine kinase)—marker found in the blood to help determine if there is muscle damage. This is often completed before starting certain cholesterol medications and also to help determine if patient is experiencing a side effect from cholesterol medications.

Coronary artery disease—narrowing and hardening of the small blood vessels that supply blood and oxygen to the heart because of a buildup of cholesterol, which may lead to a heart attack and is the leading cause of death worldwide.

Creatinine—a test that checks how well the kidneys are working; an increase means the kidneys are not working as well.

Diabetes—a condition in which your blood sugar is too high and you may require medication to keep the sugar in your blood under control.

Elevate—raise, make higher.

Fasting lipid panel—a test of the fats in your blood taken after 8-12 hours without eating any food, because the test results can change depending on what you eat.

Fiber—found in fruits, vegetables and grains. It is the part of the plant that your body can't digest. It is an important part of a healthy diet. It adds bulk to your diet and makes you feel full faster, helping you control your weight and can help lower cholesterol.

Fibrate—class of medication used to reduce triglycerides. They work by increasing the breakdown of triglycerides in the body.

HDL (high-density lipoprotein)—this is considered your "good cholesterol" which helps to prevent heart disease. This is the only cholesterol marker you want to stay "high."

Hepatic—related to the liver.

Hypertension—high blood pressure; high blood pressure increases the chance of heart attack, stroke, and kidney disease.

LDL (low-density lipoprotein)—this is considered the "bad cholesterol" and the most important cholesterol marker to control.

LFTs (liver function tests)—blood work used to determine if your liver is damaged or inflamed.

Lifestyle changes—your physician may have recommended changes in lifestyle to lower your cholesterol, which for some patients include reaching a goal weight, eating healthy, decreasing the amount of alcohol you consume, exercising, or quitting smoking.

Lipid panel—blood work that looks at cholesterol in the body and reports the amount of different components (LDL, HDL, TG, total cholesterol).

Monounsaturated fat—sometimes referred to as "good" fats; eating in moderation can reduce bad cholesterol levels; found in vegetable oils such as olive oil, canola oil, peanut oil, sunflower oil and sesame oil. Other sources include avocados, peanut butter, and many nuts and seeds.

Myalgia—muscle pain.

Myocardial infarction—(MI) heart attack, damage to the heart.

Myocardial ischemia—when the heart does not get enough oxygen/blood.

Myoglobinuria—myoglobin, a breakdown product of muscle, in the urine.

Myopathy—a potential side effect with statin medications; you may have muscle pain (myalgia), weakness, or cramps.

Obese—having a body mass index (BMI) over 30, which increases your risk of having high blood pressure, diabetes, and cardiovascular disease.

Omega-3—"fish oils" used to help reduce triglycerides.

Overweight—having a body mass index (BMI) over 25, which increases your risk of having high blood pressure, diabetes, and cardiovascular disease.

Pancreatitis—inflammation of the pancreas. Presents as upper belly pain, and nausea/vomiting.

PCSK9 inhibitor—injectable medication (shot) used to treat cholesterol.

Peripheral arterial disease—a type of peripheral vascular disease; decreased blood flow to the arms and legs caused by clogged arteries; pain when walking that goes away with rest is the most common symptom.

Peripheral vascular disease—decreased blood flow from the arms and legs caused by clogged arteries or veins; term often used when talking about peripheral arterial disease.

Plant stanols or sterols—substances found in plants that help block the absorption of cholesterol. Margarines, orange juice and yogurt drinks with added plant sterols can help reduce LDL cholesterol.

Plaque—a build-up of cholesterol and other things found in the blood which start to block blood vessels.

Polyunsaturated fat—sometimes referred to as "good" fats; eating in moderation can reduce bad cholesterol levels; found in vegetable oils, including soybean oil, corn oil and safflower oil, as well as fatty fish such as salmon,

FIGURE 22-1 Living room language for dyslipidemia.

mackerel, herring and trout. Other sources include some nuts and seeds such as walnuts and sunflower seeds.

Pooled Cohort Risk Assessment Equation—tool used to help determine your individual risk of developing diseases caused by a buildup of cholesterol, such as heart attacks and strokes.

Protein—a main type of nutrient that helps to build and maintain bones, muscles, and skin. You get proteins in your diet from meat, dairy products, nuts and certain grains and beans.

Rhabdomyolysis—a severe condition where the muscles are breaking down. You may have muscle weakness and pain, along with breakdown products of muscle in the urine (*myoglobinuria*), which may look like cola-colored urine.

Saturated fat—a type of fat that is usually solid at room temperature, found in animal meats, dairy, baked goods, and fried foods. Eating too much saturated fat can raise cholesterol levels. Sometimes called "bad" fats.

Smoking cessation—quitting smoking, which can lower your chance of heart disease.

Statin—class of medications commonly used to treat elevated cholesterol levels (eg, pravastatin, lovastatin, and simvastatin).

Stroke—a condition caused by bleeding or lack of blood in the brain, which may cause a loss of speech, memory, or other abilities.

TG—triglycerides; type of fat (lipid) found in your blood. When you eat, your body converts any calories it does not need to use right away into triglycerides. The triglycerides are stored in your fat cells. Later, hormones release triglycerides for energy between meals. If you regularly eat more calories than you burn, particularly "easy" calories like carbohydrates and fats, you may have high triglycerides.

TIA (transient ischemic attack)—occurs when the brain does not get enough blood/oxygen, most likely due to a blockage in a blood vessel that brings blood/oxygen to the brain.

Total cholesterol—This is the complete amount of cholesterol in the body, which is comprised of 20%-30% HDL, 60%-70% LDL, and 10%-15% TG.

Trans fat—a bad type of fat found in processed foods. Another name for trans fats is "partially hydrogenated oils." Trans fats raise your bad (LDL) cholesterol levels and lower your good (HDL) cholesterol levels. Found in many prepared foods such as baked goods, cookies, and fried foods.

Unstable angina—pain or a feeling of pressure on the chest, which is a medical emergency and may lead to a heart attack.

Veins—blood vessels that carry blood toward the heart.

FIGURE 22-1 (*Continued*)

TABLE 22-9 • Questions to Anticipate Regarding Dyslipidemia

Questions Commonly Asked by Patients
• **What is cholesterol?** Cholesterol is a fatty-type substance in the body. It is needed for the development of new cells in the body. The components that make up cholesterol are measured in mg/dL.
• **What is high cholesterol?** When the healthcare provider says your cholesterol is high, this means that you have more cholesterol in your body than you need. The extra amount of cholesterol can clog up your blood vessels and increase your risk of heart disease.
• **What causes high cholesterol?** A variety of conditions can cause high cholesterol. Eating foods high in fats and cholesterol, not being active, or being overweight can lead to high cholesterol. There are also other medical conditions that could lead to high cholesterol. Some things you cannot control can also lead to high cholesterol, like getting older and genetics.
• **What health problems are associated with high cholesterol?** There are many problems. Plaque or fatty material may build up on blood vessel walls. Stroke, heart attacks, and early death may result from high cholesterol.
• **How do I know if I have high cholesterol?** High cholesterol often has no symptoms until it becomes a major problem. For this reason, you usually do not feel it. Having your cholesterol checked by a healthcare provider is a good way to see if your numbers are high.
• **Why am I taking a cholesterol medication when my cholesterol is not that high?** Cholesterol is not the only risk factor for developing heart disease and stroke. If you have already had a heart attack or stroke, or have risk factors for having one, such as, diabetes, hypertension, elevated age, tobacco use, etc, you may be placed on cholesterol medication. Statin medications have been shown to help reduce your risk of having a heart attack or stroke, even if your cholesterol is not high.
• **Why are cholesterol medications so important?** It is important to keep your cholesterol low so that you can stay healthy. People with high cholesterol are more likely to be sent to the hospital, have strokes, heart attacks, heart failure, kidney failure, or other health issues.
• **I can't tell when my cholesterol is high. Can I just stop my medications if I feel okay?** Cholesterol medicines do not correct your levels permanently, so you have to continue taking the medications that were prescribed for you by your physician. It is extremely important that you continue taking your cholesterol medications to prevent future problems, such as heart attack and stroke, among many others.
• **I have been having muscle pain. Could this be from my cholesterol medication?** Muscle pain can be a side effect of certain cholesterol medications, most commonly statins. It can start soon after beginning these medications and usually happens on both sides of the body and in large muscle groups like your thigh and leg muscles. Muscle pain can also happen with increased physical activity or with other health conditions. It is important to discuss this with your physician so they can determine if the muscle pain is from your medication or another cause.
• **What can happen if I stop taking my cholesterol medications?** A heart attack, stroke, and other serious health conditions can arise. Plaque may grow in your blood vessels and lead to further problems in the future.
• **What should I do if I have a problem with my cholesterol medications?** Never stop taking your cholesterol medications without first talking to your healthcare provider. Speak with your physician and/or pharmacist to let them know about any problems you are having and together you can make sure your cholesterol medications are the right ones for you.

CORE ELEMENT 2—PERSONAL MEDICATION LIST[9]

The following is a sample personal medication list (PML) for a patient with dyslipidemia (Figure 22-2). This example is representative only of antihyperlipidemic medications. Additional medications for other disease states should be added and listed separately. MTM providers should remember to use plain language when creating the PML.

CORE ELEMENT 3—MEDICATION ACTION PLAN[9]

The following is a sample medication action plan (MAP) for a patient with dyslipidemia (Figure 22-3). This example is representative only of action steps for a patient with dyslipidemia. MAPs for other disease states or other MRPs should be added and listed separately. In general, only a few of the most important action steps should be listed, so as not to overwhelm the patient. Other areas for patient self-management can be addressed at later visits. MTM providers should remember to use plain language when creating the MAP.

CORE ELEMENT 4—INTERVENTION AND/OR REFERRAL

Interventions for management of dyslipidemia should always include lifestyle modifications. Patients not adequately controlled with lifestyle modifications should be started on drug therapy. Medications should be selected based on treatment goals, other disease states, and concurrent medications. Patients should be encouraged to follow up with their healthcare provider at regular intervals to assess therapy needs. Table 22-10 summarizes dietary

PERSONAL MEDICATION LIST FOR *<Insert Patient's name*, DOB: *mm/dd/yyyy>*	
Medication: Lipitor (atorvastatin) 20 mg tablet	
How I use it: Take one tablet (20 mg) every evening	
Why I use it: High cholesterol	**Prescriber:** Smith
Date I started using it: 1/6/2017	**Date I stopped using it:** *(Leave blank for patient's notes)*
Why I stopped using it: *(Leave blank for patient's notes)*	
Medication: Tricor (fenofibrate) 145 mg tablet	
How I use it: Take one tablet (145 mg) every morning	
Why I use it: High triglycerides (fats in the blood)	**Prescriber:** Smith
Date I started using it: 3/4/2017	**Date I stopped using it:** *(Leave blank for patient's notes)*
Why I stopped using it: *(Leave blank for patient's notes)*	

FIGURE 22-2 Example personal medication list for dyslipidemia medications.

	DATE PREPARED: *<Insert date>*
What we talked about: You have trouble remembering to take your cholesterol medication (rosuvastatin). It is important for you to take this medication every day to lower your cholesterol levels and to help prevent the risk of heart disease in the future.	
What I need to do: Here are some things I can do to help remember to take my rosuvastatin: • It is best if I take cholesterol medication before I go to bed, but if I can't remember it, try moving it to earlier in the day, like supper time. • Use a pillbox to help organize my medications. • Set an alarm on my watch or phone to help me remember to take this medication. • Create a medication calendar where I can check off if I took a dose.	**What I did and when I did it:** *(Leave blank for patient's notes)*
What we talked about: Need to improve diet and physical activity to help lower cholesterol levels	
What I need to do: • Limit intake of saturated fats (examples include high fat dairy products like whole milk, cheeses, butter, and cream and high fat meats) to less than 7% of total calories. • Limit intake of cholesterol to less than 200 mg per day. • Choose more fruits and vegetables • Increase fiber intake by choosing whole grain starches. • Increase my physical activity. Try walking for 30 minutes 5 times per week after dinner.	**What I did and when I did it:** *(Leave blank for patient's notes)*

FIGURE 22-3 Example medication action plan for a patient with dyslipidemia.

TABLE 22-10 • Macronutrient Recommendations for the TLC Diet

Component[a]	Recommended Intake
Total fat	25%-35% of total calories
Saturated fat	<7% of total calories
Polyunsaturated fat	Up to 10% of total calories
Monounsaturated fat	Up to 20% of total calories
Carbohydrates[b]	50%-60% of total calories
Cholesterol	<200 mg per day
Dietary fiber	20-30 grams per day
Plant sterols	2 grams per day
Protein	Approximately 15% of total calories
Total calories	To achieve and maintain desirable body weight

[a] Calories from alcohol not included.

[b] Carbohydrates should derive from foods rich in complex carbohydrates such as whole grains, fruits, and vegetables.

Abbreviation: TLC = therapeutic lifestyle changes.

Source: Reproduced, with permission, from DiPiro JT, Talbert RL, Yee GC, Matzke GR, Wells BG, Posey L, eds. *Pharmacotherapy: A Pathophysiologic Approach.* 10th ed. New York, NY: McGraw-Hill; 2017.

modifications for patients with dyslipidemia. Physical activity should also be recommended, along with dietary modification. Physical activity recommendations include 150 minutes per week, eg, 30 to 40 minutes of moderate aerobic activity such as brisk walking 3 to 5 days a week.[2,4] Table 22-11 provides an overview of medications used for the treatment of dyslipidemia. A treatment algorithm for dyslipidemia and criteria for referral for management of dyslipidemia are found in Figures 22-4 and 22-5, respectively. In addition, Table 22-12 outlines herbal remedies that may be useful in the management of dyslipidemia.

TABLE 22-11 • Medications Used in the Treatment of Dyslipidemia

Medication Class and Example Drugs	Common/Serious Side Effects[a]	Blackbox Warnings/ Contraindications	Pregnancy Category[b]
HMG-CoA reductase inhibitors (statins) atorvastatin fluvastatin lovastatin pitavastatin pravastatin rosuvastatin simvastatin[c]	Headache Myalgias Myopathy Rhabdomyolysis	• Absolute CI Breastfeeding Cholestasis Pregnancy Hepatic disease Hepatic encephalopathy Hepatitis Jaundice Rhabdomyolysis	X
Bile acid sequestrants cholestyramine colesevelam colestipol	Constipation GI obstruction Hypoprothrombinemia	• Absolute CI GI obstruction Hypertriglyceridemia Pancreatitis Biliary obstruction (colestipol)	B - colesevelam C - others
Cholesterol absorption inhibitor ezetimibe	Myalgia (if taken with statins) Fatigue Diarrhea	• None	C
PCSK9 inhibitors alirocumab evolocumab	Pharyngitis Diarrhea Myalgia Injection site reaction Infection	• Breastfeeding • Pregnancy	No human data available
Microsomal transfer protein (MTP) inhibitor lomitapide	Abdominal pain Diarrhea Dyspepsia Vomiting Nausea	• Absolute CI Hepatic disease Pregnancy Requires experienced clinician	X
Apolipoprotein B (apo B) synthesis inhibitor mipomersen	Antibody formation Erythema Influenza Injection site reaction Angioedema Glomerulonephritis	• Absolute CI Hepatic disease	B
Fibric acid derivatives fenofibrate gemfibrozil	Dyspepsia Nausea Vomiting Diarrhea Abdominal pain Myopathy Elevated LFTs	• Absolute CI Biliary cirrhosis Hepatic disease Renal failure Fenofibrate: Breastfeeding Dialysis Gallbladder disease	C

(*Continued*)

TABLE 22-11 • Medications Used in the Treatment of Dyslipidemia (*Continued*)

Medication Class and Example Drugs	Common/Serious Side Effects[a]	Blackbox Warnings/ Contraindications	Pregnancy Category[b]
Niacin niacin OTC niacin Rx	Flushing Hyperglycemia Hyperuricemia Nausea Hypophosphatemia Decreased platelets	• Absolute CI Bleeding Hepatic disease	C
Omega-3 fatty acids fish oil OTC fish oil Rx icosapent ethyl	Halitosis (fishy breath) Fishy belches Reoccurrence of atrial fibrillation	• None	C

[a] This is a general list and does not include all side effects that can occur from these drugs. Consult a drug reference source for a more inclusive list before making any recommendations. MTM providers should also consult a comprehensive drug interaction database before making pharmacotherapy recommendations.

[b] Product labeling for all prescription drugs is being updated to reflect the new FDA Pregnancy Labeling and Lactation Rule. Please check individual product labeling for the most accurate and updated pregnancy information.

[c] Simvastatin has many important drug interactions and dose limitations. Review additional information at http://www.fda.gov/Drugs/DrugSafety/ucm256581.htm

Abbreviations: CI = contraindications; GI = gastrointestinal; HMG-CoA = 3-hydroxy-3-methyl-glutaryl-coenzyme A; PCSK9 = proprotein convertase subtilisin kexin type 9; OTC = over-the-counter.

Source: References 1, 2, 3, 4, and 10.

TABLE 22-12 • Herbal Supplements for Dyslipidemia

Herbal Supplement	Recommended Dosage	Level of Effectiveness[a]	Cost[b]
Fish oil	2 to 4 grams of EPA + DHA daily	Effective (hypertriglyceridemia)	$$
Barley	Oil: 1.5 grams BID Extract: 1.5-2.5 grams BID	Likely effective	$$
Red yeast rice	1.2 grams BID	Likely effective	$$
Flaxseed	Liquid: 7 grams (15 mL) daily Oil caps: 1-2 grams daily Powder: 50 grams daily dissolved in water	Possibly effective	$
Garlic (Allium sativum)	600-900 mg caps daily 2-5 grams (1-2 cloves) of fresh garlic daily	Possibly effective	$
Soy	20-106 grams daily	Possibly effective	$$
Chitosan	1-6 grams daily	Insufficient evidence	$$
Krill oil	1-3 grams daily	Insufficient evidence	$$$
Plant stanols and sterols	2 grams daily	Insufficient evidence	$
Policosanol	5-40 mg daily	Insufficient evidence	$$

[a] Level of evidence. Likely effective: This product has a very high level of reliable clinical evidence supporting its use for a specific indication. Products rated "likely effective" are generally considered appropriate to recommend. Possibly effective: This product has some clinical evidence supporting its use for a specific indication; however, the evidence is limited by quantity, quality, or contradictory findings. Products rated "possibly effective" might be beneficial, but do not have enough high-quality evidence to recommend for most people. Insufficient evidence: There is not enough reliable scientific evidence to provide an effectiveness rating.

[b] Cost of a month supply of recommended dosage: $ = $10 or less; $$ = $11-$20 per month; $$$ = $21-$50 per month; $$$$ = >$50.

Source: Reference 11.

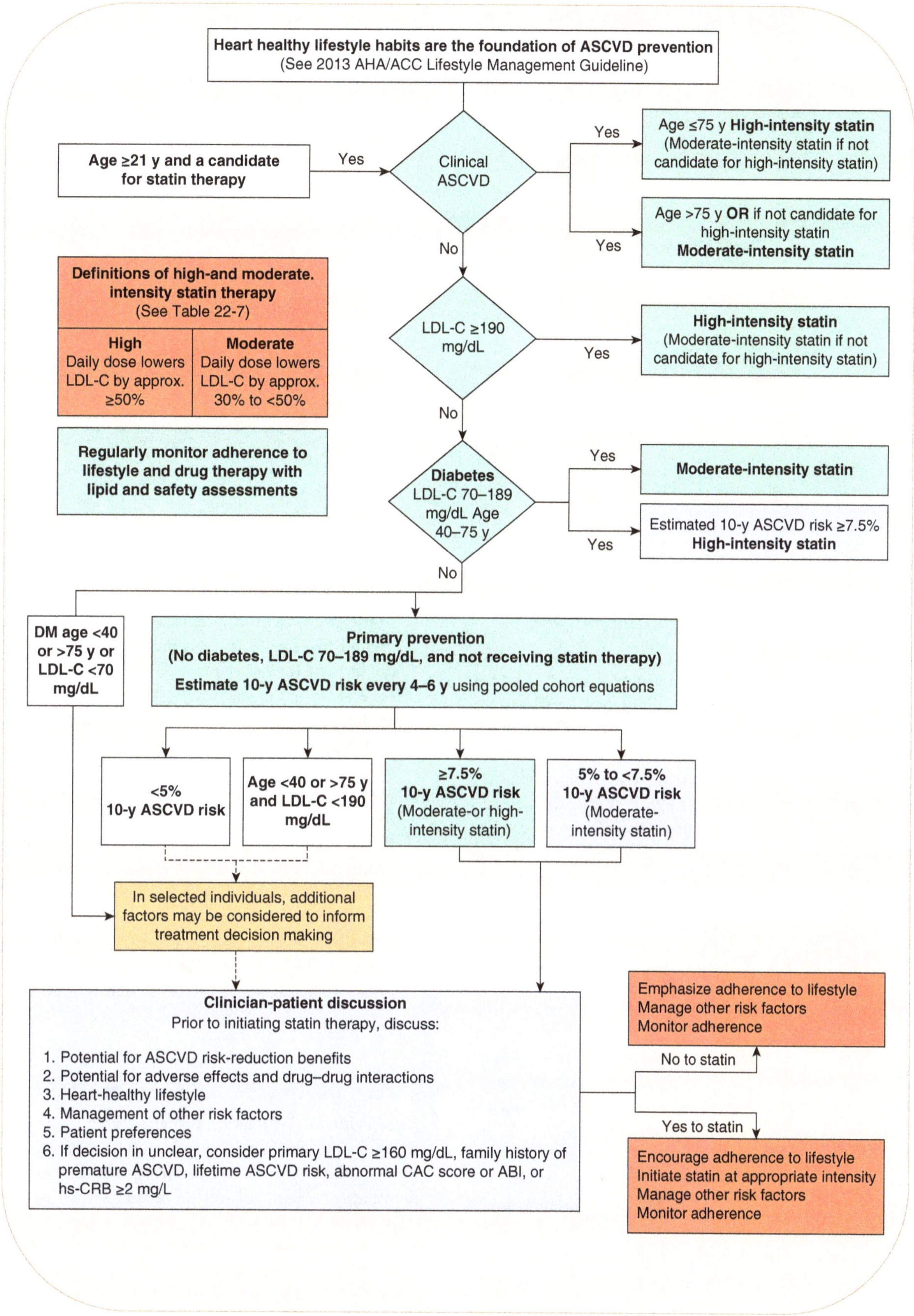

FIGURE 22-4 Statin initiation for management of dyslipidemia.[2]

Source: Reproduced, with permission, from DiPiro JT, Talbert RL, Yee GC, Matzke GR, Wells BG, Posey L, eds. *Pharmacotherapy: A Pathophysiologic Approach*. 10th ed. New York, NY: McGraw-Hill; 2017.

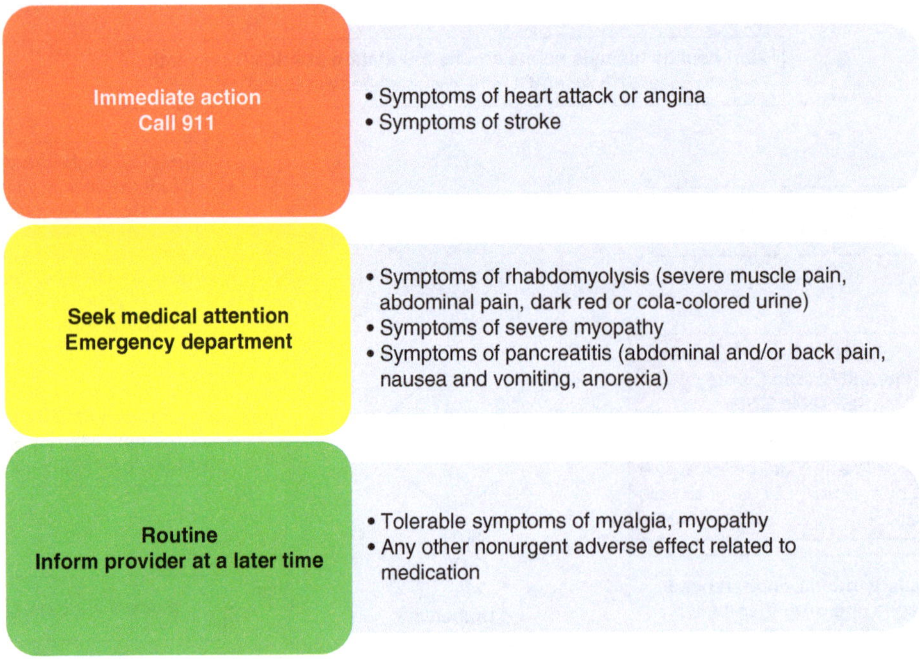

FIGURE 22-5 Referral for management of dyslipidemia.

Selection of Drug Therapy for Dyslipidemia[2,6,10-19]

Clinical guidelines from the ACC/AHA, American Association of Clinical Endocrinologists, and American Diabetes Association have all moved away from recommendations of lowering cholesterol to certain target goals to treatment focused on ASCVD risk reduction. These evidence-based guidelines all recommend that treatment should start with a statin unless there is a contraindication to statin therapy (Figure 22-4). Other lipid-lowering therapies are second- or third-line options after statin therapy. Some compelling indications that may warrant the use of an alternative therapy include intolerance to multiple statins, inadequate response to statin therapy, or highly elevated triglycerides (>500 mg/dL). The lipid-lowering effects of both statins and other therapies for dyslipidemia can be found in Table 22-13.

Monitoring after initiation of statin therapy

- Due to the risk of myalgias with statin use, baseline creatine kinase (CK) levels should be measured prior to starting therapy and then in those who develop myalgias with statin therapy to assess potential muscle damage.[2,7] For patients who develop myalgias, the following recommendations apply:
    - If CK levels are greater than 10 times the upper limit of normal (ULN) or signs/symptoms of rhabdomyolysis are present, statin therapy should be discontinued. CK levels should then be measured after stopping statin to ensure levels have declined to baseline. A trial with a lower intensity statin therapy may be attempted or alternative lipid lowering agents may be used.[2]
    - If muscle symptoms are tolerable and CK elevations are mild (<10 times ULN), statin therapy can be continued at the same dose or reduced, using muscle-related symptoms as a guide.[2]
    - In patients who develop muscle symptoms, an evaluation of thyroid function is recommended because hypothyroidism can increase the risk of myopathies and myalgias.[2]
    - An evaluation for exacerbating factors should be conducted, such as drug or food interactions that reduce statin metabolism, eg, grapefruit juice consumption. MTM providers also need to evaluate the use of OTC herbal remedies such as red yeast rice, which contains lovastatin and may increase risk of myopathies.
    - If muscle symptoms are intolerable, the statin should be discontinued regardless of CK levels until the patient is asymptomatic. Once the patient is asymptomatic, the same statin can then be restarted at the same dose to test the reproducibility of symptoms. Alternatively, the statin can be started at a lower dose with or without other lipid-lowering medications, or another statin can be used instead of the offending agent.

Nonstatin Treatment Considerations[1-2,4,7,14-15]

- In individuals with severe or very severe triglyceride elevations (>500 mg/dL), lifestyle modifications in addition to drug therapy aimed at lowering serum triglycerides (eg, fenofibrate, niacin, fish oil) is recommended to reduce risk of pancreatitis.
- For individuals that have suboptimal response to statin therapy (eg, <50% reduction in LDL with high-intensity statins or <30% to 50% reduction in LDL with moderate-intensity statin therapy) adjustments may be needed.
    - First confirm adherence with the statin therapy. If adherence seems appropriate, then intensify statin therapy if possible and tolerated by the patient.

TABLE 22-13 • Effects of Drug Therapy on Lipids and Lipoproteins

Drug	Mechanism of Action	Effects on Lipids	Effects on Lipoproteins	Comment
Cholestyramine, colestipol, and colesevelam	↑ LDL catabolism Cholesterol ↓ absorption	↓ Cholesterol	↓ LDL ↑ VLDL	Problem with compliance; binds many coadministered acidic drugs
Niacin	↓ LDL and VLDL ↓ synthesis	↓ Triglyceride and ↓ cholesterol	↓ VLDL, ↓ LDL, ↑ HDL	Problems with patient acceptance; good in combination with bile acid resins; extended release niacin causes less flushing and is less hepatotoxic than sustained release
Gemfibrozil, fenofibrate, clofibrate	↑ VLDL clearance ↓ VLDL synthesis	↓ Triglyceride and cholesterol	↓ VLDL, ↓ LDL, ↑ HDL	Clofibrate causes cholesterol gall stones; modest LDL lowering; raises HDL; gemfibrozil inhibits glucuronidation of simvastatin, lovastatin, and atorvastatin
Lovastatin, pravastatin, simvastatin, fluvastatin, atorvastatin, rosuvastatin	↑ LDL catabolism; inhibit LDL synthesis	↓ Cholesterol	↓ LDL	Highly effective in heterozygous familial hypercholesterolemia and in combination with other agents
Ezetimibe	Blocks cholesterol absorption across the intestinal border	↓ Cholesterol	↓ LDL	Few adverse effects; effects additive to other drugs
Mipomersen	Inhibitor of Apolipoprotein B-100	↓ Cholesterol, LDL, non-HDL	↓ LDL, non-HDL	Increase in transaminases, risk of hepatosteatosis and hepatotoxicity; must be given by SQ injection. Only indicated for familial hypercholesterolemia. To be used along with other lipid lowering therapies (statins)
Lomitapide	Microsomal triglyceride transfer protein inhibitor	↓ Cholesterol	↓ LDL, non-HDL	Hepatotoxicity must be monitored via Juxtapid Risk Evaluation and Mitigation Strategy program; only indicated for familial hypercholesterolemia; to be used along with other lipid lowering therapies (statins)
Alirocumab Evolocumab	PCSK9 inhibitor	↓ Cholesterol, ↓ Lpa	↓ Cholesterol and LDL	Given by SQ injection, injection site pain, low risk of hepatoxicity

Abbreviations: HDL = high-density lipoprotein; LDL = low-density lipoprotein; Lpa = lipoprotein A; PCSK9 = proprotein convertase subtilisin kexin type 9; SQ = subcutaneous; VLDL = very low-density lipoprotein.

Source: Reproduced, with permission, from DiPiro JT, Talbert RL, Yee GC, Matzke GR, Wells BG, Posey L, eds. *Pharmacotherapy: A Pathophysiologic Approach*. 10th ed. New York, NY: McGraw-Hill; 2017.

- If patient is fully adherent and on maximum tolerated dose of high-intensity statin therapy without a greater than 50% reduction in LDL from baseline, the use of additional cholesterol lowering medications such as ezetimibe may be considered.[2,19,20]
- The use of a new class of medications, proprotein convertase subtilisin/kexin type 9 (PCSK9) inhibitors, may also be considered. These injectable medications have shown great reduction in LDL cholesterol and a recent study demonstrated a reduction in CV events when added to statin therapy; however, this study found no reduction in deaths.[21] Since data is still limited and the cost of these agents is very high, they should be used in select populations who are intolerant or fail to respond to statin therapy.

- Use of nonstatin therapies in addition to statins, other than those discussed previously, has shown very little benefit in reducing morbidity and mortality and typically should not be recommended in the absence of a compelling indication such as triglycerides over 500 mg/dL.

CORE ELEMENT 5—DOCUMENTATION AND FOLLOW-UP

Clear and succinct documentation of MRPs and recommendations is a key component of the MTM consult. Examples of potential MRPs in patients with dyslipidemia are provided in Table 22-14. Sample communications and recommendations to providers to address medication-related issues are found in Figure 22-6.

TABLE 22-14 • Medication-Related Problems (MRPs) in Patients With Dyslipidemia

Category of MRP	Example Medication-Related Problem
Nonadherence	• Suboptimal control of dyslipidemia due to nonadherence with lifestyle modifications (eg, restriction of dietary fats, physical activity) • Suboptimal control of dyslipidemia due to patient missing doses of antihyperlipidemic medication • Patient unable to afford currently prescribed medication(s)
Unnecessary medication	• Duplicate therapy (eg, two statins) • Multiple therapies may not be needed; current therapy may increase potential adverse effects with little benefit
Need for additional medication	• Desired reduction in LDL not achieved despite appropriate statin therapy
Ineffective medication	• Maximal dose of a statin without achieving appropriate LDL reduction • Statin monotherapy in patients with severe or very severe elevations (>1000 mg/dL) in triglycerides
Dosage too low	• Based on medical history, patient requires an increase in statin intensity • Based on 10-year risk for developing ASCVD, patient requires increase in statin intensity
Dosage too high	• Patient on medication that increases risk of adverse effects with simvastatin • Patient with renal impairment on rosuvastatin not adjusted for renal function
Adverse drug event	• Myalgias, myopathy, or rhabdomyolysis with statin therapy or other lipid-lowering therapies • Patient not taking niacin due to flushing (may also be classified as nonadherence) • Significant elevations in liver enzymes with statin therapy (eg, 3 times upper limit of normal)

Scenario: Patient given samples of rosuvastatin but cannot afford Rx once samples are finished
MRP: Nonadherence

- **Assessment:**
  Patient with uncontrolled dyslipidemia on rosuvastatin 10 mg. Unable to meet recommended statin therapy goals secondary to nonadherence with rosuvastatin. Switching to atorvastatin would be more affordable for patient and meet recommendations for appropriate intensity statin therapy.
- **Plan:**
  Consider discontinuation of rosuvastatin and addition of atorvastatin 20 mg every night at bedtime to meet statin therapy needs.

Scenario: Diabetes patient with elevated cholesterol not currently on a statin
MRP: Need for additional therapy

- **Assessment:**
  According to the pooled cohort risk equation, this patient with diabetes has a 10-year risk for developing ASCVD of 12.9%. According to ACC/AHA guidelines patient should be treated with high-intensity statin therapy, along with appropriate lifestyle modifications.
- **Plan:**
  Consider initiation of atorvastatin 80 mg every night at bedtime.
  Monitor fasting lipid panel in 6 weeks to evaluate adherence to therapy.

Scenario: Patient with history of stroke on pravastatin 10 mg daily
MRP: Dosage too low

- **Assessment:**
  According to history of stroke, patient meets requirements for defined ASCVD. The ACC/AHA guidelines recommend patients over age 21 with history of ASCVD be treated with high-intensity statin therapy for secondary prevention. Patient is currently treated with pravastatin 10 mg, which is considered low-intensity therapy.
- **Plan:**
  Recommend discontinue pravastatin.
  Consider initiation of rosuvastatin 20 mg every night at bedtime.
  Monitor fasting lipid panel in 6 weeks to evaluate adherence to therapy.
  Follow up with patient in 2 to 4 weeks to evaluate tolerability of therapy.

FIGURE 22-6 Sample provider communications for dyslipidemia.
Source: References 2 and 6.

Recommendations may be communicated via secure fax, telephone, or other means of written or secure electronic communication. The examples that follow are for illustrative purposes. Actual communications to providers should be individualized based on the type of recommendation, patient specific characteristics, and the nature of the relationship with the provider.

Follow-up to assess levels of lipoprotein, effects of interventions, and potential adverse effects is essential in patients with dyslipidemia. The interval for follow-up will depend on a number of factors, including when therapy was initiated and patient specific factors such as age, comorbid conditions, and ability to return for follow-up. Suggested intervals for follow-up are provided in Table 22-15.

TABLE 22-15 • Suggested Intervals for Follow-Up in Patients with Dyslipidemia

Follow-up and Monitoring in Patients with Dyslipidemia
Treatment response
• Fasting lipid profile 4 to 12 weeks after initiating therapy.
• If patient is not meeting treatment goals at initial follow-up and adjustments in dose or changes in therapy occur, another fasting lipid profile should be assessed in 4 to 12 weeks.
• Once the patient has achieved the treatment goal(s), follow-up intervals may be reduced to every 3 to 12 months. The primary focus of these visits is encouragement of long-term adherence with therapy.
• Fasting lipid profiles should be measured at least annually.
Toxicity
• Consider monitoring CK level at baseline prior to initiation of therapy.
• LFTs should be monitored at baseline prior to initiation of therapy and as clinically indicated thereafter. Routine monitoring of LFTs is not recommended.
• Monitor for adverse drug effects 6 to 8 weeks after starting a new agent or dose increase.
• Monitor every 6 to 12 months in stable patients.

Abbreviations: CK = creatine kinase; LFTs = liver function tests.

Source: Reference 2.

REFERENCES

1. Talbert RL. Hyperlipidemia. In: DiPiro JT, Talbert RL, Yee GC, Matzke GR, Wells BG, Posey L, eds. *Pharmacotherapy: A Pathophysiologic Approach*. 10th ed. New York, NY: McGraw-Hill; 2017. Available at http://accesspharmacy.mhmedical.com/content.aspx?bookid=1861&sectionid=146057587. Accessed April 28, 2017.
2. Stone NJ, Robinson J, Lichtenstein AH, et al. 2013 ACC/AHA guideline on the treatment of blood cholesterol to reduce atherosclerotic cardiovascular risk in adults. *Circulation*. 2014;129(25 suppl 2):S1-S45.
3. Goff DC, Lloyd-Jones DM, Bennett G, et al. 2013 ACC/AHA guideline on the assessment of cardiovascular risk: a report of the American College of Cardiology/American Heart Association Task Force on Practice Guidelines. *Circulation*. 2014;129(25 suppl 2):S49-S73.
4. Eckel RH, Jakicic JM, Ard JD, et al. 2013 AHA/ACC guideline on lifestyle management to reduce cardiovascular risk: a report of the American College of Cardiology American/Heart Association Task Force on Practice Guidelines. *Circulation*. 2014;129(25 suppl 2):S76-S99.
5. American College of Cardiology ASCVD risk estimator. ACC website. Available at http://tools.acc.org/ASCVD-Risk-Estimator/. Accessed January 3, 2017.
6. Drozda JP Jr, Ferguson TB Jr, Jneid H, et al. 2015 ACC/AHA focused update of secondary prevention lipid performance measures: a report of the American College of Cardiology/American Heart Association Task Force on Performance Measures. *J Am Coll Cardiol*. 2016;67(5):558-587.
7. Jellinger PS, Smith DA, Mehta AE, et al. American Association of Clinical Endocrinologists' guidelines for management of dyslipidemia and prevention of atherosclerosis (AACE). *Endocr Pract*. 2012;18(suppl 1):1-78.
8. Grundy SM, Cleeman JI, Bairey Merz CN, et al. Implications of recent clinical trials for the National Cholesterol Education Program Adult Treatment Panel III Guidelines. *Circulation*. 2004;110(2):227-239.
9. CMS. *Medicare Part D Medication Therapy Management Program Standardized Format*. CMS website. Available at https://www.cms.gov/Medicare/Prescription-Drug-Coverage/PrescriptionDrugCovContra/Downloads/MTM-Program-Standardized-Format-English-and-Spanish-Instructions-Samples-v032712.pdf. Accessed June 7, 2017.
10. Clinical Pharmacology [database online]. Tampa, FL: Gold Standard, Inc.; 2017. Available at http://www.clinicalpharmacology.com. Accessed June 7, 2017.
11. Natural Medicines [database online]. Somerville, MA: Therapeutic Research Center; 2017. Available at https://naturalmedicines.therapeuticresearch.com/. Accessed June 7, 2017.
12. Ridker PM, Danielson E, Fonseca FA, et al. Rosuvastatin to prevent vascular events in men and women with elevated C-reactive protein. *N Engl J Med*. 2008;359(21):2195-2207.
13. Berglund L, Brunzell JD, Goldberg AC, et al. Evaluation and treatment of hypertriglyceridemia: an Endocrine Society clinical practice guideline. *J Clin Endocrinol Metab*. 2012;97(9):2969-2989.
14. Miller M, Stone NJ, Ballantyne C, et al. Triglycerides and cardiovascular disease: a scientific statement from the American Heart Association. *Circulation*. 2011;123(20):2292-2333.
15. Boden WE, Probstfield JL, Anderson T, et al. AIM-HIGH Investigators. Niacin in patients with low HDL cholesterol levels receiving intensive statin therapy. *N Engl J Med*. 2011;365:2255-2267.
16. HPS2-THRIVE. Niacin causes serious unexpected side-effects, but no worthwhile benefits, for patients who are at increased risk of heart attacks and strokes [press release]. Published March 9, 2013. Available at http://www.hps2-thrive.org/press_release.htm. Accessed June 7, 2017.
17. Praluent (alirocumab) [package insert]. Bridgewater, NJ: Sanofi-Aventis LLC; July 2015. Available at https://www.accessdata.fda.gov/drugsatfda_docs/label/2015/125559Orig1s000lbledt.pdf Accessed June 7, 2017.
18. Repatha (evolocumab) injection [package insert]. Thousand Oaks, CA: Amgen Inc; November 2016. Available at http://pi.amgen.com/united_states/repatha/repatha_pi_hcp_english.pdf. Accessed June 7, 2017.
19. American Diabetes Association. Standards of medical care in diabetes—2017. *Diabetes Care*. 2017;40(suppl 1):S11-S24.
20. Cannon, CP, et al, Ezetimibe added to statin therapy after acute coronary syndromes. *N Engl J Med*. 2015;372:2387-2397.
21. Sabatine MS, Giugliano RP, Keech AC, et al. Evolocumab and clinical outcomes in patients with cardiovascular disease. *N Engl J Med*. 2017;376:1713-1722.

Review Questions

1. Which lipid marker remains valid if the patient is not fasting at the time the lipid panel is completed?
   a. LDL
   b. HDL
   c. TG
   d. VLDL

2. All of the following are consistent with the definition of ASCVD **EXCEPT:**
   a. congestive heart failure.
   b. myocardial infarction.
   c. abdominal aortic aneurysm.
   d. peripheral arterial disease.

3. Which statin is most appropriate for a 58-year-old patient diagnosed with type 2 diabetes mellitus and a 10-year ASCVD risk of 15%?
   a. Simvastatin 40 mg daily
   b. Pravastatin 80 mg daily
   c. Atorvastatin 20 mg daily
   d. Rosuvastatin 20 mg daily

4. Which is the best description of rhabdomyolysis in living room language?
   a. A serious condition due to degradation of muscle tissue caused by statins; associated with myalgias and myoglobinuria
   b. A severe condition where the muscles are breaking down, presenting with muscle weakness and pain, along with cola-colored urine
   c. A potential side effect with HMG CoA reductase inhibitors; patient may experience muscle pain (myalgia), weakness, or cramps
   d. Something bad that happens, a bad reaction, an unexplained or unwanted effect

5. A 42-year-old patient with dyslipidemia is new to MTM service. After performing a medication therapy review with the patient, the pharmacist completes a medication action plan (MAP). Which statement best represents the type of information that should be included in the patient's MAP?
   a. Take simvastatin 20 mg tablet nightly for cholesterol.
   b. Side effects experienced with this medication may include myalgias, myopathy, and rhabdomyolysis.
   c. Remember to take simvastatin every night; use a pillbox or alarm reminder to help remember.
   d. Pharmacist will call Dr. Smith to discuss switching simvastatin to a stronger medication for cholesterol.

6. All findings would indicate the need for referral to the emergency department **EXCEPT:**
   a. The patient is experiencing severe chest pain that is radiating to his/her arm.
   b. The patient is suffering from myopathy.
   c. The patient reports his/her urine has turned to a cola color.
   d. The patient has severe head pain and complains of one-sided weakness.

7. Which MRP category is matched appropriately with an example of that category?
   a. Nonadherence – Patient has 52% LDL reduction on high-intensity statin.
   b. Adverse drug event – Patient is taking duplicate therapy (eg, two statins).
   c. Unnecessary medication – Patient is experiencing myalgias, myopathy, or rhabdomyolysis with statin therapy or other lipid-lowering therapies.
   d. Dosage too low — Patient with clinical ASCVD is on moderate-intensity statin.

8. A 65-year-old patient with a diagnosis of diabetes who is currently taking no medications for lipids presents with a fasting lipid profile as follows: LDL 199 mg/dL, TG 286 mg/dL, HDL 41 mg/dL, and TC 228 mg/dL. What would be the most appropriate therapy for this patient?
   a. Niacin 1000 mg daily
   b. Atorvastatin 80 mg nightly
   c. Tricor 135 mg daily
   d. Simvastatin 80 mg nightly

9. A 42-year-old Hispanic female with a history of smoking and peripheral arterial disease presents with a BP 154/82 mm Hg, TC 256 mg/dL, LDL 152mg/dL, and HDL 52 mg/dL. Her current medication includes lisinopril 20 mg daily. Which is the correct assessment of her 10-year risk of ASCVD and intensity of statin therapy?
   a. Ten-year risk is 8.4%; moderate-intensity statin therapy is required.
   b. Ten-year risk is 0.4%; no statin is required.
   c. Ten-year risk is 20%; moderate-intensity statin therapy is required.
   d. Calculation of 10-year ASCVD risk is not required to determine statin needs; patient requires high-intensity statin therapy.

10. A patient is initiated on simvastatin 40 mg nightly. What is an appropriate time to recommend a follow-up fasting lipid panel?
   a. 4 to 6 months
   b. 4 to 12 weeks
   c. Annually
   d. 6 to 12 months

ANSWERS

1. b	2. a	3. d
4. b	5. c	6. b
7. d	8. b	9. d
10. b		

23

Gastroesophageal Reflux Disease MTM Data Set

Andrew Y. Hwang, PharmD, BCPS

KEY POINTS

- The need for lifestyle modifications for management of gastroesophageal reflux disease (GERD) should be assessed at each encounter with the patient.
- Medication therapy management (MTM) providers should evaluate medications for GERD at each encounter, specifically assessing efficacy, need for continued therapy (ie, the patient should be taking the lowest effective dose for symptom relief), and potential adverse effects.
- MTM providers should educate patients on the importance of watching for alarm symptoms of GERD and when to seek medical attention.

INTRODUCTION

Approximately 18% to 28% of adults in the United States experience symptoms of heartburn or regurgitation at least once weekly.[1] While most cases are not serious, these symptoms are referred to as "gastroesophageal reflux disease" or GERD.[2] GERD is a condition that develops when the reflux of stomach contents causes troublesome symptoms and/or complications. Furthermore, symptoms are considered "troublesome" if they adversely impact well-being and/or quality of life. Episodic heartburn that occurs infrequently or is not painful enough to be considered bothersome by the patient is not included in the definition of GERD.[3,4] Table 23-1 highlights the definitions and common abbreviations associated with the discussion of GERD.

A key feature in the development of GERD is abnormal reflux. Gastric contents from the stomach enter the esophagus, irritate the lining of the esophagus, and cause symptoms. Some patients also have other factors that contribute to presentation of symptoms, including defective lower esophageal sphincter (LES) pressure or function. Other secondary causes can contribute to presentation of GERD symptoms; these and other factors are highlighted in Table 23-2.[3] Additionally, endogenous substances produced by the body may promote esophageal damage on reflux into the esophagus. These include gastric acid, pepsin, bile acids, and pancreatic enzymes. Therefore, the composition and volume of the refluxate, as well as duration of exposure, are all aggravating factors that play a role in damaging the lining of the esophagus and causing symptoms and complications of GERD and the associated syndromes (Table 23-3).[3]

Therapeutic Goals and Treatment Outcomes for GERD

Objective measurable endpoints of GERD treatment are difficult to assess, and success of treatment is often based on subjective data such as symptomatology. Long-term goals of therapy are geared toward (1) alleviating or eliminating symptoms, (2) decreasing the frequency or recurrence and duration of GERD, (3) promoting healing of the injured mucosa, and (4) preventing the development of complications. Short-term goals are geared toward the relief of symptoms, such as heartburn or regurgitation, to ensure that symptoms do not impair quality of life.[3]

CORE ELEMENT 1—COMPREHENSIVE MEDICATION REVIEW FOR PATIENTS WITH GERD

Table 23-4 presents a list of suggested questions to use when conducting a medication therapy review with a patient with GERD. The number and types of questions will depend on several factors,

TABLE 23-1 • GERD: Common Definitions and Abbreviations

Definitions	*Barrett esophagus*: Complication of GERD when tissue lining the esophagus is replaced by tissue similar to the lining of the intestine *Erosive esophagitis*: Erosion of the squamous epithelium of the esophagus *Esophagitis*: Inflammation of the lining of the esophagus *Gastroesophageal reflux disease*: A condition that develops when the reflux of stomach contents causes troublesome symptoms and/or complications *Nonerosive reflux disease*: GERD symptoms without esophagitis *Refluxate*: Material that rises from the stomach into the esophagus; contains food, acid, pepsin, and bile
Abbreviations	*GERD*: Gastroesophageal reflux disease *GI*: Gastrointestinal *H_2RAs*: Histamine type 2 receptor antagonists *LES*: Lower esophageal sphincter *NERD*: Nonerosive reflux disease *PPI*: Proton pump inhibitor

including the amount of time for the interview, number of concurrent medication-related problems (MRPs), urgency of MRPs, and reliability of the patient in providing accurate information, among other factors. In time-limited interactions or in complex cases with multiple medical issues, the MTM provider may choose to target questions that help to identify or rule out issues of an urgent nature (see questions to ask for prevention/assessment of medical emergencies). MTM providers should remember to use living room language[5] during the interview (Table 23-5), and to be prepared for questions that patients may ask regarding GERD (Table 23-6).

CORE ELEMENT 2—PERSONAL MEDICATION LIST[6]

Figure 23-1 presents a sample personal medication list (PML) for a patient with GERD. This example is representative only of GERD medications. Additional medications for other disease states should be added and listed separately. MTM providers should remember to use plain language when creating the PML.

TABLE 23-2 • Secondary Causes and Contributing Factors that Worsen Symptoms of GERD

Pathophysiological features	Defective lower esophageal sphincter (LES) pressure or function Abnormal esophageal anatomy Improper esophageal clearance of gastric fluids Reduced mucosal resistance to acid Delayed or ineffective gastric emptying Inadequate production of epidermal growth factor Reduced salivary buffering of acid		
Medications	Decreased LES pressure	Anticholinergics Barbiturates Caffeine Dihydropyridine calcium channel blockers Dopamine Estrogen	Ethanol Nicotine Nitrates Progesterone Tetracycline Theophylline
	Direct irritants to the esophageal mucosa	Bisphosphonates Aspirin Nonsteroidal anti-inflammatory drugs	Iron Quinidine Potassium chloride
Foods	Decreased LES pressure	Fatty meal Peppermint Spearmint Chocolate	Coffee, cola, tea Garlic Onions Chili peppers
	Direct irritants to the esophageal mucosa	Spicy foods Orange juice Tomato juice Coffee	
Other contributing factors	Family history Obesity Smoking Respiratory diseases		

TABLE 23-3 • Symptoms and Complications of GERD and Associated GERD Syndromes

Symptom-based syndromes[a] (exist with or without esophageal injury)	Typical symptoms	Atypical symptoms	Alarm symptoms
	Heartburn Hypersalivation Regurgitation Belching	Chronic cough Asthma-like symptoms Hoarseness Dental enamel erosion Chest pain	Dysphagia Odynophagia GI bleeding Weight loss Vomiting
Tissue injury-based syndromes (exist with or without symptoms)	Esophagitis Barrett esophagus Strictures Esophageal adenocarcinoma		

[a] Symptoms are not a predictor of damage.

Source: Reference 3.

TABLE 23-4 • Suggested Questions for the GERD Patient

How long have you had heartburn/GERD?

- When did you first start having problems?
- How often do you have a burning feeling behind your breastbone or heartburn?
- How often do you have stomach contents (liquid or food) moving upward to your throat or mouth (regurgitation)?
- How often do you have pain in the center of your stomach?
- How often do you experience nausea, if any?
- How often do you have difficulty getting a good night's sleep because of heartburn and/or regurgitation?

What do you already know about heartburn/GERD?

What has your physician told you about lifestyle or food changes that you can make to help control your heartburn/GERD?

What medications do you take for your heartburn/GERD symptoms?

- How long have you been taking the medication(s)?
- What side effects, if any, do you experience from the medication(s)?
- How often do you miss a dose of your heartburn/GERD medication? If you miss a dose of your medication, do you feel any different?
- Do you experience heartburn even after taking your medication? If yes, what else do you take to stop the symptoms?
- How often do you take additional medication for your heartburn, other than what the physician told you take?

What other medications have you taken in the past for your heartburn/GERD symptoms?

Have you ever stopped taking any of your prescribed heartburn/GERD medications without telling your physician? If so, why?

Apart from the medications you take for your heartburn/GERD, have you ever had any procedure, such as surgery, to treat your heartburn/GERD?

What over-the-counter (OTC) medications or herbals do you use for your heartburn/GERD?

Other than medicines, what else have you tried for your heartburn/GERD (eg, lifestyle changes)?

Have you ever experienced the following signs/symptoms (atypical symptoms or alarm symptoms)?

- Difficulty or painful swallowing
- A cough not related to a cold
- Bloody or tarry stools
- Weight loss
- Vomiting
- Chest pain. If yes, how often do you experience chest pain in a week, month, etc?

Questions to Ask for Prevention/Assessment of Medical Emergencies

Have you noticed any of the following: black or tarry stools, excessive weight loss, vomiting (with or without blood), difficulty/painful swallowing?

Have you ever been hospitalized due to chest pain?

TABLE 23-5 • GERD: Living Room Language

Abdomen	Stomach, stomach area, belly, tummy
Absorption	Take in, soak up
Acute	Sudden start, short term, quick
Administer	Give, manage, take care of
Aggravate	Make worse, harm, anger, hurt
Alleviate	Lessen, ease, soften, improve, make better
Antacid	Medication, such as Maalox, Mylanta, Tums, that neutralizes acid in the stomach
Barrett esophagus	A condition in which the skin lining the food pipe is replaced by a different type of skin
Behavior modification	Developing new habits, changing what you do, stopping bad habits
Belching	Expelling gas from the stomach through the mouth, burping
Body mass index (BMI)	A measure of body fat based on height and weight
Cessation	Stopping, quitting, ending
Chronic	Constant, never ending, does not go away, long-term, long-lasting
Chronic health condition	Constant health problem, something that affects your health for a long period of time
Comprehensive	Complete, covers everything important, thorough, all
Contraindication	Dangerous to give, not good for, when a drug or procedure may be harmful
Control	Manage, have power over, take care of
Diagnosis	Ascertaining the cause of an illness, condition, disease, medical answer
Diagnostic test	A test done to determine the disease
Discontinue	Stop, end, quit
Disease	Illness, sickness
Dysphagia	Difficulty swallowing
Endoscopy	A procedure in which a flexible tube with a camera on one end is passed into the esophagus, stomach, and upper small intestine
Episode	Event, set amount of time, brief time
Erosions	Small pits, small holes in teeth or bones, eating away, loss of
Esophageal cancer	Cancer of the food pipe
Esophagus	Food pipe that connects the mouth to the stomach
Excessive	Too much
Experience	Feel, have, go through
Frequently	Often, commonly, normally, regularly, many times
Gastroesophageal reflux disease (GERD)	Chronic disease that occurs when the stomach acid or sometimes bile flows back into the food pipe
Histamine-2 receptor blocker (H_2RA)	Medication that decreases or lowers how much acid you produce; these medications work longer than antacids
Inflammation	Swelling, injury, sore
Laparoscopic fundoplication	Procedure where the fundus or upper part of the stomach is wrapped around the esophagus or food pipe to create a new valve where the esophagus meets the stomach
Lifestyle changes	Your physician may have recommended changes in lifestyle to help reduce your GERD symptoms, which for some patients include reaching a goal weight, decreasing the amount of alcohol you consume, exercising, or quitting smoking
Lower esophageal sphincter (LES)	A ring of muscle that connects the food pipe and the stomach
Manage	Control, direct, be in charge of, take care of, watch
Medication or medicine	Drug, pill, or substance to treat, prevent or help with symptoms of a disease or illness
Minimize	Make smaller
Monitor	Watch, check on, watch for changes
Neutralize	Cancel, counteract, or balance

(Continued)

TABLE 23-5 • GERD: Living Room Language (*Continued*)

Nonerosive reflux disease (NERD)	Chronic disease when you have symptoms of GERD or heartburn, but there are no changes to the food pipe
Obstruction	Barrier, blockage, hurdle
Occasionally	Sometimes, not often, once in a while
Odynophagia	Pain when swallowing
On an empty stomach	Do not eat or drink
Persistent	There all the time, constant, doesn't go away, not giving up
Pharyngitis	Sore throat or pain and swelling of the throat
Prevention	Stop, bar, avoid
Progression	Move forward, go on, get worse, advance
Proton pump inhibitor (PPI)	Medication that blocks acid production and heals the food pipe or esophagus
Pyrosis	Heartburn or a burning sensation in the chest sometimes spreading to the throat, along with a sour taste in the mouth
Recur	Come back, get again, happen again
Reduce	Lower, cut, trim, dilute
Regurgitation	Backflow or flow in the opposite direction from normal
Relief or relieve	Feel or make better, ease, not as bad, ease or lessening from pain or discomfort
Stricture	An abnormal narrowing of the food pipe
Suppress	Hold back, stop, slow down
Syndrome	Illness, sickness, set of signs that often go together
Vomit	Throw up
Warning sign	Signals to alert you that something might be wrong

TABLE 23-6 • GERD: Questions Commonly Asked by Patients

What is GERD?	GERD is a chronic disease that occurs when the stomach acid or sometimes bile flows back into the food pipe. Also, acid in contact with the esophagus, or food pipe, causes soreness, resulting in heartburn or chest pains. The acid may also cause small holes (or ulcers) in the lining of the esophagus or food pipe.
What causes GERD?	There can be many causes of GERD; some of these are related to your stomach, others are related to food, medications, and lifestyle choices. For example, as far as lifestyle choices, increased body weight can put pressure on the stomach, causing acid to rise. Smoking also increases acid released into the stomach, which can then cause symptoms. Sometimes no reason or cause can be found for symptoms.
Is there any testing that can be done for GERD?	Your physician can have you undergo endoscopy, which allows a view of the inside of your esophagus, stomach, and upper small intestine.
Why are GERD medications important?	GERD medications help decrease the amount of acid your body produces, thereby decreasing the effect that this extra acid has on the lining of your food pipe and stomach. GERD medications can help decrease the acid and protect the stomach and food pipe from further damage.
What can happen if I stop taking my medications?	It is not recommended to stop taking your medications without first telling your physician. However, if you do stop, you may find that your heartburn symptoms return or worsen with time.
How long will I have to take medications? Will I always have to take medication for my GERD?	GERD is a chronic or lifelong condition; however, some patients may be able to control their symptoms with changes in diet or lifestyle, while others will require medications. The length of treatment will depend on you and your symptoms. The goal for you is to not allow GERD or heartburn symptoms to interfere with your life. Therefore, some patients may have to be on medications for life, if it is the medication that helps control their symptoms.
When should I call my physician about my symptoms or go to the ER?	If the pain you experience changes in location (eg, if it radiates into your arms, neck, jaw, teeth, or back), intensity, or duration; if you begin to feel sick to your stomach, start vomiting or sweating, experience left-arm pain or jaw pain, develop pain in your back, shortness of breath, feeling as if you are going to pass out or begin vomiting fluid that is green, yellow, or looks like coffee grounds or blood, immediately go the nearest hospital emergency room or call 911.

PERSONAL MEDICATION LIST FOR <*Insert patient's name, DOB: mm/dd/yyyy*>	
Medication: Omeprazole 20 mg oral capsule	
How I use it: Take one capsule (20 mg) by mouth in the morning	
Why I use it: GERD (heartburn)	**Prescriber:** Jane Doe
Date I started using it: 1/6/2017	**Date I stopped using it:** (*Leave blank for patient's notes)*
Why I stopped using it: (*Leave blank for patient's notes)*	
Additional Information: Remember to take this medication on an empty stomach at least 30 minutes prior to meals	
Medication: Ranitidine 150 mg oral tablet	
How I use it: Take one tablet (150 mg) by mouth in the evening	
Why I use it: GERD (heartburn)	**Prescriber:** Jane Doe
Date I started using it: 10/9/2016	**Date I stopped using it:** (*Leave blank for patient's notes)*
Why I stopped using it: *(Leave blank for patient's notes)*	
Additional Information: *(Leave blank for patient's notes)*	

FIGURE 23-1 GERD personal medication list.

CORE ELEMENT 3—MEDICATION ACTION PLAN[6]

Figure 23-2 provides sample medication action plans (MAPs) for patients with GERD. These examples are representative only of action steps for a patient with GERD. MAPs for other disease states or other medication-related problems (MRPs) should be added and listed separately. In general, only a few of the most important action steps should be listed, so as not to overwhelm the patient. Other areas for patient self-management can be addressed at later visits. MTM providers should remember to use plain language when creating the MAP.

CORE ELEMENT 4—INTERVENTION AND/OR REFERRAL

Interventions for GERD management are targeted at relieving symptoms, reducing the frequency of symptoms, promoting healing of mucosal injury, and preventing complications. Treatment primarily includes lifestyle modifications and addition or alteration in drug therapy to achieve treatment goals. Following lifestyle modifications, providers should start with an empiric trial of acid suppression therapy for 4 to 8 weeks in patients with typical symptoms, and in the absence of atypical symptoms or symptoms suggesting complicated disease.[3] Table 23-7 summarizes lifestyle modifications and other nonpharmacologic options in the management of patients with GERD,[3,7] and Table 23-8 provides an overview of treatment options for GERD.[3,8,9] Additionally, further recommendations for providing pharmaceutical care to patients with GERD are highlighted in Table 23-9.[3] Table 23-10 outlines herbal remedies that may be useful in the management of GERD,[10-12] and Table 23-11 gives examples of situations in which patients should be referred to emergency services, their primary-care provider or appropriate specialist.[13]

CORE ELEMENT 5—DOCUMENTATION AND FOLLOW-UP

Clear and succinct documentation of MRPs and recommendations is a key component of the MTM consult. Examples of potential MRPs in patients with GERD are provided in Table 23-12. Sample communications and recommendations to providers for addressing medication-related issues are found in Figure 23-3. Recommendations may be communicated via fax, telephone, or other means of written or secure electronic communication. The examples presented below are for illustrative purposes. Actual communications to providers should be individualized according to the type of recommendation,

	DATE PREPARED: *Insert date*
What we talked about: Common foods that may make reflux (GERD or heartburn) worse	
What I need to do: Avoid or limit use of these foods to help reduce reflux: citrus, chocolate, caffeine, alcohol, fatty/fried foods, garlic, onions, mint, spicy, or tomato-based foods.	**What I did and when I did it:** *(Leave blank for patient's notes)*
What we talked about: Lifestyle changes that may improve the symptoms of GERD	
What I need to do: To help reduce reflux at night, consider raising the head of my bed 6 to 8 inches by securing wood blocks under the bedposts. Using extra pillows will not help. Adopt mealtime habits to help reduce reflux: eat smaller, more frequent meals, avoid foods and drinks that worsen symptoms, and avoid lying down for 3 hours after a meal. Stop smoking because smoking can make reflux worse. Begin a plan to lose weight, as losing weight can help reduce reflux symptoms.	**What I did and when I did it:** *(Leave blank for patient's notes)*
What we talked about: How to take your heartburn medication (omeprazole)	
What I need to do: Take omeprazole capsule on an empty stomach, at least 30 minutes before meals. If given once daily, take it in the morning.	**What I did and when I did it:** *(Leave blank for patient's notes)*

FIGURE 23-2 GERD: example medication action plan.

TABLE 23-7 • GERD: Nonpharmacological Management Options

Lifestyle changes	Recommended modifications in all patients • Elevate the head of the bed by 6-8 inches (for patients with nocturnal GERD) • Avoid eating 2-3 hours before bedtime (for patients with nocturnal GERD) • Weight reduction (reduces symptoms) in obese patients Recommended modifications that should be individualized to specific patients • Avoid foods that might decrease LES pressure • Include protein-rich meals in diet (augments LES pressure) • Avoid foods that have a direct irritant effect on the esophageal mucosa • Engage in behaviors that may reduce esophageal acid exposure Eat small meals, and avoid eating immediately prior to sleeping (3 hours before sleep) Stop smoking Avoid alcohol Avoid tight-fitting clothes Take medications that have a direct irritant effect on the esophageal mucosa in the upright sitting or standing position and with plenty of liquid, if they cannot be avoided
Other	Acupuncture Surgery: laparoscopic fundoplication

Abbreviations: GERD = gastroesophageal reflux disease; LES = lower esophageal sphincter.

Source: References 3 and 7.

TABLE 23-8 • Medications for Management of GERD

Medication Class and Example Drugs[a]	Common or Serious Side Effects[b]	Blackbox Warnings or Contraindications	Pertinent Precautions	Pregnancy Category[c]
Antacids Aluminum (Alutab®) Magnesium (Phillips' Milk of Magnesia®) Al-Mg combination products Calcium carbonate (Tums®) Alginic acid (Gaviscon®)	Diarrhea (Mg) Constipation (Al) Alterations in mineral metabolism Acid-base disturbances	Renal disease	Diverticulitis Fecal impaction GI bleeding GI obstruction Hepatic disease	C
H_2-receptor antagonists Cimetidine (Tagamet®) Famotidine (Pepcid®) Nizatidine (Axid®) Ranitidine (Zantac®)	Headache Nausea Dry mouth Somnolence Fatigue Dizziness Constipation Diarrhea	None	Hepatic impairment Renal impairment Immunosuppression	B
Proton pump inhibitors Dexlansoprazole (Dexilant®) Esomeprazole (Nexium®) Lansoprazole (Prevacid®) Omeprazole (Prilosec®) Omeprazole and sodium bicarbonate (Zegerid®) Pantoprazole (Protonix®) Rabeprazole (Aciphex®)	Headache Dizziness Diarrhea Constipation Nausea Vitamin B_{12} deficiency Hypomagnesemia Bone fractures	Proton pump inhibitor hypersensitivity	Abdominal pain Dysphagia GI bleeding Hepatic disease Osteoporosis Pseudo-membranous colitis	B (except omeprazole–category C)

(Continued)

TABLE 23-8 • Medications for Management of GERD (*Continued*)

Medication Class and Example Drugs[a]	Common or Serious Side Effects[b]	Blackbox Warnings or Contraindications	Pertinent Precautions	Pregnancy Category[c]
Promotility agent Metoclopramide (Reglan®)	Drowsiness Acute dystonic reactions Fatigue Restlessness Headache Dizziness Somnolence Nausea Vomiting	Tardive dyskinesia [B] Hypersensitivity GI obstruction, perforation, or hemorrhage Pheochromocytoma Seizure disorder GI bleeding	Abrupt discontinuation Breast cancer Cardiac disease Depression Diabetes mellitus Heart failure Hepatic disease Hypertension Malignant hyperthermia Parkinsons disease Renal disease	B

[a] Bethanechol and sucralfate have not been included in this chart as they are not routinely recommended for the management of GERD.

[b] This is a general list and does not include all side effects that can occur from these drugs. Consult a drug reference source for a more inclusive list before making any recommendations. MTM providers should also consult a comprehensive drug interaction database before making pharmacotherapy recommendations.

[B] Denotes a blackbox warning.

[c] Product labeling for all prescription drugs is being updated to reflect the new FDA Pregnancy Labeling and Lactation Rule. Please check individual product labeling for the most accurate and updated pregnancy information.

Source: References 3, 8, and 9.

TABLE 23-9 • Recommendations for Providing Pharmaceutical Care to Patients with GERD

- Assess the patient's symptoms to determine whether patient-directed therapy is appropriate or whether patient should be evaluated by a clinician. Determine the type of symptoms, frequency, and exacerbating factors. Refer any patient with alarm or atypical symptoms to a clinician for further diagnostic workup.
- Obtain a thorough history of prescription, nonprescription, and natural drug product use.
- Counsel the patient on lifestyle modifications that will improve symptoms.
- Recommend appropriate drug therapy based on patient presentation.
- Develop a plan to assess effectiveness of acid-suppression therapy after an appropriate amount of time (8–16 weeks). Recommend alternative therapy if necessary.
- Assess improvement in quality-of-life measures such as physical, pathologic, and social functioning and well-being.
- Evaluate patient for the presence of adverse drug reactions, allergies, and drug interactions.
- Stress the importance of compliance with the therapeutic regimen, including lifestyle modifications. Recommend a therapeutic regimen that is easy for the patient to accomplish.
- Provide patient education with regard to disease state, lifestyle modifications, and drug therapy. Patients should be counseled on
  - What causes GERD and what things to avoid
  - When to take their medications
  - What potential adverse effects or drug interactions may occur
  - What alarm signs they should report to their clinician

Source: Reference 3.

TABLE 23-10 • GERD: Herbal Supplements

Common Name (Scientific Name)	Recommended Dose	Grade[a]	Cost[b]
Caraway (*Carum carvi*)	*Fruit*: 1- 6 g of dried caraway fruit daily *Tea*: 1-2 teaspoons of pressed seeds in 150 mL of boiling water; cover and allow to steep for 10-15 minutes and consume 2-4 cups daily between meals *Oil*: 50-100 mg daily, in combination with peppermint oil, or 1-4 drops of caraway oil on a lump of sugar or in a teaspoonful of water	Possibly effective	$$

(*Continued*)

TABLE 23-10 • GERD: Herbal Supplements (*Continued*)

Common Name (Scientific Name)	Recommended Dose	Grade[a]	Cost[b]
Chamomile (*Matricaria recutita*)	*Tea*: 1-4 cups taken daily (from teabags) *Dried flower heads:* 2-8 g 3 times daily *Tablets/capsules*: 400-1600 mg daily in divided doses (standardized to 1.2% apigenin and 0.5% essential oil per dose)	Possibly effective	$
Lemon Balm (*Melissa officinalis*)	*Tea*: 1 cup taken several times daily as needed *Extract*: Single doses of 300, 600, and 900 mg have been studied	Possibly effective	$$
Licorice (*Glycyrrhiza glabra*)	*Powdered root*: 1-4 g per day, divided into 3 or 4 doses *Fluid extract*: 2 mL - 4 mL per day *DGL (deglycyrrhizinated licorice) Extract*: 350 mg -1,140 mg three times daily (20 minutes prior to meals)	Possibly effective	$$
Melatonin (*N*-acetyl-5-methoxytryptamine)	*Tablets/Capsules*: 5 mg in the evening	Insufficient evidence	$
Peppermint (*Mentha x piperita, M. arvensis, M. halpocalyx*)	*Oil:* 90 mg 2-3 times daily, in combination with caraway oil	Possibly effective	$$
Turmeric (*Curcuma longa*)	*Capsules*: 250 mg of dried root powder containing 0.02 mL of volatile oil and 0.024 g of total curcuminoids have been used 4 times daily for 7 days	Insufficient evidence	$$

[a] Level of evidence: "Likely effective"—this product has a very high level of reliable clinical evidence supporting its use for a specific indication. Products rated "likely effective" are generally considered appropriate to recommend; "possibly effective"—this product has some clinical evidence supporting its use for a specific indication; however, the evidence is limited by quantity, quality, or contradictory findings. Products rated "possibly effective" might be beneficial, but do not have enough high-quality evidence to be recommended for most people; "insufficient evidence"—there is not enough reliable scientific evidence to provide an effectiveness rating.

[b] Cost: $ = ≤$10/month supply in recommended dosage, $$ = $11-$20/month.

Source: References 10, 11, and 12.

TABLE 23-11 • GERD: Situations for Referral

Symptom or Sign	Immediate Action: Call 911	Nonimmediate: Seek Medical Attention (call MD) or Go to ER	Routine: Inform MD at Later Time
Abdominal discomfort (bloating, cramps, etc)	Associated with fever, continuous GI bleeding, or other concerning symptoms	Persistent discomfort not associated with other symptoms	More than occasional discomfort but not persistent
Abdominal pain	Abrupt-onset severe pain, distention, or abdominal pain with fever and vomiting	Moderate diffuse or localized pain, unrelieved by antacids or laxatives	Persistent mild to moderate discomfort, without associated symptoms
Bleeding, rectal (melena)	Persistent, or accompanied by sweating, tachycardia, significant orthostatic BP drop	Recent self-limited bleeding: tarry stool or melena without other signs or symptoms	
Chest pain, pressure, or tightness	New or abrupt onset, unrelieved by current medications *or* accompanied by sweating and other signs/symptoms	Relieved by antacids or nitroglycerin, without other symptoms, but recurring more often than usual	Gradual or persistent change in usual pattern or frequency
Nausea and vomiting	Persistent vomiting, with or without abdominal pain, bleeding, or fever	Intermittent recurrent nausea and vomiting	Occasional mild to moderate vomiting with or without other symptoms
Sore throat	Accompanied by respiratory distress or painful swallowing	Mild to moderate symptoms of upper respiratory infection not responding to standard conservative treatments	Sore throat or hoarseness without other signs of upper respiratory infection

(*Continued*)

TABLE 23-11 • GERD: Situations for Referral (*Continued*)

Symptom or Sign	Immediate Action: Call 911	Nonimmediate: Seek Medical Attention (call MD) or Go to ER	Routine: Inform MD at Later Time
Swallowing difficulty	New-onset or progressive choking feeling	Decreased intake due to painful swallowing, with potential risk of dehydration or malnutrition	Increase in frequency or duration of trouble swallowing over time
Vomiting blood (hematemesis)	New-onset vomiting with clots or accompanied with other signs or symptoms (eg, drop in blood pressure)	New or recurrent blood-streaked vomiting without other significant symptoms	

Source: References 3 and 7.

TABLE 23-12 • GERD: Medication-Related Problems (MRPs)

Category of MRP	Example of a Medication-Related Problem
Nonadherence	Patient reports no longer taking proton pump inhibitor, with continued complaints of dyspepsia and regurgitation Patient reports taking H_2-receptor antagonist as needed with continued complaints of dyspepsia and regurgitation Patient reports taking proton pump inhibitor with meal and other meds, instead of on an empty stomach, as directed
Unnecessary medication	Patient reports that H_2-receptor antagonist (ie, ranitidine) was started following hospital stay; however, patient has no current symptoms Patient taking two different proton pump inhibitors
Need for additional medication	Patient has daily heartburn not relieved with antacids Patient had good relief of GERD symptoms with trial of proton pump inhibitor, but symptoms have recurred off medication (indicates need for maintenance therapy)
Ineffective medication or dose too low	Patient has continued symptoms of dyspepsia despite taking once-daily H_2-receptor antagonist Patient not responding to therapy for another disorder because the increased gastric pH caused by proton pump inhibitor is decreasing absorption of another medication (eg, iron salts)
Dosage too high	Patient taking H_2-receptor antagonist 5 times daily as needed for symptom relief Patient taking a dose of H_2-receptor antagonist that is not dosed appropriately for renal function
Adverse drug event	Patient reports muscle spasms/tremors while taking promotility agent (ie, metoclopramide)

Scenario 1: Nonadherence	
Assessment	• During the comprehensive medication review, your patient reported the following: No longer taking prescribed therapy: • Omeprazole 20 mg oral capsule • Prescribed 1 capsule by mouth once daily Continued symptoms of regurgitation and dyspepsia at least 3-4 times per week
Plan	The above information is provided to inform you of your patient's nonadherence with prescribed therapy. If appropriate, please consider speaking with your patient at the next office visit regarding the importance of taking prescribed therapy daily to avoid development of symptoms and further GI-related issues.
Scenario 2: Ineffective medication	
Assessment	• During the comprehensive medication review, your patient reported the following: Currently taking the following with regard to this recommendation: • Ranitidine 150 mg tablet • Patient reports taking 1 tablet by mouth once daily Continued symptoms of dyspepsia despite taking once-daily H_2-receptor antagonist
Plan	If appropriate, please consider increasing the frequency of H_2-receptor antagonist dosing to twice daily or changing therapy to a proton pump inhibitor to help reduce GERD symptoms and optimize therapy.
Scenario 3: Unnecessary Medication/Duplication of Therapy (Two Different Prescribers)	
Assessment	• During the comprehensive medication review, your patient reported taking the following medications: Omeprazole 40 mg capsule • Patient reports taking 1 capsule by mouth once daily • Prescribed by: John Doe, MD Pantoprazole sodium 40 mg tablet • Patient reports taking 1 tablet by mouth once daily • Prescribed by: Jane Doe, MD
Plan	Please consider discontinuing one of the above proton pump inhibitors.

FIGURE 23-3 GERD: sample provider communications.

TABLE 23-13 • Therapeutic Approach to GERD in Adults

Patient Presentation	Recommended Treatment Regimen	Comments
Intermittent, mild heartburn	**Lifestyle modifications PLUS patient-directed therapy** Antacids Maalox or Mylanta 30 mL as needed or after meals and at bedtime Gaviscon 2 tablets after meals and at bedtime Calcium carbonate 500 mg, 2-4 tablets as needed *and/or* Nonprescription H_2-receptor antagonists (taken ≤2 times daily) Cimetidine 200 mg Famotidine 10 mg Nizatidine 75 mg Ranitidine 75 mg *or* Nonprescription proton pump inhibitor (taken once daily) Esomeprazole 20 mg Lansoprazole 15 mg Omeprazole 20 mg Omeprazole/sodium bicarbonate 20 mg/1000 mg	Lifestyle modifications should be individualized for each patient. Weight loss in obese patients and elevation of the head of the bed have been proven most beneficial. If symptoms are unrelieved with lifestyle modifications and nonprescription medications after 2 weeks, patient should seek medical attention.
Symptomatic relief of GERD	**Lifestyle modifications PLUS prescription-strength acid-suppression therapy** H_2-receptor antagonists (for 6-12 weeks) Cimetidine 400 mg 4 times daily or 800 mg twice daily Famotidine 20 mg twice daily Nizatidine 150 mg twice daily Ranitidine 150 mg twice daily *or* Proton pump inhibitors (for 4-8 weeks); all are given once daily Dexlansoprazole 30 mg Esomeprazole 20-40 mg Lansoprazole 15 mg Omeprazole 20 mg Omeprazole/sodium bicarbonate 20 mg Pantoprazole 40 mg Rabeprazole 20 mg	For typical symptoms, treat empirically with prescription-strength acid-suppression therapy. If symptoms recur, consider maintenance therapy. *Note*: Most patients will require standard doses for maintenance therapy. Mild GERD can usually be treated effectively with H_2-receptor antagonists. Patients with moderate to severe symptoms should receive a proton pump inhibitor as initial therapy.
Healing of erosive esophagitis or treatment of patients presenting with moderate to severe symptoms or complications	**Lifestyle modifications *plus*** Proton pump inhibitors for 4-16 weeks (up to twice daily) Dexlansoprazole 60 mg daily Esomeprazole 20-40 mg daily Lansoprazole 30 mg daily Omeprazole 20 mg daily Pantoprazole 40 mg daily Rabeprazole 20 mg daily *or* High-dose H_2-receptor antagonist (for 8-12 weeks) • Cimetidine 400 mg 4 times daily or 800 mg twice daily • Famotidine 20-40 mg twice daily • Nizatidine 150 mg 2-4 times daily • Ranitidine 150 mg 4 times daily	For atypical or alarm symptoms, obtain endoscopy (if possible) to evaluate mucosa. Give a trial of a proton pump inhibitor. If symptoms are relieved, consider maintenance therapy. Proton pump inhibitors are the most effective maintenance therapy for patients with atypical symptoms, complications, and erosive disease. Patients not responding to pharmacologic therapy, including those with persistent atypical symptoms, should be evaluated via ambulatory reflux monitoring to confirm the diagnosis of GERD (if possible).
Interventional therapies	Antireflux surgery	

Source: Data compiled from DiPiro JT, Talbert RL, Yee GC, et al. *Pharmacotherapy: A Pathophysiologic Approach*, 10th ed. New York, NY: McGraw-Hill; 2017.

patient-specific characteristics, and the nature of the relationship with the provider.

Follow-up to assess relief of symptoms, effects of interventions, and potential adverse effects is essential in patients with GERD. The interval for follow-up will depend on a number of factors, including severity of symptoms at time of intervention, type of intervention, and patient-specific factors such as age, comorbid conditions, and ability to return for follow-up. A concise representation for general guidelines for the medical management of patients with GERD is provided in Table 23-13.[3] Many patients with GERD may require maintenance therapy with a proton pump inhibitor or other agent for management of recurrent symptoms. Maintenance therapy should be provided with the least potent agent at the lowest possible dose that adequately controls symptoms.

REFERENCES

1. El-Serag HB, Sweet S, Winchester CC, Dent J. Update on the epidemiology of gastro-oesophageal reflux disease: A systematic review. *Gut.* 2014;63: 871-880.
2. Wallace JL, Sharkey KA. Pharmacotherapy of gastric acidity, peptic ulcers, and gastroesophageal reflux disease. In: Brunton LL, Chabner BA, Knollmann BC, eds. *Goodman & Gilman's: The Pharmacological Basis of Therapeutics*, 12th ed. New York, NY: McGraw-Hill; 2011: Chap 45.
3. May D, Thiman M, Rao SSC. Chapter 32. Gastroesophageal reflux disease. In: DiPiro JT, Talbert RL, Yee GC, Matzke GR, Wells BG, Posey LM, eds. *Pharmacotherapy: A Pathophysiologic Approach*, 10th ed. New York, NY: McGraw-Hill; 2017.
4. The American Gastroenterological Association (AGA) Institute Medical Position Panel. American Gastroenterological Association medical position statement on the management of gastroesophageal reflux disease. *Gastroenterology.* 2008;135:1383-1391.
5. *Plain Language Thesaurus for Health Communications.* National Center for Health Marketing; October 2007. Available at https://www.benaroyaresearch.org/sites/default/files/Plain_Language_Thesaurus_for_Health_Communications.pdf. Accessed May 2, 2017.
6. *Medicare Part D Medication Therapy Management Program Standardized Format.* Available at https://www.cms.gov/Medicare/Prescription-Drug-Coverage/PrescriptionDrugCovContra/Downloads/MTM-Program-Standardized-Format-English-and-Spanish-Instructions-Samples-v032712.pdf. Accessed May 2, 2017.
7. Katz PO, Gerson LB, Vela MF. Guidelines for the diagnosis and management of gastroesophageal reflux disease. *Am J Gastroenterol* 2013;108:308-328.
8. Clinical Pharmacology [database online]. Tampa, FL: Gold Standard, Inc.; 2017. Report available at http://clinicalpharmacology.com. Accessed May 2, 2017.
9. LexiComp Online [database online]. Hudson, OH: Lexicomp, Inc.; 2017. Report available at http://online.lexi.com. Accessed May 2, 2017.
10. Natural Medicines [database online]. Somerville, MA: Therapeutic Research Center; 2017. Report available at https://naturalmedicines.therapeuticresearch.com. Accessed May 2, 2017.
11. Kiefer D, Cherney K. *Herbs and Supplements for Acid Reflux (GERD).* Available at http://www.healthline.com/health/gerd/melatonin. Accessed May 2, 2017.
12. Patrick L. Gastroesophageal reflux disease (GERD): A review of conventional and alternative treatments. *Altern Med Rev.* 2011;16:116-133.

Review Questions

1. Which of the following is the most appropriate definition for gastroesophageal reflux disease (GERD)?
   a. Inflammation of the lining of the esophagus.
   b. A condition that develops when reflux of the stomach content causes troublesome symptoms and/or complications.
   c. Erosion of the squamous epithelium of the esophagus.
   d. A condition in which tissue lining the esophagus is replaced by tissue similar to the lining in the intestine.

2. Which of the following is a potential secondary cause and/or contributing factor that may worsen symptoms of GERD?
   a. Eating a high protein, low-fat meal
   b. Drinking water
   c. Eating chocolate
   d. Taking calcium supplements

3. A patient comes to the pharmacy complaining of belching and regurgitation. She states that her diet has been consistent with her favorites of grape juice, noodles (containing carrots, onions, and sweet bell peppers) and pasta. She is currently taking acetaminophen for general pain and amlodipine for hypertension (therapy started 1 month ago). Which of the following foods and/or medication is likely causing the patient's GERD symptoms?
   a. Grape juice
   b. Carrots
   c. Acetaminophen
   d. Amlodipine

4. Which of the following is an appropriate therapeutic goal for management of GERD?
   a. Alleviating or eliminating symptoms
   b. Decreasing frequency and duration of GERD symptoms
   c. Preventing the development of complications
   d. All of the above are appropriate therapeutic goals

5. A patient approaches you in a clinic setting and asks "What is a PPI?" How would you respond utilizing living room language?
   a. A PPI is a medication that decreases gastric hyperacidity by working on the proton pumps in the gut.
   b. A PPI is a medication that neutralizes acid in the stomach, thereby reducing GERD symptoms.
   c. A PPI is a medication that prevents the stomach from producing acid and can heal the food pipe or esophagus.
   d. A PPI is medication that binds to proton pumps in the stomach and inhibits acid production in a very potent manner.

6. A patient asks for additional tips and recommendations to help in managing GERD symptoms. Which of the following is an appropriate statement to include in the medication action plan?
   a. Begin a plan to lose weight, as this may help to reduce symptoms.
   b. Prop your head up with pillows to help decrease reflux at night.
   c. Take proton pump inhibitor with foods that may increase acid or reflux.
   d. Take antacids as often as needed to treat breakthrough symptoms of GERD.

7. A patient notes that omeprazole was continued after hospital discharge. On further questioning, the patient states that she does not experience any GERD symptoms and wants to stop taking the medication. Following the MTM encounter, you decide to communicate this finding to the physician. Which of the following would be the best categorization for this medication-related problem?
   a. Unnecessary medication
   b. Nonadherence
   c. Dosage too high
   d. Adverse drug event

8. Which of the following is an alarm symptom that would constitute immediate referral or a possible emergency in a patient with GERD?
   a. Persistent sore throat with hoarseness
   b. Mild and occasional regurgitation
   c. New-onset dysphagia with choking feeling
   d. More than occasional abdominal discomfort and cramps

9. A patient with typical GERD symptoms takes a 2-week trial of OTC omeprazole. Following the trial, the patient reports no improvement in symptoms, despite taking omeprazole at the recommended dosage for 2 weeks. Which of the following is the most appropriate recommendation?
   a. Follow up with her physician for further evaluation.
   b. Take an additional 2 weeks of omeprazole.
   c. Take an additional capsule of omeprazole in the evening.
   d. Stop the omeprazole and switch to ranitidine 75 mg one tablet daily.

10. For patients with symptomatic GERD, which of the following is an appropriate treatment option?
    a. Once-daily dosing of H_2-receptor antagonists
    b. Twice-daily dosing of proton pump inhibitors
    c. Once-daily dosing of proton pump inhibitors
    d. Twice-daily dosing of antacids

ANSWERS

1. b	2. c	3. d
4. d	5. c	6. a
7. a	8. c	9. a
10. c		

24

Headache MTM Data Set

Stacey D. Curtis, PharmD and Kristin W. Weitzel, PharmD, CDE, FAPhA

KEY POINTS

- When assessing a patient who is experiencing headache for the first time, it is important to ask appropriate questions to determine the type of headache (eg, tension, migraine).
- Medication therapy management (MTM) providers should assess for any underlying conditions that may contribute to headache, and refer patients in whom a headache may be a symptom of a more serious problem (eg, severely elevated blood pressure).
- When possible, MTM providers should encourage patients experiencing moderate to severe migraine to take migraine-specific medications such as "triptans" for relief of pain. These medications are more effective than analgesic pain relievers for migraine headache.
- MTM providers should educate patients to take triptans as soon as possible at the start of migraine pain for maximal effect.
- MTM providers should stay alert for patients who have frequent, very severe, or long-lasting migraine headaches. These patients may benefit from preventive therapy to decrease migraine frequency or severity.

INTRODUCTION TO HEADACHE

Headache is a pain that arises from either the neck or the head. In 2013, the International Headache Society (IHS) updated its classification system and diagnostic criteria for headache disorders, cranial neuralgias, and facial pain.[1] The IHS classifies headache into two categories: *primary* (migraine, tension-type, and cluster headache) and *secondary* (symptomatic of organic disease) headache disorders.

Migraines affect more women than men in adulthood. Adults between the ages of 30 and 39 years have the highest incidence of migraine headache. Economically, migraines cost 13 billion dollars per year because of missed workdays and lower productivity.[1,2] Similar to migraines, tension-type headaches are more common in women than men and have the highest incidence in patients in their fourth decade of life. Cluster headaches are uncommon, but can be extremely severe, with acute attacks, or "cluster" periods, that can last weeks and up to months. Unlike migraines and tension headaches, cluster headaches are more common in men and occur in the third to fifth decade of life.[1,2] Information presented in this chapter will focus on migraine treatment, as this headache type has a significant number of available pharmacotherapy options and is encountered relatively frequently in practice (Table 24-1).

Headaches can be classified in various ways, and are diagnosed and classified according to presenting symptoms, medical history, and physical exam (Table 24-2). A neurologic exam can be used, but only if proper assessment cannot be done with a patient history or physical examination. Migraine headaches are commonly associated with provoking factors, or triggers (Table 24-3).

Other terms associated with headache are as follows:

- *Aura*—transient neurological symptoms (visual, sensory, and/or speech) that precede a headache in some subsets (eg, migraine with aura). Aura symptoms often include visual changes such as flashing lights, flickering lines, loss of vision, tingling, or numbness.
- *Primary headache*—headache not associated with another disease state or health condition.
- *Secondary headache*—headache caused by another disease state or health condition.
- *Rebound headache*—increasing headache frequency due to overuse of medication; also referred to as medication-overuse headache.

Prognosis and Outcomes for Headache

Although headaches may be a chronic condition, they are manageable in most cases. Severity and frequency of headaches usually decline as patients get older. However, there is a risk for ischemic stroke in patients who experience chronic migraines.[1,2] Additionally, patients experiencing chronic daily headache or chronic migraine have greater headache-related disability. In these cases, patients may spend a significant amount of time with debilitating pain and associated symptoms.[6]

TABLE 24-1 • International Headache Society Classification System: Focus on Migraine Headache

Migraine without aura
Migraine with aura Migraine with typical aura (lasting <1 hour) with or without headache
Migraine with brainstem aura Hemiplegic migraine (familial, sporadic) Retinal migraine (repeated attacks of monocular visual disturbance)
Chronic migraine (occurring on ≥15 days/month for >3 months)
Complications of migraine Status migrainous (debilitating attack lasting for >72 hours) Persistent aura without infarction (symptoms persisting for >1 week) Migrainous infarction (aura symptoms associated with an ischemic brain lesion) Migraine aura-triggered seizure
Probable migraine with or without aura
Episodic syndromes that may be associated with migraine Recurrent gastrointestinal (GI) disturbance (cyclical vomiting syndrome or abdominal migraine) Benign paroxysmal vertigo Benign paroxysmal torticollis
Tension-type headache
Cluster headache and other trigeminal autonomic cephalalgias
Other primary headaches
Headache attributed to head and/or neck trauma
Headache attributed to cranial or cervical vascular disorder
Headache attributed to nonvascular intracranial disorder
Headache attributed to a substance or its withdrawal
Headache attributed to infection
Headache attributed to disorder of homeostasis
Headache or facial pain attributed to disorder of cranium, neck, eyes, ears, nose, sinuses, teeth, mouth, or other facial or cervical structure
Headache attributed to psychiatric disorder
Cranial neuropathies and facial pains
Other headache disorders, not elsewhere classified or unspecified

Source: Data from reference 1.

TABLE 24-2 • IHS Diagnostic Criteria for Migraine

Migraine without aura
At least five attacks
Headache attack lasts 4-72 hours (untreated or unsuccessfully treated)
Headache has at least two of the following characteristics: Unilateral location Pulsating quality Moderate or severe intensity Aggravation by or avoidance of routine physical activity (e.g., walking or climbing stairs)
During headache at least one of the following: Nausea, vomiting, or both Photophobia and phonophobia Not attributed to another disorder
Migraine with aura (classic migraine)
At least two attacks
Migraine aura fulfills criteria for typical aura, hemiplegic aura, retinal migraine, or brainstem aura
Not attributed to another disorder
Typical aura
Fully reversible visual, sensory, or speech symptoms (or any combination) but no motor weakness
Homonymous or bilateral visual symptoms, including positive features (eg, flickering lights, spots, lines) or negative features (eg, loss of vision) or unilateral sensory symptoms including positive features (eg, pins and needles) or negative features (ie, numbness), or any combination
At least two of the following: At least one symptom that develops gradually over a minimum of 5 minutes or different symptoms that occur in succession or both Each symptom lasts for at least 5 minutes and for no longer than 60 minutes Headache that meets criteria for migraine without aura begins during the aura or follows aura within 60 minutes

Abbreviation: IHS = International Headache Society.

Source: Data from reference 1.

Therapeutic Goals for Headache

Proper management of symptoms is vital for the treatment of primary headaches to reduce pain acutely and decrease frequency of headache recurrence. For migraine therapy, short-term goals include restoring the ability to function normally after acute attacks, reducing dependence on acute medications, and avoiding adverse effects. Long-term goals include reducing overall migraine frequency, reducing exposure to migraine triggers, reducing the need for preventive medications, and improving overall quality of life (Table 24-4). Treatment goals for tension headaches are similar to those for migraines. For cluster headaches, the primary goal is to reduce the incidence of attacks during cluster periods. For secondary headaches, the general approach to therapy is to treat the underlying condition, instead of treating the headache itself (Table 24-5).[2]

Therapeutic Failure

Drug therapy for headaches is deemed a therapeutic failure if the patient does not gain normal functionality after acute treatment, or if an individual experiences consistent or enhanced recurrence of headache symptoms.[1,2]

TABLE 24-3 • Commonly Reported Triggers of Migraine

Food triggers
Alcohol
Caffeine/caffeine withdrawal
Chocolate
Fermented and pickled foods
Monosodium glutamate (eg, in Chinese food, seasoned salt, and instant foods)
Nitrate-containing foods (eg, processed meats)
Saccharin/aspartame (eg, diet foods or diet sodas)
Tyramine-containing foods
Environmental triggers
Glare or flickering lights
Heat
High altitude
Loud noises
Medication overuse
Strong smells and fumes
Tobacco smoke
Weather changes
Behavioral-physiologic triggers
Emotional stress
Excess or insufficient sleep
Fatigue
Hormonal fluctuations
Insufficient nutrition
Menstruation, menopause
Neck pain
Sexual activity
Skipped meals
Strenuous physical activity (eg, prolonged overexertion) or not enough
Stress or poststress

Source: References 2, 3, 4, and 5.

CORE ELEMENT 1—COMPREHENSIVE MEDICATION REVIEW FOR PATIENTS WITH HEADACHE

Table 24-6 lists some suggested questions to use when conducting a medication therapy review in a patient with headache. The number and types of questions will depend on several factors, including the amount of time for the interview, number of concurrent medication-related problems (MRPs), urgency of MRPs, and the reliability of the patient in providing accurate information, among others. In time-limited interactions or in complex cases with multiple medical issues, the MTM provider may choose to target questions that help to identify or rule out issues of an urgent nature (see red flags for immediate medical referral in Table 24-7). MTM providers should remember to use living room language during the interview (Figure 24-1), and to be prepared for questions that patients may ask regarding their headaches (Table 24-8).

In some cases, a headache can be a symptom of a severe, acute neurologic event (eg, subarachnoid hemorrhage or meningitis). MTM providers should be aware of the warning signs of acute headaches caused by a more serious underlying pathology and be prepared to refer these patients to medical care immediately if needed (Table 24-7).

TABLE 24-4 • Goals of Therapy in Migraine Management

Goals of long-term migraine treatment
Reduce migraine frequency, severity, and disability
Reduce reliance on poorly tolerated, ineffective, or unwanted acute pharmacotherapies
Improve quality of life
Prevent headache
Avoid escalation of headache medication use
Educate and enable patients to manage their disease
Reduce headache-related distress and psychological symptoms
Goals for acute migraine treatment
Treat migraine attacks rapidly and consistently without recurrence
Restore the patient's ability to function
Minimize the use of backup and rescue medications[a]
Optimize self-care for overall management
Be cost-effective in overall management
Cause minimal or no adverse effects

[a] Rescue medications are defined as medications used at home when other treatments fail that permit the patient to get relief without a visit to the physician's office or emergency department.

Source: References 3, 7, and 8.

TABLE 24-5 • When to Consider Secondary Headache

Subacute and/or progressive headache(s) that worsen over a long period of time (months)
A new or different headache or a statement by the headache patient that "this is the worst headache ever"
Any headaches of maximum severity at onset
Headaches of new onset after the age of 50 years old
Headaches arising from a cough, sneeze, or exertion (physical or sexual)
Headaches presenting with systemic effects (fever, confusion, visual alteration, etc) or associated with other disease states, such as meningitis or cancer
Neurological signs that may suggest a secondary cause (meningismus, confusion, papilledema, etc)
History of seizures

Source: References 1 and 2.

TABLE 24-6 • Suggested Questions to Ask When Conducting a Medication Review in a Patient with Headache

How often do you experience headaches?
How long have you experienced headaches? When did they first begin?
How long do your headaches last?
Where is most of your pain located? Does it radiate to other parts of your body?
Using a scale of 1 to 10 to describe the pain, with 10 being the worst possible pain, how bad is the pain from your headaches?
What makes the pain worse?
What makes the pain better?
Do you have any other symptoms with your headaches (nausea, vomiting, sensitivity to light and sound, etc)? If so, what symptoms do you experience?
Are you able to go about your everyday routine when you experience your headaches?
Do you know if anything triggers your headache? If so, what?
What medications do you take for your headaches? How do you take them?
How well do your medications work to treat your headaches?
What other medications have you taken in the past for your headache?
(If patient is female) What effect does your menstrual cycle have on your headaches?
Have you ever stopped taking any of your prescribed headache medications without telling your physician? If so, why?
What over-the-counter (OTC) medications or herbals do you use for your headache?
Other than medicines, what have you tried for your headache (eg, lifestyle changes)?
What has your physician discussed with you regarding OTC medications that you should avoid because they can worsen your headache?

Source: References 1, 2, 8, and 9.

Acute headache—sudden attack of head pain.

Anticonvulsants—medications for seizures, but can be used to prevent headaches; also referred to as *antiseizure* or *antiepileptic medications.*

Antidepressants—medications that can be used to prevent headaches.

Aura—a set of neurologic symptoms that can happen before a migraine.

Bilateral—two-sided.

Cluster headache—a very painful type of headache that involves one side of the head.

Migraine—a type of headache that usually has medium to really severe pain; usually the pain is on one side of the head, and it may worsen with activity and you may be sensitive to light and/or sound.

Narcotics—a synonym for opiates; powerful pain relievers.

NSAIDs—nonsteroidal anti-inflammatory drugs; a class of pain relievers that can be used to treat the pain from headaches; can be prescription or OTC.

Opioids—a class of pain relievers that can be used to treat the pain from headaches; a prescription is required for these types of medications.

Pain scale—a numerical scale that is used to assess pain level; usually uses the numbers 1 through 10, where 10 is the worst possible pain.

Primary headache—a headache that is not caused by another health condition.

Prophylaxis—prevention.

Rebound headache—also known as *medication overuse headache*, this is a headache that can be caused by using too many pain reliever medications for headache symptoms.

Secondary headache—headache caused by another health issue.

Stroke—a condition caused by bleeding or lack of blood in the brain, which may cause a loss of speech, memory, or other abilities; some types of headache may increase risk of stroke.

Tension headache—the most common type of headache; pressure is usually on both sides of the head and the pain may come from the back of the neck, or other muscles.

Triggers—dietary, lifestyle, or other factors that can cause a patient to have a headache; may include certain foods, changes in sleep patterns or altitude, caffeine intake, etc.

Triptans—a class of medications usually used to treat moderate to severe migraine headaches (sumatriptan, etc.)

Unilateral—one-sided.

FIGURE 24-1 Living room language for headache.

TABLE 24-7 • Warning Signs in Headache: Red Flags for Immediate Medical Referral

Head or neck injury
New-onset headache, new type of pain (eg, "worst ever" headache)
New type of headache pain or changes in headache pattern
Progressively worsening headache
Abrupt onset of maximal pain
Headache brought on by exertion
New-onset headache in patients aged > 50 years
Coexisting neurological symptoms (eg, confusion, weakness)
Coexisting systemic symptoms (eg, fever, weight loss)
Secondary risk factors such as a history of cancer or human immunodeficiency virus infection

Source: Reference 10.

CORE ELEMENT 2—PERSONAL MEDICATION LIST[11]

A sample personal medication list (PML) for a patient with headache is given in Figure 24-2. This example is representative of medications related to headache. Additional medications for other disease states should be added and listed separately. MTM providers should remember to use plain language when creating the PML.

CORE ELEMENT 3—MEDICATION ACTION PLAN[11]

A sample medication action plan (MAP) for patients with headache is provided in Figure 24-3. This example is representative only of action steps for the patient with headache. MAPs for other disease states or other MRPs should be added and

TABLE 24-8 • Questions to Anticipate from Patients Regarding Headache

What is aura?

- A common symptom often coming before migraines. It may come on as a strange light, an unpleasant smell, or confusing thoughts. Sometimes you can have an aura and then not get the migraine.

What are the differences among headache types?

- The most common types of headaches are migraines, cluster headaches, and tension headaches.
- *Migraine* is a chronic disorder characterized by a series of headaches. The pain is usually on one side of the head and is of a pulsating nature. Headaches can last anywhere between 2 and 72 hours. Migraines can be further classified as those with or without aura.
- *Cluster headaches* are also one-sided. However, they usually last only between 15 and 180 minutes and can occur up to 8 times per day. The pain from a cluster headache is excruciating, sometimes being described as the worst pain a human can endure. Patients are usually described as restless or agitated during an acute attack. Symptoms associated with cluster headaches are tearing and watering of the eyes, nasal congestion, runny nose, forehead and facial sweating, and other eye-related symptoms, such as swelling or visual changes.
- *Tension-type headaches* are the most common type of headache. The pain from these headaches can radiate from the lower back of the head, the neck, or the eyes. Typical tension-type headaches last 4-6 hours. They are more common in women.

What causes a headache?

- Headaches can be caused by a person's genetic predisposition (family history of headaches), lifestyle factors (changes in sleep, stress), other triggers (diet, etc), other diseases, some medications (eg, bupropion), or other factors.

What health problems are associated with headache?

- Headaches are a common symptom of many other health conditions. If a headache is caused by another condition, it is referred to as a *secondary headache*. Headaches can be associated with head/neck trauma, cranial/cervical disorders such as stroke or intracranial hemorrhage, substance abuse or withdrawal, infection such as meningitis, and psychiatric disorders such as anxiety.

Do I have to take my headache medications every day?

- Medication used for acute headache attacks needs to be taken only during acute attacks. Prophylactic or preventive medication is taken every day to decrease frequency and severity of headaches.

Can I just stop my medications if I feel okay?

- Medication used for acute headache attacks can be discontinued after symptoms have been relieved. Prophylactic medications should be continued until your physician says otherwise.

What can happen if I stop taking my headache medications?

- Stopping your preventive medications all at once is not recommended. Do not discontinue these medications without talking to a healthcare provider. Acute headache treatments can usually be stopped without problems. If stopping your acute medications leads to increasing headache, you may be experiencing rebound headache and should be evaluated by a healthcare provider.

Can I take too much of my headache medication?

- Yes. Taking higher than recommended doses of acute or preventive medications can lead to an overdose and/or side effects. Additionally, rebound headaches may occur if certain acute medications are taken on a regular basis. Patients experiencing increased frequency or severity of headaches or needing higher doses should be evaluated by their healthcare providers.

When should I call my physician about my headaches?

- Call your physician when your headache symptoms are worse than normal, for example, if the headache is more painful than usual, or if it is located in a different area. Also call your physician if you experience new symptoms with your headache, such as fever or vision changes.

What should I do if I have a problem with my headache medications?

- Don't stop taking your headache medications without first talking to your physician. Speak with your physician and/or pharmacist to let them know about any problems you are having and together you can make sure your headache medications are the right ones for you.

PERSONAL MEDICATION LIST FOR *<Insert patient's name, DOB: mm/dd/yyyy>*	
Medication: Imitrex (sumatriptan) 50 mg	
How I use it: Take 1-2 tablets (50-100 mg) at onset of headache and repeat dose after 2 hours if pain is not relieved.	
Why I use it: Acute migraine	**Prescriber:** Parker
Date I started using it: 2/9/2017	**Date I stopped using it:** *(Leave blank for patient's notes)*
Why I stopped using it: *(Leave blank for patient's notes)*	
Medication: Chlorpromazine 10 mg	
How I use it: Take 1 tablet (10 mg) orally with sumatriptan at onset of migraine as needed for nausea.	
Why I use it: Nausea/vomiting	**Prescriber:** Parker
Date I started using it: 2/9/2017	**Date I stopped using it:** *(Leave blank for patient's notes)*
Why I stopped using it: *(Leave blank for patient's notes)*	

FIGURE 24-2 Sample personal medication list for headache patients.

<table>
<tr><td colspan="2">DATE PREPARED: <Insert date></td></tr>
<tr><td colspan="2">What we talked about:
You reported having headaches more often after taking acetaminophen 2 tablets twice daily for 3 weeks. It sounds as though you are experiencing rebound headache, which is seen in patients who overuse acute headache medications.</td></tr>
<tr><td>What I need to do:
Here are some things that I can do to help lessen this effect:
• Slowly cut down on the amount of acetaminophen needed for my headaches.
• If an acute headache arises, use ibuprofen 1 or 2 tablets instead of acetaminophen.
• After cutting back on the acetaminophen, limit my acute medication for headache to 2 or 3 times per week.
• If the number of headaches does not decrease, or if I find that I need to take an acute medication more than 2 or 3 times per week, make a return appointment. I may need a preventive medication.</td><td>What I did and when I did it:
(Leave blank for patient's notes)</td></tr>
<tr><td colspan="2">What we talked about:
Need to see how well the new prescription for sumatriptan is working to decrease migraine severity and pain.</td></tr>
<tr><td>What I need to do:
Keep a headache diary over the next 4 weeks that describes
• When (how often) I have a headache
• How bad the headache is
• How long the headache lasts
• Any triggers I can think of
• How the new medication works to relieve the headache
Bring this headache diary to my next visit so that we can see how well the medication is working and if any changes are needed.</td><td>What I did and when I did it:
(Leave blank for patient's notes)</td></tr>
</table>

FIGURE 24-3 Sample medication action plan for a patient with headache.

listed separately. In general, only a few of the most important action steps should be listed, so as not to overwhelm the patient. Other areas for patient self-management can be addressed at later visits. MTM providers should remember to use plain language when creating the MAP.

CORE ELEMENT 4—INTERVENTION AND/OR REFERRAL

Interventions for headache are mainly pharmacologic, but some nonpharmacologic interventions can help to decrease headache severity or frequency. Acutely, application of ice or moving to a quiet, darkened room may provide relief for a migraine. Chronically, patient awareness of and decreased exposure to known headache triggers can help to decrease headache frequency. Female patients should be aware that changes in estrogen levels can trigger, intensify, or alleviate migraine headaches. It is important to advise patients to keep a journal to track possible triggers on onset of symptoms. Medications should be selected for either prevention or management of acute headache pain and are most effective if taken at the onset of migraine.[2]

Tables 24-9 and 24-10 provide an overview of drug therapy for acute and preventive treatment of headaches, respectively; Table 24-11 includes information on choice of therapy in comorbid conditions or special populations. In addition, Table 24-12 outlines

TABLE 24-9 • Medications for Management of Acute Headache

Medication Class and Drug Examples	Common/Serious Side Effects[b]	Blackbox Warnings/Contraindications	Pregnancy Category[c]	Headache Subtype
Serotonin agonists	Paresthesias	Acute myocardial infarction	C	M
"triptans"	Fatigue	Angina		
Almotriptan	Dizziness	Atherosclerosis		T
Eletriptan[a]	Flushing	Cardiac disease		
Frovatriptan	Warm sensations	MAOI therapy		C
Naratriptan	Somnolence	Hemiplegic and basilar migraines		
Rizatriptan		Stroke		
Sumatriptan		Hypertension		
Zolmitriptan		Hepatic disease		
		Coronary artery disease		

(Continued)

TABLE 24-9 • Medications for Management of Acute Headache (*Continued*)

Medication Class and Drug Examples	Common/Serious Side Effects[b]	Blackbox Warnings/Contraindications	Pregnancy Category[c]	Headache Subtype
NSAIDs Diclofenac Ibuprofen Ketorolac Naproxen	Bleeding GI upset Rebound headache	Coronary artery bypass graft GI bleeding GI perforation Myocardial infarction Stroke NSAID hypersensitivity Salicylate hypersensitivity	C	M T
Antiplatelets Aspirin	Tinnitus Bleeding	Salicylate hypersensitivity Bleeding disorders Children < 16 years old	D	M T
Acetaminophen (APAP)—various single-ingredient and combination products	Liver toxicity Rash	Alcoholism Hepatic disease Hepatitis	C	M T
Isometheptene combinations Isometheptene/ dichloralphenazone/APAP	Dizziness Skin rash Drowsiness Hepatitis	Cardiac disease Glaucoma Hepatic disease Hypertension MAOI therapy Renal disease Renal failure	C	M
Butalbital combinations Butalbital/APAP/caffeine Butalbital/ASA/caffeine	Nausea/vomiting Diarrhea Constipation Dizziness Drowsiness	Agranulocytosis Anemia Hematological disease Hemophilia Hepatic disease Hypoprothrombinemia Nasal polyps Peptic ulcer disease Porphyria Thrombotic thrombocytopenic purpura Vitamin K deficiency Von Willebrand disease	C (with APAP) C or D (with aspirin)	M
Ergot alkaloids Dihydroergotamine Ergotamine tartrate	Nausea/vomiting Abdominal pain Paresthesias Diarrhea Chest tightness	Coronary artery disease Hypertension Peripheral vascular disease Angina Arteriosclerosis Cardiac disease Myocardial infarction Stroke Buerger's disease Hypersensitivity Renal failure/impairment	X	M C

[a] Eletriptan is associated with significantly more drug interactions than other triptan agents.

[b] This is a general list and does not include all side effects that can occur from these drugs. Consult a drug reference source for a more inclusive list before making any recommendations. MTM providers should also consult a comprehensive drug interaction database before making pharmacotherapy recommendations.

[c] Product labeling for all prescription drugs is being updated to reflect the new FDA Pregnancy Labeling and Lactation Rule. Please check individual product labeling for the most accurate and updated pregnancy information.

Abbreviations: APAP = acetaminophen; ASA = acetylsalicylic acid (aspirin); C = cluster (headache subtype); GI = gastrointestinal; M = migraine; MAOI = monoamine oxidase inhibitor; NSAID = nonsteroidal anti-inflammatory drug; T = tension headache.

Source: References 2, 12, and 13.

TABLE 24-10 • Medications for Migraine Prophylaxis

Medication Class and Drug Examples	Common/Serious Side Effects[a]	Blackbox Warnings/Contraindications	Pregnancy Category[b]	Headache Subtype
Anticonvulsants Topiramate Valproate	**Topiramate** Paresthesias Fatigue Anorexia Diarrhea Weight loss Hyperesthesia Memory difficulty Taste perversion Language problems Nausea **Valproate** Alopecia Tremor Asthenia Somnolence Weight gain	**Topiramate** Children, infants, neonates Elderly Glaucoma Depression COPD Renal disease **Valproate** Hepatitis Hepatic failure Pregnancy Children, infants, neonates Pancreatitis	D	M
Antidepressants Amitriptyline Venlafaxine	**Amitriptyline** Dry mouth Dizziness Drowsiness Rash **Venlafaxine** Headache Insomnia Drowsiness Dizziness Weight loss Diaphoresis Nausea Ejaculation dysfunction Nausea Orthostatic hypotension	**Amitriptyline** Increased risk of suicidal thoughts and behavior in children and young adults, particularly during the first few months of therapy Exacerbates underlying myocardial dysfunction TCA hypersensitivity MAOI therapy **Venlafaxine** Increased risk of suicidal thoughts and behavior in children and young adults, particularly during the first few months of therapy Increased risk of bleeding events if used with aspirin, NSAIDS, warfarin, or other anticoagulants Tachycardia MAOI therapy	C	M T
β-Blockers Atenolol Metoprolol Nadolol Propranolol Timolol	Mask hypoglycemia in diabetics Worsen insulin sensitivity, breathing disorders, and PVD Bradycardia Dizziness Exercise intolerance Fatigue Orthostatic hypotension (especially mixed α- and β-blockers)	Abrupt discontinuation Asthma (avoid nonselective BB) AV block Bradycardia Cardiogenic shock Acute heart failure Hypotension Pheochromocytoma (if not on α-blocker) Sick sinus syndrome	C D (atenolol)	M

(Continued)

TABLE 24-10 • Medications for Migraine Prophylaxis (*Continued*)

Medication Class and Drug Examples	Common/Serious Side Effects[a]	Blackbox Warnings/Contraindications	Pregnancy Category[b]	Headache Subtype
Calcium channel blockers Verapamil	Bradycardia Constipation	Acute MI AV block Cardiogenic shock Hypotension Heart failure/left ventricular systolic dysfunction Sick sinus syndrome Ventricular tachycardia Wolff-Parkinson-White syndrome	C	M
Nonsteroidal anti-inflammatory drugs Ibuprofen Ketoprofen Naproxen sodium	Bleeding GI upset Rebound headache	Coronary artery bypass graft GI bleeding GI perforation Myocardial infarction Stroke NSAID hypersensitivity Salicylate hypersensitivity	C	M T

[a] This is a general list and does not include all side effects that can occur from these drugs. Consult a drug reference source for a more inclusive list before making any recommendations. MTM providers should also consult a comprehensive drug interaction database before making pharmacotherapy recommendations.

[b] Product labeling for all prescription drugs is being updated to reflect the new FDA Pregnancy Labeling and Lactation Rule. Please check individual product labeling for the most accurate and updated pregnancy information.

Abbreviations: AV = atrioventricular; BB = β-blocker; C = cluster (headache subtype); COPD = chronic obstructive pulmonary disease; GI = gastrointestinal; M = migraine; MAOI = monoamine oxidase inhibitor; MI = myocardial infarction; NSAID = nonsteroidal anti-inflammatory drug; T = tension headache; TCA = tricyclic antidepressant.

Source: References 2, 12, and 13.

TABLE 24-11 • Considerations in Individualizing Headache Therapy

Comorbid Condition and Special Populations	Considerations for Drug Therapy
Hypertension, angina	**Acute** **Avoid:** Long-term use of nonsteroidal anti-inflammatory drugs, serotonin agonists **Prophylaxis (preferred agents)** β-Blockers: atenolol, metoprolol, nadolol, propranolol, timolol Verapamil
Anxiety, depression, fibromyalgia	**Prophylaxis** Tricyclic antidepressants
Epilepsy	**Prophylaxis** Valproate, topiramate
Essential tremor	**Prophylaxis** Propranolol
Comorbid conditions accompanied by weight gain (eg, fibromyalgia)	**Prophylaxis** Topiramate
Elderly	**Avoid:** Tricyclic antidepressants, anticonvulsants, or other agents with anticholinergic effects that may increase fall risk
Pregnancy and/or lactation	**Avoid:** Ergots, valproate, topiramate; assess risks and benefits of other treatments before use

Source: References 1, 2, and 14.

TABLE 24-12 • Herbal Supplements for Headache

Herbal	Typical Dose	Grade[a]	Cost[b]
Butterbur	75-150 mg specialized rhizome extract daily in ≤2 divided doses for ≤4 months	Possibly effective	$$-$$$
Coenzyme Q10	100 mg ≤3 times daily for 3 months 1-3 mg/kg of CoQ10 in liquid gel capsules daily 150 mg of CoQ10 has been taken daily	Possibly effective	$$-$$$
Feverfew	50-150 mg powder once daily for ≤4 months 2.08-18.75 mg extract 3 times daily for 3-4 months 300 mg with white willow 300 mg twice daily for 3 months	Possibly effective	$
Peppermint oil	10% applied across the forehead and temples at onset of tension headache and repeat in 15-30 minutes	Possibly effective	$$

[a] Level of evidence: "Likely effective"—this product has a very high level of reliable clinical evidence supporting its use for a specific indication. Products rated "likely effective" are generally considered appropriate to recommend; "possibly effective"—this product has some clinical evidence supporting its use for a specific indication; however, the evidence is limited by quantity, quality, or contradictory findings. Products rated "possibly effective" might be beneficial, but do not have enough high-quality evidence to be recommended for most people; "insufficient evidence"—there is insufficient reliable scientific evidence to provide an effectiveness rating.

[b] Cost: $ = ≤$10/month supply in recommended dosage; $$ = $11-$20/month; $$$ = $21-$50/month; $$$$ = >$50/month.

Source: Data compiled from reference 15.

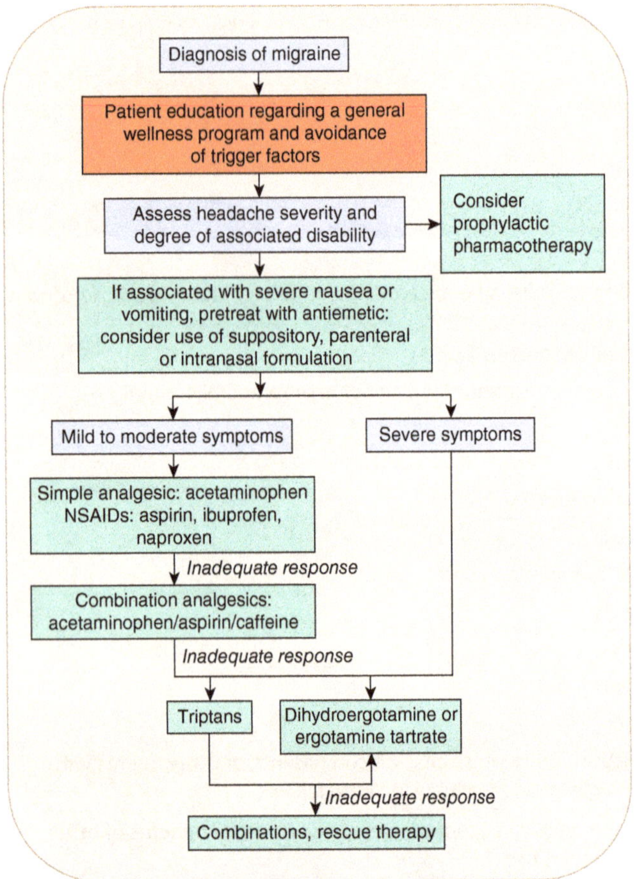

FIGURE 24-4 Treatment algorithm for migraine headaches.
Source: Reproduced, with permission, from DiPiro JT, Talbert RL, Yee GC, Matzke GR, Wells BG, Posey LM, eds. *Pharmacotherapy: A Pathophysiologic Approach*, 10th ed. New York, NY: McGraw-Hill; 2017.

herbal remedies that may be useful in the management of headache. Algorithms for acute migraine attacks, migraine prophylaxis, and guidelines for patient referral are provided in Figures 24-4, 24-5, and 24-6, respectively.

CORE ELEMENT 5—DOCUMENTATION AND FOLLOW-UP

Clear and succinct documentation of MRPs and recommendations is a key component of the MTM consult. Examples of potential MRPs in patients with headache are provided in Table 24-13. Sample communications and recommendations to providers to address medication-related issues are found in Figure 24-7. Recommendations may be communicated via fax, telephone, or other means of written or secure electronic communication. The examples below are for illustrative purposes. Actual communications to providers should be individualized according to the type of recommendation, patient specific characteristics, and the nature of the relationship with the provider.

Follow-up to assess headache and potential adverse effects is essential in patients with headache disorders. The interval for follow-up will depend on a number of factors, including severity of headache, type of intervention, and patient-specific factors such as age, comorbid conditions, and ability to return for follow-up. In many cases, the initial follow-up interval will be at least 4 to 6 weeks after the first visit. Patients will need time to experience migraines to determine whether a trial of acute therapy is successful. Additionally, most prophylactic medications will require at least 4 weeks to take effect. Patient counseling on proper medication use and adherence is necessary for positive therapeutic outcomes.

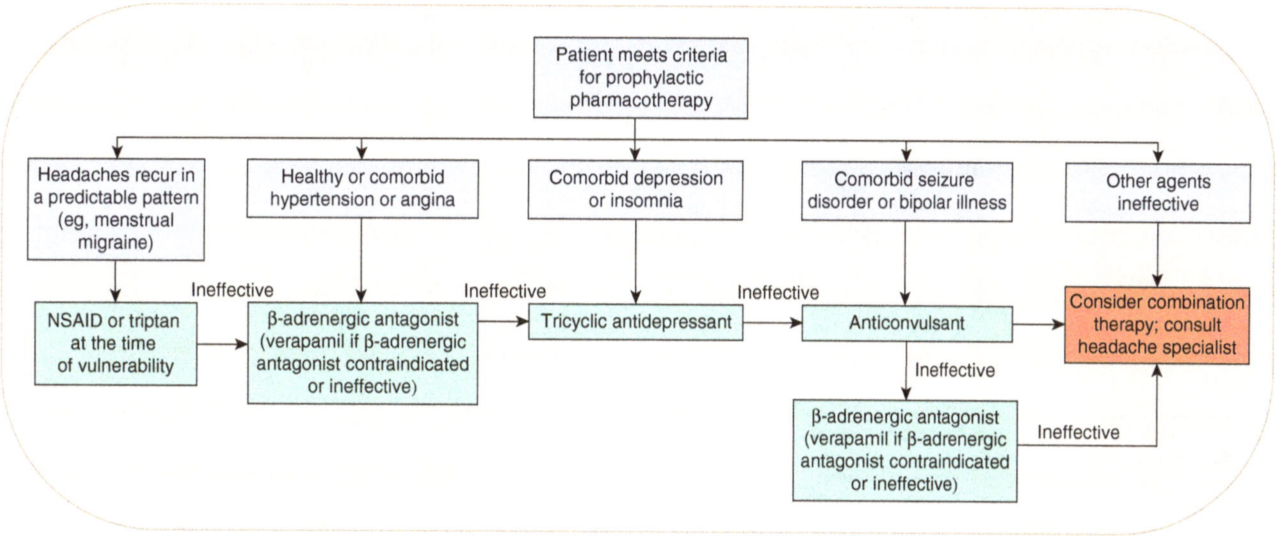

FIGURE 24-5 Treatment algorithm for prophylactic management of migraine headaches.
Source: Reproduced, with permission, from DiPiro JT, Talbert RL, Yee GC, Matzke GR, Wells BG, Posey LM: *Pharmacotherapy: A Pathophysiologic Approach*, 10th ed. New York, NY: McGraw-Hill; 2017.

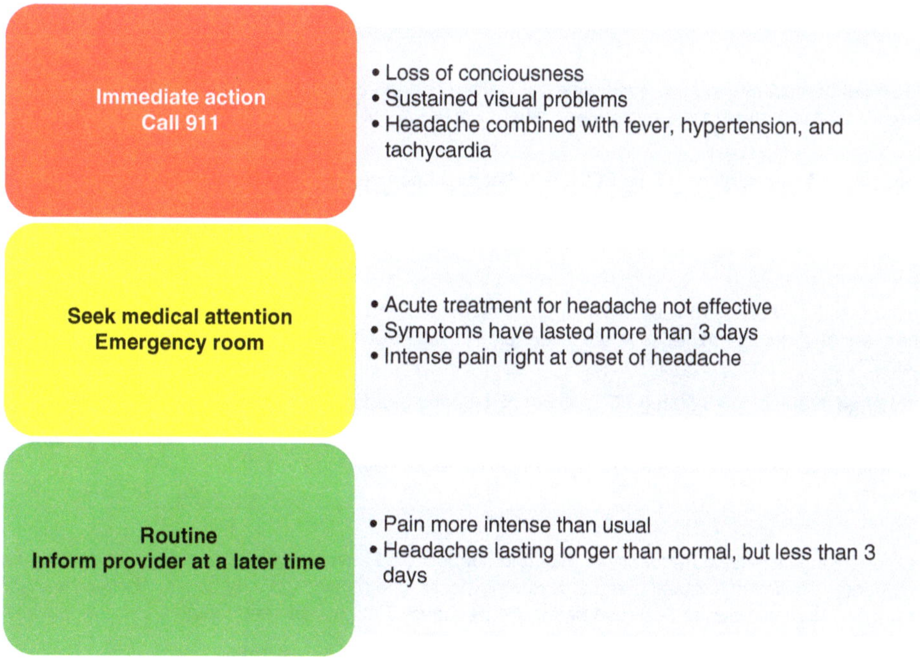

FIGURE 24-6 Referral for management of headache.
Source: References 1 and 8.

TABLE 24-13 • Medication-Related Problems (MRPs) in Patients with Headache

Category of MRP	Sample Medication-Related Problem
Nonadherence	Suboptimal control of headache frequency due to patient not taking prescribed preventive therapy Patient not taking triptan therapy due to lack of insurance coverage/cost of medication
Unnecessary medication	Duplicate therapy (eg, ergotamine and sumatriptan)
Need for additional medication	Lack of preventive therapy when it is indicated to decrease frequency and/or severity of migraines No antiemetic therapy when nausea is a significant component of patient's migraine
Ineffective medication	Patient taking only nonprescription acetaminophen for moderate to severe migraine headache Patient taking propranolol as needed for acute headache treatment

(*Continued*)

TABLE 24-13 • Medication-Related Problems (MRPs) in Patients with Headache (*Continued*)

Category of MRP	Sample Medication-Related Problem
Dosage too low	Suboptimal pain relief on low dose of triptan
Dosage too high	Patient experiencing rebound headaches due to overuse of acute migraine medication Patient with excessive sedation from valproate
Adverse drug event	Nausea from dihydroergotamine Gastric ulceration from high-dose NSAID[a] therapy

[a] Nonsteroidal anti-inflammatory drug.

Scenario: Patient given topiramate for migraine prophylaxis, but forgets to take it.
MRP: Nonadherence.

Assessment:

Patient with uncontrolled migraine on topiramate 25 mg daily. Lack of migraine control likely secondary to nonadherence with topiramate. Patient missing doses of topiramate due to forgetting to take medication. Establishing a routine and adherence reminders will help patient to remember to take topiramate.

Plan:

Recommend patient obtain pillbox, place in a convenient place, and set a daily alarm to remind her to take topiramate.

Scenario: Patient taking only nonprescription ibuprofen for acute moderate to severe migraine.
MRP: Ineffective medication.

Assessment:

Patient with uncontrolled relief of moderate to severe migraine pain taking nonprescription ibuprofen. Lack of migraine control likely secondary to use of nonspecific analgesic for moderate to severe migraine. Patient would benefit from migraine-specific therapy due to severity of migraines.

Plan:

Recommend medication change to sumatriptan 50 mg PO at onset of migraine headache.

Scenario: Patient taking isometheptene combination product and experiencing severe dizziness and drowsiness after each dose.
MRP: Adverse effect.

Assessment:

Patient with migraine experiencing dizziness/drowsiness after each isometheptene combination product dose when used for acute pain relief. Patient would benefit from a trial of another migraine agent less likely to cause these effects.

Plan:

Consider drug therapy change to sumatriptan 50 mg PO at onset of migraine headache.

Scenario: Patient taking zolmitriptan 2.5 mg by mouth as needed for migraine. She has increased her zolmitriptan from once per week to 3 days per week on average in the last 6 months. Patient is not on prophylactic migraine therapy.
MRP: Need for additional medication.

Assessment:

Patient with migraine experiencing increasing frequency of migraine headaches. Patient interview reveals no underlying serious causes of increased headache frequency. Continued frequent use (>2 days/week) of rescue medication may cause rebound headache. Patient would benefit from a trial of a preventive medication to decrease headache frequency. Patient has used topiramate for prophylaxis in the past with good response and tolerability.

Plan:

Consider addition of topiramate starting with 25 mg daily by mouth, titrated in 25 mg/week increments to a target of 100 mg daily given in two divided doses.

FIGURE 24-7 Sample provider communications for headache.

REFERENCES

1. Headache Classification Committee of the International Headache Society (IHS). The International Classification of Headache Disorders, 3rd ed. *Cephalalgia* 2013;33(9):629-808.
2. Minor DS, Harrell T. Headache disorders. In: DiPiro JT, Talbert RL, Yee GC, Matzke GR, Wells BG, Posey L. eds. *Pharmacotherapy: A Pathophysiologic Approach*, 10th ed. New York, NY: McGraw-Hill; 2017. Available at http://accesspharmacy.mhmedical.com/content.aspx?bookid=1861&sectionid=146063736.
3. Buse DC, Rupnow FT, Lipton RB. Assessing and managing all aspects of migraine: Migraine attacks, migraine-related functional impairment, common comorbidities, and quality of life. *Mayo Clin Proc.* 2009;84:422-435.
4. Martin PR. Behavioral management of migraine headache triggers: Learning to cope with triggers. *Curr Pain Headache Rep.* 2010;14:221-227.
5. Martin PR. Behavioral management of the triggers of recurrent headache: A randomized controlled trial. *Behav Res Ther.* 2014;64:1-11.
6. Manack AN, Buse DC, Lipton RB. Chronic migraine: Epidemiology and disease burden. *Curr Pain Headache Rep* 2011;15:70-78.

7. Matchar DB, Young WB, Rosenberg JA, et al. *Evidence-Based Guidelines for Migraine Headache in the Primary Care Setting: Pharmacological Management of Acute Attacks*. The US Headache Consortium; 2000.

8. Da Silva AN, Tepper SJ. Acute treatment of migraines. *CNS Drugs*. 2012;10:823-839.

9. Peng KP, Wang SJ. Migraine diagnosis: Screening items, instruments, and scales. *Acta Anaesthesiol* (Taiwan). 2012;50:69-73.

10. Bartleson JD. When and how to investigate the patient with headache. *Semin Neurol*. 2006;26:163-170.

11. *Medicare Part D Medication Therapy Management Program Standardized Format*. Available at https://www.cms.gov/Medicare/Prescription-Drug-Coverage/PrescriptionDrugCovContra/Downloads/MTM-Program-Standardized-Format-English-and-Spanish-Instructions-Samples-v032712.pdf. Accessed on May 17, 2017.

12. Clinical Pharmacology [database online]. Tampa, FL: Gold Standard, Inc.; 2017. Available at http://clinicalpharmacology.com.

13. Lexi-Comp Online™. Lexi-Drugs Online™. Hudson, Ohio: Lexi-Comp, Inc.; 2017.

14. Ruoff GE. Migraine comorbidity: Consequent pharmacologic strategies for treatment. *Headache & Pain*. 2004;15(1):9-15.

15. Natural Medicines [database online]. Somerville, MA: Therapeutic Research Center; 2017. Available at https://naturalmedicines.therapeuticresearch.com/. Accessed May 17, 2017.

Review Questions

1. Which of the following is correct regarding migraine headaches?
   a. Migraine headaches affect men more often than women.
   b. Migraine headaches tend to occur in clusters.
   c. Migraine headaches are commonly associated with provoking factors (triggers).
   d. Although there are different types of headache, the treatment options are the same for all of them.

2. When assessing the headache patient, it is important to be aware of characteristics and symptoms of different types of headaches. Which of the following is consistent with a migraine headache?
   a. Bilateral location of pain
   b. Pulsating quality of pain
   c. Mild intensity
   d. Physical exertion or activity improves pain

3. Which of the following is correct regarding goals of therapy for migraine headache?
   a. The goals of treatment are the same for acute and long-term migraine management.
   b. Patients should maximize the use of backup and rescue medications to avoid preventive medications in migraine therapy.
   c. It is possible to reduce migraine severity, but not frequency.
   d. Optimal migraine therapy should avoid escalation of headache medication use.

4. Using living room language, a secondary headache is best defined as
   a. migraine headache that is associated with a score of 5 or higher on the pain scale.
   b. headache caused by another health issue.
   c. a very painful type of headache that is unilateral in nature.
   d. a headache that responds to antiseizure prophylactic therapy.

5. A 67-year-old female is a patient in your medication therapy management service. At her most recent visit, you developed a medication action plan for her, as she was experiencing rebound headache due to overuse of ibuprofen for migraine headache. Which of the following would you include in her medication action plan?
   a. Recommendation for her physician to change her migraine medication to a triptan.
   b. An alert for her about potential drug interactions with ibuprofen.
   c. Instructions for her to slowly reduce the amount of ibuprofen that she is taking to reduce her rebound headaches.
   d. A list of all of her medications, how she takes each one, prescriber names, and dates of use.

6. Which of the following patients should be referred emergently for evaluation of headache symptoms?
   a. A patient with a history of uncontrolled hypertension who is experiencing acute, severe headache and rapid heart rate.
   b. A patient whose headache is lasting longer than usual, but less than 3 days.
   c. A patient who is experiencing nausea after taking a dose of her/his headache medicine.
   d. A patient whose pain is more intense than usual, although it is still relieved by their headache medicine.

7. A 66-year-old female comes to her initial MTM visit with all of her medications for a medication review. You notice that she has samples of rizatriptan, frovatriptan, and intranasal dihydroergotamine from her physician's office, as well as prescriptions for sumatriptan 50 mg and dichloralphenazone/isometheptene/acetaminophen capsules to be taken by mouth. She states that she takes "a few" of these together when she has a migraine. She is not experiencing any negative effects from these medications, but does seem confused about her medication regimen. Her list of medication-related problems would most likely include:
   a. need for additional medication.
   b. unnecessary medication.
   c. dosage too low.
   d. adverse drug event.

8. Patients with severe migraine symptoms should initiate acute treatment with:
   a. triptans.
   b. acetaminophen/aspirin/caffeine.
   c. isometheptene combinations.
   d. opioids.

9. Which of the following would be the most appropriate prophylactic migraine therapy in a patient who also has comorbid depression?
   a. Propranolol
   b. Verapamil
   c. Ibuprofen
   d. Amitriptyline

10. All of the following herbal supplements have some evidence of benefit for migraine treatment EXCEPT:
    a. Valerian root
    b. Feverfew
    c. Peppermint oil
    d. Coenzyme Q10

ANSWERS

1. c	2. b	3. d
4. b	5. c	6. a
7. b	8. a	9. d
10. a		

25

Heart Failure MTM Data Set

Shawn D. Anderson, PharmD, BCACP, and Katherine Vogel Anderson, PharmD, BCACP

KEY POINTS

- The management of heart failure (HF) with preserved ejection fraction (EF) is different from the management of HF with reduced EF.
- Optimal pharmacotherapy is determined by EF and symptoms.
- Symptoms of HF are managed with pharmacotherapy and lifestyle interventions.
- Medication therapy management (MTM) is imperative for achieving target doses of life-saving drugs in HF with reduced EF.
- MTM providers should assess adherence with medications for HF at each visit, and identify reasons for nonadherence.
- MTM providers should educate patients on lifestyle interventions for management of HF.

INTRODUCTION

Heart failure (HF) is defined as a clinical syndrome with typical signs and symptoms precipitated by abnormal function or structure of the heart. This abnormality impairs the ability of the ventricle to fill with or eject blood, and results in the inability of the heart to meet the metabolic demands of the body.[1-5] The inability of the heart to eject blood optimally is termed *heart failure with reduced ejection fraction* (HFrEF) or *systolic dysfunction*. This is due to a reduction in myocardial contractility. HF may also be precipitated by impaired relaxation of the heart that prevents the ventricle from filling properly. This is termed *HF with preserved ejection fraction* (HFpEF), or diastolic dysfunction. The acronyms HFrEF and HFpEF both refer to disorders of the left ventricle of the heart. Less commonly, patients may develop right-heart failure (RHF). This term is used to describe a syndrome related to a reduced output of the right ventricle.[5] It is important to note that HF subtypes described above do not always occur in isolation. That is, patients with HFrEF can also have diastolic dysfunction and/or signs or symptoms of RHF. The three major HF types are summarized in Table 25-1, and potential etiologies are listed in Table 25-2. Medications and substances that may cause or worsen HF are found in Table 25-3.

Regardless of the initial insult leading to HF, the underlying pathophysiology and clinical manifestations are similar. The initial insult leads to a reduction in blood flow (cardiac output), which activates compensatory responses. At first, the compensatory responses are beneficial and increase cardiac output; however, long-term activation leads to complex changes and progression of HF[1-4] (Table 25-4).

Guidelines have established stages of HFrEF that emphasize the progressive nature of the disease—from those at risk of developing HF to those with end-stage HF.[1] HF stages are shown in Figure 25-1. HF stages have not been established with HFpEF or RHF, except to comment on severity of diastolic dysfunction for HFpEF or severity of right heart systolic dysfunction.[1,4,5]

HF signs and symptoms vary throughout the progression of disease and are usually classified by functional class (Table 25-5). Typically, HF follows a gradual worsening of signs and symptoms with acute episodes of decompensation. This classical view of HF progression, and the clinical course, is pictured in Figure 25-2.

Signs and symptoms of HF are not always correlated with EF.[3] For example, a patient with an EF of <30% may be asymptomatic, while a patient with a preserved EF may have symptoms at rest.

TABLE 25-1 • Heart Failure Definitions

Heart failure with reduced ejection fraction	Clinical syndrome typically with signs and symptoms of heart failure and an EF of ≤40%
Heart failure with preserved ejection fraction	Clinical syndrome with signs and symptoms of heart failure and an EF of >40%
Right-heart failure	Clinical syndrome of "right-sided" HF signs and symptoms and objective evidence of RV dysfunction

Abbreviations: EF = ejection fraction; RV = right ventricle.

Source: References 1, 4, and 5.

TABLE 25-2 • Causes of Heart Failure

Systolic dysfunction (decreased contractility) Reduction in muscle mass (eg, myocardial infarction) Dilated cardiomyopathies Ventricular hypertrophy Pressure overload (eg, systemic or pulmonary hypertension, and aortic or pulmonic valve stenosis) Volume overload (eg, valvular regurgitation, shunts, and high-output states)
Diastolic dysfunction (restriction in ventricular filling) Increased ventricular stiffness Ventricular hypertrophy (eg, hypertrophic cardiomyopathy; other examples above) Infiltrative myocardial diseases (eg, amyloidosis, sarcoidosis, and endomyocardial fibrosis) Myocardial ischemia and infarction Mitral or tricuspid valve stenosis Pericardial disease (eg, pericarditis and pericardial tamponade)

Source: Reference 6.

TABLE 25-3 • Drugs that May Precipitate or Exacerbate Heart Failure

Negative inotropic effect Antiarrhythmics (eg, disopyramide, flecainide, propafenone) β-Blockers (eg, propranolol, metoprolol, carvedilol) Calcium channel blockers (eg, verapamil, diltiazem) Itraconazole
Cardiotoxic Doxorubicin Epirubicin Daunomycin Cyclophosphamide Trastuzumab Bevacizumab Mitoxantrone Ifosfamide Mitomycin Lapatinib Sunitinib Imatinib Ethanol Amphetamines (eg, cocaine, methamphetamine)
Sodium and water retention NSAIDs COX-2 inhibitors Rosiglitazone and pioglitazone Glucocorticoids Androgens and estrogens Salicylates (high-dose) Sodium-containing drugs (eg, carbenicillin disodium, ticarcillin disodium)

Abbreviations: COX-2 = cyclooxygenase-2; NSAIDs = nonsteroidal anti-inflammatory drugs.

Source: Reference 3.

TABLE 25-4 • Beneficial and Detrimental Effects of the Compensatory Responses in Heart Failure

Compensatory Response	Beneficial Effects of Compensation	Detrimental Effects of Compensation
Increased preload (through Na^+ and water retention)	Optimize stroke volume via Frank-Starling mechanism	Pulmonary and systemic congestion and edema formation Increased MVO_2
Vasoconstriction	Maintain BP in face of reduced CO Shunt blood from nonessential organs to brain and heart	Increased MVO_2 Increased afterload decreases stroke volume and further activates the compensatory responses
Tachycardia and increased contractility (due to SNS activation)	Helps maintain CO	Increased MVO_2 Shortened diastolic filling time β_1-receptor downregulation, decreased receptor sensitivity Precipitation of ventricular arrhythmias Increased risk of myocardial cell death
Ventricular hypertrophy and remodeling	Helps maintain CO Reduces myocardial wall stress Decreases MVO_2	Diastolic dysfunction Systolic dysfunction Increased risk of myocardial cell death Increased risk of myocardial ischemia Increased arrhythmia risk Fibrosis

Abbreviations: BP = blood pressure; CO = cardiac output; MVO_2 = myocardial oxygen demand; SNS = sympathetic nervous system.

Source: Reference 2.

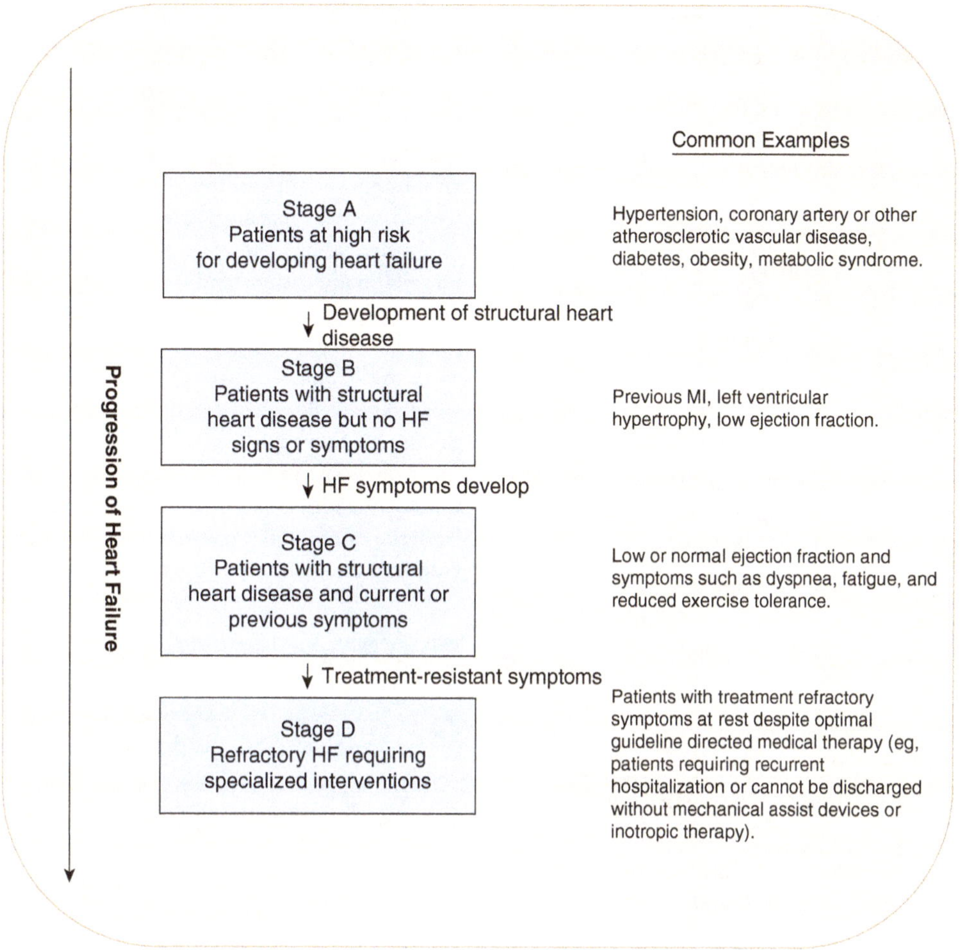

FIGURE 25-1 American College of Cardiology/American Heart Association (ACC/AHA) Heart Failure Staging System.
Abbreviations: HF = heart failure; MI = myocardial infarction.

TABLE 25-5 • New York Heart Association Functional Classification

Functional class
I. Patients with cardiac disease but without limitations of physical activity. Ordinary physical activity does not cause undue fatigue, dyspnea, or palpitation.
II. Patients with cardiac disease that results in slight limitations of physical activity. Ordinary physical activity results in fatigue, palpitation, dyspnea, or angina.
III. Patients with cardiac disease that results in marked limitation of physical activity. Although patients are comfortable at rest, less than ordinary activity will lead to symptoms.
IV. Patients with cardiac disease that results in an inability to carry on physical activity without discomfort. Symptoms of congestive heart failure are present even at rest. With any physical activity, increased discomfort is experienced.

Source: Reproduced, with permission, from DiPiro JT, Talbert RL, Yee GC, Matzke GR, Wells BG, Posey LM, eds. *Pharmacotherapy: A Pathophysiologic Approach*, 10th ed. New York, NY: McGraw-Hill; 2017.

Moreover, signs and symptoms cannot always be attributed to the disease of a particular ventricle. A patient with an EF of 40% and a qualitatively normal-functioning right ventricle can have typical left-heart symptoms such as dyspnea, and can have right-heart signs and symptoms such as peripheral edema and ascites. Common signs and symptoms of HF, along with standard diagnostic tests are reviewed in Table 25-6.

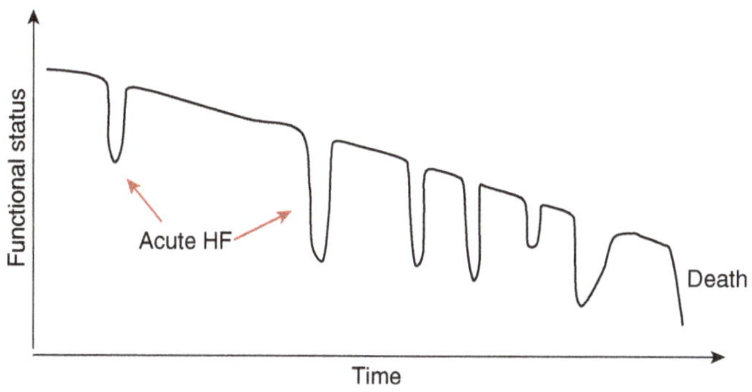

FIGURE 25-2 Classical clinical course of heart failure.

TABLE 25-6A • Heart Failure Signs and Symptoms[a]

Left-heart failure symptoms	Right-heart failure symptoms
Dyspnea, particularly on exertion Orthopnea Paroxysmal nocturnal dyspnea Exercise intolerance Tachypnea Cough Fatigue Hemoptysis Mental status changes	Abdominal pain Anorexia Nausea Bloating Poor appetite, early satiety Ascites Dizziness Syncope
Left-heart failure signs	**Right-heart failure signs**
Pulmonary rales Pulmonary edema Cool extremities Pleural effusion Cheyne-Stokes respiration Tachycardia Narrow pulse pressure Cardiomegaly Murmur of mitral regurgitation	Peripheral edema Jugular venous distension Hepatojugular reflux Hepatomegaly Murmur of tricuspid regurgitation

TABLE 25-6B • Diagnostic Testing Commonly Used in Heart Failure

Labs: B-type natriuretic peptide or NT-proBNP, serum sodium, creatinine, liver function test, complete blood count
Electrocardiogram
Chest x-ray
Echocardiogram
Stress testing: myocardial perfusion study, cardiac CT scan, cardiac MRI
Left- and/or right-heart catheterization

[a] Signs and symptoms are not mutually exclusive to left- or right-side HF.

Abbreviations: BNP = B-type natriuretic peptide; NT-proBNP = amino-terminal fragment of proBNP, which is cosecreted with BNP; CT = computed tomography; MRI = magnetic resonance imaging.

Source: References 1, 3, 4, 5, 6, and 7.

HF is a clinical syndrome, and there is no singular test to diagnose the disease. HF is often suspected based on presenting signs or symptoms, but there are other disorders that may also present with similar symptoms (eg, pulmonary embolism, acute exacerbation of chronic bronchitis).[1,4,5] As such, a complete history and physical are essential at initial presentation. This may possibly uncover common reversible causes of HF (eg, hypothyroidism) or known precipitants of new or worsening HF, such as medications or illicit drugs. The most useful diagnostic test for HF is the echocardiogram. The echocardiogram assesses the structure and function of the heart, including, but not limited to, quantifying the EF of the left ventricle, identifying and assessing the severity of diastolic dysfunction, qualitatively assessing right ventricular function, and assessing the structure and function of heart valves.[3]

Goals of Therapy for Heart Failure

Following a diagnosis of HF, treatment will depend on the etiology, severity of disease, and type of HF. Goals of therapy are to improve or maintain quality of life, reduce or eliminate signs or symptoms, prevent acute HF hospitalizations, and improve survival by slowing disease progression.[1,4,5] Certain etiologies may be treated nonpharmacologically (eg, with valvular replacement, or revascularization). However, HF treatment will most likely involve lifestyle modifications and medications to meet goals of therapy. The majority of this chapter will focus on medication therapy for HFrEF.

A well-conducted patient interview will help the MTM provider determine whether the HF regimen is meeting goals of therapy. A thorough assessment classifies symptom severity and functional class to help guide medication therapy for both symptomatic management and survival benefit. The knowledge gained from the careful interview identifies MRPs, which the MTM provider can then address to optimize the HF regimen.

CORE ELEMENT 1—COMPREHENSIVE MEDICATION REVIEW FOR PATIENTS WITH CHRONIC HEART FAILURE

A list of suggested questions to use when conducting a medication therapy review in a patient with chronic HF is presented in Table 25-7. Keep in mind that patients with HF likely have other comorbidities (eg, ischemic heart disease, hypertension), and referring to suggested questions regarding those disease states is recommended. The number and types of questions will depend on several factors, including the amount of time for the interview, number of concurrent MRPs, urgency of MRPs, and the reliability of the patient in providing accurate information, among others. In time-limited interactions or in complex cases with multiple medical issues, the MTM provider may choose to target questions that help to identify or rule out issues of an urgent nature (see questions to ask for prevention/assessment of medical emergencies). For HF patients, it is wise to recommend that they seek medical attention for symptoms at rest (if such symptoms are new), symptomatic hypotension, altered mental status, symptoms of acute coronary syndromes or uncontrolled arrhythmias, and defibrillator firings.[4] MTM providers should remember to use living room language during the interview (Figure 25-3), and to be prepared for questions that patients may ask regarding their condition (Table 25-8).

CORE ELEMENT 2—PERSONAL MEDICATION LIST[8]

Figure 25-4 presents a sample personal medication list (PML) for a patient with chronic HF. This example is representative only of chronic HF medications. Additional medications for other disease states should be added and listed separately. MTM providers should remember to use plain language when creating the PML.

TABLE 25-7 • Suggested Questions to Ask When Conducting a Medication Review in a Patient with Chronic Heart Failure

Questions Assessing Identification and Control of Chronic Heart Failure

Describe your heart failure symptoms.

- What activity brings on symptoms?
- Do your symptoms get worse when you lie down?
- What makes it better?
- What makes it worse?
- How often does it occur?
- How much of a change is this from the best you have felt recently?
- How much do the symptoms of heart failure limit you from doing activities you enjoy?

How long have you had problems with heart failure?

Have you had a heart attack? Open-heart surgery? Stents placed in your heart? When?

What medications do you take to treat heart failure or for heart protection?

What medications do you take for blood pressure?

What medications do you take for heart rate or rhythm?

What have your daily weights been?

Questions Assessing General Medication Use and Adherence

How do you take your medications? Morning or evening?

How often do you miss a dose of your medications?

Have you ever stopped taking any of your prescribed medications without telling your physician? If so, why?

What over-the-counter medications or herbals do you use?

How much sodium (salt) are you consuming per day?

How much liquid are you drinking per day?

Questions Assessing Additional Risk Factors

What tobacco products do you use?

How is your blood pressure? Heart rate?

  How often do you check your blood pressure? Heart rate?

  What is a "typical" blood pressure for you? Heart rate?

How is your cholesterol?

How is your blood sugar?

What kinds of physical activity do you do on a regular basis?

Questions to Ask for Prevention/Assessment of Medical Emergencies

Crisis planning: What are the warning signs of acute heart failure? What is your action plan?

Do you have any new symptoms of heart failure at rest?

Is your blood pressure low?

  What are your symptoms with this blood pressure?

Is your heart rate slow or fast?

  What are your symptoms with this heart rate?

Are you thinking clearly, or are you more confused?

Have you been taking more water/fluid pill lately with less effect?

Has your defibrillator fired?

After the defibrillator fired, how did you feel?

TABLE 25-8 • Questions to Anticipate Regarding Chronic Heart Failure

- **What is heart failure?**
  Heart failure is a condition associated with reduced heart function or the inability of the heart to relax. Heart failure may make you feel tired, especially with activity, or become short of breath easily. There are many other signs or symptoms of heart failure that you should be aware of, such as swelling in the abdomen or legs, or difficulty breathing while lying down.
- **What causes heart failure?**
  There are many causes of heart failure; the most common is coronary artery disease. Having high blood pressure for a long time may also cause heart failure. Whatever the cause, it should be treated appropriately, as untreated heart failure can worsen.
- **How can a heart attack cause heart failure?**
  A heart attack may damage the heart and make it weaker. If the heart is weaker, it cannot meet the demands of the body. The body will attempt to fix this problem by stimulating the heart and blood vessels, and also by increasing blood volume. However, these changes will damage the heart in the long term and cause symptoms of heart failure.
- **What health problems are associated with heart failure?**
  Heart failure can be associated with coronary artery disease, high blood pressure, and other more common chronic conditions, such as diabetes and obesity. There are many other health problems associated with heart failure, highlighting the need to treat risk factors early before heart failure develops.
- **Why are medications so important?**
  Medications used to treat chronic heart failure can improve symptoms and quality of life and allow you to live longer. Most of these medications block the harmful effects of the body trying to make the heart work harder. Taking medications as prescribed is one of the best things you can do to prevent further health problems and early death.
- **What can happen if I stop taking my medications?**
  If you stop taking your medicines suddenly, your heart failure symptoms may get worse. You also increase you risk of dying from heart failure or an abnormal heart rhythm.
- **When should I seek medical attention for my heart failure?**
  Since many patients have coronary artery disease and heart failure, you should call 911 if you have angina or chest pain that does not get better after your first dose of nitroglycerin, or if it is not completely relieved after three doses. Waiting to call 911 may cause a delay in getting the appropriate emergency treatment. You should also seek emergency medical attention for symptoms at rest if this is new, if you have low blood pressure with symptoms, changes in your ability to think, or your heart is beating very quickly or abnormally, and if your defibrillator fires. If your heart failure symptoms are worsening, but not to the point of requiring immediate medical attention, you should contact your clinician as soon as possible to see you in clinic earlier and adjust your medications.
- **What should I do if I have a problem with my medications?**
  Never stop taking your medications without first talking to your primary clinician. Speak with your clinician (eg, physician, nurse practitioner and/or pharmacist) to let them know about any problems you are having and together you can make sure your medications are the right ones for you.
- **Can heart failure be cured?**
  Although medications, certain heart procedures, and certain devices can improve heart function and reduce heart symptoms, most patients will always have heart failure.

ACE inhibitor—a medicine used to help the heart function more efficiently. May also be used to lower blood pressure and protect the heart and the kidney.

Acute coronary syndrome—decreased blood flow to the heart which may lead to a heart attack.

Adverse event—something bad that happens, bad reaction, unexplained or unwanted effects.

Aldosterone antagonist—a medicine that blocks the harmful effects of aldosterone. Aldosterone is a hormone produced in the body to increase blood volume and blood pressure.

Angina—chest pain or discomfort caused by decreased blood flow to the heart muscle.

Angioedema—a rare side effect of ACE inhibitors and a medical emergency involving rapid swelling of the lips, tongue, and throat that may affect breathing.

Angiotensin II receptor blocker—a medicine that acts similarly to an ACE inhibitor without certain side effects.

Antiarrhythmic—a medicine that may be used to control the way your heart rhythm functions or to prevent defibrillator firings.

Antihypertensive medication—a medicine that lowers blood pressure.

Arrhythmia—irregular heartbeat, skipped heartbeat, heart problem; an example is atrial fibrillation.

Arteries—blood vessels that carry blood away from the heart.

Ascites—extra fluid that accumulates in the abdomen or belly.

B-Type natriuretic peptide (BNP)—a hormone released from the heart when the heart is under stress. This hormone can be measured to diagnose and guide treatment for heart failure.

β-Blocker—a medicine used to help the heart function more efficiently. May also lower blood pressure, control heart rate, prevent abnormal heart rhythms, and prevent chest pain.

Bradycardia—a slow heartbeat, <60 times in a minute.

Calcium channel blocker—a medicine used to lower blood pressure. Some of these medicines also control heart rate. Can be used to prevent chest pain.

Cardiac—related to the heart.

Cardiac catheterization—procedure that allows a physician to examine the heart and heart vessels.

Cardiac resynchronization therapy—a device implanted under the skin to pace and resynchronize the heart. The device can improve your heart failure symptoms and allow you to live longer.

Cardiologist—physician specialized in heart diseases and disorders.

Chronic—constant, long-lasting, persistent.

Coronary angiography—a procedure that allows a physician to see blockages in the heart vessels.

Coronary artery bypass surgery—open-heart surgery that helps restore good blood flow to the heart.

Coronary artery disease—narrowing and hardening of the small blood vessels that supply blood and oxygen to the heart.

Creatinine test—a test that checks how well the kidneys are working; an increase means that the kidneys are not working well.

Diastolic—related to the heart relaxing.

Digoxin—a medication used to improve heart failure symptoms or possibly to control heart rate.

Direct renin inhibitor—a medicine used to lower blood pressure by decreasing the activity of renin, which is a substance in the body that may lead to increases in blood pressure.

Direct vasodilator—a medicine used to treat or prevent chest pain or lower blood pressure; it works by relaxing blood vessels.

Diuretic—a medicine used to reduce or prevent fluid buildup. Also may be referred to as a "fluid pill." It works by increasing the amount of urine.

Dyspnea on exertion—difficulty breathing with activity.

ECG—a test that measures electrical activity in the heart and looks for any damage to or problems with your heart.

Echocardiogram—a test that uses sound waves to view the heart and heart valves. This test can estimate heart function and pressures.

Edema—swelling because of the buildup of too much fluid.

Ejection fraction (EF)—the amount of blood pumped out of the heart with each beat. Normal is approximately 60%.

Electrolytes—a type of necessary salt found in blood, such as sodium, potassium, and calcium.

Fasting lipid panel—a test of the fats in your blood taken after 8-12 hours without eating any food.

Funny channel blocker—a medication that is used to help the heart function more efficiently by slowing the heart rate.

Heart failure with preserved EF (HFpEF)—syndrome that causes typical heart failure signs and symptoms associated with a normal EF, but abnormal heart relaxation.

Heart failure with reduced EF (HFrEF)—syndrome that causes typical heart failure signs and symptoms associated with a low EF.

Heart rate—how many times your heart beats each minute.

Heart valve surgery—surgery to either repair or replace a heart valve to allow for normal functioning.

Hyperkalemia—high potassium; very high potassium is a medical emergency and could cause a deadly change in the way your heart beats.

Hypertension—high blood pressure.

Hypokalemia—low potassium, which may cause muscle weakness and cramping.

Hypotension—low blood pressure.

Implantable cardioverter-defibrillator (ICD)—a device implanted under the skin that may shock the heart if it is not functioning properly.

Ischemic heart disease—heart problems caused by a lack of blood flow to the heart.

Jugular venous distension—enlargement of the jugular vein in the neck that may be seen when you lie at an angle. This would suggest that you are holding on to extra fluid.

Lifestyle changes—your physician may have recommended changes in lifestyle to lower your blood pressure, which for some patients include reaching a goal weight, decreasing the amount of alcohol you consume, exercising, or quitting smoking.

Lifestyle modifications—very similar to lifestyle changes, but may be more specific to heart failure, such as reducing fluid intake and limiting sodium (salt).

Low-sodium diet—a diet with <2 g (2000 mg) of salt per day.

Myocardial infarction—heart attack, damage to the heart.

Neprilysin inhibitor—a medication that enhances the effects of "good" hormones in the body. This medication is combined in one tablet with an angiotensin II receptor blocker.

Nitrate—a medicine used to relieve chest pain; may be used in combination with another drug to treat heart failure.

NT-pro-B-type natriuretic peptide (NT-pro-BNP)—a breakdown product of BNP. This product can be measured to diagnose and guide heart failure treatment.

Obese—having a body mass index (BMI) of >30, which may increase the risk of developing or worsening heart failure.

Orthopnea—difficulty breathing while lying down due to excess fluid in the lungs.

Orthostatic hypotension—dizziness or lightheadedness on standing because of low blood pressure.

Pacemaker—a device that is implanted under the skin that can pace the heart to prevent it from beating too slowly.

Peripheral edema—swelling that occurs in the feet, ankles, and legs.

Phosphenes—visual images seen as lights, stars, or bright spots without light entering the eye.

Positive inotrope—a medication administered through the veins to improve heart function short-term. This medication may be used outside of the hospital in rare occasions for patients with severe heart failure.

Renin—a substance in the body that may lead to increases in blood pressure.

Revascularization—a procedure that restores good blood flow to the heart.

Right-heart failure—a clinical syndrome with typical right-sided signs and symptoms of heart failure such as swelling in the belly or legs.

Serum potassium—a test that checks the amount of potassium in the blood (see *Hyperkalemia* and *Hypokalemia*).

Sleep apnea— a sleep disorder that often involves pauses in breathing during the night; this may worsen heart failure.

Smoking cessation—quitting smoking.

Sodium—salt, which can increase blood pressure and/or cause fluid retention.

Statin—a medicine used to lower cholesterol; can also lower the risk of heart disease.

Syncope—losing consciousness or fainting.

Systolic—related to the heart contracting.

Tachycardia—a rapid heartbeat, >100 times in a minute.

Veins—blood vessels that carry blood toward the heart.

FIGURE 25-3 Living room language for patients with chronic heart failure.

PERSONAL MEDICATION LIST FOR *<Insert patient's name, DOB: mm/dd/yyyy>*	
Medication: Coreg (carvedilol) 25 mg tablet	
How I use it: Take one pill (25 mg) every 12 hours	
Why I use it: Heart failure	**Prescriber:** Jones
Date I started using it: 12/22/2016	**Date I stopped using it:** *(Leave blank for patient's notes)*
Why I stopped using it: *(Leave blank for patient's notes)*	
Medication: Lasix (furosemide) 40 mg tablet	
How I use it: Take 1 tablet (40 mg) every morning. I can take an additional tablet (40 mg) in the afternoon if I gain >3 lb in 24 hours or >5 lb in 1 week and have signs or symptoms of worsening heart failure.	
Why I use it: To reduce heart failure signs (swelling in feet and legs) and symptoms (shortness of breath); water pill	**Prescriber:** Jones
Date I started using it: 12/22/2016	**Date I stopped using it:** *(Leave blank for patient's notes)*
Why I stopped using it: *(Leave blank for patient's notes)*	

FIGURE 25-4 Sample personal medication list for chronic heart failure medications.

CORE ELEMENT 3—MEDICATION ACTION PLAN[8]

A sample medication action plan (MAP) for a patient with chronic HF is shown in Figure 25-5. This example is representative only of action steps for a patient with chronic HF. MAPs for other disease states or other MRPs should be added and listed separately. In most cases, only a few of the most important action steps should be listed, so as not to overwhelm the patient. Other areas for patient self-management can be addressed at later visits. MTM providers should remember to use plain language when creating the MAP.

CORE ELEMENT 4—INTERVENTION AND/OR REFERRAL

Interventions for the management of chronic HF are determined by type of HF (ie, HFrEF, HFpEF, RHF) and severity of symptoms. As mentioned previously, HFrEF is the focus of this chapter, since the majority of clinical evidence exists with this type of HF. In the setting of HFrEF, MTM is, for the most part,

	DATE PREPARED: *<Insert date>*
What we talked about: You reported having chronic heart failure with reduced ejection fraction. Your ejection fraction is 35% and has been this for the last 3 years. You last saw your nurse practitioner 4 weeks ago. The clinic made no changes at that time since you are taking a maximized heart failure medication regimen. You have symptoms of shortness of breath with moderate activity and will sometimes have swelling in your belly. We talked about steps you can take to keep the heart failure from getting worse.	
What I need to do: Here are some things I can do to help keep from heart failure symptoms getting worse: • Take all medications as directed to prevent heart failure symptoms from getting worse. • Watch how much fluid I take in. Try to keep it less than 2 L/day to minimize heart failure symptoms. • Stick to a low-salt diet so I won't worsen heart failure symptoms, <2000 mg of sodium (salt) daily.	**What I did and when I did it:** *(Leave blank for patient's notes)*
What we talked about: The importance of seeing how well my new medicine (eplerenone [Inspra]) is working for my heart failure	
What I need to do: • Check and record blood pressure at home. Notify the clinic if my blood pressure is >180/120 mmHg or <100/60 mmHg. • Check and record heart rate at home. Notify the clinic if my heart rate is >100 bpm or <60 bpm. • Check and record weight at home. I should weigh myself first thing in the morning after voiding with minimal clothing. Since I mostly have worsening symptoms with a fluid-weight gain of 4 lb, I should notify the clinic if my weight changes by more than 3-4 lb in 24 hours or 4 lb in 1 week. • Bring log book every time I come to clinic.	**What I did and when I did it:** *(Leave blank for patient's notes)*

FIGURE 25-5 Example medication action plan for a patient with chronic heart failure with reduced ejection fraction.

TABLE 25-9 • Modifiable Risk Factors in Chronic Heart Failure

Risk Factor	Treatment Consideration
Tobacco use	Encourage smoking cessation and avoidance of secondhand smoke. Utilize a stepwise strategy (ask, advise, assess, assist, arrange, avoid) for smoking cessation.
Hypertension	Refer to Chapter 27 and follow most recent guidelines
Hypercholesterolemia and dyslipidemia	Refer to Chapter 22 and follow most recent guidelines
Diabetes	Refer to Chapter 21 and follow most recent guidelines
Obesity	Initial weight loss of 5%-10% from baseline through physical activity and reduced caloric intake. Goal is to maintain or achieve a BMI between 18.5 and 24.9 kg/m^2.
Alcohol consumption	Once a patient develops HFrEF, abstinence is often recommended since alcohol is considered cardiotoxic. If no HF, light alcohol consumption is reasonable to prevent cardiovascular disease. Men: ≤2 drinks/day Women and lighter persons: ≤1 drink/day (1 drink equals 12 oz beer, 5 oz wine, or 1.5 oz of 80-proof whiskey)
Sedentary lifestyle	Most patients should participate in 30-60 minutes of moderate-intensity aerobic activity at least 5 days per week. High-risk patients should participate in a medically supervised cardiac rehabilitation program.
Psychological (stress, anxiety, depression)	Refer to Chapter 20 (depression). It is reasonable to screen for mental illness and refer to mental health provider, if indicated.

Abbreviations: BMI = body mass index; HF = heart failure; HFrEF = heart failure with reduced ejection fraction.

Source: References 1, 3, 4, and 5.

evidence-based. To help guide treatment, the American Heart Association classifies HFrEF into stages (see Figure 25-1) and functional class (see Table 25-5).[1] Symptom management is accomplished by diuretics and digoxin. Most medications that prolong survival in HFrEF also reduce symptoms, but take longer than diuretics or digoxin to realize their effects. For HFrEF, patients should take medications that have been shown to improve survival, regardless of symptoms or success of lifestyle modification.

Management of HFpEF is briefly discussed in the guidelines.[1,4,5] For HFpEF, symptoms are managed by controlling heart rate and/or rhythm, blood pressure, and volume status with both medications and lifestyle modifications. There are no specific medications that must be used to accomplish these goals for HFpEF, but most HF experts prefer using a beta-blocker and angiotensin converting enzyme inhibitor (ACEI). An aldosterone antagonist may also be considered to reduce the risk of hospitalization, if no contraindications exist and the patient is not at high risk of hyperkalemia. Finally, compelling indications must still be considered when selecting medications for treatment of HFpEF.

It should be noted that right-heart failure is not extensively discussed in HF guidelines[5] but is often managed by cardiologists and HF specialists. For RHF, symptom management is often accomplished with diuretics and treatment of the underlying condition (eg, pulmonary arterial hypertension [PAH]).[5,7] There are no life-prolonging therapies specifically developed for RHF, but pulmonary vasodilators may be utilized to improve symptoms if PAH is the primary cause.[5,6]

Regardless of the type of HF, patients should follow strict lifestyle modifications to prevent worsening of symptoms and to reduce the need for increased doses of diuretics. Patients not adequately controlled with lifestyle modifications should be started on drug therapy. Table 25-9 summarizes modifiable risk factors that contribute to progression of HF.

Many patient factors should be considered when selecting HF medications. These factors include, but are not limited to, compelling indications, comorbid disease states, concomitant medications, cost, and adherence. Patients should be encouraged to monitor vital signs (blood pressure, heart rate, weight) at home and to follow up in clinic at regular intervals so that progress toward treatment goals can be assessed. As a standard rule in medication management for HF, medications are started at evidence-based, low doses and then slowly titrated according to vital signs and tolerability. In HFrEF, target doses have been established for all medications that have proven survival benefits. Table 25-10 provides an overview of target doses for medications for HF. Considerations for HF drug therapy such as compelling indications and individualization of drug therapy are found in Tables 25-11 and 25-12, respectively. Although HF guidelines do not recommend using herbal remedies, many patients take herbal products without recommendations from clinicians. A few herbal remedies with an acceptable effectiveness-to-safety profile are outlined in Table 25-13. HF treatment algorithms for HFrEF stages A and B, HFrEF stage C, and HFpEF are found in Figures 25-6, 25-7, and 25-8, respectively.

Despite advances in medication management, device therapies, disease management programs, and HF transitional care programs,

TABLE 25-10 • Medications for Management of Chronic Heart Failure

Medication Class and Drug Examples	Common/Serious Side Effects[a]	Target or Typical Doses	Black Box Warnings/ Contraindications	Pregnancy Category[b]
ACE inhibitors (ACEIs) Captopril Enalapril Fosinopril Lisinopril Quinapril Ramipril Trandolapril	Angioedema Dry cough Hypotension Headache Hyperkalemia Dizziness Fatigue Azotemia Renal failure	**Target doses** Captopril 50 mg tid Enalapril 10 mg bid Fosinopril 80 mg once daily Lisinopril 20 mg once daily Quinapril 80 mg once daily Ramipril 10 mg once daily Trandolapril 4 mg once daily	Pregnancy Angioedema Serum K > 5.0 mEq/L Serum creatinine > 2.5 mg/dL Cough Severe aortic stenosis Bilateral renal artery stenosis	D
Aldosterone antagonists Eplerenone Spironolactone	Hyperkalemia Diarrhea Fatigue Dizziness Orthostatic hypotension Spironolactone: Gynecomastia Sexual dysfunction Menstrual irregularity	**Target doses** Eplerenone 50 mg once daily Spironolactone 25 mg once daily	Anuria CrCl < 30 mL/min for eplerenone in HFrEF Serum creatinine >2.5 mg/dL for spironolactone in HFrEF Serum K^+ > 5.0 mEq/L	B (eplerenone) C (spironolactone)
Angiotensin II receptor blockers (ARBs) Candesartan Losartan Valsartan	Dizziness Fatigue Headache Hypotension Diarrhea Hyperkalemia Arthralgia Azotemia Renal failure	**Target doses** Candesartan 32 mg once daily Losartan 100 mg once daily Valsartan 160 mg bid	Pregnancy Serum K^+ > 5.0 mEq/L Serum creatinine >2.5 mg/dL Severe aortic stenosis Bilateral renal artery stenosis	D
Angiotensin II receptor–neprilysin inhibitor (ARNI) Sacubitril/valsartan	Cough Dizziness Hypotension Hyperkalemia Azotemia Renal failure Angioedema	**Target doses** Sacubitril/valsartan 97/103 mg bid	Pregnancy Breastfeeding Angioedema Serum K^+ > 5.0 mEq/L Severe aortic stenosis Bilateral renal artery stenosis Renal failure Use within 36 hours of an ACEI	May cause fetal harm
β-blockers Bisoprolol Carvedilolol Metoprolol succinate	Mask hypoglycemia in diabetics, Worsen insulin sensitivity, breathing disorders, and PVD Bradycardia Dizziness Exercise intolerance Fatigue Orthostatic hypotension (especially mixed α- and β-blockers)	**Target doses** Bisoprolol 10 mg once daily Carvedilol 50 mg bid Metoprolol succinate 200 mg once daily	Abrupt discontinuation Asthma (avoid nonselective BB or high-dose selective BB) AV block Bradycardia Cardiogenic shock Hypotension Pheochromocytoma (if not on α-blocker) Sick sinus syndrome	C

(*Continued*)

TABLE 25-10 • Medications for Management of Chronic Heart Failure (*Continued*)

Medication Class and Drug Examples	Common/Serious Side Effects[a]	Target or Typical Doses	Black Box Warnings/ Contraindications	Pregnancy Category[b]
Calcium channel blockers Dihydropyridines Amlodipine Felodipine Nifedipine	Dizziness Flushing Gingival hyperplasia Headache Nausea Peripheral edema Postural hypotension **IR preparations** Reflex tachycardia	**Typical doses** Amlodipine 5-10 mg once daily Felodipine 5-10 mg once daily Nifedipine CR 30-120 mg once daily	Avoid short-acting dihydropyridines that may worsen angina or HFrEF (ie, immediate-release nifedipine or nicardipine)	C
Calcium channel blockers Non-dihydropyridines Diltiazem Verapamil	Bradycardia Hypotension Peripheral edema **Diltiazem** Headache Nausea **Verapamil** Constipation	**Typical doses** Diltiazem SR 120-480 mg once daily Verapamil SR 180-480 mg once daily	Acute MI AV block Cardiogenic shock Hypotension Heart failure with reduced EF Sick sinus syndrome Ventricular tachycardia Wolff-Parkinson-White syndrome	C
Cardiac glycosides Digoxin	Atrial and ventricular arrhythmias Heart block Anorexia Nausea/vomiting Diarrhea Hyperkalemia Blurred or yellow-vision	**Typical doses** Digoxin 0.125 mg every other day or once daily to 0.25 mg once daily Dose to maintain a trough serum drug concentration between 0.5 and 0.8 ng/dL	Ventricular fibrillation Acute MI Bradycardia Hypokalemia Hypomagnesemia Hyperkalemia Hypercalcemia	C
Direct renin inhibitor Aliskiren	Angioedema Cough Diarrhea Dizziness Headache Hyperkalemia Hypotension Renal failure	**Typical doses** Aliskiren 150-300 mg once daily	Pregnancy Angioedema Serum K > 5.0 mEq/L Serum creatinine > 2.5 mg/dL Severe aortic stenosis Bilateral renal artery stenosis	D
Direct vasodilators Hydralazine	Hypotension Dizziness Headache Flushing Weakness Nausea Constipation Swelling of lower legs Tachycardia Lupus-like symptoms	**Target doses** Hydralazine 75 mg tid	Coronary artery disease Rheumatic heart disease Systemic lupus erythematosus	C
I_f "funny" channel blocker Ivabradine	Bradycardia Hypotension Dizziness Phosphenes Atrial fibrillation	**Target doses** Ivabradine 7.5 mg bid	Acute heart failure Bradycardia Heart block Hypotension Sick sinus syndrome	May cause fetal harm

(*Continued*)

TABLE 25-10 • Medications for Management of Chronic Heart Failure (*Continued*)

Medication Class and Drug Examples	Common/Serious Side Effects[a]	Target or Typical Doses	Black Box Warnings/ Contraindications	Pregnancy Category[b]
Loop diuretics Bumetanide Furosemide Torsemide Ethacrynic acid	Hypotension Hyperglycemia Hyperuricemia Hypomagnesemia Hypokalemia Hypocalcemia Azotemia Hypovolemia Loss of appetite Pancreatitis Photosensitivity	**Typical doses** Bumetanide 0.5-2 mg once or twice daily Furosemide 20-80 mg once or twice daily Torsemide 10-40 mg once or twice daily Ethacrynic acid 75-150 mg once or twice daily	Anuria Sulfonamide hypersensitivity except for ethacrynic acid Hypokalemia	C
Nitrates Isosorbide dinitrate Isosorbide mononitrate	Headache Dizziness Hypotension Flushing Nausea	**Target doses** Isosorbide dinitrate 40 mg tid	Concomitant use with PDE inhibitors Constrictive pericarditis Restrictive cardiomyopathy Tolerance may occur at high doses or with administration without a nitrate-free interval	C
Thiazide diuretics Chlorthalidone Hydrochlorothiazide Metolazone	Hypotension Hyperglycemia Hypokalemia Hypercalcemia Hyponatremia Hypomagnesemia Hyperuricemia Azotemia Pancreatitis Photosensitivity	**Typical doses** Chlorthalidone 25-100 mg once daily Hydrochlorothiazide 25-200 mg once daily Metolazone 2.5-5 mg once daily	Anuria Sulfonamide and thiazide diuretic hypersensitivity CrCl < 30 mL/min (except metolazone) Hypokalemia	B
Vasopressin antagonist Tolvaptan	Xerostomia Constipation Polydipsia Hypovolemia Hypernatremia Hyperkalemia Hyperglycemia Polyuria Variceal bleeding in patients with history of cirrhosis	**Typical doses** Tolvaptan 15-60 mg once daily	Alcoholism Hepatic disease Malnutrition Anuria Hypovolemia	C

[a] This is a general list and does not include all side effects that can occur from these drugs. Consult a drug reference source for a more inclusive list before making any recommendations. MTM providers should also consult a comprehensive drug interaction database before making pharmacotherapy recommendations.

[b] Product labeling for all prescription drugs is being updated to reflect the new FDA Pregnancy Labeling and Lactation Rule. Please check individual product labeling for the most accurate and updated pregnancy information.

Abbreviations: ACEI = angiotensin-converting enzyme inhibitor; ARB = angiotensin II receptor blocker; ARNI = angiotensin II receptor/neprilysin inhibitor; AV = atrioventricular; BB = β-blocker; bid = twice daily; CR = controlled release; CrCl = creatinine clearance; EF = ejection fraction; IR = immediate release; K^+ = serum potassium; MI = myocardial infarction; PDE = phosphodiesterase; PVD = peripheral vascular disease; SR = sustained release; tid = 3 times daily.

Source: References 1, 4, 5, and 9.

TABLE 25-11 • Compelling Indications in Heart Failure

Compelling Indication[a]	Preferred Drug Options
Post–myocardial infarction	β-Blocker. For HFrEF, carvedilol is the drug of choice ACEI or ARB **Avoid:** IR DHP CCBs, β-blockers with ISA activity (acebutolol, penbutolol, pindolol)
Atrial arrhythmias	β-Blocker or non-DHP CCBs. For HFrEF, use bisoprolol, carvedilol, or metoprolol succinate. Digoxin may be added for additional rate control **Avoid:** IR DHP CCBs (reflex tachycardia), non-DHP CCBs in HFrEF (negative inotrope), β-blockers with ISA activity (acebutolol, penbutolol, pindolol)
Ventricular arrhythmias	β-Blocker. For HFrEF, use bisoprolol, carvedilol, or metoprolol succinate. Amiodarone or sotalol may be added to prevent arrhythmia burden and/or defibrillator firings **Avoid:** IR DHP CCBs, non-DHP CCBs, digoxin, β-blockers with ISA activity (acebutolol, penbutolol, pindolol)
Chronic kidney disease	ACEI or ARB if ACEI intolerant for renal protection
High coronary disease risk	β-Blocker. For HFrEF, use bisoprolol, carvedilol, or metoprolol succinate. ACEI or ARB **Avoid:** IR DHP CCBs, β-blockers with ISA activity (acebutolol, penbutolol, pindolol)
Diabetes mellitus	ACEI or ARB for both heart protection and renal protection
Secondary stroke prevention	Diuretic plus ACEI or ARB if BP is elevated in HFpEF For HFrEF, there is no prospective evidence to suggest that treatment of stroke takes priority over HFrEF. However, strict BP control is still a goal of treatment. Follow HFrEF treatment algorithm for medication therapy. If BP still elevated after maximized HF regimen, add a DHP CCB, a diuretic or both.
Angina pectoris/ischemic heart disease	β-Blocker is first-line therapy. For HFrEF, use bisoprolol, carvedilol, or metoprolol succinate. May add a CCB if angina persists. Avoid IR CCBs in all patients and avoid non-DHP CCBs in HFrEF. Add a long-acting nitrate if angina persists. Ranolazine should be used cautiously in HFrEF due to potential negative inotropy. Regardless of angina, all patients should take an ACEI or ARB unless contraindicated or not tolerated.

[a] If a patient with HF has a condition for which the use of certain medications has been shown to be beneficial in controlling the disease or its sequelae, this is considered a compelling indication.

Abbreviations: ACEI = angiotensin-converting enzyme inhibitor; ARB = angiotensin II receptor blocker; BP = blood pressure; CCB = calcium channel blocker; DHP = dihydropyridine; HFrEF = heart failure with reduced ejection fraction; HFpEF = heart failure with preserved ejection fraction; IR = immediate release; ISA = intrinsic sympathomimetic activity.

Source: References 1, 3, and 5.

TABLE 25-12 • Considerations in Individualizing Heart Failure Therapy

Condition or Special Population	Drug Options
Aortic stenosis	Patients with moderate-to-severe AS may not be able to tolerate arterial vasodilators. β-Blockers such as bisoprolol and metoprolol succinate are preferred in HFrEF. Alpha activity with carvedilol may not be tolerated. Add diuretics cautiously for symptomatic management. May continue ACEI or ARB if new diagnosis and patient is tolerating. However, keep at low doses. **Avoid:** Non-DHP and DHP CCBs
Blacks	There are no specific recommendations in HFpEF. BP may respond better to diuretics and DHP CCBs. For HFrEF, maximize BB and ACEI or ARB. Consider FDC HYD/ISDN if patient has low EF and at least NYHA class II symptoms.
Bradycardia	Maximize other HF therapies that do not affect heart rate. Consider referral for advanced device therapies if patient has HFrEF (eg, CRT).
Chronic kidney disease	CKD is a poor prognostic indicator of survival in HF. Patients may not be able to tolerate target doses. Patients are also at higher risk of hyperkalemia and AKI with concomitant diuretic use. Use ACEI or ARB if ACEI intolerant.

(Continued)

TABLE 25-12 • Considerations in Individualizing Heart Failure Therapy (*Continued*)

Condition or Special Population	Drug Options
Diabetes	Although BBs may worsen glucose control, these medications should be used in HFrEF. Carvedilol may have neutral effects on A1c. Non-DHP CCB can be used in HFpEF if no recent history of an MI. ACEI or ARB if ACEI intolerant Diabetes places patient at higher risk of hyperkalemia with use of AAs
Elderly	Although evidence is not as robust in the elderly, treatment strategies are similar for HFrEF and HFpEF. Elderly may be more prone to orthostasis with BBs, ACEIs and diuretics.
Hypertension	HFrEF: Utilize HF-approved BBs and ACEIs or ARBs if ACEI intolerant. Consider aldosterone antagonists, ARNI and/or FDC HYD/ISDN if patient meets criteria. Add diuretic if patient is symptomatic. DHP CCB may be added.
Low blood pressure or hypotension	Assess diuretic use initially and reduce dose if symptoms are under good control. Patients with severe HFrEF may have low BP. Attempt to initiate low doses of BBs, ACEIs, and AAs and titrate as long as patient does not have symptomatic hypotension.
Pulmonary disease	β-Blockers may be used in either HFpEF or HFrEF if patient can tolerate. Use a β_1-selective agent if patient has bronchospastic disease.
Women	Although evidence is not as robust in women, treatment strategies are similar for HFrEF and HFpEF. Digoxin for symptomatic HF may have less benefit in women than men.

AA = aldosterone antagonist; ACEI = angiotensin-converting enzyme inhibitor; AKI = acute kidney injury; ARB = angiotensin II receptor blocker; ARNI = angiotensin II receptor/neprilysin inhibitor; AS = aortic stenosis; BB = β-blocker; BP = blood pressure; CCB = calcium channel blocker; CKD = chronic kidney disease; CRT = chronic resynchronization therapy; DHP = dihydropyridine; FDC HYD/ISDN = fixed-dose combination of hydralazine and isosorbide dinitrate; HF = heart failure; HFpEF = heart failure with preserved ejection fraction; HFrEF = heart failure with reduced ejection fraction; IR = immediate release; MI = myocardial infarction; NYHA = New York Heart Association.

Source: References 1, 4, 5,10, 11, 12, and 13.

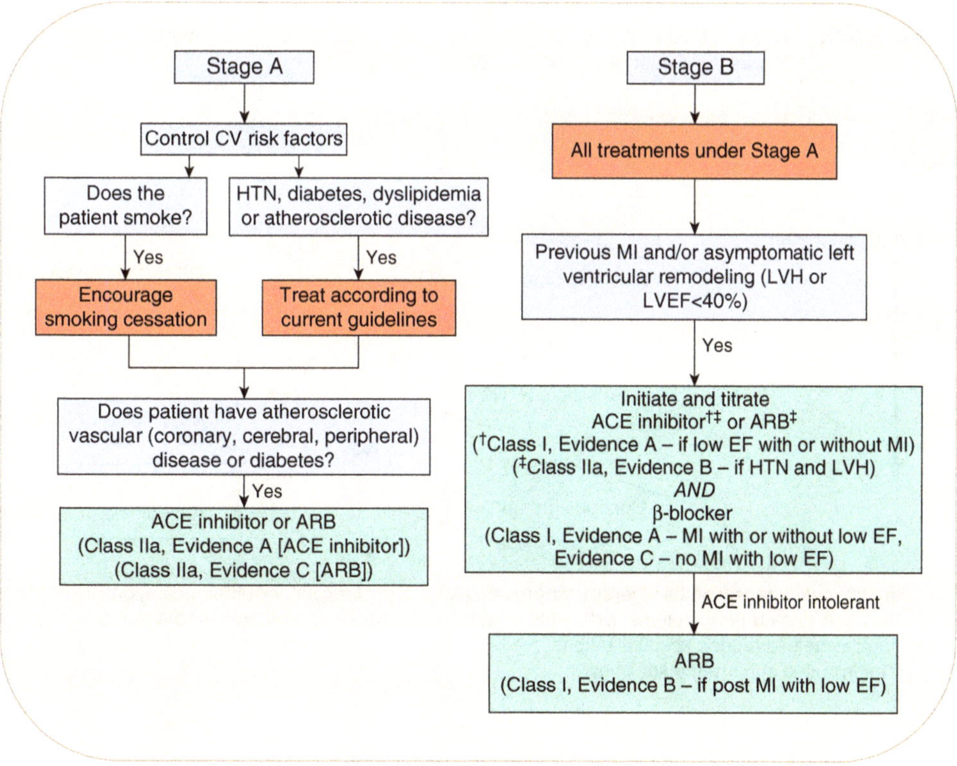

FIGURE 25-6 Treatment algorithm for patients with ACC/AHA stages A and B heart failure.

Abbreviations: ACE = angiotensin-converting enzyme; ARB = angiotensin receptor blocker; CV = cardiovascular; EF =ejection fraction; HTN = hypertension; LVEF = left ventricular ejection fraction; LVH = left ventricular hypertrophy; MI = myocardial infarction.

Source: References 1 and 2.

TABLE 25-13 • Herbal Supplements for Chronic Heart Failure

Supplement	Typical Dose[a]	Grade[b]	Cost[c]
Hawthorn	160-900 mg of extract per day in 2-3 divided doses[c]	Possibly effective	\$-\$\$\$
L-Arginine	2 g tid	Insufficient evidence	\$\$\$
Coenzyme Q10	100 mg tid	Possibly effective	\$-\$\$\$

[a] Hawthorn: Dosing standardization corresponds to 3.5-19.8 mg flavonoids or 30-168.8 mg oligomeric procyanidins; L-arginine—no established standardization for oral products. Dosage range of 5.6 - 12.6 g daily in divided doses has been studied.

[b] Level of evidence: "Likely effective"—this product has a very high level of reliable clinical evidence supporting its use for a specific indication. Products rated "likely effective" are generally considered appropriate to recommend; "possibly effective"—this product has some clinical evidence supporting its use for a specific indication; however, the evidence is limited by quantity, quality, or contradictory findings. Products rated "possibly effective" might be beneficial, but do not have enough high-quality evidence to recommend for most people; "insufficient evidence"—there is not enough reliable scientific evidence to provide an effectiveness rating.

[c] Cost: \$ = ≤\$10/month supply in recommended dosage; \$\$ = \$11-\$20/month; \$\$\$ = \$21-\$50/month; \$\$\$\$ = >\$50/month.

Source: Data compiled from reference 14.

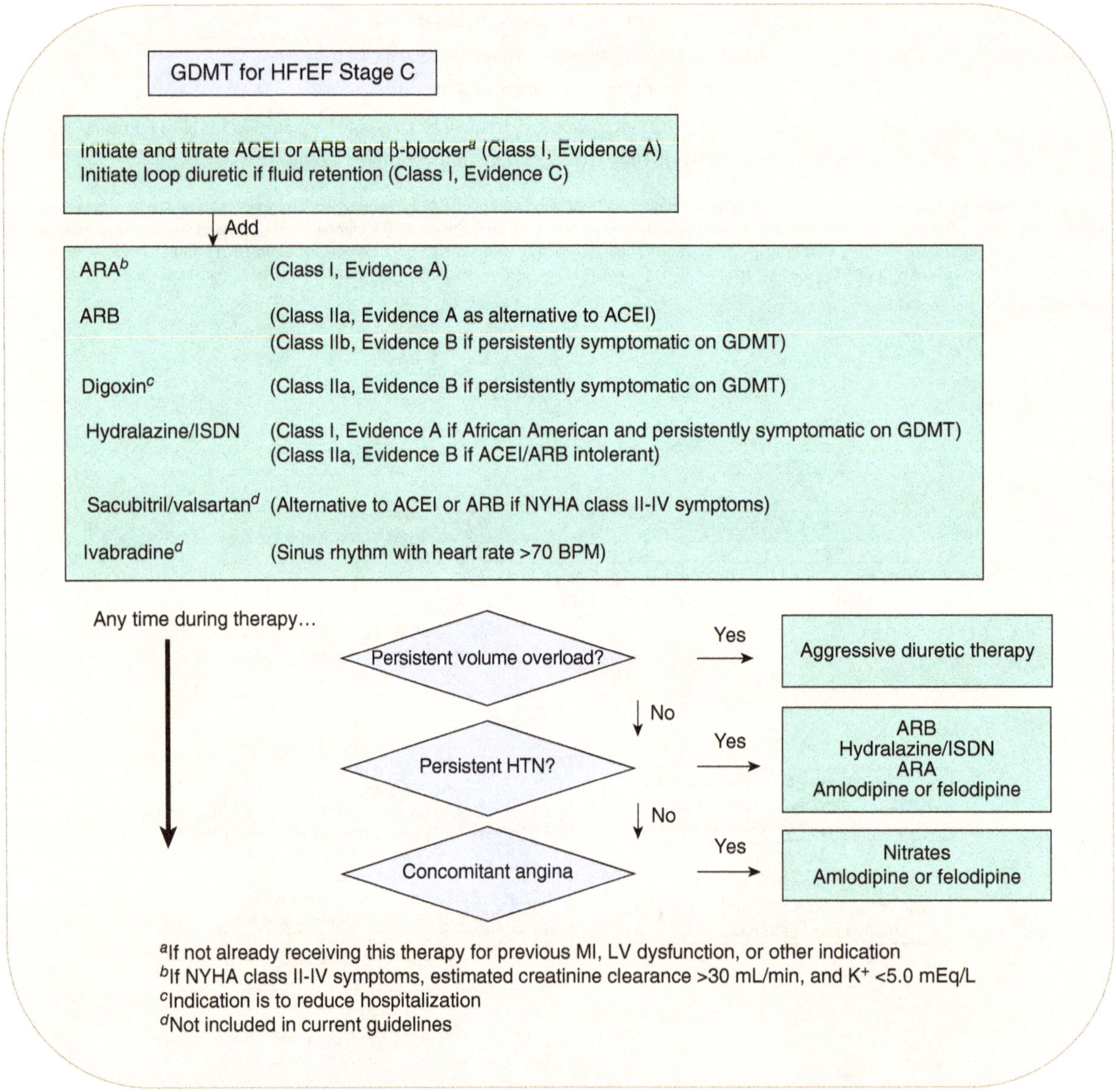

FIGURE 25-7 Guideline-directed treatment algorithm for patients with ACC/AHA stage C heart failure.

Abbreviations: ACEI = angiotensin-converting enzyme inhibitor; ARA = aldosterone receptor antagonist; ARB = angiotensin receptor blocker; BB = β-blocker; BPM = beats per minute (bpm); GDMT = guideline-directed medical therapy; HFrEF = heart failure with reduced ejection fraction; HTN = hypertension; ISDN = isosorbide dinitrate; K^+ = potassium; LV = left ventricular; MI = myocardial infarction; NYHA = New York Heart Association.

Source: References 1 and 2.

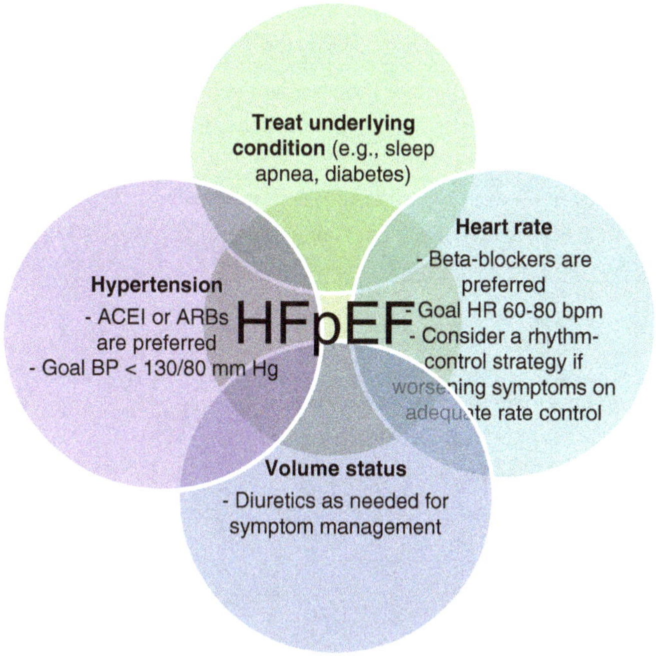

FIGURE 25-8 Current treatment strategy for heart failure with preserved ejection fraction.
Source: References 1, 4, and 5.

readmission to the hospital for worsening HF is quite common.[4] A HF admission places the patient at higher risk of HF readmission and mortality[1,4,5] As such, clinicians must be aware of indications that a patient should seek emergent medical care. Figure 25-9 highlights clinical scenarios where hospital admission would either be recommended or considered.

CORE ELEMENT 5—DOCUMENTATION AND FOLLOW-UP

Clear, concise, and evidence-based documentation of MRPs and recommendations is a key component of the MTM consult. Examples of potential MRPs in patients with HF are provided in Table 25-14. Sample communications and recommendations to providers to address medication-related issues are found in Figure 25-10. Recommendations may be communicated via fax, telephone, or other means of written or secure electronic communication. The examples below are for illustrative purposes. Actual communications to providers should be individualized according the type of recommendation, patient specific characteristics, and the nature of the relationship with the provider.

There are no specific intervals for follow-up recommended in chronic HF, except after a HF admission. Since recently admitted patients are at increased risk of death and readmission, the recommended follow-up is usually within 7 days. Those considered at very high risk should be seen even earlier in clinic for reassessment (eg, 48 hours after discharge). In addition, follow-up intervals should be shorter in patients with more severe disease and symptoms, and in those with symptom instability.[1,4,5] In some cases, early follow-up may be done over the telephone or other telecommunication device (eg, televideo).

From a MTM perspective, many medications used in HF need close follow-up to evaluate tolerability and safety. Suggested medication-related follow-up intervals are provided in Table 25-15.

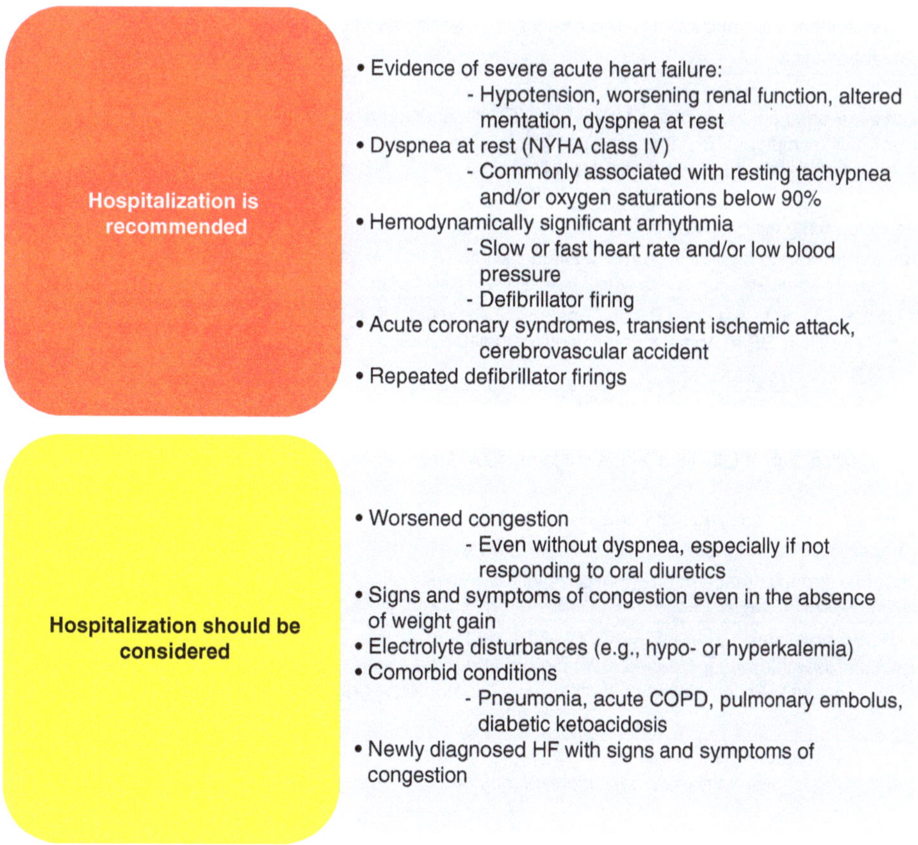

FIGURE 25-9 Referral for worsening heart failure signs and symptoms.
Source: Reference 4.

TABLE 25-14 • Medication-Related Problems (MRPs) in Patients with Chronic Heart Failure

Category of MRP	Sample Medication-Related Problem
Nonadherence	Worsening HF signs and symptoms due to nonadherence with lifestyle modifications (eg, sodium restrictions) Presenting to the emergency department due to nonadherence with HF medications (eg, BB, diuretic)
Unnecessary medication	Duplicate therapy (eg, ACEI and an ARB in HFpEF)
Need for additional medication	A Black patient not taking an optimal regimen for HFrEF (add hydralazine/ISDN combination) Suboptimal heart rate control in HFpEF and atrial fibrillation in a patient taking maximum BB dose (add low-dose digoxin)
Ineffective medication	Patient using metoprolol tartrate for HFrEF A patient taking high-dose furosemide with worsening ascites, dyspnea on exertion, and hepatomegaly (reduced oral absorption of furosemide)
Dosage too low	Worsening ascites and dyspnea on exertion on torsemide 5 mg once every morning
Dosage too high	Patient with CKD taking target dose of spironolactone and experiencing hyperkalemia Symptomatic bradycardia on metoprolol succinate 150 mg daily
Adverse drug event	Orthostatic hypotension on carvedilol Hypokalemia and worsening renal function with a loop diuretic

Abbreviation: ACEI = angiotensin-converting enzyme inhibitor; ARB = angiotensin receptor blocker; BB = β-blocker; CKD = chronic kidney disease; HF = heart failure; HFpEF = heart failure with preserved ejection fraction; HFrEF = heart failure with reduced ejection fraction; ISDN = isosorbide dinitrate.

Scenario: Patient given instructions to limit sodium intake and fluid intake, but is unsure of the amounts. Patient now has worsening orthopnea.
MRP: Nonadherence to lifestyle/dietary modifications

Assessment:
Poor patient understanding on the amount of sodium and fluid limitations resulted in worsening HF symptoms. Patient is willing and able to follow recommendation if provided reinstruction.

Plan:
Limit daily sodium intake to <2000 mg daily.

Limit total daily fluid intake to 1.5 L or approximately 48 oz.

If symptoms have not improved on dietary modifications, please call the clinic within one week.

Source: HFSA 2010 Comprehensive Heart Failure Practice Guideline. *J Cardiac Fail.* 2010;16:e1-e194.

Scenario: Patient on target dose of a BB and ACEI with NYHA class II symptoms and an EF < 30%.
MRP: Need for additional medication

Assessment:
Patient is doing well from a HF perspective. Per the EMPHASIS-HF trial, addition of eplerenone may benefit patients with an EF of <30% with NHYA class II symptoms. Vitals, symptoms, EF, and current medication regimen at target doses allow for patient to start low-dose eplerenone. Patient likely at low risk of hyperkalemia due to preserved renal function and no history of diabetes.

Plan:
Consider starting eplerenone 25 mg every morning.

Reassess renal function, serum K^+ and signs/symptoms of HF in 1 week.

Source: EMPHASIS-HF Study Group. Eplerenone in patients with systolic heart failure and mild symptoms. *N Engl J Med.* 2011;364:11-21.

Scenario: Patient with HFrEF and on target dose BB and enalapril 2.5 mg bid. HF symptoms are stable at NYHA class III. Patient has preserved renal function and serum K+ is WNL. BP at home is consistently 100-110 mmHg systolic. BP in clinic today is 108/64 mmHg.
MRP: Dose too low

Assessment:
Patient is stable from a HF standpoint. Higher ACEI doses have been shown to reduce risk of readmission for worsening HF. The target dose of enalapril in HFrEF is 10 mg twice daily. Vitals, labs, and symptoms allow for increase in ACEI closer to target dose.

Plan:
Increase enalapril to 5 mg bid. Continue to monitor home BP.

Reassess renal function, serum K^+ and signs/symptoms of HF in 1 week.

Follow up for assessment for further increase in enalapril dose in 2-4 weeks.

Source: HFSA 2010 Comprehensive Heart Failure Practice Guideline. *J Cardiac Fail.* 2010;16:e1-e194.

Scenario: Patient has HFpEF and is taking a nonDHP CCB, ACEI, and furosemide. One month ago patient had worsening signs/symptoms of HF and a 6-lb weight gain. Furosemide was increased to 40 mg bid and patient was to follow up in 1 week. The patient rescheduled the appointment and is returning 3 weeks later with complaints of symptomatic hypotension and a 12-lb weight loss.
MRP: Adverse effect

Assessment:
Patient is likely having symptoms of overdiuresis. Excess diuresis may cause worsening renal function and electrolyte disturbances.

Plan:
Hold furosemide and ACEI and present to urgent care for evaluation and labs to assess renal function and electrolytes.

FIGURE 25-10 Sample provider communications for heart failure.

TABLE 25-15 • Suggested Monitoring Intervals for Chronic HF Medications

Tolerability and safety
Assessment includes but is not limited to: vital signs, signs/symptoms of HF, signs/symptoms of hypotension or bradycardia.
β-Blockers: Reassess 2 weeks after starting or increasing dose. Increase dose at biweekly intervals. For unstable patients (eg, low BP or moderate or severe symptoms at baseline), consider evaluating tolerability in 2 weeks and titrate after 1 month.
ACEI, ARB, or ARNI: Repeat labs (BUN, SCr, K^+) and reassess 1-2 weeks after starting or titrating. Titrate no sooner than every 2 weeks. Repeat labs and reassess at least every 4 months thereafter.
Aldosterone antagonist: Repeat labs (BUN, SCr, and K^+) and reassess at 1 and 4 weeks after initiating or increasing dose, and at 8 and 12 weeks and 6, 9, and 12 months, then every 4 months thereafter. Consider titration of aldosterone antagonists at 4 to 8-week intervals.
Diuretics: Repeat labs (BUN, SCr, K^+) and reassess 1-2 weeks after starting or titrating. Repeat labs and reassess at least every 4 months thereafter.
FDC HYD/ISDN: Reassess 2 weeks after starting or increasing dose. Increase dose at biweekly intervals. For unstable patients (eg, low BP), consider evaluating tolerability in 2 weeks and titrate after 1 month.
Digoxin: There is no specific laboratory monitoring frequency for digoxin after initiating or increasing dose. However, it would be reasonable to repeat labs (BUN, SCr, K^+, Mg^{2+}, and trough digoxin level) and reassess 1 month after starting or titrating. Once at a therapeutic range (0.5-0.8 ng/mL), repeat labs and reassess at least every 6 months.
Ivabradine: Reassess heart rate and tolerability 2 weeks after starting or changing dose. Consider dose change at biweekly intervals. Clinical trials obtained an electrocardiogram (ECG) at each follow-up, which may not be absolutely necessary if other measurement techniques are considered accurate (eg, manual palpation or blood pressure monitor)

Abbreviations: ACEI = angiotensin-converting enzyme inhibitor; ARB = angiotensin receptor blocker; ARNI = angiotensin II receptor/neprilysin inhibitor; BP = blood pressure; BUN = blood urea nitrogen; FDC HYD/ISDN = fixed-dose combination hydralazine/isosorbide dinitrate; HF = heart failure; SCr = serum creatinine.

Source: References 1, 3, and 4.

REFERENCES

1. Yancy CW, Jessup M, Bozkurt B, et al. 2013 ACCF/AHA guideline for the management of heart failure. *Circulation*. 2013;128:e240-e327.
2. Yancy CW, Jessup M, Bozkurt B, et al. *2017 ACC/AHA/HFSA Focused Update of the 2013 ACCF/AHA Guideline for the Management of Heart Failure*. Available at http://www.onlinejcf.com/article/S1071-9164(17)30107-0/fulltext. Accessed May 5, 2017.
3. Parker RB, Nappi JM, Cavallari LH. Chronic heart failure. In: DiPiro JT, Talbert RL, Yee, GC, Matzke GR, Wells BG, Posey LM, eds. *Pharmacotherapy: A Pathophysiologic Approach*, 10th ed. New York: McGraw-Hill; 2017, Chapter 14.
4. Heart Failure Society of America, Lindenfeld J, Albert NM, Boehmer JP, et al. HFSA 2010 Comprehensive Heart Failure Practice Guideline. *J Cardiac Fail*. 2010;16:e1-194.
5. Ponikowski P, Voors AA, Anker SD, et al. 2016 ESC guidelines for the diagnosis and treatment of acute and chronic heart failure: The Task Force for the Diagnosis and Treatment of Acute and Chronic Heart failure of the European Society of Cardiology (ESC). Developed with the special contribution of the Heart Failure Association (HFA) of the ESC. *Eur J Heart Fail*. 2016;18:891-975.
6. Mann DL. Management of patients with heart failure with reduced ejection fraction. In: Mann DL, Zipes DP, Libby P, Bonow RO, Braunwald E, eds. *Braunwald's Heart Disease: A Textbook of Cardiovascular Medicine*, 10th ed. Philadelphia, PA: Elsevier; 2015:512-546.
7. Simon MA. Assessment and treatment of right ventricular failure. *Nat Rev Cardiol*. 2013; 10:204-218.
8. *Medicare Part D Medication Therapy Management Program Standardized Format*. Available at https://www.cms.gov/Medicare/Prescription-Drug-Coverage/PrescriptionDrugCovContra/Downloads/MTM-Program-Standardized-Format-English-and-Spanish-Instructions-Samples-v032712.pdf. Accessed May 7, 2017.
9. Clinical Pharmacology [database online]. Tampa, FL: Gold Standard, Inc.; 2017. Available at http://www.clinicalpharmacology.com. Accessed May 7, 2017.
10. Nadir MA, Wei L, Elder DH, et al. Impact of renin-angiotensin system blockade therapy on outcome in aortic stenosis. *J Am Coll Cardiol*. 2011;58:570-576.
11. Bakris GL, Fonseca V, Katholi RE, et al. Metabolic effects of carvedilol vs metoprolol in patients with type 2 diabetes mellitus and hypertension: a randomized controlled trial. *JAMA*. 2004;292:2227-2236.
12. Rathore SS, Wang Y, Krumholz HM. Sex-based differences in the effect of digoxin for the treatment of heart failure. *N Engl J Med*. 2002;347: 1403-1411.
13. Adams KF Jr, Patterson JH, Gattis WA, et al. Relationship of serum digoxin concentration to mortality and morbidity in women in the Digitalis Investigation Group trial: a retrospective analysis. *J Am Coll Cardiol*. 2005;46:497-504.
14. Natural Medicines [database online]. Somerville, MA: Therapeutic Research Center; 2017. Available at https://naturalmedicines.therapeuticresearch.com/. Accessed May 8, 2017.

Review Questions

1. *Heart failure* (HF) is defined as a clinical syndrome with signs and symptoms precipitated by abnormal function or structure of the heart. What is the definition of HF with reduced ejection fraction (EF)?
   a. Signs and symptoms of HF with an EF of >40%.
   b. Signs and symptoms of HF with an EF of ≤40%.
   c. Signs and symptoms of right-sided HF with an EF of ≤40%.
   d. Signs and symptoms of right-sided HF with an EF of >40%.

2. Symptoms of HF may be "left-sided" or "right-sided." All of the following are left-sided symptoms of HF EXCEPT:
   a. Orthopnea
   b. Tachypnea
   c. Cough
   d. Ascites

3. When a diagnosis of HF is made, treatment depends on etiology, disease severity, and type of HF. Which of the following is an important treatment goal in the management of HF?
   a. Decrease blood pressure to <140/90 mmHg.
   b. Maintain current cardiovascular status.
   c. Prevent hospitalization.
   d. Lower LDL-cholesterol to <70 mg/dL.

4. It is important to use living room language when talking to a patient about HF. What is appropriate living room language for describing dyspnea?
   a. Difficulty breathing with activity
   b. Chest pain when breathing in
   c. Rapid breathing
   d. A feeling of chest pressure

5. A 65-year-old male is newly diagnosed with HF with reduced EF. His cardiologist prescribes metoprolol succinate 12.5 mg once daily. What is an appropriate step to include in the medication action plan?
   a. At this stage, I do not have to monitor sodium intake.
   b. I should check and record my blood sugar 3 times per week.
   c. I should check and record my blood pressure daily.
   d. I should get blood drawn one month after starting this medication.

6. When is it appropriate to refer a patient with HF to seek medical attention?
   a. When blood pressure is below the goal, but patient has no symptoms of hypotension
   b. When the patient gains one pound in a 14-day time period
   c. When the patient inadvertently consumes more sodium than recommended at breakfast
   d. When the patient experiences new symptoms of HF at rest

7. A 65-year-old female with a 3-year history of HF with preserved EF is a regular customer at your pharmacy. She brings in a new prescription for valsartan. On review of her records, you discover that she is on lisinopril. Which potential medication-related problem could occur with the addition of valsartan?
   a. Nonadherence
   b. Need for additional therapy
   c. Unnecessary medication
   d. Ineffective medication

8. A 70-year-old male with HF with reduced EF (New York Heart Association Class II) has been taking metoprolol succinate 200 mg once daily. As the result of an insurance formulary change, the patient will have to switch to carvedilol. The patient is stable, with no symptoms. What is an equivalent dose of carvedilol?
   a. Carvedilol 6.25 mg twice daily
   b. Carvedilol 12.5 mg twice daily
   c. Carvedilol 25 mg twice daily
   d. Carvedilol 50 mg twice daily

9. A 70-year-old female is diagnosed with HF with reduced EF. She has a past medical history significant for diabetes, hypertension, and seasonal allergies. Which medication should be avoided for this patient?
   a. Glipizide
   b. Lisinopril
   c. Chlorthalidone
   d. Pioglitazone

10. A patient with HF with reduced EF is on a maximized HF regimen including target dose carvedilol, enalapril, and spironolactone. She is starting sacubitril/valsartan. How should this patient safely transition to sacubitril/valsartan?
    a. Start sacubitril/valsartan as soon as received.
    b. Stop carvedilol, wait 24 hours after last carvedilol dose, then start sacubitril/valsartan.
    c. Stop spironolactone, wait 36 hours after last spironolactone dose, then start sacubitril/valsartan.
    d. Stop enalapril, wait 36 hours after last enalapril dose, then start sacubitril/valsartan.

ANSWERS

1. b	2. d	3. c
4. a	5. c	6. d
7. c	8. d	9. d
10. d		

26

HIV MTM Data Set

Jamie Kisgen, PharmD, BCPS-AQ ID

KEY POINTS

- Early, aggressive treatment of HIV is now the mainstay of therapy in order to prevent the long-term infectious and noninfectious causes of morbidity and mortality.
- Adherence is one of the major predictors of success and failure when treating HIV patients. Medication therapy management (MTM) providers should be vigilant for nonadherence and work with the patient and the physician to design a regimen that is manageable, tolerable, and efficacious.
- MTM providers should recognize the importance of careful screening for drug interactions and adverse effects when initiating and monitoring human immunodeficiency virus (HIV) medications.

INTRODUCTION TO HUMAN IMMUNODEFICIENCY VIRUS INFECTION

Human immunodeficiency virus (HIV) is a single-stranded RNA retrovirus that causes *acquired immunodeficiency syndrome* (AIDS) and other HIV-related disorders. HIV is subdivided into two distinct types: HIV-1 and HIV-2.[1] Type 1 is more common, more virulent, and easier to transmit than HIV-2. HIV-2 is found mostly on the western coast of Africa, whereas HIV-1 is common throughout the world. The primary modes of transmission are sexual, parenteral, and perinatal. The most common mode of transmission is sexual intercourse, primarily anal and vaginal. The estimated risk of HIV transmission, based on type of patient exposure, is highlighted in Table 26-1. Some of the factors that influence the probability of transmission are type of exposure, use of condoms, stage of index partner, viral load of index partner, presence of sexually transmitted diseases, and use of antiretrovirals (ARV).[1,2]

Complications of HIV

Despite the advent of new antiretroviral therapies (ART), more aggressive treatment guidelines, and public education, many patients continue to develop complications from the virus. Approximately 20% of patients with HIV are undiagnosed and, therefore, may not present until they have an AIDS-defining condition.[3] A patient whose immune system becomes compromised and develops full-blown AIDS usually presents with an opportunistic infection or an infection-related cancer. The definitive diagnosis of AIDS is a CD4 count of less <200 cells/mm^3, a CD4 percentage less than 14, or documentation of an AIDS-defining condition. Table 26-2 provides an outline of the staging of HIV and a list of AIDS-defining conditions.

Of note, HIV is a chronic infection that causes an increase in cytokine levels and inflammation throughout the body. The constant state of inflammation is damaging to cells, vessels, and organs, and can increase the risk of noninfectious complications. Examples include myocardial infarction, HIV-associated nephropathy (HIVAN), and certain types of cancers. Some noninfectious complications are correlated with the degree of CD4 suppression, while others are independent of CD4 count. Table 26-3 lists common infectious and noninfectious complications of HIV, and usual CD4 count associated with the condition. Not only are HIV-related comorbidities a concern; ARV agents themselves can increase the risk of developing complications. Other host risk factors also need to be considered when evaluating the patient for possible complications. As HIV patients age, so does the risk of developing hypertension, diabetes, kidney disease, and other common conditions that affect patients without HIV. These conditions can be difficult to manage individually, not to mention in patients with HIV on potent ARV agents. Careful screening and follow-up are essential

TABLE 26-1 • Estimated Risk of HIV Transmission Based on Exposure to an Infected Source

Type of Exposure[a]	Estimated Risk
Blood transfusion	92.5% (925 in 1000)
Needle sharing during injection drug use	0.63% (1 in 159)
Percutaneous exposure (ie, needlestick, sharp)[a]	0.23% (1 in 435)
Receptive anal intercourse	1.38% (1 in 73)
Insertive anal intercourse	0.11% (1 in 910)
Receptive vaginal intercourse	0.08% (1 in 1250)
Insertive vaginal intercourse	0.04% (1 in 2500)
Receptive or insertive oral intercourse	Low, accurate estimate unavailable
Biting, spitting, throwing body fluids, or sharing sex toys	Negligible

[a] Factors that may impact risk of transmission include an active, untreated sexually transmitted disease, acute HIV infection, end-stage AIDS, viral load of source patient, and use of prophylaxis measures (eg, active antiretroviral [ARV] treatment, male circumcision, condoms, preexposure prophylaxis).

Source: Reference 2.

to identify noninfectious complications of HIV early in the process and minimize the impact of complications on the patient with HIV. MTM providers can play an important role in screening for these complications and ensuring that patients with HIV receive the proper treatment and appropriate follow-up.

HIV Treatment Goals

Although new agents continue to be developed and approved for HIV, none of the current therapies are able to eradicate the infection from the body. Therefore, current treatment focuses on reducing the risk of HIV-associated morbidity and mortality, maximizing viral suppression, restoring the immune system, and decreasing HIV transmission, while limiting drug-related adverse effects and maintaining quality of life.[7] Sustained suppression of the virus also prevents the selection of drug resistance, preserves CD4 cell numbers, and decreases the incidence of non-AIDS-defining diseases (ie, cardiovascular disease, kidney disease, and malignancies). Achievement of these goals requires commitment of the patient to adhere to the drug therapy and dedication of health-care professionals in supporting the patient's success.

Not all patients are willing and able to initiate ART immediately after diagnosis. Potential concerns of initiating therapy

TABLE 26-2 • Surveillance Case Definition for HIV Infection Stage Based on $CD4^+$ T-Lymphocyte Counts, United States, 2014

General Case/Stage Definition						
A. Age on Date of $CD4^+$ T-Lymphocyte Test						
	<1 Year		1-5 Years		≥6 Years	
Stage	Cells/µL ($\times 10^6$/L)	%	Cells/µL ($\times 10^6$/L)	%	Cells/µL ($\times 10^6$/L)	%
1	≥1500	≥34	≥1000	≥30	≥500	≥26
2	750-1499	26-33	500-999	22-29	200-499	14-25
3 (AIDS)	<750	<26	<500	<22	<200	<14

B. AIDS Indicator Conditions	
Bacterial infections, multiple or recurrent (specific to children <6 years), intestinal (duration >1 month)	
Candidiasis of bronchi, trachea, or lungs	Lymphoma, Burkitt
Candidiasis, esophageal	Lymphoma, immunoblastic
Cervical cancer, invasive (specific to adults, adolescents, children >6 years)	Lymphoma, primary, or brain
Coccidioidomycosis, disseminated or extrapulmonary	*Mycobacterium avium* complex or *M. kansasii*, disseminated or extrapulmonary
Cryptococcosis, extrapulmonary	*Mycobacterium tuberculosis*, any site (pulmonary or extrapulmonary)
Cryptosporidiosis, chronic intestinal (duration >1 month)	*Mycobacterium*, other species or unidentified species, disseminated or extrapulmonary
Cytomegalovirus disease (other than liver, spleen, or nodes), onset at age > 1 month	*Pneumocystis jirovecii* pneumonia (PCP)
Cytomegalovirus retinitis (with loss of vision)	Pneumonia, recurrent (specific to adults, adolescents, children >6 years)
Encephalopathy, HIV-related	Progressive multifocal leukoencephalopathy
Herpes simplex: chronic ulcer(s) (duration >1 month); or bronchitis, pneumonitis, or esophagitis, onset at age > 1 month	*Salmonella* septicemia, recurrent
	Toxoplasmosis of brain, onset at age >1 month
	Wasting syndrome due to HIV
Histoplasmosis, disseminated or extrapulmonary	Kaposi's sarcoma
Isosporiasis, chronic intestinal (duration >1 month)	

Source: Centers for Disease Control and Prevention.[4]

TABLE 26-3 • Infectious and Noninfectious Complications of HIV

CD4 Cell Count	Infectious Complications	Noninfectious Complications
Can occur at any CD4 count	Proctitis and anorectal ulcers from STDs	Fat malabsorption Protease inhibitor-related gastrointestinal effects Insulin resistance and diabetes Dyslipidemia and lipodystrophy Cardiovascular disease and atherosclerosis Reduced bone mineral density Myopathy (including autoimmune-mediated)
>500 cells/mm³	Acute retroviral syndrome Candida vaginitis	Aseptic meningitis Guillain-Barré syndrome PGL
200-500 cells/mm³	Bacterial pneumonia (including *Streptococcus pneumoniae*) Herpes zoster/Varicella zoster Kaposi's sarcoma Neurosyphilis (<350 cells/mm³) Oral hairy leukoplakia Thrush (oropharyngeal candidiasis) Tuberculosis (pulmonary)	Anemia (HIV- or drug-induced) B-Cell lymphoma Cervical and anal cancer or dysplasia (associated with human papillomavirus) Hodgkin's lymphoma Idiopathic thrombocytopenic purpura Lymphocytic interstitial pneumonitis
<200 cells/mm³	Coccidioidomycosis Herpes simplex virus (disseminated) Histoplasmosis PCP PML Tuberculosis (miliary/extrapulmonary)	Cardiomyopathy HIV-associated dementia HIV-induced enteropathy (chronic diarrhea with occasional weight loss) Non-Hodgkin lymphoma Peripheral neuropathy Progressive polyradiculopathy Wasting
<100 cells/mm³	Candida esophagitis Cryptosporidiosis *Isospora belli* Microsporidiosis Toxoplasmosis	
<50 cells/mm³	Cryptococcal meningioencephalitis CMV MAC	Primary CNS lymphoma

Abbreviations: CMV = cytomegalovirus; CNS = central nervous system; HIV = human immunodeficiency virus; MAC = *Mycobacterium avium* complex; PCP = *Pneumocystis jirovecii* pneumonia; PGL = persistent generalized lymphadenopathy; PML = progressive multifocal leukoencephalopathy; STD = sexually transmitted disease.

Source: References 5 and 6.

include toxicity from the therapy, cost of therapy and nonadherence to ART, which not only prevents immune system recovery, but also increases the risk of resistance. Screening patients for treatment readiness, risks for side effects, and available financial resources is paramount in the baseline assessment. The process can sometimes be very overwhelming for patients, and it may take time to weigh all the pros and cons and identify barriers of therapy. MTM providers can make significant contributions to care by discussing the risks and benefits of therapy, educating on potential side effects, and providing encouragement when needed.

Because of the resistant nature of HIV, combination therapy with at least two, and preferably three, active ARV medications is essential for adequate virologic response while minimizing the risk of drug resistance. There are several known predictors of virologic success that can aid clinicians in determining which patients will respond well to therapy. These include high potency of ARV regimen selected, excellent adherence to the treatment regimen, low baseline viremia, higher baseline CD4 count (>200 cells/μL), and rapid reduction of viremia in response to treatment.[7] Selection of the initial combination regimen based on pretreatment resistance testing, side effect profile, patient lifestyle, and comorbidities are important strategies in achieving treatment goals.

After initiating therapy, some of the measurable treatment goals are to improve the CD4 count from baseline, as well as attain virologic suppression of HIV. *Virologic suppression* is defined as an HIV RNA level below the level of detection of the assay (eg, <20 copies/mL). Despite the advent of new therapies that have less pill burden, easier dosing schedules, and fewer side effects, virologic failure still occurs. *Virologic failure* is defined as the inability to achieve or maintain suppression of viral replication to an HIV RNA level of <200 copies/mL.[7] Common causes of virologic failure include higher pretreatment or baseline HIV RNA level, low CD4 count, history of AIDS diagnosis, comorbidities (eg, active substance abuse, depression), transmitted or acquired drug resistance, poor medication adherence, missed clinic appointments, and adverse drug reactions. In some cases a virologic "blip" occurs, which is a temporary increase in the viral load after virologic suppression. A blip, however, is not a sign of virologic failure and should return to undetectable with the next blood draw. In cases of virologic failure, careful assessment of risk factors and potential causes is important before altering therapy. MTM providers can assist with identification of reasons for virologic failure, and provide education and guidance to patients and clinicians.

CORE ELEMENT 1—COMPREHENSIVE MEDICATION REVIEW FOR PATIENTS WITH HIV

Suggested questions to ask when conducting a medication therapy review in a patient with HIV are listed in Table 26-4. The number and types of questions will depend on several factors, including the amount of time for the interview, number of concurrent medication-related problems (MRPs), urgency of MRPs, and the reliability of the patient in providing accurate information, among others. In time-limited interactions or in complex cases with multiple medical issues, the MTM provider may choose to target questions that help to identify or rule out issues of an urgent nature (see questions to ask for prevention/assessment of medical emergencies). MTM providers should remember to use living room language during the interview (Figure 26-1), and to be prepared for questions that patients may ask regarding HIV (Table 26-5).

TABLE 26-4 • Questions to Ask When Conducting a Medication Review in a Patient with HIV

Questions Commonly Asked by Clinicians Interviewing HIV Patients
Background: How long have you had HIV? When were you diagnosed? What do you know about the risks associated with HIV?
HIV medications: What medications do you take for HIV? How do you take them? In a given week, how often do you miss a dose of your HIV medication? What other medications have you taken in the past for HIV? Have you ever stopped taking any of your HIV medications without telling your physician? If so, why? Have you recently experienced any of the following signs/symptoms? Fever, rash, nausea, vomiting, diarrhea, abdominal pain, malaise, or respiratory symptoms (eg, cough, shortness of breath)
Opportunistic infection medications: Do you take any medications to prevent infections (eg, Bactrim or Zithromax)? If so, what are they and how do you take them? How long have you been on these medications? Has your physician discussed with you why it is important to take these medications? Are you up-to-date on your vaccines? When was the last time you had a flu shot, pneumonia shot, and tetanus shot?
Other conditions: Do you have any other medical conditions? If so, what medications do you take to treat these conditions?
OTC/herbal medications: What over-the-counter (OTC) medications or herbals do you use? What has your physician discussed with you regarding OTC medications that you should avoid because they can interact with your medications (eg, St. John's wort)?
Questions to Ask for Prevention/Assessment of Medical Emergencies
Have you recently experienced any of the following signs or symptoms? • *Any signs of infection*—fever, shortness of breath, weight loss, night sweats, cough, unexplained new onset rash or lesion, confusion, stiff neck • *Fanconi syndrome*—passing large amounts of urine, which can lead to dehydration, bone pain, and weakness (Look for in patients on tenofovir) • *Hypersensitivity syndrome*—fever, rash, malaise, swelling, shortness of breath, especially if the patient recently started on a medication known to cause hypersensitivity (ie, abacavir, nonnucleoside reverse transcriptase inhibitors) • *Neuropsychiatric side effects*—abnormal dreams, dizziness, depression, or suicidal thoughts (especially within 2-4 weeks after starting efavirenz) • *Pancreatitis*—pain, nausea and vomiting, and a swollen abdomen • *Stevens-Johnson syndrome* (SJS)—skin rash characterized by red, blistered spots on the skin; blisters in the mouth, eyes, genitals, or other moist areas of the body; peeling skin that results in painful sores

Acquired immunodeficiency syndrome (AIDS)—a disease of the immune system due to infection with HIV. HIV destroys the CD4 T lymphocytes (CD4 cells) of the immune system, leaving the body open to life-threatening infections and cancers. AIDS is the most advanced stage of HIV infection.
Acute retroviral syndrome—flu-like symptoms of acute HIV infection that may appear 2-4 weeks after initial infection. Common symptoms such as fever, headache, fatigue, and swollen lymph nodes can last from a few days to 4 weeks, and then disappear.
Adherence—taking your medications exactly as prescribed. Poor adherence to an HIV treatment regimen can increase the risk for developing drug-resistant HIV and lead to the medicines not working.
Adverse drug reaction—also called a *side effect*. This is an unintended or undesirable effect of a medication.
AIDS-defining condition—an HIV-related illness that has been determined by the CDC as meeting the diagnostic criteria for AIDS. Most of the conditions are infections or cancers and are usually life-threatening in a person with HIV.
AIDS Drug Assistance Programs (ADAPs)—federally funded programs that provide medications and other HIV-related services to low-income, uninsured, and underinsured people with HIV/AIDS.
Alanine aminotransferase (ALT)—an enzyme found mostly in the liver. ALT may be measured as part of a liver function test and helps to determine whether a patient's liver may have been damaged.
Antibiotic—a drug used to kill or suppress the growth of microorganisms, such as bacteria and fungi.
Antiretroviral (ARV)—a drug used to prevent HIV from multiplying (eg, protease inhibitors).
Antiretroviral therapy (ART)—the recommended treatment for HIV infection. ART usually involves a combination of three or more ARV drugs from at least two different HIV drug classes to prevent HIV from multiplying.
Antiviral—a medicine used to prevent the growth or replication of viruses.
Aspartate aminotransferase (AST)—an enzyme found mostly in the heart, muscle, and liver cells. AST may be measured as part of a liver function test and helps to determine whether the liver may have been damaged.
Asthenia—lack of energy or strength; weakness.
Bilirubin—a component of the liver function blood test. This is a substance produced by the body after breaking down red blood cells. It can accumulate in the body when the liver is damaged or diseased and can cause jaundice. This can also be elevated by certain drugs (eg, atazanavir).
Blip—see *Virologic blip*.
Blood glucose—blood sugar.
BMI—body mass index; a measure of weight in relation to height that assigns people to a weight class of underweight, normal weight, overweight, or obese according to their amount of excess weight.
Boosting agent—a medication that is used to increase the amount of another medication that gets into the body. This allows for either less frequent dosing, fewer pills per dose, or both. Two agents commonly used for boosting are ritonavir and cobicistat.
Cachexia—when the body loses a significant amount of body weight and muscle mass. This is commonly seen in patients with chronic HIV/AIDS.
Candidiasis—a fungal infection caused by the yeast. *Candida*. This is typically found in the mouth, vagina, and anus, but can also be found in other areas of the body as well (eg, esophagus and lungs).
CCR5 antagonist—a medicine used to prevent HIV from entering the CD4 cell.
CD4 count—a laboratory test that measures the number of CD4 T lymphocytes (CD4 cells) in a sample of blood. This is commonly used as a marker of how well your immune system is working and is usually measured every 3-6 months. Normal is 500-1200 cells/μL.
CD4 percentage—a laboratory test that measures the percentage of white blood cells that are CD4 T lymphocytes (CD4 cells). This is commonly used as a marker of how well a patient's immune system is working, especially in children.
CD4 T-lymphocyte (CD4) *cell* ("*T-cell*")—a type of white blood cell that helps coordinate the immune system to fight an infection. HIV weakens the immune system by attacking and killing CD4 cells.
Central nervous system (CNS)—the part of the nervous system comprising the brain and spinal cord. HIV infection or use of some antiretroviral (ARV) drugs can cause damage to the CNS.
Chlamydia—a common sexually transmitted disease (STD) caused by a bacterial infection. Some patients may not present with symptoms; however, all patients and their partners should be treated to prevent complications and further transmission. STDs also increase the risk of HIV transmission.
Chronic—constant, never-ending, does not go away.
Chronic kidney disease—when the kidneys are not able to work well, which may cause high blood pressure and other serious health problems.
Colitis—inflammation of the colon (large bowel or intestines). Common symptoms include nausea, diarrhea, or abdominal pain/discomfort. This can occur in HIV patients with chronic disease or in the setting of an OI.
Creatinine test—a test that checks how the kidneys are working; an increase means that the kidneys are not working well.
Drug interaction—when one or more medications (or in some cases food) impact the drug actions in the body and have the potential to either affect the response to the drug and/or cause additional side effects.
Electrolyte—a type of necessary salt found in blood, such as sodium, potassium, and calcium.
Fanconi syndrome—a kidney disorder that can affect how the body maintains the appropriate balance of nutrients, including electrolytes, proteins, and glucose. This can be caused by certain HIV medications (eg, tenofovir).
Fusion inhibitor—a medicine used to prevent HIV entry into the CD4 cell.
Genital warts—a sexually transmitted disease caused by a viral infection (human papillomavirus or HPV). The warts can appear on the surface of the penis, anus, vagina, or cervix and are typically raised, pink-colored bumps.
Genotypic resistance assay (*genotype*)—a test that looks at certain pieces of the HIV virus. These pieces can tell us whether a particular ARV medication might work against a specific patient's virus. This is commonly done before the patient starts ARV medications or if the medicines are not working (ie, the virus might be resistant to the medication) against the virus.
Gonorrhea—a common sexually transmitted disease caused by a bacterial infection. Some patients may not present with symptoms; however, all patients and their partners should be treated to prevent complications and further transmission. STDs also increase the risk of HIV transmission.
Hematocrit—a blood test that studies the amount of red blood cells that a patient has; a very low amount could be a sign of anemia.
Hepatitis—inflammation of the liver, usually from a viral infection (ie, hepatitis B or C).
HIV-associated nephropathy (HIVAN)—a kidney disease that is associated with HIV; typically found with advanced and/or untreated HIV.
*HLA-B*5701 testing*—a blood test that is used to determine whether a patient is at risk for a severe drug reaction (hypersensitivity) to the medication abacavir. Patients with a positive test should not receive the drug abacavir.
Hormonal contraceptives—birth control medicine; may interact with some of the HIV medications.
Human immunodeficiency virus (HIV)—the virus that causes AIDS. It occurs as two types: HIV-1 and HIV-2. A person can get either type by direct contact with infected body fluids such as blood, semen, and genital secretions.
Hyperkalemia—high potassium level; very high potassium is a medical emergency and could cause a deadly change in the way the heart beats.

FIGURE 26-1 Living room language for HIV.
Source: Data compiled from reference 8.

Hypokalemia—low potassium, which may cause muscle weakness and cramping.
Immune reconstitution syndrome (IRIS)—an exaggerated inflammatory response by the body's immune system against an infection. This usually happens when the immune system starts to recover after initiation of HIV therapy, especially in patients who have low CD4 counts. This could be due to a known infection that has already been treated or a new infection that was "unmasked" by the immune system as it begins to "wake up."
Incomplete virologic response—when the amount of virus in the blood remains above 200 copies/mL in two separate blood draws after the patient has been on HIV treatment for at least 24 weeks (6 months).
Insulin resistance—when the body's ability to respond to insulin decreases and more insulin is required to have the same effect. This can lead to high blood sugar and eventually to prediabetes or type 2 diabetes. Some forms of ART (eg, protease inhibitors) may increase the risk of insulin resistance.
Integrase inhibitor—a group of medicines used to prevent HIV from multiplying.
Jaundice—a yellowing of the skin, fingernails, and/or eyes that occurs when the body accumulates too much bilirubin. This can be caused by liver injury/disease, certain blood diseases, problems with the gallbladder, and some ARV agents, including atazanavir.
Lipoatrophy—when the body loses fat from specific areas, including the face, arms, and buttocks. Several older ARV medications are known to cause lipoatrophy.
Liver function test—a blood test that is used to measure key substances related to the liver. This is used to identify, evaluate, and monitor for liver damage or disease.
Mycobacterium avium complex (MAC)—a bacterium that typically infects patients with a weakened immune system. In HIV patients it usually occurs when the CD4 count is < 50 cells/μL. Infection can occur throughout the body, including in the skin, lungs, and gut.
Nadir—the lowest CD4 count measured for a patient.
Nephrolithiasis—also known as "kidney stones." These usually consist of calcium and can occur in patients receiving certain HIV medications (eg, atazanavir, indinavir).
Nonnucleoside reverse transcriptase inhibitors (NNRTIs)—a group of medicines used to prevent HIV from multiplying.
Nucleoside reverse transcriptase inhibitors (NRTIs)—a group of medicines used to prevent HIV from multiplying.
Obese—having a body mass index (BMI) of >30, which increases the risk of having high blood pressure, diabetes, and cardiovascular disease.
Opportunistic infection (OI)—an infection that occurs more often or is more severe in patients with weakened immune systems (cancer, organ transplant, HIV, etc) than in patients with healthy immune systems.
Osteopenia—when the bone mass or bone mineral density (BMD) is lower than normal. If this continues to worsen, it can lead to osteoporosis. This is commonly seen in patients taking certain ARVs for an extended period of time (eg, tenofovir).
Osteoporosis—a disease in patients with progressive bone loss and diminished bone mineral density (BMD) who are at an increased risk of fracture. Patients on long-term ARVs may be at increased risk for developing osteoporosis and should be monitored carefully.
Overweight—having a body mass index (BMI) of >25, which increases the risk of developing high blood pressure, diabetes, and cardiovascular disease.
Pancreatitis—inflammation of the pancreas. Common symptoms include pain, nausea and vomiting, and a swollen belly.
Peripheral neuropathy—damage to the peripheral nervous system, which includes the nerves outside of the brain and spinal cord. Symptoms include pain, numbness, tingling, swelling, and muscle weakness.
Phenotypic resistance assay (phenotype)—a test that measures the ability of the HIV virus to grow in different concentrations of ARV drugs. It is generally used in patients who have been on many different HIV medicines in the past or have a very resistant virus.
Pneumocystis jirovecii pneumonia (PCP)—a lung infection caused by the fungus *Pneumocystis jirovecii*. This fungus is common in the environment and typically causes illness only in people with weakened immune systems. It is considered an AIDS-defining condition.
Pneumonia—inflammation of the lungs, which is usually caused by a bacterial, viral, or fungal infection.
Postexposure prophylaxis (PeP)—medications that are given to a patient right after a high-risk exposure to HIV or hepatitis B (eg, sexual assault, needlestick exposure). These medications help reduce the risk of infection.
Preexposure prophylaxis (PrEP)—medicine given before potential HIV exposure to reduce the risk of getting HIV.
Primary prophylaxis—medicine used to prevent the development of an infection, in someone who is at risk but has never had this infection before (eg, PCP prophylaxis in a patient with CD4 count < 200 cells/μL).
Protease inhibitors (PIs)—a group of medicines used to prevent HIV from multiplying.
Rapid HIV antibody test—a test that can find antibodies to HIV in the blood or mouth in <30 minutes.
Relapse—recurrence of a disease after a period when symptoms disappeared or diminished.
Resistance testing—a blood test used to identify which ARVs will work best against a patient's virus. See *Genotype* and *Phenotype* for examples.
Secondary prophylaxis—medicine(s) used to prevent a disease or infection from returning (ie, to prevent relapse), after someone has completed initial treatment, but remains at risk for developing it again because the immune system is still too weak (eg, PCP secondary prophylaxis is given to a patient who finishes a 3-week course for treatment because the CD4 count is still < 200 cell/μL).
Serum bilirubin—a blood test that measures the amount of bile products in the blood. This is commonly used as a measure of liver function and is sometimes monitored closely in patients receiving atazanavir, as this drug may cause the bilirubin level to rise.
Serum potassium—a test that determines the amount of potassium in your blood (see *Hyperkalemia* and *Hypokalemia*).
Sexually transmitted diseases (STDs)—infections passed during sex (also called *sexually transmitted infections*). Most STDs increase the risk of HIV transmission.
Stevens-Johnson syndrome (SJS)—a severe and sometimes life-threatening reaction to a medication. It is characterized by a skin rash with red, blistered spots on the skin, and blisters in the mouth, eyes, genitals, or other moist areas of the body. Peeling of the skin that results in painful sores is also commonly observed.
Syphilis—a common sexually transmitted disease caused by a bacterial infection (*Treponema pallidum*). Some patients may not present with symptoms; however, all patients and their partners should be treated to prevent complications and further transmission. STDs also increase the risk of HIV transmission.
Systemic—pertaining to the whole body. This could refer to an infection that affects the whole body.
T cell (or T lymphocyte)—a term that commonly refers to CD4 count.
Therapeutic drug monitoring—a blood test used to measure the levels of ARVs in the body. This helps determine the best possible dose to provide safe and effective treatment.
Toxoplasmosis—a parasite that comes from bird poop or raw/undercooked meat. In most people this rarely causes any problems. It may cause a lung, skin, or brain infection in a patient with a very weak immune system (eg, CD4 count <100 cells/μL).
Tropism testing—when HIV attaches to the CD4 cell, it does this by binding one of two areas on the outside. The two areas are designated as CCR5 and CXCR4. This is a test to see which area the virus likes to attach to. Some HIV viruses can attach to only one of these areas or sometimes both. This is important to know if the patient will be using a medicine that works against CCR5, such as maraviroc.
Undetectable viral load—when the amount of HIV in a person's blood is too low to be detected with a blood test.

FIGURE 26-1 *(Continued)*

Unprotected sex—sex without using a condom.
Urinalysis—physical, chemical, and microscopic examination of urine.
Viral load—a blood test used to count the amount of HIV virus in a patient's blood. This is also used to see how well ARV medications are working. This is routinely measured before the patient begins taking the medicine and then after 3 and 6 months.
Viremia—the presence of a virus in the blood.
Virologic blip—a temporary, detectable increase in the amount of HIV in a patient's blood (viral load). This may occur after the HIV medications have already suppressed the virus completely. This is not considered virologic failure because it is temporary.
Virologic failure—when the current HIV treatment is unable to decrease the amount of virus to <200 copies/mL. Some of the causes of failure include resistance, toxicity from the medication, or poor adherence by the patient.
Virologic rebound—when the amount of HIV virus in the blood increases from undetectable (<20 copies/mL of blood) to >200 copies/mL.
Virologic suppression—when the amount of HIV virus in a patient's blood is no longer detectable using currently available blood tests (eg, <20-75 copies/mL of blood, depending on the test used).
Wasting syndrome—an AIDS-defining condition. This is characterized by an unintentional loss of >10% of a patient's body weight. The patient may also have at least 30 days of diarrhea or weakness and fever.
Western blot—a blood test that is used to confirm the diagnosis of HIV.
Wild-type virus—the natural form of HIV that has no mutations.
Yeast infection—see *Candidiasis*.

FIGURE 26-1 (*Continued*)

TABLE 26-5 • Questions to Anticipate from Patients Regarding HIV

What is HIV?
HIV (human immunodeficiency virus) is the virus that causes HIV infection. The virus attacks and eventually destroys the body's CD4 cells (T cells). These white blood cells are important infection-fighting cells. When they are depleted, it is difficult for the immune system to fight off infections. Eventually HIV infection can lead to acquired immune deficiency syndrome, or AIDS.

Is there a cure for HIV?
No. None of the currently available ART are able to rid the body of the virus. The goal of current HIV treatment is to keep the virus to very low levels so that patients can have a healthy immune system and live longer.

What is AIDS?
AIDS (acquired immunodeficiency syndrome) is the most advanced stage of HIV infection. A diagnosis of AIDS occurs when the CD4 count drops below 200 cells/µL, the CD4 count percentage drops below 14, or the patient presents with an AIDS-defining condition.

What are examples of an AIDS-defining condition?
Examples of AIDS-defining conditions are *Pneumocystis jirovecii* pneumonia (PCP), Kaposi sarcoma, lymphoma, mycobacterium avium complex (MAC), progressive multifocal leukoencephalopathy (PML), tuberculosis, and toxoplasmosis. The complete list is available from the CDC (www.cdc.gov/mmwr/preview/mmwrhtml/rr5710a2.htm). (See also Table 26-2.)

How long does it take for HIV to cause AIDS?
Untreated, the average time between HIV infection and AIDS is 8-11 years. This may vary from patient to patient, depending on the patient's health, other diseases, and genetics.

What are "T cells" or CD4 cells, and why are they so important?
"T cells" (also known as CD4 cells) are white blood cells that help the body's immune system fight infections.

What is a normal CD4 count or T-cell number?
The CD4 count for a normal healthy person is 500-1200 cells/µL. The CD4 count is one means of measuring how well the immune system is working.

What is a viral load, and why is it so important?
The *viral load* is the amount of measured HIV virus copies per milliliter of blood. With treatment, the goal is to have an "undetectable" viral load. However, an "undetectable" viral load does not mean that the patient is cured of the virus; it simply means that the amount of virus circulating is below what the test can detect (ie, <20-75 copies/mL of blood, depending on the assay used).

What are opportunistic infections?
Opportunistic infections (OIs) are infections that occur more often or are more severe in patients with weak immune systems (in cancer, organ transplant, HIV, etc) compared to those with healthy immune systems. Examples include *Pneumocystis jirovecii* pneumonia, *Mycobacterium avium* complex (MAC), and toxoplasmosis.

Other than infections, is there anything else I need to worry about?
Yes. Since HIV virus is an infection, the body's response to this infection leads to a chronic inflammatory state that can be harmful to all the organs in the body. This chronic inflammatory state can lead to other conditions such as heart disease (heart attack, stroke), kidney disease, neurologic disease (dementia, PML), and cancers (lymphoma, sarcoma).

Will I have to take these medications forever?
Yes, none of the medications available today are able to completely eliminate the virus from your body. The goal of current HIV therapy is to suppress the virus so patients can maintain a healthy immune system and therefore live longer.

What can happen if I stop taking my HIV medications?
The virus will continue to multiply unchecked and attack more of your CD4 cells (T cells). This will weaken your immune system and increase your chance of having an infection and other chronic conditions. If you don't take all of your medications together as prescribed, you may also develop resistance to the medications and limit your available treatment options for the future.

When should I call my physician about my HIV medications?
Call your physician if you are experiencing serious or unexplained side effects from your medications.

What should I do if I have a problem with my HIV medications?
Never stop taking your HIV medications without first talking to physician. Speak with your physician and/or pharmacist to let them know about any problems you are having so that together you can make sure that your HIV medications are the right ones for you.

PERSONAL MEDICATION LIST FOR *<Insert patient's name, DOB: mm/dd/yyyy>*	
Medication: Descovy (emtricitabine/tenofovir alafenamide) 200 mg/25 mg tablet	
How I use it: Take one tablet (200 mg/25 mg) every day	
Why I use it: HIV	**Prescriber:** Smith
Date I started using it: 1/7/2017	**Date I stopped using it:** *(Leave blank for patient's notes)*
Why I stopped using it: *(Leave blank for patient's notes)*	
Medication: Prezcobix (darunavir/cobicistat) 800 mg/160 mg tablet	
How I use it: Take one tablet (800 mg/150 mg) every day with food	
Why I use it: HIV	**Prescriber:** Smith
Date I started using it: 1/7/2017	**Date I stopped using it:** *(Leave blank for patient's notes)*
Why I stopped using it: *(Leave blank for patient's notes)*	
Medication: Bactrim DS (trimethoprim/sulfamethoxazole) 160 mg/800 mg tablet	
How I use it: Take one tablet (160 mg/800 mg) every morning	
Why I use it: Infection (PCP) prevention	**Prescriber:** Smith
Date I started using it: 12/17/2016	**Date I stopped using it:** *(Leave blank for patient's notes)*
Why I stopped using it: *(Leave blank for patient's notes)*	

FIGURE 26-2 Example of a personal medication list for HIV patients.

DATE PREPARED: *<Insert date>*	
What we talked about: You reported missing the evening dose of the Isentress (raltegravir) 2-3 times per week. This is the only medication you take at night; all other medications are taken in the morning.	
What I need to do: Here are some things that I can do to help remember to take the medication: 1. Use a pillbox that has a morning slot and an evening slot for each day of the week. 2. Use my cellphone to set up a daily reminder to take my Isentress (raltegravir) at the same time each night (eg, 9:00 pm). Try to link taking my medicine with something I do every night, like walking my dog or brushing my teeth.	**What I did and when I did it:** *(Leave blank for patient's notes)*
What we talked about: You reported having an upset stomach (nausea, belly pain) every time you take your azithromycin 1200 mg on Wednesdays. You understand the importance of taking this medication to prevent you from getting an infection, but it is difficult to take it every week because of its side effects. We have contacted your physician and recommended a change in your medicine, and she has agreed.	
What I need to do: Here are some things that I can do to lessen these side effects: 1. Split the dose and take one tablet (600 mg) on Monday and one tablet (600 mg) on Thursday. 2. Take the medication with food to minimize stomach upset. 3. Call my physician or pharmacist if I continue to have upset stomach and I am unable to tolerate the azithromycin.	**What I did and when I did it:** *(Leave blank for patient's notes)*

FIGURE 26-3 Example medication action plan for a patient with HIV.

CORE ELEMENT 2—PERSONAL MEDICATION LIST

A sample personal medication list (PML) for a patient with HIV is presented in Figure 26-2. This example is representative only of HIV medications. Additional medications for other disease states should be added and listed separately. MTM providers should remember to use plain language when creating the PML.

CORE ELEMENT 3—MEDICATION ACTION PLAN

A sample medication action plan (MAP) for a patient with HIV is provided in Figure 26-3. This example is representative only of action steps for a patient with HIV. MAPs for other disease states or other medication-related problems (MRPs) should be added and listed separately. In general, only a few of the most important action steps should be listed, so as not to overwhelm the patient. Other areas for patient self-management can be addressed at later visits. MTM providers should remember to use plain language when creating the medication action plan.

CORE ELEMENT 4—INTERVENTION AND/OR REFERRAL

Interventions for HIV patients may include improving adherence, identifying drug-drug interactions, and recognizing and mitigating adverse drug events. Long-term and sustained adherence can be difficult to achieve, since many regimens can be complex and difficult to tailor to a given patient's lifestyle. When tailoring a regimen, clinicians should consider all aspects of the patient's life, including eating habits, sleeping habits, work schedule, and willingness to participate. Pill burden and pill fatigue are common problems that need to be identified in patients who have been receiving ART for an extended period. Even with new therapeutic regimens, drug adverse effects remain another major concern in HIV patients, and should be discussed at each encounter. Drug adverse effects impact not only adherence but also quality of life and willingness to continue lifelong treatment. Tables 26-6 and 26-7 review recommendations for initiating ART. Tables 26-8 and 26-9 provide an overview of the individual ARV agents and list the preferred agents for treatment naïve patients, respectfully. Treatment and prophylaxis of opportunistic infections are reviewed in Tables 26-10 through 26-12.

Herbal Supplements for HIV

Despite the number of medications and overall cost associated with ART HIV patients commonly use herbal supplements to treat HIV or mitigate some of the symptoms associated with

TABLE 26-6 • Guideline Rating Scheme for Recommendations for HIV Therapy

Rating of Recommendations	Rating of Evidence
A = Strong	I = Data from randomized controlled trials (RCTs)
B = Moderate	II = Data from well-designed nonrandomized trials or observational cohorts
C = Optional	III = Expert opinion

Source: Reference 7.

the disease or the medications. The best available scientific data regarding herbal supplements for HIV are either unclear or conflicting.[12] Not only are the data limited at this point, but the potential harm associated with use of herbal products can be substantial. Some of the many concerns with herbal medications for HIV patients include drug interactions, allergic reactions, additional cost, polypharmacy, and additive adverse effects. For example, St. John's wort is a potent inducer of cytochrome P450 3A4 and has a significant impact on the metabolism of protease inhibitors and nonnucleoside reverse transcriptase inhibitors that can lead to treatment failure and resistance. Garlic is another herbal medication that has been shown to significantly affect the levels

TABLE 26-7 • Current Guidelines for Initiating Antiretroviral Therapy in Treatment of Naive Patients with HIV

Antiretroviral therapy (ART) is recommended for all HIV-infected individuals, irrespective of the patient's pretreatment CD4 count, in order to reduce the risk of morbidity and mortality associated with HIV infection (AI). Effective ART also has been shown to prevent transmission of HIV from an infected individual to a sexual partner; therefore, ART should be offered to patients who are at risk of transmitting HIV to sexual partners (AI). Before starting ART, it is important to determine if the patient is willing and able to commit to treatment. They should understand the benefits and risks of therapy and the importance of adherence. In some cases, patients may choose to postpone therapy, and providers, on a case-by-case basis, may elect to defer therapy on the basis of clinical and/or psychosocial factors.

Source: Reference 7.

TABLE 26-8 • Medications for Management of HIV

Medication	Drug-Specific Side Effects[a]	Blackbox Warnings / Contraindications	Pregnancy Category[b]
Nucleoside/Nucleotide Reverse Transcriptase Inhibitors (NRTIs)			
Class adverse effects: Nausea, vomiting, diarrhea **Class blackbox warning: Lactic acidosis (especially d4T, ZDV, ddI) and severe hepatomegaly with steatosis**			
Abacavir (ABC) Ziagen Epzicom (ABC/3TC) Triumeq (ABC/DTG /3TC)	Hypersensitivity reaction, including fever, rash, abdominal pain, malaise, or respiratory symptoms. Patients who test positive for HLA-B*5701 are at highest risk. If reaction occurs, stop promptly and follow up with physician. Hyperlipidemia Some cohort studies have shown increased risk of myocardial infarction	Serious hypersensitivity reactions Highest risk in patients who test positive for HLAB*5701 Moderate or severe hepatic impairment	C
Didanosine (ddI) Videx EC	Pancreatitis, peripheral neuropathy, retinal changes, optic neuritis, insulin resistance/diabetes	Fatal and nonfatal pancreatitis Fatal lactic acidosis in pregnant women who received the combination of didanosine and stavudine Allopurinol Ribavirin	B
Emtricitabine (FTC) Emtriva Atripla (TDF/FTC/ EFV) Complera (TDF/FTC/RPV) Descovy (FTC/TAF) Genvoya (EVG/COBI /FTC/TAF) Odefsey (FTC/RPV /TAF) Stribild (EVG/COBI/ TDF/FTC) Truvada (TDF/FTC)	Hyperpigmentation/skin discoloration, rash, headache, cough, asthenia, dizziness, fatigue, pancreatitis, fat maldistribution	Acute exacerbation of hepatitis if co-infected with Hepatitis B and drug is discontinued Previous hypersensitivity	B

(*Continued*)

TABLE 26-8 • Medications for Management of HIV (*Continued*)

Medication	Drug-Specific Side Effects[a]	Blackbox Warnings / Contraindications	Pregnancy Category[b]
Lamivudine (3TC) Epivir Combivir (3TC/AZT) Epzicom (ABC/3TC) Triumeq (ABC/DTG /3TC)	Headache, cough, fever, malaise, fatigue, pancreatitis, fat maldistribution	Acute exacerbation of hepatitis if coinfected with hepatitis B and drug is discontinued Previous hypersensitivity	C
Stavudine (d4T) Zerit	Headache, rash, peripheral neuropathy, pancreatitis, severe lipoatrophy, hyperlipidemia	Fatal and nonfatal pancreatitis has occurred with didanosine (especially during pregnancy) Previous hypersensitivity	C
Tenofovir alafenamide (TAF) Descovy (FTC/TAF) Genvoya (EVG/COBI /FTC/TAF) Odefsey (FTC/RPV/TAF)	Renal insufficiency (less than TDF), Fanconi syndrome, decrease in bone mineral density (less than TDF), headache	Acute exacerbation of hepatitis if coinfected with hepatitis B and drug is discontinued	Insufficient data
Tenofovir disoproxil fumarate (TDF) Viread Atripla (TDF/FTC/ EFV) Complera (TDF/FTC/RPV) Stribild (EVG/ COBI/TDF/FTC) Truvada (TDF/FTC)	Rash, headache, asthenia, renal insufficiency, Fanconi syndrome, osteopenia, decrease in bone mineral density, angioedema	Acute exacerbation of hepatitis if coinfected with hepatitis B and drug is discontinued	B
Zidovudine (AZT) Retrovir Combivir (3TC/AZT)	Bone marrow suppression (macrocytic anemia or neutropenia), headache, insomnia, asthenia, nail pigmentation, lactic acidosis/ severe hepatomegaly with hepatic steatosis, hyperlipidemia	Hematologic toxicity, including neutropenia and severe anemia, myopathy Previous hypersensitivity	C
Nonnucleoside Reverse Transcriptase Inhibitors (NNRTIs)			
Class adverse effects: Rash (including Stevens-Johnson syndrome), elevated transaminases **Class drug interactions: Avanafil, rifapentine, St. John's wort**			
Efavirenz (EFV) Sustiva Atripla (TDF/FTC/ EFV)	Dizziness, nausea, headache, fatigue, insomnia, vomiting, neuropsychiatric symptoms (somnolence, insomnia, abnormal dreams, dizziness, depression, psychosis, and suicidal ideation). Symptoms usually subside or diminish after 2-4 weeks; bedtime dosing and avoiding food with administration can decrease these effects), hyperlipidemia, potentially teratogenic in humans	Previous hypersensitivity Boceprevir Ergot derivatives Midazolam All other NNRTIs St. John's wort Triazolam Avoid in women of childbearing potential trying to conceive or not using effective contraception	D
Etravirine (ETR) Intelence	Peripheral neuropathy, diarrhea, hypersensitivity syndrome	Carbamazepine Phenobarbital Phenytoin Rifampin St. John's wort	B

(*Continued*)

TABLE 26-8 • Medications for Management of HIV (*Continued*)

Medication	Drug-Specific Side Effects[a]	Blackbox Warnings / Contraindications	Pregnancy Category[b]
Nevirapine (NVP) Viramune Viramune XR	Hypersensitivity, symptomatic hepatitis, including fatal hepatic necrosis (often associated with skin rash or hypersensitivity)	Fatal and nonfatal hepatotoxicity and fatal and nonfatal skin reactions Use as part of occupational and nonoccupational postexposure prophylaxis Hepatic impairment (Child-Pugh B or C) St. John's wort Avoid if baseline CD4 count <250 for females, <400 for males due to hepatotoxicity	B
Rilpivirine (RPV) Edurant Complera (TDF/FTC/RPV) Odefsey (FTC/RPV/TAF)	Depression, insomnia, headache	Carbamazepine Dexamethasone (multiple doses) Oxcarbazepine Phenobarbital Phenytoin Primidone Proton-pump inhibitors Rifabutin, rifampin St. John's wort	B
Protease Inhibitors (PIs)			
Class adverse effects: Gastrointestinal (nausea, vomiting, diarrhea), headache, hyperglycemia, hyperlipidemia (less with ATV), elevated transaminases, fat distribution (lipohypertrophy) **Class drug interactions: All are hepatically metabolized by CYP3A enzymes, some are inhibitors or inducers of CYP enzymes and PGP; common interactions include: atorvastatin, bosentan, calcium channel blockers, clarithromycin, colchicine, corticosteroids (inhaled, intranasal, and systemic), garlic, hormonal contraceptives, itraconazole, maraviroc, quinidine, red yeast rice extract, rivaroxaban, ticagrelor, voriconazole, warfarin** **Class contraindications: Alfuzosin, avanafil, amiodarone, conivaptan, dronedarone, eplerenone, ergot derivatives, lovastatin, midazolam, nimodipine, ranolazine, rifampin, rifapentine, triazolam, sildenafil (except for erectile dysfunction), simvastatin, St. John's wort, salmeterol, tolvaptan, triazolam**			
Atazanavir (ATV) Reyataz Evotaz (ATV/COBI) *Preferred with ritonavir or cobicistat*	Skin rash (20%), jaundice, scleral icterus, asymptomatic indirect hyperbilirubinemia, nephrolithiasis, cholelithiaisis, increased PR interval (use with caution in patients with conduction defects or medications that can cause PR prolongation), and Stevens-Johnson syndrome/toxic epidermal necrolysis	Previous hypersensitivity See additional contraindications above (*Note:* If patient on proton-pump inhibitor, the dose should not exceed a dose comparable to omeprazole 20 mg daily.)	B
Darunavir (DRV) Prezista Prezcobix (DRV/COBI) *Must be given with ritonavir or cobicistat*	Rash (10%, sulfa moiety), including Stevens-Johnson syndrome and erythema multiforme, diarrhea, nausea, headache, hepatotoxicity	Previous hypersensitivity See additional contraindications above	C
Fosamprenavir (FPV) Lexiva	Skin rash (12%–19%, sulfa moiety), including Stevens-Johnson syndrome/toxic epidermal necrolysis, nephrolithiasis, myocardial infarction, neutropenia	Hypersensitivity to amprenavir or fosamprevanvir Flecainide Propafenone	C

(*Continued*)

TABLE 26-8 • Medications for Management of HIV (*Continued*)

Medication	Drug-Specific Side Effects[a]	Blackbox Warnings / Contraindications	Pregnancy Category[b]
Indinavir (IDV) Crixivan	Altered taste, heartburn, nephrolithiasis (approximately 12.4%), asymptomatic indirect hyperbilirubinemia (approximately 14%), asthenia, blurred vision, Stevens-Johnson syndrome, toxic epidermal necrolysis, bleeding	Previous hypersensitivity Alprazolam	C
Lopinavir/ Ritonavir (LPV/r) Kaletra	Pancreatitis, asthenia, central nervous system depression, PR and QT prolongation, Torsades de pointes, atrioventricular block, Stevens-Johnson syndrome, toxic epidermal necrolysis	Previous hypersensitivity to lopinavir or ritonavir	C
Nelfinavir (NFV) Viracept	Fatigue, flatulence, increased bleeding episodes in patients with hemophilia, prolonged QT interval, torsades de pointes	See contraindications above	B
Saquinavir (SQV) Invirase *Must be given with ritonavir*	Abdominal pain, pneumonia, atrioventricular block, PR and QT prolongation, torsades de pointes, Stevens-Johnson syndrome, psychiatric disorder, suicidal ideation, bone marrow suppression	Patients with atrioventricular block (without pacemaker), prolonged QT, drugs that prolong QT interval (ie, Class I and III antiarrhythmics, macrolides) Previous hypersensitivity Severe hepatic impairment Trazodone	B
Tipranavir (TPV) Aptivus *Must be given with ritonavir*	Skin rash (3%–21%, sulfa moiety), fatigue, fever, pancreatitis, hepatotoxicity, rare cases of fatal and nonfatal intracranial hemorrhages have been reported	Hepatitis and hepatic decompensation, including fatalities Fatal and nonfatal intracranial bleeding Hepatic impairment (Child-Pugh B or C) Flecainide Propafenone	C
	Entry Inhibitors		
Enfuvirtide (T-20) Fuzeon	Local injection site reactions: pain, erythema, induration nodules, pruritus in almost 100%, increased incidence of bacterial pneumonia, nausea, diarrhea, fatigue, hypersensitivity	Previous hypersensitivity to enfuvirtide	B
Maraviroc (MVC) Selzentry	Upper respiratory tract infections, cough, pyrexia, rash, dizziness	Hepatotoxicity, which may be preceded by systemic allergic reaction Severe renal impairment (CrCl <30 mL/min) End-stage renal disease Concomitant potent CYP3A inhibitors or inducers that have not been tested	B
	Integrase Inhibitors		
Dolutegravir (DTG) Tivicay Triumeq (ABC/DTG /3TC)	Rash, constitutional symptoms, insomnia, headache, depression and suicidal ideation (typically seen in patients with preexisting psychiatric conditions)	Previous hypersensitivity to dolutegravir Dofetilide	B

(*Continued*)

TABLE 26-8 • Medications for Management of HIV (*Continued*)

Medication	Drug-Specific Side Effects[a]	Blackbox Warnings / Contraindications	Pregnancy Category[b]
Elvitegravir (EVG) Genvoya (EVG/COBI /FTC/TAF) Stribild (EVG/COBI/TDF/ FTC)	Proteinuria (~39%), nausea, diarrhea, headache, fatigue, pancreatitis, muscle weakness, myalgia, rhabdomyolysis; cobicistat can cause a false increase in serum creatinine and decrease in CrCl (*Note*: See tenofovir and emtricitabine for other common side effects with this combination.)	Lactic acidosis and severe hepatomegaly with steatosis Acute exacerbation of hepatitis If coinfected with hepatitis B and drug is discontinued Not approved for Hepatitis B coinfection Alfuzosin Ergot derivatives Lovastatin Midazolam Rifabutin, rifampin, rifapentine Salmeterol Sildenafil (for PAH) Simvastatin St. John's wort Triazolam	B
Raltegravir (RAL) Isentress	Nausea, headache, diarrhea, pyrexia, muscle weakness, creatine phosphokinase elevation, rhabdomyolysis, rash (including Stevens-Johnson syndrome), hypersensitivity, and toxic epidermal necrolysis	None	C
Pharmacokinetic Enhancer			
Cobicistat (COBI) Tybost Evotaz (ATV/COBI) Genvoya (EVG/COBI /FTC/TAF) Prezcobix (DRV/COBI) Stribild (EVG/COBI/TDF/FTC)	Decrease in creatinine clearance due to inhibition of tubular secretion of serum creatinine; no impact on actual glomerular filtration rate	See class contraindications under the Protease Inhibitor section	B

[a] This is a general list and does not include all side effects that can occur from these drugs. Consult a drug reference source for a more inclusive list before making any recommendations. MTM providers should also consult a comprehensive drug interaction database before making pharmacotherapy recommendations.

[b] Product labeling for all prescription drugs is being updated to reflect the new FDA Pregnancy Labeling and Lactation Rule. Please check individual product labeling for the most accurate and updated pregnancy information.

Source: References 7, 9, and 10.

of protease inhibitors and should be avoided. At this time, there is limited evidence to support the use of herbal supplements in patients with HIV. Patients should discuss risks and benefits with a physician or pharmacist prior to taking any herbal supplement. Clinicians should consult appropriate references to determine the potential impact of each herbal supplement before assuming it will cause harm to a patient. Many patients perform their own research and may know more about a given product than expected.

CORE ELEMENT 5—DOCUMENTATION AND FOLLOW-UP

Clear and succinct documentation of MRPs and recommendations is a key component of the MTM consult. Examples of potential MRPs in patients with HIV are provided in Table 26-13. Since adherence is the most common MRP identified with HIV therapy, a review of common causes and potential solutions for nonadherence is provided in Table 26-14.

Additional Online Resources

The following websites provide information on HIV and AIDS:

- AIDSinfo: www.aidsinfo.nih.gov
- AIDS Education and Training Centers National Resource Center: www.aids-etc.org
- National HIV/AIDS Clinicians' Consultation Center (NCCC): www.nccc.ucsf.edu
- Stanford University HIV Drug Resistance Database: https://hivdb.stanford.edu
- U.S. Department of Health and Human Services: Health Resources and Services Administration – HIV/AIDS Programs. http://hab.hrsa.gov/
    - Common application for HIV patient assistance program http://hab.hrsa.gov/patientassistance/index.html

TABLE 26-9 • Treatment of Human Immunodeficiency Virus Infection: Preferred Antiretroviral Regimens Recommended in Antiretroviral-Naive Persons[a]

General		
	Preferred Regimens	**Selected Limitations**
PI-based	Darunavir + ritonavir + tenofovir disoproxil fumarate + emtricitabine (AI)	Rash (darunavir has sulfonamide moiety); GI; food requirement; CYP3A4 drug interactions
InSTI-based	Raltegravir + tenofovir disoproxil fumarate + emtricitabine (AI)	Twice daily (not once daily); interactions with polyvalent antacids; creatine kinase increases
	Elvitegravir + cobicistat + tenofovir disoproxil fumarate + emtricitabine (co-formulated) (AI)	Only if creatinine clearance (CrCl) ≥70 mL/min food requirement; interactions with polyvalent antacids; CYP3A4 drug interactions; cobicistat inhibits creatinine secretion increasing serum creatinine (SCr)—without affecting actual glomerular function
	Elvitegravir + cobicistat + tenofovir alafenamide fumarate + emtricitabine (co-formulated) (AI)	Only if CrCl ≥30 mL/min; same as above
	Dolutegravir + abacavir + lamivudine (coformulated) (AI)	Only if HLA-B*5701-negative; interactions with polyvalent antacids; dolutegravir inhibits creatinine secretion increasing SCr—without affecting actual glomerular function
	Dolutegravir + tenofovir disoproxil fumarate + emtricitabine (AI)	Same as above without HLA-B*5701-negative requirement
Selected Alternative Regimens (Some Potential Disadvantages vs Preferred Regimens)		
NNRTI-based	Efavirenz + tenofovir disoproxil fumarate + emtricitabine (coformulated) (BI)	CNS side effects with efavirenz; CYP450 drug interactions; empty stomach dosing; teratogenic in nonhuman primates—avoid in women planning to conceive
	Rilpivirine + tenofovir disoproxil fumarate + emtricitabine (coformulated) (BI)	Not recommended when HIV-RNA >100 000 copies/mL (>100 000 × 10^3/L) or CD4 <200 cells/μL (<200 × 10^6/L); no proton-pump inhibitors (rilpivirine); food requirement; antacid interactions
PI-based	Atazanavir + ritonavir (or cobicistat) + tenofovir disoproxil fumarate + emtricitabine (BI)	GI; food requirement; CYP3A4 drug interactions; hyperbilirubinemia leading to drug discontinuation especially in those with Gilbert syndrome; only for CrCl ≥ 70 mL/min as cobicistat inhibits creatinine secretion, increasing SCr—distinguish vs renal dysfunction
	Darunavir + ritonavir (or cobicistat) + abacavir + lamivudine (BII for ritonavir and BIII for cobicistat)	Only if HLA-B*5701-negative; see issues above
	Darunavir + cobicistat + tenofovir disoproxil fumarate + emtricitabine (BII)	Only for CLcr ≥70 mL/min as cobicistat inhibits creatinine secretion increasing Scr - distinguish vs renal dysfunction; see issues above
Selected Regimens or Components that Should Not Be Used at Any Time		
Regimen or Component		**Comment**
Any or all NRTI regimens (AIBII)		Inferior virologic efficacy
Didanosine + tenofovir (AII)		Inferior virologic efficacy, CD4 declines
Didanosine + stavudine (AII)		Toxicity including subcutaneous fat loss, peripheral neuropathy, and lactic acidosis
Two NNRTI combinations (AI)		Higher adverse events, drug interactions
Emtricitabine + lamivudine or zidovudine + stavudine (AIIAIII)		Analogs of same nucleobase; no additive benefit (or antagonistic)
Unboosted PIs (ie, darunavir, saquinavir, tipranavir) (AII)		Inadequate bioavailability
Etravirine + selected boosted PIs (AII)		Possible induction of PI metabolism, doses not established
Nevirapine in ARV naïve with higher CD4 counts (>250 for women, >400 for men) (BI)		High incidence of symptomatic hepatotoxicity

[a] Evidence-based rating definition; rating strength of recommendation: A—strong recommendation; B—moderate recommendation; C—optional recommendation. Rating quality of evidence supporting the recommendation: I—evidence from at least one correctly randomized, controlled trial with clinical outcomes and/or validated laboratory endpoints; II—evidence from at least one well-designed clinical trial without randomization or observational cohorts with long-term clinical outcomes; III—expert opinion. Lamivudine and emtricitabine are considered interchangeable.

Source: Reference 7.

TABLE 26-10 • Selected Therapies for Common Opportunistic Pathogens in HIV-Infected Individuals

Clinical Disease	Preferred Initial Therapies for Acute Infection in Adults (Strength of Recommendation in Parentheses)	Common Drug- or Dose-Limiting Adverse Reactions
Fungi		
Candidiasis, oral	Fluconazole 100 mg orally for 7-14 days (AI)	Elevated liver function tests, hepatotoxicity, nausea, and vomiting
	or	
	Nystatin 500,000 units oral swish (~5 mL) 4 times daily for 7-14 days (BII)	Taste, patient acceptance
Candidiasis, esophageal	Fluconazole 100-400 mg orally or IV daily for 14-21 days (AI)	Same as above
	or	
	Itraconazole 200 mg/day orally for 14-21 days (AI)	Elevated liver function tests, hepatotoxicity, nausea, and vomiting
Pneumocystis jirovecii pneumonia	Trimethoprim–sulfamethoxazole IV or orally 15-20 mg/kg daily as trimethoprim component in three to four divided doses for 21 days[a] (AI); moderate or severe therapy should be started IV	Skin rash, fever, leukopenia Thrombocytopenia
	or	
	Pentamidine IV 4 mg/kg daily for 21 days[a] (AI)	Azotemia, hypoglycemia, hyperglycemia, arrhythmias
Mild episodes		
	Atovaquone suspension 750 mg (5 mL) orally twice daily (bid) with meals for 21 days[a] (BI)	Rash, elevated liver enzymes, diarrhea
Cryptococcal meningitis	Liposomal amphotericin B 3-4 mg/kg daily IV for a minimum of 2 weeks with flucytosine 100 mg/kg daily orally in four divided doses (AI) *followed by*	Nephrotoxicity, hypokalemia, anemia, fever, chills Bone marrow suppression
	Fluconazole 400 mg/day, orally for 8 weeks or until CSF cultures are negative (AI)[a]	Same as above
Histoplasmosis	Liposomal amphotericin B 3 mg/kg daily IV for 2 weeks (AI) *followed by*	Same as above
	Itraconazole 200 mg orally thrice daily (tid) for 3 days then twice daily, for 12 months (AII)[a]	
Coccidioidomycosis	Liposomal amphotericin B 4-6 mg/kg/day IV until clinical improvement (usually after 500-1,000 mg) then switch to azole (AIII)[a]	Same as above
	or	
	Fluconazole 400-800 mg once daily (meningeal disease) (AII)[a]	Same as above
Protozoa		
Toxoplasmic encephalitis	Pyrimethamine 200 mg orally once, then 50-75 mg/day	Bone marrow suppression
	plus	
	Sulfadiazine 1-1.5 g orally 4 times daily	Rash, drug fever
	and	
	Leucovorin 10-25 mg orally daily for 6 weeks (AI)[a]	
Isosporiasis	Trimethoprim and sulfamethoxazole: 160 mg trimethoprim and 800 mg sulfamethoxazole orally or IV 4 times daily for 10 days (AII)[a]	Same as above
Bacteria		
Mycobacterium avium complex	Clarithromycin 500 mg orally twice daily, *plus* ethambutol 15 mg/kg daily orally (AI) for at least 12 months	GI intolerance, optic neuritis, peripheral neuritis, elevated liver tests

(*Continued*)

TABLE 26-10 • Selected Therapies for Common Opportunistic Pathogens in HIV-Infected Individuals (*Continued*)

Clinical Disease	Preferred Initial Therapies for Acute Infection in Adults (Strength of Recommendation in Parentheses)	Common Drug- or Dose-Limiting Adverse Reactions
Salmonella enterocolitis or bacteremia	Ciprofloxacin 500-750 mg orally (or 400 mg IV) bid 14 days (longer duration for bacteremia or advanced HIV) (AIII)	GI intolerance, headache, dizziness
Campylobacter enterocolitis (mild to moderate)	Ciprofloxacin 500-750 mg orally (or 400 mg IV) bid for 7-10 days (or longer with bacteremia) (BIII)	Same as above
Shigella enterocolitis	Ciprofloxacin 500-750 mg orally (or 400 mg IV) bid for 7-10 days (or 14 days for bacteremia) (AIII)	Same as above
Viruses		
Mucocutaneous herpes simplex	Acyclovir 5 mg/kg IV every 8 hours until lesions regress, then acyclovir 400 mg orally tid until complete healing (famciclovir or valacyclovir is alternative) (AIII)	GI intolerance, crystalluria
Primary varicella zoster	Acyclovir 10-15 mg/kg every 8 hours IV for 7-10 days (severe cases), then switch to oral valacyclovir 1 g tid after defervescence (famciclovir or acyclovir is alternative) (AIII)	Obstructive nephropathy, CNS symptoms
Cytomegalovirus (retinitis)	Intravitreal ganciclovir (2 mg) one to four doses over 7-10 days (for sight-threatening lesions) *plus* valganciclovir 900 mg twice daily for 14-21 days then once daily until immune recovery from ART (AIII)[a]	Neutropenia, thrombocytopenia
Cytomegalovirus esophagitis or colitis	Ganciclovir 5 mg/kg IV every 12 hours for 21-42 days; may switch to valganciclovir 900 mg orally every 12 hours when oral therapy can be tolerated (BI)	Same as above

[a] Maintenance therapy is recommended.

Abbreviations: ART = antiretroviral therapy; CSF, cerebrospinal fluid; HIV = human immunodeficiency virus.

Source: Reproduced, with permission, from DiPiro JT, Talbert RL, Yee GC, Matzke GR, Wells BG, Posey LM, eds. *Pharmacotherapy: A Pathophysiologic Approach*. 10th ed. New York, NY: McGraw-Hill; 2017.

TABLE 26-11 • Primary Prophylaxis for Common Opportunistic Infections

Infection	Indication	Preferred Regimen[a]
Pneumocystis jirovecii pneumonia (PCP)	CD4 < 200 cells/µL or CD4% < 14% or oropharyngeal candidiasis	Trimethoprim/sulfamethoxazole 1 double-strength (DS) PO once daily or 1 single-strength (SS) PO once daily (AI)
Toxoplasmosis gondii encephalitis	CD4 < 100 cells/µL and toxoplasma IgG-positive	Trimethoprim/sulfamethoxazole 1 DS PO once daily (AII)
Disseminated *Mycobacterium avium* complex (MAC) disease	CD4 < 50 cells/µL (after ruling out active MAC infection)	Azithromycin 1200 mg PO weekly or 600 mg PO 2x/week *or* clarithromycin 500 mg PO bid

[a] Alternative regimens are available for patients with allergies or intolerance to preferred regimens; consult the CDC guidelines for recommended alternatives at www.aidsinfo.nih.gov.

Source: Reference 11.

Sample communications and recommendations to providers to address medication-related issues are found in Figure 26-4. Recommendations may be communicated via fax, telephone, or other means of written or secure electronic communication. The examples below are for illustrative purposes. Actual communications to providers should be individualized based on the type of recommendation, patient specific characteristics, and the nature of the relationship with the provider.

TABLE 26-12 • Criteria for Discontinuing Primary Prophylaxis

Infection	Criteria
Pneumocystis jirovecii pneumonia (PCP)	CD4 > 200 cells/µL for >3 months in response to ART[a] Reinitiate if CD4 falls to <200
Toxoplasmosis gondii encephalitis	CD4 > 200 cells/µL for >3 months in response to ART Reinitiate if CD4 falls to <100-200
Disseminated *Mycobacterium avium* complex (MAC) disease	CD4 > 100 cells/µL for ≥3 months in response to ART Reinitiate if CD4 falls to <50

[a] Antiretroviral therapy.

Source: Reference 11.

TABLE 26-13 • Medication-Related Problems (MRPs) in Patients with HIV

Category of MRP	Example of a Medication-Related Problem
Nonadherence	Suboptimal immunologic or virologic response because of patient missing doses of HIV medication (especially with BID regimens) Patient not taking HIV medication because of cost Patient not taking HIV medication because of "pill fatigue" Patient forgets to take medication because of interruptions in daily routine (eg, travel, work schedule)
Unnecessary medication	Infection prophylaxis no longer indicated (eg, PCP prophylaxis no longer needed if CD4 > 200 cells/μL for > 3 months)
Need for additional medication	Indication for infection prophylaxis due to immunologic failure (eg, CD4 count < 200 cells/μL = PCP prophylaxis) Uncontrolled diarrhea despite lifestyle modification; consider adding OTC agent (ie, loperamide) or a prescription agent (ie, atropine/diphenoxylate - Lomotil) or crofelemer (Fulyzaq)
Ineffective medication	Adequate trial of new HIV medications without significant virologic and/or immunologic response (consider resistance testing)
Dosage too low	Drug interaction requiring dose adjustment or addition of boosting medication (eg, PPI and atazanavir) Dose adjustment due to renal function improvement
Dosage too high	Patient taking tenofovir that is not dosed appropriately for renal function Patient taking dose of abacavir inappropriate for mild hepatic impairment Combination of potent 3A4 inhibitor (eg, darunavir) with maraviroc
Contraindicated drug or dose	Drug-drug interaction (eg, rifampin and protease inhibitors) Drug dose that is too high to overcome interaction (eg, atazanavir and omeprazole dose >20 mg/day)
Adverse drug event	Patient unable to function adequately because of neuropsychiatric side effects of efavirenz Patient not taking HIV medications because of GI intolerance (could also be classified under nonadherence)

TABLE 26-14 • Strategies for Improving Adherence to HIV Medications

Barrier Identified	Intervention
Forgetting to take the medication	Identify likely cause (eg, complexity of regimen, busy work schedule, travel, storage location of medications, knowledge deficit) Tailor administration to daily activities (eating a meal, brushing teeth, walking a dog, drinking coffee/tea) Suggest adherence reminders (smartphone, alarm, calendar, etc) Suggest using a pillbox or getting medications in blister packs Discuss how patients should catch up if they miss a dose, document when doses are missed, and share this with their provider at the next visit Consider contacting the provider to simplify regimen
Lack of patient understanding	Educate on importance of adherence and how that can affect response to therapy, as well as lead to resistance Discuss how resistance can have an impact on future therapy and increase complexity of drug regimen If literacy is a concern, consider visual aids to demonstrate concepts
Side effects	Educate in the beginning what side effects to expect and how to manage them if they occur, including lifestyle modifications and OTC products if applicable; include expected duration of side effects Work with the patient and the provider to tailor regimens for tolerability and ease of administration. If side effects are unmanageable using lifestyle modifications and OTC products, contact provider and suggest alternative if available or adjunct prescription therapy to treat side effect. (eg, atropine/diphenoxylate for uncontrolled diarrhea) Counsel patient to contact provider if side effects are severe/unmanageable
Lack of social support	Provide encouragement and support as an MTM provider Discuss importance of revealing status to friends/family to enlist support Refer patient to HIV-related social network
Physical and economic factors	Collaborate with a local social worker Refer patient to state AIDS Drug Assistant Program (ADAP) Offer manufacturer coupons Identify situations where patient may qualify for waiver of copay Discuss drug assistance programs with patient and provider Find a pharmacy that can deliver the medication directly to the patient

Source: Reference 13.

Scenario: Patient complains of severe nausea and lack of appetite shortly after taking weekly dose of azithromycin 1200 mg for MAC prophylaxis. CD4 count 38 cells/μL.
MRP: Adverse drug event

Assessment:
Patient still needs MAC prophylaxis on the basis of latest CD4 count. Azithromycin twice weekly is an alternative regimen that may cause less nausea than once-weekly azithromycin or clarithromycin. It also has a lower pill burden and less risk of nonadherence, as compared to twice daily clarithromycin.
Plan:
Consider splitting weekly dose of 1200 mg into twice-weekly dose of 600 mg on Monday and Thursday to decrease GI side effects.

Scenario: Patient has been on ART for 6 months. Patient has also been on primary prophylaxis for PCP with one Bactrim (sulfamethoxazole/trimethoprim) DS tablet daily. The CD4 count at baseline was 150 cells/μL. Repeat CD4 count at 3 months was 212 (16%) and at 6 months was 250 (18%).
MRP: Unnecessary medication

Assessment:
On the basis of CD4 count at 3 months and 6 months, the patient no longer needs PCP prophylaxis with sulfamethoxazole/trimethoprim. This would decrease overall pill burden and risk of adverse drug events.
Plan:
Consider discontinuing PCP prophylaxis and monitor CD4 count in 3 months to ensure still > 200 cells/μL. Restart PCP prophylaxis if CD4 count drops below 200 cells/μL.

Scenario: Patient has been on Truvada (emtricitabine/tenofovir) 1 tablet daily and Reyataz (atazanavir) 300 mg daily for 3 years. CD4 count 2 months ago was 550 cells/μL and viral load was undetectable. He was seen by a GI specialist 2 weeks ago for frequent GERD symptoms and started on omeprazole 20 mg PO daily.
MRP: Dosage too low, need for additional medication

Assessment:
Omeprazole significantly decreases the oral bioavailability of atazanavir and increases the risk for virologic failure and drug resistance. Since the patient has responded well to therapy, it would be ideal to continue the current regimen. Options include discontinuing the PPI, changing to an H_2-antagonist (no more than 20 mg of famotidine equivalent/day), or adding on ritonavir to boost the levels of atazanavir. Ritonavir-boosted atazanavir is now preferred in the guidelines over unboosted atazanavir for all patients.
Plan:
Discuss need for continued PPI use. If PPI needs to be continued, consider adding ritonavir (Norvir) 100-mg tablet daily to be given with atazanavir. The dose of PPI should not exceed 20 mg of omeprazole equivalent/day and needs to be given 12 hours before the atazanavir and ritonavir. Consider repeat viral load and CD4 count in 2-8 weeks to assess impact of drug interaction.

Scenario: Patient has been taking Truvada (emtricitabine/tenofovir) 1 tablet by mouth daily and Isentress (raltegravir) 400 mg PO BID for 2 years without any complaints. According to the patient, his most recent viral load is undetectable and his CD4 count was "at goal." At his last visit, though, his primary physician said his kidneys have "gotten worse" and has referred him to a "kidney specialist."
MRP: Possible dosage too high

Assessment:
If renal function has declined, there is a concern for excessive dose of Truvada. This drug combination must be adjusted to every 48 hours if the creatinine clearance (CrCl) is < 50 mL/min and discontinued if the CrCl is < 30 mL/min. Tenofovir may also worsen renal function and should be monitored carefully.
Plan:
Contact healthcare provider and assess current renal function. If necessary, adjust dose for renal function (if CrCl < 50 mL/min) or switch to alternative regimen. May consider switching to Descovy (TAF/FTC) as this combination has less risk for nephrotoxicity. Abacavir may be an alternative to tenofovir as it does not have significant renal elimination. May need to review most recent genotype/phenotype and HLA-5701-B results to assess options. Consider rechecking serum creatinine, BUN, and urine analysis in 2-8 weeks.

FIGURE 26-4 Sample provider communications for HIV.

During an MTM interview, a healthcare provider may come across a patient who requires immediate referral to either the physician or emergency room. In other cases, education and follow-up at a later time is all that is required. MTM providers have an excellent opportunity to catch urgent issues before they become life-threatening, and with proper referral and management, they can make a big difference. Table 26-15 provides examples of situations where immediate referral is necessary and when follow-up can occur at a later point. Since frequent monitoring and follow-up are essential for success in HIV patients, the guidelines outline recommended intervals for follow-up to assess adverse effects and response to therapy (Table 26-16).

TABLE 26-15 • Referral for Management of HIV

Contact Provider Immediately or Go to Nearest Emergency Room
Any signs of infection: fever, shortness of breath, weight loss, night sweats, cough, unexplained new onset rash or lesion, confusion, stiff neck
Signs or symptoms of Fanconi syndrome: passing large amounts of urine, which can lead to dehydration, bone pain, and weakness (Look for in patients on tenofovir.)
Signs or symptoms of hypersensitivity syndrome: fever, rash, malaise, swelling, shortness of breath, especially if the patient recently started on a medication known to cause hypersensitivity (ie, abacavir, NNRTIs)
Signs or symptoms of pancreatitis: pain, nausea and vomiting, and a swollen abdomen
Signs or symptoms of Stevens-Johnson syndrome: skin rash characterized by red, blistered spots; blisters in the mouth, eyes, genitals, or other moist areas of the body; peeling skin that results in painful sores
Neuropsychiatric side effects: abnormal dreams, dizziness, depression, or suicidal thoughts (especially within 2-4 weeks after starting efavirenz)
Patients on nevirapine: signs or symptoms of hepatitis, increased transaminases combined with rash or other systemic symptoms, severe skin or hypersensitivity reactions, any rash with systemic symptoms (especially within the first 6 weeks and ≤18 weeks of initiation)
Patients on maraviroc: signs and symptoms of a systemic allergic reaction (eg, pruritic rash, eosinophilia, or elevated IgE)
Routine—Inform Provider at a Later Time
Mild side effect from medication (eg, mild diarrhea or upset stomach)
Missing one or two doses of medication

TABLE 26-16 • Suggested Intervals for Follow-up and Monitoring in Patients with HIV

Adherence and tolerability:

Monitor for adherence and adverse drug effects 2-8 weeks after starting a new regimen

Monitor every 3-6 months in stable patients (if clinically stable and if viral load is suppressed, can consider monitoring every 6-12 months)

Basic chemistry, liver function, and CBC with differential:

On entry into care

Every 3-6 months before antiretroviral therapy (ART) initiation

Before ART initiation or modification

2-8 weeks after ART initiation or modification

Every 3-6 months

Viral load:

- Upon entry into care
- Before ART initiation or modification
- 2 to 8 weeks after ART initiation or modification
- If HIV RNA is detectable at 2 to 8 weeks, repeat every 4 to 8 weeks until suppression to <200 copies/mL, then every 3 to 6 months
- Every 3 to 6 months
  - May extend testing to every 6 months in adherent patients with consistently suppressed viral load and stable immunologically for at least 2 years
- Treatment failure

CD4 count:

- On entry into care
- Before ART initiation or modification
- Every 3-6 months for the following patients:
  - During first 2 years of ART
  - If viremia develops while patient is on ART
  - CD4 count < 300 cells/mm^3
- After 2 years on ART with consistently suppressed viral load:
  - CD4 count 300–500 cells/mm^3: every 12 months
  - CD4 count >500 cells/mm^3: CD4 monitoring is optional
- Treatment failure

Resistance testing:

- On entry into care (genotype preferred)
- Before ART initiation (optional if already performed at entry into care and treatment naive)
- Treatment failure
- Coreceptor tropism assays should be performed whenever the use of a CCR5 antagonist is being considered

Source: Reference 7.

REFERENCES

1. Anderson PL, Kakuda TN, Fletcher CV. Human Immunodeficiency virus infection. In: DiPiro JT, Talbert RL, Yee GC, Matzke GR, Wells BG, Posey LM, eds. *Pharmacotherapy: A Pathophysiologic Approach*, 10th ed. New York, NY: McGraw-Hill; 2017.
2. CDC HIV/AIDS. *HIV Risk Behaviors*. Available at https://www.cdc.gov/hiv/risk/estimates/riskbehaviors.html. Accessed May 5, 2017.
3. Chen M, Rhodes PH, Hall HI, et al. Prevalence of undiagnosed HIV infection among persons aged ≥13 years—National HIV Surveillance System, United States, 2005-2008. *MMWR* 2012;61;57-64.
4. Anonymous. Revised surveillance case definition for HIV infection–United States, 2014. *MMWR Recomm Rep*. 2014;63(RR-03):1-10.
5. Chu C, Selwyn PA. Complications of HIV infection: a systems-based approach. *Am Fam Physician*. 2011;83:395-406.
6. Bartlett JG, Gallant JE, Pham P. *Medical Management of HIV Infection*. Baltimore, MD: Johns Hopkins University School of Medicine; 2009-2010.
7. Panel on Antiretroviral Guidelines for Adults and Adolescents. Guidelines for the Use of Antiretroviral Agents in HIV-1-Infected Adults and Adolescents. Department of Health and Human Services. (Last updated July 14, 2016.) Available at https://aidsinfo.nih.gov/contentfiles/lvguidelines/adultandadolescentgl.pdf. Accessed May 5, 2017.
8. *AIDSinfo Glossary of HIV/AIDS-Related Terms*, 8th ed.; August 2015. Available at https://aidsinfo.nih.gov/contentfiles/GlossaryHIVrelatedTerms_English.pdf. Accessed May 6, 2017.
9. Clinical Pharmacology [database online]. Tampa, FL: Elsevier. 2017 Available at http://www.clinicalpharmacology.com (cited 5/6/2017).
10. Micromedex® Solutions (electronic version). Ann Arbor, MI: Truven Health Analytics. Available at http://www.micromedexsolutions.com (cited 5/6/2017).
11. Panel on Opportunistic Infections in HIV-Infected Adults and Adolescents. Guidelines for the Prevention and Treatment of Opportunistic Infections in HIV-Infected Adults and Adolescents: Recommendations from the Centers for Disease Control and Prevention, the National Institutes of Health, and the HIV Medicine Association of the Infectious Diseases Society of America. Available at http://aidsinfo.nih.gov/contentfiles/lvguidelines/adult_oi.pdf. Accessed May 4, 2017.
12. Natural Medicines [database online]. Somerville, MA: Therapeutic Research Center; 2017. Available at https://naturalmedicines.therapeuticresearch.com/. Accessed May 7, 2017.
13. Kibicho J, Owczarzak J. Pharmacists' strategies for promoting medication adherence among patients with HIV. *J Am Pharm Assoc*. 2011;51:746-755.

Review Questions

1. Which of the following absolute CD4 cell counts is consistent with a diagnosis of AIDS?
   a. < 350 cells/mm^3
   b. < 250 cells/mm^3
   c. < 200 cells/mm^3
   d. < 100 cells/mm^3

2. Which of the following is commonly associated with virologic failure?
   a. High baseline CD4 count
   b. Low baseline viral load
   c. Missed clinic appointments
   d. Excellent adherence

3. How would you explain the definition of virologic suppression using living room language?
   a. A confirmed HIV RNA level below the limit of assay detection.
   b. A temporary, detectable increase in the amount of HIV in your blood (viral load).
   c. When the amount of HIV virus in your blood goes from undetectable to >200 copies/mL.
   d. When the amount of HIV virus in your blood is no longer detectable using currently available blood tests.

For questions 4 and 5, please use the following case.

A 39-year-old male with HIV has been on antiretroviral therapy for 6 months and you are contacting him for a scheduled MTM session over the phone. He tells you that he takes atazanavir 300 mg, one capsule every morning; ritonavir 100 mg: one tablet every morning; emtricitabine/tenofovir: 1 tablet every morning; and sulfamethoxazole/trimethoprim DS, one tablet every morning. He states that he has also been taking over-the-counter (OTC) omeprazole 20 mg twice daily for heartburn for the past 2 weeks. His most recent viral load was <20 copies/mL (baseline 5200 copies/mL) and his CD4 count was 198 cells/mm^3 (baseline 123 cells/mm^3).

4. Which of the following MRPs have you identified with this patient?
   a. Unnecessary medication
   b. Nonadherence
   c. Contraindicated drug or dose
   d. Dosage too low

5. Which of the following is the most appropriate assessment of his virologic response to therapy?
   a. Incomplete virologic response
   b. Virologic failure
   c. Virologic blip
   d. Virologic suppression

6. A 45-year-old HIV patient has been on multiple antiretroviral regimens in the past. She currently takes raltegravir 400 mg twice daily, tenofovir 300 mg once daily, darunavir 600 mg twice daily, and ritonavir 100 mg twice daily. During your MTM session, you find that she is skipping her evening dose of raltegravir, darunavir, and ritonavir, which she attributes to her variable schedule working at a restaurant. Which of the following would be most appropriate to include on the medication action plan as a way to improve adherence?
   a. Change jobs to avoid conflict with her HIV medications.
   b. Take all of her doses at the same time so that it is easier for her to remember.
   c. Use an alarm on her cellphone to remind her to take her dose every night.
   d. Contact the healthcare provider and switch her to Atripla for convenience.

7. In which of the following situations should you contact the healthcare provider immediately or send the patient with HIV to the nearest emergency room?
   a. Passing large amounts of urine for the last 2 days and new-onset bone pain
   b. Missing two doses of HIV medications
   c. Having an upset stomach for 2 days after starting new HIV regimen
   d. Having two or three loose stools per day for the past 4 days after starting a ritonavir-based regimen

8. Which of the following treatment regimens is considered "Recommended" for treatment-naive patients, regardless of baseline viral load, CD4 count, or renal function?
   a. Raltegravir and abacavir/lamivudine
   b. Elvitegravir/cobicistat/tenofovir alafenamide/emtricitabine
   c. Rilpivirine and tenofovir/emtricitabine
   d. Efavirenz/tenofovir/emtricitabine

9. A 26-year-old female is newly diagnosed with HIV. Her current viral load is 15 000 and her CD4 count is 115. Which of the following opportunistic infections require primary prophylaxis for this patient?
   a. *Pneumocystis jirovecii* pneumonia
   b. *Toxoplasmosis gondii* encephalitis
   c. Disseminated *Mycobacterium avium* complex disease
   d. *Pneumocystis jirovecii* pneumonia and *Toxoplasmosis gondii* encephalitis

10. Which of the following medications is most likely to cause abnormal dreams, which usually occurs within the first 2-4 weeks of therapy?
   a. Etravirine
   b. Tenofovir
   c. Atazanavir
   d. Efavirenz

ANSWERS

1. c	2. c	3. d
4. c	5. d	6. c
7. a	8. b	9. a
10. d		

27

Hypertension MTM Data Set

Karen Whalen, PharmD, BCPS, CDE

KEY POINTS

- Blood pressure goals should be individualized, especially for older persons who may have difficulty tolerating complicated pharmacotherapy regimens.
- The medication therapy management (MTM) provider should review the medication profile to screen for other medications that may be contributing to hypertension.
- Because blood pressure medications may make patients feel worse than the disorder of hypertension itself, nonadherence is a likely problem. MTM providers need to be vigilant for nonadherence to medications and recommend changes in pharmacotherapy, if needed, to promote adherence.
- Regular follow-up and monitoring are key to helping patients achieve blood pressure goals and reduce the risk of end-organ damage.

INTRODUCTION TO HYPERTENSION

Primary (essential) *hypertension* is persistently elevated arterial blood pressure (BP) in the absence of an identifiable cause.[1,2] The relationship between BP and risk of cardiovascular disease is significant and independent of other risk factors.

Blood pressure should be classified on the basis of at least two readings taken on at least two separate occasions (Table 27-1). When systolic and diastolic blood pressure levels fall into different categories, the higher category should be selected in classifying blood pressure.

Other Terms Associated with Hypertension

- *Hypertensive crises*
  - *Hypertensive emergency*: BP > 180/120mmHg with ongoing or progressive target organ damage
  - *Hypertensive urgency*: Systolic blood pressure (SBP) > 180 mmHg or diastolic blood pressure (DBP) > 110 mmHg without evidence of progressive target organ damage
- *Isolated systolic hypertension*: SBP ≥ 140 mmHg and DBP ≤ 90 mmHg; this is common in the elderly.
- *Masked hypertension*: Home BP is significantly higher than anticipated on the basis of the in-clinic BP measurement (opposite of white-coat hypertension).
- *Orthostatic hypotension*: Decrease in SBP of >20 mmHg or decrease in DBP of >10 mmHg when changing from a supine to a standing position.
- *Pseudohypertension*: A falsely elevated BP secondary to calcified arteries that are not compressed by the cuff when taking the BP measurement.
- *Secondary hypertension*: Hypertension attributable to an identifiable cause, such as chronic kidney disease, medication, or diet (Table 27-2).
- *White-coat hypertension*: A normal BP at home, but elevated BP in clinic; related to seeing medical personnel in white coats or other medical attire (opposite of masked hypertension).

> Treatment of secondary causes of hypertension may reduce the need for antihypertensive medications or necessitate a change in drug therapy.

TABLE 27-1 • Classification of Blood Pressure in Adults (Age ≥ 18 Years)[a]

Classification	Systolic Blood Pressure (mmHg)		Diastolic Blood Pressure (mmHg)
Normal	<120	and	<80
Prehypertension[b]	120-139	or	80-89
Stage 1 hypertension	140-159	or	90-99
Stage 2 hypertension	≥160	or	≥100

[a] Classification is determined by averaging two or more properly measured seated BP values from two or more clinical encounters. If systolic and diastolic BP values yield different classifications, the highest category is used for the purpose of determining a classification.

[b] For certain patients, BP values within the prehypertension range are considered above goal.

Source: Reproduced, with permission, from DiPiro JT, Talbert RL, Yee GC, Matzke GR, Wells BG, Posey LM, eds. *Pharmacotherapy: A Pathophysiologic Approach*, 10th ed. New York: McGraw-Hill; 2017.

Complications of Hypertension

Hypertension is often called the "silent killer" because patients are usually asymptomatic and may not feel ill when their blood pressure is high. Unfortunately, even if there are no outward symptoms, the elevated pressure still causes damage to target organs. In general, there may also be a lack of awareness of the dangers of uncontrolled hypertension. Therefore, patients need to be educated on the importance of controlling blood pressure and adherence to blood pressure medication. Blood pressure should be assessed routinely, and treatment modified as needed to achieve blood pressure

TABLE 27-2 • Secondary Causes of Hypertension

Disease	Drugs and Other Products Associated with Hypertension[a]
Chronic kidney disease Cushing syndrome Coarctation of the aorta Obstructive sleep apnea Parathyroid disease Pheochromocytoma Primary aldosteronism Renovascular disease Thyroid disease	Prescription drugs Amphetamines (amphetamine, dexmethylphenidate, dextroamphetamine, lisdexamfetamine, methylphenidate, phendimetrazine, phentermine) Antivascular endothelin growth factor agents (bevacizumab, sorafenib, sunitinib) Corticosteroids (cortisone, dexamethasone, fludrocortisone, hydrocortisone, methylprednisolone, prednisolone, prednisone, triamcinolone) Calcineurin inhibitors (cyclosporine, tacrolimus) Decongestants (pseudoephedrine, phenylephrine) Ergot alkaloids (bromocriptine, dihydroergotamine, methysergide) Erythropoiesis-stimulating agents (erythropoietin, darbepoetin) Estrogen-containing oral contraceptives Nonsteroidal anti-inflammatory drugs: cyclooxygenase-2-selective (celecoxib) and -nonselective (aspirin [at higher doses], choline magnesium trisalicylate, diclofenac, diflunisal, etodolac, fenoprofen, flurbiprofen, ibuprofen, indomethacin, ketoprofen, ketorolac, meclofenamate, mefenamic acid, meloxicam, nabumetone, naproxen, naproxen sodium, oxaprozin, piroxicam, salsalate, sulindac, tolmetin) Others: desvenlafaxine, venlafaxine, bupropion Situations: β-blocker or centrally acting α-agonists (when abruptly discontinued); β-blocker without α-blocker first when treating pheochromocytoma; use of a monoamine oxidase inhibitor (isocarboxazid, phenelzine, tranylcypromine) with tyramine-containing foods or certain drugs Street drugs and other products Cocaine and cocaine withdrawal Ephedra alkaloids (eg, Ma huang), "herbal ecstasy," other analogs Nicotine and withdrawal, anabolic steroids, narcotic withdrawal, ergot-containing herbal products, St. John's wort Food substances Sodium Ethanol Licorice

[a] Agents of most clinical importance.

Source: Reproduced, with permission, from DiPiro JT, Talbert RL, Yee GC, Matzke GR, Wells BG, Posey LM, eds. *Pharmacotherapy: A Pathophysiologic Approach*, 10th ed. New York: McGraw-Hill; 2017.

TABLE 27-3 • Complications of Hypertension

Type of Complication	Examples
Cardiovascular disease	Angina pectoris Atherosclerosis Atrial fibrillation Coronary heart disease Left ventricular hypertrophy Heart failure Myocardial infarction Sudden death
Cerebrovascular disease	Cognitive decline Intracerebral hemorrhage Ischemic stroke Transient ischemic attack (TIA) Vascular dementia
Ophthalmologic disorders	Age-related macular degeneration Hypertensive retinopathy
Peripheral vascular disease	Atherosclerosis Edema Peripheral arterial disease
Renal disorders	Arteriosclerosis Chronic kidney disease Microalbuminuria/proteinuria

Source: References 1 and 2.

goals and reduce the risk of end-organ complications. Table 27-3 provides an overview of the complications of hypertension.

Therapeutic Goals for Blood Pressure

Adequate control of blood pressure helps to prevent complications of hypertension and reduces the development or progression of cardiovascular, cerebrovascular, and renal morbidity and mortality. Table 27-4 outlines recommended goals for blood pressure. It is important to note that less stringent goals are acceptable in older patients.

Accurate blood pressure readings are key to assessing achievement of therapeutic goals. Tables 27-5 and 27-6 detail appropriate measurement of blood pressure within and outside of the clinical setting, respectively. Table 27-7 highlights potential reasons for inaccurate blood pressure measurements.

TABLE 27-4 • Therapeutic Goals for Blood Pressure

Therapeutic Goal	Patient Population
Blood pressure < 140/90 mmHg	Most patients Patients with diabetes Patients with chronic kidney disease
Blood pressure <150/90 mmHg	Patients ≥ 80 years of age Frail elderly unable to achieve lower blood pressure goals without risk of falls or serious adverse events
Blood pressure < 130/80 mmHg[a]	Patients with chronic kidney disease and albuminuria (>30 mg /24 hours) Patients with diabetes

[a] Optional lower goal; may be appropriate for certain patients (eg, younger patients) who can tolerate therapy without undue burden.

Source: References 1, 4, 5, and 6.

TABLE 27-5 • Assessment of Blood Pressure in the Clinical Setting

Technique of measuring BP using a manual or automated sphygmomanometer: Equipment for measuring blood pressure must meet certain national standards to ensure maximum quality and precision with measurement. Patients should refrain from nicotine or caffeine ingestion and exercise for 30 minutes prior to taking the measurement. Patients should be seated with the lower back supported in a chair, feet flat on the floor, legs uncrossed, and bare arm supported and resting near heart level. A properly sized cuff should be used, encircling at least 80% of the upper arm in length and 40% in width. If the cuff is too small, BP can be overestimated. Measurement should begin after a 5-minute rest.
For manual determinations: Palpate the radial pulse. Inflate the cuff to 20-30 mmHg above the level at which the radial pulse is obliterated. Place the stethoscope over the brachial artery. Deflate the cuff at a rate no greater than 2-3 mmHg per second. Listen for the first sounds (Korotkoff sounds). This denotes the systolic BP. Listen for the disappearance of sound. This denotes the diastolic BP.
Measuring BP while patients are lying down or standing up is indicated under special circumstances: Suspected orthostatic hypotension Diabetic autonomic neuropathy Volume depletion Dehydration
Downfalls of clinic BP monitoring: Inherent biologic blood pressure variability Inaccurate or suboptimal technique used White-coat effect

Source: References 1, 2, and 7.

Therapeutic Failure

Drug treatment for hypertension is deemed a therapeutic failure if the patient does not reach the desired blood pressure goal (Table 27-4) after an adequate trial of lifestyle modifications combined with therapeutic doses of antihypertensive medication(s). New or worsening end-organ damage is also indicative of therapeutic failure.

Resistant hypertension is defined as the failure to achieve goal BP in patients who are adhering to full doses of an appropriate three-drug regimen that includes a diuretic.[1]

CORE ELEMENT 1—COMPREHENSIVE MEDICATION REVIEW FOR PATIENTS WITH HYPERTENSION

A list of suggested questions to use when conducting a medication therapy review in a patient with hypertension is given in Table 27-8. The number and types of questions will depend on several factors,

TABLE 27-6 • Assessment of Blood Pressure Outside the Clinical Setting

Ambulatory Blood Pressure Monitoring (ABPM)[a]
An automated device is preprogrammed to document BP at set time intervals (eg, every 15-30 minutes) during a 24-hour period, with most devices providing average day, night, and 24-hour pressures.
BP values are usually lower than clinic-measured values.
ABPM correlates better than office measurements with cardiovascular events and target organ injury, since it detects important aspects of the circadian BP cycle, such as the morning BP surge, measures of dipping, and nocturnal BP.
The ability to record nighttime BP is an advantage of ambulatory monitors, and is helpful in identifying "nondippers" (patients with BP that does not drop by >10% at night). These patients may be at increased risk for complications of hypertension.
Clinical situations in which ABPM is useful:
Masked hypertension
Suspected white-coat hypertension
Irregular blood pressure values or significant diurnal variation
Assessment of antihypertensive treatment response in the setting of complex regimens or clinical trials
Resistance to antihypertensive treatment
Hypotensive symptoms with antihypertensive medications
Self (Home)-Monitoring[a]
The patient uses a home monitoring device to collect BP measurements, preferably during the early-morning hours for most days and then at different times of the day on alternating days of the week.
Self-monitoring offers a practical approach to assess differences between clinic and out-of-office BP prior to considering ABPM.
Patients must be sufficiently educated on the proper use of their self-monitoring/home BP devices.
Self-monitoring allows patients to assess their own response to antihypertensive medications, which may increase compliance.

[a] Monitoring devices for ambulatory and self-monitoring must also be validated and meet quality standards.

Source: References 1, 2, 8, and 9.

including the amount of time for the interview, number of concurrent medication-related problems MRPs, urgency of MRPs, and the reliability of the patient in providing accurate information, among others. In time-limited interactions or in complex cases with multiple medical issues, the MTM provider may choose to target questions that help to identify or rule out issues of an urgent nature (see questions to ask for prevention/assessment of medical emergencies). MTM providers should remember to use living room language during the interview (Figure 27-1), and to be prepared for questions that patients may ask regarding their hypertension (Table 27-9).

TABLE 27-7 • Causes of Inaccurate Blood Pressure Readings

Biologic variability in blood pressure (eg, time of day, emotions)
Inadequate training and/or suboptimal measurement technique
Inappropriate environment (eg, ambient temperature too high or low)
Lack of a rest period prior to measurement
Masked hypertension
Presence of auscultatory gap
Pseudohypertension
Patients with irregular ventricular heart rates (atrial fibrillation, atrial flutter)
Use of caffeine/alcohol/nicotine prior to measurement
Use of inaccurate measuring devices (eg, wrist or finger monitors)
White-coat effect

Source: References 1, 2, 8, and 9.

CORE ELEMENT 2— PERSONAL MEDICATION LIST[10]

A sample personal medication list (PML) for a patient with hypertension is shown in Figure 27-2. This example is representative only of antihypertensive medications. Additional medications for other disease states should be added and listed separately. MTM providers should remember to use plain language when creating the PML.

CORE ELEMENT 3—MEDICATION ACTION PLAN[10]

Some sample medication action plans (MAPs) for patients with hypertension are provided in Figure 27-3. These examples are representative only of action steps for a patient with hypertension. MAPs for other disease states or other MRPs should be added and listed separately. In general, only a few of the most important action steps should be listed, so as not to overwhelm the patient. Other areas for patient self-management can be addressed at later visits. MTM providers should remember to use plain language when creating the MAP.

CORE ELEMENT 4—INTERVENTION AND/OR REFERRAL

Interventions for blood pressure management may include lifestyle modifications and/or drug therapy. Patients not adequately controlled with lifestyle modifications should be started

TABLE 27-8 • Questions to Ask When Conducting a Medication Review in a Patient with Hypertension

Suggested Questions for the Patient with Hypertension
How long have you had high blood pressure? When were you diagnosed?
Who else in your family has high blood pressure?
What do you know about the risks of uncontrolled blood pressure?
How often do you check your blood pressure at home? • What do you use to check your blood pressure? • How often do you check your blood pressure? • What is a "typical" blood pressure for you? • According to your physician, what should your blood pressure be (or what is a "good" blood pressure)? • Do you record your numbers in a diary or log book? If so, request to see. • If your blood pressure is high when you check it at home, what do you do? Has your physician given you any instructions to follow if your blood pressure is high?
Have you ever experienced the following signs/symptoms of low blood pressure (hypotension)? • Blurry vision • Confusion • Dizziness or lightheadedness • Falling or blacking out when going from a sitting/lying down to standing position • Fatigue (feeling tired) • Nausea (sick to your stomach) • Weakness
What medications do you take for your high blood pressure? How do you take them?
How often do you miss a dose of your blood pressure medication?
What other medications have you taken in the past for your high blood pressure?
Have you ever stopped taking any of your prescribed blood pressure medications without telling your physician? If so, why?
What over-the-counter (OTC) medications or herbals do you use for your blood pressure?
Other than medicines, what have you tried for your blood pressure (eg, lifestyle changes)?
Has your physician recommended reducing your salt intake in your diet? If so, what measures have you taken?
What exercise regimen do you follow?
What has your physician discussed with you regarding OTC medications that you should avoid because they can increase your blood pressure?
Questions to Ask for Prevention/Assessment of Medical Emergencies
Crisis planning: What are the warning signs of a heart attack or stroke, and what is your action plan?
Have you fallen, felt dizzy, or had blurred vision or racing heart when getting up from sitting or lying down?
Have you ever been hospitalized for high blood pressure?
What is a "typical" blood pressure for you?
Where would your physician like your blood pressure to be?

on drug therapy. Antihypertensives should be selected on the basis of patient characteristics such as age, race, compelling indications, and other comorbid disease states. Many patients will require more than one medication to control their blood pressure. Table 27-10 summarizes lifestyle modifications, and Tables 27-11 and 27-12 provide an overview of first-line and alterative antihypertensive medications, respectively. The current treatment algorithm for hypertension is provided in Figure 27-4. In addition, compelling indications for antihypertensive therapy are found in Figure 27-5, and considerations for individualization of drug therapy are listed in Table 27-13. Table 27-14 outlines herbal remedies that may be useful in the management of hypertension. Finally, the criteria for referral for management of hypertension are found in Figure 27-6.

CORE ELEMENT 5—DOCUMENTATION AND FOLLOW-UP

Clear and succinct documentation of MRPs and recommendations is a key component of the MTM consult. Examples of potential MRPs in patients with hypertension are provided in Table 27-15. Because blood pressure medications may make patients feel worse than the disorder of hypertension itself,

Abdominal aortic aneurysm—widening or ballooning of the large blood vessel that supplies blood to the gut, hip area, and legs that occurs because of weakness in the wall of the blood vessel. This may cause the blood vessel to burst and cut off blood flow to areas of the body.

ACE inhibitor—a medicine used to help lower blood pressure; may also help prevent changes or damage to the heart and kidneys.

Acute coronary syndrome—term used to cover any symptoms caused by decreased blood flow to the heart, such as a heart attack or chest pain.

Adverse event—something bad that happens, bad reaction, unexplained or unwanted effects.

Aldosterone—a chemical produced by the body that causes a person to absorb salt; too much of this may be a cause of high blood pressure.

Aldosterone antagonist—a medicine that lowers blood pressure by causing the body to absorb less salt.

α-Blocker—a medicine used to lower blood pressure; it works by relaxing blood vessels.

Aneurysm—widening or ballooning of a portion of a blood vessel carrying blood away from the heart; this occurs because of weakness in the wall of the blood vessel.

Angina—chest pain or discomfort caused by decreased blood flow through the heart, which could be a sign of heart attack.

Angioedema—a rare side effect of ACE inhibitors and a medical emergency involving rapid swelling of the lips, tongue, and throat that may affect breathing.

Angiotensin II—a compound in the blood that causes the blood vessels to narrow, which increases blood pressure; ACE inhibitors and ARBs decrease the effects of angiotensin II on blood pressure.

Antihypertensive medication—a medicine that lowers blood pressure.

ARB—angiotensin II receptor blocker, a medicine used to help lower blood pressure, it may also help prevent changes or damage to the heart and kidneys.

Arrhythmia—irregular heartbeat, skipped heartbeat, heart problem; an example is atrial fibrillation.

Arteries—blood vessels that carry blood away from the heart.

Atherosclerosis—hardening or clogging of the arteries due to a buildup of fatty material. This could lead to decreased blood flow to important areas of the body and may cause a heart attack.

β-Blocker—a medicine used to help lower blood pressure and the rate at which the heart beats. It works by decreasing the body's reaction to stress.

Blood glucose—blood sugar; if you have high blood pressure, your physician will check your blood sugar to be sure that you do not also have diabetes, as the two conditions are often seen together.

BMI—body mass index; a measure of weight in relation to height that assigns people to a weight class of underweight, normal weight, overweight, or obese, according to the amount of excess weight.

Bradycardia—a slow heartbeat, less than 60 times in a minute.

Calcium channel blocker—a medicine used to lower blood pressure or treat chest pain; it works by decreasing the force of the heart pumping and relaxing blood vessels.

Cardiac—related to the heart.

Cardiologist—physician specialized in heart disease and disorders.

Chronic—constant, never-ending, does not go away.

Chronic kidney disease—when the kidneys are unable to work well, which may cause high blood pressure and other serious health problems.

Coarctation of the aorta—narrowing of the largest artery in the body, which may cause high blood pressure.

Coronary artery disease—narrowing and hardening of the small blood vessels that supply blood and oxygen to the heart because of a buildup of cholesterol, which may lead to a heart attack and is the leading cause of death worldwide.

Creatinine—a test that checks how well the kidneys are working; an increase means that the kidneys are not working well.

Cushing syndrome—a group of symptoms and changes in normal body processes that may result if a class of drugs known as *glucocorticoids* are taken over a long period of time; this may be a cause of high blood pressure.

DASH diet—a diet high in fruits, vegetables, and low-fat dairy products, which has been proved to lower blood pressure.

Diastolic—the bottom blood pressure number, smaller number; the pressure in the arteries when the heart relaxes.

Direct renin inhibitor—a medicine used to lower blood pressure by decreasing the activity of renin, which is a substance in the body that may lead to increases in blood pressure.

Direct vasodilator—a medicine used to lower blood pressure; it works by relaxing blood vessels.

Diuretic—water pill.

Edema—swelling due to a buildup of too much fluid.

EKG—a test that looks for any damage to or problems with the heart.

Electrolytes—a type of necessary salt found in blood, such as sodium, potassium, and calcium.

Elevate—raise, make higher.

Essential or primary hypertension—high blood pressure without a known cause.

Fasting lipid panel—A test of the fats in the blood taken after 8-12 hours without eating any food, because the test results can change depending on what the patient eats.

Gingival hyperplasia—overgrowth of gum tissue in the mouth, which could be caused by calcium channel blockers.

Heart rate—how many times the heart beats each minute.

Hyperkalemia—high potassium; very high potassium is a medical emergency and could cause a deadly change in the way the heart beats.

Hyperparathyroidism—a condition that may cause high blood pressure; one of the reasons why a physician tests a patient's calcium is to check for this condition.

Hypertension—high blood pressure that increases the chance of heart attack, stroke, and kidney disease.

Hypertensive crisis—a combination of very high blood pressure and the shutdown of a major part of the body such as the brain, heart, or kidneys, which is a medical emergency.

Hypokalemia—low potassium, which may cause muscle weakness and cramping.

Hypotension—low blood pressure.

Insomnia—difficulty sleeping, despite good conditions and sufficient time for sleep, which affects a person's ability to function during the day; it is a possible side effect of many blood pressure medicines.

FIGURE 27-1 Living room language for hypertension.

Left ventricular hypertrophy—when the left side of the heart becomes large, which may change the way the heart beats and could lead to heart failure.

Lifestyle changes—your physician may have recommended changes in lifestyle to lower your blood pressure, which for some patients include reaching a goal weight, decreasing the amount of alcohol consumed, exercising, or quitting smoking.

Low-sodium diet—a diet with <2 g (2000 mg) of salt each day, which may lower blood pressure.

Myocardial infarction—heart attack, damage to the heart.

Obese—having a body mass index (BMI) of >30, which increases the risk of developing high blood pressure, diabetes, and cardiovascular disease.

Obstructive uropathy—when the flow of urine is blocked, which may cause high blood pressure.

Oral contraceptives—birth control medication, which may be a cause of high blood pressure.

Orthostatic hypotension—dizziness or lightheadedness on standing because of low blood pressure.

Overweight—having a body mass index (BMI) of >25, which increases the risk of developing high blood pressure, diabetes, and cardiovascular disease.

Packaged and processed foods—foods with added salt, which may increase blood pressure; examples include frozen dinners, canned soups, and other foods that require little or no preparation.

Peripheral arterial disease—a disease characterized by decreased blood flow to the arms and legs caused by clogged blood vessels.

Peripheral edema—swelling, usually of the legs, that may be a side effect of calcium channel blockers.

Prehypertension—blood pressure that is higher than the desired goal of <120/80; the top number is between 120 and 139, or the bottom number is between 80 and 89; this may lead to high blood pressure in the future.

Primary aldosteronism—condition in which the body produces too much of a chemical called *aldosterone*, which causes the body to absorb more salt; this may be a cause of high blood pressure.

Renal artery stenosis/renovascular disease—narrowing of the artery that brings blood to the kidneys, which makes it difficult for blood to flow; this may be a cause of high blood pressure.

Renin—a substance in the body that may lead to increases in blood pressure.

Retinopathy—damaged blood vessels in the eyes, which may be caused by high blood pressure and could lead to loss of eyesight.

Secondary hypertension—high blood pressure where the cause has been identified; the blood pressure may lower if that cause is treated.

Serum potassium—a test that checks the amount of potassium in the blood (see *Hyperkalemia* and *Hypokalemia*).

Sleep apnea—a sleep disorder that often involves pauses in breathing during the night; this may cause high blood pressure.

Smoking cessation—quitting smoking, which can lower the risk of heart disease.

Sodium—salt, which can increase blood pressure if consumed.

Spot urine albumin-to-creatinine ratio—a test that checks how well the kidneys are working. An increase means that the kidneys are not working well.

Stage 1 hypertension—high blood pressure, where the top number is between 140 and 159, or the lower number is between 90 and 99.

Stage 2 hypertension—very high blood pressure, where the top number is above 159, or the lower number is above 99.

Stroke—a condition caused by bleeding or lack of blood in the brain, which may cause a loss of speech, memory, or other abilities.

Systolic—the top blood pressure number, the larger number; the pressure in the arteries when the heart contracts.

Tachycardia—a fast pace for the heart to beat, more than 100 times in a minute.

Topically—applied to the skin.

Unstable angina—pain or a feeling of pressure on the chest, which is a medical emergency and may lead to a heart attack.

Veins—blood vessels that carry blood toward the heart.

FIGURE 27-1 *(Continued)*

PERSONAL MEDICATION LIST FOR *<Insert patient's name, DOB: mm/dd/yyyy>*	
Medication: Chlorthalidone 25-mg tablet	
How I use it: Take one tablet (25 mg) by mouth every morning	
Why I use it: Blood pressure (water pill)	**Prescriber:** Jones
Date I started using it: 1/6/2017	**Date I stopped using it:** *(Leave blank for patient's notes)*
Why I stopped using it: *(Leave blank for patient's notes)*	
Medication: Lisinopril 10-mg tablet	
How I use it: Take one tablet (10 mg) by mouth every night at bedtime	
Why I use it: Blood pressure	**Prescriber:** Jones
Date I started using it: 10/9/16	**Date I stopped using it:** *(Leave blank for patient's notes)*
Why I stopped using it: *(Leave blank for patient's notes)*	

FIGURE 27-2 Sample personal medication list for hypertension medications.

TABLE 27-9 • Questions to Anticipate Regarding Hypertension

What is blood pressure? Blood pushes on the walls of the arteries when your heart beats. Blood pressure is the force of that push. A blood pressure reading is two numbers. An example of a reading is 120 over 80. Blood pressure is measured in millimeters of mercury (mmHg).
What is high blood pressure? One or both of the blood pressure numbers in the reading can be too high. The top number is your systolic blood pressure. This is the pressure when your heart contracts. It is considered high in most cases if it is over 140 mmHg. The bottom number is your diastolic blood pressure. This is the pressure when your heart relaxes. Diastolic pressure greater than 90 is high in most cases.
What causes high blood pressure? The cause of high blood pressure in most people is uncertain. A variety of conditions can be the cause. Not being active or being overweight can lead to high blood pressure. If a person has a diet high in salt and fats, this could also cause high pressure. Some things you cannot control can also lead to high blood pressure, like getting older and genetics.
What health problems are associated with high blood pressure? There are many problems. Plaque or fatty material may build up on blood vessel walls. Heart, kidney, and eye diseases are often seen with high blood pressure. Stroke and early death often come along with high blood pressure, too.
How do I know if I have high blood pressure? High blood pressure does not have any symptoms. For this reason, you rarely feel it. Having your blood pressure checked by a healthcare provider is a good way to see if your numbers are high.
Why are blood pressure medications so important? It is important to keep your blood pressure normal so that you can stay healthy. People with high blood pressure are more likely to be sent to the hospital, and to have strokes, heart attacks, heart failure, kidney failure, or other health issues.
I can't tell when my blood pressure is high. Can I just stop my medications if I feel okay? Blood pressure medicines do not correct your high blood pressure permanently, so you have to continue taking the medications that were prescribed for you by your physician. It is extremely important that you continue taking your blood pressure medications to prevent future complications that can result from high blood pressure, such as heart failure, heart attack, stroke, kidney disease, and eye disease, among many others.
What can happen if I stop taking my blood pressure medications? A heart attack, stroke, and other serious health problems can arise. If you stop taking your medicine suddenly, your blood pressure can get too high. Also, when you restart your medicine, your dose may have to be lowered for a period of time to prevent side effects. Your prescriber will tell you how to slowly work your way back up to your usual dose.
When should I call my physician about high blood pressure? Call your physician if you are not responding to the prescribed treatment (your blood pressure is still high), or if you are having side effects. Call your physician if you experience any of the following symptoms of high blood pressure: dizziness, nosebleed, upset stomach, nausea, appetite changes, severe headache, severe anxiety, shortness of breath, or vision disturbances such as blurred vision. Call your physician if you experience the following symptoms of low blood pressure: dizziness, fainting, lightheadedness on standing, or chest pain.
What should I do if I have a problem with my blood pressure medications? Never stop taking your blood pressure medications without first talking to your physician. Speak with your physician and/or pharmacist to let them know about any problems you are having, and together you can make sure that your blood pressure medications are the right ones for you.

	DATE PREPARED: *<Insert date>*
What we talked about: You reported having some dizziness on standing. This is sometimes known as *orthostatic hypotension*. It means that your heart may be having trouble adjusting its pumping abilities to the change in pressure when you stand up. This is common in people who take multiple medications for high blood pressure.	
What I need to do: Here are some things you can do to help lessen this effect: 1. Get up *slowly*. Most people get up quickly, and this doesn't give the heart enough time to adjust to the change in position. Slowly move from a laying position to a sitting position (think over 10 or more seconds). Then, slowly stand up, supporting yourself with your bed, a chair, or a nightstand. 2. Unless you have limits on your fluid intake, keep yourself well hydrated. 3. Avoid walking in hot weather. 4. Breathe in through pursed lips (think "kissy lips") when you are moving from sitting to standing.	**What I did and when I did it:** *(Leave blank for patient's notes)*
What we talked about: Need to see how well new medicine (lisinopril) is working for blood pressure	
What I need to do: 1. Check blood pressure at home at least 3 times weekly. 2. Write down my blood pressure in the logbook. Notify the clinic if my blood pressure is higher than 180/120 mmHg or lower than 100/60 mmHg. 3. Bring logbook and my blood pressure machine the next time I come to clinic.	**What I did and when I did it:** *(Leave blank for patient's notes)*

FIGURE 27-3 Sample medication action plan for a patient with hypertension.

TABLE 27-10 • Lifestyle Modifications to Prevent and Manage Hypertension

Modification	Recommendation	Approximate Systolic Blood Pressure Reduction (mmHg)[a]
Weight loss	Maintain normal body weight (body mass index, 18.5-24.9 kg/m^2)	5-20 per 10-kg weight loss
DASH-type dietary patterns	Consume a diet rich in fruits, vegetables, and low-fat dairy products with a reduced content of saturated and total fat	8-14
Reduced salt intake	Reduce daily dietary sodium intake as much as possible, ideally to ≈65 mmol/day (1.5 g/day sodium, or 3.8 g/day sodium chloride)	2-8
Aerobic physical activity	Three or four sessions per week, lasting an average of 40 min/session, and involving moderate- to vigorous-intensity physical activity	4-9
Moderation of alcohol intake	Limit consumption to ≤2 drink equivalents per day in men and ≤1 drink equivalent per day in women and lighter-weight persons[b]	2-4

[a] Effects of implementing these modifications are time- and dose-dependent and could be greater for some patients.

[b] One drink equivalent is equal to 1.5 oz (approximately 45 mL) of 80-proof distilled spirits (eg, whiskey), a 5-oz (approximately 150 mL) glass of wine (12%), or 12 oz (approximately 350 mL) of beer.

Source: Reproduced, with permission, from DiPiro JT, Talbert RL, Yee GC, Matzke GR, Wells BG, Posey LM, eds. *Pharmacotherapy: A Pathophysiologic Approach*, 10th ed. New York: McGraw-Hill; 2017.

TABLE 27-11 • First-Line and Other Common Antihypertensive Agents

Class	Subclass	Drug (Brand Name)	Usual Dose Range (mg/day)	Daily Frequency	Comments
ACEI		Benazepril (Lotensin) Captopril (Capoten) Enalapril (Vasotec) Fosinopril (Monopril) Lisinopril (Prinivil, Zestril) Moexipril (Univasc) Perindopril (Aceon) Quinapril (Accupril) Ramipril (Altace) Trandolapril (Mavik)	10-40 12.5-150 5-40 10-40 10-40 7.5-30 4-16 10-80 2.5-10 1-4	1 or 2 2 or 3 1 or 2 1 1 1 or 2 1 1 or 2 1 or 2 1	May cause hyperkalemia in patients with CKD or in those receiving a potassium-sparing diuretic, aldosterone antagonist, ARB, or direct renin inhibitor; can cause acute kidney failure in patients with severe bilateral renal artery stenosis or severe stenosis in artery to solitary kidney; do not use in pregnancy or in patients with a history of angioedema; starting dose should be reduced 50% in patients who are on a thiazide, are volume depleted, or are very elderly because of risks of hypotension
ARB		Azilsartan (Edarbi) Candesartan (Atacand) Eprosartan (Teveten) Irbesartan (Avapro) Losartan (Cozaar) Olmesartan (Benicar) Telmisartan (Micardis) Valsartan (Diovan)	40-80 8-32 600-800 150-300 50-100 20-40 20-80 80-320	1 1 or 2 1 or 2 1 1 or 2 1 1 1	May cause hyperkalemia in patients with CKD or in those receiving a potassium-sparing diuretic, aldosterone antagonist, ACEI, or direct renin inhibitor; can cause acute kidney failure in patients with severe bilateral renal artery stenosis or severe stenosis in artery to solitary kidney; do not cause a dry cough like an ACEI may; do not use in pregnancy; starting dose should be reduced 50% in patients who are on a thiazide, are volume depleted, or are very elderly due to risks of hypotension

(*Continued*)

TABLE 27-11 • First-Line and Other Common Antihypertensive Agents (*Continued*)

Class	Subclass	Drug (Brand Name)	Usual Dose Range (mg/day)	Daily Frequency	Comments
Calcium channel blocker	Dihydropyridine	Amlodipine (Norvasc)	2.5-10	1	Short-acting dihydropyridines should be avoided, especially immediate-release nifedipine and nicardipine; dihydropyridines are more potent peripheral vasodilators than nondihydropyridines and may cause more reflex sympathetic discharge (tachycardia), dizziness, headache, flushing, and peripheral edema; have additional benefits in Raynaud syndrome
		Felodipine (Plendil)	5-20	1	
		Isradipine (DynaCirc)	5-10	2	
		Isradipine SR (DynaCirc SR)	5-20	1	
		Nicardipine sustained release (Cardene SR)	60-120	2	
		Nifedipine long-acting (Adalat CC, Nifedical XL, Procardia XL)	30-90	1	
		Nisoldipine (Sular)	10-40	1	
	Nondihydropyridine	Diltiazem sustained release (Cardizem SR)	180-360	2	Extended-release products are preferred for hypertension; these agents reduce heart rate; may produce heart block, especially in combination with β-blockers; these products are not AB rated as interchangeable on an equipotent milligram-per-milligram basis, due to different release mechanisms and different bioavailability parameters; Cardizem LA, Covera-HS, and Verelan PM have delayed drug release for several hours after dosing, when dosed in the evening can provide chronotherapeutic drug delivery starting shortly before patients awake from sleep; nondihydropyridines have additional benefits in patients with atrial tachyarrhythmia
		Diltiazem sustained release (Cardizem CD, Cartia XT, Dilacor XR, Diltia XT, Tiazac, Taztia XT)	120-480	1	
		Diltiazem extended release (Cardizem LA)	120-540	1 (morning or evening)	
		Verapamil sustained release (Calan SR, Isoptin SR, Verelan)	180-480	1 or 2	
		Verapamil controlled onset, extended release (Covera-HS)	180-420	1 (in the evening)	
		Verapamil chronotherapeutic oral drug absorption system (Verelan PM)	100-400	1 (in the evening)	
Diuretic	Thiazide	Chlorthalidone (Hygroton)	12.5-25	1	Hydrochlorothiazide is a "thiazide-type" agent; chlorthalidone, indapamide, and metolazone are "thiazide-like" agents. Dose in the morning to avoid nocturnal diuresis; thiazides are more effective antihypertensives than loop diuretics in most patients; use usual doses to avoid adverse metabolic effects; hydrochlorothiazide, chlorthalidone, and indapamide are preferred; chlorthalidone is approximately 1.5 times as potent as hydrochlorothiazide and has a much longer half-life; have additional benefits in osteoporosis; use with caution in patients with a history of gout
		Hydrochlorothiazide (Esidrix, HydroDiuril, Microzide, Oretic)	12.5-50	1	
		Indapamide (Lozol)	1.25-2.5	1	
		Metolazone (Zaroxolyn)	2.5-10	1	
	Loop	Bumetanide (Bumex)	0.5-4	2	Dose in the morning and late afternoon (when twice daily) to avoid nocturnal diuresis; higher doses may be needed for patients with severely decreased GFR or heart failure; preferred over thiazides in patient with concomitant renal dysfunction and resistant hypertension
		Furosemide (Lasix)	20-80	2	
		Torsemide (Demadex)	5-10	1	

(*Continued*)

TABLE 27-11 • First-Line and Other Common Antihypertensive Agents (*Continued*)

Class	Subclass	Drug (Brand Name)	Usual Dose Range (mg/day)	Daily Frequency	Comments
	Potassium sparing	Amiloride (Midamor) Amiloride/hydrochlorothiazide (Moduretic) Triamterene (Dyrenium) Triamterene/hydrochlorothiazide (Dyazide)	5-10 5-10/50-100 50-100 37.5-75/25-50	1 or 2 1 1 or 2 1	Weak diuretics that are generally used in combination with a thiazide to minimize hypokalemia; do not significantly lower BP unless used with a thiazide; should generally be reserved for patients experiencing diuretic-induced hypokalemia; avoid in patients with CKD (estimated creatinine clearance [CrCl] <30 mL/min [<0.5 mL/s]); may cause hyperkalemia, especially in combination with an ACEI, ARB, direct renin inhibitor, or potassium supplements
	Aldosterone antagonist	Eplerenone (Inspra) Spironolactone (Aldactone) Spironolactone/hydrochlorothiazide (Aldactazide)	50-100 25-50 25-50/25-50	1 or 2 1 or 2 1	Dose in the morning and late afternoon (when twice daily) to avoid nocturnal diuresis; eplerenone contraindicated in patients with an estimated CrCl <50 mL/min (<0.83 mL/s), elevated serum creatinine (>1.8 mg/dL [159 μmol/L] in women, >2 mg/dL [177 μmol/L] in men), and type 2 diabetes with microalbuminuria; spironolactone often used as add-on therapy in resistant hypertension; avoid spironolactone in patients with CKD (estimated CrCl <30 mL/min [<0.5 mL/s]); may cause hyperkalemia, especially in combination with an ACEI, ARB, direct renin inhibitor, or potassium supplements
β-Blocker	Cardioselective	Atenolol (Tenormin) Betaxolol (Kerlone) Bisoprolol (Zebeta) Metoprolol tartrate (Lopressor) Metoprolol succinate extended release (Toprol XL)	25-100 5-20 2.5-10 100-400 50-200	1 1 1 2 1	Abrupt discontinuation may cause rebound hypertension; inhibit β_1-receptors at low to moderate dose, higher doses also block β_2-receptors; may exacerbate asthma when selectivity is lost; have additional benefits in patients with atrial tachyarrhythmia or preoperative hypertension
	Nonselective	Nadolol (Corgard) Propranolol (Inderal) Propranolol long acting (Inderal LA, Inderal XL, InnoPran XL) Timolol (Blocadren)	40-120 160-480 80-320 10-40	1 2 1 1	Abrupt discontinuation may cause rebound hypertension; inhibit β_1- and β_2-receptors at all doses; can exacerbate asthma; have additional benefits in patients with essential tremor, migraine headache, portal hypertension, thyrotoxicosis
	Intrinsic sympathomimetic activity	Acebutolol (Sectral) Carteolol (Cartrol) Pindolol (Visken)	200-800 2.5-10 10-60	2 1 2	Abrupt discontinuation may cause rebound hypertension; partially stimulate β-receptors while blocking against additional stimulation; no clear advantage for these agents; contraindicated in patients post-MI

(*Continued*)

TABLE 27-11 • First-Line and Other Common Antihypertensive Agents (*Continued*)

Class	Subclass	Drug (Brand Name)	Usual Dose Range (mg/day)	Daily Frequency	Comments
	Mixed α- and β-blockers	Carvedilol (Coreg) Carvedilol phosphate (Coreg CR) Labetalol (Normodyne, Trandate)	12.5-50 20-80 200-800	2 1 2	Abrupt discontinuation may cause rebound hypertension; additional α-blockade produces vasodilation and more orthostatic hypotension
	Cardioselective and vasodilatory	Nebivolol (Bystolic)	5-20	1	Abrupt discontinuation may cause rebound hypertension; additional vasodilation does not result in more orthostatic hypotension

Source: Reproduced, with permission, from DiPiro JT, Talbert RL, Yee GC, Matzke GR, Wells BG, Posey LM, eds. *Pharmacotherapy: A Pathophysiologic Approach*, 10th ed. New York: McGraw-Hill; 2017.

nonadherence is a likely problem. MTM providers need to be vigilant for nonadherence to medications and recommend changes in pharmacotherapy, if needed, to promote adherence. Sample communications and recommendations to providers to address medication-related issues are found in Figure 27-7. Recommendations may be communicated via fax, telephone, or other means of written or secure electronic communication. The examples below are for illustrative purposes. Actual communications to providers should be individualized based on the type of recommendation, patient specific characteristics, and the nature of the relationship with the provider.

Follow-up to assess blood pressure, effects of interventions, and potential adverse effects is essential in patients with hypertension. The interval for follow-up will depend on a number of factors, including severity of hypertension, type of intervention, and patient-specific factors such as age, comorbid conditions, and ability to return for follow-up. Suggested intervals for follow-up are provided in Table 27-16.

TABLE 27-12 • Alternative Antihypertensive Agents

Class	Drug (Brand Name)	Usual Dose Range (mg/day)	Daily Frequency	Comments
α_1-Blocker	Doxazosin (Cardura) Prazosin (Minipress) Terazosin (Hytrin)	1-8 2-20 1-20	1 2 or 3 1 or 2	Give first dose at bedtime; patients should rise from sitting or lying down slowly to minimize risk of orthostatic hypotension; additional benefits in men with benign prostatic hyperplasia
Direct renin inhibitor	Aliskiren (Tekturna)	150-300	1	May cause hyperkalemia in patients with CKD and diabetes or in those receiving a potassium-sparing diuretic, aldosterone antagonist, ACEI, or ARB; may cause acute kidney failure in patients with severe bilateral renal artery stenosis or severe stenosis in artery to solitary kidney; do not use in pregnancy
Central α_2-agonist	Clonidine (Catapres) Clonidine patch (Catapres-TTS) Methyldopa (Aldomet)	0.1-0.8 0.1-0.3 250-1,000	2 1 weekly 2	Abrupt discontinuation may cause rebound hypertension; most effective if used with a thiazide to diminish fluid retention; clonidine patch is replaced once per week
Peripheral adrenergic antagonist	Reserpine (generic only)	0.05-0.25	1	Used in many of the landmark clinical trials; should be used with a thiazide to diminish fluid retention
Direct arterial vasodilator	Minoxidil (Loniten) Hydralazine (Apresoline)	10-40 20-100	1 or 2 2 to 4	Should be used with thiazide and β-blocker to diminish fluid retention and reflex tachycardia

Source: Reproduced, with permission, from DiPiro JT, Talbert RL, Yee GC, Matzke GR, Wells BG, Posey LM, eds. *Pharmacotherapy: A Pathophysiologic Approach*, 10th ed. New York: McGraw-Hill; 2017.

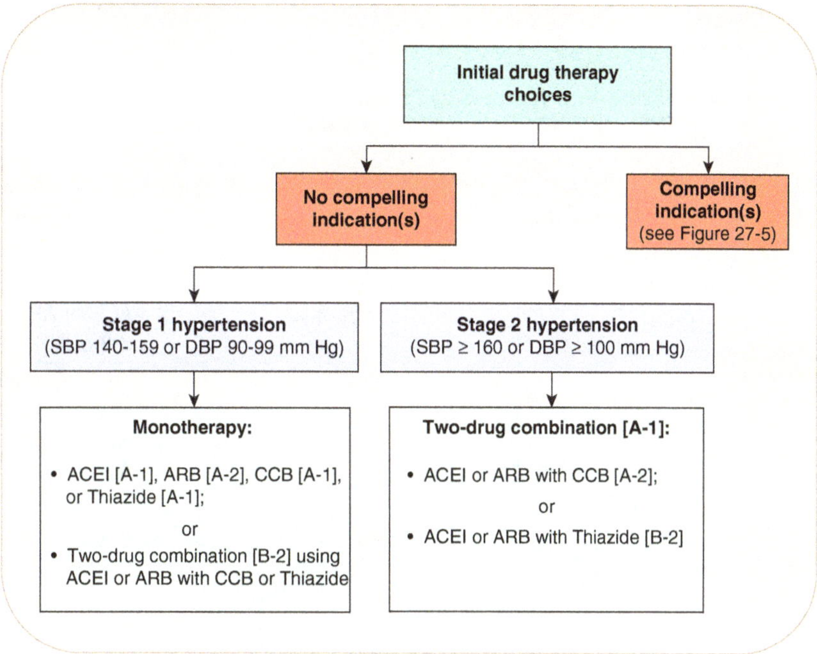

FIGURE 27-4 Algorithm for treatment of hypertension. Drug therapy recommendations are graded with strength of recommendation and quality of evidence in brackets. Grading for strength of recommendations is as follows: A, B, and C are good, moderate, and poor evidence to support recommendation, respectively. Quality of evidence: (1) evidence from more than one properly randomized controlled trial; (2) evidence from at least one well-designed clinical trial with randomization, from cohort or case-controlled studies, or dramatic results from uncontrolled experiments or subgroup analyses; (3) evidence from opinions of respected authorities, based on clinical experience, descriptive studies, or reports of expert communities.

Source: Reproduced, with permission, from DiPiro JT, Talbert RL, Yee GC, Matzke GR, Wells BG, Posey LM, Schwinghammer T, eds. *Pharmacotherapy: A Pathophysiologic Approach*, 10th ed. New York: McGraw-Hill; 2017.

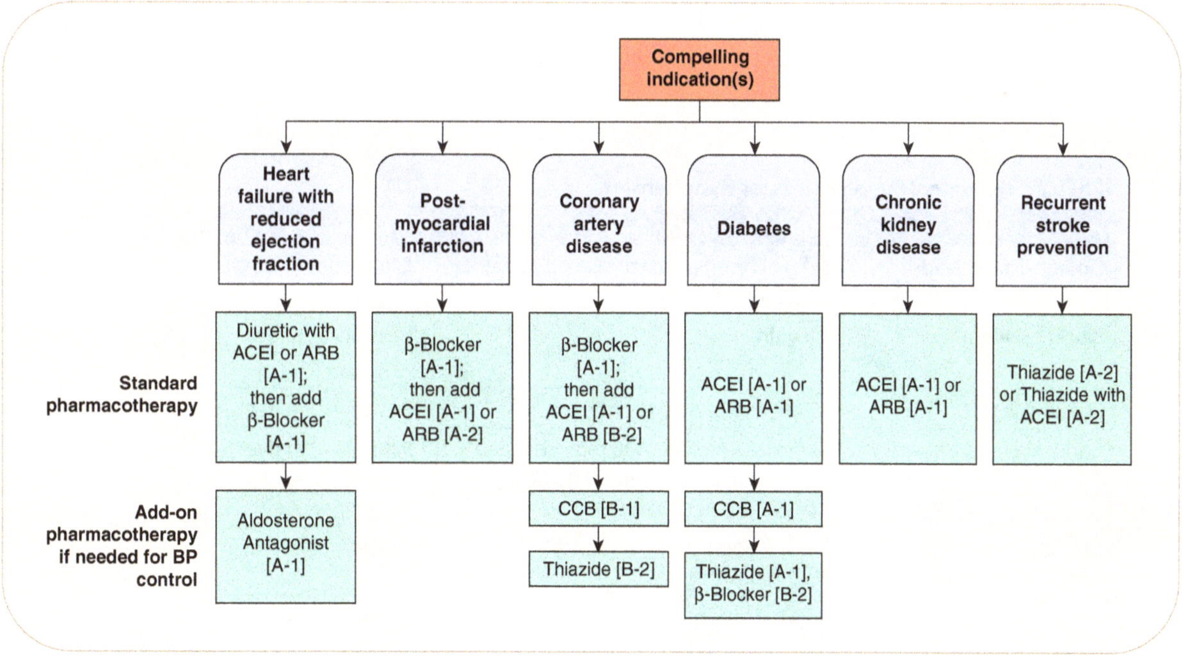

FIGURE 27-5. Compelling indications for individual drug classes. Compelling indications for specific drugs are evidenced-based recommendations from outcome studies or existing clinical guidelines. The order of drug therapies serves as a general guidance that should be balanced with clinical judgment and patient response. Add-on pharmacotherapy recommendations are when additional agents are needed to lower BP to goal values. Blood pressure control should be managed concurrently with the compelling indication. Drug therapy recommendations are graded with strength of recommendation and quality of evidence in brackets. Strength of recommendations: A, B, and C are good, moderate, and poor evidence to support recommendation, respectively. Quality of evidence: (1) evidence from more than one properly randomized controlled trial; (2) evidence from at least one well-designed clinical trial with randomization, from cohort or case-controlled analytic studies or multiple time series, or dramatic results from uncontrolled experiments or subgroup analyses; (3) evidence from opinions of respected authorities, based on clinical experience, descriptive studies, or reports of expert communities.

Source: Reproduced, with permission, from DiPiro JT, Talbert RL, Yee GC, Matzke GR, Wells BG, Posey LM, Schwinghammer T, eds. *Pharmacotherapy: A Pathophysiologic Approach*, 10th ed. New York: McGraw-Hill; 2017.

TABLE 27-13 • Considerations in Individualizing Antihypertensive Therapy

A. Comorbid Conditions and Treatment Considerations		B. Preferred Drug Options for Specific Populations	
Comorbid Condition[a]	**Drug Therapy Considerations**	**Special Populations**	**Preferred Drug Options**
Asthma	Avoid: Noncardioselective β-blockers	African-Americans	Diuretics (use as initial therapy unless contraindicated) CCB
Benign prostatic hypertrophy	α_1-Blocker (do not use as monotherapy for hypertension)		
Erectile dysfunction	Avoid: Centrally acting agents (eg, clonidine)	Whites	ACEI or ARB β-Blocker
Essential tremor	β-Blocker (nonselective)	Elderly	Thiazide-like diuretic CCB (long-acting) ACEI or ARB Avoid: α_1-Blockers, combined α, β-blockers, central α_2-agonists
Heart failure	ACEI or ARB β-Blocker (bisoprolol, metoprolol succinate), carvedilol		
Hyperthyroidism	β-Blocker	Pregnancy	β-Blocker (labetalol) Methyldopa Avoid: ACEIs, ARBs, direct renin inhibitors
Migraine	β-Blocker (nonselective) CCB		
Osteoporosis	Thiazide diuretic Avoid: Loop diuretics	Lactation	Methyldopa, hydralazine β-Blocker if indicated (propranolol, labetalol) Avoid: ACEIs, ARBs, diuretics
Peripheral vascular disease	ACEI or ARB CCB Avoid: β-Blockers, unless there is another compelling indication (eg, aortic aneurysm, post-MI, angina)		
Raynaud syndrome	CCB (dihydropyridine)		

[a] Not a compelling indication.

Abbreviations: ACEI = angiotensin-converting enzyme inhibitor; ARB = angiotensin receptor blocker; CCB = calcium channel blocker; MI = myocardial infarction.

Source: References 1, 2, 4, and 5.

TABLE 27-14 • Herbal Supplements for Hypertension

Herbal	Typical Dose	Effectiveness[a]	Cost[b]
Omega-3 fatty acids	3-4 g of omega-3 fatty acids ≤3× daily (tid), taken with meals	Likely effective	$$
Blond psyllium	3.5 g tid	Possibly effective	$
Coenzyme Q10	75-360 mg of CoQ10 daily	Possibly effective	$$
Garlic (*Allium sativum*)	Garlic tablets 300-1500 mg in divided doses daily or dehydrated garlic powder tablet 600 mg daily	Possibly effective	$
Hibiscus tea (*Hibiscus sabdariffa*)	1-2 teaspoon (3-6 g) in 1 cup (250 mL) water	Possibly effective	$
L-Arginine	4-24 g daily	Possibly effective	$

[a] Level of evidence: "Likely effective"—this product has a very high level of reliable clinical evidence supporting its use for a specific indication. Products rated "likely effective" are generally considered appropriate to recommend; "possibly effective"—this product has some clinical evidence supporting its use for a specific indication; however, the evidence is limited by quantity, quality, or contradictory findings. Products rated "possibly effective" might be beneficial, but do not have enough high-quality evidence to be recommended for most people; "insufficient evidence"—there is not enough reliable scientific evidence to provide an effectiveness rating.

[b] Cost: $ = ≤$10/month supply in recommended dosage; $$ = $11-$20/month; $$$$ = >$50/month.

Source: Data compiled from reference 11.

Action	Criteria
Immediate action **Call 911**	• Blood pressure >180/120 mm Hg with target organ damage HTN (Hypertensive Emergency) • Symptoms of heart attack or angina • Symptoms of stroke
Seek medical attention **Emergency Room**	• Severe elevation in blood pressure (SBP >180 mm Hg or DBP > 110 mm Hg) without evidence of target organ damage (Hypertensive Urgency) • Symptoms may include headache or anxiety
Routine **Inform provider at a later time**	• Blood pressure above goal (but <180/110 mm Hg) without signs or symptoms of hypertensive urgency or emergency • Non-urgent side effects from antihypertensives (e.g., dry cough)

FIGURE 27-6 Referral for management of hypertension.

Scenario: Patient given samples of valsartan, but cannot afford Rx once samples are finished.
MRP: Nonadherence.

Assessment:
Patient with uncontrolled blood pressure on valsartan 80 mg. Lack of BP control likely secondary to nonadherence with valsartan. Patient nonadherent with valsartan because of cost issues. Switching valsartan to an ACE inhibitor would provide for more affordable BP control and renal protection in this patient with type 2 diabetes mellitus.
Plan:
Consider discontinuation of valsartan and addition of lisinopril 10 mg daily with titration to blood pressure goal of <140/90 mmHg.

Scenario: Opportunity to reduce antihypertensive pill burden.
MRP: Nonadherence (or the potential to minimize nonadherence by simplifying regimen).

Assessment:
On the basis of pharmacy claims and/or patient report, your patient is currently receiving
○ Lisinopril ___ mg daily
○ Hydrochlorothiazide ____ mg daily
Please note: There is a lisinopril/hydrochlorothiazide combination product available that is supplied in the following strengths: 10 mg/12.5 mg, 20 mg/12.5 mg, and 20 mg/25 mg. This combination is available for the cost of a generic copay.
Plan:
If appropriate, please consider switching your patient to the combination product to help reduce pill burden and optimize current therapy.

Scenario: Diabetes patient with elevated blood pressure not on ACE inhibitor or ARB.
MRP: Need for additional therapy.

Assessment:
Blood pressure above goal of <140/90 mmHg in this patient with type 2 diabetes and albuminuria. Lifestyle modifications have not resulted in adequate response. ACE inhibitor may help achieve BP goals and provide renal protection.
Plan:
Consider initiation of ramipril 2.5 mg PO daily.
Patient to check blood pressure with home machine 3 times weekly and bring logbook to next visit.

Scenario: Patient on hydrochlorothiazide (HCTZ) for 3 months with no significant BP response.
MRP: Ineffective medication.

Assessment:
Uncontrolled blood pressure on HCTZ 25 mg daily. Patient reports adherence to therapy. No significant BP response with HCTZ despite adequate trial. Patient may benefit from switch to another class of BP medication. Goal BP <140/90 mmHg.
Plan:
Recommend discontinue HCTZ.
Consider initiation of lisinopril 10 mg daily.
Patient to monitor BP at least 3 times weekly and record.
Follow-up for BP check in 2 weeks.

FIGURE 27-7 Sample provider communications for hypertension.

TABLE 27-15 • Medication-Related Problems (MRPs) in Patients with Hypertension

Category of MRP	Sample Medication-Related Problem
Nonadherence	Suboptimal control of blood pressure due to nonadherence with lifestyle modifications (eg, restriction of salt, smoking cessation) Suboptimal control of blood pressure due to patient missing doses of antihypertensive medication Patient not taking antihypertensive medication due to cost
Unnecessary medication	Duplicate therapy (eg, two ACE inhibitors)
Need for additional medication	Monotherapy for hypertension with suboptimal blood pressure control Patient with diabetes and albuminuria not on ACE inhibitor or ARB for hypertension
Ineffective medication	Adequate trial of new antihypertensive without significant clinical response Monotherapy with α_1-blocker
Dosage too low	Suboptimal blood pressure control on low dose of antihypertensive agent
Dosage too high	Patient with orthostatic hypotension Patient with bradycardia from β-blocker
Adverse drug event	Cough from ACE inhibitor Patient not taking calcium channel blocker due to constipation (could also be classified under nonadherence)

Abbreviations: ACE = angiotensin-converting enzyme; ARB = angiotensin receptor blocker.

TABLE 27-16 • Suggested Intervals for Follow-up and Monitoring in Patients with Hypertension

Blood pressure response
2-4 weeks after initiating or making changes in therapy
After blood pressure goal is met and is stable, assuming that no signs or symptoms of acute target organ disease are present, patients should be monitored every 3-6 months.
Patients with stage 2 hypertension, comorbid conditions, history of poor control, nonadherence, progressive target organ damage, or symptoms of adverse drug effects should be followed more frequently.
Toxicity
Monitor for adverse drug effects 2-4 weeks after starting a new agent or dose increase.
Monitor every 6-12 months in stable patients.
Serum potassium and creatinine should be monitored 1-2 times each year.

References 1 and 2

REFERENCES

1. Chobanian AV et al. *The Seventh Report of the Joint National Committee on Prevention, Detection, Evaluation, and Treatment of High Blood Pressure.* https://www.nhlbi.nih.gov/files/docs/guidelines/jnc7full.pdf. Publication 04-5230, August 2004.
2. Saseen JJ, MacLaughlin EJ. Hypertension. In: DiPiro, JT, Talbert RL, Yee GC, Matzke GR, Wells BG, Posey LM, Schwinghammer T, eds. *Pharmacotherapy: A Pathophysiologic Approach*, 10th ed. New York, NY; 2017, Chapter 13. Available at http://www.accesspharmacy.com.lp.hscl.ufl.edu/content.aspx?aid=7969921. Accessed May 11, 2017.
3. Wilson L, Saseen JJ. Hypertension. In: Tisdale JE, Miller DA, eds. *Drug-Induced Diseases: Prevention, Detection, and Management*, 3rd ed. Bethesda, MD: American Society of Health-Systems Pharmacists, Inc.; 2016.
4. Weber MA, Schiffrin EL, White WB, et al. Clinical practice guidelines for the management of hypertension in the community: A statement by the American Society of Hypertension and the International Society of Hypertension. *J Clin Hypertens.* 2014;16:14-26.
5. James PA, Oparil S, Carter BL, et al. 2014 evidence-based guideline for the management of high blood pressure in adults report from the panel members appointed to the Eighth Joint National Committee (JNC 8). *JAMA.* 2014;311:507-520.
6. American Diabetes Association. Cardiovascular disease and risk management. Section 9. In Standards of Medical Care in Diabetes—2017. *Diabetes Care.* 2017;40(Suppl 1):S75-S87.
7. Pickering TG, Hall JE, Appel LJ, et al. Recommendations for blood pressure measurement in humans and experimental animals: Part 1: Blood pressure measurement in humans: A statement for professionals from the Subcommittee of Professional and Public Education of the American Heart Association Council on High Blood Pressure Research. *Circulation.* 2005;111:697-716.
8. Pickering TG, White WB. ASH Position Paper: Home and ambulatory blood pressure monitoring. When and how to use self (home) and ambulatory blood pressure monitoring. *J Clin Hypertens.* 2008;10:850-855.
9. O'Brien E, Pickering T, Asmar R, et al. Working Group on Blood Pressure Monitoring of the European Society of Hypertension International Protocol for Validation of Blood Pressure Measuring Devices in Adults. *Blood Press Monit.* 2002;7:3-18.
10. *Medicare Part D Medication Therapy Management Program Standardized Format.* Available at https://www.cms.gov/Medicare/Prescription-Drug-Coverage/PrescriptionDrugCovContra/Downloads/MTM-Program-Standardized-Format-English-and-Spanish-Instructions-Samples-v032712.pdf. Accessed May 11, 2017.
11. Natural Medicines [database online]. Somerville, MA: Therapeutic Research Center; 2017. Available at https://naturalmedicines.therapeuticresearch.com/. Accessed May 11, 2017.

Review Questions

1. A 55-year-old Hispanic male is seen in the MTM clinic for management of his hypertension. The average of his last several blood pressure readings is 166/94 mmHg. Which of the following is the most appropriate classification of his hypertension?
   a. Stage 1 hypertension
   b. Stage 2 hypertension
   c. Isolated systolic HTN
   d. Hypertensive urgency

2. All of the following can affect the accuracy of blood pressure measurements EXCEPT:
   a. use of a digital blood pressure monitor for the blood pressure measurement.
   b. temperature of the room in which blood pressure is measured.
   c. ingestion of caffeine prior to the blood pressure measurement.
   d. skill of the practitioner performing the blood pressure measurement.

3. An 82-year-old white male has a history of hypertension, dyslipidemia, and gout. Which of the following is an appropriate blood pressure goal for this patient?
   a. <130/80 mmHg
   b. <140/80 mmHg
   c. <140/90 mmHg
   d. <150/90 mmHg

4. Which of the following best describes how you would explain the use of a β-blocker to a patient using living room language?
   a. A medication for your hypertension.
   b. A blood pressure medicine that works by slowing down how fast the heart beats and decreasing the body's reaction to stress.
   c. A blood pressure medicine that works by blocking response to stimuli from the sympathetic nervous system.
   d. A blood pressure medicine that exerts its mechanism by blocking β-receptors in the heart.

5. All of the following are appropriate for inclusion on the medication action plan of a patient with high blood pressure EXCEPT:
   a. Monitor your hypertension 3 times weekly with a sphygmomanometer.
   b. Write down your blood pressure readings and bring them to your next visit.
   c. Avoid adding salt to your food at the table.
   d. Take your blood pressure medicine every morning.

6. Which of the following would indicate the need for emergent referral of a patient with hypertension?
   a. A blood pressure of 180/112 mmHg with a severe headache
   b. Orthostatic hypotension from an α-blocker
   c. A blood pressure of 165/99 mmHg with anxiety
   d. Newly diagnosed hypertension with a blood pressure of 162/100 mmHg

7. A patient with hypertension and worsening blood pressure control is referred for a comprehensive medication review. He currently takes lisinopril 20 mg daily, HCTZ 25 mg daily, and amlodipine 5 mg daily for his blood pressure and reports adherence. During the review it is discovered that the patient has been taking OTC naproxen twice daily for back pain. Which of the following is the most appropriate categorization of the medication-related problem?
   a. Adverse effect
   b. Dosage too high
   c. Need for additional medication
   d. Ineffective medication

8. A 65-year-old white male was recently diagnosed with diabetes and hypertension. His blood pressure today is 152/102 mmHg. Which of the following is the most appropriate for management of his blood pressure?
   a. Initiate lisinopril 10 mg daily.
   b. Initiate lisinopril 10 mg daily plus HCTZ 12.5 mg daily.
   c. Initiate amlodipine 10 mg daily.
   d. Initiate terazosin 2 mg HS.

9. A 42-year-old female has a history of hypertension, severe migraines, and generalized anxiety disorder. She currently takes lisinopril 20 mg daily for her blood pressure. Her BP today is 145/92, and her pulse is 82. Which of the following is most appropriate for management of her hypertension?
   a. Add atenolol.
   b. Add hydrochlorothiazide.
   c. Add valsartan.
   d. Add verapamil.

10. During a comprehensive medication review with a patient who has diabetes, the MTM provider notes that she takes only metoprolol for her blood pressure. The current blood pressure is 148/86 mmHg. Which of the following is the most appropriate communication to the patient's physician?
    a. The metoprolol is not working for her blood pressure. Please change it.
    b. Please consider the addition of ramipril 2.5 mg daily.
    c. A β-blocker is not a good choice in diabetes. Please switch to an ACE (angiotensin-converting enzyme) inhibitor.
    d. Recommend continuing metoprolol at current dose.

ANSWERS

1. b	2. a	3. d
4. b	5. a	6. a
7. a	8. b	9. d
10. b		

28

Incontinence MTM Data Set

Katherine Vogel Anderson, PharmD, BCACP, and Sarah E. Honaker, PharmD

KEY POINTS

- Medication therapy management (MTM) providers should screen for medications that may contribute to urinary incontinence.
- A combination of behavioral and drug therapies is the mainstay of treatment of urinary incontinence. Adherence to behavioral therapies should be assessed at each MTM encounter.
- Medications for urinary incontinence are often difficult to tolerate because of the anticholinergic effects; elderly patients may be particularly susceptible to these adverse effects.
- MTM providers should work with the patient and the prescriber to find the most acceptable regimen and help manage the adverse effects of medications for urinary incontinence.

INTRODUCTION TO INCONTINENCE

The simplistic definition of urinary incontinence (UI) is involuntary loss of urine.[1-3] The exact prevalence of urinary incontinence is difficult to determine, but it is estimated that 22% of American adults suffer from some type of incontinence. UI is more common in women than in men. Data suggest that about one-quarter of young women, half of all postmenopausal women, and three-quarters of elderly women in nursing homes have some form of UI. Only 9% of men, regardless of age, have some variation of UI.[1,2]

The lower urinary tract includes the bladder, urethra, urinary sphincter, and surrounding connective tissue, nerves, and blood vessels. Under normal circumstances, the bladder detrusor muscle relaxes during filling and contracts during emptying, while the urinary sphincter contracts during filling to prevent urine leakage and relaxes during emptying. These actions are mediated by the parasympathetic nervous system. Acetylcholine activity at muscarinic receptors throughout the urinary tract mediates urinary function. Usually, the bladder and sphincter work in unison. However, if anything disrupts this balance, then UI may result (see Table 28-1). Medications that influence the function of the lower urinary tract are presented in Table 28-2, and reversible causes of UI are outlined in Figure 28-1. There are several different types of UI; urge incontinence is the most common.

Incontinence Definitions[3]

- *Urge UI* (also known as *overactive bladder* [OAB])—involuntary leakage of urine accompanied by, or immediately preceded by, urgency; usually due to overactive, involuntary bladder contractions; the most common type of UI
- *Stress UI*—Involuntary leakage of urine on exertion; usually due to a change in intra-abdominal pressure while coughing, sneezing, or exercising
- *Overflow UI*—An uncommon type of UI that results when the bladder is full, but unable to empty, causing urine to leak
- *Functional UI*—Inability of a normally continent person to reach the toilet in time; usually due to cognitive disorder (e.g., dementia), or limited mobility (e.g., following surgery)
- *Mixed UI*—Involuntary loss of urine associated with urgency and/or exertion

Urinary incontinence has both physical and psychological complications, which are schematically represented in Figure 28-2.

TABLE 28-1 • Differentiating Bladder Overactivity from Urethral Underactivity

Symptoms	Bladder Overactivity	Urethral Underactivity
Urgency (strong, sudden desire to void)	Yes	Not common
Frequency with urgency	Yes	Rarely
Leaking during physical activity (eg, coughing, sneezing, lifting)	No	Yes
Amount of urinary leakage with each episode of incontinence	Large if present	Usually small
Ability to reach the toilet in time following an urge to void	No or just barely	Yes
Nocturnal incontinence (presence of wet pads or undergarments in bed)	Yes	Rare
Nocturia (waking to pass urine at night)	Usually	Seldom

Source: Reproduced, with permission, from DiPiro JT, Talbert RL, Yee GC, Matzke GR, Wells BG, Posey LM, eds. *Pharmacotherapy: A Pathophysiologic Approach*, 10th ed. New York, NY: McGraw-Hill; 2017.

Patients with UI may feel socially isolated or fear participation in normal activities because of fear of an incontinent episode.[2,5]

Therapeutic Goals for UI

When treating UI, the goals of therapy are to reduce and/or eliminate symptoms, improve quality of life, and prevent complications. The best treatment plan begins with a thorough evaluation, so that reversible causes of UI may be identified and treated.[5,6] If no reversible causes of UI are identified, a combination of nonpharmacologic and pharmacologic types of treatment may be prescribed. As OAB is the most common type of UI, the rest of this chapter will focus on MTM for patients with OAB. It is important to note that UI is not a disease; rather, it is a symptom complex that is seldom life-threatening.[6] As such,

Use the mnemonic **"DIAPERS"** to remember reversible causes:[4]

D – Delirium
I – Infection
A – Atrophic vaginitis
P – Psychiatric disorders or Pharmacological causes
E – Excessive urine output (eg, diabetes, heart failure)
R – Restricted mobility (eg, Parkinson disease, osteoarthritis, rheumatoid arthritis, stroke)
S – Stool impaction

FIGURE 28-1 Reversible causes of urinary incontinence.

TABLE 28-2 • Medications that Influence Lower-Urinary-Tract Function

Medication	Effect
Diuretics, acetylcholinesterase inhibitors	Polyuria resulting in urinary frequency, urgency
α-Receptor antagonists	Urethral muscle relaxation and stress urinary incontinence
α-Receptor agonists	Urethral muscle contraction (increased urethral closure forces) resulting in urinary retention (more common in men)
Calcium channel blockers	Urinary retention due to reduced bladder contractility
Narcotic analgesics	Urinary retention due to reduced bladder contractility
Sedative hypnotics	Functional incontinence caused by delirium, immobility
Antipsychotic agents	Anticholinergic effects resulting in reduced bladder contractility and urinary retention
Anticholinergics	Urinary retention due to reduced bladder contractility
Antidepressants, tricyclic	Anticholinergic effects resulting in reduced bladder contractility, and α-antagonist effects resulting in urethral smooth muscle contraction (increased urethral closure forces) both contributing to urinary retention
Alcohol	Polyuria resulting in urinary frequency, urgency
ACEIs[a]	Cough as a result of ACEIs may aggravate stress urinary incontinence

[a] Angiotensin-converting enzyme inhibitors.

Source: Reproduced, with permission, from DiPiro JT, Talbert RL, Yee GC, Matzke GR, Wells BG, Posey LM, eds. *Pharmacotherapy: A Pathophysiologic Approach*, 10th ed. New York, NY: McGraw-Hill; 2017.

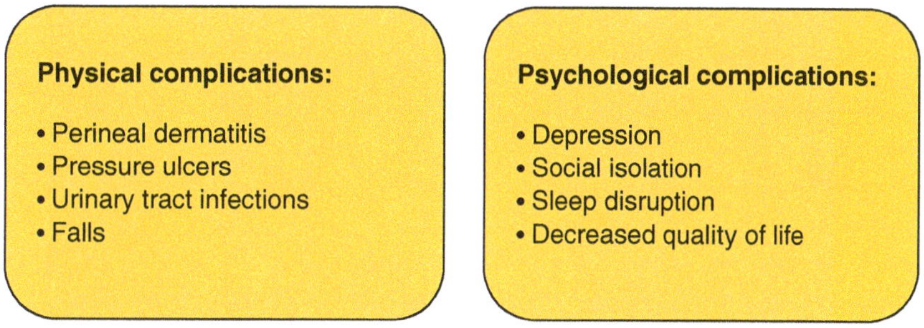

FIGURE 28-2 Complications of urinary incontinence.

after diagnosis and/or treatment of secondary causes of UI, a patient may choose not to be treated with medications at all.[6]

Although men may be less affected by UI, both men and women are treated in a similar manner. However, if it is determined that the male patient has UI caused by benign prostatic hyperplasia (BPH), the treatment modalities presented in this chapter could potentially worsen BPH symptoms. Instead, BPH symptoms should be managed with an α-blocker and/or a 5-α-reductase inhibitor.

Therapeutic Failures

Treatment of UI is a balance of risk and benefit. Medications used to treat UI may be difficult to tolerate, given the anticholinergic side effect profile. Of particular importance is the use of these drugs in the elderly, who are more susceptible to falls and mental status changes. In particular, patients with Alzheimer disease who are taking a cholinesterase inhibitor are at increased risk of mental status changes when an anticholinergic medication is added.[5,6]

Treatment failures occur when patients do not achieve desired symptom relief, or when they are unable to tolerate treatment due to adverse events (Table 28-3).[6]

CORE ELEMENT 1—COMPREHENSIVE MEDICATION REVIEW FOR PATIENTS WITH OVERACTIVE BLADDER

A list of suggested questions to use when conducting a medication therapy review in a patient with overactive bladder (OAB) is presented in Table 28-4. The number and types of questions will depend on several factors, including the amount of time for the interview, number of concurrent medication-related problems (MRPs), urgency of MRPs, and the reliability of the patient in providing accurate information, among others. In time-limited interactions or in complex cases with multiple medical issues, the MTM provider may choose to target questions that help to identify or rule out issues of an urgent nature (see questions to ask for

TABLE 28-3 • Adverse Event Incidence Rates with Approved Drugs for Bladder Overactivity[a]

Drug	Dry Mouth	Constipation	Dizziness	Vision Disturbance
Oxybutynin IR	71	15	17	10
Oxybutynin XL	61	13	6	14
Oxybutynin TDS	7	3	NR	3
Oxybutynin gel	10	1	3	3
Tolterodine	35	7	5	3
Tolterodine LA	23	6	2	4
Trospium chloride IR	20	10	NR	1
Trospium chloride XR	11	9	NR	2
Solifenacin	20	9	2	5
Darifenacin ER	24	18	2	2
Fesoterodine ER	27	5	NR	3
Mirabegron ER	3	3	3	NR

[a] All values constitute mean data, predominantly using product information from the manufacturers.

Abbreviations: ER/XR = extended release; IR = immediate release; LA = long-acting; NR = not reported; TDS = transdermal system.

Source: Reproduced, with permission, from DiPiro JT, Talbert RL, Yee GC, Matzke GR, Wells BG, Posey LM, eds. *Pharmacotherapy: A Pathophysiologic Approach*, 10th ed. New York, NY: McGraw-Hill; 2017.

TABLE 28-4 • Questions to Ask When Conducting a Medication Review in a Patient with Overactive Bladder

Suggested Questions for the Patient with Overactive Bladder
How long have you been experiencing overactive bladder? When were you diagnosed? Have you spoken to your physician about exercises and treatments to prevent your overactive bladder symptoms? What medications are you taking for your overactive bladder? Have you experienced any side effects from your overactive bladder medication(s)? Have you ever stopped taking your prescribed medications for overactive bladder without telling your physician? If so, why? What over-the-counter (OTC) medications or herbals do you use for OAB? What has your physician discussed with you regarding OTC medications or supplements that you should avoid because they can worsen your overactive bladder?
Questions to Ask for Prevention/Assessment of Medical Emergencies
Have you experienced any blood in your urine? Have you experienced any severe side effects of your overactive bladder medication(s) such as swelling of the face, lips, and tongue that may affect breathing? Have you experienced any noticeable changes in your brain function, including memory, since starting your overactive bladder medication(s)?

prevention/assessment of medical emergencies). MTM providers should remember to use living room language during the interview (Figure 28-3), and to be prepared for questions that patients might ask regarding UI (Table 28-5).

CORE ELEMENT 2—PERSONAL MEDICATION LIST[8]

A sample personal medication list (PML) for a patient with OAB is provided in Figure 28-4. This example is representative only of medications for OAB. Additional medications for other disease states should be added and listed separately. MTM providers should remember to use plain language when creating the PML.

CORE ELEMENT 3—MEDICATION ACTION PLAN[8]

Sample medication action plans (MAPs) for patients with OAB are presented in Figure 28-5. These examples are representative only of action steps for the patient with OAB. MAPs for other disease

Adverse event—something bad that happens, bad reaction, unexplained or unwanted effects.
Angioedema—a rare side effect of some overactive bladder medications and a medical emergency involving rapid swelling of the lips, tongue, and throat that may affect breathing.
Antimuscarinic—a type of medication used for urinary incontinence by relaxing bladder muscles and increasing the amount that the bladder can hold.
BMI—body mass index; a measure of weight in relation to height that assigns people to a weight class of underweight, normal weight, overweight, or obese according to the amount of excess weight.
Chronic—constant, never-ending, does not go away.
Chronic kidney disease—when the kidneys are unable to work well, which may cause high blood pressure and other serious health problems.
Creatinine test—a test that checks how well the kidneys are working; an increase indicates that the kidneys are not working well.
Diuretic—water pill.
Electrolytes—a type of necessary salt found in blood, such as sodium, potassium, and calcium.
Elevate—raise, make higher.
Functional incontinence—urinary incontinence due to a physical problem such as arthritis or dementia preventing one from getting to the bathroom in time.
Hypertension—high blood pressure that increases the chance of heart attack, stroke, and kidney disease.
Hypotension—low blood pressure.
Lifestyle changes—your physician may have recommended changes in lifestyle to help your urinary incontinence, which for some patients include reaching a goal weight, decreasing the amount of caffeine consumed, or quitting smoking.
Obese—having a body mass index (BMI) of >30, which increases the risk of developing high blood pressure, diabetes, cardiovascular disease, and incontinence.
Obstructive uropathy—when the flow of urine is blocked, which may cause high blood pressure.
Orthostatic hypotension—dizziness or lightheadedness on standing because of low blood pressure.
Overactive bladder (OAB)—urinary incontinence consisting of an urgent need to go to the bathroom, possibly without making it in time and leaking urine.
Overflow incontinence—urinary incontinence, more common in men caused by a more limited ability to empty the bladder completely, causing leakage once the bladder is full.
Overweight—having a body mass index (BMI) of >25, which increases the risk of developing high blood pressure, diabetes, cardiovascular disease, and incontinence.
Stress incontinence—urinary incontinence as a result of increased pressure in the gut, such as laughing, coughing, and exercising.
Topically—applied to the skin.
Urge incontinence—see *Overactive bladder*.
Urinary incontinence—the loss of bladder control, which can range from leaking urine when coughing, laughing, or sneezing to having a sudden uncontrollable urge to urinate without getting to a toilet in time.

FIGURE 28-3 Living room language for incontinence.

TABLE 28-5 • Questions to Anticipate Regarding Overactive Bladder

- **What is urinary incontinence?**
  Urinary incontinence is the loss of bladder control, which can range from leaking urine when coughing, laughing, or sneezing to having a sudden uncontrollable urge to urinate without getting to a toilet in time.
- **What is overactive bladder (urge incontinence)?**
  Overactive bladder is a type of urinary incontinence consisting of an urgent need to go to the bathroom, possibly without making it in time and leaking urine.
- **What causes overactive bladder?**
  Symptoms of overactive bladder can be the result of many different causes. Urine production may be increased as a result of increased fluid intake, poor kidney function, diuretics ("water pills"), and diabetes. Other factors may be neurological disorders such as Parkinson disease, stroke, and multiple sclerosis, or bladder problems such as tumors or bladder stones, enlarged prostate, and drinking caffeine or alcohol.
- **Why are overactive bladder medications important?**
  It is important to control overactive bladder with medications if other options have failed and your symptoms are affecting your daily activities.
- **Can I just stop my medications if I feel okay?**
  Abruptly stopping medications can sometimes lead to a worsening of symptoms; this is why it is important to speak with your physician first.
- **When should I call my physician?**
  Call your physician if you experience severe side effects of your medications, such as changes in cognitive (thinking) function and memory or sudden swelling of the face, lips, tongue, and neck. You should also let your physician know if your medication for overactive bladder is not working after 4-8 weeks. Any blood in your urine, fever, lower back pain, or other abnormalities should be reported as well.
- **What should I do if I have a problem with my medications?**
  Do not abruptly stop taking your overactive bladder medication without consulting your physician. Speak with your physician and/or pharmacist to let them know about any problems you are having, and together you can make sure your medications are the right ones for you.

Source: Reference 7.

PERSONAL MEDICATION LIST FOR *<Insert patient's name, DOB: mm/dd/yyyy>*	
Medication: Ditropan XL (oxybutynin) 5 mg	
How I use it: Take one tablet (5 mg) every morning	
Why I use it: To prevent accidents with urine	**Prescriber:** Jones
Date I started using it: 10/27/2016	**Date I stopped using it:** (*Leave blank for patient's notes*)
Why I stopped using it: (*Leave blank for patient's notes*)	

FIGURE 28-4 Sample personal medication list for OAB patients.

DATE PREPARED: *<Insert date>*	
What we talked about: You reported that you have trouble with an overactive bladder. It is important to address this issue with your physician.	
What I need to do: Here are some things I can do to help control my overactive bladder symptoms: 1. Speak with my physician about possible ways to help control symptoms such as bladder training, bladder control strategies, pelvic floor muscle training, and fluid management. 2. If these options do not help, speak with my physician about possible medications that can help control my overactive bladder.	**What I did and when I did it:** (*Leave blank for patient's notes*)
What we talked about: It is important to know the benefit and possible side effects of oxybutynin for overactive bladder.	
What I need to do: 1. Speak with my physician or pharmacist about possible side effects, such as constipation that I may experience while taking oxybutynin for my overactive bladder. 2. Keep a diary of my bladder control issues to bring to my next appointment. 3. Inform my physician or pharmacist if I begin to experience any side effects that interfere with my daily activities.	**What I did and when I did it:** (*Leave blank for patient's notes*)

FIGURE 28-5 Sample medication action plans for a patient with OAB.

states or other MRPs should be added and listed separately. In general, only a few of the most important action steps should be listed, so as not to overwhelm the patient. Other areas for patient self-management can be addressed at later visits. MTM providers should remember to use plain language when creating the MAP.

CORE ELEMENT 4—INTERVENTION AND/OR REFERRAL

Interventions for management of OAB include lifestyle modifications and/or drug therapy. Patients not adequately controlled with lifestyle modifications should be started on drug therapy. Medications should be selected on the basis of patient characteristics such as age, cost, patient preference, and other comorbid disease states. Patients should be encouraged to keep a log of urinary symptoms and to follow up at regular intervals so that OAB control may be assessed. Table 28-6 summarizes lifestyle modifications, and Table 28-7 highlights nonpharmacologic therapy. Tables 28-8 and 28-9 and provide an overview of OAB drug therapy. Table 28-10 outlines herbal remedies that may be useful in the management of OAB. The OAB treatment algorithm, the AUA recommendations for treatment of OAB, and criteria for referral for management of OAB are found in Figure 28-6, Table 28-11, and Figure 28-7, respectively.

TABLE 28-6 • Lifestyle Modifications for Management of OAB

Modification	Recommendation
Cigarette smoking	Cigarette smoking is associated with incontinence. Although data are lacking to assess the effect of smoking cessation on OAB, it is still recommended to stop smoking.
Weight management	Obesity is associated with incontinence. Data show that weight loss is associated with a reduction in OAB symptoms.
Fluid intake	Only for patients with an abnormally high fluid intake (>3000 mL/day) should fluid restriction be advised.
Caffeine	Caffeine can cause detrusor overactivity. Reduction in caffeine intake can reduce the number of incontinence episodes.

Source: References 6 and 9.

TABLE 28-7 • Nonpharmacologic Management of Urinary Incontinence

Intervention	Description	Patient Characteristics
Lifestyle modifications		
Behavioral changes (eg, fluid and caffeine modifications, smoking cessation, weight loss, constipation prevention)	Self-management strategies targeted toward reducing or eliminating risk factors that cause or exacerbate UI	Used as first-line therapies or in combination with pharmacologic treatment in patients with stress, urgency, and mixed incontinence
Scheduling regimens		
Timed voiding	Toileting on a fixed schedule where interval does not change, typically every 2 hours during waking hours	Used for patients with cognitive or physical impairments
Habit retraining	Scheduled toiletings with adjustments of voiding intervals (longer or shorter) on the basis of the patient's voiding pattern	Used for institutionalized or homebound patients with cognitive or physical impairments
Prompted voiding	Scheduled toiletings that require prompts to void from a caregiver, typically every 2 hours; patient assisted in toileting only if response is positive; used in conjunction with operant conditioning techniques for rewarding patients for maintaining continence and appropriate toileting	Used for patients who are functionally able to use toilet or toilet substitute, able to feel urge sensation, and able to request toileting assistance appropriately; used primarily in institutional settings or in homebound patients with an available caregiver
Bladder training	Scheduled toiletings with progressive voiding intervals; includes teaching urgency suppression strategies using relaxation and distraction techniques, self-monitoring, and use of reinforcement techniques; sometimes combined with drug therapy	Used for stress, urgency, and mixed incontinence in patients who are cognitively intact, able to toilet, and motivated to comply with training program
Pelvic floor muscle rehabilitation		
Pelvic floor muscle exercises (eg, Kegel exercises)	Regular practice of pelvic floor muscle contractions; may involve use of pelvic floor muscle contraction for prevention of stress leakage and urge inhibition	Used for stress, urgency, and mixed incontinence in patients who can isolate and correctly contract pelvic floor muscles; requires cognitively intact and highly motivated patient
Biofeedback	Use of electronic or mechanical instruments to display visual or auditory information about neuromuscular or bladder activity; used to teach correct pelvic floor muscle contraction or urge inhibition; home trainers available	Used for stress, urgency, and mixed incontinence in patients who have the capability to learn voluntary control through observation and are motivated; used in conjunction with pelvic floor muscle exercises
Vaginal weight training	Active retention of increasing vaginal weights; typically used in combination with pelvic floor muscle exercises at least twice per day	Women with stress incontinence who are cognitively intact, can correctly contract pelvic floor muscles, are able to stand, and have sufficient vaginal vault and introitus to retain cone, and are highly motivated; contraindicated in patients with moderate to severe pelvic organ prolapse

(*Continued*)

TABLE 28-7 • Nonpharmacologic Management of Urinary Incontinence (*Continued*)

Intervention	Description	Patient Characteristics
External neuromodulation		
Nonimplantable electrical stimulation	Application of electric current through vaginal, anal, surface, or fine-needle electrodes; used to inhibit bladder overactivity and improve awareness, contractility, and efficacy of pelvic floor muscle contraction; handheld stimulators for home use are available	Used for stress, urgency, and mixed incontinence in patients who are highly motivated; contraindicated in patients with diminished sensory perception; urinary retention, history of cardiac arrhythmia, cardiac pacemakers, or implantable defibrillators; also contraindicated in patients who are pregnant or attempting pregnancy; vaginal or anal electrodes are contraindicated in moderate or severe pelvic organ prolapse
Percutaneous tibial nerve stimulation	Application of a pulsed electrical current through a fine needle electrode placed externally near the tibial nerve	Used for treatment of overactive bladder with urinary urgency, frequency, and urgency incontinence; contraindicated in patients with pacemakers or implantable defibrillators, and in patients prone to excessive bleeding, or women who are pregnant
Extracorporeal magnetic electrical stimulation	Pulsed magnetic stimulation to pelvic floor musculature causing depolarization of motor neurons, thus inducing pelvic floor muscle contraction; stimulation is provided through a specially designed chair that contains a device for producing a pulsing magnetic field	Used for treatment of stress, urgency, and mixed incontinence; contraindicated in patients with demand cardiac pacemakers or metallic joint replacements; may be a useful treatment option when other approaches fail or are not feasible
Alternative medicine therapies		
Acupuncture	Involves insertion of disposable sterile fine stainless-steel needles into points on the skin that are thought to suppress or stimulate spinal and/or supraspinal reflexes to the bladder and/or urethra	Used for stress, urgency, and mixed incontinence and UI due to spinal cord injury
Anti-incontinence devices		
Bed or pant alarms	Sensor devices that respond to wetness; used to awaken or alert individuals via noise or vibrating mechanism	Primarily used for nocturnal enuresis in children; system available for monitoring incontinence in homecare and institutional environments
Pessaries	Intravaginal devices designed to support the bladder neck, relieve minor to moderate pelvic organ prolapse, and change pressure transmission to the urethra	Used for female stress incontinence and mild to moderate pelvic organ prolapse; in postmenopausal women, topical estrogen therapy is typically prescribed to prevent ulceration and breakdown of vaginal tissue; requires good manual dexterity to manipulate device
Urethral insert (women only)	Intraurethral device	Used in female patients with stress incontinence who are cognitively intact and have good manual dexterity
Urethral compression device (men only)	Penile clamp	Used in adult male patients with stress incontinence who are cognitively intact and have good manual dexterity
External collection devices (men only)	Condom catheter with leg bag	Used in men with urgency, stress, and overflow incontinence and in those with functional impairments
Catheters	Disposable, intermittent urethral catheters and indwelling urethral and suprapubic catheters	Used for overflow incontinence; used in patients who are bedbound or with significant mobility impairments and severe incontinence; those with terminal illness; those with sacral pressure ulcers until healing occurs
Supportive interventions		
Toileting substitutes and other environmental modifications	Female and male urinals, bedside commodes, elevated toilet seats	Used for patients with mobility impairments that make reaching toilet in timely fashion difficult

(*Continued*)

TABLE 28-7 • Nonpharmacologic Management of Urinary Incontinence (*Continued*)

Intervention	Description	Patient Characteristics
Absorbent products	Variety of reusable and disposable liners, pads, male drip collectors, male guard, collector undergarment, fitted brief, and pant systems; some products contain a polymer that absorbs and wicks urine away from the body	Used for all types of incontinence
Physical therapy	Gait and/or strength training	Used for older patients with mobility impairments that make reaching a toilet in timely fashion difficult

Source: Reproduced, with permission, from DiPiro JT, Talbert RL, Yee GC, Matzke GR, Wells BG, Posey LM, eds. *Pharmacotherapy: A Pathophysiologic Approach*, 10th ed. New York, NY: McGraw-Hill; 2017.

TABLE 28-8 • Medications for Management of OAB

Medication Class and Drug Examples	Common/Serious Side Effects[a]	Blackbox Warnings / Contraindications	Pregnancy Category[b]
Antimuscarinics Darifenacin (D) Fesoterodine (FE) Flavoxate (FL) Solifenacin (S) Tolterodine (TO) Trospium (TR)	Constipation Confusion Xerostomia Headache Immune hypersensitivity reaction Angioedema Solifenacin, Tolterodine: QT prolongation Angioedema	Achalasia (FL) Bladder obstruction (FL) Closed-angle glaucoma (D, FE, S, TO, TR) Gastroparesis (D, FE, S, TO, TR) GI bleeding (FL) GI obstruction (D, FE, S, TO, TR) Ileus (FL) Urethral stricture (FL) Pyloric stenosis (D, FE, S, TO, TR) Urinary retention Urinary-tract obstruction (FL)	All C except flavoxate, which is category B
Mixed action Oxybutynin	Application site rash and pruritus (topical) Constipation Diarrhea Xerostomia UTI Nasopharyngitis Angioedema	Closed-angle glaucoma Gastroparesis GI obstruction Pyloric stenosis Urinary retention	B
Acetylcholine release inhibitor/neuromuscular blocking agent OnabotulinumtoxinA	Urinary retention UTI Dysuria Hematuria Autonomic dysreflexia	Botulism Infection Urinary retention UTI	C
β_3-Agonist Mirabegron	Hypertension Headache UTI Nasopharyngitis	None	C

[a] This is a general list and does not include all side effects that can occur from these drugs. Consult a drug reference source for a more inclusive list before making any recommendations. MTM providers should also consult a comprehensive drug interaction database before making pharmacotherapy recommendations.

[b] Product labeling for all prescription drugs is being updated to reflect the new FDA Pregnancy Labeling and Lactation Rule. Please check individual product labeling for the most accurate and updated pregnancy information.

Abbreviations: GI = gastrointestinal; UTI = urinary tract infection.

Source: Data compiled from reference 10.

TABLE 28-9 • Dosing of Anticholinergic/Antimuscarinic Medications Approved for OAB or UUI

Drug	Brand Name	Initial Dose	Usual Range	Special Population Dose	Comments
Oxybutynin IR	Ditropan	2.5 mg twice daily	2.5-5 mg twice daily-four times daily		Titrate in increments of 2.5 mg/day every 1-2 months; available in oral solution
Oxybutynin XL	Ditropan XL	5-10 mg once daily	5-30 mg once daily		Adjust dose in 5 mg increments at weekly interval; swallow whole
Oxybutynin TDS	Oxytrol Oxytrol for Women (OTC)		3.9 mg/day; apply one patch twice weekly		Apply every 3-4 days; rotate application site
Oxybutynin gel 10%	Gelnique		One sachet (100 mg) topically daily		Apply to clean, dry, intact skin on abdomen, thighs, or upper arms/shoulders; contains alcohol
Oxybutynin gel 3%	Gelnique 3%		Three pumps (84 mg) topically daily		Same as above
Tolterodine IR	Detrol		1-2 mg twice daily	1 mg twice daily if patient is taking CYP3A4 inhibitors, or with renal/hepatic impairment	
Tolterodine LA	Detrol LA		2-4 mg once daily	2 mg once daily in those who are taking CYP3A4 inhibitors or with renal/hepatic impairment	Swallow whole; avoid in patients with CrCl ≤10 mL/min
Trospium chloride IR	Sanctura		20 mg twice daily	20 mg once daily in patients aged ≥75 years or CrCl ≤ 30 mL/min (≤0.5 mL/s)	Take 1 hour before meals or on empty stomach; patients aged ≥75 years should take at bedtime
Trospium chloride ER	Sanctura XR		60 mg once daily	Avoid in patients aged ≥75 years or creatinine clearance ≤30 mL/min (≤0.5 mL/s)	Take 1 hour before meals or on empty stomach; swallow whole
Solifenacin	VESIcare	5 mg daily	5-10 mg once daily	5 mg daily if patient is taking CYP3A4 inhibitors or with creatinine clearance ≤30 mL/min (≤0.5 mL/s) or moderate hepatic impairment; avoid in severe hepatic impairment	Swallow whole
Darifenacin ER	Enablex	7.5 mg once daily	7.5-15 mg once daily	7.5 mg daily if patient is taking potent CYP3A4 inhibitors or with moderate hepatic impairment; avoid in severe hepatic impairment	Titrate dose after ≥2 weeks; swallow whole
Fesoterodine ER	Toviaz	4 mg once daily	4-8 mg once daily	4 mg daily if patient is taking potent CYP3A4 inhibitors or with CrCl ≤ 30 mL/min (≤0.5 mL/s); avoid in severe hepatic impairment	Prodrug (metabolized to 5-hydroxymethyl tolterodine); swallow whole
β_3-Adrenergic agonist					
Mirabegron ER	Myrbetriq	25 mg once daily	25-50 mg once daily	25 mg once daily if CrCl = 15-29 mL/min (0.25-0.49 mL/s) or moderate hepatic impairment; avoid in patients with ESRD or severe hepatic impairment	Swallow whole

Abbreviations: CrCl = creatinine clearance; CYP = cytochrome P450 enzyme; ER = extended release; ESRD = end-stage renal disease; IR = immediate release; LA = long-acting; OAB = overactive bladder; OTC = over the counter; TDS = transdermal system; UUI = urge urinary incontinence; XL = extended release.

Source: Reproduced, with permission, from DiPiro JT, Talbert RL, Yee GC, Matzke GR, Wells BG, Posey LM, eds. *Pharmacotherapy: A Pathophysiologic Approach*, 10th ed. New York, NY: McGraw-Hill; 2017.

TABLE 28-10 • Herbal Supplements for OAB

Supplement	Recommended Dosage	Grade[a]	Cost[b]
Chondroitin sulfate	200-400 mg twice daily-three times daily or 800-1200 mg once daily	Insufficient evidence	$
Cranberry	500 mg capsule three times daily (reduce odor from incontinence)	Insufficient evidence	$$

[a] Level of evidence: "Likely effective"—this product has a very high level of reliable clinical evidence supporting its use for a specific indication. Products rated "likely effective" are generally considered appropriate to recommend; "possibly effective"—this product has some clinical evidence supporting its use for a specific indication; however, the evidence is limited by quantity, quality, or contradictory findings. Products rated "possibly effective" might be beneficial, but do not have enough high-quality evidence to be recommended for most people; "insufficient evidence"—insufficient reliable scientific evidence to provide an effectiveness rating.

[b] Cost: $ = ≤$10/month supply in recommended dosage; $$ = $11-$20/month.

Source: Data compiled from reference 11.

CORE ELEMENT 5—DOCUMENTATION AND FOLLOW-UP

Clear and succinct documentation of MRPs and recommendations is a key component of the MTM consult. Examples of potential MRPs in patients with OAB are provided in Table 28-12. Sample communications and recommendations to providers to address medication-related issues are found in Figure 28-8. Recommendations may be communicated via fax, telephone, or other means of written or secure electronic communication. The examples below are for illustrative purposes. Actual communications to providers should be individualized according to the type of recommendation, patient-specific characteristics, and the nature of the relationship with the provider.

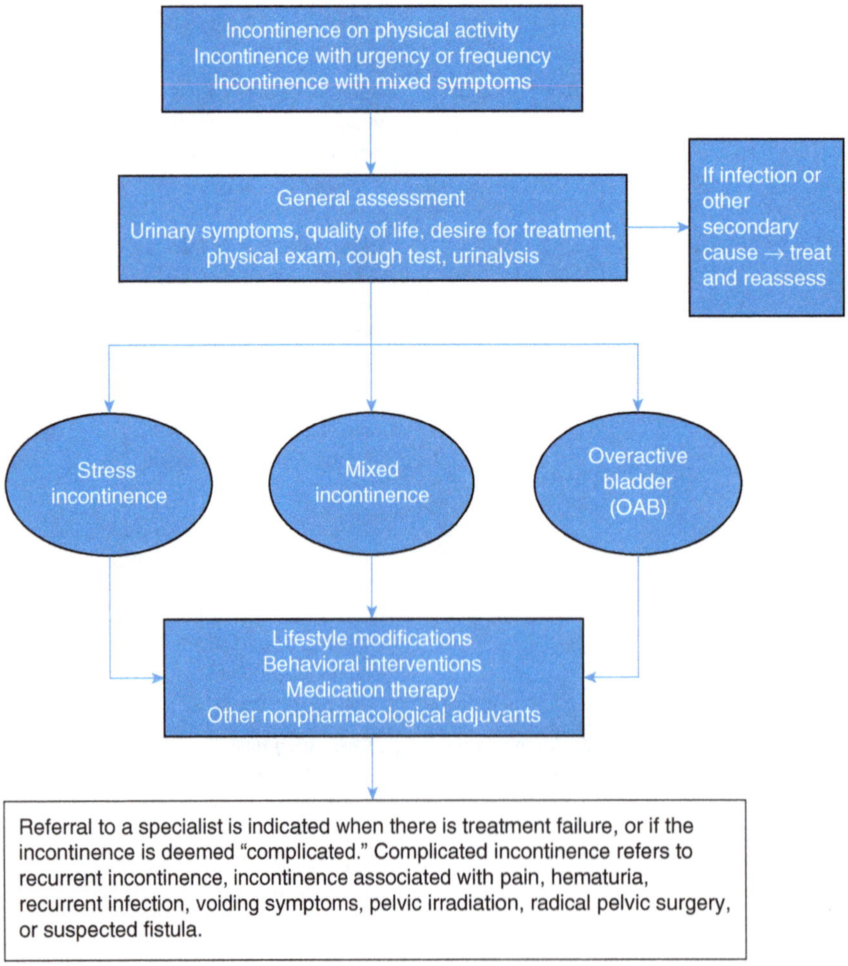

FIGURE 28-6 Treatment algorithm for urinary incontinence.
Source: References 3 and 6.

TABLE 28-11 • AUA Recommendations for Overactive Bladder

First-Line Treatment
Behavioral therapies—bladder training, bladder control strategies, pelvic floor muscle training, fluid management.
Behavioral therapies *may* be combined with antimuscarinic therapies.
Second-Line Treatments
Oral *antimuscarinics* are second-line therapy, after behavior modification. If both immediate-release (IR) and extended-release (ER) formulations are available, the ER should be prescribed.
Transdermal oxybutynin—either the patch or the gel—may be used.
If a patient cannot tolerate one antimuscarinic because of side effects, then a dose modification *or* a different antimuscarinic medication may be tried.
Do *not* use antimuscarinics in patients with narrow-angle glaucoma (unless approved by an ophthalmologist); use antimuscarinics with *caution* in patients with impaired gastric emptying or with a history of urinary retention.
If a patient has constipation or dry mouth, it is better to treat these symptoms (with fluid management, dose modification, or a bowel regimen) *rather than* abandon therapy with an antimuscarinic.
Use *caution* if prescribing antimuscarinics to patients on other anticholinergic drugs.
Frail elderly patients are particularly susceptible to anticholinergic side effects.
A patient refractory to *both* behavioral *and* medical therapies should be referred to a specialist.
Third-Line Treatments
Sacral neuromodulation (SNS) is recommended for patients who are *not* candidates for antimuscarinic therapies *and* who are able to undergo surgery.
Peripheral tibial nerve stimulation (PTNS) is appropriate for carefully selected patients.
Onabotulinumtoxin A—if used, this treatment should be applied only for patients who are refractory to first- and second-line therapies. Such patients *must* be able to return for postvoid residual evaluations *and* be willing to self-catheterize if necessary.
• *Indwelling catheters* are a treatment of last resort.

Source: Reproduced, with permission, from Gormley EA, Lightner DJ, Faraday M, Vasavada SP. Diagnosis and treatment of overactive bladder (non-neurogenic) in adults: AUA/SUFU guideline amendment. *J Urol.* 2015;198:1572-1580.

Follow-up to assess compliance, efficacy, side effects, and possible alternative treatments should be offered to the patient with OAB. The interval for follow-up will depend on a number of factors, including medication regimen, severity of symptoms, type of intervention, and patient-specific factors such as age, comorbid conditions, and ability to return to clinic. Patients should be encouraged to persist with a particular treatment for 4 to 8 weeks before attributing treatment failure to lack of symptom improvement and/or intolerable adverse effects. Suggested intervals for follow-up are provided in Table 28-13.

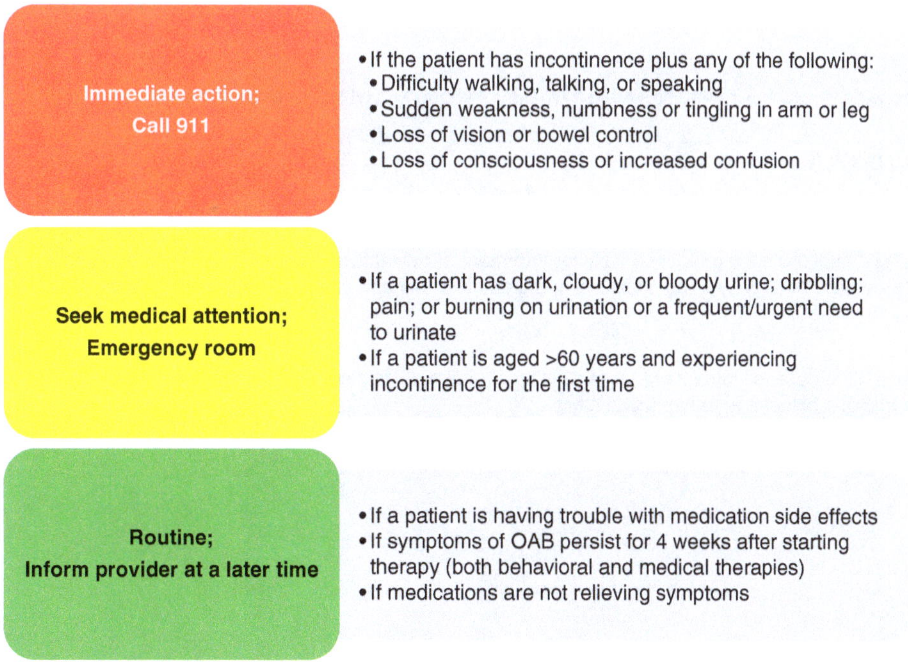

FIGURE 28-7 Referral for management of OAB.
Source: Reference 7.

TABLE 28-12 • Medication-Related Problems (MRPs) in Patients with OAB

Category of MRP	Sample Medication-Related Problem
Nonadherence	Suboptimal symptom control of OAB due to nonadherence with lifestyle modifications (eg, cigarette smoking, high caffeine intake) Suboptimal control of OAB due to patient missing doses of antimuscarinic medications Patient not taking antimuscarinic therapy because of cost
Unnecessary medication	Duplicate therapy (eg, two antimuscarinics)
Need for additional medication	Lifestyle and behavioral modifications have not decreased incontinence symptoms
Ineffective medication	Adequate trial of new antimuscarinic without significant clinical response Anticholinergic side effects are intolerable, so treatment is discontinued
Dosage too low	Suboptimal OAB control on low dose of antimuscarinic agent
Dosage too high	Patient with chronic kidney disease taking extended-release tolterodine that is not dosed appropriately for renal function
Adverse drug event	Mental status change due to anticholinergic side effects Fall secondary to dizziness after starting antimuscarinic therapy

Scenario: Patient is experiencing dry mouth as a side effect of Toviaz (fesoterodine)
MRP: Adverse drug event

Assessment:

Patient taking Toviaz for OAB and experiencing dry mouth. Severity of dry-mouth symptoms should be assessed to determine if it abates over time or requires action such as switching medications or treating dry mouth with another agent.

Plan:

Encourage patient to continue Toviaz for 2-4 more weeks; instruct patient to call provider if symptoms are intolerable.

Follow up to evaluate severity of dry-mouth symptoms.

If no improvement, consider switching patient to another agent such as Vesicare (solifenacin) if appropriate.

Scenario: Patient noncompliant with immediate-release oxybutynin
MRP: Nonadherence

Assessment:

Patient reports being prescribed oxybutynin 5 mg 4 times daily for overactive bladder, but is taking only one tablet daily because of forgetfulness and excessive pill burden. Other agents for overactive bladder require once-daily dosing, such as extended-release oxybutynin, Enablex, and Vesicare.

Plan:

If appropriate, please consider switching immediate-release oxybutynin 5 mg to oxybutynin extended-release 5 mg once daily for control of overactive bladder.

Scenario: Patient taking Detrol (tolterodine) 3 times daily
MRP: Dosage too high

Assessment:

Patient currently receiving Detrol 2 mg tablet 3 times daily for treatment of overactive bladder. The maximum dosage limit recommended by the manufacturer is 2 mg twice daily (4 mg/day). The additional 2 mg/day that this patient is receiving could contribute to increased adverse effects without an increased benefit.

Plan:

Please consider decreasing the dose to Detrol 2 mg twice daily for control of overactive bladder. Additionally, if higher dosing is needed for symptom control, consider a trial of a different agent for this patient.

FIGURE 28-8 Sample provider communications for OAB.

TABLE 28-13 • Suggested Intervals for Follow-up in Patients with OAB

Drug	Adverse Drug Reaction	Monitoring Parameters	Comments
Antimuscarinic			
Oxybutynin IR Oxybutynin XL Oxybutynin TDS Oxybutynin gel 10% Oxybutynin gel 3% Tolterodine IR Tolterodine LA Trospium chloride IR Trospium chloride ER Solifenacin Darifenacin ER Fesoterodine ER	Anticholinergic adverse effects: dry mouth, constipation, headache, dyspepsia, dry eyes, blurred vision, cognitive impairment, tachycardia, sedation, orthostatic hypotension Application-site reactions (topical agents): pruritus, erythema	Contraindications and precautions: urinary retention, gastric retention, severely decreased GI motility, angioedema, myasthenia gravis, uncontrolled narrow-angle glaucoma Worsening of renal/hepatic condition or concomitant drug therapy, which may necessitate dosage reduction or drug cessation Mental status change or risk for falls in elderly or frail patients	In general, ER, LA, XL, and topical products are associated with fewer anticholinergic adverse effects, particularly dry mouth Possible transference of drug from topical application Avoid open fire or smoke until alcohol-based gel has dried
β_3-Adrenergic agonist			
Mirabegron ER	Hypertension, nasopharyngitis, urinary tract infection, headache	Precautions: urinary retention, severe uncontrolled hypertension Worsening of renal/hepatic condition, which may necessitate dosage reduction or drug cessation Increased effect of narrow-therapeutic-index drugs that are CYP2D6 substrates QT prolongation	Mirabegron is a CYP2D6 inhibitor

Abbreviations: CYP = cytochrome P450 enzyme; ER/XL = extended-release; IR = immediate release; LA = long-acting; OAB = overactive bladder; TDS = transdermal system; UUI = urge urinary incontinence.

Source: Reference 2. From Table 85-6 in DiPiro JT, Talbert RL, Yee GC, Matzke GR, Wells BG, Posey LM, eds. *Pharmacotherapy: A Pathophysiologic Approach*, 10th ed. New York, NY: McGraw-Hill; 2017. Available at www.acccesspharmacy.com.

REFERENCES

1. AHRQ. *Evidence-based Practice Center Systematic Review Protocol: Diagnosis and Comparative Effectiveness of Treatments for Urinary Incontinence in Adult Women.* Available at https://effectivehealthcare.ahrq.gov/ehc/products/169/834/urinary-incontinence-treatment-report-130909.pdf. Accessed May 8, 2017.
2. Rovner ES, Wyman J, Lam S. Urinary incontinence. In: DiPiro JT, Talbert RL, Yee GC, Matzke GR, Wells BG, Posey L, et al., eds. *Pharmacotherapy: A Pathophysiologic Approach*, 10th ed. New York, NY: McGraw-Hill; 2017. Available at http://accesspharmacy.mhmedical.com.lp.hscl.ufl.edu/content.aspx?bookid=1861&sectionid=133892819. Accessed May 8, 2017.
3. Abrams P, Anderson KE, Birder L, Brubaker L, et al. Fourth International Consultation on Incontinence Recommendations of the International Scientific Committee: Evaluation and treatment of urinary incontinence, pelvic organ prolapse, and fecal incontinence. *Neurol Urodyn.* 2010;29:213-240.
4. Marshall LL, Bailey W. Urinary incontinence management in geriatric patients. *Consult Pharm.* 2008;23:681-694.
5. Ouslander JG. Management of overactive bladder. *New Engl J Med.* 2004;350:786-799.
6. Gormley EA, Lightner DJ, Faraday M, Vasavada SP. Diagnosis and treatment of overactive bladder (non-neurogenic) in adults: AUA/SUFU guideline amendment. *J Urol.* 2015;198:1572-1580.
7. Marinkovic SP, Rovner ES, Moldwin RM, Stanton SL et al. The management of overactive bladder syndrome. *Br Med J.* 2012;344:e2365.
8. *Medicare Part D Medication Therapy Management Program Standardized Format.* Available at https://www.cms.gov/Medicare/Prescription-Drug-Coverage/PrescriptionDrugCovContra/Downloads/MTM-Program-Standardized-Format-English-and-Spanish-Instructions-Samples-v032712.pdf. Accessed May 7, 2017.
9. Nygaard I. Idiopathic urgency urinary incontinence. *New Engl J Med.* 2010;363:1156-1162.
10. Clinical Pharmacology [database online]. Tampa, FL: Gold Standard, Inc.; 2017. Available at http://www.clinicalpharmacology.com. Accessed May 7, 2017.
11. Natural Medicines [database online]. Somerville, MA: Therapeutic Research Center; 2017. Available at https://naturalmedicines.therapeuticresearch.com/. Accessed May 7, 2017.

Review Questions

1. Which type of incontinence is the same as overactive bladder (OAB)?
   a. Urge incontinence
   b. Stress incontinence
   c. Overflow incontinence
   d. Functional incontinence

2. All of the following are reversible causes of urinary incontinence EXCEPT:
   a. Delirium
   b. Infection
   c. Atrophic vaginitis
   d. Pelvic irradiation

3. A 70-year-old female reports episodes of incontinence at nighttime to her primary care provider. She admits to drinking gingerale immediately before bedtime. She has a past medical history significant for hypertension, and takes amlodipine 5 mg once daily. Which is an appropriate recommendation for treatment of incontinence in this patient?
   a. Change from amlodipine to hydrochlorothiazide to decrease incontinence.
   b. Start oxybutynin 5 mg once daily.
   c. Limit fluid intake prior to bedtime.
   d. Begin cranberry supplements 3 times daily.

4. Which of the following best defines functional incontinence using living room language?
   a. Urinary incontinence consisting of an urgent need to go to the bathroom, possibly without making it in time and leaking urine.
   b. Urinary incontinence due to a physical problem such as arthritis or dementia preventing one from getting to the bathroom in time.
   c. Urinary incontinence as a result of increased pressure in the gut, such as laughing, coughing, or exercising.
   d. Urinary incontinence as a result of a physical disability that prevents one from successfully arriving at the bathroom before urination occurs.

5. All of the following are recommended as appropriate behavioral therapies for a patient to discuss with her/his healthcare provider regarding overactive bladder EXCEPT:
   a. fluid management.
   b. pelvic floor muscle training.
   c. taking an antispasmodic medication such as oxybutynin.
   d. bladder control strategies.

6. Which of the following is an example of when a patient should seek medical attention or go to the emergency room for OAB?
   a. Experiencing dark, cloudy, or bloody urine
   b. Experiencing dry mouth from OAB medication
   c. Experiencing symptoms of OAB for 4 weeks after starting behavioral or medical therapy
   d. Experiencing OAB for the first time, regardless of age

7. Which of the following OAB medication-related problems is matched with the correct category of MRP?
   a. Nonadherence—experiencing dry mouth while on fesoterodine
   b. Dosage too low—patient on low dosage of two antimuscarinic agents
   c. Ineffective medication—adequate trial of antispasmodic without significant symptomatic and clinical response
   d. Adverse drug event—no decrease in incontinence symptoms with behavioral modifications

8. Anticholinergic side effects often limit the tolerability of oxybutynin. Which of the following is an example of an anticholinergic side effect?
   a. Hypertension
   b. Xerostomia
   c. Diarrhea
   d. Sweating

9. A 75-year-old female takes donepezil for mild Alzheimer disease. She lives in an assisted-living facility. It is noted in her chart that she has episodes of incontinence, and the decision is made to prescribe tolterodine. Which of the following adverse drug events is of particular importance with the addition of tolterodine in this patient?
   a. Increased blood pressure
   b. Decreased glucose
   c. Increased confusion
   d. Decreased heart rate

10. How long should a patient be encouraged to take an antispasmodic before declaring a treatment failure due to lack of symptom improvement?
    a. 3-5 days
    b. 1-2 weeks
    c. 2-4 weeks
    d. 4-8 weeks

ANSWERS

1. a	2. d	3. c
4. b	5. c	6. a
7. c	8. b	9. c
10. d		

29

Osteoarthritis MTM Data Set

Eric Dietrich, PharmD

KEY POINTS

- Treatment goals for osteoarthritis (OA) should be identified prior to beginning treatment and should be individualized on a patient-by-patient basis. An acceptable balance between minimizing pain and side effects, while maximizing functionality and quality of life, should be targeted.
- Optimal treatment of OA includes both pharmacologic and nonpharmacologic therapies. Adherence to nonpharmacologic treatment should be assessed at each medication therapy management (MTM) encounter.
- Given the significant adverse effects of chronic treatment with nonsteroidal anti-inflammatory drugs (NSAIDs), reassessment of risk factors such as cardiovascular risk and risk of gastrointestinal bleeding should be conducted during each MTM encounter to ensure safety of continued treatment and potential need for additional medications to reduce risk (eg, proton-pump inhibitors for risk of gastrointestinal bleeding).
- Assessment of potential adverse effects from analgesic therapy should be determined during each MTM encounter. Importantly, bleeding from NSAIDs or constipation, sedation, and/or respiratory depression associated with opioids should be monitored frequently.

INTRODUCTION

Osteoarthritis (OA) is the most common form of arthritis. OA is characterized by damage to the joint and joint structures, commonly in weight-bearing joints such as the hips and knees (Figure 29-1). OA may also occur in non-weight-bearing joints such as the hands. OA affects approximately 27 million Americans,[1] and since the prevalence of disease increases with age, the number of individuals suffering from OA is estimated to increase significantly in the near future.[2] Women are more commonly affected than men, and they also tend to have more joints involved. The prevalence of OA is similar in both African-Americans and Caucasians, although Caucasians are more likely to experience severe disease.

The development of OA is multifactorial and results when biomechanical weaknesses and risk factors combine in a susceptible individual. Increasing age is the most significant risk factor for OA. Other risk factors include a history of trauma, obesity, involvement in certain sports, occupations with repetitive and/or strenuous movements, female gender, and genetic factors.[3]

OA can be broadly categorized as primary or secondary (Table 29-1). Primary OA does not have an identifiable cause and can be further classified as localized, generalized, or erosive. Secondary OA can be attributed to an identifiable cause such as trauma, inflammatory conditions, congenital disorders, endocrine disorders, metabolic disorders, or other conditions that contribute to or increase the risk of developing OA.[3]

The diagnosis of OA is based largely on presenting signs and symptoms, history, and physical exam. The diagnosis may be aided with imaging tests such as x-ray and/or magnetic resonance imaging (MRI), although x-ray may not be helpful early in the disease process. In more advanced disease, joint space narrowing, changes in subchondral bone, and the presence of osteophytes may be visible on imaging, while gross joint changes may be visible on physical exam.[4] Currently no laboratory data clearly diagnose OA, although

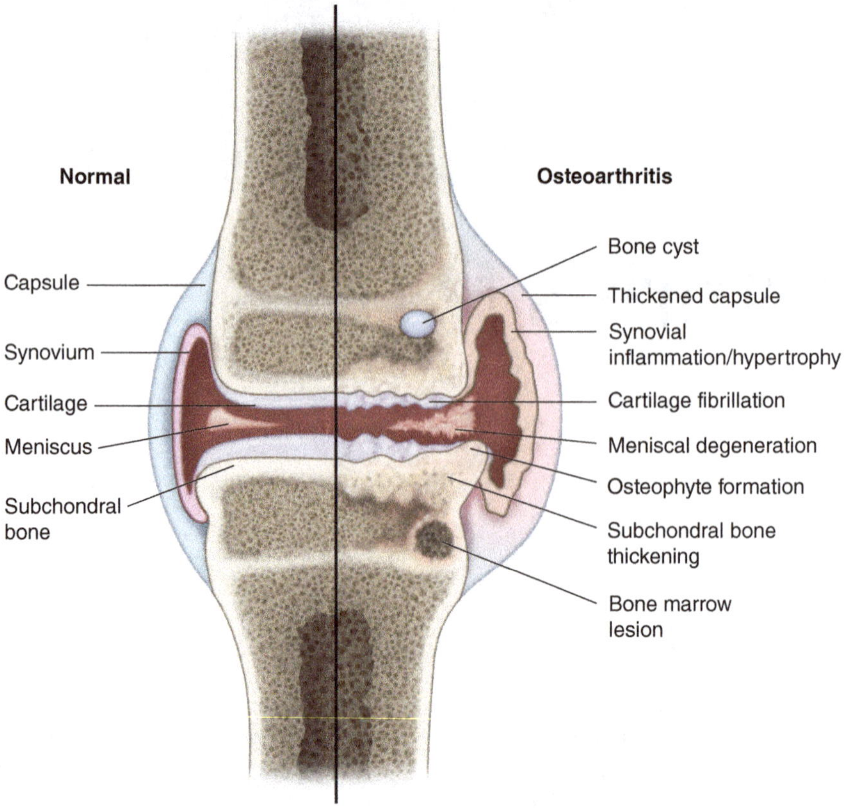

FIGURE 29-1 Characteristics of osteoarthritis in the diarthrodial joint.
Source: Reproduced, with permission, from Loeser RF. Age-related changes in the musculoskeletal system and the development of osteoarthritis. *Clin Geriatr Med*. 2010; 26(3): 371-386.

basic labs and inflammatory markers are often ordered as part of the diagnostic workup.

Complications of Osteoarthritis

Joint damage can occur before patients begin to experience signs or symptoms of OA. Untreated OA can lead to progressive joint damage, pain, impairment in daily activities, disability,[5] and reduced quality of life.[6] OA is a leading cause of chronic disability, and is the leading cause of hip and knee replacement.[7] Appropriate treatment of secondary causes of OA is important to reduce the disease burden of the secondary disease, as well as treat or limit OA progression and its associated complications.

TABLE 29-1 • Classification of Osteoarthritis

Primary Osteoarthritis	Secondary Osteoarthritis
Localized (involving one or two joints) Generalized (involving more than three joints) Erosive	Joint trauma Congenital abnormalities of the joint or joint structures Inflammatory conditions such as rheumatoid arthritis Endocrine disorders such as hyper- or hypothyroidism, acromegaly Metabolic disorders such as gout Genetic predisposition

Source: Reference 3.

Therapeutic Goals for OA

Reduction in pain, improvement in physical functioning and quality of life, and preservation of joint integrity are general treatment goals for OA. Given the variability in presentation, severity of symptoms, location and number of joints involved, and degree of disability, treatment goals must be individualized on a case-by-case basis. Goals of therapy for pain control, physical functioning, and quality of life should be discussed and outlined at diagnosis to allow for continued assessment of the success of treatment. Given the multifactorial nature of OA, treatment must also be multimodal and include both nonpharmacologic and pharmacologic interventions. Treatment success is unlikely without employing nonpharmacologic interventions.[8] Complete relief of pain for some patients may not be an attainable goal without undue treatment burden or adverse effects of drug therapy. Therefore, an acceptable balance between minimizing pain and side effects, while maximizing functionality and quality of life, should be targeted. Use of structured assessment tools to track functional status may be helpful in order to objectively show the benefits of the treatment regimen, if pain cannot be completely relieved.

Treatment Failure

Treatment failure is considered when both pharmacologic and nonpharmacologic interventions fail to meet patient-specific goals of therapy. Often these patients suffer severe disability, pain, and further joint deterioration. Adherence to nonpharmacologic treatment measures such as physical therapy, weight reduction, and exercise should be ensured prior to considering treatment failure of pharmacologic agents. However, severe pain and disability may limit the ability to comply with these interventions. Surgical intervention and/or evaluation for joint replacement are often reserved for those failing medical therapy or those who have significant disability.

CORE ELEMENT 1—COMPREHENSIVE MEDICATION REVIEW FOR PATIENTS WITH OSTEOARTHRITIS

A list of suggested questions to ask when conducting a medication therapy review in a patient with OA is presented in Table 29-2. Questions cover both nonpharmacologic and pharmacologic methods of treatment for OA. The depth and breadth of questions depend on numerous factors such as time available for the interview, number and type of medications, number of medication-related problems (MRPs), severity of identified problems, and ability to obtain accurate and reliable information. Targeted questions concerning only potentially urgent medical problems or side effects may be required in situations with significant time constraints. The suggested questions should also take into consideration the patient's comorbid medical conditions, age, and concomitant medications. It is important to use living room language during the interview (Figure 29-2) and be prepared for questions patients may ask regarding OA and its treatment (Table 29-3).

TABLE 29-2 • Questions to Ask When Conducting a Medication Review in Patients with OA

Suggested Questions for the Patient with Osteoarthritis
How long have you had OA? When were you told you had OA?
What led to being told you had OA? Do you have other diseases or factors that caused your OA?
What joints are affected by OA?
What has your physician told you about OA?
What have you and your physician identified as your goals of treatment?
What medication(s) do you take for your OA? What medications have you tried in the past?
How well do you think your medications are working? Are you meeting your goals of treatment?
How do you take your medication(s)? How often do you miss a dose of your medication(s)?
What other medications containing acetaminophen do you take? Do you monitor your intake of acetaminophen?
How much alcohol do you consume?
Have you ever experienced bleeding in the stomach or gut, or had a stomach ulcer?
Has a physician ever told you to stay away from NSAIDs (ibuprofen, naproxen, etc)?
Are you taking aspirin for heart protection or other reason?
Have you ever stopped taking any of your prescribed OA medications without telling your physician? If so, why?
What over-the-counter (OTC) medications or herbals do you use for your OA? What have you tried in the past? How do you feel these treatments are working? Have you told your physician about these medications?
How often do you have bowel movements? How have your bowel habits changed since starting your medication(s)?
Have you ever experienced constipation from your medication? Do you use anything to help prevent or limit your constipation?
What has your physician told you about driving while taking your medication?
How do you apply your medication(s) to your skin?
Other than medicines, what have you tried for your OA (eg, lifestyle changes)?
What exercise regimen do you follow?
Do you use any devices to assist you with performing daily tasks or getting around?
How does your OA limit you from performing daily activities such as dressing, bathing, preparing meals, or doing housework?
Questions to Ask for Prevention/Assessment of Medical Emergencies
Have you ever experienced any of the following potential signs/symptoms of bleeding? • Coughing up or vomiting red blood • Coughing up or vomiting material that looks like coffee grounds • Having black or tarry stools • Having abnormal stomach pain and/or burning that is new or severe • Changes in weight that are unexplained and unintentional
Have you ever experienced any of the following? • Falling asleep from your medication • Difficulty in breathing from your medication • Inability to go to the bathroom for many days

Acupuncture—therapy to reduce pain by putting small needles into specific points on the skin.
Addiction—continued use of a medication despite the fact that it causes harm and problems; feeling that the medication is "required" or "have to have it no matter what"; rare occurrence.
Adverse event—something unexpected occurs, with negative consequences; something bad happens after taking a drug that is unwanted, unexpected, or cannot be explained.
Analgesia—reduction in pain; pain relief.
Analgesic—medication that reduces pain.
Anticoagulant—medication used to the thin the blood to prevent or reduce the chance of having a clot form.
Anti-inflammatory—effects to reduce swelling, redness, and pain; overactive inflammation can damage joints.
Arthroplasty—surgery to replace or repair a joint such as the knee or hip.
As needed (or PRN)—taking a medication only when needed; taking a pain medication only in response to pain.
Blood pressure—force of blood pushing on the blood vessels.
BMI—body mass index; compares weight in relation to height to classify people as underweight, normal weight, overweight, or obese.
Cardiac—related to the heart.
Cardiovascular—organs such as heart, brain, kidneys, and others that make up the cardiovascular system.
Cartilage—material (tissue) in joints that cushions and protects bones.
Chondroprotective—protecting the structures of a joint.
Constipation—going to the bathroom (defecating) less often than is normal.
Corticosteroid—medication that reduces inflammation and swelling; may reduce pain also.
COX-2 inhibitor—pain medication that is easier on the stomach.
Dependence—when the body is used to a medication; when the medication is taken away, the body may react to the medication not being there and cause problems.
Erosion—damage to bone or joint and structure of joint.
First-line therapy—medication used first to treat a condition.
Gastrointestinal—stomach and intestines.
Gastroprotection—protecting the lining of the stomach and intestine to prevent formation of an ulcer.
Hematemesis—vomiting blood.
Hemoptysis—coughing up blood.
Intra-articular—injecting medication directly into the joint.
Joint—where bones meet; allows for arms, legs, and fingers to move freely.
Joint integrity—keeping joint working properly without damage.
Knee effusion—swelling of the knee caused by fluid in the knee joint.
Lifestyle changes—changing habits such as reducing intake of high-calorie, sweet, or high-fat foods; increasing the amount of exercise; performing stretching and strengthening activities; or other activity.
Melena=—black- or tarry-appearing stools.
MRI—magnetic resonance imaging; a type of test that looks more closely at bones, joints, and joint structures; computer-created picture.
Mucous membrane—moist lining of the eyes, lips, mouth, and nose.
Myocardial infarction—damage to the heart, heart attack.
Narcotic—pain medication that is regulated by the government because it can be dangerous if not used under the supervision of a physician; opioids are narcotics.
Nonpharmacologic—treatments such as exercise, diet, or others that are not a medication.
NSAID—nonsteroidal anti-inflammatory drug; a type of pain reliever that also reduces swelling and redness.
Obese—having a body mass index (BMI) of >30; weighing more than is recommended according to height.
Opioid—pain medication.
Osteoarthritis—damage to the joint or joint structures.
Osteophyte—growth of bone that is not normal.
Overweight—having a BMI of >25; weighing more than is recommended according to height.
Pharmacologic—medications, including prescription or over-the-counter (OTC) drugs.
Primary OA—OA where the cause cannot be identified.
Proton-pump inhibitor (PPI)—medication used to reduce the acid in the stomach and protect the stomach from medications that may cause an ulcer.
Renal function—how well the kidneys are working to filter blood.
Respiratory depression—difficulty breathing.
Scheduled dosing—taking a medication at certain times every day regardless of whether pain is present.
Secondary OA—osteoarthritis where the cause can be identified.
Second-line therapy—medication used secondarily to treat a condition, usually after the first-line therapy does not work or causes side effects.
Sedation—feeling sleepy or having trouble staying awake.
Side effect—unwanted response to a medication; can range from mild to serious; some are rare and some are more common.
Stroke—damage to the brain that occurs abruptly due to reduced blood flow in the brain; can result in paralysis or other effects, usually on one side of the body.
Tai Chi—a form of Chinese exercise.
Tolerance—when the body becomes used to a medication and a higher dose is needed to cause the same effects.
Topically—applied to the skin.
Transcutaneous electrical stimulation—stimulating muscles and nerves with small amounts of electricity.
Trauma—event that could damage joints.
Ulcer—damage to the lining of stomach or intestines that can cause discomfort, pain, or bleeding.
X-ray—type of test that studies bones and joints; creates a picture to look at bones.

FIGURE 29-2 Living room language for osteoarthritis patients.

CORE ELEMENT 2—PERSONAL MEDICATION LIST[9]

A sample personal medication list (PML) for a patient with OA is provided in Figure 29-3. This example is representative only of medications for OA. Additional medications for other disease states should be added and listed separately. MTM providers should remember to use living room language when creating the PML. Using the patient's own terminology, when accurate, may be useful to ensure the information is understandable for the patient.

TABLE 29-3 • Questions to Anticipate Regarding Osteoarthritis

- **What is osteoarthritis?**
  Osteoarthritis, or OA, occurs when joints become damaged and cause pain. Joints like the knee, hip, or those of the hand are most commonly affected.
- **What causes osteoarthritis?**
  Osteoarthritis can be caused by diseases or conditions, by traumatic events such as injuries or accidents, or by an unknown factor. Osteoarthritis is often associated with doing strenuous activities repeatedly for many years that leads to joint damage.
- **How is osteoarthritis treated?**
  Osteoarthritis is best treated with a combination of medications to reduce pain and lifestyle changes to reduce weight, increase understanding of the disease, strengthen joints, and improve overall health. You and your physician should determine your treatment goals in order to ensure that your medications and lifestyle changes are meeting your goals.
- **Besides medications, what can I do to treat my osteoarthritis and reduce my pain?**
  Reducing weight, getting exercise, performing stretching and strengthening activities, and learning more about your osteoarthritis have all been shown to help improve the symptoms of osteoarthritis.
- **Are there any natural remedies for osteoarthritis?**
  Natural or herbal products such as devil's claw, willow's bark, SAMe, and others have been studied for osteoarthritis. Be sure to tell your physician and pharmacist if you decide to use an herbal product. Be aware the consistency from product to product is not guaranteed, as the products are not regulated by the FDA like prescription medications.
- **How long does it take for my medications to start working?**
  For acetaminophen it may take 4-6 weeks to see the maximum effects, while for NSAIDs the effects can be seen after 2-3 weeks; opioid analgesics typically begin working in a matter of hours or days. For injected corticosteroids, it can take only a few days to see a benefit, while hyaluronic acid injections may take several weeks to months. Glucosamine/chondroitin may also take several months to see the full benefits.
- **How often can I receive the injection treatments?**
  In general, a joint should not be injected more than 3-5 times per year. However, for hyaluronic acid, a single treatment regimen might consist of weekly injections for 3-5 weeks. Your physician will determine how often injection therapy will be required according to your specific joint(s) involved and your type of osteoarthritis.
- **Will I become addicted to my opioid?**
  Addiction to opioids is rare and does not happen to the majority of patients who take opioids. Your physician will determine whether you have a higher-than-normal risk for becoming addicted to opioids; having a family history of addiction, past personal history of addiction, and other factors may increase your risk. Be sure to take your medication as instructed and talk to your physician if your pain is not controlled.
- **When should I call my physician about my osteoarthritis?**
  Call your physician if you are not responding to the prescribed treatment (your pain is not controlled) or if you are having side effects. Call your physician if you are experiencing any signs or symptoms of bleeding, if you have difficulty staying awake or breathing, if you have not gone to the bathroom for several days, or if you are using capsaicin cream and it comes into contact with your eyes.
- **What should I do if I have a problem or side effect from one of my medications?**
  Never stop taking your medications without first talking to your physician. Speak with your physician and/or pharmacist to let them know about any problems you are having, and together you can make sure that your medications are the right ones for you. If you experience side effects, you should call your physician right away or speak to a pharmacist to determine whether your physician should be alerted.

PERSONAL MEDICATION LIST FOR *<Insert patient's name, DOB: mm/dd/yyyy>*	
Medication: Acetaminophen 500 mg	
How I use it: Take two tablets (1000 mg) every 8 hours	
Why I use it: Pain reliever	**Prescriber:** Carter
Date I started using it: 1/6/2017	**Date I stopped using it:** (*Leave blank for patient's notes*)
Why I stopped using it: (*Leave blank for patient's notes*)	
Medication: Glucosamine-chondroitin 500 mg/400 mg	
How I use it: Take one pill (500 mg/400 mg) every 8 hours	
Why I use it: Joint function	**Prescriber:** Carter
Date I started using it: 11/10/2016	**Date I stopped using it:** (*Leave blank for patient's notes*)
Why I stopped using it: (*Leave blank for patient's notes*)	

FIGURE 29-3 Sample personal medication list for osteoarthritis patients.

CORE ELEMENT 3—MEDICATION ACTION PLAN

A sample medication action plan (MAP)[9] should be generated for each encounter with a patient and be grouped by disease state or MRP. a sample MAP for a patient with OA is shown in Figure 29-4. As this plan is developed for the patient, it should be written in plain, easy-to-understand language. Using the patient's own descriptions may be a useful method to complete the MAP, as long as the descriptions are accurate reflections of the intended information. Only important information regarding use, administration, or monitoring should be included, and it should be written in living room language. Adherence to lifestyle modifications such as diet, exercise, and weight reduction should be included, as these are key components for the successful treatment of OA.

CORE ELEMENT 4—INTERVENTION AND/OR REFERRAL

Interventions for patients with OA may include both pharmacologic and nonpharmacologic measures. Pharmacologic therapy (Table 29-4) serves as an adjunct to nonpharmacologic therapy (Table 29-5) in the provision of analgesia; currently there is no proven therapy that modifies the disease course of OA. Additional pharmacotherapy may be recommended to offset the side effects of medications for OA in specific patient populations (eg, use of proton-pump inhibitors [PPIs] to reduce the risk of gastrointestinal [GI] side effects from nonsteroidal anti-inflammatory drugs [NSAIDs]). The potential risks and benefits of each treatment option should be considered on an individual basis and discussed with the patient before initiating pharmacological therapy.[10]

Nonpharmacologic Treatment

Nonpharmacologic therapy should be recommended for all patients with OA, and should include education, lifestyle modification, and physical therapy, exercise, or strengthening and stretching exercises.[8] Specific interventions may vary according to the location and severity of disease and number of joints involved. Weight loss is especially important for overweight or obese individuals suffering from hip and/or knee OA. Physical therapy, exercise, and stretching and strengthening exercises can improve physical functioning, decrease disability, reduce pain, and strengthen and stabilize joints. For patients with knee arthritis, Tai Chi, traditional Chinese acupuncture, and transcutaneous electrical stimulation may provide benefit and are recommended by the American College of Rheumatology (ACR).[8] Exercise programs should be implemented, taking into consideration the baseline physical fitness level, disease severity, and comorbidities. Evaluation of ability to perform daily activities and the need for assistive devices should be assessed at

DATE PREPARED: *<Insert date>*

What we talked about:
You reported having some burning and tingling sensations after you applied capsaicin cream to your hands; you started the capsaicin 4 days ago for OA in your hands. This is a common side effect when starting capsaicin and often goes away with continued use.

What I need to do:	What I did and when I did it:
1. Continue using the capsaicin cream as directed by my physician or up to 4 times per day, every day. 2. Thoroughly rub cream onto my hands. 3. Wait 30 minutes after applying cream to wash hands; avoid touching mouth, eyes, nose, lips, or other sensitive areas until hands are washed. 4. Wash hands thoroughly. 5. Notify my physician if the burning and tingling in the hands is too unpleasant.	(*Leave blank for patient's notes*)

What we talked about:
Acetaminophen is not helping your knee osteoarthritis. You started it 2 weeks ago and you are taking one tablet (500 mg) as needed; only taking one or two tablets per day.

What I need to do:	What I did and when I did it:
1. Discuss dosing regimen with your physician. You may have to take a higher dose of acetaminophen or take it more often. 2. Discuss the option of taking the acetaminophen every 6 or 8 hours to help treat the pain and help prevent the pain. 3. Avoid alcohol while taking acetaminophen. 4. Do not take more than 3 g/day of acetaminophen, or 4 g if directed by the physician. Acetaminophen may be an ingredient in other products such as cough-and-cold products.	(*Leave blank for patient's notes*)

FIGURE 29-4 Sample medication action plan for a patient with osteoarthritis.

TABLE 29-4 • Medications Commonly Used in the Treatment of Osteoarthritis

Drug	Brand Name	Starting Dose	Usual Range	Other
Oral analgesics				
Acetaminophen	Tylenol	325-500 mg tid	325-650 mg every 4-6 hours or 1 g tid or qid	Contained in many combination analgesics
Tramadol Tramadol ER	Ultram Ultram ER	25 mg in the morning 100 mg daily	Titrate dose in 25-mg increments to reach a maintenance dose of 50-100 mg tid Titrate to 200-300 mg daily	May need to taper dose on discontinuation to prevent withdrawal symptoms
Hydrocodone/ acetaminophen	Lortab, Vicodin	5 mg/325 mg tid	2.5-10 mg/325-650 mg tid to 5 times daily	Maximum dose limited by total daily dose of acetaminophen
Oxycodone/ acetaminophen	Percocet	5 mg/325 mg tid	2.5-10 mg/325-650 mg tid to 5 times daily	Maximum dose limited by total daily dose of acetaminophen
Topical analgesics				
Capsaicin 0.025% or 0.075%	CapzasinHP		Apply to affected joint tid-qid	—
Diclofenac 1% gel	Voltaren		Apply 2 or 4 g per site as prescribed, qid	
Diclofenac 1.3% patch	Flector		Apply one patch bid to the site to be treated, as directed; apply 40 drops to the affected knee, applying and rubbing in 10 drops	
Diclofenac 1.5% solution	Pennsaid		Apply 40 drops to the affected knee, applying and rubbing in 10 drops at a time; repeat for a total of qid	
Diclofenac 2% solution	Pennsaid		Apply 40 mg (two pump actuations) bid	
Intra-articular corticosteroids				
Triamcinolone	Kenalog	5-15 mg per joint	10-40 mg per large joint (knee, hip, shoulder)	Often administered concomitantly with a local anesthetic
Methylprednisolone acetate	Depo-Medrol	10-20 mg per joint	20-80 mg per large joint (knee, hip, shoulder)	
Nonsteroidal anti-inflammatory drugs (NSAIDs)				
Aspirin, plain, buffered, or enteric-coated	Bayer, Ecotrin, Bufferin	325 mg tid	325-650 mg qid	Doses of 3600 mg/day are needed for anti-inflammatory activity
Celecoxib	Celebrex	100 mg daily	100 mg bid or 200 mg daily	
Diclofenac XR Diclofenac IR	Voltaren-XR Cataflam	100 mg daily 50 mg bid	100-200 mg daily 50-75 mg bid	
Diflunisal	Dolobid	250 mg bid	500-750 mg bid	
Etodolac	Lodine	300 mg bid	400-500 mg bid	
Fenoprofen	Nalfon	400 mg tid	400-600 mg tid-qid	
Flurbiprofen	Ansaid	100 mg bid	200-300 mg/day in 2-4 divided doses	
Ibuprofen	Motrin, Advil	200 mg tid	1200-3200 mg/day in 3-4 divided doses	Available OTC and Rx
Indomethacin Indomethacin SR	Indocin Indocin SR	25 mg bid 75 mg SR once daily	Titrate dose by 25-50 mg/day until pain controlled or maximum dose of 50 mg tid Can titrate to 75 mg SR twice daily if needed	
Ketoprofen	Orudis	50 mg tid	50-75 mg tid-qid	
Meclofenamate	Meclomen	50 mg tid	50-100 mg tid-qid	
Mefenamic acid	Ponstel	250 mg tid	250 mg qid	FDA approval for 1 week of therapy

(Continued)

TABLE 29-4 • Medications Commonly Used in the Treatment of Osteoarthritis (*Continued*)

Drug	Brand Name	Starting Dose	Usual Range	Other
Meloxicam	Mobic	7.5 mg daily	15 mg daily	
Nabumetone	Relafen	500 mg daily	500-1,000 mg 1-2 times/day	
Naproxen	Naprosyn	250 mg bid	500 mg bid	Available OTC and Rx
Naproxen sodium Naproxen sodium controlled-release tablets	Anaprox, Aleve Naprelan	220 mg bid	220-550 mg bid 375-750 mg bid	
Oxaprozin	Daypro	600 mg daily	600-1200 mg daily	
Piroxicam	Feldene	10 mg daily	20 mg daily	
Salsalate	Disalcid	500 mg bid	500-1000 mg bid-tid	

Abbreviations: bid = twice per day; CrCl = creatinine clearance; OTC = over-the-counter; qid = 4 times per day; SR = sustained release; tid = 3 times per day.

Source: Reproduced, with permission, from DiPiro JT, Talbert RL, Yee GC, Matzke GR, Wells BG, Posey LM, eds. *Pharmacotherapy: A Pathophysiologic Approach*, 10th ed. New York, NY: McGraw-Hill; 2017.

baseline and throughout follow-up.[8] Topical application of heat or cold treatments can provide analgesia and improve range of motion. Caution should be exercised when using heating pads because of the potential for burns if not used correctly.

Surgical intervention may be required for those refractory to standard therapy or in those who experience severe pain, reductions in physical functioning, and/or limitations in performing activities of daily living. Although expensive and invasive, hip or knee replacement surgeries can greatly benefit appropriately selected patients. Arthroscopic interventions may also be recommended to remove cartilage or debris from within the joint for patients with less severe disease.

Pharmacologic Treatment

Acetaminophen Acetaminophen is considered the first-line treatment for mild-to-moderate OA because of its efficacy and favorable side effect profile. If pain is intermittent, acetaminophen can be dosed on an as-needed basis. For continuous pain, scheduled dosing of ≤4 g/day (1000 mg every 6 hours) is more likely to be effective. An adequate trial to assess efficacy consists of approximately 4-6 weeks. Acetaminophen can cause hepatic toxicity, which can be fatal;[11] caution should be used in those with liver disease or a history of alcoholism, and use of alcohol should be discouraged.[12] Patients should be cautioned against consuming alcohol or using other products that contain acetaminophen, such as OTC cough and cold products. Rarely, acetaminophen has been associated with worsening blood pressure or reducing renal function.[13,14]

TABLE 29-5 • Nonpharmacologic Interventions in the Treatment of OA

Type of Nonpharmacologic Intervention	Strength of Recommendation
Exercise	Strong
Weight loss (if overweight)	Strong
Patient education	Strong
Use of assistive device (ie, cane)	Moderate
Use of shoe insoles	Moderate
Application of heat	Moderate
Use of fitted knee braces	Minimal
Lateral patellar taping	Minimal
Passive exercise alone	Minimal

Source: Reproduced, with permission, from DiPiro JT, Talbert RL, Yee GC, Matzke GR, Wells BG, Posey LM, eds. *Pharmacotherapy: A Pathophysiologic Approach*, 10th ed. New York, NY: McGraw-Hill; 2017.

NSAIDs Nonsteroidal anti-inflammatory drugs are considered second-line therapy for mild-to-moderate OA, because of their significant adverse effect profile. However, NSAIDs may provide more analgesia compared to acetaminophen and, therefore, be recommended as first-line therapy for moderate-to-severe OA. All NSAIDs are considered equally efficacious at equivalent doses. Failure of one NSAID does not predict failure of a subsequent NSAID. Side effects range from sodium and water retention, reductions in renal function, and increases in blood pressure to GI ulceration, renal insufficiency, and adverse cardiovascular (CV) events such as myocardial infarction or stroke. NSAIDs are contraindicated in the first 10-14 days after coronary artery bypass graft (CABG) surgery, as use may increase the risk of myocardial infarction.[12] Naproxen appears to have the lowest risk for adverse CV events of all the NSAIDs,[15] but recently celecoxib was shown to have similar risks for adverse CV events in a large randomized trial.[16] Use of ibuprofen with aspirin may attenuate the beneficial antiplatelet effects of aspirin when used for primary or secondary prevention of CV disease.[8]

Proton-pump inhibitors previously defined can be utilized to mitigate the GI risks of NSAIDs in appropriate patients (Table 29-6), and should be considered for patients at moderate to high risk for GI bleeding[17] (Table 29-7). Figure 29-5 outlines a potential algorithm for assessing and managing the risk of GI bleeding in patients requiring long-term NSAID therapy.[18] All patients should be counseled to take

TABLE 29-6 • Risk Factors[a] Associated with NSAID-Induced Ulcers and Upper Gastrointestinal Complications

Age >65 years
Previous peptic ulcer
Previous ulcer-related upper-GI complication
High-dose NSAIDs
Multiple NSAID use
Selection of NSAID (eg, COX-1 vs COX-2 inhibition)
NSAID-related dyspepsia
Aspirin (including cardioprotective dosages)
Concomitant use of NSAID plus low-dose aspirin
Concomitant use of oral bisphosphonates (eg, alendronate)
Concomitant use of corticosteroids
Concomitant use of anticoagulant or coagulopathy
Concomitant use of antiplatelet drugs (eg, clopidogrel)
Concomitant use of selective serotonin reuptake inhibitor
Chronic debilitating disorders (eg, cardiovascular disease, rheumatoid arthritis)
Helicobacter pylori infection
Cigarette smoking
Alcohol consumption

[a] Please note that combinations of risk factors are additive.

Source: References 17, 20, 21, 22, 23, and 24.

NSAIDs with food to help reduce the potential for adverse GI events. Patients at high risk for GI bleeding or those aged >75 years should potentially avoid long-term NSAIDs.[8] If a minimal number of superficial joints are affected, topical NSAID therapy with diclofenac gel can be considered to minimize risk of systemic side effects; combining topical diclofenac with oral acetaminophen can also be considered prior to initiating systemic NSAIDs. Topical diclofenac is now available as an OTC product. The American College of Rheumatology (ACR) recommends the use of topical NSAIDs over oral NSAIDs for those aged ≥75 years who suffer from hand OA, but not for patients with hip or knee OA.[8] Patients taking NSAIDs should be regularly assessed for signs of GI bleeding and monitored for changes in blood pressure. Extra caution should be utilized when recommending NSAIDs in patients receiving anticoagulation therapy (eg, warfarin, dabigatran, apixaban, rivaroxaban) or those already receiving aspirin for primary or secondary CV protection, due to a 2- to 3-fold increase in the risk for major bleeding.[19]

The cyclooxygenase-2 inhibitor celecoxib can be considered for those at high risk for GI bleeding who require an NSAID, as it possesses a lower risk for GI bleeding compared to NSAIDs. However, celecoxib carries a similar risk for CV adverse events as other systemic NSAIDs and should be used cautiously in those at high risk of CV events.[16] Similar to NSAIDs, celecoxib has a warning for use after CABG surgery.[12] It is unclear whether combining aspirin with celecoxib mitigates the CV risk of celecoxib, but until further evidence is available, the combination should not be recommended at this time.

TABLE 29-7 • Guidelines for Reducing Gastrointestinal Risk Factors[a] for Patients Receiving Chronic NSAID Therapy

Cardiovascular Risk	No or Low GI Risk (No Risk Factors)	Moderate GI Risk (1–2 Risk Factors)	High GI Risk (>2 Risk Factors or Prior Ulcer or Ulcer-Related Complication)
	Age < 65 years)	Age ≥ 65 years High-dose NSAIDs Concomitant use of aspirin, corticosteroids, or anticoagulants	Age ≥ 65 years Concomitant use of aspirin, corticosteroids, or anticoagulants Dual-antiplatelet therapy
No or low CV risk (patient does not require low-dose aspirin)	Nonselective NSAID or partially selective NSAID	Nonselective NSAID or partially selective NSAID + PPI or misoprostol Selective COX-2 inhibitor NSAID (if available)	Avoid NSAID or selective COX-2 inhibitor, if possible; use alternative therapy Nonselective NSAID or partially selective NSAID + PPI or misoprostol Selective COX-2 inhibitor NSAID (if available) + PPI or misoprostol
High CV risk (patient requires low-dose aspirin), no NSAID	No prophylaxis required	PPI or misoprostol	PPI or misoprostol
High CV risk (patient requires low-dose aspirin) and NSAID	Naproxen + PPI or misoprostol	Naproxen + PPI or misoprostol	Avoid NSAID or selective COX-2 inhibitor, if at all possible; use alternative therapy If anti-inflammatory drug is needed and CV risk is > GI risk, use naproxen and aspirin + PPI or misoprostol If anti-inflammatory drug and aspirin are needed and GI risk is > CV, use selective COX-2 inhibitor + PPI or misoprostol

[a] See Table 29-6.

Abbreviations: CV = cardiovascular; GI = gastrointestinal; NSAID = nonsteroidal anti-inflammatory drug; PPI = proton-pump inhibitor.

Source: References 17, 21, 22, 23, 25, 26, and 27.

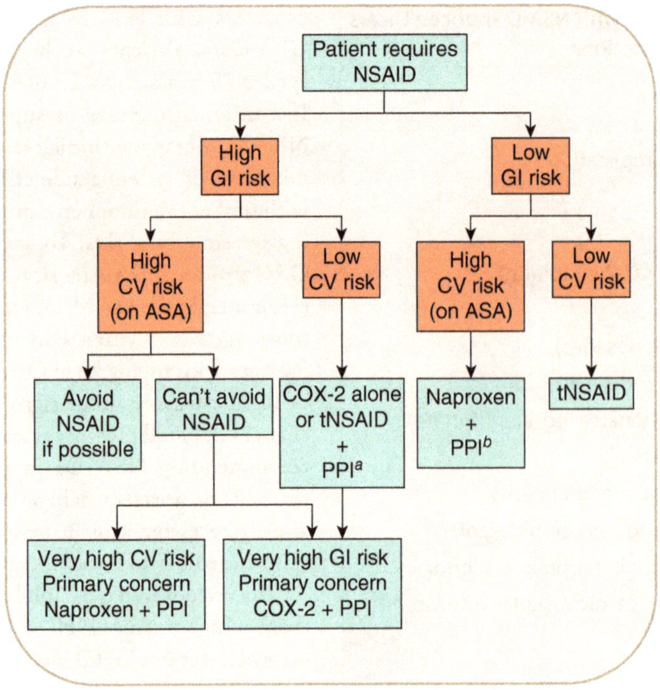

FIGURE 29-5 Algorithm for the use of long-term NSAID therapy and gastroprotective agents according to a patient's GI and cardiovascular risk.[18]

[a] In high-risk patients, a COX-2 inhibitor and a tNSAID plus proton pump inhibitor (PPI) show similar reductions in rebleeding rates, but these reductions may be incomplete.

[b] In general, most patients on acetylsalicylic acid plus naproxen would need the addition of a PPI. However, for some patients at very low GI risk, naproxen alone may be appropriate.

Source: Reproduced, with permission, from DiPiro JT, Talbert RL, Yee GC, Matzke GR, Wells BG, Posey LM, eds. *Pharmacotherapy: A Pathophysiologic Approach*, 9th ed. New York, NY: McGraw-Hill; 2014.

Opioid analgesics can be considered for patients who fail to respond to other therapies or for those patients who have contraindications to other options. Tramadol is often tried initially, as it is indicated for mild to moderate pain and may have an improved side effect profile compared to stronger opioids. For patients unresponsive to tramadol, the opioids such as oxycodone are often utilized, despite inconsistent evidence that the high incidence of adverse effects is offset by the analgesia provided.[28] Morphine should be used with caution in the elderly and those with significant renal disease, because of reduced renal clearance of potentially toxic metabolites.[12] Long-term use of opioids may lead to tolerance and dependence. Patients should be counseled that escalating doses may be required because of tolerance, and should be cautioned against abrupt discontinuation to avoid withdrawal symptoms. All patients on long-term opioids should receive a bowel regimen to prevent constipation, ideally with both a stimulant and a stool softener. Although addiction to opioids is possible, it is relatively uncommon;[29] patients should be monitored frequently for signs or symptoms of addiction to ensure the benefits of treatment continue to outweigh the potential risks.

Intra-articular Therapies Intra-articular therapy includes corticosteroids or hyaluronic acid. Injectable therapies are generally reserved for those failing or receiving minimal benefit from oral therapy. Corticosteroids can be beneficial for those with inflammatory OA or knee effusion. Analgesic benefits can appear in a matter of days, but often fail to persist past 4 weeks. The volume and dose of steroid vary relative to the condition of the joint. In general, a joint should not be injected more than 3-5 times per year. Hyaluronic acid, or viscosupplementation, is accomplished by weekly injections of a hyaluronic acid formulation for 3-5 weeks; analgesia may take up to 10 weeks for full effects,[30] but the benefit appears to continue for a matter of months. Currently there is no evidence to suggest the molecular weight of a particular hyaluronic acid formulation has an impact on the benefit.[31]

The ACR considers intra-articular corticosteroids a potential option for knee and hip OA, but recommends against their use in hand OA. Similarly, hyaluronic acid is not recommended for hand OA, and the ACR does not provide a recommendation for or against its use in hip or knee OA.[8] However, the benefit of hyaluronic acid is variable and the small potential for benefit may not outweigh the potential risks in all patients.[32] Side effects of hyaluronic acid are relatively uncommon, but may include postinjection flare-ups and rare cases of anaphylaxis or intra-articular infection. Corticosteroid injections have a similar side effect profile, and adverse events are relatively uncommon, provided the injection is administered with proper technique.

Other Prescription Products Duloxetine has gained FDA approval for the treatment of chronic pain related to OA.[12] This agent may be considered as an adjunctive therapy to provide analgesia, especially in those with concomitant anxiety, depression, or chronic musculoskeletal pain.

Capsaicin is available in a prescription-strength patch (8%).[12] As capsaicin is recommended only for hand OA by the ACR,[8] this dosage form may not be effective if the patch cannot maintain consistent adherence to the skin. See discussion in the following paragraphs for a more detailed description of capsaicin.

TABLE 29-8 • Herbal Products for Osteoarthritis

Herbal Product	Recommended Dosage	Level of Evidence[a]	Cost[b]
Willow bark (*Salix alba*)	1360 -2160 mg willow bark extract (240 mg of salicin) per day	Insufficient evidence	$$$
Avocado/soybean unsaponifiables (ASU)	300-600 mg/day; ≤300 mg/kg has also been studied	Possibly effective	$$$
Devil's claw (*Harpagophytum procumbens*)	50-100 mg of hapagoside per day (dose varies on product)	Possibly effective	$-$$
Rose hip (*Rosa canina*)	5 g daily given in two divided doses	Possibly effective	$
S-Adenosyl-ʟ-methionine (SAMe)	600-1200 mg/day, given in 1-3 divided doses	Likely effective	$$$-$$$$

[a] Level of evidence: "Likely effective"—this product has a very high level of reliable clinical evidence supporting its use for a specific indication. Products rated "likely effective" are generally considered appropriate to recommend; "possibly effective"—this product has some clinical evidence supporting its use for a specific indication; however, the evidence is limited by quantity, quality, or contradictory findings. Products rated "possibly effective" might be beneficial, but do not have enough high-quality evidence to be recommended for most people; "insufficient evidence"—there is not enough reliable scientific evidence to provide an effectiveness rating.

[b] Cost: $ = ≤$10/month supply in recommended dosage; $$ = $11-$20/month; $$$ = $21-$50/month; $$$$ = >$50/month.

Source: Data compiled from reference 36.

OTC Products Topical capsaicin can reduce pain transmission by depleting substance P from sensory nerves.[12] Capsaicin is applied 4 times a day, and analgesia may take up to 2-4 weeks to be realized. It is recommended only for those suffering from hand OA.[8] Application may result in a mild burning sensation that often abates with continued use. Patients should be counseled to wash their hands 30 minutes after administration (to allow skin to fully absorb the product) and to avoid contact between capsaicin and the eyes or mucus membranes.

Glucosamine and chondroitin are believed to have chondroprotective effects and serve as building blocks for cartilage. However, evidence demonstrating a consistent benefit is scant; the combination was not more effective than placebo in the landmark GAIT trial.[33] Accordingly, the ACR conditionally recommends against the use of glucosamine and chondroitin for hip or knee OA.[8] Glucosamine is derived from oyster, crab, lobster, or shrimp shells, and susceptible patients may experience allergic reactions when receiving the supplement; however, the true importance of this potential reaction may be overstated.[34] Glucosamine may also raise blood glucose levels, and those with elevated blood glucose or diabetes should be monitored closely. The products are regulated as dietary supplements, as opposed to medications. Thus, purity,

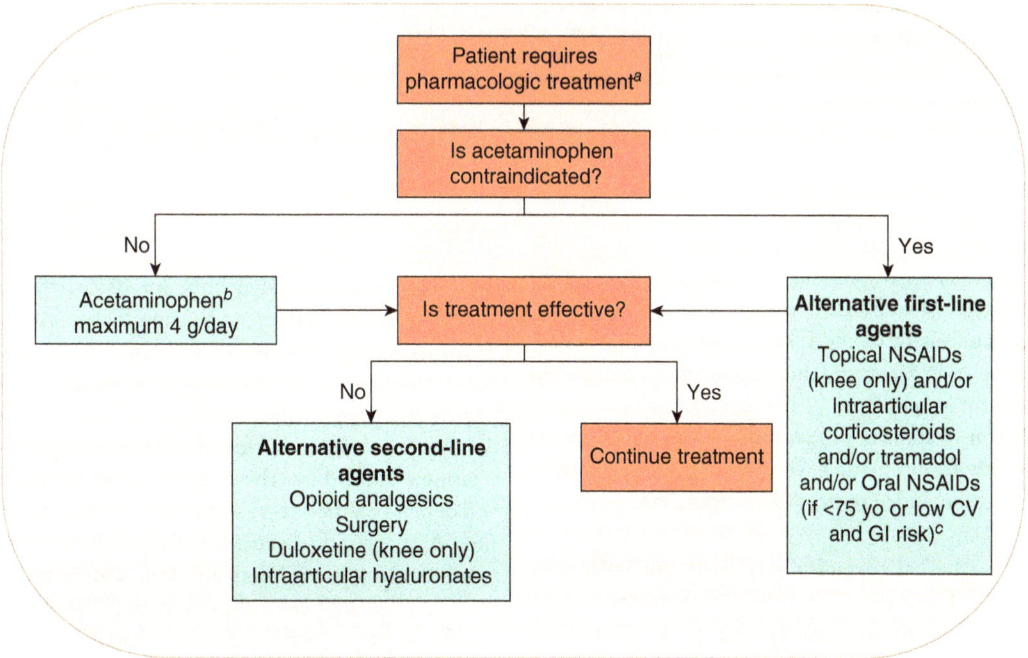

FIGURE 29-6 Treatment algorithm for hip and knee osteoarthritis.

Abbreviations: CV = cardiovascular; GI = gastrointestinal; NSAIDs = nonsteroidal anti-inflammatory drugs.

[a] Selection of a medication should consider patient-specific characteristics.

[b] The patient must be counseled regarding all acetaminophen-containing products.

[c] When used for chronic management of osteoarthritis, consider the addition of a proton pump inhibitor.

Source: Reproduced, with permission, from DiPiro JT, Talbert RL, Yee GC, Matzke GR, Wells BG, Posey LM, eds. *Pharmacotherapy: A Pathophysiologic Approach*, 10th ed. New York, NY: McGraw-Hill; 2017.

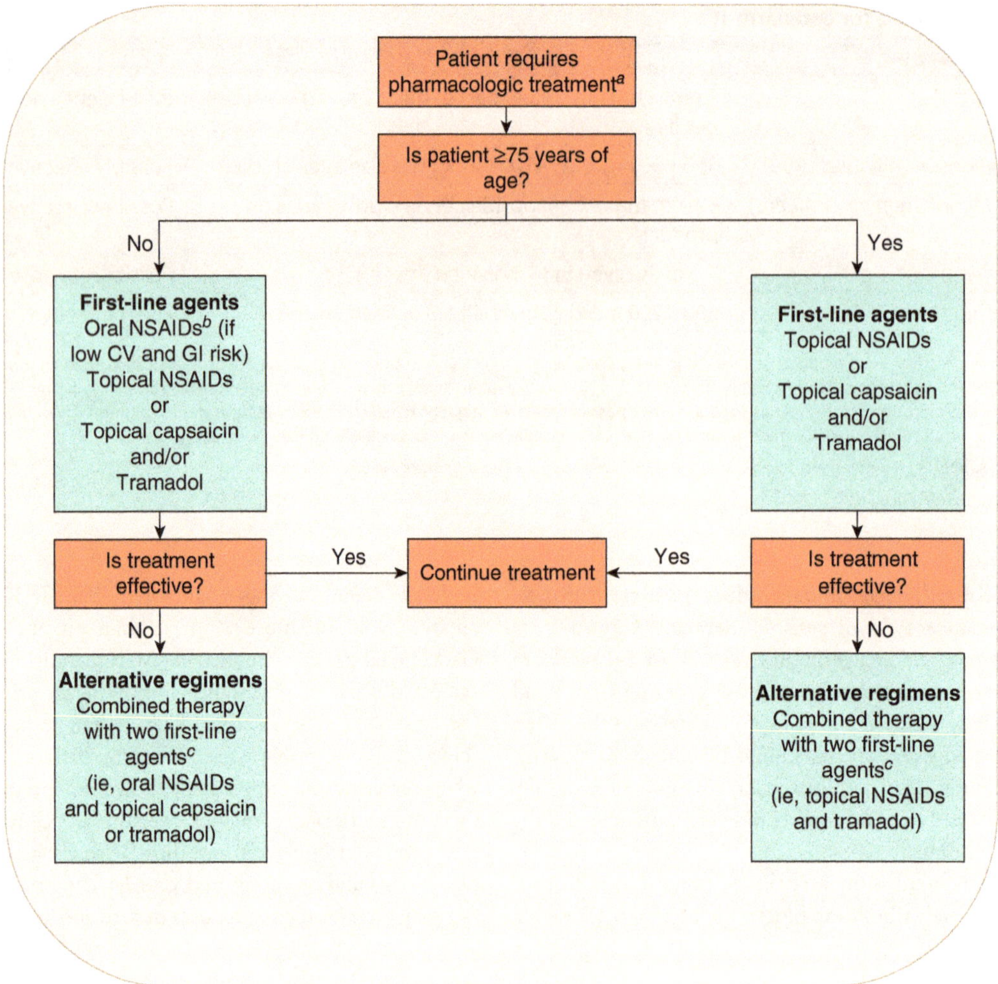

FIGURE 29-7 Treatment recommendations for hand osteoarthritis.

Abbreviations: CV= cardiovascular; GI = gastrointestinal; NSAIDs = nonsteroidal anti-inflammatory drugs.

[a] Selection of a medication should consider patient-specific characteristics.

[b] When used for chronic management of osteoarthritis, consider the addition of a proton pump inhibitor.

[c] Topical and oral NSAIDs should not be combined.

Source: Reproduced, with permission, from DiPiro JT, Talbert RL, Yee GC, Matzke GR, Wells BG, Posey LM, eds. *Pharmacotherapy: A Pathophysiologic Approach*, 10th ed. New York, NY: McGraw-Hill; 2017.

consistency, and potency may not be reliable. Despite these possible drawbacks, the potential for benefit may outweigh the small likelihood of harm. Patients who choose to use glucosamine and chondroitin should be counseled that the full analgesic benefit may take months to be completely realized. Glucosamine and chondroitin should not be used for acute pain.

Administration of vitamin D was recently shown to provide no benefit to those with symptomatic knee OA.[35] Therefore, vitamin D should not be recommended to treat OA at this time.

Herbals Numerous herbal therapies have been studied in OA with varying levels of success (Table 29-8).[36] Patients should be informed that the consistency, purity, and quality of natural products may be variable, as all products are marketed as dietary supplements and are not subject to strict FDA regulations. Those with an allergy to aspirin and those taking NSAIDs should avoid taking willow bark.[36] Patients should be counseled to tell their physicians and pharmacists about any herbal medications, since herbals may interact with other medications.

Treatment Algorithm

A general treatment algorithm for osteoarthritis is outlined in Figure 29-6 (hip and knee OA) and Figure 29-7 (hand OA). The Third Canadian Consensus Conference created a summary of evidence-based recommendations for the treatment of OA to help clinicians select appropriate therapy (Table 29-9). Nonpharmacologic therapy is recommended for all patients at all points throughout the treatment algorithm. The specific nonpharmacologic intervention will depend on the site(s) and severity of disease. Pharmacotherapy should be individualized according to the severity of disease, the number and type of joints affected, past medical history, current medications, and personal preference for therapy. Acetaminophen should be recommended for most patients as first-line therapy. Those failing acetaminophen can switch to oral NSAIDs or be considered for the addition of topical NSAIDs, depending on the location and number of affected joints. Addition of topical NSAIDs may be a preferred alternative if acetaminophen provided some benefit, and the avoidance of systemic NSAIDs is desired. Intra-articular therapy may be considered for those who fail NSAIDs

TABLE 29-9 • Recommendations for Osteoarthritis

Criterion/Category	Recommendation	Level of Evidence[a]	Grade of Recommendation[b]
1. Patient-physician communication	Patients should be fully informed about evolving information regarding the benefits and risks of their treatment options.	3	C
2. Indications	NSAIDs and coxibs are generally more effective and preferred by patients over acetaminophen, although a trial of the latter is warranted for some patients; topical NSAID formulations may confer benefit in knee OA	1	A
3. GI toxicity	For patients with risk factors for PUB, a coxib is still the anti-inflammatory drug of choice, depending on the patient's cardiovascular risks; high-risk patients who must use nonselective NSAIDs should have a PPI.	1	A
4. Renal	Before starting an NSAID or coxib, determine renal status and creatinine clearance for patients aged >65 years or for those with comorbid conditions that may affect renal function	3	C
	Advise patients that if they cannot eat or drink that day, they should withhold that day's dose of NSAID/coxib	4	D
5. Hypertension	For patients receiving antihypertensive drugs, measure blood pressure within a few weeks after initiating NSAID/coxib therapy and monitor appropriately; drug doses may need adjustment	1	A
6. Cardiovascular	Patients taking rofecoxib have been shown to have an increased risk of CV events; current data suggest that this increased CV risk may be an effect of the NSAID/coxib class; physicians and patients should weigh the benefits and risks of NSAID/coxib therapy	1	A
7. Geriatric considerations	NSAIDs/coxibs should be used with caution in elderly patients, who are at the greatest risk for serious GI, renal, and CV side effects	3	C
8. Pharmacoeconomics	Although the data are ambiguous, coxibs may be more cost-effective than traditional NSAID + proprietary PPI among high-risk patients	3	C

[a] Categories of evidence: 1A, meta-analysis of RCT; 1B, at least one RCT; 2A, at least one controlled study without randomization; 3, descriptive studies, such as comparative, correlation, or case-control studies; 4, expert committee reports or opinions and/or clinical experience of respected authorities.

[b] Grades of recommendation: A—category 1 evidence; B—category 2 evidence or extrapolated recommendation from category 1 evidence; C—category 3 evidence or extrapolated recommendation from category 1 or 2 evidence; D—category 4 evidence or extrapolated recommendation from category 2 or 3 evidence.

Abbreviations: CV = cardiovascular; GI = gastrointestinal; NSAID = nonsteroidal anti-inflammatory drug; PPI = proton pump inhibitor; PUB = perforations, ulcers, and bleeds.

Source: Reproduced, with permission, from DiPiro JT, Talbert RL, Yee GC, Matzke GR, Wells BG, Posey LM, eds. *Pharmacotherapy: A Pathophysiologic Approach*, 8th ed. New York, NY: McGraw-Hill; 2012.

or receive only partial benefit; opioids should likely be reserved for those failing all other therapies or those who cannot tolerate or have contraindications to other treatment options. Surgical intervention is a last-line option.

Referral

Osteoarthritis does not pose an emergent threat directly to patients. However, the disease may lead to a reduction in physical functioning and impact the ability to perform activities of daily living. Referral for surgical intervention would be appropriate for these patients or those with severe pain refractory to available analgesic options. Pharmacologic treatment options used for OA, such as systemic NSAIDs or opioids, may lead to serious and emergent adverse events such as bleeding or respiratory depression, respectively. Patients should be monitored for signs or symptoms of bleeding at each encounter (Figure 29-8). Sedation and respiratory depression can be magnified by concomitant use of other CNS depressants such as barbiturates, benzodiazepines, or alcohol, and patients should be directed to avoid these substances unless directed under the close supervision of their physician. Sensory and motor impairment may limit the ability to drive or operate machinery safely and may pose a risk to the patient or others. Opioids can also cause constipation, which left untreated can lead to bowel impaction and other serious negative sequelae.

CORE ELEMENT 5—DOCUMENTATION AND FOLLOW-UP

Clear and succinct documentation of MRPs and recommendations is a key component of the MTM consult. Examples of potential MRPs are shown in Table 29-10. Sample communications and recommendations to providers to address medication-related issues are found in Figure 29-9. These recommendations may be transmitted via fax, telephone, or other form of communication, and need to be adapted relative to the mechanism of delivery, as well as familiarity with the physician. Patients with OA should be followed consistently to ensure adequate control of pain and avoidance of further joint deterioration and limitation of physical functioning. Suggested intervals for follow-up are shown in Table 29-11.

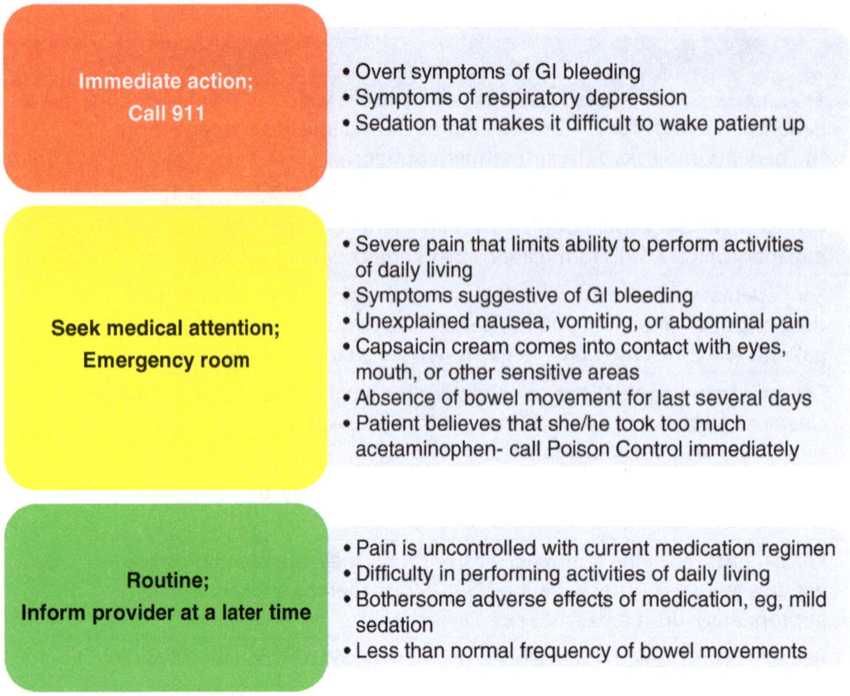

FIGURE 29-8 Referral for management of osteoarthritis.

TABLE 29-10 • Medication-Related Problems (MRPs) in Patients with Osteoarthritis

Category of MRP	Example of Medication-Related Problem
Nonadherence	Suboptimal pain relief due to nonadherence with lifestyle modifications (eg, exercise, stretching and strengthening joints) Suboptimal pain relief due to patient missing doses of anti-inflammatory medication Patient not taking pain medication due to cost
Unnecessary medication	Duplicate therapy (eg, two NSAIDs) PPI for gastroprotection without NSAID, ASA, antiplatelet agent, or history of GERD, GI bleeding, or ulcer
Need for additional medication	Patient on NSAID with risk factors for GI bleeding not receiving a PPI Patient on chronic opioid therapy not receiving bowel regimen to prevent constipation
Ineffective medication	Adequate trial of pain reliever with suboptimal reduction in pain Use of glucosamine/chondroitin for >6 months without benefit
Dosage too low	Suboptimal dose of acetaminophen; receiving only 1 tablet once daily
Dosage too high	Daily dose of acetaminophen from all sources >4 g/day Patient with significant sedation on opioid analgesic
Adverse drug event	Constipation from opioid analgesic Sedation from opioid analgesic

Abbreviations: ASA = acetylsalicylic acid (aspirin); GERD = gastroesophageal reflux disease; GI = gastrointestinal; NSAID = nonsteroidal anti-inflammatory drug; PPI = proton-pump inhibitor.

Scenario 1: Patient receiving oxycodone and reports constipation (bowel movement every 4-5 days, previous normal every 1-2 days) MRP: Adverse drug event, need for additional therapy
Assessment: Patient receiving oxycodone for OA pain reporting constipation; previously had a bowel movement every 1-2 days, now having one every 4-5 days. Patient is not receiving bowel regimen to prevent opioid-induced constipation. **Plan:** If appropriate, please consider adding a bowel regimen to treat and prevent constipation associated with chronic opioid use. Optimal regimen contains both a stool softener (e.g., docusate) and a stimulant laxative (eg, sennosides).
Scenario 2: Patient using capsaicin cream to treat hip OA and not experiencing any benefit **MRP:** Unnecessary medication
Assessment: Patient using capsaicin cream to treat OA-related hip pain. Because of the depth of the joint away from skin surface, capsaicin is unlikely to provide benefit. Additionally, patient reports having received no benefit for capsaicin treatment. **Plan:** If appropriate, please consider discontinuing capsaicin therapy, as it is not recommended by the American College of Rheumatology Guidelines for the treatment of hip OA. Oral acetaminophen in the absence of contraindications is considered a first-line treatment option for painful hip OA.
Scenario 3: Patient at high risk for GI bleeding, receiving an NSAID, and not receiving gastroprotection with a PPI **MRP:** Need for additional therapy
Assessment: Patient is at high risk for GI bleeding, due to age ≥65 years and concomitant use of aspirin 81 mg for secondary prevention of cardiovascular event. Given chronic use of NSAID therapy, patient should likely receive a PPI to reduce risk for GI bleeding. **Plan:** If appropriate, please consider initiation of PPI such as omeprazole, pantoprazole, or lansoprazole to reduce risk for GI bleeding.
Scenario 4: Patient not taking medication due to cost **MRP:** Nonadherence
Assessment: Patient prescribed Oxycontin (oxycodone ER) for relief of OA-related knee pain. Because of the cost of the prescription, patient cannot afford the medication and therefore is not taking it. **Plan:** If appropriate, please consider switching from oxycodone ER to a less expensive alternative such as morphine sulfate ER. Patient may also benefit from adjunctive analgesic agents such as duloxetine or venlafaxine to limit dose of opioid required.

FIGURE 29-9 Sample provider communications for osteoarthritis.
Source: References 8 [scenario 2], 12 (scenario 1 and 4) and 17 [scenario 3].

TABLE 29-11 • Suggested Intervals for Follow-up and Monitoring for Patients with Osteoarthritis

Pain reduction
For full analgesic effects, 4-6 weeks after initiating acetaminophen, 2-3 weeks after initiating an NSAID or opioid analgesic, 1-2 weeks after corticosteroid injection, and 4-8 weeks after hyaluronic acid injection After pain control is established, it should be reassessed on a monthly basis (or at each visit) Ability to perform activities of daily living, physical functioning, and mobility should be assessed at each visit
Toxicity
Monitor for adverse drug effects 1-4 weeks after starting a new agent or increasing the dose Monitor for adverse events 2-3 days after an intra-articular injection Monitor every 2-3 months in stable patients and at each visit Monitor for signs/symptoms of gastrointestinal bleeding at each visit Monitor for changes in bowel habits indicating constipation for patients receiving opioids at each visit

REFERENCES

1. The National Arthritis Data Workgroup. Estimates of the prevalence of arthritis and other rheumatic conditions in the United States: Part II. *Arthritis Rheum*. 2008;58:26-35.
2. Hootman JM, Helmick CG. Projections of U.S. prevalence of arthritis and associated activity limitations. *Arthritis Rheum*. 2006;54:226-229.
3. Lane NE. Clinical practice. Osteoarthritis of the hip. *New Engl J Med*. 2007;357:1413-1421.
4. Hunter DJ. In the clinic. Osteoarthritis. *Ann Intern Med*. 2007;147: ITC8-1-ITC8-16.
5. Lethbridge-Cejku M, Schiller JS, Bernadel L. Summary health statistics for U.S. adults: National Health Interview Survey, 2002. *Vital Health Stat*. 2004;222:1-151.
6. Salaffi F, Carotti M, Stancati A, Grassi W. Health-related quality of life in older adults with symptomatic hip and knee osteoarthritis: A comparison with matched healthy controls. *Aging Clin Exp Res*. 2005;17:255-263.
7. Lawrence RC, Felson DT, Helmick CG, et al. Estimates of the prevalence of arthritis and other rheumatic conditions in the United States. Part II. *Arthritis Rheum*. 2008;58:26-35.
8. Hochberg MC, Altman RD, April KT, et al. American College of Rheumatology 2012 recommendations for use of nonpharmacologic and pharmacologic therapies in osteoarthritis of the hand, hip, and knee. *Arthritis Care Res*. 2012;64:465-474.

9. *Medicare Part D Medication Therapy Management Program Standardized Format.* Available at https://www.cms.gov/Medicare/Prescription-Drug-Coverage/PrescriptionDrugCovContra/Downloads/MTM-Program-Standardized-Format-English-and-Spanish-Instructions-Samples-v032712.pdf. Accessed May 4, 2017.
10. Tannenbaum H, Bombardier C, Davis P, Russell AS, Third Canadian Consensus Conference Group. An evidence-based approach to prescribing nonsteroidal antiinflammatory drugs. Third Canadian Consensus Conference. *J Rheumatol.* 2006;33:140-157.
11. Graham GG, Scott KF, Day RO. Tolerability of paracetamol. *Drug Safety.* 2005;25:227-240.
12. Clinical Pharmacology [database online]. Tampa, FL: Gold Standard, Inc.; 2017. Available at http://clinicalpharmacology.com. Accessed May 4, 2017.
13. Fored CM, Ejerblad E, Lindblad P, et al. Acetaminophen, aspirin, and chronic renal failure. *New Engl J Med.* 2001;345:1801-1808.
14. Curhan GC, Knight EL, Rosner B, et al. Lifetime non-narcotic analgesic use and decline in renal function in women. *Arch Intern Med.* 2004;164:1519-1524.
15. Trelle S, Reichenback S, Wandel S, et al. Cardiovascular safety of non-steroidal anti-inflammatory drugs: Network meta-analysis. *Br Med J.* 2011;342:c7086.
16. Nissen SE, Yeomans ND, Solomon DH, et al. Cardiovascular safety of celecoxib, naproxen, or ibuprofen for arthritis. *New Engl J Med.* 2016;375:2519-2529.
17. Lanza FL, Chan FK, Quigley EM. Guidelines for prevention of NSAID-related ulcer complications. *Am J Gastroenterol.* 2009;104:728-738.
18. Rostom A, Moayyedi P, Hunt R. Canadian consensus guidelines on long-term nonsteroidal anti-inflammatory drug therapy and the need for gastroprotection: benefits versus risks. *Aliment Pharmacol Ther.* 2009;29:481-496.
19. Davidson BL, Verheijen S, Lensing AW, et al. Bleeding risk of patients with acute venous thromboembolism taking nonsteroidal anti-inflammatory drugs or aspirin. *JAMA Intern Med.* 2014;174:947-953.
20. Soll AH, Graham DY. Peptic ulcer disease. In: Yamada T, Alpers DH, Kalloo KN, et al, eds. *Textbook of Gastroenterology*, 5th ed. Hoboken, NJ: Wiley-Blackwell; 2009:936-981.
21. Bhatt DL, Scheiman J, Abraham NS, et al. ACCF/ACG/AHA 2008 expert consensus document on reducing the gastrointestinal risks of antiplatelet therapy and NSAID use: A report of the American College of Cardiology Foundation Task Force on clinical expert consensus documents. *Am J Gastroenterol.* 2008;103:2890-2907.
22. Chan FKL Abraham NS, Scheiman JM, Laine L. Management of patients on nonsteroidal anti-inflammatory drugs: A clinical practice recommendation from the First International Working Party on Gastrointestinal and Cardiovascular Effects of Nonsteroidal Anti-Inflammatory Drugs and Anti-platelet Agents. *Am J Gastroenterol.* 2008;103:2908-2918.
23. Cryer B. Management of patients with high gastrointestinal risk on antiplatelet therapy. *Gastroenterol Clin N Am.* 2009;38:289-303.
24. Loke YK, Trivedi AN, Singh S. Meta-analysis: Gastrointestinal bleeding due to interaction between selective serotonin uptake inhibitors and non-steroidal anti-inflammatory drugs. *Aliment Pharmacol Ther.* 2008;27:31-40.
25. Chan FKL. The David Y. Graham Lecture: Use of nonsteroidal antiinflammatory drugs in a COX-2 restricted environment. *Am J Gastroenterol.* 2008;103:221-227.
26. Scheiman JM. Balancing risks and benefits of cyclooxygenase-2 selective nonsteroidal anti-inflammatory drugs. *Gastroenterol Clin N Am.* 2009;38:305-14.
27. Arora G, Singh G, Triadafilopoulos G. Proton pump inhibitors for gastroduodenal damage related to nonsteroidal antiinflammatory drugs or aspirin: Twelve important questions for clinical practice. *Clin Gastroenterol Hepatol* 2009;7:725-736.
28. The American Academy of Pain Medicine, the American Pain Society; The use of opioids for the treatment of chronic pain: A consensus statement from the American Academy of Pain Medicine and the American Pain Society. *Clin J Pain.* 1997;13:6-8.
29. Ballantyne JC, Mao J. Opioid therapy for chronic pain. *New Engl J Med.* 2003;349:1943-1953.
30. Bannuru RR, Natov NS, Dasi UR, et al. Therapeutic trajectory following intra-articular hyaluronic acid injection in knee osteoarthritis—meta-analysis. *Osteoarth Cartil.* 2011;19:611-619.
31. Juni P, Reichenbach S, Trelle S, et al. Efficacy and safety of intraarticular hylan or hyaluronic acids for osteoarthritis of the knee: A randomized controlled trial. *Arthritis Rheum.* 2007;56:3610-3619.
32. Rutjes AWS, Juni P, da Costa BR, et al. Viscosupplementation for osteoarthritis of the knee: Systematic review and meta-analysis. *Ann Intern Med.* 2012;157:180-191.
33. Clegg DO, Reda DJ, Harris CI, et al. Glucosamine, chondroitin sulfate, and the two in combination for painful knee osteoarthritis. *New Engl J Med.* 2006;354:795-808.
34. Gray HC, Hutcheson PS, Gray RG. Is glucosamine safe in patients with seafood allergy? *J Allergy Clin Immunol.* 2004;114:459-460.
35. McAlindon T, LaVelley M, Schneider E, et al. Effect of vitamin D supplementation on progression of knee pain and cartilage volume loss in patients with symptomatic osteoarthritis: A randomized controlled trial. *JAMA.* 2013;309:155-162.
36. Natural Medicines [database online]. Somerville, MA: Therapeutic Research Center; 2017. Available at https://naturalmedicines.therapeuticresearch.com/. Accessed May 4, 2017.

Review Questions

1. Which of the following is correct regarding the development of osteoarthritis?
   a. Osteoarthritis is an immune-mediated condition that develops rapidly over a period of weeks to months.
   b. Osteoarthritis is more likely to affect younger patients than older patients.
   c. The development of osteoarthritis is multifactorial and may include factors such as a history of joint trauma and biomechanical factors.
   d. Primary osteoarthritis is attributed to a specific precipitating factor such as an inflammatory or endocrine disorder.

2. Which of the following questions is LEAST likely to be beneficial when assessing a patient's osteoarthritis?
   a. "What activities are associated with improving or worsening your symptoms?"
   b. "What do you do for exercise?"
   c. "Which joint or joints are affected?"
   d. "Do you have an x-ray of the affected joint(s)?"

3. Which of the following statements concerning treatment goals for osteoarthritis is correct?
   a. Treatment plans should aim to completely eliminate pain with one or more analgesic therapies.
   b. Treatment plans should minimize pain and side effects while maximizing functioning and quality of life.
   c. Treatment goals should be developed on an individual basis once initial first-line therapy has failed.
   d. Treatment goals should be outlined at diagnosis and should not be changed once therapy is initiated.

4. All of the following statements utilize acceptable living room language when discussing osteoarthritis with a patient EXCEPT:
   a. Hyaluronic acid may provide chondroprotective benefits.
   b. Joints are where bones meet and allow arms, legs, and fingers to move freely.
   c. Intra-articular therapy can involve injection of medication directly into a joint.
   d. Knee effusion is when the knee joint swells as a result of fluid within the knee joint.

5. When discussing osteoarthritis with a patient, which of the following should be included in a medication action plan (MAP)?
   a. The names of all the medications that the patient is taking.
   b. The strengths, administration routes, and directions for medications for the disease state of interest.
   c. The reason why the patient takes the medication and when the medication was started.
   d. Specific instructions or solutions to problems that were identified and/or discussed during the interview.

6. For patients with osteoarthritis taking a nonsteroidal anti-inflammatory drug (NSAID), which of the following symptoms should prompt immediate referral to an urgent-care clinic or emergency department?
   a. Inadequate pain relief such that patient rates it as an 8/10
   b. Coughing or vomiting up blood
   c. Loose or watery stools for 1 day
   d. Mild sedation

7. The patient is using acetaminophen 500 mg 3 times a day for relief of knee pain associated with osteoarthritis. She reports that the acetaminophen adequately controls her pain. She has a past medical history significant for hypertension. In addition to acetaminophen, she takes amlodipine 5 mg daily and pantoprazole 40 mg daily. Which of the following correctly identifies a medication-related problem in this patient?
   a. Dosage too high—acetaminophen dose is too high.
   b. Ineffective medication—acetaminophen is not adequately controlling the pain.
   c. Need for additional medication—the patient requires a bowel regimen to prevent constipation associated with analgesic.
   d. Unnecessary medication—the patient is receiving a proton-pump inhibitor without history of gastroesophageal reflux disease, gastrointestinal bleeding, ulcer, or aspirin, antiplatelet, or NSAID use.

8. Which of the following constitutes an adequate trial of acetaminophen before declaring a treatment failure in a patient with no other medications or past medical history other than knee osteoarthritis?
   a. 4 weeks at a total daily dose of 1-2 g
   b. 4 weeks at a total daily dose of 3-4 g
   c. 2 weeks at a total daily dose of 3-4 g
   d. 2 weeks at a total daily dose of 1-2 g

9. Prior to recommending therapy with a NSAID, which of the following disease states is LEAST important to consider?
   a. History of cardiovascular disease
   b. History of renal dysfunction
   c. History of gastrointestinal bleeding or ulceration
   d. History of autoimmune disorder(s)

10. Which of the following statements about glucosamine/chondroitin is incorrect?
    a. Glucosamine/chondroitin is derived from shellfish and may lead to allergic reactions in susceptible patients.
    b. Glucosamine/chondroitin is not regulated by the FDA, and therefore quality, potency, and purity may not be consistent.
    c. Glucosamine/chondroitin may raise blood sugar in susceptible patients.
    d. Glucosamine/chondroitin can be used to provide relief of acute pain.

ANSWERS

1. c	2. d	3. b
4. a	5. d	6. b
7. d	8. b	9. d
10. d		

30

Osteoporosis MTM Data Set

Karen Whalen, PharmD, BCPS, CDE, FAPhA, and Shannon A. Miller, PharmD, BCACP

KEY POINTS

- Medication therapy management (MTM) providers should screen for medications that are associated with an increased risk of osteoporosis and recommend bone mineral density testing to the primary provider, if appropriate.
- Adequate calcium and vitamin D intake is essential for prevention and treatment of osteoporosis. An evaluation of dietary calcium intake will assist in determination of required calcium supplementation.
- Calcium carbonate is the salt of choice for calcium supplementation because it has the highest percentage of elemental calcium and is the least expensive; however, calcium citrate should be considered for elderly patients with low acid production or those on acid-reducing medications.
- MTM providers should assess for appropriate administration of bisphosphonate therapy and counsel patients on the importance of appropriate administration to reduce adverse effects and maximize efficacy of therapy.
- Adherence is poor with bisphosphonate therapy and decreases efficacy. MTM providers should screen for nonadherence and recommend changes in pharmacotherapy or other methods to improve adherence.

INTRODUCTION TO OSTEOPOROSIS

Osteoporosis is associated with low bone mass and increased bone porosity, resulting in reduced bone strength and an increased risk of bone fracture.[1,2] The hip, spine, wrist, and ribs are the most commonly affected bones.[2] Women have a higher risk of developing osteoporosis compared to men. Primary causes of osteoporosis include menopause and osteoporosis of aging.[2] Hyperthyroidism and chronic medication use (Table 30-1) are examples of secondary causes. Additional medical conditions associated with osteoporosis are listed in Table 30-2. Table 30-3 lists the risk factors for osteoporosis and osteoporotic fractures. Hip fractures result in the greatest morbidity, mortality and increased healthcare costs in older seniors.[3-5]

Osteoporosis is best diagnosed with bone mineral density (BMD) measurement by central dual-energy x-ray absorptiometry (DXA). Bone mass is reported as a *T-score*, which is the BMD mean standard deviation from a young normal adult female population; the lower the score, the greater the risk of fracture (Table 30-4).[2,3] The test also reports a *Z-score*, which is the bone density in the patient compared to other people with a similar age, height and weight. The Z-score is more useful than a T-score in a young person (premenopausal). A risk assessment helps identify patients who should be referred for a BMD.[19] A low-trauma fracture after age 50 years is also consistent with a diagnosis of osteoporosis.

Complications of Osteoporosis

Fractures of the vertebrae, hip, forearm, or humerus are considered osteoporotic fractures and can result in increased morbidity and mortality and a decreased quality of life. Hip fractures are associated with the greatest morbidity and mortality, with men suffering from a greater mortality rate than women.[3,5] Patients with osteoporotic fractures experience fear, pain, loss of self-esteem from physical deformity, and a loss of independence and mobility, which often leads to depression. Severe kyphosis can cause respiratory problems and gastrointestinal complications. Once a patient experiences a low-trauma fracture, the risk for future fractures increases significantly.[3]

TABLE 30-1 • Selected Medications Associated with Increased Bone Loss and/or Fracture Risk

Medications	Comments
Anticonvulsant therapy (phenytoin, carbamazepine, phenobarbital, and valproic acid)	↓ BMD and ↑ fracture risk; increased vitamin D metabolism leading to low 25(OH) vitamin D concentrations
Antiretroviral therapy (ARVT) Nucleoside/nucleotide reverse transcriptase inhibitors (NRTIs) (zidovudine, didanosine, lamivudine, and tenofovir) Protease inhibitors (PI) (nelfinavir, indinavir, saquinavir, ritonavir, and lopinavir)	↓ BMD (NRTIs > PI), no fracture data; increased osteoclast activity and decreased osteoblast activity
Aromatase inhibitors (eg, letrozole and anastrozole)	↓ BMD and ↑ fracture risk; reduced estrogen concentrations
Canagliflozin	↓ BMD and ↑ fracture risk (FDA reviewing SLGT2 inhibitor class of medications)
Furosemide	↑ fracture risk; increased calcium renal elimination
Glucocorticoids (long-term oral therapy)	↓ BMD and ↑ fracture risk; increased bone resorption and decreased bone formation; dose and duration dependent
Gonadotropin-releasing hormone agonists or analogs (eg, leuprolide and goserelin)	↓ BMD and ↑ fracture risk; decreased sex hormone production
Heparin (unfractionated, UFH) or low-molecular-weight heparin (LMWH)	↓ BMD and ↑ fracture risk (UFH >>> LMWH) with long-term use (eg > 6 months); decreased osteoblast replication and increased osteoclast function
Medroxyprogesterone acetate depot administration	↓ BMD, no fracture data; possible BMD recovery with discontinuation; decreased estrogen concentrations
Proton pump inhibitor therapy (long-term therapy)	↓ BMD and ↑ fracture risk; possible calcium malabsorption secondary to acid suppression for carbonate salts
Selective serotonin reuptake inhibitors	↓ BMD and ↑ fracture risk; decreased osteoblast activity
Thiazolidinediones (pioglitazone and rosiglitazone)	↓ BMD and ↑ fracture risk; decreased osteoblast function
Thyroid—excessive supplementation	↓ BMD and ↑ fracture risk; risk increases with TSH concentration < 0.1 mIU/L; possible increase in bone resorption
Vitamin A—excessive intake (> 1.5 mg of retinol form)	↓ BMD and ↑fracture risk; decreased osteoblast activity and increased osteoclast activity

Abbreviations: BMD = bone mineral density; DXA, dual-energy x-ray absorptiometry; TSH, thyroid-stimulating hormone.

Source: Reproduced, with permission, from DiPiro JT, Talbert RL, Yee GC, Matzke GR, Wells BG, Posey LM, eds. *Pharmacotherapy: A Pathophysiologic Approach*, 10th ed. New York, NY: McGraw-Hill; 2017.

TABLE 30-2 • Select Medical Conditions Associated with Osteoporosis in Children and Adults

Endocrine/hormonal Primary or secondary ovarian failure Testosterone deficiency Hyperthyroidism Cushing disease Growth hormone deficiency (in children) Primary hyperparathyroidism Diabetes, type 1 and type 2	**Chronic illness** Chronic kidney disease Malignancies (eg, multiple myeloma, lymphoma, leukemia) Human immunodeficiency virus infection/acquired immunodeficiency syndrome Organ transplant
Gastrointestinal Nutritional disorders (eg, anorexia nervosa) Malabsorptive states (eg, Crohn disease, celiac disease, gastrectomy, bariatric surgery) Chronic liver disease (eg, primary biliary cirrhosis)	**Disuse/immobility** Muscular dystrophy Multiple sclerosis Stroke/cerebrovascular accident
Disorders of calcium balance Hypercalciuria Vitamin D deficiency	**Genetic** Osteogenesis imperfecta Cystic fibrosis Hemochromatosis Hypophosphatasia
Inflammatory disorders Rheumatoid arthritis	

Source: Reproduced, with permission, from DiPiro JT, Talbert RL, Yee GC, Matzke GR, Wells BG, Posey LM, eds. *Pharmacotherapy: A Pathophysiologic Approach*, 10th ed. New York, NY: McGraw-Hill; 2017.

TABLE 30-3 • Risk Factors for Osteoporosis and Osteoporotic Fractures

Low bone mineral density[a]
Female sex[a]
Advanced age[a]
Race/ethnicity[a]
History of a previous fragility (low-trauma) fracture as an adult[a] (especially clinical vertebral fracture or hip fracture)
Osteoporotic fracture in a first-degree relative (especially parental hip fracture[a])
Low body weight or body mass index[a]
Premature menopause (before 45 years old)
Secondary osteoporosis (especially rheumatoid arthritis[a,b])
Past or present systemic oral glucocorticoid therapy[a]
Current cigarette smoking[a]
Alcohol intake of three or more drinks/day[a]
Low calcium intake
Low physical activity or immobilization
Vitamin D insufficiency and deficiency
Recent falls
Cognitive impairment
Impaired vision

[a] Factors included in the World Health Organization fracture risk assessment tool (FRAX).

[b] Secondary causes included in the FRAX tool question are type 1 diabetes, osteogenesis imperfecta as an adult, long-standing untreated hyperthyroidism, hypogonadism, premature menopause (<45 years old), chronic malnutrition, malabsorption, and chronic liver disease.

Source: Reproduced, with permission, from DiPiro JT, Talbert RL, Yee GC, Matzke GR, Wells BG, Posey LM, eds. *Pharmacotherapy: A Pathophysiologic Approach*, 10th ed. New York, NY: McGraw-Hill; 2017.

Therapeutic Goals for Osteoporosis

Ideally, the goal is to prevent the development of osteoporosis. MTM providers should be aware of medications that may contribute to osteoporosis, screen for appropriate calcium intake, and assist patients in reducing other controllable risk factors for osteoporosis. Once diagnosed, the goal for a patient with low bone mass or osteoporosis is to prevent further bone loss and prevent fractures. Reduction of pain and deformity, improvement in functional capacity and quality of life, and a decrease in the risk for future falls and fractures are additional goals for patients who have a history of osteoporotic fractures.[3]

TABLE 30-4 • Diagnosis of Osteoporosis

Bone Classification[a]	T-Score[b] (Bone Mineral Density Measurement)
Normal	At −1.0 and above
Osteopenia (low bone mass)	Between −1.0 and −2.5
Osteoporosis	At −2.5 or below

[a] Based on World Health Organization classification of BMD.

[b] Mean standard deviation from a young normal adult female population.

Source: Reference 2.

Therapeutic Success

A BMD result that has maintained or increased is considered successful therapy.[2]

Therapeutic Failure

Although there is no absolute definition of treatment failure, the occurrence of a fracture while on medication for a year is considered a failure. A significant decrease in BMD on treatment (rare) is also considered a treatment failure. In this case, other causes such as noncompliance, improper administration, malabsorption, calcium or vitamin D deficiency, or a secondary cause of bone loss must be ruled out. Patients that fail treatment should be evaluated for an alternative treatment or combination therapy.[2]

CORE ELEMENT 1—COMPREHENSIVE MEDICATION REVIEW FOR PATIENTS WITH OSTEOPOROSIS

A list of suggested questions to use when conducting a medication therapy review in a patient with osteoporosis is provided in Table 30-5. The number and types of questions will depend on several factors, including the amount of time for the interview,

TABLE 30-5 • Questions to Ask When Conducting a Medication Review in a Patient with Osteoporosis

Suggested Questions for the Patient with Osteoporosis
How long have you had osteoporosis? When were you diagnosed?
What do you know about the risks of having osteoporosis?
Who else in your family has osteoporosis?
Has either parent had a hip fracture?
How old were you when you had your last menses (females)?
Have you ever experienced the following signs/symptoms: • Bone pain • Inability to move • Diagnosis with a fracture in your spine, hip, wrist, or forearm
What medications are you currently taking?
Are you able to remain upright for 30 minutes after your medication?
Have you taken oral steroids in the past?
Do you use tobacco? If so, how much and for how long?
How much alcohol do you consume per day?
How much caffeine do you consume per day?
How many carbonated beverages do you consume per day?
What medications do you take for osteoporosis? How do you take them?
How often do you miss a dose of your osteoporosis medication(s)?
What other medications have you taken in the past for your osteoporosis?
Have you ever stopped taking any of your prescribed osteoporosis medications without telling your physician? If so, why?
What over-the-counter (OTC) medications or herbals do you use for your osteoporosis?
Other than medicines, what have you tried in the past to treat osteoporosis (eg, diet, exercise)?
What exercise regimen do you follow?

(Continued)

TABLE 30-5 • Questions to Ask When Conducting a Medication Review in a Patient with Osteoporosis (*Continued*)

Questions to Ask for Prevention/Assessment of Medical Emergencies
Are you experiencing severe pain? Have you had prior fractures from osteoporosis?
Have you had any falls?
Are you experiencing bleeding in your stool or are you vomiting blood?
Are you experiencing any jaw pain? Do you have any ulcers in your mouth?
Are you experiencing any pain, redness, or swelling in your legs?
Are you experiencing any shortness of breath (for patients on raloxifene or estrogen)?
Are you experiencing numbness, weakness, confusion, trouble speaking or understanding, seeing, trouble with balance or coordination, or a severe headache without a known cause (for patients on raloxifene or estrogen)?

number of concurrent medication-related problems (MRPs), urgency of MRPs, and the reliability of the patient in providing accurate information, among others. In time-limited interactions or in complex cases with multiple medical issues, the MTM provider may choose to target questions that help to identify or rule out issues of an urgent nature. MTM providers should remember to use living room language during the interview (Figure 30-1), and to be prepared for questions that patients may ask regarding osteoporosis (Table 30-6).

CORE ELEMENT 2—PERSONAL MEDICATION LIST[20]

A sample personal medication list for a patient with osteoporosis is shown in Figure 30-2. This example is representative only of osteoporosis medications. Additional medications for other disease states should be added and listed separately. MTM providers should remember to use plain language when creating the personal medication list.

CORE ELEMENT 3—MEDICATION ACTION PLAN[20]

Sample MAPs for patients with osteoporosis are shown in Figure 30-3. These examples are representative only of action steps for the patient with osteoporosis. MAPs for other disease states or other MRPs should be added and listed separately. In general, only a few of the most important action steps should be listed, so as not to overwhelm the patient. Other areas for patient self-management can be addressed at later visits. Remember to use plain language when creating the medication action plan MAP.

Adherence—the ability to stick to something; medication adherence is the ability to follow the instructions for use.

Adverse event—something bad that happens, bad reaction; unexplained or unwanted effects.

Antiresorptive medication—medications used to treat osteoporosis that slow the rate of bone loss.

Biomarkers—a test that can be used as a marker of an event or condition; biomarkers in osteoporosis identify bone loss.

Bisphosphonate—antiresorptive medication that slows the rate of bone loss.

Bone mineral density (BMD) *test*—a test used to estimate the compactness of the bones; reflects the strength of the bones represented by calcium content.

Calcium—mineral in the body necessary for bone strength and for cells in the body to work properly.

Central dual-energy x-ray absorptiometry (DXA)—the standard test for measuring bone mineral density. It has high precision, short scan time, and a low radiation dose.

Creatinine test—a test that checks how well the kidneys are working; an increase means the kidneys are not working as well.

Cushing syndrome—a condition in which the body is exposed to high levels of the hormone cortisol; results in bone loss leading to osteoporosis.

Formation medication—medications used in osteoporosis to rebuild bone.

Fracture—a broken bone; the most common areas for a fracture in osteoporosis are the hip, wrist, and spine.

FRAX— fracture risk assessment tool; a tool used to evaluate fracture risk.

Glucocorticoid—a class of medications that has an increased risk of causing osteoporosis.

Lifestyle changes—your physician may have recommended changes in lifestyle to increase bone strength and reduce fracture risk, which for some patients includes decreasing the amount of alcohol you drink, exercising, or quitting smoking.

Low-trauma fracture—a break in a bone that occurs from a fall from standing position or less.

Osteopenia—low bone mass; patients with osteopenia may benefit from treatment to decrease the chance of osteoporosis.

Osteoporosis—a disease where bones are thin, spongy, and likely to break for little or no reason.

Postmenopausal osteoporosis—bone loss that happens after women go through the "change" (menopause); bone loss can be greatest for ≤4 years after menopause.

Primary osteoporosis—osteoporosis due to advanced age or menopause.

Secondary osteoporosis—bone loss associated with medical conditions (hyperthyroidism, Cushing syndrome, medications, etc.).

Serum 25 (OH) *vitamin D*—a test that measures how much vitamin D is in a patient's body.

Smoking cessation—Quitting smoking; this can lower your risk of bone loss.

T-score—number from a BMD test; this number compares your bones to those of a healthy young woman and determines whether you have osteoporosis.

Vertebrae—series of bones that make up the spine.

WHO—World Health Organization.

Z-score—a number generated from the bone density test that compares BMD to a person of similar age.

FIGURE 30-1 Living room language for osteoporosis.

TABLE 30-6 • Questions to Anticipate Regarding Osteoporosis

- **What is osteoporosis?**
  Osteoporosis occurs when there is too much bone loss. Bones are weak and can break as a result of a minor fall. More women than men suffer from osteoporosis.
- **Who is at risk for osteoporosis?**
  Uncontrollable risk factors: Age >50 years, female, postmenopause, family history, low body weight (small and thin), broken bones, loss of height
  Controllable risk factors: Not enough calcium and vitamin D, diet low in fruits and vegetables, too much sodium and caffeine, not getting enough activity, too much alcohol, losing weight, smoking
  Additional risk factors: Medications such as glucocorticoids and proton-pump inhibitors and other diseases that cause bone loss
- **What is BMD?**
  Bone mineral density. It is a number that tells us how much calcium and other minerals are in the bone. From the result, the number gives us an idea of how strong the bones are.
- **What causes osteoporosis?**
  Low estrogen (female), low testosterone (male), other hormone imbalances, lack of calcium, lack of vitamin D, inactivity or conditions such as paralysis, muscular dystrophy, thyroid problems, smoking, and medications that cause bone loss.
- **What health problems are associated with osteoporosis?**
  Fractures of the spine, hip, forearm, and the bone running from the shoulder to the elbow (humerus) can occur in osteoporosis. Hip fracture has the greatest impact on health and incidence of death. Depression and respiratory problems may also occur with osteoporosis.
- **How do I know if I have osteoporosis?**
  You may be asked questions to assess your risk for osteoporosis. You may also have a test done to review the calcium and minerals in your bones. If your test score is low, you may have osteoporosis or be at a higher risk for developing it.
- **Why are medications to treat osteoporosis so important?**
  Medications are important because they can prevent, slow down, or stop the progress of bone loss. Taking medications for osteoporosis as directed may even improve your bone health. The medications may also reduce the risk of broken bones.
- **What can happen if I stop taking my osteoporosis medications?**
  If you stop taking your medication, you may continue to experience bone loss and increase your risk for fractures and falls.
- **I have read that there is actually an increase in fractures with my osteoporosis medication. Why is that?**
  Atypical femoral fractures (fractures affecting the long shaft portion of the femur) have been associated with bisphosphonates. These bone-building medications affect the normal cycle of bone and may increase the risk of fracture. However, the benefit of bisphosphonates greatly outweighs the risk of atypical fracture. The incidence of an atypical fracture is low compared to risk of a typical hip fracture.
- **How long do I have to take medications for osteoporosis?**
  How long you will need to take medications for osteoporosis will depend on the initial bone test done by the physician and the results of any additional bone tests completed after the medication is started. Medications such as calcium and vitamin D will continue, but sometimes other medications may be stopped after 3-5 years.
- **When should I call my physician about my osteoporosis treatment?**
  You should call your physician if you are experiencing pain in the jaw, difficulty swallowing, vomiting blood, severe pain or pain that you have not experienced before, shortness of breath, redness or swelling in a leg, or symptoms of a stroke. You should also let your physician know if you start or stop any of your other medications, as this may affect your osteoporosis medication.
- **What should I do if I have a problem with my osteoporosis medications?**
  Contact your pharmacist or healthcare provider.

PERSONAL MEDICATION LIST FOR *<Insert patient's name, DOB: mm/dd/yyyy>*	
Medication: Calcium citrate 630 mg with vitamin D_3 500 international units (Citracal Maximum®)	
How I use it: 2 caplets (1260 mg) by mouth twice daily	
Why I use it: To help my bones	**Prescriber:** Dr. Patel
Date I started using it: 3/5/2017	**Date I stopped using it:** (*Leave blank for patient's notes*)
Why I stopped using it: (*Leave blank for patient's notes*)	
Medication: Alendronate 70 mg	
How I use it: 1 tablet (70 mg) by mouth weekly (Wednesday) on empty stomach	
Why I use it: help my bones	**Prescriber:** Dr. Patel
Date I started using it: 3/5/2017	**Date I stopped using it:** (*Leave blank for patient's notes*)
Why I stopped using it: (*Leave blank for patient's notes*)	

FIGURE 30-2 Sample personal medication list for osteoporosis medications.

	DATE PREPARED: *<Insert date>*
What we talked about: Adding the medication alendronate to prevent bone loss and reduce the risk of fractures.	
What I need to do: Take one 70 mg tablet by mouth once a week on the same day of every week. Take with at least 6 oz of plain water. Take 30 minutes before food, medications, vitamins, or supplements. Remain upright for 30 minutes. If I miss a dose, take it the next day. Skip the dose if more than 1 day has passed and wait to take at my next scheduled dose.	**What I did and when I did it:** (*Leave blank for patient's notes*)
What we talked about: Getting enough calcium to help my bones.	
What I need to do: Eat foods rich in calcium such as broccoli and milk and other dairy products. Limit the amount of alcohol, caffeine, and soda. Consider calcium supplements if daily dietary intake is not enough. Consider weight-bearing, resistance- and balance-improving exercise.	**What I did and when I did it:** (*Leave blank for patient's notes*)

FIGURE 30-3 Sample medication action plan for a patient with osteoporosis.

CORE ELEMENT 4—INTERVENTION AND/OR REFERRAL

Interventions for osteoporosis prevention and management may include lifestyle modifications and/or drug therapy. Medications should be selected on the basis of patient preference and other comorbid disease states. Patients should be encouraged to be compliant with their treatment and follow-up at regular intervals so that osteoporosis may be assessed. Table 30-7 summarizes lifestyle modifications, and Tables 30-8 and 30-9 provide an overview of osteoporosis drug therapy. Patients who have chronic kidney disease or an age-related decline in renal function should be carefully evaluated for the best treatment option.[3] The treatment algorithm for the management of osteoporosis is found in Figure 30-4. A flowchart showing referral for management of osteoporosis is given in Figure 30-5.

WHO Fracture Risk Assessment Tool

The WHO Fracture Risk Assessment Tool (FRAX®) is a tool that evaluates the risk for osteoporotic fractures (see www.shef.ac.uk/FRAX).[21] The tool takes into account individual patient risk factors for a fracture, as well as BMD. The tool provides a 10-year probability of hip fracture and a 10-year probability of a major osteoporotic fracture. This tool is useful in determining the need for therapy in patients who have a low bone mass but do not meet the criteria for osteoporosis; for example, patients with a low bone mass (T-score between -1.0 and -2.5 at the femoral neck or spine) and a 10-year probability of a hip fracture of ≥3% or a 10-year probability of a major osteoporosis-related fracture of ≥20% are candidates for bisphosphonate or other therapy.[2,21]

Herbal Supplements for Osteoporosis

Currently supplements for osteoporosis have conflicting or unclear evidence or lack data to support their use. Medications and therapies with proven efficacy should be utilized for the prevention and treatment of osteoporosis.[22]

TABLE 30-7 • Lifestyle Modifications for Management of Osteoporosis

Modification	Recommendation
Manage weight	Maintain normal body weight (body mass index: 18.5-24.9 kg/m^2) Speak to your healthcare provider before initiating a weight loss plan
Eat a well-balanced diet	Consume a diet rich in calcium (eg, milk and other dairy products, broccoli). The amount of vitamin D in food is low. Another source of vitamin D is sunlight. Many patients may need additional vitamin D supplementation. Limit caffeine to ≤2 servings per day, and limit consumption of carbonated beverages.
Increase physical activity	Weight-bearing exercise (exercise where feet support the body; eg, walking, Tai Chi, dancing) of moderate intensity for 30-40 minutes 3-4 days/week and a resistance activity (working against the weight of another object; eg, free weights, resistance tubing) for 20-30 minutes twice per week. Balance exercises will also help minimize falls.
Decrease alcohol consumption	Men: ≤2 drinks/day Women and lighter persons: ≤1 drink/day (1 drink = 12 oz beer, 5 oz wine, or 1.5 oz. of 80-proof whiskey)
Stop smoking	For bone health, smoking should stop. It is associated with an ≤80% increased relative risk for hip fractures.
Prevent falls	Educate patient on home safety to decrease falls (anchor rugs, light hallways). Recommend a falls assessment for patients with a history of a falls and/or those with walking or balance problems.

Source: Data from reference 3.

TABLE 30-8 • **Drug Dosing Table for Medications Used to Prevent and Treat Osteoporosis**

Drug	Brand Name	Dose	Comments
		Antiresorptive Medications—Nutritional Supplements	
Calcium	Various	**Adequate daily intake:** IOM: 200-1200 mg/day, varies per age; supplement dose is difference between required adequate intake and dietary intake Immediate-release doses should be <500-600 mg	Recommend food first to achieve goal intake. Available in different salts, including carbonate and citrate, absorption of other salts not fully quantified. Different formulations, including chewable, liquid, gummy, softgel, drink, and wafer; different combination products. Review package to determine number of units to create a serving size and desired amount of elemental calcium. Give calcium carbonate with meals to improve absorption.
Vitamin D D_3 (cholecalciferol) D_2 (ergocalciferol)	**OTC:** Tablets: 400, 1000, 2000 units Capsule: 400, 1000, 2000, 5000, 10 000 units Gummies: 300, 500, 1000 units Drops: 300, 400, 1000, 2000 units/mL or drop Solution: 400, 5000 units/mL Spray: 1000, 5000 units/spray Creams and lotions: 500 and 1000 units per ¼ teaspoonful. **Prescription:** Capsule: 50 000 units Solution: 8000 units/mL	**Adequate daily intake:** IOM—400-800 units/day to achieve adequate intake; NOF—800-1000 units orally daily; if low 25(OH) vitamin D concentrations, malabsorption, or altered metabolism. higher doses (>2000 units daily) might be required **Vitamin D deficiency:** 50 000 units orally once to twice weekly for 8-12 weeks; repeat as needed until therapeutic concentrations	Vegetarians and vegans need to read label to determine whether it is a plant-based product. Slight advantage of vitamin D_3 over D_2 for increasing serum 25(OH) vitamin D concentrations. For drops, ensure measurement is correct for desired dose. Ability of sprays, lotions, and creams to resolve deficiencies or maintain adequate intakes is unknown.
		Antiresorptive Prescription Medications	
Bisphosphonates			
Alendronate	Fosamax Fosamax Plus D Binosto (effervescent tab)	Treatment: 10 mg orally daily or 70 mg orally weekly Prevention: 5 mg orally daily or 35 mg orally weekly	Generic available for weekly tablet product. The 70-mg dose is available as a tablet, effervescent tablet, oral liquid, or combination tablet with 2800 or 5600 units of vitamin D_3. Administered in the morning on an empty stomach with 6-8 oz plain water. Do not eat and remain upright for at least 30 minutes following administration. Do not coadminister with any other medication or supplements, including calcium and vitamin D.
Ibandronate	Boniva	Treatment: 150 mg orally monthly, 3 mg intravenous quarterly Prevention: 150 mg orally monthly	Generic available for oral product. Administration instructions same as for alendronate, except must delay eating and remain upright for at least 60 minutes.
Risedronate	Actonel Atelvia (delayed-release)	Treatment and Prevention: 5 mg orally daily, 35 mg orally weekly, 150 mg orally monthly	Generic available for immediate-release product. A 35-mg dose is also available as a delayed-release product. Administration instructions same as for alendronate, except delayed-release product is taken immediately following breakfast.
Zoledronic acid	Reclast	Treatment: 5 mg intravenous infusion yearly Prevention: 5 mg intravenous infusion every 2 years	Can premedicate with acetaminophen to decrease infusion reactions. Contraindicated if CrCl < 35 mL/min. Also marketed under the brand name Zometa (4 mg) for treatment of hypercalcemia and prevention of skeleton-related events from bone metastases from solid tumors with different dosing.

(Continued)

TABLE 30-8 • Drug Dosing Table for Medications Used to Prevent and Treat Osteoporosis (*Continued*)

Drug	Brand Name	Dose	Comments
RANK Ligand Inhibitors			
Denosumab	Prolia	Treatment: 60 mg subcutaneously every 6 months	Administered by a healthcare practitioner. Correct hypocalcemia before administration. Also marketed under the brand name Xgeva (70 mg/mL) for treatment of hypercalcemia and prevention of skeletal-related events from bone metastases from solid tumors with different dosing.
Estrogen Agonist/Antagonist and Tissue Selective Estrogen Complex			
Raloxifene	Evista	60 mg daily	Generic available.
Bazedoxifene with conjugated equine estrogens (CEE)	Duavee	20 mg plus 0.45 mg CEE daily	For postmenopausal women with a uterus; no progestogen needed. Bazedoxifene monotherapy available in some countries.
Calcitonin			
Calcitonin (salmon)	Fortical	200 units (1 spray) intranasally daily, alternating nares every other day 100 units subcutaneously daily	Generic available. Refrigerate nasal spray until opened for daily use, then room temperature. Prime with first use.
Formation Medications			
Recombinant human PTH 1-34 units			
	Forteo	20 μg subcutaneously daily for ≤2 years	First dose at night. Refrigerate before and after each use. Use new needle with each dose. Inject thigh or stomach. Discard after 28 days or if cloudy.

Abbreviations: CEE = conjugated equine estrogen; IOM = Institute of Medicine; NOF = National Osteoporosis Foundation; NSAID = nonsteroidal anti-inflammatory drug; OTC = over the counter; PTH= parathyroid hormone.

Source: Data from reference 3.

TABLE 30-9 • Calcium and Vitamin D Recommended Daily Allowances and Upper Limits

Group and Ages	Elemental Calcium (mg)	Calcium Upper Limit (mg)	Vitamin D (Units)[a]	Vitamin D Upper Limit (Units)
Infants				
Birth to 6 months	200	1000	400	1000
6-12 months	260	1500	400	1500
Children				
1-3 years	700	2500	600	2500
4-8 years	1000	2500	600	3000
9-18 years	1300	3000	600	4000
Adults				
19–50 years	1000	2500	600[b]	4000
51-70 years (men)	1000	2000	600[b]	4000
51-70 years (women)	1200	2000	600[b]	4000
>70 years	1200	2000	800[b]	4000

[a] Other guidelines recommend intake to achieve a 25(OH) vitamin D concentration of >30 ng/mL (μg/L; >75 nmol/L),[2,14,15] which is higher than the IOM goal of >20 ng/mL (μg/L; >50 nmol/L).[18]

[b] 2014 National Osteoporosis Foundation Guidelines recommend 400-800 units for adults aged <50 years and 800-1000 units for adults aged ≥50 years.[2]

Source: Reproduced, with permission, from DiPiro JT, Talbert RL, Yee GC, Matzke GR, Wells BG, Posey LM, eds. *Pharmacotherapy: A Pathophysiologic Approach*, 10th ed. New York, NY: McGraw-Hill; 2017.

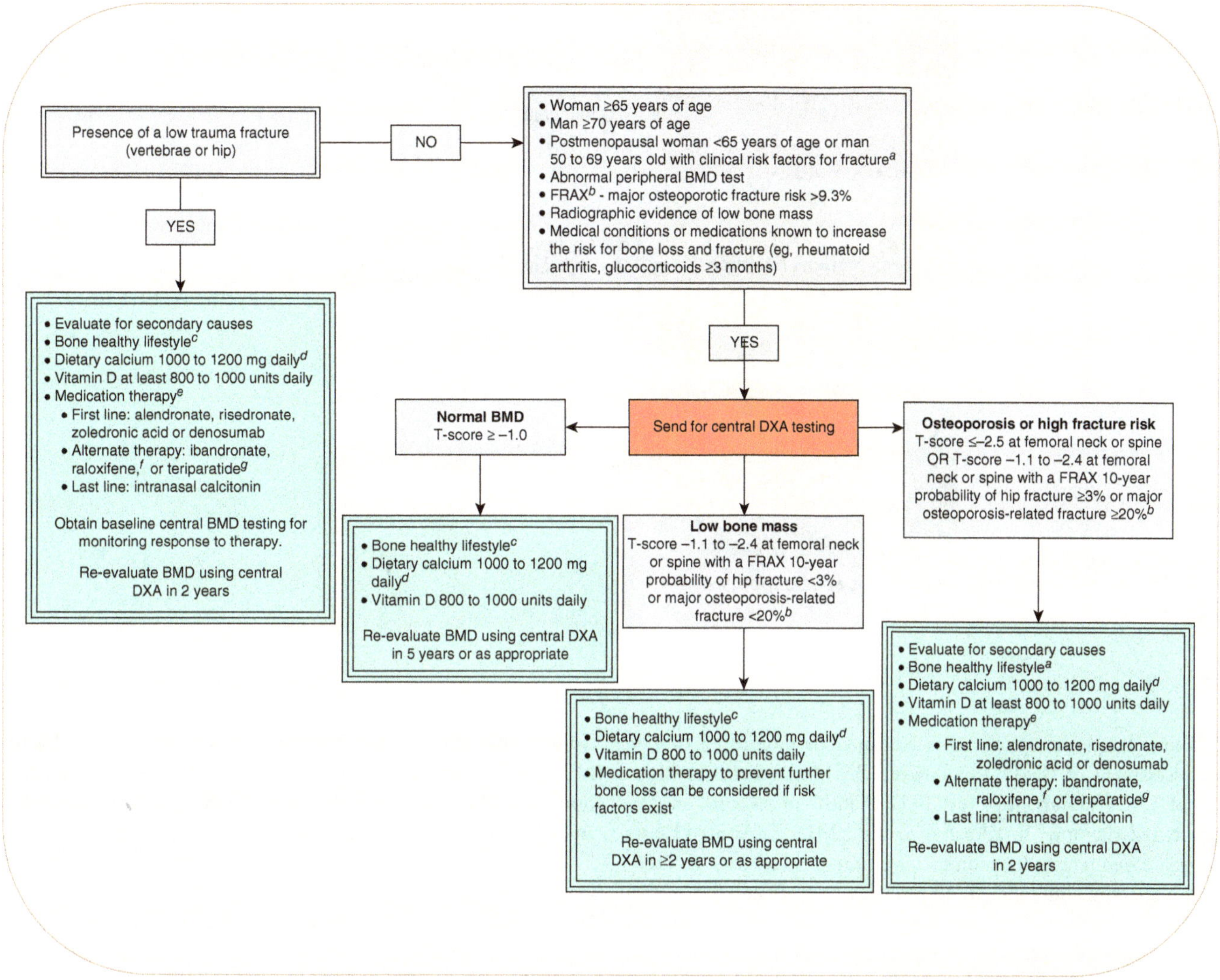

FIGURE 30-4 Algorithm for management of osteoporosis in postmenopausal women and men aged ≥50 years.

Abbreviations: BMD = bone mineral density; DXA = dual-energy x-ray absorptiometry.

[a] Major clinical risk factors for fracture: current smoker, low body weight or body mass index, history of osteoporosis or low-trauma fracture in a first-degree relative, personal history of fracture as an adult (aged >50 years), excessive alcohol intake.

[b] FRAX = World Health Organization fracture risk assessment tool.

[c] Bone-healthy lifestyle includes smoking cessation, limited alcohol intake, well-balanced diet with adequate calcium and vitamin D intake, weight-bearing/resistance exercises, and fall prevention.

[d] Dietary caution preferred. If diet is inadequate, supplement as necessary.

[e] Sometimes men with hypogonadism also receive testosterone replacement; sometimes women with menopausal symptoms receive low-dose hormone therapy for a short time.

[f] Raloxifene can be a good option in women who are at high risk for breast cancer.

[g] Teriparatide can be considered a first-line option in patients who are at very high risk for fracture (eg, T-score ≤ 3.5 or multiple low-trauma fractures) or who are intolerant to other medications.

Source: References 2, 13, 14, and 15. From Figure 92-3 in DiPiro JT, Talbert RL, Yee GC, Matzke GR, Wells BG, Posey LM, eds. *Pharmacotherapy: A Pathophysiologic Approach*, 10th ed. New York, NY: McGraw-Hill; 2017. Available at www.accesspharmacy.com.

CORE ELEMENT 5—DOCUMENTATION AND FOLLOW-UP

Clear and succinct documentation of MRPs and recommendations is a key component of the MTM consult. Examples of potential MRPs in patients with osteoporosis are provided in Table 30-10. Sample communications and recommendations to providers to address medication-related issues are found in Figure 30-6. Recommendations may be communicated via fax, telephone, or other means of written or secure electronic communication. The examples below are for illustrative purposes. Actual communications to providers should be individualized according to the type of recommendation, patient-specific characteristics, and the nature of the relationship with the provider.

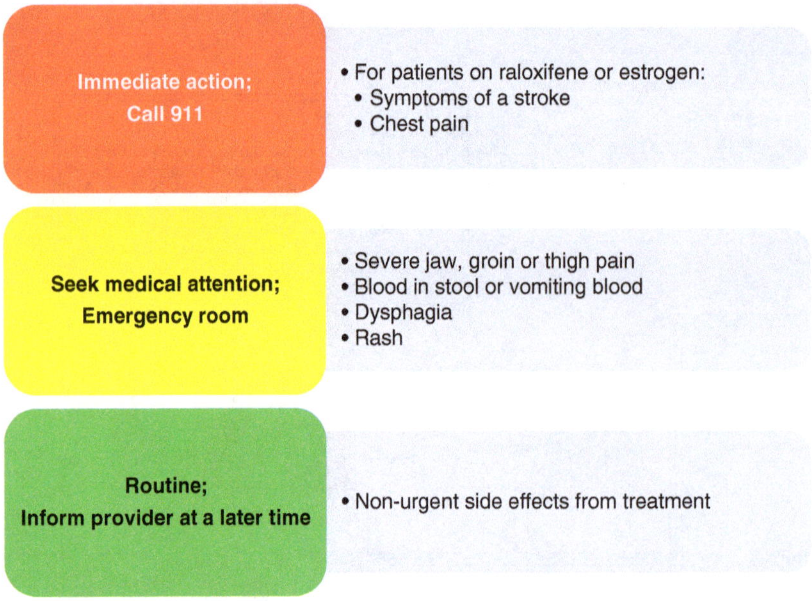

FIGURE 30-5 Referral for management of osteoporosis.

The outcome of osteoporosis treatment is monitored though the assessment of BMD. A follow-up BMD may occur at intervals of 12-24 months, or every 6-12 months in patients on glucocorticoid therapy.[2] In addition to the BMD, Table 30-11 lists suggested frequencies for monitoring efficacy and toxicity of osteoporosis therapy, and Table 30-12 provides an overview of monitoring parameters for various osteoporosis medications. The optimal duration of bisphosphonate therapy for osteoporosis is uncertain. Some experts recommend that continuation of oral bisphosphonates be reevaluated after 5 years, with a drug holiday considered in women with higher bone mineral density and lower risk of fracture. MTM providers should stay current with the latest recommendations regarding duration of osteoporosis therapy, as this may afford an opportunity to streamline therapy in some patients.

Quality Measures

Many payers of MTM services are accountable for providing high-quality healthcare to their beneficiaries, the patients. These payers, usually healthcare plans, are "graded" on a 5-star rating system (where 1 reflects low quality and 5 reflects the highest

TABLE 30-10 • Medication-Related Problems (MRPs) in Patients with Osteoporosis

Category of MRP	Sample Medication-Related Problem
Nonadherence	Patient not taking osteoporosis medication because of complexity of administration Patient not taking osteoporosis medication because she/he does not perceive a benefit Patient not taking osteoporosis medication because of cost
Unnecessary medication	Duplicate therapy (eg, calcium supplementation with good documentation of adequate dietary intake)
Need for additional medication	Patient with a T-score of -2.5 and not on a medication for treatment of osteoporosis Patient on a bisphosphonate without adequate calcium or vitamin D intake (diet or supplementation)
Ineffective medication	Adequate trial of an osteoporosis medication with a decrease in BMD Elderly patient taking calcium carbonate when calcium citrate would be preferred
Dosage too low	Patient taking bisphosphonate with other medications and obtaining inadequate absorption (could also be classified as ineffective medication)
Dosage too high	Patient taking dosage of bisphosphonate that is inappropriate for decreased renal function Increased risk of kidney stones with oversupplementation of calcium
Adverse drug event	Constipation from calcium supplementation Esophagitis from bisphosphonate

Scenario: Patient cannot remember to take weekly alendronate dose **MRP:** Nonadherence
Assessment: Patient nonadherent with alendronate because of forgetfulness. Adherence is a major concern with osteoporosis patients. Options include reminder calls/texts, or change medication to a monthly or annual frequency. Follow-up calls have shown improvement in adherence. **Plan:** Select the best day of the week for the patient to take the alendronate. Set up a weekly reminder call to the patient the day before taking alendronate.
Scenario: Patient taking weekly alendronate with food **MRP:** Ineffective medication
Assessment: Absorption is decreased when taken with food or beverage other than plain water. Options include taking alendronate 30 minutes before food or beverage or changing to an intravenous bisphosphonate. **Plan:** Reeducate patient to take alendronate 30 minutes before food. Take with a full glass of plain water only. Reemphasize additional education points, including remaining upright for 30 minutes after taking alendronate. Follow up with patient in 2 weeks to determine whether patient has been successful taking on an empty stomach, and ask about side effects.
Scenario: Patient with osteoporosis not taking a calcium supplement with vitamin D **MRP:** Need for additional therapy
Assessment: Vitamin D increases the absorption of calcium and decreases the rate of bone loss. A dose of vitamin D > 400 units is necessary for fracture and fall prevention. Sources of vitamin D include sunlight, diet, and supplementation. Sunlight alone will not meet the vitamin D requirements. The options include adding vitamin D to the current regimen or changing the calcium supplement to include vitamin D. **Plan:** Discontinue current calcium supplementation. Start calcium citrate with vitamin D_3 (Citracal = calcium citrate with vitamin D maximum) two caplets by mouth twice daily. Follow up in one week to assess compliance and side effects (constipation, gas, upset stomach).
Scenario: 70-year-old female taking calcium carbonate 500 mg twice daily **MRP:** Ineffective medication
Assessment: Calcium carbonate has decreased absorption in patients with low acid production. Elderly patients or patients receiving treatment for GERD may experience decreased absorption. Calcium citrate does not need an acidic environment for absorption. **Plan:** Discontinue calcium carbonate. Start calcium citrate with vitamin D_3 (Citracal = calcium citrate with vitamin D maximum) two caplets by mouth twice daily. Follow up in one week to assess compliance and side effects (constipation, gas, upset stomach).

FIGURE 30-6 Sample provider communications for osteoporosis.

quality standard) by the Centers for Medicare and Medicaid Services (CMS). Plans are assessed across multiple categories, ranging from specific disease state measures to customer service measures. Providers of MTM services have an opportunity to ensure the safe and effective use of medications and to improve the management of many health conditions. Therefore, payers view MTM as a valuable service for addressing medication usage and disease management, with a potential to improve star ratings. Table 30-13 displays an example of a quality measure impacted by MTM providers conducting medication reviews in patients with osteoporosis.[23]

TABLE 30-11 • Suggested Intervals for Follow-up and Monitoring in Patients with Osteoporosis

Efficacy
Repeat BMD test not earlier than 12-24 months after baseline
Repeat BMD test not earlier than 6-12 months for patients on glucocorticoid therapy
Annual height and weight
Annual serum calcium and 25(OH) vitamin D
Assessment of chronic back pain
Optional: biochemical markers of bone turnover
Toxicity
Monitor for adverse drug effects 2-4 weeks after starting a new agent or dose increase
Monitor every 6-12 months in stable patients

Source: References 2 and 3.

TABLE 30-12 • Drug Monitoring Table for Osteoporosis Medications

Drug	Adverse Drug Reaction	Monitoring Parameter	Comments
Antiresorptive Medications—Nutritional Supplements			
Calcium	Constipation, gas, upset stomach, kidney stones	Dietary calcium intake, constipation	Education about a bowel healthy lifestyle (eg, adequate water, fiber, and exercise).
Vitamin D	Hypercalcemia, hypercalciuria, weakness, headache, somnolence, nausea; rare—cardiac rhythm disturbance	Serum 25(OH) vitamin D concentration, symptoms	Adverse effects rarely experienced until 25(OH) vitamin D concentrations >100-150 ng/mL (μg/L; > 250-375 nmol/L), which are seldom achieved with recommended therapeutic doses.
Antiresorptive Prescription Medications			
Bisphosphonates			
Bisphosphonates	Dyspepsia (oral), transient or chronic musculoskeletal pain, nausea, transient flu-like illness (injectable) Rare: GI perforation, ulceration, and/or bleeding (oral); osteonecrosis of the jaw; atypical femoral shaft fracture, severe musculoskeletal pain	Bone density, fractures, GI symptoms, muscle aches; serum calcium for zoledronic acid	Pregnancy category C for alendronate, risedronate, and ibandronate. Pregnancy category D for zoledronic acid. Adherence is suboptimal, thus should be assessed frequently. Assess correct use of products with refills.
RANK Ligand Inhibitor			
Denosumab	Back pain, arthralgia, eczema, cellulitis, and infection Rare: osteonecrosis of the jaw, atypical femoral shaft fracture	Serum calcium, bone density, fractures	Pregnancy category X. REMS: Medication guide and monitoring plan due to risks of serious infections, dermatologic adverse reactions, and suppression of bone turnover.
Estrogen Agonist/Antagonist and Tissue Selective Estrogen Complex			
Raloxifene	Hot flushes, leg pain, spasms, or cramps, peripheral edema, venous thromboembolism (warm swollen leg, chest pain, shortness of breath, coughing up blood, and change in vision)	Bone density, fractures, hot flushes, leg cramps, and blood clots	Pregnancy category X. Warning for fatal stroke-rare events seen predominantly in women at high risk for stroke.
Bazedoxifene with conjugated equine estrogens	Similar to raloxifene and estrogens	Bone density, fractures, leg cramps, blood clots	Pregnancy category X.
Calcitonin			
Calcitonin (salmon)	Nasal: rhinitis, epistaxis Injection: nausea, flushing, local inflammation	Bone density, fractures, nasal symptoms	Pregnancy category C.
Formation Medications			
Recombinant human PTH (1-34 units)			
Teriparatide	Orthostasis with first few injections, pain at injection site, nausea, headache, dizziness, leg cramps, rare increase in uric acid, slightly increased calcium stays with regular adverse effects	Bone density, fractures, trough serum calcium concentration 1 month after therapy initiation	Pregnancy category C. If serum calcium is high (>10.6 mg/dL [>2.65 mmol/L]), calcium intake should be decreased. Warning about osteosarcoma in rats and therefore contraindicated in patients at high risk for this adverse event. REMS: Medication guide and communication plan due to the increased risk of osteosarcoma and to inform healthcare providers of the 2-year maximum lifetime treatment.

Abbreviations: PTH = parathyroid hormone; REMS = risk evaluation and mitigation strategy.

Source: Reproduced, with permission, from DiPiro JT, Talbert RL, Yee GC, Matzke GR, Wells BG, Posey LM, eds. *Pharmacotherapy: A Pathophysiologic Approach*, 10th ed. New York, NY: McGraw-Hill; 2017.

TABLE 30-13 • Medicare Star Ratings Measure[a] Related to Osteoporosis

Measure	Measure Target
Osteoporosis Management in Women who had a Fracture	Percent of women aged 67-85 years who had a fracture *and* had a bone mineral density or had prescribed medications for osteoporosis within 6 months of the fracture For a 5-star rating: ≥70% For a 4-star rating: ≥51% to <70%

[a] Medicare Part C measure.

REFERENCES

1. National Osteoporosis Foundation. *Learn About Osteoporosis*. Available at nof.org/learn/basics. Accessed May 11, 2017.
2. Cosman F, de Beur SJ, LeBoff MS, et al. Clinician's guide to prevention and treatment of osteoporosis. *Osteoporos Int*. 2014;25:2359-2381.
3. O'Connell MB, Vondracek SF. Chapter 92: Osteoporosis and osteomalacia. In: DiPiro JT, Talbert RL, Yee GC, Matzke GR, Wells BG, Posey LM, eds. *Pharmacotherapy: A Pathophysiologic Approach*, 10th ed. New York, NY: McGraw-Hill Education; 2017.
4. Centers for Disease Control and Prevention (CDC). *Injury Prevention and Control: Home and Recreational Safety*. Available at http://www.cdc.gov/homeandrecreationalsafety/falls/adulthipfx.html. Accessed May 11, 2017.
5. Vondracek SF, Linnebur SA. Diagnosis and management of osteoporosis in the older senior. *Clin Intervent Aging*. 2009;4:121-136.
6. Miller PD. Unrecognized and unappreciated secondary causes of osteoporosis. *Endocrinol Metab Clin N Am*. 2012;41:613-628.
7. Mirza F, Canalis E. Management of endocrine disease: Secondary osteoporosis: Pathophysiology and management. *Eur J Endocrinol*. 2015;173:R131-R151.
8. Borgelt LM, Vondracek SF. Osteoporosis and osteomalacia. In: Tisdale JE, Miller DA, eds. *Drug-induced Diseases Prevention, Detection, and Management*, 2nd ed. Bethesda, MD: American Society of Health-System Pharmacists; 2010:991-1004.
9. Mazziotti G, Canalis E, Giustina A. Drug-induced osteoporosis: Mechanisms and clinical implications. *Am J Med*. 2010;123:877-884.
10. McLendon AN, Woodis CB. A review of osteoporosis management in younger premenopausal women. *Womens Health*. 2014;10:59-77.
11. O'Sullivan S, Grey A. Adverse skeletal effects of drugs—beyond glucocorticoids. *Clin Endocrinol*. 2015;82:12-22.
12. US Food and Drug Administration. *Invokana and Invokamet (Canagliflozin): Drug Safety Communication—New Information on Bone Fracture Risk and Decreased Bone Mineral Density*; 2015. Available at http://www.fda.gov.lp.hscl.ufl.edu/Safety/MedWatch/SafetyInformation/SafetyAlertsforHumanMedicalProducts/ucm461876.htm. Accessed May 11, 2017.
13. The North American Menopause Society. Management of osteoporosis in postmenopausal women: 2010 position statement of the North American Menopause Society. *Menopause*. 2010;17:25-54.
14. Watts NB, Adler RA, Bilezikian JP, et al. Osteoporosis in men: An Endocrine Society clinical practice guideline. *J Clin Endocrinol Metab*. 2012;97:1802-1822.
15. Watts NB, Bilezikian JP, Camacho PM, et al. American Association of Clinical Endocrinologists medical guidelines for clinical practice for the diagnosis and treatment of postmenopausal osteoporosis. *Endocr Pract*. 2010;16(Suppl 3):1-37.
16. Ward LM, Konji VN, Ma J. The management of osteoporosis in children. *Osteoporos Int*. 2016;27:2147-2179.
17. Cosman F. Combination therapy for osteoporosis: A reappraisal. *Bonekey Rep*. 2014;3:518.
18. Institute of Medicine. *Dietary Reference Intakes for Adequacy: Calcium and Vitamin D. Institute of Medicine (US) Committee to Review Dietary Reference Intakes for Vitamin D and Calcium*. Washington, DC: National Academies Press (US); 2011. 345-401.
19. Raisz LG. Screening for osteoporosis. *New Engl J Med*. 2005;353(2):164-170.
20. *Medicare Part D Medication Therapy Management Program Standardized Format*. Available at https://www.cms.gov/Medicare/Prescription-Drug-Coverage/PrescriptionDrugCovContra/Downloads/MTM-Program-Standardized-Format-English-and-Spanish-Instructions-Samples-v032712.pdf. Accessed May 11, 2017
21. *FRAX Fracture Risk Assessment Tool*. Available at www.shef.ac.uk/FRAX. Accessed May 11, 2017.
22. Natural Medicines [database online]. Somerville, MA: Therapeutic Research Center; 2017. Available at https://naturalmedicines.therapeuticresearch.com/. Accessed May 11, 2017.
23. CMS. *2017 Part C & D Star Ratings Measures*. Available at https://www.cms.gov/Medicare/Prescription-Drug-Coverage/PrescriptionDrugCovGenIn/Downloads/2017-Measure-List.pdf. Accessed May 12, 2017.

Review Questions

1. Which of the following represents a risk factor for osteoporosis?
   a. Vitamin B insufficiency
   b. Hypothyroidism
   c. Premature menopause
   d. Obesity

2. Which of the following is consistent with a diagnosis of osteoporosis?
   a. A low trauma fracture before age 40
   b. A 10-year risk of hip fracture of 2.5%
   c. A T- score between 1.0 and 2.0
   d. A T-score at 2.5 or below

3. Which of the following represents an appropriate therapeutic goal for treatment of osteoporosis?
   a. Avoid use of injectable medications.
   b. Discontinue oral medications after one year.
   c. Prevent fractures of hip, wrist, and spine.
   d. Reduce pain level by 50% from baseline.

4. Which of the following statements best defines primary osteoporosis using living room language?
   a. Osteoporosis caused by medications that the patient is taking (eg, steroids).
   b. Osteoporosis caused by advanced age or "going through the change" (menopause).
   c. Osteoporosis that occurs after the climacteric.
   d. Osteoporosis caused by diseases such as hyperthyroidism or Cushing disease.

5. Which of the following instsructions should be included in the medication action plan for a patient taking a bisphosphonate?
   a. Instructions to take with 6 oz of any liquid
   b. Instructions to take with a meal
   c. Directions for missed doses
   d. Importance of remaining upright for 5 minutes after the dose

6. A patient taking a bisphosphonate reports pain in her throat and trouble swallowing food. Sometimes she spits up blood. Which of the following is the correct course of action?
   a. She should stop all her medications and schedule an appointment with her physician.
   b. She should see her physician immediately or go to the emergency room.
   c. She should call 911.
   d. Explain to her that this is a normal side effect and it will go away in a couple of weeks.

7. The patient is taking a bisphosphonate weekly and reports that she is compliant. On review of her medications the healthcare provider notes that she is not taking additional calcium or vitamin D. An interview with the patient reveals an inadequate dietary intake of calcium. What type of medication-related problem does this patient have?
   a. Nonadherence
   b. Ineffective medication
   c. Unnecessary medication
   d. Need for additional medication

8. The patient is a 70-year-old female who has been diagnosed with osteoporosis. Which of the following is the most appropriate first-line therapy?
   a. Alendronate
   b. Calcium
   c. Raloxifene
   d. Calcitonin

9. How much calcium and vitamin D should this patient receive daily from her diet and supplements?
   a. Calcium 1200 mg and vitamin D 400 IU
   b. Calcium 500 mg and vitamin D 1000 IU
   c. Calcium 1000 mg and vitamin D 800 IU
   d. Calcium 1200 mg and vitamin D 800 IU

10. Which of the following medication classes are associated with increased bone loss or increased fracture risk?
    a. Sulfonylureas
    b. Thiazide diuretics
    c. Histamine blockers
    d. Proton pump inhibitors

ANSWERS

1. c	2. d	3. c
4. b	5. c	6. b
7. d	8. a	9. d
10. d		

31

Pain Management MTM Data Set

Robin Moorman Li, PharmD, BCACP, CPE, and Juan Hincapie Castillo, PharmD

KEY POINTS

- Proper assessment is vital when treating a patient suffering from pain and must include the physical effects of pain as well as the psychological and social impact of pain.
- Pain management may include nonpharmacological, nonopioid, opioid, and adjuvant therapies. Several of these options are often used together to achieve better pain management.
- Many concerns are associated with opioid therapy, and it is important for medication therapy management (MTM) providers to understand the advantages and disadvantages of this treatment option when managing patients suffering from pain.
- Constipation is a very common side effect associated with opioid therapy, and proper education, treatment, and monitoring by MTM providers is imperative.

INTRODUCTION

The International Association for the Study of Pain defines pain as "an unpleasant sensory and emotional experience associated with actual or potential tissue damage, or described in terms of such damage."[1] The term *pain management* is very broad and includes not only the pharmacological management of a variety of different types of pain, but also the use of nonpharmacological treatments, complementary treatments, and other types of treatments to reduce or stop pain. Prior to developing a treatment plan for a patient with pain, MTM providers must understand the difference between nociceptive and neuropathic pain as well as differences in the treatment of acute and chronic pain.

Pathophysiology

The understanding of the pathophysiology of pain continues to evolve. When a tissue injury occurs, various physiological and chemical changes happen peripherally and centrally. Patients may experience short-term pain (ie, acute pain) or continued pain leading to persistent or chronic pain. Pain can be classified by inferred pathophysiology into one of two categories: physiological pain or pathological pain.[2] Physiological pain includes *nociceptive pain* and inflammatory pain. Nociceptive pain is characterized as "pain that arises from actual or threatened damage to nonneural tissue and is due to the activation of nociceptors,"[1] and inflammatory pain involves activation of the immune system resulting from tissue injury.[3] Pathological pain is a maladaptive process, which occurs when the nervous system is not functioning properly; it can present as neuropathic pain or centralized pain.[2] *Neuropathic pain* is characterized as the "abnormal processing of sensory input by the peripheral or central nervous system (CNS)."[1] Centralized sensitization is a dysfunction in the CNS in which the pain processing process leads to hypersensitivity and spontaneous pain.[3] It is very important for the MTM provider to understand the distinction between nociceptive and neuropathic pain so that therapeutic interventions can be tailored to address the appropriate type of pain.

Nociceptive Pain

Nociceptive pain is a natural response to the injury that is causing the painful stimulus. Nociceptive pain can be further divided into two distinct categories: *somatic pain* and *visceral pain*. Somatic pain is a type of pain that is derived from muscle, skin, bone, or connective tissue. Somatic pain typically includes aching or throbbing pain that is easily pinpointed to an exact location. Unlike somatic pain, visceral pain is difficult to pinpoint, as it originates from internal organs such as the pancreas or the gastrointestinal tract. It is often described as a generalized aching without a specific focal point. Visceral pain has been associated with *referred pain*, where the pain is perceived at a different location than the actual site of injury.[4]

Neuropathic Pain

Neuropathic pain can occur both in the peripheral nervous system (eg, painful diabetic peripheral neuropathy, trigeminal neuralgia, radicular pain, or neuropathic cancer pain) or in the CNS (eg, central poststroke pain, spinal cord injury neuropathic pain, multiple sclerosis).[5] Many patients describe the sensations associated with neuropathic pain as burning, radiating, or tingling, with some experiencing numbness. There are two common types of symptoms associated with neuropathic pain: *allodynia* and *hyperalgesia*. Allodynia is pain produced by a stimulus that is normally not painful, such as brushing a cotton ball on the forearm. Hyperalgesia is an exaggerated response to a stimulus that is usually minimally painful. For example, a simple pinch to the arm would normally cause a very mild discomfort, but instead it causes extreme pain to someone who is experiencing hyperalgesia.[6] These heightened responses can also be associated with central sensitization that can occur across many organ systems and lead to overlap in various syndromes, such as fibromyalgia, irritable bowel syndrome, chronic daily headaches, and chronic pelvic pain.[7]

Clinical Presentation of Pain

Acute pain is a normal process that alerts the body to injury, and it is typically associated with nociceptive pain. Acute pain is usually self-limiting and should resolve after a few days or weeks, or in some situations a few months, as the healing process progresses. It is essential to address acute pain because uncontrolled acute pain can lead to emotional, psychological, and physical distress that can progress to chronic pain.[8]

When pain persists for months or even years beyond the time for the normal healing process, pain is considered chronic in nature. Based on guidelines, continued pain after ninety days can be classified as chronic pain.[8] Patients who have chronic disease states such as rheumatoid arthritis as well as patients who suffer from various forms of cancer may present with chronic pain. Additionally, patients can develop chronic pain in the absence of any identifiable injury. In contrast to acute pain, chronic pain can include nociceptive pain, neuropathic pain, or a combination of both.[3] In a chronic pain situation, a maladaptive process leads not only to physical changes within the nervous system but also emotional and psychological stresses on the patient. This results in a negative impact on a patient's quality of life. The term *chronic pain syndrome* includes the physical pain as well as the psychological, emotional, and social components often seen in patients who suffer from chronic pain.[8] The MTM provider should understand the clinical differences between acute and chronic pain (Table 31-1) because the treatment approach varies considerably.

TABLE 31-1 • Characteristics of Acute and Chronic Pain

Characteristic	Acute Pain	Chronic Pain
Relief of pain	Highly desirable	Highly desirable
Dependence and tolerance to medication	Unusual	Common
Psychological component	Usually not present	Often a major problem
Organic cause	Common	May not be present
Environmental/ family issues	Small	Significant
Insomnia	Unusual	Common component
Treatment goal	Cure	Functionality
Depression	Uncommon	Common

Source: Reproduced, with permission, from DiPiro JT, Talbert RL, Yee GC, Matzke GR, Wells BG, Posey L, eds. *Pharmacotherapy: A Pathophysiologic Approach*, 10th ed. New York, NY: McGraw-Hill; 2017.

Therapeutic Goals

Inadequate management of chronic pain can lead to physical, psychological, and emotional suffering, which results in reduced quality of life, more disability, lost productivity, and increased healthcare costs. A patient-centered approach must be utilized when working with patients who suffer from chronic pain. Management of chronic pain can be very difficult because it includes not only the pain aspect but also psychological and emotional components. As emphasized in The Centers for Disease Control and Prevention (CDC) Guidelines for Prescribing Opioids for Chronic Pain, treatment goals must be established to include pain relief, improvements in overall activity, and minimal adverse effects of pharmacologic therapy.[9] Treatment goals should be individualized, realistic, and include the understanding that the pain may never completely resolve. It is important to have a clear and direct discussion with patients about their specific goals of therapy and how these align with achievable and safe clinical outcomes.

CORE ELEMENT 1—PAIN MANAGEMENT HEALTH ASSESSMENT AND CONDUCTING THE COMPREHENSIVE MEDICATION REVIEW

In the MTM setting, management of chronic pain associated with chronic conditions is a much more common scenario than management of acute pain. Pain management can be a very broad topic to cover in most time-limited settings, so MTM providers should focus on assessment of the current pain management regimen.[10] Table 31-2 provides a list of questions for use in this process. Although time-consuming, a proper and thorough pain assessment can provide helpful information in managing pain patients. For example, an evaluation of current treatments can offer some objective information for a very subjective condition (ie, the interviewer can get an idea of pain control based on current utilization trends of pain medications). Asking the patient to merely provide a single numerical rating of his/her pain with no context does not provide sufficient information to alter therapy. The use of living room language (Figure 31-1) is imperative in MTM settings to ensure proper communication between the patient and the MTM provider. In preparation for the interview, MTM providers should be ready to answer a variety of pain-related questions that could arise during the session (Table 31-3).

TABLE 31-2 • Suggested Questions to Ask When Conducting a Medication Review in a Patient with Pain

- What type of pain are you experiencing?
- Where is the pain located? Does the pain travel (radiate) to other parts of the body?
- How long have you been experiencing this pain?
- Based on a scale of 0-10: 0 is no pain at all; 10 is the worst imaginable pain: how would you rate your pain at this moment? Is this a good day or a bad day?
- How does your pain level change throughout the day?
- What is the highest pain level you have experienced in the last week?
- What is the lowest pain level you have experienced in the last week?
- What medications do you take for pain relief?
- Have you ever experienced the following side effects associated with your pain medications:
  - Dizziness
  - Daytime drowsiness
  - Difficulty passing a bowel movement (constipation)
  - Difficulty urinating
  - Changes in mood
  - Confusion
  - Nausea or vomiting
  - Itching
  - Other side effects?
- How well are these medications working?
- What other medications have you tried in the past for pain relief?
- How did the medications you took in the past help you with pain relief?
- How was your pain medication originally prescribed by your physician?
- How often have you had to increase the amount of pain medication to help control your pain?
- What are your goals in relation to your pain management? (pain level goal, activity goals, etc)
- Pain can fluctuate sometimes; how much medication do you need to get enough pain relief on a daily basis?
- How many doses of your breakthrough pain medication are you taking during the day?
- Have you noticed an improvement in your daily activities since you started the medication?
- Do you keep a log of your pain control from day to day? If so, have you noticed any changes lately?
- What over-the-counter medications or herbals do you take for pain relief?
- What nondrug therapies have you tried for pain control?

Questions to Ask for Prevention/Assessment of Medical Emergency

- Crisis Planning: Have you discussed what possible symptoms you might experience if you accidently take more of your pain medication than prescribed?
- What types of responses should you monitor when your pain medication is increased?
- What are the signs of higher levels of pain outside the normal range? This might be a sign of a worsening condition or a new injury which needs evaluation by your physician. Have you discussed this type of situation with your physician? What is your action plan?

Acute pain—a normal pain experience that is related to injury.

Addiction—any activity, substance, object, or behavior that becomes the major focus of a person's life, resulting in physical, mental, and/or social withdrawal from normal activities.

Adjuvant medication—medications that are used for other purposes but can be used to help some painful conditions.

Allodynia—pain caused by something that normally does not cause pain (eg, light touch).

Analgesia—pain relief.

Analgesic—a medication that relieves pain.

Antidepressant—drugs that originally were used to treat mood but also have the ability to provide pain relief.

Arthritis—a chronic condition that involves joint inflammation and pain.

Breakthrough pain—an occasional pain that comes and goes and is above the baseline pain that is being controlled with regularly scheduled pain medication.

Chronic pain—a painful experience that continues to occur beyond the normal healing process.

Controlled substance—substances that require a higher level of monitoring due to their potential for abuse.

Endorphins—naturally occurring substances produced by the body to relieve pain.

Epidural analgesia—analgesics administered via a catheter that deliver medication directly to the spine.

Equianalagesic dose—a dose of one pain medication that produces the same amount of pain relief as another.

Hyperalgesia—increased response to something that is normally only mildly painful.

Inflammation—the body's response to injury; symptoms may include redness, swelling, pain, and increased temperature.

Muscle relaxant—medications used to treat muscle spasms.

Neuralgia—pain occurring along a nerve or nerves in the body.

Neuropathic pain—resulting from nerve injury or dysfunction of the nervous system where pain is often described as burning, radiating, or electric shock-like. Examples include diabetic peripheral neuropathy, postherpetic neuralgia, and phantom limb pain.

Nociceptive pain—pain that is usually in one area, constant, and aching in quality. Examples include breaking a bone, burns, or muscle pain.

Nociceptor—nerves that sense and respond to tissue irritation or injury by sending pain signals to the brain.

Opioid—the most common class of medication used to treat pain

Opioid rotation—switching from one pain medication to another as a way to get better pain control.

Pain—an unpleasant feeling or emotional experience caused by actual or possible tissue damage.

Pain management—a branch of medicine that is focused on controlling pain and decreasing suffering caused by pain.

Physical dependence—occurs when withdrawal symptoms are experienced by a patient when a drug is reduced or removed quickly.

Physiological tolerance—reduction in drug effect that requires an increase in dosage to achieve desired effect (eg, pain relief).

Postherpetic neuralgia (PHN)—pain that occurs due to nerve damage after the viral infection with varicella zoster (chicken pox/shingles virus).

Radiculopathy—general term used to describe pain that arises from an inflamed or compressed nerve in the spinal column.

Refractory pain—pain that is resistant to usual treatments.

Shingles—an acute infection caused by a virus (Herpes zoster); symptoms include a painful skin rash with blisters in a narrow area on one side of the body, which can cause ongoing nerve pain.

Withdrawal—unpleasant symptoms that occur after discontinuing certain medications quickly.

FIGURE 31-1 Living room language for patients with pain.

TABLE 31-3 • Questions to Anticipate Regarding Pain Management

Is the pain ever going to stop?
Pain is very subjective. What one patient feels is painful, another patient may see as just a feeling of discomfort. Acute pain tends to go away after healing has occurred, but this process can take longer for some patients. Chronic pain, on the other hand, continues to stay and rarely goes away completely. It is important to remember that chronic pain is not only physical pain, but can also lead to emotional and psychological pain. Focusing on various treatments including medicine, physical therapy, counseling, and complementary therapies can help in decreasing or controlling the overall pain.

Am I going to get addicted to my pain medications?
This is a common concern with pain medications, and although there is a risk for addiction, risk assessment can help identify factors associated with the development of an addiction disorder. With the use of this type of medication, it is important to take your medications as prescribed and continue to have regular follow-up appointments with your physician. There is often confusion with common words used in pain management, such as addiction, dependence, and tolerance. Addiction to pain medications is characterized by behaviors that can include compulsive use, cravings, loss of control over the use of the drug, or continuing use despite harm. Dependence occurs with many types of medications. When a pain medication is stopped abruptly for any reason, the patient can develop unpleasant withdrawal symptoms, indicating there is dependence. Tolerance is also common in patients who are taking pain medications for a long time. Tolerance means that over time the body adjusts to the pain medication and the pain-relieving effects might decrease, leading to the need for more medicine to get the same pain relief.

Can I just have surgery to eliminate this pain?
Surgery is recommended only for select patients. It is important to have this discussion with your physician to determine if surgery is right for you. Pain can have many causes, so even if you do have surgery, the pain might not go away completely.

Is taking a long-acting pain medication better than taking a short-acting one?
Clinical studies have not proven that the use of long-acting pain medications is any better than the use of short-acting ones. Each patient suffering from pain is different, and each treatment plan should be made especially for the patient and the type of pain the patient has. It is important to give specific answers to each pain-related question your physician asks you, so he/she can create the best treatment plan for you.

Why does my physician require a urine drug screen multiple times a year?
Your physician might request a urine drug screen if your medication regimen includes certain pain medications. It is recommended that all patients who are taking these types of medications undergo evaluation on a regular basis. A urine drug screen is one of the ways to do this, along with regular follow-up appointments.[9]

CORE ELEMENT 2—PERSONAL MEDICATION LIST

The following is an example of a personal medication list (PML) for a pain management patient (Figure 31-2).[10] This example is representative only of medications for pain management.

PERSONAL MEDICATION LIST FOR *<Insert patient's name, DOB: mm/dd/yyyy>*	
Medication: MS Contin (Morphine Sulfate ER) 60 mg	
How I use it: Take one tablet (60 mg) by mouth every 12 hours	
Why I use it: Chronic back pain (maintenance)	**Prescriber:** Parker
Date I started using it: 06/23/2016	**Date I stopped using it:** *(Leave blank for patient's notes)*
Why I stopped taking it: *(Leave blank for patient's notes)*	
Medication: Morphine Sulfate IR 15 mg	
How I use it: Take one tablet (15 mg) by mouth every 4 to 6 hours as needed for breakthrough pain	
Why do I use it: Pain (breakthrough)	**Prescriber:** Parker
Date I started using it: 07/25/2016	**Date I stopped using it:** *(Leave blank for patient's notes)*
Why I stopped taking it: *(Leave blank for patient's notes)*	

FIGURE 31-2 Example personal medication list for pain management medications.

Additional medications for other disease states should be added and listed separately. MTM providers should remember to use plain language when creating the PML. In addition, it is important to avoid using abbreviations such as sig codes when recording how to take the medication and indicate whether the medication is for control of maintenance or breakthrough pain. If the patient has multiple pain conditions, list the type of pain the medication is targeting (eg, pregabalin for diabetic peripheral neuropathy).

CORE ELEMENT 3—MEDICATION ACTION PLAN

The following is a sample medication action plan (MAPs) for a pain management patient (Figure 31-3).[10] This example is representative only of action steps for a patient suffering from chronic nonmalignant pain. Patients with chronic pain often have other comorbid disease states, so it is important that MAPs for those disease states be added and listed separately. Patients can become overwhelmed when asked to face too many health concerns at one time, so it is essential to prioritize the concerns identified and only address the most significant issues in a particular session. Lower priority items can be reevaluated and addressed during subsequent follow-up sessions. MTM providers should remember to use clear, "living room" language when developing the MAP.

CORE ELEMENT 4—INTERVENTION AND/OR REFERRAL

Interventions for chronic nonmalignant pain can include lifestyle modifications, nonpharmacologic therapy, complementary therapy, and appropriate pharmacotherapy.[10] Since chronic pain management requires an individualized approach, the intervention(s) should include a very detailed description of the treatment

	DATE PREPARED: *<Insert date>*
What we talked about: You reported stopping scheduled acetaminophen 3 weeks ago since you did not feel it was effective in controlling your pain. You felt morphine is the only agent that is decreasing your pain, and your average pain levels have started to increase over the last week, increasing from 4/10 to 7/10. You have increased morphine IR without your physician's knowledge or approval in order to improve your pain control, and you are now experiencing some daytime sleepiness.	
What I need to do: Here are some things I can do to help improve my pain level and decrease my daytime sleepiness. 1. Begin taking the acetaminophen as the physician prescribed. 2. Do not increase morphine IR without my physician's approval. 3. Make sure to continue exercise program to strengthen my muscles.	**What I did and when I did it:** *(Leave blank for patient's notes)*
What we talked about: You have had a hard time moving your bowels, and your last bowel movement was 2 days ago. A common side effect from pain medication (morphine) is constipation. It is important to take a laxative medication on a scheduled basis to help you with regular bowel movements. The best medicine for patients on chronic pain medications includes Senna S, which is an over-the-counter medication you can buy at any pharmacy.	
What I need to do: 1. Start Senna S 1 tablet by mouth twice daily as needed for constipation (purchase today after our session). 2. Increase fruits and vegetable intake. 3. Drink plenty of fluids. 4. Continue exercise program.	**What I did and when I did it:** *(Leave blank for patient's notes)*

FIGURE 31-3 Example medication action plan for a patient with chronic nonmalignant pain.

modalities recommended to help control the pain. In addition, an explanation of how these modalities work together for pain management should be included because chronic pain is often multifactorial. Nonpharmacologic therapies are commonly used to help overall pain control. Although the efficacy of nonpharmacologic therapies has not been well studied, there is some evidence showing benefit as adjunctive therapy for arthritic pain.[11] Table 31-4 outlines nonpharmacologic options for pain management. Chronic pain can also negatively impact psychological and emotional state, so it is important to encourage the patient to seek assistance from a psychologist and/or psychiatrist as necessary.

Pharmacologic Therapies for Pain Management

Pharmacologic intervention depends on the type of pain as well as the clinical presentation of the pain. A patient may experience pain as the result of multiple pain syndromes. This often necessitates a treatment approach that includes multiple pharmacologic therapies, a technique known as rational polypharmacy.

TABLE 31-4 • Pain Management: Nonpharmacologic Treatment Options

Category	Examples
Physical	Acupuncture Exercise (general and light resistance) TENS (transcutaneous electrical nerve stimulation) Strength training Qigong
Psychosocial	Self-management education Meditation Guided imagery Listening to music Relaxation Cognitive-behavioral therapy

Source: Reference 8.

Nonopioids. It is important to try to use nonopioid agents to help control pain and reduce or eliminate the need for opioids, if possible. When opioids are needed to control pain, nonopioid therapies can decrease the total opioid dose required to relieve pain. This approach is known as *opioid sparing*. Table 31-5 lists various nonopioid analgesics. The choice of agent is usually based on the type of pain as well as pharmacokinetic properties of the drug, potential for drug interactions, side effect profile, and availability or cost, since efficacy comparisons are inconsistent.[3] The use of herbal therapies has also become more popular with many patients. Table 31-6 includes a select list of herbal products that have been used for symptoms associated with chronic pain. While patients might consider using herbal products for additional pain relief, it is important to warn them of possible drug-herbal interactions and variation of evidence for effectiveness.

Opioids. Opioids are commonly used for both acute and chronic management of nociceptive pain. Opioids have been used in the treatment of neuropathic pain; however, current guidelines list them as a weak recommendation based on current evidence.[14] Safety and efficacy data regarding the long-term use of opioids are limited.[9] Current opioid guidelines recognize some benefit of using opioids in select patients who have been carefully assessed and will be closely monitored.[9] Tables 31-7, 31-8, and 31-9 provide information on select opioid analgesics used in chronic nonmalignant pain.

Monitoring Patients During Opioid Use. The CDC Guideline for Prescribing Opioids for Chronic Pain is developed for prescribers who manage patients with chronic pain in the primary care setting. The guideline does not pertain to patients who are receiving active cancer treatment or undergoing palliative care or end-of-life care. The guideline provides recommendations for proper assessment, patient selection, treatment goals, risk stratification, and monitoring parameters for patients who are currently taking or may soon be receiving opioid therapy.[9] For patients prescribed opioids, a comprehensive evaluation and ongoing assessment at regular intervals should be conducted to ascertain the efficacy of therapy, including evaluation of functional status, degree of pain relief, occurrence of undesirable side effects, and monitoring for abuse behaviors.[9] When considering

TABLE 31-5 • Adult FDA-Approved Nonopioid Analgesics (Includes Only FDA-Approved Agents for Pain)

Class and Generic Name (Brand Name)	Approximate Half-life (h)	Usual Dosage Range (mg)	Maximal Dose (mg/day)
Salicylates			
Acetylsalicylic acid[a]—aspirin (various)	0.25	325-1000 every 4-6 h	4000
Choline and magnesium trisalicylate (various)	9-17	1000-1500 every 12 h	3000
		750 every 8 h (elderly)	
Diflunisal (Dolobid, various)	8-12	500-1000 initial, 250-500 every 8-12 h	1500
Salsalate (various)	1	1000 every 12 h or 500 every 6 h	3000
Para-aminophenol			
Acetaminophen[a] (Oral—Tylenol, various; Parenteral—Ofirmev)	2-3	325-1000 every 4-6 h	4000[b] Dosing for peds lower based on weight
Fenamates			
Meclofenamate (various)	0.8-3.3	50-100 every 4-6 h	400
Mefenamic acid (Ponstel)	2	Initial 500, 250 every 6 h (max. 7 days)	1000[c]
Pyranocarboxylic acid			
Etodolac (various) (immediate release)	7.3	200-400 every 6-8 h	1000, 1200 with extended-release product
Acetic acid			
Diclofenac potassium (Cataflam, various, Flector [patch], Voltaren Gel, Pennsaid [solution])	1.9	In some patients, initial 100, 50, three times per day Patch available—to be applied twice daily to painful area (intact skin only), Gel and solution dosing joint specific	150[d]
Propionic acids			
Ibuprofen[a] (Motrin, Caldolor, various)	2-2.5	200-400 every 4-6 h Injectable, 400-800 every 6 h (infused over 30 min)	3200[e] 2400[e] 1200[f]
Fenoprofen (Nalfon, various)	3	200 every 4-6 h	3200
Ketoprofen (various)	2	25-50 every 6-8 h	300 200 with extended-release product
Naproxen (Naprosyn, Anaprox, various)	12-17	500 initial	1000[c]
		500 every 12 h or 250 every 6-8 h	
Naproxen sodium[a] (Aleve, various, combined with esomeprazole [Vimovo])	12-17	In some patients, 440 initial[f] 220 every 8-12 h[f]	660[f]
Pyrrolizine carboxylic acid			
Ketorolac—parenteral (Toradol, various)	5-6	30[g]-60 (single IM dose only)	30[g]-60
		15[g]-30 (single IV dose only)	15[g]-30
		15[g]-30 every 6 h (IV dose) (max. 5 days)	60[g]-120
Ketorolac—oral, indicated for continuation with parenteral only (various)	5-6	10 every 4-6 h (max. 5 days, which includes parenteral doses)	40
		In nonelderly patients, initial oral dose of 20	
Ketorolac—nasal spray, indicated for acute, moderate, to moderately severe pain		1 spray (15.75 mg) in each nostril every 6-8 h in adults <65 yr and weight ≥50 kg	126

(Continued)

TABLE 31-5 • **Adult FDA-Approved Nonopioid Analgesics (Includes Only FDA-Approved Agents for Pain)** ***(Continued)***

Class and Generic Name (Brand Name)	Approximate Half-life (h)	Usual Dosage Range (mg)	Maximal Dose (mg/day)
Pyrazoles			
Celecoxib (Celebrex)	11	Initial 400 followed by another 200 on first day, then 200 twice daily (note some recommend maintenance doses of 200 mg/day due to cardiovascular concerns)	400

[a] Available both as an over-the-counter preparation and as a prescription drug.

[b] Some experts believe 4000 mg may be too high. OTC max dose 3000 mg daily, lower with weight based dosing in pediatric patients.

[c] Up to 1250 mg on the first day.

[d] Up to 200 mg on the first day.

[e] Some individuals may respond better to 3200 mg as opposed to 2400 mg, although well-controlled trials show no better response; consider risk versus benefits when using 3200 mg/day.

[f] Over-the-counter dose.

[g] Dose for elderly and those under 50 kg (110 lb).

Source: Reproduced, with permission, from DiPiro JT, Talbert RL, Yee GC, Matzke GR, Wells BG, Posey L, eds. *Pharmacotherapy: A Pathophysiologic Approach*, 10th ed. New York, NY: McGraw-Hill; 2017.

Abbreviations: FDA = Food and Drug Administration; h = hours; IM = intramuscular; IV = intravenous.

TABLE 31-6 • **Herbal Supplements Used in Pain Management**

Herbal Product (Scientific Name)	Recommended Dosage	Medical Condition	Cost[b]
	Likely Effective[a]		
Camphor (Cinnamomum camphora)	Topical analgesic in strengths ranging from 3% to 11%. Use topically up to 3 to 4 times/day.	Pain (Listed as possibly effective for osteoarthritis pain)	$
Capsicum (Capsicum annum)	Topical analgesic in strengths ranging from 0.025% to 0.075% capsaicin concentrations.	Pain, postherpetic neuralgia, diabetic peripheral neuropathy (Listed as possibly effective for back pain.)	$$
	Possibly Effective[a]		
Comfrey (Symphytum officinale)	Topical analgesic Traumaplant®, 2-3 grams of cream, applied to skin 3 times daily, for up to 14 days has been used Kytta-Salbe® f, 2 grams of cream applied to skin 4 times daily for 7 to 9 days has been used	Back pain, osteoarthritis	$$
Devil's claw (Harpagophytum procumbens)	600-1200 mg (standardized to contain 50-100 mg of harpagoside) by mouth in 3 split doses daily	Back pain, osteoarthritis	$
Willow bark (Salix – multiple species)	OA: 120-240 mg willow bark extract for 4 weeks has been used Back pain: extract 393-1600 mg providing salicin 120-240 mg has been used daily for 4 weeks	Back pain	$

[a] Level of evidence: Likely effective. This product has a very high level of reliable clinical evidence supporting its use for a specific indication. Products rated "likely effective" are generally considered appropriate to recommend. Possibly effective: This product has some clinical evidence supporting its use for a specific indication; however, the evidence is limited by quantity, quality, or contradictory findings. Products rated "possibly effective" might be beneficial, but do not have enough high-quality evidence to recommend for most people; "insufficient evidence"—there is not enough reliable scientific evidence to provide an effectiveness rating.

[b] Cost: $ = $10/month supply in the recommended dosage; $$ = $11-$20/month.

Abbreviation: OA = osteoarthritis.

Source: References 12 and 13.

TABLE 31-7 • Opioid Analgesics, Central Analgesics, Opioid Antagonists

Class and Generic Name (Brand Name)	Chemical Source	Relative Histamine Release	Route[a]	Equianalgesic Dose in Adults (mg)	Approximate Onset (min)/ Half-life (h)
Phenanthrenes (morphine-like agonists)					
Morphine (Embeda[j] various)	Naturally occurring	+++	IM/IV	10	10-20/2
			PO	30	
Hydromorphone (Dilaudid, Exalgo, various)	Semisynthetic	+	IM	1.5	10-20/2-3
			PO	7.5	
Oxymorphone (Numorphan, Opana)	Semisynthetic	+	IM	1	10-20/2-3
			PO	10	
Levorphanol (various)	Semisynthetic	+	IM	Variable	10-20/12-16
			PO	Variable	
Codeine (various)	Naturally occurring	+++	IM	15-30[b]	
			PO	15-30[b]	10-30/3
Hydrocodone (available as combination, single entity extended release—Hysingla ER, Zohydro ER)	Semisynthetic	N/A	PO	5-10[b]	30-60/4
Oxycodone (OxyContin[j], Oxecta[j], Xtampza, Xartemis XR [oxycodone & acetaminophen])	Semisynthetic	+	PO	15-30[c]	30-60/2-3
Phenylpiperidines (meperidine-like agonists)					
Meperidine (Demerol, various)	Synthetic	+++	IM/IV	75	10-20/3-5
			PO	300[c]; not recommended	
Fentanyl (Sublimaze, Duragesic, Lazanda, Abstral, Fentora, Subsys, OTFC, Ionsys, various)	Synthetic	+	IM	0.125[d]	7-15/3-4
			Transdermal, buccal, transmucosal, sublingual, nasal inhaled	Variable[e]	
				Variable[e]	
Diphenylheptanes (methadone-like agonists)					
Methadone	Synthetic	+	IM/IV	Variable[f] (acute)	
(Dolophine, various)			PO	Variable[f] (acute)	30-60/12-190
			IM	Variable[f] (chronic)	
			PO	Variable[f] (chronic)	
Agonist–antagonist derivatives					
Pentazocine (Talwin, various)	Synthetic	N/A	IM	Not recommended	
			PO	50[b]	15-30/2-3
Butorphanol (Stadol, various)	Synthetic	N/A	IM	2	10-20/3-4
			Intranasal	1[b] (one spray)	
Nalbuphine (Nubain, various)	Synthetic	N/A	IM/IV	10	<15/5
Buprenorphine (Buprenex, Butrans, Suboxone, Belbuca, Subutex, various)	Synthetic	N/A	IM Transdermal Sublingual	0.3 Variable Variable	10-20/2-3

(Continued)

TABLE 31-7 • Opioid Analgesics, Central Analgesics, Opioid Antagonists (*Continued*)

Class and Generic Name (Brand Name)	Chemical Source	Relative Histamine Release	Route[a]	Equianalgesic Dose in Adults (mg)	Approximate Onset (min)/ Half-life (h)
Antagonist					
Naloxone (Narcan, various)	Synthetic	N/A	IV	0.4-2[g]	1-2 (IV), 2-5 (IM)/0.5-1.3
Methylnaltrexone (Relistor)	Synthetic	N/A	SC	Variable	
Naltrexone (Revia)	Synthetic	N/A	PO		
Alvimopan (Entereg)	Synthetic	N/A	PO	12 mg QD-Q12[b]	N/A; 15-dose max
Naloxegol (Movantik)	Synthetic	N/A	PO	12.5-25 mg QD[b]	120/6-11
Central analgesics					
Tramadol (Ultram, Rybix, Ryzolt, ConZip, various)	Synthetic	N/A	PO	50-100[b,h,i]	<60/5-7
Tapentadol (Nucynta)	Synthetic	N/A	PO	50-100[b,h,i]	Within 60/4

[a] The IM route should be avoided whenever possible—produces significant pain with administration and rate and extent of absorption is highly variable. If IV route is unavailable, then administer subcutaneously (SC).

[b] Starting dose only (equianalgesia not shown).

[c] Starting doses lower (oxycodone 5-10 mg, meperidine 50-150 mg).

[d] Equivalent PO morphine dose = variable.

[e] For breakthrough pain only. Equianalgesic dose conversion should be avoided for Transmucosal Immediate Release Fentanyl (TIRF) products.

[f] The equianalgesic dose of methadone when compared with other opioids will decrease progressively the higher the previous opioid dose. Caution should be exercised when initiating in opioid-naïve patients.

[g] Starting doses to be used in cases of opioid overdose.

[h] First day of dosing may administer second dose 1 hour after first dose.

[i] Onset of action may differ for long-acting formulations. Ceiling dose recommendations exist and may differ from immediate release dosing recommendations.

[j] FDA approved as abuse-deterrent formulation.

Abbreviations: IM = intramuscular; IV = intravenous; N/A = not available; PO = oral.

Source: Reproduced, with permission, from DiPiro JT, Talbert RL, Yee GC, Matzke GR, Wells BG, Posey L, eds. *Pharmacotherapy: A Pathophysiologic Approach*, 10th ed. New York, NY: McGraw-Hill; 2017.

TABLE 31-8 • Dosing Guidelines for Select Opioids

Agent(s)	Doses (Use Lowest Effective Dose, Titrate Up or Down Based on Patient Response, Opioid-Tolerant Patients May Need Dose Modification)	Notes
NSAIDs/acetaminophen/aspirin	Use lowest effective dose for the shortest duration possible (see Table 31-5)	Used in mild-to-moderate pain
		May use in conjunction with opioid agents to decrease doses of each
		Regular alcohol use and acetaminophen may result in liver toxicity
		Care must be exercised to avoid overdose when combination products containing these agents are used
		Underlying renal impairment, hypovolemia, and heart failure may predispose to nephrotoxicity
Morphine	PO 5-30 mg every 4 h[a]	Drug of choice in severe pain
	IM 5-20 mg every 4 h[a]	Use immediate-release product with SR product to control breakthrough pain in cancer patients
	IV 5-15 mg every 4 h[a]	Typical patient-controlled analgesia IV dose is 1 mg with a 10-minute lock out interval
	SR 15-30 mg every 12 h (may need to be every 8 h in some patients)	Every 24-hour products available, use caution in renally compromised patients
	Rectal 10-20 mg every 4 h[a]	

(*Continued*)

TABLE 31-8 • Dosing Guidelines for Select Opioids (*Continued*)

Agent(s)	Doses (Use Lowest Effective Dose, Titrate Up or Down Based on Patient Response, Opioid-Tolerant Patients May Need Dose Modification)	Notes
Hydromorphone	PO 2-4 mg every 4-6 h[a]	Use in severe pain
	XR 8 mg to 64 mg every 24 h IM 1-2 mg every 4-6 h[a]	More potent than morphine; otherwise, no advantages
	IV 0.5-2 mg every 4 h[a]	Typical patient controlled analgesia IV dose is 0.2 mg with a 10-minute lock out interval
	Rectal 3 mg every 6-8 h[a]	Every 24-hour product (Exalgo) available
Oxymorphone	IM 1-1.5 mg every 4-6 h[a]	Use in severe pain
	IV 0.5 mg every 4-6 h[a]	No advantages over morphine
	PO immediate-release 5-10 mg every 4-6 h[a]	Use immediate-release product with controlled-release product to control breakthrough pain in cancer or chronic pain patients
	PO extended-release 5-10 mg every 12 h[a]	Manufacturer recommends 5 mg every 12 h in opioid-naïve patients Take ER on empty stomach
Levorphanol	PO 2-3 mg every 6-8 h[a] (Levo-Dromoran)	Use in severe pain
	PO 2 mg every 3-6 h[a] (Levorphanol Tartrate)	Extended half-life useful in cancer patients
	IM 1-2 mg every 6-8 h[a]	In chronic pain, wait 3 days between dosage adjustments
	IV 1 mg every 3-6 h[a]	
Codeine	PO 15-60 mg every 4-6 h[a]	Use in mild to moderate pain
	IM 15-60 mg every 4-6 h[a]	Weak analgesic; analgesic prodrug
Hydrocodone	PO 5-10 mg every 4-6 h[a]	Use in moderate/severe pain
Oxycodone	PO 5-15 mg every 4-6 h[a]	Use in moderate/severe pain
	Controlled release 10-20 mg every 12 h	
		Use immediate-release product with controlled-release product to control breakthrough pain in cancer or chronic pain patients CR reformulated to deter abuse
Meperidine	IM 50-150 mg every 3-4 h[a]	Use in severe pain
	IV 5-10 mg every 5 min prn[a]	Oral not recommended
		Do not use in renal failure
		May precipitate tremors, myoclonus, and seizures
		Monoamine oxidase inhibitors can induce hyperpyrexia and/or seizures or opioid overdose symptoms
Fentanyl	IV 25-50 mcg/h	Used in severe pain
	IM 50-100 mcg every 1-2 h[a]	**Do not use transdermal in acute pain**
	Transdermal 25 mcg/h every 72 h	Transmucosal for breakthrough cancer pain in patients already receiving or tolerant to opioids
	Transmucosal (Actiq/OTFC Lozenge and Onsolis buccal film) 200 mcg may repeat × 1, 30 min after first dose is started, then titrate	**Always start with lowest dose despite daily opioid intake; product specific titration recommendations exist**
	Transmucosal (Fentora Buccal Tablet) 100 mcg, may repeat × 1, 30 min after first dose is started, then titrate	
	Intranasal (Lazanda Spray) 100 mcg (one spray) in one nostril. Wait 2 h prior to redosing	

(*Continued*)

TABLE 31-8 • Dosing Guidelines for Select Opioids (*Continued*)

Agent(s)	Doses (Use Lowest Effective Dose, Titrate Up or Down Based on Patient Response, Opioid-Tolerant Patients May Need Dose Modification)	Notes
Fentanyl	Sublingual (Subsys Spray) 100 mcg (1 spray). Wait 4 h prior to redosing	
	Sublingual (Abstral Tablet) 100 mcg tablets placed sublingually. Must wait 2 h prior to redosing	
Methadone	PO 2.5-10 mg every 8-12 h[a]	Effective in severe chronic pain
	IM 2.5-10 mg every 8-12 h[a]	
		Some chronic pain patients can be dosed every 12 h
		Equianalgesic dose of methadone when compared with other opioids will decrease progressively the higher the previous opioid dose; avoid dose titrations more frequently than weekly in chronic pain maintenance
Pentazocine	PO 50-100 mg every 3-4 h[b] (max. 600 mg daily, for those 50-mg tablet containing 0.5 mg of naloxone)	Second-line agent for moderate-to-severe pain; may precipitate withdrawal in opiate-dependent patients; parenteral doses not recommended
	PO 25 mg every 4 h[b] (max. 150 mg daily, for those 25 mg tablet containing 325 mg of acetaminophen)	
Butorphanol	IM 1-4 mg every 3-4 h[b]	Second-line agent for moderate-to-severe pain
	IV 0.5-2 mg every 3-4 h[b]	May precipitate withdrawal in opiate-dependent patients
	Intranasal 1 mg (1 spray) every 3-4 h[b]	
	If inadequate relief after initial spray, may repeat in other nostril × 1 in 60-90 min	
	Max. 2 sprays (one per nostril) every 3-4 h[b]	
Nalbuphine	IM/IV 10 mg every 3-6 h[b] (max. 20 mg dose, 160 mg daily)	Second-line agent for moderate-to-severe pain; may precipitate withdrawal in opiate-dependent patients Used frequently in low doses to treat/prevent opioid-induced pruritus
Buprenorphine	IM 0.3 mg every 6 h[b]	Second-line agent for moderate-to-severe pain
	Slow IV 0.3 mg every 6 h[b]	May precipitate withdrawal in opiate-dependent patients
		Transdermal delivery systems (5, 7.5, 10, 15, 20 mcg/h) available for every 7-day administration; detailed manufacturer dosing conversion recommendations exist
	May repeat × 1, 30-60 min after initial dose	Naloxone may not be effective in reversing respiratory depression
Naloxone	IV IM 0.4-2 mg	When reversing opiate side effects in patients needing analgesia, dilute and titrate (0.1-0.2 mg every 2-3 min) so as not to reverse analgesia
Tramadol	PO 50-100 mg every 4-6 h[a]	Maximum dose for nonextended-release, 400 mg/24 h; maximum for extended release, 300 mg/24 h
	If rapid onset not required, start 25 mg/day and titrate over several days	Decrease dose in patient with renal impairment and in the elderly
	Extended release PO 100 mg every 24 h	
Tapentadol	PO 50-100 mg every 4-6 h[a]	First day of therapy may administer second dose after the first within 1 h; maximum dose first day 700 mg, max. dose thereafter 600 mg (max. dose for CR 500 mg)

[a] May start with an around-the-clock regimen and switch to prn if/when the painful signal subsides or is episodic.

[b] May reach a ceiling analgesic effect.

Abbreviations: CR = controlled release; ER = extended release; IM = intramuscular; IV = intravenous; NSAID = nonsteroidal anti-inflammatory drug; PO = oral; prn = as needed; SR = sustained release; HCL = hydrochloride.

Source: Reproduced, with permission, from DiPiro JT, Talbert RL, Yee GC, Matzke GR, Wells BG, Posey L, eds. *Pharmacotherapy: A Pathophysiologic Approach*, 10th ed. New York, NY: McGraw-Hill; 2017.

TABLE 31-9 • Pharmacodynamic and Pharmacokinetic Properties of Commonly Prescribed Opioids

Hydroxylated Phenanthrene	Receptor Binding	Relative Mu Receptor Binding Affinity	Equivalent Doses	$T_{1/2}$	Duration of Action	Volume of Distribution (Vd)	Metabolism	Available Doses[a]
Morphine (Brand names: MSIR, Roxanol, MSContin, Avinza, Kadian)	Binds to both μ1 & μ2 ~equally Weak κ agonist M-6-G δ-receptor agonist	+	30 mg PO	2-4 hr	IR: 4 hr	3-4 L/kg	Phase II glucuronidation to morphine-3-glucuronide (not active for analgesia but will cause side effects) and morphine-6- glucuronide (active) Both major metabolites accumulate in renal failure Morphine (parent) accumulates in hepatic failure	IV: 2 mg/mL, 4 mg/mL, 5 mg/mL, 8 mg/mL, 10 mg/0.7 mL, 10 mg/mL, 15 mg/mL, 25 mg/mL, 50 mg/mL IR: 15 mg, 30 mg Solution: 2 mg/mL, 4 mg/mL, 20 mg/mL SA: MSContin 15 mg, 30 mg, 60 mg, 100 mg, 200 mg; Avinza 30 mg, 60 mg, 90 mg, 120 mg; Kadian 20 mg, 30 mg, 50 mg, 60 mg, 80 mg, 100 mg, 200 mg
Codeine	Prodrug, metabolized to morphine μ-receptor agonist with low binding affinity	+/– Metabolites responsible for analgesic properties	200 mg po	2.5-3.5 hr	4-6 hr	3.5 L/kg	2D6 mediated O-demethylation to morphine (active) Phase II glucuronidation to codeine-6-glucuronide 3A4 mediated N-demethylation to norcodeine (inactive)	IV: 15 mg/mL, 30 mg/mL IR: phosphate 30 mg, 60 mg; sulfate 15 mg, 30 mg, 60 mg SA: (not available in U.S.) 50 mg, 100 mg, 150 mg, 200 mg
Diacetyl-morphine	not available	not available	not available	3-5 min	not available	60-100L	Peripheral metabolism to 6-acetylmorphine, morphine, morphine-3-glucuronide, normorphine, 6-acetylmorphine 3-glucuronide, normorphine glucuronide	not available in the U.S.
Dehydroxylated phenanthrene	**Receptor Binding**	**Relative Mu Receptor Binding Affinity**	**Equivalent Doses**	**$T_{1/2}$**	**Duration of Action**	**Volume of Distribution (Vd)**	**Metabolism**	**Available Doses[a]**
Levorphanol (Brand name: Levo-Dromoran)	μ-agonist κ1, κ3 >>κ2 Noncompetitive NMDA receptor antagonist SNRI activity	++	4 mg	~30 hr	6-15 hr	10-13 L/kg	Phase II glucuronidation to levorphanol-3-glucuronide	IV: 2 mg/mL IR: 1 mg, 2 mg, 3 mg

Hydromorphone (Brand name: Dilaudid)	μ receptor agonist	++	7.5 mg PO	1-3 hr	IR: 4-5 hr	4 L/kg	Phase II glucuronidation to hydromorphone-3-glucuronide and to some extent hydromorphone-6-glucuronide H3G accumulates in renal failure	IV: 1 mg/mL, 2 mg/mL, 4 mg/mL, 10 mg/mL IR: 2 mg, 4 mg, 8 mg
Hydrocodone (Brand names: Vicodin, Lortab, Lorcet, Vicoprofen)	μ receptor agonist with low binding affinity	+	30 mg PO	3.8 hr	4-6 hr	3.4-4.7 L/kg	O-demethylation, N-demethylation and 6-keto reduction to 6-α- and 6-β-hydroxymetabolites CYP3A4 mediated N-demethylation to norhydrocodone is the primary metabolic pathway. Nearly 60% of hydrocodone's metabolism is mediated through the combined CYP 2D6 and CYP 3A4 pathways resulting in the formation of hydromorphone and norhydrocodone[2]. Metabolism and excretion patterns of hydrocodone in urine found that norhydrocodone was the most abundant metabolite and frequently detected in combination with hydrocodone within 2 hours of drug administration.[b,c]	Combination with APAP: 2.5/500 mg, 5/325 mg, 7.5/325 mg, 10/325 mg, 5/500 mg, 7.5/500 mg, 10/500 mg, 7.5/750 mg, 10/650 mg, 10/660 mg Combination with IBU: 5/200 mg, 7.5/200 mg
Oxycodone (Brand names: Oxy IR, OxyContin, Roxicodone, Percocet, Roxicet, Tylox)	μ receptor agonist with low binding affinity Greater kappa agonist binding affinity than morphine suggesting it may be the opioid of choice for visceral pain because the viscera have relatively more kappa receptors than peripheral tissues	+	20 mg PO	IR: 2-3 hr SA: ~5 hr	IR: 3-6 hr SA: 12 hr	2.6 L/kg	*3A4 mediated N-demethylation to noroxycodone *2D6 mediated O-demethylation to oxymorphone (active)	IR: 5 mg, 15 mg, 30 mg Solution: 1 mg/mL, 20 mg/mL SA: 10 mg, 20 mg, 40 mg, 60 mg, 80 mg, 160 mg Combination with APAP: 5/325 mg, 5/500 mg, 7.5/325 mg, 7.5/500 mg, 10/325 mg, 10/350 mg
Oxymorphone (Brand name: Opana, Opana ER)	μ receptor agonist with low binding affinity	*	10 mg PO	IV: 2 hr IR: 7-9 hr SA: 9-11 hr	IV: 3-6 hr IR: 4-6hr SA: ~12 hr	1.9-4.2 L/kg	Phase II glucuronidation to oxymorphone-3-glucuronide	IV: 1 mg/mL IR: 5 mg, 10 mg SA: 5 mg, 10 mg, 20 mg, 40 mg

(Continued)

TABLE 31-9 • Pharmacodynamic and Pharmacokinetic Properties of Commonly Prescribed Opioids (*Continued*)

Dehydroxylated phenanthrene	Receptor Binding	Relative Mu Receptor Binding Affinity	Equivalent Doses	$T_{1/2}$	Duration of Action	Volume of Distribution (Vd)	Metabolism	Available Doses[a]
Buprenorphine (Brand names: Buprenex, Subutex, Suboxone)	Binds to μ1>>>>μ2 ~90% more; does not block the alpha receptor as much as morphine; means no withdrawal, not addicting κ receptor antagonist	++++	0.3 mg IV	2.2 hr	6-8 hr	97-187 L/kg	3A4 mediated N-dealkylation to norbuprenorphine (weakly active) Phase II glucuronidation of both the parent compound and norbuprenorphine	IV/IM: 0.3 mg/mL SL: 2 mg, 8 mg SL combination with naltrexone: 2 mg/0.5 mg, 8 mg/2 mg
Phenylpiperidine	**Receptor Binding**	**Relative Mu Receptor Binding Affinity**	**Equivalent Doses**	**$T_{1/2}$**	**Duration of Action**	**Volume of Distribution (Vd)**	**Metabolism**	**Available Doses[a]**
Fentanyl (Brand names: Sublimaze, Actiq, Duragesic)	μ receptor agonist	+++	0.1 mg IV/IM	IV: 2-4 hr Transdermal patch: 17-22 hr Transmucosal lozenge: 7 hr	IV: 0.5-1 hr IM:1-2 hr Transdermal: 48-72 hr	6 L/kg	3A4 mediated oxidative N-dealkylation to norfentanyl	IV: 0.05 mg/mL Transdermal patch: 12 mcg/hr, 25 mcg/hr, 50 mcg/hr, 75 mcg/hr, 100 mcg/hr Transmucosal lozenge: 200 mcg, 400 mcg, 600 mcg, 800 mcg, 1200 mcg, 1600 mcg
Meperidine (Brand name: Demerol)	μ receptor agonist δ receptor agonist	**	300 mg PO	Parent: 2.5-4 hr Liver Disease: 7-11 hr Normeperidine: 15-30 hr	2-5 hr	3.7 L/kg	Phase II hydrolysis to meperidinic acid N-demethylation to normeperidine (neurotoxic); normeperidine accumulates in hepatic failure	IM/SC: 25 mg/mL, 50 mg/mL, 100 mg/mL Solution/Syrup: 10 mg/mL IR: 50 mg, 100 mg

Diphenylheptanes	Receptor Binding	Relative Mu Receptor Binding Affinity	Equivalent Doses	$T_{1/2}$	Duration of Action	Volume of Distribution (Vd)	Metabolism	Available Doses[a]
Propoxyphene (Brand names: Darvon, Darvon-N, Darvon Compound 32, Darvon Compound 65, Darvocet A, Darvocet N)	μ receptor agonist	++	130 mg* or 200 mg** PO (*HCl salt **napsylate salt)	Parent: 6-12 hr Norpropoxyphene: 30-36 hr	4-6 hr	16 L/kg	3A4 mediated N-demethylation to norpropoxyphene with is excreted by the kidneys *metabolite accumulates in renal failure	IR: 65 mg, 100 mg Combo with APAP: 50/325 mg, 65/650 mg, 100/325 mg, 100/650 mg
Methadone (Brand name: Dolophine, Methadose)	μ receptor agonist Noncompetitive NMDA receptor antagonist SNRI activity	++	7.5 mg PO	8-59 hr	15-60 hr	Vdss 1-8 L/kg	3A4, 2B6, 2C19 mediated N-demethylation to 2-ethylidene-1,5-dimethyl-3,3-diphenylpyrrolidene (EDDP)	IV/IM: 10 mg/mL Solution: 1 mg/mL, 2 mg/mL, 10 mg/mL Tablets: 5 mg, 10 mg
Analgesic Miscellaneous								
Tapentadol (Brand name: Nucynta)	Strong mu receptor agonist with low binding affinity SNRI activity	– *18x less potent than morphine	75-100 mg	4 hr	4-6 hr	540 ± 98 L	Phase II glucuronidation to O-glucuronide 2C9/2C19 mediated methylation to N-desmethyl-tapentadol	50 mg, 75 mg, 100 mg

[a] Most common dosage forms listed; not all-inclusive.

[b] Cone EJ, Heltsley R, Black DL, Mitchell JM, Lodico CP, Flegel RR. Prescription opioids. II. Metabolism and excretion patterns of hydrocodone in urine following controlled single-dose administration. *J Anal Toxicol.* 2013;37(8):486-494.

[c] Valtier S, Bebarta VS. Excretion profile of hydrocodone, hydromorphone and norhydrocodone in urine following single dose administration of hydrocodone to healthy volunteers. *J Anal Toxicol.* 2012;36(7):507-514.

MSIR [package insert]. Perdue Pharma, Stamford, CT; Oct 2004;

MS Contin [package insert]. Perdue Pharma, Stamford, CT; March 2009.

Buprenex [package insert]. Richmond, VA: Reckitt Benckiser Pharmaceuticals 20Inc; April 2005.

Suboxone/Subutex [package insert]. Richmond, VA: Reckitt Benckiser Pharmaceuticals Inc; 2006.

Lacy CF, Armstrong LL, Goldman LP, Lance LL, eds. *Drug Information Handbook.* 17th ed. Hudson, OH: Lexi-Comp; 2008.

Methadose [package insert]. Hazelwood, Mo: Mallinckrodt Inc; 2009.

Duragesic [package inset]. Raritan, NJ: PriCara; July 2009.

OxyContin [package insert]. Stamford, CT: Purdue Pharma; April 2010.

Molina DK, Hargrove VM. What is the lethal concentration of hydrocodone: a comparison of postmortem hydrocodone concentrations in lethal and incidental intoxications. *Am J Forensic Med Pathol.* 2011;32(2):108-111.

Koska AJ 3rd, Kramer WG, Romagnoli A, et al. Pharmacokinetics of high-dose meperidine in surgical patients. *Anesth Analg.* 1981;60(1):8-11.

Nucynta [package insert]. Raritan, NJ: Pricara; March 2010.

Rook EJ, Huitema AD, van den Brink W, van Ree JM, Beijnen JH. Pharmacokinetics and pharmacokinetic variability of heroin and its metabolites: review of the literature. *Curr Clin Pharmacol.* 2006;1(1):109-118.

Mayyas F, Fayers P, Kaasa S, Dale O. A systematic review of oxymorphone in the management of chronic pain. *J Pain Symptom Manage.* 2010;39(2):296-308.

Gold MS, Redmond DE Jr, Kleber HD. Clonidine blocks acute opioid-withdrawal symptoms. *Lancet.* 1978;312(8090):599-602.

the concerns surrounding opioid therapy, an MTM session is a great opportunity to ensure the patient receives recommended monitoring. During the consult, if a patient is experiencing minor periodic increases in pain or side effects which have been moderately controlled, it is appropriate to monitor the patient and inform the provider at a later time. However, if the patient is reporting severe uncontrolled pain despite taking medications as prescribed, is showing signs of medication overuse or abuse, or is experiencing unmanageable side effects, it is important to intervene with the appropriate physician and counsel the patient to seek prompt medical attention for identified concerns.

Adverse Effects of Opioid Therapy. During an MTM session, it is important to recognize the possible side effects associated with opioids (Table 31-10). A very common side effect is opioid-induced constipation. The prevalence of opioid-induced constipation in patients treated for noncancer pain ranges from 41% to 81%.[16] If opioids are part of the current medication regimen, it is likely that patients may complain of constipation. If they do not openly share this concern during the MTM session, it is crucial that this common opioid-induced adverse effect is discussed with the patient and a MAP is created to ensure continuous monitoring and adequate management. Opioid-induced constipation can occur at any time when a patient is taking an opioid, so education and continual monitoring for this side effect is very important. Table 31-11 provides suggested questions to assess issues with constipation during an MTM session. Table 31-12 provides an overview of common over-the-counter (OTC) treatment options for constipation. The use of a stimulant laxative and a stool softener is a common initial regimen for opioid-induced constipation.[16] Although bulk-forming agents are available OTC for the treatment of constipation, these agents can increase the risk of a bowel obstruction, especially if the patient is not adequately hydrated. Therefore, bulk-forming agents are not recommended for the treatment or prevention of opioid-induced constipation. In addition, all laxatives and surfactants are contraindicated in bowel obstructions.[17] If the patient continues to experience constipation despite use of OTC options, or if a bowel obstruction is suspected, the patient should be referred to the provider and encouraged to seek prompt medical attention.[18]

TABLE 31-10 • Major Adverse Effects of Opioid Analgesics

Effect	Manifestation
Mood changes	Dysphoria, euphoria
Somnolence	Sedation, inability to concentrate
Stimulation of chemoreceptor trigger zone	Nausea, vomiting
Respiratory depression	Decreased respiratory rate
Decreased gastrointestinal motility	Constipation
Increase in sphincter tone	Biliary spasm, urinary retention (varies among agents)
Histamine release	Urticaria, pruritus, rarely exacerbation of asthma because of bronchospasm (varies among agents)
Tolerance	Larger doses for same effect
Dependence	Withdrawal symptoms upon abrupt discontinuation
Addiction	Genetic predisposition leads to loss of control of drug use, continued use despite harm, compulsion to use, cravings
Hypogonadism	Fatigue, depression, loss of analgesia, sexual dysfunction, amenorrhea (women)
Sleep	Disrupts sleep-wake cycle, causes dose-dependent rapid eye movement (REM) suppression

Source: Reproduced, with permission, from DiPiro JT, Talbert RL, Yee GC, Matzke GR, Wells BG, Posey L, eds. *Pharmacotherapy: A Pathophysiologic Approach*, 10th ed. New York, NY: McGraw-Hill; 2017.

TABLE 31-11 • Screening for Opioid-Induced Constipation: Example Assessment Questions

Frequency and consistency of bowel movements
When was your last bowel movement?
How difficult was it to pass the bowel movement?
What was the consistency of the stool?
Changes in bowel habits
How frequently do you have a bowel movement?
Has the frequency decreased recently?
Do you experience pain while having a bowel movement?
How often do you feel that you need to have a bowel movement but are unable to because of pain?
After a bowel movement, do you feel you have passed the entire stool?
Treatment
What type of medicines, herbals, or dietary options have you tried recently to help with constipation?
Did you experience relief with the treatment?
Other information
How much fluid do you drink during the day?
What type of activity do you participate in during the day?

Source: Reference 17.

Respiratory depression is another common side effect of opioids. It can be fatal and is a common cause of opioid-related deaths.[19] Risk factors for developing respiratory depression secondary to opioid use include doses of opioids exceeding 50 morphine milligram equivalents (MME)/day, history of overdose, concurrent use of benzodiazepines, renal or hepatic impairment, diagnosis of sleep apnea, history or current use of other drugs or alcohol, current methadone use, high risk of drug-drug interactions because of polypharmacy, comorbid psychiatric disorders, or cognitive impairment issues.[8,19] Naloxone, which is an opioid antagonist, is effective in reversing opioid-induced respiratory depression.[20] The FDA has approved two naloxone single-use products which are intended for use in the community (Table 31-13). These products include the intranasal delivery formulation (Narcan®)[21] and a hand-held auto injector (Evzio®).[22,23] The MTM session offers the opportunity to

TABLE 31-12 • Medications for Management of Constipation

Intervention	Dose	Comment
Stimulant laxatives		These agents directly stimulate peristalsis and may reduce colonic absorption of water.
Prune juice	120-240 mL/d	Work in 6-12 h.
Senna (Senokot)	2-8 tablets PO bid	
Bisacodyl	5-15 mg/d PO, PR	
Osmotic laxatives		These agents are not absorbed. They attract and retain water in the gastrointestinal tract.
Lactulose	15-30 mL PO q4–8h	Lactulose may cause flatulence and bloating.
Magnesium hydroxide (Milk of Magnesia)	15-30 mL/d PO	Lactulose works in 1 day, magnesium products in 6 h.
Magnesium citrate	125-250 mL/d PO	
Stool softeners		These agents work by increasing water secretion and as detergents, increasing water penetration into the stool.
Sodium docusate (Colace)	50-300 mg/d PO	Work in 1-3 days.
Calcium docusate	240 mg/d PO	
Suppositories and enemas		
Bisacodyl	10-15 PR qd	
Sodium phosphate enema	PR qd	Fixed dose, 4.5 oz, Fleet's.

Source: Reproduced, with permission, from Kasper D, Fauci A, Hauser S, Longo D, Jameson J, Loscalzo J, et al., eds. *Harrison's Principles of Internal Medicine*, 19th ed. New York, NY: McGraw-Hill; 2014.

evaluate the risk for opioid-induced respiratory depression and to suggest obtaining a naloxone device in case the patient experiences opioid-induced respiratory depression. Both the patient and the caregiver(s) should receive proper education on the use and storage of these devices. Education should include signs and symptoms of an overdose, how to perform rescue breathing, the importance of calling emergency services immediately, and the proper use of naloxone. During this education, it is imperative to reiterate the importance of calling emergency services if naloxone is used, even if the patient responds to the naloxone, since further medical evaluation and care is needed. Further detailed information on how to educate a patient on naloxone can be found at http://store.samhsa.gov/shin/content//SMA16-4742/SMA16-4742.pdf.[20]

Adjuvants. Along with nonopioid analgesics, *adjuvant* medications are often utilized in the treatment of pain. These agents are technically not classified as analgesics, but they have pharmacological properties that help manage different types of pain, especially neuropathic pain. Adjuvants can have some opioid-sparing effects, and they should be considered when clinically indicated. Table 31-14 highlights adjuvant medications used in chronic pain management.

TABLE 31-13 • Single Use Naloxone Products Intended for Distribution in the Community

Naloxone Product	Product Description	Available Strengths	Instructions
Evzio Auto-Injector	Hand-held auto-injector with electronic voice that provides user instructions for use	2 mg per 0.4 mL	Inject in the muscle or skin of the outer thigh. May repeat injection with a new injector every 2-3 minutes if patient is not responding until emergency services arrive
Narcan Nasal Spray	Nasal spray	4 mg: most commonly used 2 mg: restricted to patients who are at risk for experiencing severe opioid withdrawal reactions and it is determined there is a low risk for accidental or intentional opioid exposures within the household	1. Do not prime or test this device prior to administration 2. Place patient in supine position and support the back of the neck 3. Tilt the head back 4. Place tip of device in one nostril and press firmly on the device plunger 5. Remove device from nostril 6. Seek medical attention immediately after administering dose 7. May repeat after 2-3 minutes if response is not seen 8. If additional dose is administered, alternate nostrils

Source: References 21, 22, and 23.

TABLE 31-14 • Adjuvant Analgesics

Drug	Pain Syndrome	Dosing	Comments
Anticonvulsants			
Gabapentin; 100, 300, 400 mg caps; 600, 800 mg tabs; 250 mg/5 mL PO solution	Neuropathic pain	Initial 100 mg PO TID; increase by 100 mg TID Q3d; 300-3600 mg/d divided TID	Adjust dose for renal dysfunction (Cr_{Cl} <60 mL/min); no significant documented drug–drug interactions; do not stop abruptly; monitor for changes in mood, suicidal ideation
Pregabalin (Lyrica®); 25, 50, 75, 100, 150, 200, 225, 300 mg caps	Neuropathic pain	Initial 150 mg PO divided BID/TID; max 450 mg divided BID/TID	
Lamotrigine (Lamictal®); 25, 50, 100, 200 mg tab; 2, 5, 25 mg chewable tabs; 25, 50, 100, 200, 300 mg XR tabs; 25, 50, 100 mg ODTs	Neuropathic pain	Initial 25 mg QOD ×2 wk; then 25 mg QD ×2 wk; then ↑ by 25-50 mg/d Q1-2 wk; up to 50-400 mg/d typical	Do not DC abruptly
Topiramate (Topamax®) 15, 25 mg sprinkle caps, 25, 50, 100, 200 mg tabs	Neuropathic pain	Initial 25-50mg QD; ↑ by 25-50mg Qwk; 200 mg BID studied; max 1600 mg/d	Limited data
Valproic acid 125, 250, 500 mg softgel IR and XR; 250/5 mL PO solution	Neuropathic pain	Initial 125 mg TID; maint 500-1000 mg TID	Monitor levels (<100 mcg/mL); CYP450 inhibitor; monitor for drug interactions
Antidepressants			
Duloxetine (Cymbalta®); 20, 30, 60 mg caps	Diabetic neuropathy, fibromyalgia	Initial 20 mg/d initial; typical 20-60 mg/d (QD or divide BID)	May increase BP; monitor for changes in mood, suicidal ideation
Venlafaxine (Effexor®); 25, 37.5, 50, 75, 100 mg tabs; 37.5, 50, 75, 150, 225 mg XR tabs; 37.5, 50, 75, 150 mg XR caps	Neuropathic pain	Initial 37.5-75 mg/d; may ↑ dose Q4d by 75 mg/d; typical 75-225 mg/d divided BID/TID	Causes ↑ BP; monitor
Amitriptyline; 10, 25, 50, 75, 100, 150 mg tabs	Neuropathic pain	Initial 25 mg PO HS; 10 mg if frail, elderly; typical 25-100 mg HS; 1-2wk (up to 4) for effects; titrate every few days to ↓ AE	Anticholinergic effects ↑ with SSRIs, avoid tramadol: ↑ seizure risk; anticholinergic fx: amitriptyline > nortriptyline > desipramine
Nortriptyline; 10, 25, 50, 75 mg caps; 10 mg/5mL PO solution			
Desipramine; 10, 25, 50, 75, 100, 150 mg tabs			
Corticosteroids			
Dexamethasone; 0.5, 0.75, 1, 1.5, 2, 4, 6 mg tabs; 0.5/5 mL, 1 mg/mL PO solution; solution for injection Methylprednisolone 4, 8, 16, 32 mg tabs, solution and suspension for injection	Spinal cord compression, ↑ ICP	Load 40-100 mg IV dex or equivalent (methylpred 40-80 mg IV) or 10-20 mg IV Q6h for initial 24-72 h	High dose ≤72h; if no benefit, dose can be rapidly tapered; if pain improves, taper to lowest effective dose Usefulness limited to 2-3 mo before steroid-induced side effects outweigh benefit
	Nerve compression, visceral distension, ↑ ICP	Dex 4-8 mg PO Q8-12h; methylpred 20-40 mg PO Q8-12h	
	Bone pain, nausea, anorexia	Dex 4-12 mg/d	
Miscellaneous			
Lidocaine patch (Lidoderm®) 5%	Postherpetic neuralgia	1 patch for 12h/d; 1-3 patches	Clinical experience supports use in painful peripheral neuralgia
Pamidronate (Aredia®) 3, 6, 9 mg/mL injection solution; 30, 90 mg powder for reconstitution	Bone pain	90 mg IV Q4wk, may ↓ interval to Q3wk; ↓ dose renal dysfunction	↓ impact of disease progression in patients with osteolytic lesions 2/2 multiple myeloma, breast cancer, prostate cancer
Zoledronic acid (Zometa®, Reclast®); 4, 5 mg/100 mL, 4 mg/5 mL injection solution		4 mg IV Q4wk; may ↓ interval to Q3wk; ↓ dose renal dysfunction	

Source: Reproduced, with permission, from Attridge RL, Miller ML, Moote R, Ryan L, eds. *Internal Medicine: A Guide to Clinical Therapeutics*. New York, NY: McGraw-Hill; 2013.

CORE ELEMENT 5—DOCUMENTATION AND FOLLOW-UP

Clear and succinct documentation of medication-related problems (MRPs) and recommendations is a key component of the MTM consult. Table 31-15 includes common MRPs in patients who suffer from chronic pain. Various opportunities for recommendations may be noted during the MTM consult. Communicating these recommendations clearly to the prescriber is important because this could improve the overall management of the patient's pain. Figure 31-4 provides sample communications and recommendations to prescribers that may be shared via fax, telephone, or other secure electronic communication method. The examples are for illustrative purposes only. Actual communications to providers should be individualized based on the type of recommendation, patient specific characteristics, and the nature of the relationship with the provider.

Follow-Up

Chronic pain should be treated similarly to other disease states with continual follow-up to assess pain control, adverse effects, activity levels, and emotional health. The required interval for follow-up depends on many factors including comorbid conditions, recent stability of overall pain control, recent medication changes, and availability for follow-up. Because of the subjective nature of pain, it is reasonable to consider a follow-up session via telephone based on the needs of the patient. When opioids are incorporated into the treatment plan, appropriate evaluation, documentation, screening, and risk stratification is indicated at initiation and throughout the duration of opioid therapy. Use of opioid therapy should be assessed during each MTM session to determine if the patient understands the therapy and to evaluate for possible overuse. Overuse of an opioid may be related to a substance abuse problem. However, it could be associated with the development of tolerance to the current regimen or even undertreatment of pain. Ongoing, frequent assessment is imperative for chronic pain management.[9]

Maintenance of a pain diary will further enhance the quality of follow-up care. Pain diaries can be used for any patient who suffers from chronic pain, and they are especially useful for patients who are poor historians or those who have had difficulty achieving pain control after multiple interventions. The diary should include the average pain score, pain levels associated with activities of daily living, a record of any short-acting medications used for breakthrough pain if applicable, and any other actions taken to help alleviate the pain. Various examples of pain diaries may be found on the internet including the Daily Pain Diary (http://pain-focus.com/pcpost/keep-pain-diary/.) Use of a pain diary can be recommended to the patient during an MTM session. This tool will help identify trends in pain levels throughout the day that enable the MTM provider customize a pain management regimen. Regardless of the follow-up method, it is important to continuously evaluate the patient to ensure safe and effective pain control.

TABLE 31-15 • Potential Medication-Related Problems (MRPs) in Patients with Chronic Pain

Category of MRP	Example Medication-Related Problem
Nonadherence	• Suboptimal control of chronic pain because of nonadherence to recommended physical therapy sessions or other nonpharmacologic interventions • Suboptimal control of chronic pain because of nonadherence with nonopioid therapy • Suboptimal control of chronic pain because of nonadherence with adjuvant therapy • Suboptimal control of chronic pain because of opioid overuse (opioid-induced hyperalgesia) or underuse
Unnecessary medication	• Duplicate therapy (eg, two NSAIDs, two long-acting opioids)
Need for additional medication	• Suboptimal pain control on monotherapy with opioid; need to utilize nonpharmacologic, nonopioid, and adjuvant therapy for adequate pain control
Ineffective medication	• Muscle relaxant prescribed for nociceptive pain; no evidence of muscle spasms • Bulk laxative (psyllium) being used for prevention of opioid-induced constipation
Dosage too low	• Suboptimal pain control on low dose of gabapentin
Dosage too high	• Patient with daytime sedation secondary to high dose opioid(s)
Adverse drug event	• Constipation secondary to chronic opioid use • Black tarry stools secondary to chronic use of NSAIDs

Abbreviation: NSAIDs = nonsteroidal anti-inflammatory drugs.

Scenario: Patient on ibuprofen 800 mg TID for moderate chronic knee pain secondary to severe osteoarthritis. Has stopped taking ibuprofen due to severe dyspepsia. **MRP:** Nonadherence, adverse drug event
• Assessment: Patient with long-standing moderate pain secondary to severe OA in bilateral knees experiencing severe dyspepsia with ibuprofen. Patient has not tried acetaminophen as nonopioid option in the past. Acetaminophen can be helpful in managing pain secondary to osteoarthritis and will not cause the gastrointestinal adverse effects associated with NSAIDs. Note: No indication of hepatic dysfunction. • Plan: Consider discontinuing ibuprofen and start acetaminophen 500 mg 1 tablet by mouth QID (scheduled). May increase to a maximum dose of 3000 mg per day dependent on the patient's health status.
Scenario: Patient reports severe constipation; last bowel movement approximately 2 days ago (normal schedule 1 bowel movement daily) and increased straining over the last few weeks. **MRP:** Adverse drug event
• Assessment: Patient with opioid-induced constipation on morphine CR 15 mg by mouth every 12 hours—started therapy 1 month ago. Patient currently not on a bowel regimen. A daily bowel regimen consisting of a stimulant and stool softener should be considered in the treatment plan to prevent opioid-induced constipation. The dosage will need to be adjusted as the opioid dose changes. • Plan: Consider addition of docusate sodium/senna (OTC) 1 tablet by mouth twice daily; Nonpharmacological measures: Increase fluid and fiber intake.
Scenario: Patient reports taking oxycodone 5 mg IR po BID for diabetic peripheral neuropathy. Pain continues to average 9/10 when taking oxycodone monotherapy. **MRP:** Ineffective medication
• Assessment: Patient is taking a short-acting opioid for diabetic peripheral neuropathy, which is considered a third-line option (weak recommendation) based on current guidelines. In addition, oxycodone IR would need to be dosed every 4 to 6 hours for optimal efficacy. Patients can also develop tolerance to opioids and require dose escalation over time. Consider use of pregabalin, which is first-line per evidence-based guidelines (strong recommendation). Pregabalin has been shown to improve quality of life and decrease sleep interference. Proper titration of this agent could improve overall control of pain associated with DPN. • Plan: Consider discontinuing oxycodone and starting pregabalin (Lyrica) 25 mg by mouth 3 times daily and titrate weekly up to maximum total dose of 300 mg per day based on tolerance and efficacy.

FIGURE 31-4 Sample provider communications for chronic pain.[14,16]

REFERENCES

1. International Association for the Study of Pain. Available at http://www.iasp-pain.org/Taxonomy#Pain. Accessed May 4, 2017.
2. Woolf C. What is this thing called pain? *J Clin Invest.* 2010;120(11):3742-3744.
3. Herndon CM, Strickland JM, Ray JB. Pain management. In: DiPiro JT, Talbert RL, Yee GC, Matzke GR, Wells BG, Posey L, eds. *Pharmacotherapy: A Pathophysiologic Approach*, 10th ed. New York, NY: McGraw-Hill; 2017.
4. Scullion BF, Ryan L. Pain management. In: Attridge RL, Miller ML, Moote R, Ryan L, eds. *Internal Medicine: A Guide to Clinical Therapeutics.* New York, NY: McGraw-Hill; 2013.
5. National Institute for Health and Care Excellence (NICE Guideline). Neuropathic pain in adults: pharmacological management in nonspecialist settings. Clinical guideline updated February 2017. https://www.nice.org.uk/guidance/CG173. Accessed May 5, 2017.
6. Nickel FT, Seifert F, Lanz S, et al. Mechanisms of neuropathic pain. *European Neuropsychopharmacology.* 2012;22(2):81-91.
7. Woolf C. Central Sensitization: Implications for the diagnosis and treatment of pain. *Pain.* 2011;152(suppl):S2-S15.
8. Manchikanti L, Falco F, Singh V, et al. An update of comprehensive evidence-based guidelines for interventional techniques in chronic spinal pain. Part 1: Introduction and general considerations. *Pain Physician.* 2013;16:S1-S48.
9. Dowell D, Haegerich TM, Chou R. CDC guideline for prescribing opioids for chronic pain—United States, 2016. *MMWR Recomm Rep.* 2016; 65(No. RR-1):1-49.
10. CMS. *Medicare Part D Medication Therapy Management program Standardization Format.* CMS website. Available at https://www.cms.gov/medicare/prescription-drug-coverage/prescriptiondrugcovcontra/downloads/mtm-program-standardized-format-english-and-spanish-instructions-samples-v032712.pdf. Accessed on May 5, 2017.
11. Park J, Hughes AK. Nonpharmacological approaches to the management of chronic pain in community-dwelling older adults: a review of empirical evidence. *J Am Geriatr Soc.* 2012;60:555-568.
12. Natural Medicines [database online]. Somerville, MA: Therapeutic Research Center; 2017. Available at https://naturalmedicines.therapeuticresearch.com/. Accessed May 5. 2017.
13. Herbal Supplements Monthly Cost Estimates. Available at http://www.vitacost.com/. Accessed May 5, 2017.
14. Finnerup N, Attal N, Haroutounian S, et al. Pharmacotherapy for neuropathic pain in adults: systematic review, meta-analysis, and updated NeuPSIG recommendations. *Lancet Neurol.* 2015;14:162-173.
15. Fudin J, Perkins R, Lipman A. Opioids. In: Cohen H. *Casebook in Clinical Pharmacokinetics and Drug Dosing.* 1st ed. New York: McGraw Hill; 2015.
16. Nelson A, Camilleri M. Chronic opioid induced constipation in patients with nonmalignant pain: challenges and opportunities. *Ther Adv Gastroenterol.* 2015;8206-8220.
17. Larkin PJ, Sykes NP, Centeno C, et al. The management of constipation in palliative care: clinical practice recommendations. *Palliat Med.* 2008;22:796-807.
18. Emanuel EJ. Palliative and end-of-life care. In: Kasper D, Fauci A, Hauser S, Longo D, Jameson J, Loscalzo J, et al., eds. *Harrison's Principles of Internal Medicine*, 19th ed. New York, NY: McGraw-Hill; 2014.
19. Coe M, Walsh S. Distribution of naloxone for overdose prevention to chronic pain patients. *Preventive Medicine.* 2015;80:41-43.
20. Opioid Overdose Prevention Toolkit. Substance Abuse and Mental Health Services Administration website. http://store.samhsa.gov/shin/content//SMA16-4742/SMA16-4742.pdf. Updated 2016. Accessed May 5, 2017.
21. Narcan nasal spray [Package Insert]. Radnor, PA: Adapt Pharm, Inc. February 2017.
22. Evzio [Package Insert]. Richmond, VA: Kaleo, Inc. October 2016.
23. Evzio Frequently Asked Questions. Evzio website. https://evzio.com/hcp/. Updated February 2017. Accessed April 26, 2017.

Review Questions

1. Which is the proper definition of pain as defined by the International Association for the Study of Pain?
   a. An unpleasant sensory and emotional experience associated with actual or potential tissue damage
   b. A distressing sensation in a specific part of the body that lasts longer than 3 months
   c. A transient increase in pain over a background pain that typically has a rapid onset of action
   d. An unpleasant sensory experience that has a sudden onset and decreases over time

2. During an MTM visit, a patient reports a burning, tingling sensation in bilateral feet. Which type of pain is the patient describing?
   a. Somatic pain
   b. Nociceptive pain
   c. Neuropathic pain
   d. Visceral pain

3. What is a therapeutic goal associated specifically with the treatment of chronic pain management in comparison to acute pain management?
   a. Decrease overall healthcare costs.
   b. Address and improve psychological and emotional components.
   c. Improve overall quality of life.
   d. Prevent disability associated with uncontrolled pain.

4. Which definition best describes allodynia using living room language?
   a. Pain caused by something that normally does not cause pain, such as light touch.
   b. Pain caused by a lesion or disease of the somatosensory nervous system.
   c. Exaggerated response to a slightly painful stimulus.
   d. Pain caused by damage to nonneural tissue and activation of nociceptors.

5. When developing a medication action plan for a pain patient with a complicated health history, what is the most appropriate first step?
   a. List all disease states with a new therapy recommendation for each disease.
   b. Prioritize the issues, and address only issues that are associated with medication therapy.
   c. Prioritize the issues, and explain to the patient that the lower priority items will be addressed at subsequent visits.
   d. Stress to the patient that this session will only address any pain-related issues and other medication issues can be addressed by another provider.

6. Which counseling statement is correct for a patient who just received a dose increase for opioid therapy?
   a. "Please make sure to drive slowly for the next few days since the increase in medication might decrease your reaction time."
   b. "Since your medication has been increased, please watch for any signs of increased daytime sleepiness, dizziness, or confusion which can occur with an increased dose."
   c. "Due to the dose increase, you will immediately experience severe constipation and will need to treat accordingly."
   d. "Since your medication has been increased, your pain should be completely eliminated."

7. A 72-year-old male presents for an MTM session. He reports that his pain has increased dramatically over the last week. He denies any recent injuries, but he mentions experiencing increased weakness and numbness in his legs and states he is finding it difficult to urinate. What is the best treatment option for this patient?
   a. Recommend an increase in pain medication to help control the symptoms in his legs.
   b. Recommend addition of an adjuvant medication that can help any neuropathic pain he might be experiencing.
   c. Recommend the patient call his physician immediately to be evaluated.
   d. Recommend a decrease in opioid therapy since this is the likely cause of his difficulty urinating.

8. A 68-year-old female reports blurred vision, dry mouth, and increased confusion. She experienced some back pain recently, and her physician prescribed cyclobenzaprine to help decrease her muscle spasms. She reports her back pain has decreased, but she is worried that her back pain will increase if she stops taking this new medication. What potential medication-related problem is this patient experiencing?
   a. Need for additional medication
   b. Nonadherence
   c. Adverse drug event
   d. Dosage too low

9. Which opioid is metabolized by the cytochrome P450 enzyme system?
   a. Fentanyl
   b. Oxymorphone
   c. Morphine
   d. Hydromorphone

10. Which statement is correct regarding naloxone use in an opioid overdose situation?
    a. Evzio Auto-Injector should only be administered one time when a patient is demonstrating symptoms of an overdose.
    b. Contact emergency services immediately when a patient has been administered naloxone for an overdose.
    c. Narcan Nasal Spray can only be used in one nostril for all doses of naloxone administered during an opioid overdose.
    d. There are multiple doses in the Evzio-Auto-injector, so be ready to reuse the original injector if the patient does not recover adequately after the first dose.

ANSWERS

1. a	2. c	3. b
4. a	5. c	6. b
7. c	8. c	9. a
10. b		

32

Peripheral Neuropathy MTM Data Set

Kevin Cowart, PharmD, MPH, and Karen R. Sando, PharmD, BCACP, BC-ADM

KEY POINTS

- Diabetic peripheral neuropathy is the most common type of peripheral neuropathy.
- Control of the underlying condition (ie, diabetes) may help slow the progression of diabetic peripheral neuropathy.
- Multiple medications can be used throughout the course of therapy for diabetic peripheral neuropathy.
- Medication therapy management (MTM) providers should work with the patient and prescribers to ensure that medications for diabetic peripheral neuropathy are properly titrated to symptom relief.
- MTM providers should educate patients regarding the importance of proper foot care.

INTRODUCTION

According to the International Association for the Study of Pain (IASP), neuropathic pain is defined as pain arising as a direct consequence of a lesion or disease affecting the somatosensory system.[1] Peripheral neuropathy specifically describes damage to the peripheral nervous system. The nerve damage can cause changes in pain perception, enhanced sensory transmission, nerve structure reorganization, and loss of pain inhibition.[2]

Causes of Peripheral Neuropathy

Several different disease states and conditions have been known to cause peripheral neuropathy (Table 32-1).[3] Of those, diabetic peripheral neuropathy (DPN) is the most common. Estimates of the incidence and prevalence of DPN vary greatly; DPN may occur in 20% of those with long-standing type 1 diabetes and up to 50% of those with type 2 diabetes.[4] Risk factors associated with the development of DPN include poor glucose control, hypertension, dyslipidemia, height (as a proxy for nerve length), smoking, and obesity.[4] The remainder of this chapter will focus on DPN.

Complications of Diabetic Peripheral Neuropathy

If left untreated or suboptimally treated, DPN can lead to serious and debilitating complications such as foot ulceration, lower limb amputation, Charcot neuroarthropathy, falls, and fractures.[4] It is estimated that 15% of all patients with diabetes will develop a foot ulcer during their lifetime; 60% to 70% of foot ulcers are attributed to DPN.[5] Ulcers can further be associated with cellulitis, osteomyelitis, or severe nonhealing infections that can lead to amputation of a toe, foot, or leg.[5] Risk factors for the development of ulcer complications include poor glycemic control, history of previous ulcers/amputations, poor foot hygiene and care, concurrent peripheral vascular disease, decreased sensitivity, and lack of education.[5] In general, the cost of treating DPN and associated complications averages $10.91 billion annually.[6]

Therapeutic Goals for Diabetic Peripheral Neuropathy

Control and relief of painful symptoms is the primary therapeutic goal in the management of DPN.[4] Prevention of foot ulcerations, falls, and improving quality of life are also important goals to consider.[4] Despite recent advances in understanding the pathogenesis of DPN, there are no treatment options that target the natural history of DPN or reverse the disease process once it is established. No compelling evidence exists to support glycemic control or lifestyle management as therapeutic modalities for addressing DPN symptoms.[4] However, improving glycemic control is important to slow progression of DPN and prevent

TABLE 32-1 • Types of Peripheral Neuropathy

Cancer-related nerve infiltration or compression
Chemotherapy-induced neuropathy
Complex regional pain syndrome
HIV-associated neuropathy
Nerve injury because of trauma
Painful diabetic neuropathy
Phantom limb pain
Postherpetic neuralgia
Trigeminal neuralgia

Source: Reference 3.

development of other microvascular complications associated with diabetes (eg, retinopathy and nephropathy).[4] Pain management with pharmacologic interventions is the main treatment for DPN symptoms.[4]

CORE ELEMENT 1—COMPREHENSIVE MEDICATION REVIEW FOR PATIENTS WITH DIABETIC PERIPHERAL NEUROPATHY

The following is a list of questions to ask when conducting a medication review in a patient with DPN (Table 32-2). The number and types of questions will depend upon the reliability of the patient in providing complete and accurate information as well as the amount of time available for the consult and the number and extent of any medication-related problems (MRPs). During the consult, it is important for MTM providers to use living room language (Figure 32-1) and be prepared for any questions the patient may ask about DPN (Table 32-3).

In addition to asking questions, it is appropriate for the MTM provider, with time permitting, to conduct a foot examination. The assessment can provide objective data concerning the extent and potential progression of the DPN. The examination should include physical inspection of both feet and palpation of pedal pulses (Table 32-4). A number of objective tests can also assist in determining the severity of DPN, including a pinprick test, a light touch test for sensation, a vibration test, ankle reflexes, and a pressure perception test.[4] The 10-gram monofilament sensation test is a quick (~60 seconds) and easy test that can be accomplished during the consult (Figure 32-2).[7,8] Absence of sensation is an indication of DPN.

CORE ELEMENT 2—PERSONAL MEDICATION LIST[10]

The following is an example of a personal medication list (PML) for a patient with DPN (Figure 32-3). This example is representative only of medications used to treat the symptoms of DPN and does not include medications used to treat the underlying cause of the neuropathy. Additional medications should be added and listed separately. When completing the personal medication list, MTM providers should remember to use living room language.

TABLE 32-2 • Questions to Ask When Conducting a Medication Review in a Patient with Diabetic Peripheral Neuropathy

	Suggested Questions to Ask Patients
General	• How long have you had diabetic peripheral neuropathy? • When were you diagnosed? • What do you know about diabetic peripheral neuropathy?

Footcare	• When was the last time you saw a podiatrist (foot physician)?
	  • What tests were performed?
	  • What were the results?
	• How often do you check your feet at home?
	  • How do you check your feet?
	  • What have you found in the past? Recently?
	• What kind of footwear do you use?
	• How do you care for your feet on a daily basis?

Symptoms	• Have you ever experienced the following symptoms? (Follow up each positive response with a symptom analysis: frequency, duration, severity, etc)
	  • Pain
	  • Burning
	  • Tingling
	  • Electric shocks
	  • Numbness
	  • Loss of sensation
	  • Ulcers/broken skin
	  • Deformities
	  • Amputation

Medications	• What medications (prescription and OTC) do you use for diabetic peripheral neuropathy?
	  • How do you take them?
	  • How often do you miss a dose?
	  • What other medications have you tried in the past?
	• Have you ever stopped taking a medication for diabetic peripheral neuropathy without telling your provider?
	  • Why did you stop taking the medication?

CORE ELEMENT 3—MEDICATION ACTION PLAN[10]

The following is a sample medication action plan (MAP) for a patient with DPN. (Figure 32-4). This example is representative only of action steps for a patient with DPN. MAPs for other disease states or other MRPs be added and listed separately. In general, only a few of the most important action steps should be listed, so as not to overwhelm the patient. Other areas for patient self-management can be addressed at later visits. MTM providers should remember to use plain language when creating the MAP.

Adverse event—an unexplained, unwanted reaction.

Allodynia—a painful response to an action that does not usually cause pain.

Amputation—removal of a body part.

Analgesic—a medication that relieves pain.

Calcium channel α_2-δ *ligands*—medications used in the symptomatic relief of diabetic peripheral neuropathy; an example is pregabalin.

Causalgia—constant burning pain.

Charcot joint—foot deformity seen in patients with diabetic peripheral neuropathy.

Chronic—constant; does not go away.

Diabetic peripheral neuropathy—dysfunction of the nerves that can cause pain and symptoms of numbness and tingling in the feet, legs, and arms in patients with diabetes.

Dysesthesias—painful or unpleasant symptoms of tingling, burning, or electric shocks.

Hyperalgesia—increased pain from something that is normally painful.

Hyperesthesia—abnormal increase in sensitivity to stimuli, for instance touching the skin.

Hyperpathia—exaggerated response to something painful, especially a repeated stimulus.

Monofilament—a type of thread used in foot exams to test for sensation.

Myalgia—muscle pain.

Neuralgia—nerve pain.

Neuropathy—disease or dysfunction of the nerves.

NSAID—anti-inflammatory agent to treat pain and swelling.

Opioid—controlled pain reliever medication.

Paresthesia—numbness or tingling.

Podiatrist—foot physician.

SNRI (serotonin-norepinephrine reuptake inhibitor)—typically used for mood or anxiety disorders, but can also be used in the symptomatic relief of diabetic peripheral neuropathy; an example is duloxetine.

TCA (tricyclic antidepressant)—drugs that originally were used to treat mood but also have the ability to provide pain relief for diabetic peripheral neuropathy.

Ulcer—an open sore caused by broken skin that can potentially lead to infection.

FIGURE 32-1 Living room language for diabetic peripheral neuropathy.

TABLE 32-3 • Questions to Anticipate Regarding Diabetic Peripheral Neuropathy

- **What is diabetic peripheral neuropathy?**
  Diabetic peripheral neuropathy is a dysfunction in the nerves that run throughout the body. This can cause pain, burning, tingling, loss of sensation, and can lead to complications such as ulcers, deformities, and possible amputation.
- **What causes diabetic peripheral neuropathy?**
  There are several risk factors that can increase your risk for developing diabetic peripheral neuropathy such as uncontrolled blood sugar levels, how long a person has had diabetes, smoking, and excessive alcohol intake, among others.
- **How do I know if I have diabetic peripheral neuropathy?**
  Sometimes a person can have diabetic peripheral neuropathy and not know it. Most often people discover they have it based upon symptoms. They complain of pain, numbness, tingling, burning, and electric shock feelings.
- **Why do I need to take medication for diabetic peripheral neuropathy?**
  Treatments may relieve the bothersome symptoms, and they also keep the neuropathy from getting worse. Without adequate treatment, the chance of complications increases.
- **Why should I wear special shoes?**
  The purpose of proper foot care is to avoid the complications of diabetic peripheral neuropathy like ulcers that can lead to loss of toes or feet. You want to protect your feet as much as possible from injury.
- **Is there a cure for diabetic peripheral neuropathy?**
  At this time, there is no cure for diabetic peripheral neuropathy; however, treatment can help relieve painful symptoms associated with the condition.
- **When should I call my physician about diabetic peripheral neuropathy?**
  Call your physician if your symptoms greatly increase, you are in severe pain, you are not responding to the medications that you are taking for diabetic peripheral neuropathy, you are having bothersome side effects from the medications, or if you notice any open wounds or injury to your feet.
- **What should I do if I have a problem with my medications for diabetic peripheral neuropathy?**
  Never stop taking your medications without speaking to your provider first. Let your pharmacist and provider know about the problems you are having, and they can work together to make sure you are on the right medications.

TABLE 32-4 • Foot Exam for Diabetic Peripheral Neuropathy

Test	Components
Prior to performing the foot exam, have the patient remove both shoes and socks	
Dermatologic exam	Observe and record the following: • Skin status (color, thickness, drying, cracking) • Temperature • Fungal infection (toenails, between toes) • Calluses • Blisters • Ulcers
Vascular exam	• Both pedal pulses (posterior tibial and dorsalis pedis) should be taken and recorded • Capillary refill time should also be performed and recorded for each digit
Neurological exam	Pressure perception test (most common test) • Place a Semmes-Weinstein 10-gram monofilament with light touch at 10 places on the bottom of each foot (see Figure 32-1) to determine if patient can perceive its placement Pinprick test • Use a ball-point pen cap (or similar) to assess whether the patient experiences pain when the skin is touched • Ask, "Is it painful?" Light touch test • Gently brush a piece of cotton or a tissue across the bottom of the feet to assess if action causes pain Vibration test • Place a 128 Hz tuning fork on big toe to assess pain or vibratory sense
Musculokeletal exam	Observe and record the following • Deformities (Charcot joint, clawed toes, bunion) • Amputations • Joint mobility

Source: References 4, 7, and 8.

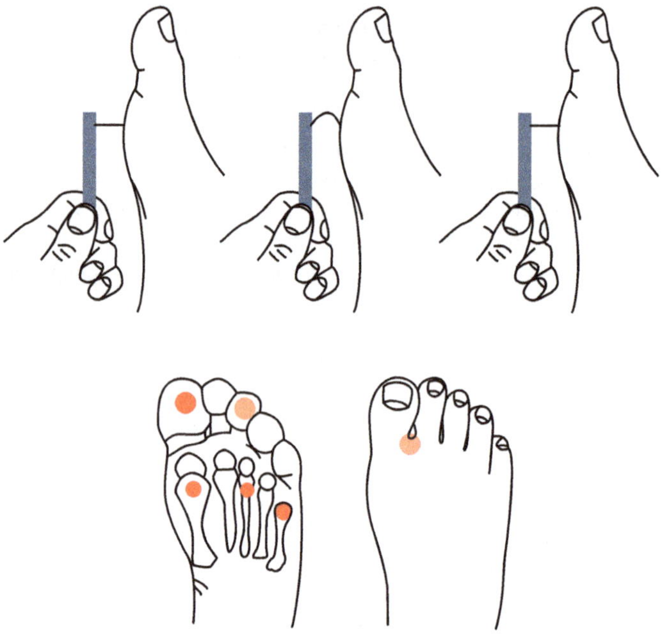

FIGURE 32-2 Monofilament test.

Source: Reproduced, with permission, from Boulton AJM, Armstrong DC, Albert SF, et al. Comprehensive foot examination and risk assessment: a report of the Task Force of the Foot Care Interest Group of the American Diabetes Association, with endorsement by the American Association of Clinical Endocrinologists. *Diabetes Care.* 2008;31(8):1679-1685.

CORE ELEMENT 4—INTERVENTION AND/OR REFERRAL

Interventions for diabetic peripheral neuropathy should include both pharmacological and nonpharmacological therapies. Control of the underlying disease state (ie, diabetes) is essential to help prevent worsening of symptoms. Patient education is a key component to treatment. Nondrug therapy should focus on proper foot hygiene and care (Table 32-5).[11] Percutaneous electrical nerve stimulation may also be helpful (Level B evidence).[12] During the consult, if the MTM provider notes an ulcer, bleeding callus or wound, cellulitis, or new deformity, it is important that the provider refer the patient to seek prompt medical attention.[4]

Drug therapy for DPN should be selected based on specific patient characteristics (age, duration of underlying cause, lifestyle factors, and social history), symptoms, and other comorbid conditions and medications.[4] It is important that patients understand that everyone is different and may respond differently to medications. As a result, multiple medications may be utilized to control symptoms throughout the course of therapy. Table 32-6 summarizes prescription and over-the-counter (OTC) medications commonly used for relief of symptoms in DPN.

The only agents with regulatory approval for neuropathic pain associated with diabetes in the United States, Europe, and Canada are pregabalin and duloxetine.[4] Tapentadol has regulatory approval in the United States.[4] The American Diabetes Association recommends either pregabalin or duloxetine as initial drug therapy for symptomatic treatment of neuropathic pain in diabetes.

PERSONAL MEDICATION LIST FOR *<Insert Patient's name, DOB: mm/dd/yyyy>*	
Medication: Lyrica (pregabalin) 100 mg	
How I use it: Take one capsule (100 mg) by mouth 3 times a day	
Why I use it: Diabetic peripheral neuropathy (pain)	**Prescriber:** Jones
Date I started using it: 12/20/2015	**Date I stopped using it:** *(Leave blank for patient's notes)*
Why I stopped using it: *(Leave blank for patient's notes)*	
Medication: Venlafaxine ER 75 mg	
How I use it: Take 1 tablet (75 mg) by mouth in the morning	
Why I use it: Diabetic peripheral neuropathy (pain)	**Prescriber:** Jones
Date I started using it: 5/13/2016	**Date I stopped using it:** *(Leave blank for patient's notes)*
Why I stopped using it: *(Leave blank for patient's notes)*	

FIGURE 32-3 Example personal medication list for a patient with diabetic peripheral neuropathy.

DATE PREPARED: <Insert date>	
What we talked about: Importance of checking feet on a daily basis to avoid complications like ulcers and infections that can lead to a loss of toes or feet.	
What I need to do: • Look at my feet daily • Buy a mirror and place under my foot so that I can see the bottom • Look for any areas of broken or cracked skin • Contact my provider if I notice any injuries • Moisturize my feet routinely to keep skin from drying out • Make sure I wear proper shoes at all times and avoid walking around barefoot	**What I did and when I did it:** *(Leave blank for patient's notes)*
What we talked about: The importance of giving my new medication (Lyrica) a chance to work. The Lyrica was just prescribed 1 week ago. It often takes some time before the medicine starts working.	
What I need to do: • Continue taking the Lyrica as prescribed • Keep a diary of my symptoms • Do not stop taking the medication without first speaking with my provider • Follow-up with my provider as scheduled in 3 weeks	**What I did and when I did it:** *(Leave blank for patient's notes)*

FIGURE 32-4 Example medication action plan for a patient with diabetic peripheral neuropathy.

Gabapentin may also be effective as an initial approach. Tricyclic antidepressants are not approved for neuropathic pain associated with diabetes in the United States and should be used with caution, given the higher risk of side effects. Opioids such as tapentadol or tramadol are not recommended as first- or second-line agents for treating painful neuropathy associated with diabetes, given the risk of addiction and other complications. According to the American Academy of Neurology, capsaicin and topical lidocaine may be considered for the treatment of painful diabetic neuropathy.[12] Table 32-7 provides some additional considerations when recommending therapy for DPN. In addition, some herbal products may also be beneficial for symptoms associated with DPN (Table 32-8).

CORE ELEMENT 5—DOCUMENTATION AND FOLLOW-UP

Clear and succinct documentation of MRPs and recommendations is a key component of the MTM consult. Examples of potential MRPs in patients with DPN are provided in Table 32-9. Sample communications and recommendations to providers to address medication-related issues are found in Table 32-10.

TABLE 32-5 • Proper Foot Care for Patients with Diabetic Peripheral Neuropathy

Proper Care

• Check feet daily
• Wash feet daily with lukewarm water and mild soap
  • Dry feet well, especially between toes
  • Use a soft towel and blot—do not rub
• Keep skin moist
• If you get a cut, scrape, or blister:
  • Wash gently with soap and water
  • Apply antibiotic cream several times daily
  • If not healed in a few days, call provider
• Cut toenails straight across (if allowed by provider)
• If you have sweaty feet:
  • Keep feet dry with a nonmedicated powder before putting on socks and shoes
• Loosen blankets and sheets at foot of bed to avoid pressure on toes, heels, or any bony processes
• Have your provider check your feet at every visit and at least annually by a podiatrist

Things to Avoid
• Do not use any instruments on your feet (except nail clippers) without notifying provider • Do not self-treat any calluses or corns unless approved by provider • Do not soak your feet • Do not use hot water, heating pad, or massager on your feet • Do not go barefoot • Do not walk in wet shoes • Avoid hot or cold surfaces with bare feet
Footwear
• Shop for shoes at the end of the day when your feet are a little swollen • Change socks and shoes everyday • Look inside your shoes every day for gravel or torn things • Do not wear shoes without socks • Do not wear sandals or open-toed shoes • Avoid high heels or shoes with a pointy toe-box • Wear well-padded white socks/stockings (if possible) • Avoid socks with inside seams

Source: Reference 11.

Recommendations may be communicated via fax, telephone, or other means of written or secure electronic communication. The following examples are for illustrative purposes. Actual communications to providers should be individualized based on the type of recommendation, patient specific characteristics, and the nature of the relationship with the provider.

While there is not a standard time frame for follow-up in patients with DPN, many of the medications used for symptomatic relief require titration and 2 to 8 weeks of treatment before symptom reduction is seen.[15,16] Therefore, frequent monitoring is important. Patients are encouraged to follow up within 4 weeks of treatment initiation or change in therapy to monitor for efficacy and appropriateness.

TABLE 32-6 • Medications Used in the Symptomatic Treatment of Diabetic Peripheral Neuropathy

Medication Class and Example Drugs	Common/Serious Side Effects[a]	Blackbox Warnings/Contraindications	Pregnancy Category[b]
Anticonvulsants gabapentin pregabalin	Dizziness Peripheral edema Sedation	Renal insufficiency	C
External analgesic capsaicin	Paresthesias Skin irritation	Sensitivity to capsicum plant (hot peppers) Broken skin or skin abrasion	B
Local anesthetic lidocaine patch	Local erythema Rash	Sensitivity to local amide anesthetics	B
Opioids methadone morphine oxycodone tapentadol[c] tramadol[d]	Constipation Drowsiness Dizziness Nausea and/or vomiting Seizures (tapentadol, tramadol)	History of substance abuse Suicide risk Driving impairment at initiation tramadol -Seizure disorder -Concurrent SSRI, SNRI, or TCA use	C (oxycodone B)
SNRI duloxetine venlafaxine	Dizziness Nausea and/or vomiting Somnolence	Concurrent tramadol use duloxetine -hepatic dysfunction -renal insufficiency -alcohol abuse venlafaxine -cardiac disease -withdrawal syndrome if stopped abruptly	C
Tricyclic Antidepressants amitriptyline desipramine nortriptyline	Blurred vision Dry mouth Sedation Urinary retention Weight gain	Cardiac disease Concurrent tramadol use Glaucoma Seizures Suicide risk	C (nortriptyline D)

[a] This is a general list and does not include all side effects that can occur from these drugs. Consult a drug reference source for a more inclusive list before making any recommendations. MTM providers should also consult a comprehensive drug interaction database before making pharmacotherapy recommendations.

[b] Product labeling for all prescription drugs is being updated to reflect the new FDA Pregnancy Labeling and Lactation Rule. Please check individual product labeling for the most accurate and updated pregnancy information.

[c] Tapentadol also acts as an inhibitor of norepinephrine reuptake.

[d] Tramadol also acts as a weak inhibitor of norepinephrine and serotonin reuptake.

Abbreviations: SNRI = serotonin-norepinephrine reuptake inhibitor; SSRI = selective serotonin reuptake inhibitor; TCA = tricyclic antidepressant.

Source: Data compiled from reference 4.

TABLE 32-7 • Considerations in Individualizing Medications Used in the Symptomatic Relief of Diabetic Peripheral Neuropathy

Category of Medication	Benefit
Anticonvulsants	Improvement in sleep No significant drug interactions
Opioids	Rapid onset of action
SNRI	Improvement of depression
Topical lidocaine	No systemic side effects
Tricyclic antidepressants	Improvement of depression Improvement of insomnia Inexpensive

Source: Reference 13.

TABLE 32-8 • Herbal Products Used in the Symptomatic Treatment of Diabetic Peripheral Neuropathy

Herbal	Recommended Dose	Level of Evidence[a]	Cost[b]
Acetyl-L-Carnitine	1500-3000 mg daily	Possibly effective	$$$
Alpha-Lipoic Acid (ALA)	600-1800 mg daily	Possibly effective	$
Cayenne (Capsicum)	Topical cream (0.075% capsaicin)	Likely effective	$
Coenzyme Q-10	400 mg daily	Possibly effective	$$
Evening primrose oil	360-480 mg gamma-linolenic acid	Insufficient evidence	$$$
Gamma-Linolenic Acid	Up to 480 mg daily	Possibly effective	$$
Vitamin B12	500-1000 mcg daily	Insufficient evidence	$
Vitamin E	400 IU daily	Insufficient evidence	$
Zinc	660 mg ($ZnSO_4$) daily	Insufficient evidence	$

[a] Level of evidence: "likely effective"—this product has a very high level of reliable clinical evidence supporting its use for a specific indication. Products rated "likely effective" are generally considered appropriate to recommend; "possibly effective"—this product has some clinical evidence supporting its use for a specific indication; however, the evidence is limited by quantity, quality, or contradictory findings. Products rated "possibly effective" might be beneficial, but do not have enough high-quality evidence to be recommended for most people; "insufficient evidence" indicates that there is insufficient reliable scientific evidence to provide an effectiveness rating.

[b] Cost: $ = $10/month supply in the recommended dosage; $$ = $11-$20/month; $$$ = $21-$50/month.

Source: Data compiled from reference 14.

TABLE 32-9 • Medication-Related Problems (MRPs) in Patients with Diabetic Peripheral Neuropathy

Category of MRP	Examples
Nonadherence	• Continued symptoms and/or progression of symptoms because of nonadherence to medication • Suboptimal symptom relief because of missed doses • Patient not taking medication as prescribed because of cost or complexity of regimen
Unnecessary medication	• Duplicate therapy (eg, two tricyclic antidepressants)
Need for additional therapy	• Patient on maximum doses of appropriate medication (eg, pregabalin) but still experiencing symptoms • Progression of symptoms with appropriate treatment such as pregabalin or duloxetine
Ineffective medication	• Patient not responding to prescribed medication even after adequate titration and trial period
Dosage too low	• Suboptimal symptom relief because of low dose of medication (eg, gabapentin 300 mg by mouth daily with no titration)
Dosage too high	• Patient experiencing side effects on dose of gabapentin that is not adjusted for renal function
Adverse drug event	• Bothersome peripheral edema from gabapentin • Oversedation from tricyclic or opioid use • Patient stopped taking nortriptyline because of excess weight gain

TABLE 32-10 • Communications to Providers for Diabetic Peripheral Neuropathy

Scenario: New onset of pain and tingling in both feet
MRP: Need for additional medication

- **Assessment:**
  Patient with a 5-year history of type 2 diabetes presents for annual medication review with complaints of pain and tingling in both feet. Ranks pain as a 5/10. Foot exam negative for any skin/structure irregularities, positive bilateral pedal pulses noted, and normal monofilament exam. Current A1C of 8.2% on metformin and glipizide.
- **Plan:**
  Consider initiation of Lyrica (pregabalin) 50 mg by mouth 3 times daily. May titrate to 100 mg by mouth 3 times daily after 1 week based on symptoms and tolerability.
  Educate on importance of maximizing glucose control to prevent progression of symptoms.

(Continued)

TABLE 32-10 • Communications to Providers for Diabetic Peripheral Neuropathy *(Continued)*

Scenario: Suboptimal relief of diabetic peripheral neuropathy symptoms **MRP:** Need for additional medication
• **Assessment:** Patient with a 10-year history of type 2 diabetes and a 1-year history of diabetic peripheral neuropathy currently on gabapentin 600 mg by mouth 3 times daily. Patient reports increasing symptoms of DPN, including burning and loss of sensation. Physical exam reveals score of 2/5 on monofilament test (down from 4/5 at last evaluation 3 months ago). Patient also complains of feeling down and depressed. May benefit from addition of antidepressant to assist with both DPN and depression symptoms. • **Plan:** Consider addition of duloxetine 30 mg by mouth once daily with titration to 60 mg by mouth once daily after 1 week.
Scenario: New onset ulcer formation **MRP:** Need for referral
• **Assessment:** Patient with 10-year history of diabetic peripheral neuropathy evaluated today for follow-up MTM consultation. Currently taking Lyrica 150 mg by mouth twice daily. Upon physical exam, new ulcer on right great toe noted. • **Plan:** Recommend prompt evaluation and treatment by provider.

REFERENCES

1. Finnerup NB, Haroutounian S, Kamerman P, et al. Neuropathic pain: an updated grading system for research and clinical practice. *Pain*. 2016;157(8):1599-1606.
2. Herndon DM, Strickland JM, Ray JB. Pain management. In: DiPiro JT, Talbert RL, Yee GC, Matzke GR, Wells BG, Posey L, eds. *Pharmacotherapy: A Pathophysiologic Approach*. 10th ed. New York: McGraw-Hill Medical Education; 2017. Available at http://accesspharmacy.mhmedical.com/content.aspx?bookid=1861&sectionid=146063604. Accessed May 3, 2017.
3. Burzynski JA, Strassels S. Persistent pain. In: Linn WD, Wofford MR, O'Keefe M, Posey L, eds. *Pharmacotherapy in Primary Care*. New York: McGraw-Hill; 2016. Available at http://accesspharmacy.mhmedical.com/content.aspx?bookid=439&sectionid=39968657. Accessed May 3, 2017.
4. Pop-Busui R, Boulton AJM, Feldman EL, et al. Diabetic neuropathy: a position statement by the American Diabetes Association. *Diabetes Care*. 2017;40(1):136-154.
5. Adler AI, Boyko EJ, Ahroni JH, et al. Risk factors for diabetic peripheral sensory neuropathy. *Diabetes Care*. 1997;20(7):1162-1167.
6. Gordois A, Scuffham P, Shearer A, et al. The health care costs of diabetic peripheral neuropathy in the US. *Diabetes Care*. 2003:26(6):1790-1795.
7. Perkins BA, Olaleye D, Zinman B, Bril V. Simple screening tests for peripheral neuropathy in the diabetes clinic. *Diabetes Care*. 2001;24(2):250-256.
8. Armstrong DG, Lavery LA. Diabetic foot ulcers: prevention, diagnosis and classification. *Am Fam Physician*. 1998;57(6):1325-1332.
9. Boulton AJM, Armstrong DC, Albert SF, et al. Comprehensive foot examination and risk assessment: a report of the Task Force of the Foot Care Interest Group of the American Diabetes Association, with endorsement by the American Association of Clinical Endocrinologists. *Diabetes Care*. 2008;31(8): 1679-1685.
10. CMS. *Medicare Part D Medication Therapy Management Program Standardized Format*. Available at https://www.cms.gov/Medicare/Prescription-Drug-Coverage/PrescriptionDrugCovContra/Downloads/MTM-Program-Standardized-Format-English-and-Spanish-Instructions-Samples-v032712.pdf. Accessed May 8, 2017.
11. Foot care for people with diabetes. *Am Fam Physician*. 1999;60:1002-1003.
12. Bril V, England J, Franklin GM, et al. Evidence-based guideline: treatment of painful diabetic neuropathy. *Neurology*. 2011;76(20):1758-1765.
13. O'Connor AB, Dworkin RH. Treatment of neuropathic pain: an overview of recent guidelines. *Am J Med*. 2009;122(suppl 10):S22-32.
14. Diabetic neuropathy and peripheral neuropathy. In: *Natural Medicines* [database online]. Somerville, MA: Therapeutic Research Center; 2017. Available at https://naturalmedicines.therapeuticresearch.com/. Accessed May 13, 2017.
15. St. Onge EL, Miller SA. Pain associated with diabetic peripheral neuropathy. *P&T*. 2008;33(3):166-176.
16. Huizinga MM and Peltier A. Painful diabetic neuropathy: a management-centered review. *Clinical Diabetes*. 2007;25(1):6-15.

Review Questions

1. Which type of peripheral neuropathy is considered the most common?
   a. Phantom limb pain
   b. Diabetic peripheral neuropathy
   c. Post-herpetic neuralgia
   d. Trigeminal neuralgia

2. What is a risk factor for development of diabetic peripheral neuropathy?
   a. Low body mass index
   b. Depression
   c. Poor glucose control
   d. Small stature

3. What is a complication of diabetic peripheral neuropathy?
   a. Retinopathy
   b. Nephropathy
   c. Tinea pedis
   d. Foot ulceration

4. Using living room language, which term is best described by the phrase "constant burning pain"?
   a. Allodynia
   b. Causalgia
   c. Dysesthesias
   d. Paresthesia

5. Which objective test uses a 10-g monofilament to determine if the patient can perceive its placement?
   a. Pinprick test
   b. Light touch test
   c. Vibration test
   d. Pressure perception test

6. In which situations should a patient with diabetic peripheral neuropathy seek prompt medical attention?
   a. Upon physical exam, feet are observed as dry.
   b. Upon physical exam, an ulcer is noted on side of large toe on left foot.
   c. Patient describes symptoms of burning in feet as worse than last visit.
   d. Patient states that prescribed medications are no longer working for neuropathic pain.

7. A 68-year-old male has a past medical history of hypertension (20 years), gastroesophageal reflux disease (5 years), type 2 diabetes (15 years), and diabetic peripheral neuropathy (2 years). Current medications include metformin 1000 mg twice daily, insulin glargine 20 units subcutaneously at bedtime, duloxetine 120 mg daily, lisinopril 40 mg daily, and omeprazole 20 mg every morning. Patient was last seen in the office 3 months ago with no complaints and an A1C of 7.4%. No changes were made to his regimen, and he presents today describing increased numbness in his feet. Monofilament test reveals a score of 1/5 (down from 3/5 at last visit), and his current A1C is 7.6%. Which medication-related problem most accurately describes the situation concerning his medication for DPN?
   a. Dose too high
   b. Dose too low
   c. Adverse drug event
   d. Need for additional therapy

8. A 47-year-old female who was recently diagnosed with diabetic peripheral neuropathy (burning and tingling in both feet) has a past medical history significant for type 2 diabetes, HTN, hyperlipidemia, seizures, insomnia, and alcohol abuse. She currently takes 12 different medications and is concerned with adding additional medications due to potential drug interactions. Which medication would be the most appropriate initial option for relief of her symptoms?
   a. Gabapentin
   b. Tramadol
   c. Duloxetine
   d. Oxycodone

9. A 53-year-old male presents with a history of type 1 diabetes, dyslipidemia, osteoarthritis, and renal insufficiency. He reports a new "pins and needles" type of pain in his feet. He currently takes insulin glulisine via insulin pump, losartan, tramadol, and pravastatin. Regarding the treatment of his symptoms of diabetic peripheral neuropathy, which agent should be avoided?
   a. Gabapentin
   b. Pregabalin
   c. Lidocaine patch
   d. Duloxetine

10. Which herbal product has the strongest amount of evidence for use in the treatment of diabetic peripheral neuropathy?
    a. Vitamin E
    b. Evening primrose oil
    c. Alpha-lipoic acid
    d. Zinc

ANSWERS

1. b	2. c	3. d
4. b	5. d	6. b
7. d	8. a	9. d
10. c		

33

Rheumatoid Arthritis MTM Data Set

Robin Moorman Li, PharmD, BCACP, CPE, and Kathryn J. Smith, PharmD

KEY POINTS

- Rheumatoid arthritis (RA) is a chronic, systemic, inflammatory disease that requires early detection and proper treatment to prevent permanent joint damage.
- Pharmacologic therapy must be utilized in patients with RA however, including nonpharmacological options in the treatment plan can lead to improved quality of life.
- Although traditional nonbiologic disease-modifying antirheumatic drugs remain in use, biologic agents are gaining popularity, and new agents are in development.
- Serious adverse effects can occur with both the nonbiologic and the biologic disease-modifying antirheumatic drugs. Medication therapy management (MTM) providers can play a key role in proper education and routine monitoring of patients taking these medications.

INTRODUCTION TO RHEUMATOID ARTHRITIS

Rheumatoid arthritis (RA) is a chronic, systemic, inflammatory disease. The disease process is characterized by inflammation of the joints and surrounding tissues, leading to joint destruction over time. The cause of inflammation that leads to RA is unknown. However, RA may have a genetic component.[1] Additionally, major histocompatibility complex molecules may have a role in determining patients who will develop RA. Patients with human lymphocyte antigen (HLA) DR4 are 3.5 times more likely to develop RA.[2] RA usually involves symmetrical joints, but patients may also experience vasculitis, eye inflammation, rheumatoid nodules, cardiopulmonary disease, and lymphadenopathy. RA affects approximately 1.3 million people over the age of 18 in the United States and is 3 times more common in women than men.[3] The onset of the disease is most commonly seen in the fifth or sixth decade of life.[1]

Pathophysiology

RA is an autoimmune disease caused by chronic inflammation of the joint lining. This leads to proliferation of tissue that invades the cartilage and bone. The ongoing inflammatory process causes joint damage and ultimately leads to joint destruction if left untreated. The immune system of patients with RA is no longer able to distinguish self from foreign cells, resulting in the immune system attacking the patient's own body. Additionally, vasoactive substances are released as part of the immune response and cause swelling, warmth, redness, and pain at the site of inflammation.[2] Patients may also develop antibodies, which are called rheumatoid factors. Patients who have circulating rheumatoid factors may have a more aggressive form of the disease than those who do not.[2]

Clinical Presentation

The joints involved in RA are commonly small joints within the wrists, hands, and feet, with patients typically presenting with symmetric joint involvement. Larger joints may also be affected, including shoulders, knees, elbows, and hips. The cervical area of the spine may also be affected, but the lumbar area of the spine is usually not.[4] Figure 33-1 depicts some of the differences in clinical presentation between RA and osteoarthritis (OA). Highlighting these distinctions can be very helpful when educating a patient in an MTM session.

Diagnosis of Rheumatoid Arthritis

Unfortunately, no one specific test confirms the diagnosis of RA. The diagnosis of RA includes an evaluation of a number of signs and symptoms (Figure 33-2), laboratory tests, and possible

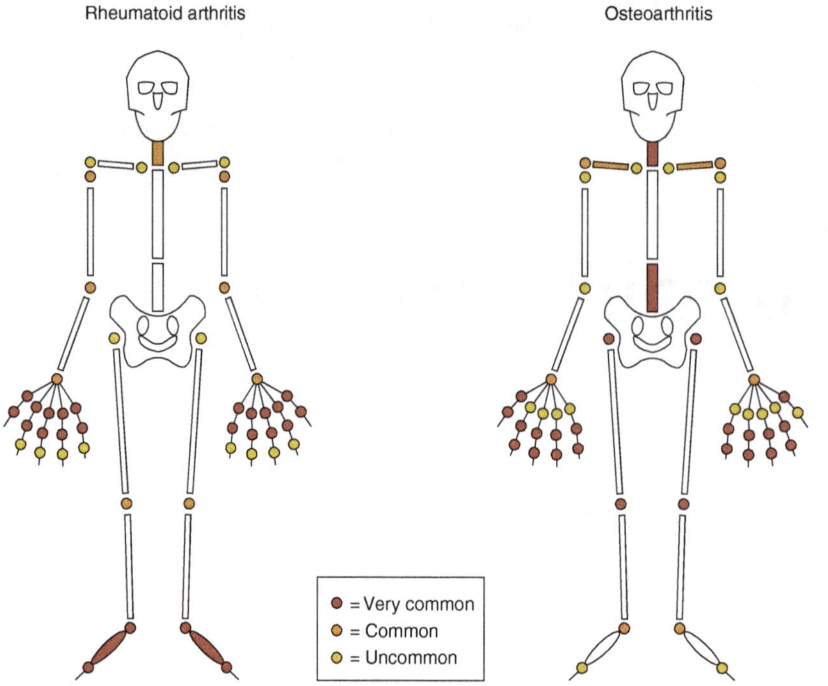

FIGURE 33-1 Patterns of joint involvement in rheumatoid arthritis and osteoarthritis.[2]

radiographic evidence of joint destruction commonly seen later in the disease process.[2]

Laboratory tests used in diagnosis may include testing for rheumatoid factor (RF), which is detectable in about 60% to 70% of patients. Other tests that may aid in diagnosis include the erythrocyte sedimentation rate (ESR) and C-reactive protein (CRP).[2] It is important to remember that these tests are not specific for RA and are only used alongside physical signs and symptoms to support the diagnosis of RA. Table 33-1 lists many diseases associated with a positive RF.

Given that a positive RF laboratory test can be associated with a variety of disease states, anti-cyclic citrullinated peptide antibodies (ACPAs), a more specific serological marker, are commonly used to help confirm the diagnosis of RA. The laboratory test ordered to detect these ACPAs is anti-cyclic citrullinated peptide (anti-CCP).[5] ACPAs have also been helpful in predicting the severity of disease because presence of these antibodies is commonly associated with increased joint destruction. The utility of anti-CCP in assessing response to various pharmacological therapies is still under investigation.[6]

The American College of Rheumatology/EULAR RA classification tool is useful for assessing severity of disease and can be used to aid treatment decisions.[7] The criteria, last updated in 2010, have been specifically developed to aid clinicians in the

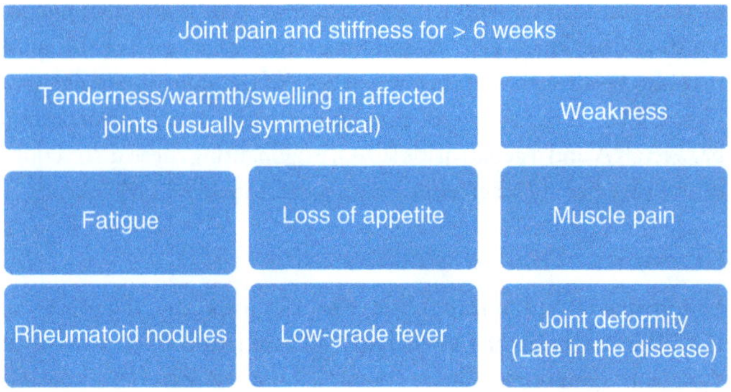

FIGURE 33-2 Signs and symptoms associated with rheumatoid arthritis.[2]

TABLE 33-1 • Diseases Associated with a Positive Rheumatoid Factor

Rheumatic diseases
Rheumatoid arthritis
Sjögren syndrome (with or without arthritis)
Systemic lupus erythematosus
Progressive systemic sclerosis
Polymyositis/dermatomyositis
Infectious diseases
Bacterial endocarditis
Tuberculosis
Syphilis
Infectious mononucleosis
Infectious hepatitis
Leprosy
Other causes
Aging
Interstitial pulmonary fibrosis
Cirrhosis of the liver
Chronic active hepatitis
Sarcoidosis

Source: Reproduced, with permission, from DiPiro JT, Talbert RL, Yee GC, Matzke GR, Wells BG, Posey L, eds. *Pharmacotherapy: A Pathophysiological Approach*. 10th ed. New York, NY: McGraw-Hill; 2017.

identification of patients in the early stages of the disease process. Earlier identification of RA allows for a timelier diagnosis, increases the likelihood of slowing progression of the disease process, and helps ensure preserved functionality through early initiation of treatment. Before using these criteria, patients must be evaluated by an expert assessor. The assessor must be thorough, identifying clinical synovitis in at least one joint, not including the joints typically affected by osteoarthritis. Examples of joints commonly affected in osteoarthritis include the distal interphalangeal joints, the first metatarsophalangeal joint, and the first carpometacarpal joint. In addition, the synovitis cannot be attributed to another disease process, such as gout or psoriatic arthritis.[7]

Complications of Rheumatoid Arthritis

The most common complication associated with RA is joint destruction leading to deformation and disability; however, there are many other possible complications associated with the disease (Table 33-2).

Therapeutic Goals for Rheumatoid Arthritis

In 2015 the American College of Rheumatology (ACR) released an updated guideline for the treatment of RA. The guideline strongly recommends use of a "treat-to-target" strategy, focused on the goal of achieving at least 50% clinical improvement within 3 months, or remission or low disease activity at 6 months.[8] It is important to recognize that no therapy will reverse joint damage which has already occurred.[2] Functional goals of therapy may include preservation of joint function, decreased joint stiffness and pain, and improvement in overall quality of life. Multiple assessment tools are available to assess disease activity.[9] Table 33-3 lists these assessment tools.[2]

TABLE 33-3 • Assessment Tools Used to Measure Rheumatoid Arthritis Disease Activity and Definitions for Low Disease Activity and Remission

Assessment Tool	Low Disease Activity	Remission
Clinical Disease Activity Index (CDAI) (range 0-76)	>2.8-10	<2.8
Disease Activity Score (DAS28) (range 0-9.4)	>2.6-3.2	<2.6
Patient Activity Scale (PAS) or PASII (range 0-10)	>2.5-3.7	0-2.5
Routine Assessment of Patient Index Data 3 (RAPID-3) (range 0-10)	>1.0-2.0	0-1.0
Simplified Disease Activity Index (SDAI) (range 0-86)	>3.3-<11.0	<3.3

Source: Reproduced, with permission, from DiPiro JT, Talbert RL, Yee GC, Matzke GR, Wells BG, Posey L, eds. *Pharmacotherapy: A Pathophysiological Approach*. 10th ed. New York, NY: McGraw-Hill; 2017.

Therapeutic Failure

Therapeutic failure for RA is difficult to assess because the terminology used in clinical studies is variable, making it difficult to extrapolate to clinical practice.[10] In the MTM setting, proper assessment of pain level, currently affected joints, quality of life, physical function, and overall response to the medication aids in the assessment of efficacy of current treatment. If the patient is not reporting adequate disease control, a referral for evaluation by a rheumatologist should be considered.

TABLE 33-2 • Possible Complications Associated with Rheumatoid Arthritis

Complication	Comments
Deformity of the hands, feet, and ankles	Chronic inflammation can lead to deformity which can decrease grip strength in the hands. Deformities in the feet can lead to changes such as development of hammer toes.
Deformity of the cervical vertebrae: C1-C2	A rare complication, but can lead to instability of the joint which increases the risk of cord compression.
Bilateral shoulder, hip, and knee pain	Chronic inflammation in these areas leads to increased pain.
Osteoporosis	RA can increase the risk of osteoporosis, and use of corticosteroids for RA can contribute to the development of osteoporosis.
Rheumatoid nodules	Normally asymptomatic, these nodules occur mainly in the extensor surfaces of the elbows, forearms, and hands. Some patients have experienced rheumatoid nodules on the feet, lungs, and, rarely, the meninges.
Vasculitis	Normally seen in long standing RA; could lead to ulcers in lower extremities.
Ocular manifestations	Dry itchy eyes; associated with Sjögren syndrome.
Lung disease	Increased risk of pulmonary fibrosis; risk increases with smoking.
Cardiac disease	Cardiovascular mortality is increased in RA; however, proper treatment with methotrexate has been shown to decrease this risk.
Felty syndrome	Associated with splenomegaly and neutropenia. A patient who has Felty syndrome and leukopenia has a higher chance of developing an infection.

Source: Reference 2.

CORE ELEMENT 1—COMPREHENSIVE MEDICATION REVIEW FOR PATIENTS WITH RHEUMATOID ARTHRITIS

Table 33-4 includes a list of suggested questions to use when conducting a medication therapy review in a patient with RA. The number and types of questions will depend upon several factors, including the amount of time for the interview, number of concurrent medication-related problems (MRPs), urgency of MRPs, and the reliability of the patient in providing accurate information. MTM providers should remember to use living room language during the interview (Figure 33-3) and be prepared for questions regarding RA (Table 33-5).

CORE ELEMENT 2—PERSONAL MEDICATION LIST

The following is a sample personal medication list (PML) for a patient with RA (Figure 33-4).[11] This example is representative only of RA medications. Additional medications for other disease states should be added and listed separately. MTM providers should remember to use plain language when creating the PML.

TABLE 33-4 • Suggested Questions for the Patient with Rheumatoid Arthritis

• How long have you had RA? When were you diagnosed? • Who else in your family has rheumatoid arthritis? • What do you know about the risks of uncontrolled RA? • How often do you see your rheumatologist? • How does your rheumatologist monitor your RA? • What medications do you take for your RA? How do you take them? • How long has it been since a medication was added or a dose was adjusted? • How do you monitor whether your RA medications are working? • How often do you miss a dose of your RA medication? • What other medications have you taken in the past for RA? • Have you ever stopped taking any of your prescribed RA medications without telling your physician? If so, why? • What over-the-counter medications or herbals do you use? • Other than medicines, what have you tried for your RA (eg, physical therapy)? • What changes in lifestyle has your physician recommended? • What exercise regimen do you follow?
Questions to Ask for Prevention/Assessment of Medical Emergency
• Crisis Planning: What steps are you to take if you suspect you are developing an infection? What is your action plan? • Have you ever been treated for serious infections since you have been taking medications to control your RA? • What are the signs of infection? • What do you do when you are experiencing a flare-up of your RA? • How often do you have a flare-up?

Adverse events—any abnormal, harmful, undesired or unexpected effects from a medication.

Anti-TNF biologic—a medication made from a living organism that works to decrease a protein in the body which is responsible for inflammation. TNF stands for tumor necrosis factor.

Arthritis—inflammation or swelling of the joints.

Autoimmune disease—a disorder in which your immune system attacks your own body.

Biologic agents—medications that are made from a living organism and target areas in the immune system or processes that cause inflammation.

Biosimilar agents—medications that are very similar in effects, safety, and quality in comparison to biologic agents that have been on the market and used for a period of time.

Comorbidities—other health conditions that you have.

Disease-modifying antirheumatic drugs (DMARDs)—medications used to slow the worsening of rheumatoid arthritis by interfering with the immune system. These agents help prevent the joint destruction seen with RA.

Flare-up—a time during which the symptoms of rheumatoid arthritis might be higher than normal. Over time the symptoms again subside with a period of better disease control.

Hepatitis—a disorder characterized by inflammation of the liver.

Inflammation—swelling that is generally painful, red, and warm.

Intravenously—inside the vein.

Malignancy—a cancerous growth.

Monotherapy—treating a condition with only one medication.

Nodules—pea-sized lumps found under the skin.

Non-TNF biologic—a medication made from a living organism that works to decrease inflammation from a different process in comparison to the anti-TNF biologic (see *anti-TNF biologic*).

Occupational therapy—therapy to maintain the ability to participate in activities of daily living (ie, cooking or cleaning).

Physical therapy—treatment of disability based on exercise activities, massage therapy, and use of heat (hot pads) or water (soaks).

Prognosis—the likely course of a disease or ailment; the outlook.

Remission—having no signs of active disease.

Rheumatoid arthritis—a long-term disease that leads to inflammation of the joints and surrounding tissues.

Rheumatoid vasculitis—inflammation of the blood vessels.

Rheumatologist —a physician that specializes in the diagnosis and treatment of rheumatic diseases (ie, arthritis, muscle, bone or joint diseases).

Subcutaneous—under the skin.

Swelling—build-up of fluid.

Symmetrical—referring to the same area on both sides of the body (eg, symmetrical joint pain involves the same joints on both sides of the body).

Synovectomy—removal of the joint lining.

Tuberculosis (TB)—a bacterial infection characterized by the growth of lumps in the lungs or other tissues.

FIGURE 33-3 Living room language for rheumatoid arthritis.

CORE ELEMENT 3—MEDICATION ACTION PLAN

The following is a sample MAP for a patient with RA (Figure 33-5).[11] This example is representative only of action steps for RA, and MAPs for other disease states or MRPs

TABLE 33-5 • Questions to Anticipate Regarding Rheumatoid Arthritis

- **What is rheumatoid arthritis?**
  Rheumatoid arthritis, also called RA, is a long-term condition that causes pain and swelling in your joints.
- **What causes RA?**
  The exact cause of RA is unknown, but there may be a genetic component to it.
- **What health problems are associated with RA?**
  There are many health conditions that can occur without proper management of RA. These include joint pain/stiffness, eye problems, problems with your blood vessels, and heart problems.
- **How do I know if I have RA?**
  Your primary care physician can evaluate you and send you to a rheumatologist if he/she thinks you have RA.
- **Why are rheumatoid arthritis medications so important?**
  These medications are important because they will help slow down the progression of the disease. Without these, your joints might not be able to function properly.
- **Can I just stop my medications if I feel okay?**
  No. Never stop taking your medications without speaking with your physician or pharmacist. Although you may feel okay, the medications are still necessary to make sure that you stay feeling okay.
- **What can happen if I stop taking my RA medications?**
  If you stop taking your medications, you may have an RA flare. During flare-ups, you might experience stiff/achy joints, fatigue, and severe headaches.
- **When should I call my physician about my RA?**
  Call your physician if you are not responding to the prescribed treatment (ie, you are still having symptoms), or if you are having side effects from your medications.
- **What should I do if I have a problem with my RA medications?**
  Never stop taking your medications without first talking to your physician. Speak with your physician and/or pharmacist to let them know about any problems you are having, and together you can make sure your RA medications are the right ones for you.

PERSONAL MEDICATION LIST FOR <*Insert Patient's name*, DOB: *mm/dd/yyyy*>	
Medication: Methotrexate 2.5 mg tablet	
How I use it: 6 tablets (15 mg) every week on Saturday	
Why I use it: Rheumatoid arthritis	**Prescriber:** Smith
Date I started using it: 7/1/2014	**Date I stopped using it:** *(Leave blank for patient's notes)*
Why I stopped using it: *(Leave blank for patient's notes)*	
Medication: Celebrex (celecoxib) 200 mg capsule	
How I use it: One capsule (200 mg) twice a day with food	
Why I use it: Pain from rheumatoid arthritis	**Prescriber:** Smith
Date I started using it: 9/25/2014	**Date I stopped using it:** *(Leave blank for patient's notes)*
Why I stopped using it: *(Leave blank for patient's notes)*	
Medication: Folic Acid 1 mg	
How I use it: One tablet (1 mg) by mouth every morning	
Why I use it: Supplement for methotrexate	**Prescriber:** Smith
Date I started using it: 7/1/2014	**Date I stopped using it:** *(Leave blank for patient's notes)*
Why I stopped using it: *(Leave blank for patient's notes)*	

FIGURE 33-4 Example personal medication list for rheumatoid arthritis medications.

should be added and listed separately. In general, only a few of the most important action steps should be listed to ensure that the patient does not become overwhelmed with the stress of implementing multiple recommendations. Other areas for patient self-management can be addressed at later visits. MTM providers should remember to use plain language when creating the MAP.

CORE ELEMENT 4—INTERVENTION AND/OR REFERRAL

Interventions for management of RA may include both lifestyle modifications and nonpharmacological treatment, such as rest and occupational therapy (Table 33-6), as well as pharmacological therapy with disease-modifying antirheumatic drugs (DMARDs) (Table 33-7). In addition, nonsteroidal anti-inflammatory drugs (NSAIDs) (Table 33-8) or corticosteroids may be used for symptom control. The 2015 ACR guidelines provide guidance for DMARD selection based on early or established RA and current level of disease activity.[8] See Figure 33-6 for an algorithm for

DATE PREPARED: <*Insert date*>	
What we talked about: You reported having some soreness and redness in your mouth. This is known as "mucositis." It means that the lining of your mouth has become inflamed due to a lack of folate. This is common in people who take methotrexate and are not receiving enough folic acid supplementation.	
What I need to do: Here are some things I can do to help lessen this effect: • Practice good dental care (do not be too aggressive when brushing; use mouth rinses and brush teeth twice daily). • Avoid hot or spicy foods and beverages. • Take folic acid every day. Try to associate taking folic acid with a daily activity (ie, eating breakfast or brushing teeth).	**What I did and when I did it:** *(Leave blank for patient's notes)*

FIGURE 33-5 Example medication action plan for a patient with rheumatoid arthritis.

TABLE 33-6 • Nonpharmacologic Options for Management of Rheumatoid Arthritis

Modification	Reasoning
Rest	Rest will alleviate stress on inflamed joints and alleviate pain. It is also essential in the prevention of progressive joint destruction.
Occupational therapy	Occupational therapy will aid the patient in maintaining skills required to participate in activities of daily living.
Physical therapy	Physical therapy can aid in maintaining patient exercise capabilities and range of motion of affected joints.
Use of assistive devices	Use of canes, walkers, and splints can help patients maintain mobility and reduce stress on affected joints.
Weight reduction	Weight reduction can reduce stress on inflamed and painful joints. Weight loss should be monitored by a health care provider.
Surgery	Surgical management such as tendon repair, joint replacements, and tenosynovectomy should be reserved for patients with severe disease.

Source: Reference 2.

TABLE 33-7 • Usual Doses for Antirheumatic Drugs

Drug	Brand Name	Starting Dose	Usual Range or Maintenance Dose	Comments
Nonsteroidal anti-inflammatory drugs			See Table 33-8	
Methotrexate	Trexall Rasuvo (SC) Otrexup (SC)	Oral: 7.5 mg once weekly or 2.5 mg q 12 h for 3 days/wk or 10-15 mg once weekly SC or IM	Oral SC or IM: 7.5-15 mg q wk	May be given with folic acid 1-5 mg/day to reduce adverse reactions
Leflunomide	Arava	Oral: loading dose: 100 mg daily for 3 days, then 20 mg/day or 10-20 mg daily without loading dose	Oral: 10-20 mg daily	Not recommended in liver disease (ALT >2 times ULN)
Hydroxychloroquine	Plaquenil	Oral: 200-300 mg BID	Oral: After 1-2 mo may decrease to 200 mg daily or 200 mg BID	Take with food or milk; use with caution in renal or hepatic impairment
Sulfasalazine	Azulfidine	Oral: 0.5-1 g/day	Oral: Increase weekly to 1 g BID (max. dose is 3 g/day if inadequate response after 12 weeks of 2 g/day)	Not recommended in renal or hepatic impairment
Etanercept	Enbrel		50 mg SubQ once weekly or 25 mg twice weekly	
Infliximab	Remicade	3 mg/kg IV at 0, 2, 6 weeks then 3 q 8 weeks	3-10 mg/kg IV q 4-8 weeks	Given in combination with methotrexate therapy
Adalimumab	Humira		40 mg SubQ q 2 weeks (may increase to 40 mg once weekly if not taking methotrexate)	
Certolizumab	Cimzia	400 mg SubQ at 0, 2, 4 weeks	200 mg SubQ every other week	
Golimumab	Simponi		50 mg SubQ once monthly	
Rituximab	Rituxan	1000 mg IV twice, 2 weeks apart	Initial dose may be repeated every 16-24 weeks based on response	

(Continued)

TABLE 33-7 • Usual Doses for Antirheumatic Drugs (*Continued*)

Drug	Brand Name	Starting Dose	Usual Range or Maintenance Dose	Comments
Abatacept	Orencia	IV: <60 kg: 500 mg 60-100 kg: 750 mg >100 kg: 1000 mg at 0, 2, and 4 weeks or initial IV dose followed by 125 mg SubQ within 24 hours	IV: dose based on weight q 4 weeks SubQ: 125 mg once weekly	
Tocilizumab	Actemra	4 mg/kg IV q 4 weeks	4-8 mg/kg q 4 weeks (max 800 mg/infusion)	
Tofacitinib	Xeljanz		5 mg BID	5 mg once daily in moderate-to-severe renal insufficiency, moderate hepatic impairment, or concomitant CYP3A4 or CYP2C19 inhibitors
Minocycline	Dynacin Minocin		Oral: 100-200 mg daily	Use with caution in renal impairment
Anakinra	Kineret		100 mg SC once daily	
Auranofin	Ridaura		Oral: 3 mg daily to BID	
Gold thiomalate	Myochrysine	IM: 10 mg test dose first week, then 25 mg second week; then 25-50 mg/wk until toxicity or cumulative 1 g dose given	IM: 25-50 mg every other week for 2-20 weeks then every 3-4 weeks	CL_{cr} 50-80 mL/min (0.83-1.33 mL/s): give 50% recommended dose; CL_{cr} <50 mL/min (<0.83 mL/s) avoid use
Azathioprine	Imuran Azasan	Oral: 1 mg/kg/day (50-100 mg) for 6-8 weeks. May increase by 0.5 mg/kg q 4 weeks to 2.5 mg/kg/day	Oral: 50-150 mg daily	
D–Penicillamine	Cuprimine Depen	Oral: 125-250 mg daily	Oral: may ↑ by 125-250 mg q 1-2 months, max. 750 mg daily	Caution with renal impairment
Cyclophosphamide			Oral: 1-2 mg/kg/day	
Cyclosporine	Gengraf Neoral Sandimmune	Oral: 2.5 mg/kg/day divided twice daily	Oral: may ↑ by 0.5-0.75 mg/kg/day at 8 and 12 weeks to max dose 4 mg/kg/day	
Corticosteroids			Oral, IV, IM, IA, and soft-tissue injections: variable	

Abbreviations: ALT = alanine aminotransferase; BID = twice daily; CL_{cr} = creatinine clearance; CYP = cytochrome P450; IA = intra-articular; IM = intramuscular; IV = intravenous; q = every; SC = subcutaneous; ULN = upper limits of normal.

Source: Reproduced, with permission, from DiPiro JT, Talbert RL, Yee GC, Matzke GR, Wells BG, Posey L, eds. *Pharmacotherapy: A Pathophysiological Approach*. 10th ed. New York, NY: McGraw-Hill; 2017.

treatment of RA. Many medications used in the management of RA have serious adverse effects and require close clinical monitoring. Table 33-9 provides guidance on common monitoring parameters to use during an MTM session for a patient taking medications for RA.[2] Herbal remedies or dietary supplements have also been used by some patients to help control some of symptoms associated with RA (Table 33-10). Lastly, the criteria for referral for management of RA are outlined in Figure 33-7.

CORE ELEMENT 5—DOCUMENTATION AND FOLLOW-UP

Clear and succinct documentation of MRPs and recommendations is a key component of the MTM consult. Examples of potential MRPs in patients with RA are provided in Table 33-11. Sample communications and recommendations to providers aimed at addressing various medication-related issues are found

TABLE 33-8 • Dosage Regimens for NSAIDs

	Recommended Anti-inflammatory Total Daily Dosage		
Drug	***Adult***	***Children***	**Dosing Schedule**
Aspirin	2.6-5.2 g	60-100 mg/kg	Four times daily
Celecoxib	200-400 mg	—	Daily to twice daily
Diclofenac	150-200 mg		Three times per day to four times daily Extended release twice daily
Diflunisal	0.5-1.5 g	—	Twice daily
Etodolac	0.2-1.2 g (max. 20 mg/kg)	—	Twice daily to four times daily
Fenoprofen	0.9-3.0 g	—	Four times daily
Flurbiprofen	200-300 mg	—	Twice daily to four times daily
Ibuprofen	1.2-3.2 g	20-40 mg/kg	Three times per day to four times daily
Indomethacin	50-200 mg	2-4 mg/kg (max. 200 mg)	Twice daily to four times daily Extended release daily
Meclofenamate	200-400 mg	—	Three times per day to four times per day
Meloxicam	7.5-15 mg	—	Daily
Nabumetone	1-2 g	—	Daily to twice daily
Naproxen	0.5-1.0 g	10 mg/kg	Twice daily Extended release daily
Naproxen sodium	0.55-1.1 g	—	Twice daily
Nonacetylated salicylates	1.2-4.8 g	—	Twice daily to six times per day
Oxaprozin	0.6-1.8 g (max. 26 mg/kg)	—	Daily to three times a day
Piroxicam	10-20 mg	—	Daily
Sulindac	300-400 mg	—	Twice daily
Tolmetin	0.6-1.8 g	15-30 mg/kg	Twice daily to four times daily

Abbreviation: NSAIDs = nonsteroidal anti-inflammatory drugs.

Source: Reproduced, with permission, from DiPiro JT, Talbert RL, Yee GC, Matzke GR, Wells BG, Posey L, eds. *Pharmacotherapy: A Pathophysiological Approach*. 10th ed. New York, NY: McGraw-Hill; 2017.

in Figure 33-8. Recommendations may be conveyed via fax, telephone, written communication, or other means of secure electronic communication. The examples below are for illustrative purposes only. Actual communications to providers should be individualized based on the type of recommendation, patient specific characteristics, and the nature of the relationship with the provider.

Follow-up

Patients who suffer from RA should have frequent follow-up visits to assess disease control and progression, pain control, side effects, activity levels, and emotional health. Adherence to a proper medication regimen is imperative to control daily symptoms and delay or prevent irreversible joint damage. MTM providers should suggest that between visits, rheumatoid arthritis patients maintain a record of any associated symptoms and/or adverse effects of treatment. This enhances the quality of follow-up care and improves the ability to recommend suitable interventions for RA.

QUALITY MEASURES

Many payers of MTM services are accountable for providing high quality care to their beneficiaries, the patients. These payers, usually healthcare plans, are "graded" on a 5-star rating system (where 1 reflects low quality and 5 reflects the highest quality standard) by the Centers for Medicare & Medicaid Services. Plans are assessed across multiple categories, ranging from specific disease state measures to customer service measures. Providers of MTM services have an opportunity to assure the safe and effective use of medications and to improve the management of many health conditions. Therefore, payers view MTM as a valuable service for addressing medication usage and disease management, with a potential to improve star ratings. For example, for RA, a quality measure for Medicare Advantage plans evaluates the percentage of patients with RA who have received at least one prescription for a DMARD during the previous year.[14] For plans to achieve a 5-star rating, at least 82% of patients with RA must have received a DMARD within the last year (≥76% to <82% for a 4-star rating).

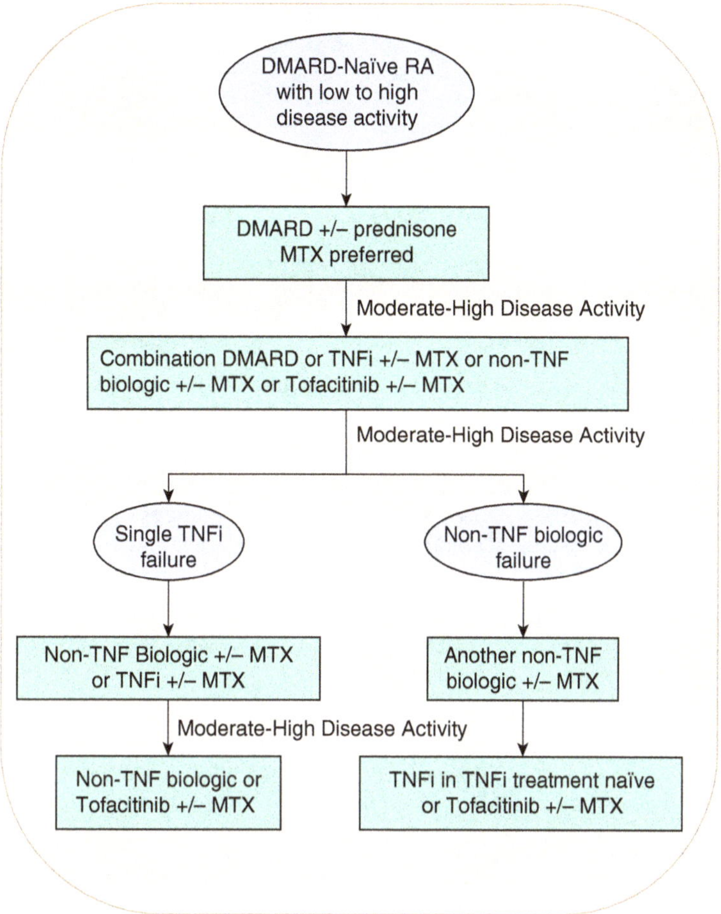

FIGURE 33-6 Algorithm for treatment of rheumatoid arthritis in early (<6 months) or established (≥6 months) RA with low to high disease activity.

Abbreviations: DMARD = disease-modifying antirheumatic drug; MTX = methotrexate.

Source: Reproduced, with permission, from DiPiro JT, Talbert RL, Yee GC, Matzke GR, Wells BG, Posey L, eds. *Pharmacotherapy: A Pathophysiologic Approach*. 10th ed. New York: McGraw-Hill Medical Education; 2017.

TABLE 33-9 • Clinical Monitoring of Drug Therapy in Rheumatoid Arthritis

Drug	Adverse Drug Reaction	Initial Monitoring	Maintenance Monitoring	Symptoms to Inquire About[a]
NSAIDs and salicylates	GI ulceration and bleeding, renal damage	SCr or BUN, CBC q 2-4 wk p starting therapy × 1-2 mo salicylates: serum salicylate levels if therapeutic dose and no response	Same as initial plus stool guaiac q 6-12 mo	Blood in stool, black stool, dyspepsia, nausea/vomiting, weakness, dizziness, abdominal pain, edema, weight gain, SOB
Corticosteroids	Hypertension, hyperglycemia, osteoporosis[b]	Glucose, blood pressure q 3-6 mo	Same as initial	Blood pressure if available, polyuria, polydipsia, edema, SOB, visual changes, weight gain, headaches, broken bones or bone pain
Gold (intramuscular or oral)	Myelosuppression, proteinuria, rash, stomatitis	Baseline and until stable: UA, CBC w/plt preinjection	Same as initial—every other dose	Symptoms of myelosuppression, edema, rash, oral ulcers, diarrhea
Hydroxychloroquine	Macular damage, rash, diarrhea	Baseline: color fundus photography and automated central perimetric analysis	Ophthalmoscopy q 9-12 mo and Amsler grid at home q 2 wk	Visual changes including a decrease in night or peripheral vision, rash, diarrhea

(Continued)

TABLE 33-9 • Clinical Monitoring of Drug Therapy in Rheumatoid Arthritis (*Continued*)

Drug	Adverse Drug Reaction	Initial Monitoring	Maintenance Monitoring	Symptoms to Inquire About[a]
Methotrexate	Myelosuppression, hepatic fibrosis, cirrhosis, pulmonary infiltrates or fibrosis, stomatitis, rash	Baseline: AST, ALT, alk phos, alb, t. bili, hep B and C studies, CBC w/plt, SCr	CBC w/plt, AST, alb q 1-2 mo	Symptoms of myelosuppression, SOB, nausea/vomiting, lymph node swelling, coughing, mouth sores, diarrhea, jaundice
Leflunomide	Hepatitis, GI distress, alopecia	Baseline: ALT, CBC with platelets	CBC with platelets and ALT monthly initially and then every 6-8 wk	Nausea/vomiting, gastritis, diarrhea, hair loss, jaundice
Penicillamine	Myelosuppression, proteinuria, stomatitis, rash, dysgeusia	Baseline: UA, CBC w/plt, then q week × 1 month	Same as initial—q 1-2 mo, but q 2 wk if dose change	Symptoms of myelosuppression, edema, rash, diarrhea, altered taste perception, oral ulcers
Cyclophosphamide	Alopecia, infertility, GI distress, hemorrhagic cystitis, myelosuppression, nephrotoxicity, cardiotoxicity	UA, CBC w/plt q week × 1 month	Same as initial—q 2-4 wk	Nausea/vomiting, gastritis, diarrhea, hair loss, urination difficulties, chest pain, rash, respiratory difficulties
Cyclosporine	Hepatotoxicity, nephrotoxicity, hypertension, headache, malignancy, infections, GI distress	SCr, blood pressure q month	Same as initial	Nausea/vomiting, diarrhea, symptoms of infection, symptoms of elevated blood pressure
Sulfasalazine	Myelosuppression, rash	Baseline: CBC w/plt, then q week × 1 month	Same as initial—q 1-2 mo	Symptoms of myelosuppression, photosensitivity, rash, nausea/vomiting
Tocilizumab	Local injection-site reactions, infection	AST/ALT, CBC w/plt, lipids	AST/ALT, CBC w/plt, lipids q 4-8 weeks	Symptoms of infection
Anakinra	Local injection-site reactions, infection	Neutrophil count	Neutrophil count monthly for 3 months then quarterly up to 1 year	Symptoms of infection
Etanercept, adalimumab, golimumab, certolizumab	Local injection-site reactions, infection	Tuberculin skin test hepatitis C screening	None	Symptoms of infection
Infliximab, rituximab, abatacept	Immune reactions, infection	Tuberculin skin test hepatitis C screening	None	Postinfusion reactions, symptoms of infection
Tofacitinib	Infection, malignancy, GI perforations, upper respiratory tract infections, headache, diarrhea, nasopharyngitis	Tuberculin skin test, hepatitis C screening, neutrophil count, lymphocytes, Hgb, AST/ALT	Neutrophils, Hgb, FLP at 4-8 weeks after treatment start, then lymphocytes, neutrophils, and Hgb q 3 months	Symptoms of infection or myelosuppression, SOB, blood in stool, black stool, dyspepsia

[a] Altered immune function increases infection; this should be considered particularly in those patients taking azathioprine, methotrexate, and corticosteroids or other drugs as a symptom of myelosuppression.

[b] Osteoporosis is unlikely to manifest itself early in treatment, but all patients should be taking appropriate steps to prevent bone loss.

Abbreviations: alb = albumin; alk phos = alkaline phosphatase; ALT = alanine aminotransferase; AST = aspartate aminotransferase; BUN = blood urea nitrogen; CBC = complete blood count; FLP = fasting lipid panel; GI = gastrointestinal; hep = hepatitis; Hgb = hemoglobin; NSAIDs = nonsteroidal anti-inflammatory drugs; p = after; plt = platelet; q = every; SCr = serum creatinine; SOB = shortness of breath; t. bili = total bilirubin; UA = urinalysis.

Source: Reproduced, with permission, from Dipiro JT, Talbert RL, Yee GC, Matzke GR, Wells BG, Posey LM. *Pharmacotherapy: A Pathophysiological Approach*. 10th ed. New York: McGraw Hill; 2017.

TABLE 33-10 • Herbal Products Rated as Possibly Effective for Treating RA

Herbal Product	Recommended Dosage	Effectiveness[a]	Cost[b]
Borage seed oil	1-3 grams gamma-linolenic acid in borage by mouth daily	Possibly effective	$$$
Cat's claw (*Uncaria guianensis*)	Capsules containing 20 mg of radix Uncariae tomentosae (Krallendorn) with 14.7 mg/gram of pentacyclic oxindole alkaloids and no tetracyclic oxindole alkaloids). One capsule by mouth three times daily	Possibly effective	$$
Fish oil	10 grams by mouth daily	Possibly effective	$$
Lactobacillus: Lactobacillus casei 01 strain	Lactobacillus casei (strain 01) 100 million colony-forming units (CFUs) once by mouth daily	Possibly effective	$$$
Tripterygium wilfordii (aka: Thunder God Vine)	180-570 mg of ethyl acetate extract of Tripterygium wilfordii by mouth daily	Possibly effective	$$$

[a] Level of evidence: "likely effective"—this product has a very high level of reliable clinical evidence supporting its use for a specific indication. Products rated "likely effective" are generally considered appropriate to recommend; "possibly effective"—this product has some clinical evidence supporting its use for a specific indication; however, the evidence is limited by quantity, quality, or contradictory findings. Products rated "possibly effective" might be beneficial, but do not have enough high-quality evidence to be recommended for most people; "insufficient evidence" indicates that there is insufficient reliable scientific evidence to provide an effectiveness rating.

[b] Cost: $ = ≤$10/month supply in recommended dosage; $$ = $11-$20/month; $$$ = $21-$50/month; $$$$ = >$50/month.

Source: References 12 and 13.

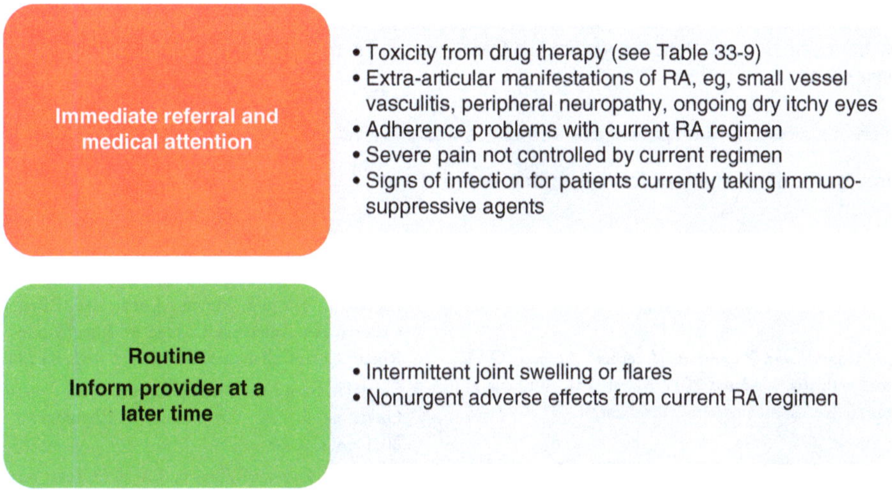

FIGURE 33-7 Referral for management of rheumatoid arthritis.

TABLE 33-11 • Medication-Related Problems (MRPs) in Patients with Rheumatoid Arthritis

Category of MRP	Example Medication-Related Problem
Nonadherence	• Suboptimal control of rheumatoid arthritis symptoms because of nonadherence with lifestyle modifications (eg, refusal to participate in physical therapy regimen) • Suboptimal control of rheumatoid arthritis because of patient missing doses of disease-modifying antirheumatic medication or biologic agent • Patient not taking medication because of cost
Unnecessary medication	• Duplicate therapy (eg, two NSAIDs)
Need for additional medication	• Infliximab therapy without methotrexate • Lack of folic acid supplementation with methotrexate
Ineffective medication	• Pain not controlled with NSAID • Flare-up of rheumatoid arthritis while on DMARD
Dosage too low	• Suboptimal immunosuppression on low dose of antirheumatic agent
Dosage too high	• GI bleeding because of NSAID use for pain associated with RA
Adverse drug event	• Infusion reactions (flu-like symptoms, malaise) with biologic agents such as abatacept, anakinra, tocilizumab, or infliximab • Infection resulting from biologic agent use

Abbreviations: DMARD = disease-modifying antirheumatic drug; GI = gastrointestinal; NSAID = nonsteroidal anti-inflammatory drug; RA = rheumatoid arthritis.

Scenario: Patient given a prescription for Enbrel (etanercept) 3 weeks ago, but insurance is rejecting the prescription due to a required prior authorization. The patient decided not to bother with the hassle of a prior authorization and increased the use of naproxen which seemed to help the joint pain.

MRP: Nonadherence

- **Assessment:**

  Patient with uncontrolled rheumatoid arthritis who was recently prescribed etanercept. Patient attempted to fill prescription and was told a prior authorization was required. Patient now exceeding recommended dosing of OTC naproxen to control joint pain.
- **Plan:**
  1. Prior authorization form supplied. Please sign and fax to indicated number.
  2. Patient to be scheduled for follow-up once medication is received for proper education on use of SureClick pen.

Scenario: Stomatitis secondary to methotrexate

MRP: Adverse drug reaction

- **Assessment:**

  Patient is currently taking methotrexate 2.5 mg 6 tablets by mouth once weekly. Patient is not taking folic acid, which has been found to be effective in preventing side effects secondary to methotrexate use such as stomatitis.

Plan:
- If appropriate, please consider initiating folic acid 5 mg the morning after MTX weekly dose.

Scenario: Duplication of therapy: Patient taking two NSAIDs

MRP: Unnecessary medication

- **Assessment:**

  Patient recently was prescribed Celebrex (celecoxib) 200 mg 1 capsule po daily per rheumatology. Patient also taking Mobic (meloxicam) 15 mg 1 tablet po daily from primary care. Patient does not feel that meloxicam is effective for RA symptoms. Two NSAIDs puts patient at risk for GI and other adverse effects.
- **Plan:**

  Consider discontinuation of meloxicam since patient did not feel this was effective.

FIGURE 33-8 Sample provider communications for rheumatoid arthritis.

REFERENCES

1. CDC: Centers for Disease Control and Prevention [Internet]. Atlanta (GA). Arthritis types: rheumatoid arthritis. [updated 2017 March 13]. Available at https://www.cdc.gov/arthritis/basics/rheumatoid-arthritis.html. Accessed May 2, 2017.
2. Wahl K, Schuna AA. Rheumatoid arthritis. In: Dipiro JT, Talbert RL, Yee GC, Matzke GR, Wells BG, Posey LM. *Pharmacotherapy: A Pathophysiological Approach*. 10th ed. New York: McGraw Hill; 2017. Available at http://accesspharmacy.mhmedical.com/content.aspx?bookid=1861&sectionid=133893255. Accessed May 2, 2017.
3. Hunter T, Boytsov N, Zhang X, et al. Prevalence of rheumatoid arthritis in the United States adult population in healthcare claims databases, 2004-2014. *Rheumatol Int.* 2017;37(9):1551-1557. Accessed May 2, 2017.
4. Gelber AC, Levine SM, Rosen A. Inflammatory rheumatic diseases. In: Gelber AC, Levine SM, Rosen A, eds. *Pathophysiology of Disease: An Introduction to Clinical Medicine*. 7th ed. New York: McGraw-Hill; 2014. Available at http://accesspharmacy.mhmedical.com.lp.hscl.ufl.edu/content.aspx?bookid=961&sectionid=53555705. Accessed May 3, 2017.
5. Jilani AA, Mackworth-Young CG. The role of citrullinated protein antibodies in predicting erosive disease in rheumatoid arthritis: a systematic literature review and meta-analysis. *Inter J Rheumatol.* 2015. http://dx.doi.org/10.1155/2015/728610.
6. Debaugnies F, Servais G, Badot V, et al. Anti-cyclic citrullinated peptide antibodies: a comparison of different assays for the diagnosis of rheumatoid arthritis. *Scand J Rheumatol.* 2013;42:108-114.
7. Aletaha D, Neogi T, Silman AJ, et al. 2010 Rheumatoid Arthritis Classification Criteria. An American College of Rheumatology/European League Against Rheumatism Collaborative Initiative. *Arthritis Rheum.* 2010;62(9):2569-2581.
8. Singh JA, Saag KG, Bridges SL, et al. 2015 American College of Rheumatology Guideline for the Treatment of Rheumatoid Arthritis. *Arthritis Rheum.* 2016;68(1):1-26.
9. Smolen JS, Ladewe R, Bijisma J, et al. EULAR recommendations for the management of rheumatoid arthritis with synthetic and biological disease-modifying antirheumatic drugs: 2016 update. *Ann Rheum Dis.* 2017;76(6):960-977.
10. Rantalaiho V, Kautiainen H, Jarvenpaa S, et al. Failure in long-term treatment is rare in actively treated patients with rheumatoid arthritis, but may be predicted by high health assessment score at baseline and by residual disease activity at 3 and 6 months: the 5-year follow-up results of the randomized clinical NEO-RACo Trial. *J Rheumatol.* 2014;41(12):2379-2385.
11. Medicare Part D Medication Therapy Management program standardization format. Available at https://www.cms.gov/medicare/prescription-drug-coverage/prescriptiondrugcovcontra/downloads/mtm-program-standardized-format-english-and-spanish-instructions-samples-v032712.pdf. Accessed May 2, 2017.
12. Natural Medicines [database online]. Somerville, MA: Therapeutic Research Center; 2017. Available at https://naturalmedicines.therapeuticresearch.com/. Accessed May 3, 2017.
13. Herbal Supplements Monthly Cost Estimates. Available at: http://www.vitacost.com/. Accessed May 3, 2017.
14. CMS. *2017 Part C and D Star Ratings Measures*. Available at https://www.cms.gov/Medicare/Prescription-Drug-Coverage/PrescriptionDrugCovGenIn/Downloads/2017-Measure-List.pdf. Accessed May 12, 2017.

Review Questions

1. Diagnosis of rheumatoid arthritis is most commonly seen in which decade of life?
   a. Second decade
   b. Third decade
   c. Fourth decade
   d. Fifth decade

2. What is the most specific serological marker used to help confirm the diagnosis and predict the severity of rheumatoid arthritis?
   a. Positive rheumatoid factor
   b. Elevated erythrocyte sedimentation rate
   c. Elevated C-reactive protein
   d. Anti-cyclic citrullinated peptide antibodies

3. What is a therapeutic goal associated specifically with the treatment of rheumatoid arthritis, but not usually associated with osteoarthritis?
   a. Prevention of disease progression
   b. Clinical remission
   c. Preservation of joint function
   d. Improvement of overall quality of life

4. Using living room language, which term is best described by the phrase, "a time in which the symptoms of rheumatoid arthritis might be higher than normal"?
   a. A remission
   b. Inflammation
   c. A flare up
   d. An adverse event

5. What is an important component of a medication action plan (MAP) for a patient with rheumatoid arthritis?
   a. Address only a few important action steps for the patient.
   b. Use technical language to ensure the reviewing physician is comfortable with this plan.
   c. Create a MAP for every disease state the patient has during this visit to ensure completeness.
   d. Combine two medication-related problems to decrease the list.

6. Which scenario associated with rheumatoid arthritis requires a referral to a physician?
   a. A patient currently taking methotrexate reports mild joint swelling and moderate fatigue.
   b. A patient currently taking etanercept reports a runny nose, but denies a fever.
   c. A patient currently taking methotrexate reports she was exposed to someone who currently has shingles.
   d. A patient currently taking etanercept reports a fever, malaise, nausea, and pain when urinating.

7. A 68-year-old female patient has been diagnosed with rheumatoid arthritis for 2 years. Her primary care physician has been managing her disease, and she reports for an MTM session. During the visit, she reports her joint pain has been "terrible" and her joints in her hands have remained swollen for a few months. Her physician recently treated her with high-dose prednisone, but she reports her symptoms returned shortly after stopping the steroids. Her current treatment for her rheumatoid arthritis includes: methotrexate 2.5 mg 4 tablets by mouth weekly, folic acid 1 mg 1 tablet by mouth daily, and acetaminophen 325 mg 2 tablets by mouth 3 times a day. Her pain rating today is an 8/10, and her pain normally averages a 7-8/10 on most days. What medication-related problem is associated with the methotrexate?
   a. Adverse drug reaction
   b. Dose too low
   c. Dose too high
   d. Wrong drug

8. Which nonbiologic DMARD can cause hepatic fibrosis?
   a. Hydroxychloroquine
   b. Minocycline
   c. Methotrexate
   d. Sulfasalazine

9. Which biologic DMARD is available in an oral formulation?
   a. Tofacitinib
   b. Tocilizumab
   c. Golimumab
   d. Rituximab

10. Which biologic DMARD is administered subcutaneously every 2 weeks for the treatment of rheumatoid arthritis?
    a. Anakinra
    b. Adalimumab
    c. Etanercept
    d. Golimumab

ANSWERS

1. c	2. d	3. b
4. c	5. a	6. d
7. b	8. c	9. a
10. b		

34

Schizophrenia MTM Data Set

Charles F. Caley, PharmD, BCPP

KEY POINTS

- Appropriate evaluation of schizophrenia includes assessment of positive symptoms, negative symptoms, and cognitive deficit severity. Medication therapy management (MTM) providers working with patients with schizophrenia should be adequately trained in the use of common rating scales.
- MTM providers should educate patients to be realistic about the expected outcomes of antipsychotic therapy, ie, even when medication is taken as prescribed, there will be occasional days where symptoms of schizophrenia may be bothersome.
- Nonadherence is a common medication-related problem in patients with schizophrenia. MTM providers should be vigilant for nonadherence and work with the patient and provider to find a regimen that promotes adherence and minimizes adverse effects and drug cost.
- Metabolic syndrome and extrapyramidal symptoms are concerning adverse effects of antipsychotic drug therapy. MTM providers should monitor for these adverse effects and recommend appropriate changes in therapy to help minimize their consequences.

INTRODUCTION TO SCHIZOPHRENIA

As a brain illness with a lifetime prevalence of approximately 1%, schizophrenia is believed to result from abnormalities in neurodevelopment.[1,2] The current diagnostic criteria for schizophrenia are published by the American Psychiatric Association in the DSM–5 (*Diagnostic and Statistical Manual of Mental Disorders*, 5th edition).[2] Presently, the diagnostic criteria for schizophrenia focus on the long-term presence of specific symptoms (eg, auditory hallucinations, paranoia, disorganized speech) that ultimately result in profound functional impairment. While many practitioners conceptualize this serious illness as one that involves excessive dopamine activity in the limbic system of the brain, schizophrenia is much more than that. Beyond the characteristic "positive" symptoms of schizophrenia, patients with this illness typically also have "negative" symptoms (eg, amotivation, alogia) and cognitive deficits (eg, poor concentration, poor memory, slowed processing speed, impaired social cognition). These two additional areas of concern are believed to result from deficient dopamine activity in the prefrontal cortex. Schizophrenia is an illness with a complex and varied etiology, and, as such, can present in a heterogenous way.[1] Table 34-1 describes categorical symptoms of the illness.

While it tends to be an acute exacerbation of positive symptoms that leads to inpatient hospitalization, it is the negative symptoms and cognitive deficits that are most likely to impair a patient's self-care efforts, as well as their social integration, once they are on a stable course of effective pharmacotherapy.

Other Terms Associated with Schizophrenia

- *Psychosis* - term typically used in reference to hallucinations, delusions, disorganization
- *Drug-induced psychosis* - psychosis caused by a medication (see Table 34-2)
- *Schizoaffective disorder* - schizophrenia with a co-occurring mood disorder, either major depression or bipolar disorder
- *Treatment refractory schizophrenia* - schizophrenia that is not responsive to routine, adequate treatment trials of antipsychotic monotherapy; indication for clozapine treatment

Complications of Schizophrenia

Individuals with schizophrenia are at risk for experiencing other psychiatric conditions, so having schizophrenia does not preclude

TABLE 34-1 • Schizophrenia Symptom Clusters

Positive	Negative	Cognitive
Suspiciousness Unusual thought content (delusions) Hallucinations Conceptual disorganization	Affective flattening Alogia Anhedonia Avolition	Impaired attention Impaired working memory Impaired executive function

Source: Reproduced, with permission, from DiPiro JT, Talbert RL, Yee GC, Matzke GR, Wells BG, Posey L, eds. *Pharmacotherapy: A Pathophysiologic Approach.* 10th ed. New York, NY: McGraw-Hill; 2017.

them from acquiring other mental health conditions. Common comorbid psychiatric conditions with schizophrenia include mood disorders, anxiety disorders, sleep disorders, or substance abuse. Thus, a patient's psychiatric pharmacotherapy may potentially include combinations of an antipsychotic, antidepressant, anxiolytic, mood stabilizer and/or a hypnotic. In addition, comorbid medical disorders, along with their respective pharmacotherapies, are also common, and metabolic syndrome, diabetes, obstructive sleep apnea, gastroesophageal reflux, and heart disease are seen frequently in the clinic. Patients with schizophrenia also have high rates of modifiable risk factors for other diseases, such as smoking, poor diet, lack of exercise, and high alcohol consumption. Taken together, outpatients with schizophrenia are an ideal group to receive comprehensive medication evaluation services from an experienced MTM provider.

Therapeutic Goals for Schizophrenia

The severity of schizophrenia is not measured in a manner that routinely generates clinical data like disease states such as hypertension or diabetes. When the severity of schizophrenia symptoms reaches a certain intensity, the level of function begins to decline. When symptoms remain persistently uncontrolled, then the level of function will likely deteriorate to the point that the patient becomes gravely disabled and is admitted for an inpatient hospitalization for an acute psychotic episode. Thus, the severity of schizophrenia is typically conceptualized in practice as being in one of three phases: acute (typically in the hospital), subacute (typically in day-long treatment program), or maintenance (stabilized outpatient).

However, there is an effort within psychiatry to make symptom severity measurement, using rating scales, be the standard by which symptom intensity of schizophrenia is assessed. The most widely used rating scale for schizophrenia is known as the Positive and Negative Syndrome Scale, or PANSS.[6] This instrument is an anchored, 30-item scale, and each item is scored between 1 (no symptoms) and 7 (extremely severe). It assesses the severity of 7 positive symptoms, 7 negative symptoms, and 16 symptoms representing general psychopathology. Administration of this rating scale in a clinical interview takes about 45 minutes. It relies on collateral information and requires a practitioner to be experienced in working with this patient population. Mathematically, the highest possible score is 210, but a patient with an acute psychotic episode typically scores between 90 and 120. It is important to discuss the details of this rating scale because the efficacy of antipsychotic treatment is assessed in terms of percent reductions in the total rating scale score. The minimally accepted PANSS total score reduction when studying antipsychotic efficacy has been 20%. For many patients, this is an achievable outcome of treatment. Some patients may experience even greater score reductions (30%-40%), and a very small number of patients do even better than this. Conclusions about response to an antipsychotic also incorporate the extent to which psychosocial functioning improves. Patients who fail at least two adequate antipsychotic treatment trials may then be considered for clozapine treatment.

TABLE 34-2 • Substances that May Cause or Worsen Psychosis

- Anticholinergic toxicity (eg, benztropine)
- Bupropion
- Dopamine agonists (eg, levodopa, bromocriptine, ropinirole)
- Drugs of abuse (ie, dextromethorphan, phencyclidine, ketamine, marijuana/synthetic marijuana, methamphetamine, ecstasy [MDMA])
- Psychostimulants (ie, methylphenidate, amphetamine)
- Triazolam
- Varenicline

Unfortunately, the use of full versions of rating scales employed during clinical trials is not practical in the clinical setting, given the time needed to complete them. An alternative to the full PANSS rating scale is the Brief Clinical Assessment for Monitoring Antipsychotic Response in Schizophrenia (Table 34-3)[7] that evaluates the severity of four positive symptoms and four negative symptoms. In addition, cognition scales exist to briefly evaluate the severity of any cognitive deficits associated with the patient's illness.[8] The use of rating scales to assess symptom severity is best when the rater has experience working with the schizophrenia population, experience scoring a rating scale, and when there is collateral information supplied by the patient's family, support network, and mental health provider.

During routine treatment without rating scale scores, practitioners need to identify: (1) target symptoms of schizophrenia the patient has or has had, (2) how persistent target symptoms are, (3) how bothersome the target symptoms are, and (4) to what extent target symptoms adversely influence day-to-day functioning.

CORE ELEMENT 1—COMPREHENSIVE MEDICATION REVIEW FOR PATIENTS WITH SCHIZOPHRENIA

The following is a list of suggested questions to use when conducting a medication therapy review in a patient with schizophrenia (Table 34-4). The number and types of questions will depend upon several factors, including the amount of time for the interview, experience of the MTM provider in working with patients who have schizophrenia, number of concurrent medication-related problems (MRPs), urgency of MRPs, and the reliability of the patient in providing accurate information, among others. In time-limited interactions or in complex cases with multiple medical issues, the MTM provider may choose to target questions that help to identify or rule out issues of an urgent nature (see "Questions to Ask for Prevention/Assessment of Medical Emergencies" in Table 34-4). MTM providers should remember to use living room language during the interview (Figure 34-1) and be prepared for questions that patients may ask regarding their schizophrenia (Table 34-5).

TABLE 34-3 • Brief Clinical Assessments for Monitoring Antipsychotic Response in Schizophrenia

Four-Item Positive Symptom Rating Scale (PSRS)								
Use each item's anchor points to rate the patient.								
1. Suspiciousness	NA	1	2	3	4	5	6	7
2. Unusual thought content	NA	1	2	3	4	5	6	7
3. Hallucinations	NA	1	2	3	4	5	6	7
4. Conceptual disorganization	NA	1	2	3	4	5	6	7
Each item is scored from 1 (not present) to 7 (extremely severe)								SCORE: ______
Brief Negative Symptom Assessment (BNSA)								
Use each item's anchor points to rate the patient.								
1. Prolonged time to respond	1	2	3	4	5	6		
2. Emotion: unchanging facial expression, blank, expressionless face	1	2	3	4	5	6		
3. Reduced social drive	1	2	3	4	5	6		
4. Poor grooming and hygiene	1	2	3	4	5	6		
Each item is scored from 1 (normal) to 6 (severe)				SCORE: ______				

Note: To enhance consistency in ratings, the structured probes in the *Administration Manual* should be used each time the scales are used. The complete manual for the PSRS and the BNSA can be accessed from the appendices in the *Texas Medication Algorithm Project Procedural Manual for Schizophrenia* at the Texas Department of State Health Services website available at http://www.dshs.state.tx.us/mhprograms.

Abbreviation: NA = not able to be assessed.

Source: Reproduced, with permission, from DiPiro JT, Talbert RL, Yee GC, Matzke GR, Wells BG, Posey L. eds. *Pharmacotherapy: A Pathophysiologic Approach.* New York, NY: McGraw-Hill; 2017.

TABLE 34-4 • Questions to Ask When Conducting a Medication Review in a Patient with Schizophrenia

Suggested Questions for the Patient with Schizophrenia
• When were you first diagnosed with schizophrenia? How many schizophrenia-related hospitalizations have you had? What other mental health conditions do you have? • Do any of your family members have any mental health conditions? • What medical conditions do your family members have? Is there any history of high blood pressure, heart disease, or diabetes? • (For female patients of childbearing potential) Are you planning on having children in the future? Are there any medications that you take now that you feel you absolutely need in order for your symptoms to be controlled? • What do you know about the risks of schizophrenia when it is not well controlled? • Which symptoms of schizophrenia are most bothersome to you? Do you have any symptoms that cause you to feel unsafe? (If so, have patient describe.) • What medications do you take for schizophrenia? How/when do you take them? Describe your symptoms and functioning in life when you are receiving treatment that you think is working well for you. • How often do you miss a dose of your antipsychotic medication? • What other medications have you taken in the past for schizophrenia? • Have you ever received long-acting injectable antipsychotic treatment? If the circumstances were right, would you ever be willing to receive an injectable long-acting antipsychotic? • Have you ever stopped taking any of your prescribed medications without telling your physician? If so, why? • What over-the-counter medications or herbal medications do you use? • What other treatments have you tried (eg, lifestyle changes)? • Do you smoke cigarettes? (If so, how much?) Do you drink caffeinated beverages or use energy drinks or energy "shots"? (If so, how much?) Do you drink alcohol? (If so, how much? If so, do you ever skip a dose, or doses, of your schizophrenia medications?) Do you use street drugs? (If so, what and how much? If so, do you ever skip a dose, or doses, of your schizophrenia medications?) • What exercise regimen do you follow?
Questions to Ask for Prevention/Assessment of Medical Emergencies
• Crisis planning: What are the warning signs of your symptoms when they are not in control, and what is your action plan? (May be helpful to have patient discuss what their symptoms were like just prior to his/her last inpatient hospital admission.) • Have you ever felt like you were not safe? Have you ever tried to hurt yourself? Describe what that was like for you. • Have you ever felt anxious or depressed? Describe what that was like for you. • Have you ever not been able to sleep well? How have you been sleeping in the past week?

Abnormal Involuntary Movement Scale (AIMS)—a questionnaire that is used to check for unusual movements known as "tardive dyskinesia."

Acute psychotic episode—worsening of positive symptoms such as hearing voices and paranoia; these are the symptoms that usually lead to going into the hospital.

Adequate antipsychotic treatment trial—receiving enough medication (Table 34-7) for a long enough period of time (approximately 6 weeks), in order for the medication to have a good chance to work.

Affect—facial and body expressions that reflect how you are feeling.

Akathisia—feeling very restless and uncomfortable inside, a possible side effect of medication.

Alogia—poor speech productivity; a negative symptom.

Ambivalence—having thoughts that are contradictory; a type of negative symptom.

Amotivation—no motivation to get things done; a type of negative symptom.

Anticholinergic side effects—dry mouth, constipation, urinary retention, impaired ejaculation, blurry vision, memory difficulties, rapid heart rate.

Apathy—a lack of interest or concern; a type of negative symptom.

Attention—being able to concentrate on something, especially while other things are on-going.

Atypical antipsychotic—the main type of medication used to treat schizophrenia, also known as a second-generation antipsychotic.

Auditory hallucinations—hearing voices; a type of positive symptom.

BMI—body mass index; a measure of weight in relation to height.

BPRS—an 18-item questionnaire known as the Brief Psychiatric Rating Scale; typically used in clinical research to evaluate the severity of schizophrenia symptoms.

Cognitive deficit—a decrease in the ability to do one or more of the following: pay attention, concentrate, process information, remember, problem solve, organize, and/or plan.

Delusion—a fixed belief that is not true; a type of positive symptom

Disorganized thoughts—lack of organized thinking.

Dopamine—a chemical produced by the body that has importance to the positive symptoms of schizophrenia.

Dyskinesia—unusual, involuntary movement.

Dystonia—a potential extrapyramidal side effect of antipsychotic treatment that presents as contraction of a group of muscles that can be painful or impair function; typically seen at the beginning of treatment.

Extrapyramidal—a reference to a part of the brain involved with the control of movement.

Extrapyramidal side effects—a group of four possible side effects of antipsychotic treatment that include akathisia, dystonia, parkinsonism, and tardive dyskinesia.

First-generation antipsychotic—a group of medications used to treat schizophrenia in the past before there were second-generation antipsychotics, for example, Haldol®, Thorazine®.

Flat affect—expressionless, especially when discussing topics that have potential for an emotional quality.

Glutamate—a chemical produced by the body that is believed to be involved in the cause of schizophrenia.

Grandiose—a type of delusion reflecting a belief that the person possesses an extreme measure of wealth, power, or influence.

Hallucination—misperception of one's surroundings as having either auditory or visual stimuli when nothing is around, either hearing voices or "seeing things."

Memory—a part of thinking that allows us to recall information that has been learned before.

Metabolic syndrome—having three or more of the following: increased waist circumference, increased blood pressure, increased blood sugar, increased serum triglyceride level, and/or decreased HDL cholesterol level.

Mood—reported emotional state.

Negative symptom—alogia, amotivation, flat affect, ambivalence, withdrawal.

Orthostasis—a reduction in blood pressure resulting from postural changes, for example, when you stand up from a sitting position, or when getting out of bed.

PANSS—a 30-item questionnaire known as the Positive and Negative Syndrome Scale; typically used in clinical research to evaluate the severity of schizophrenia symptoms.

Paranoia—a type of delusion where a person fears that they are not safe.

Parkinsonism—a potential extrapyramidal side effect of antipsychotic treatment that can present with one or more of the following: tremor, stooped posture, slowness of movement, reduced arm swing while walking, facial masking.

Positive symptom—hallucinations, delusions, ideas of influence, loose associations.

Psychosis—changes in thought, perception and behavior; common observations of a person who is "psychotic" include paranoia/suspiciousness, hearing voices, being distracted, actively avoiding social contact.

Refractory schizophrenia—schizophrenia that does not respond well to adequate antipsychotic treatment trials.

Residual symptoms—despite having a good effect, antipsychotics do not completely control schizophrenia symptoms; milder symptoms of schizophrenia remain.

Schizoaffective disorder—a diagnosis of having both schizophrenia and a mood disorder (either Major Depression or Bipolar Disorder) at the same time.

Schizophrenia—a brain illness that affects a person's thinking, mood, behavior, and motivation, resulting in serious impairment in ability to function.

Second-generation antipsychotic—an antipsychotic medication that blocks the activity of the neurochemicals serotonin and dopamine, also known as an atypical antipsychotic.

Serotonin—a chemical produced by the body that has central importance to the symptoms of schizophrenia.

Somatic—a type of delusion reflecting a belief that there is something wrong with one's body, such as an illness.

Suspicious—cautious distrust of something or someone, similar to paranoia.

Tardive dyskinesia—a potential extrapyramidal side effect of antipsychotic treatment that presents as unusual involuntary movements typically involving the muscles around the mouth and face; important concern about this adverse effect is the possibility that it may become irreversible if allowed to persist.

Typical antipsychotic—an antipsychotic that works by blocking the activity of the neurochemical dopamine, also known as a first-generation antipsychotic.

Withdrawal—not interacting with other people, either through active avoidance because of paranoia, or passively withdrawing because of amotivation.

FIGURE 34-1 Living room language for schizophrenia.

TABLE 34-5 • Questions Commonly Asked by Patients Regarding Schizophrenia

- **What is psychosis?**
  Psychosis is a term that usually refers to a disorder of thinking, behavior, and mood. The symptoms that are usually characteristic of psychosis include auditory hallucinations (hearing voices), paranoia or suspiciousness, and being very agitated and irritable. If these symptoms become too intense, then it could be the reason why the person experiencing them becomes hospitalized. Hospitalization for psychosis will happen if the symptoms place the person experiencing them, or others, at risk for harm.
- **What causes schizophrenia?**
  Schizophrenia is a brain illness that involves psychosis. However, schizophrenia also includes negative symptoms such as amotivation and passive social withdrawal as well as changes in thinking that include difficulty with memory and attention.
- **What health problems are associated with schizophrenia?**
  A person with schizophrenia may also experience other mental health conditions such as depression, anxiety, or substance abuse. Schizophrenia can also be associated with several medical conditions such as metabolic syndrome, gastroesophageal reflux (heartburn), or sleep problems.
- **How do I know if I have schizophrenia?**
  When schizophrenia is first diagnosed, people typically are either not convinced that they have this illness or they have difficulty accepting this diagnosis. It usually takes time for people to know that they have schizophrenia. Schizophrenia is an illness that is characterized by changes in how surroundings are interpreted, disorganized thinking, poor motivation, and possibly hearing voices. Admission to the hospital when these types of symptoms become more intense is another sign of this illness.
- **Why are antipsychotic medications so important?**
  Antipsychotic medications are able to keep the intensity of schizophrenia symptoms at a level that allows the individual with schizophrenia to not be distracted by them and to focus his/her attention on functioning day-to-day.
- **Can I just stop my antipsychotic medication if I feel okay?**
  No. Antipsychotics do not cure the illness of schizophrenia like an antibiotic might cure an infection. Antipsychotic medications control symptoms, so if you are feeling okay while taking the antipsychotic, then that means the medication is working.
- **What can happen if I stop taking my antipsychotic medication?**
  An acute psychotic episode. Individuals with schizophrenia who stop taking their antipsychotic medications eventually have more symptoms and are at great risk for an inpatient hospitalization.
- **When should I call my physician about schizophrenia?**
  Call your physician if you become more bothered by your symptoms, especially if you begin to feel unsafe. Call your physician if you believe you might be experiencing side effects from your antipsychotic.
- **What should I do if I have a problem with my antipsychotic medication?**
  Never stop taking your antipsychotic medications without first talking to your physician. Speak with your physician and/or pharmacist to let them know about any problems you are having, and together you can make sure your antipsychotic medications are the right ones for you.

PERSONAL MEDICATION LIST FOR *<Insert Patient's name*, DOB: *mm/dd/yyyy>*	
Medication: Haloperidol 5 mg tablet	
How I use it: Take 1 tablet (5 mg) 3 times daily	
Why I use it: Symptoms of schizophrenia	**Prescriber:** Alias
Date I started using it: 10/9/2016	**Date I stopped using it:** *(Leave blank for patient's notes)*
Why I stopped using it: *(Leave blank for patient's notes)*	
Medication: Clozapine 100 mg tablet	
How I use it: Take 4 tablets (400 mg) every night at bedtime	
Why I use it: Symptoms of schizophrenia	**Prescriber:** Alias
Date I started using it: 1/6/2017	**Date I stopped using it:** *(Leave blank for patient's notes)*
Medication: Benztropine 0.5 mg tablet	
How I use it: Take 1 tablet (0.5 mg) 2 times daily	
Why I use it: To treat movement side effects	**Prescriber:** Alias
Date I started using it: 10/9/2016	**Date I stopped using it:** *(Leave blank for patient's notes)*
Why I stopped using it: *(Leave blank for patient's notes)*	

FIGURE 34-2 Example personal medication list for antipsychotic medications.

CORE ELEMENT 2—PERSONAL MEDICATION LIST

The following is a sample personal medication list (PML) for a patient with schizophrenia (Figure 34-2).[10] This example is representative only of antipsychotic and related medications. Additional medications for other disease states should be added and listed accordingly. Remember to use plain language when creating the PML.

CORE ELEMENT 3—MEDICATION ACTION PLAN

The following is a sample medication action plan (MAP) for a patient with schizophrenia (Figure 34-3).[10] These examples are representative only of action steps for the patient with schizophrenia. MAPs for other disease states or other MRPs should be added and listed separately. In general, only a few of the most important action steps should be listed so as not to overwhelm the patient. Other areas for patient self-management can be addressed at later visits. Remember to use plain language when creating the MAP.

CORE ELEMENT 4—INTERVENTION AND/OR REFERRAL

Interventions for schizophrenia nearly always include pharmacotherapy, either atypical or typical antipsychotics, and should also include psychotherapeutic efforts. Table 34-6 provides an overview

DATE PREPARED: *<Insert date>*

What we talked about:

You discussed how there are days when you hear no voices and are not suspicious of other people, and there are days when the voices and suspiciousness are noticeable and bothersome. It is important to keep taking your <atypical antipsychotic> as intended even though your symptoms change from time to time. If you end up having more days where your symptoms are bothersome, then that may mean you need a higher dose of your <atypical antipsychotic> from your psychiatrist. If this happens, please inform your psychiatrist.

What I need to do:	What I did and when I did it:
Here are some things I can do to help lessen this effect: • Remember that symptoms of an illness can be influenced by life stress. • Remember that even when I take my medication as prescribed, I will have days when symptoms are bothersome—this does not mean my medication is not working. • Use the coping skills I have learned from my psychiatrist/therapist. • Contact my psychiatrist if the symptoms continue to get worse, or if I become concerned about my safety.	*(Leave blank for patient's notes)*

What we talked about:

Need to keep track of how your weight changes over time

What I need to do:	What I did and when I did it:
1. Check weight at home at least once per week. 2. Record weight and date in log book. 3. Bring log book with me to all clinic appointments.	*(Leave blank for patient's notes)*

FIGURE 34-3 Example medication action plan for a patient with schizophrenia.

of psychotherapeutic interventions. In addition, an important element of treatment for a patient is to have routine mental health care appointments and to develop a support network of family, friends, peers, and advocates such as those who are affiliated with the National Alliance on Mental Illness (www.nami.org). Antipsychotic treatment should be selected on the basis of patient characteristics such as age, antipsychotic treatment history, concurrently prescribed medications, history of treatment adherence, and comorbid disease states. Patients should be encouraged to be aware that antipsychotic treatment may not completely control all of their symptoms and to develop a sense of which symptoms are persisting once they have been stabilized on antipsychotic treatment. Awareness of the symptoms can allow the patient to apply coping skills designed to minimize any distress that residual symptoms may cause.

TABLE 34-6 • Psychotherapeutic Approaches to the Treatment of Schizophrenia

Individual	Group	Cognitive Behavioral
Supportive/counseling Personal therapy Social skills therapies Vocational sheltered employment rehabilitation therapies	Interactive/social	Cognitive behavioral therapy Compliance therapy

Source: References 3, 5, 11, and 12.

Many patients require more than one psychotropic medication to control their schizophrenia. Table 34-7 summarizes antipsychotic therapies, and a treatment algorithm for schizophrenia is found in Figure 34-4. Table 34-8 lists the relative propensity of antipsychotic treatments to cause specific adverse effects, and drug interactions are addressed in Table 34-9. Compelling indications for antipsychotic therapy include the diagnoses of schizophrenia (all types) and schizoaffective disorder. Antipsychotics can also be used in the management of bipolar disorder (acute mania, depression) and major depression with psychotic features. Lastly, there are no herbal remedies that have meaningful therapeutic utility in the management of schizophrenia. Table 34-10 addresses considerations the MTM practitioner should make when attempting to individualize antipsychotic therapy.

Patients who are treatment responsive but have difficulty remaining treatment adherent and who are willing to receive intramuscular injections are good candidates for long-acting injectable antipsychotics. Access to this antipsychotic dosage form can often be achieved through awareness of community pharmacies that dispense these medications as well as area mental health treatment facilities that offer injection services.

Patients who do not respond to at least two adequate trials of antipsychotic monotherapy may receive clozapine treatment. Clozapine was the first second-generation antipsychotic (SGA) introduced in the United States, and it has proven efficacy for treatment refractory schizophrenia.[13] Clozapine also has clinical utility for patients with a history of violence (including suicide attempts), substance abuse disorder, and those who cannot tolerate other antipsychotics because of extrapyramidal symptoms (EPS). Use of this agent is associated with a high rate of metabolic syndrome. In addition, use of clozapine necessitates mandatory, regular monitoring for agranulocytosis and neutropenia, and continued assessment for tardive dyskinesia.

Complications of Antipsychotic Treatment

MTM providers should be aware of adverse effects of antipsychotic therapy (see Table 34-9). Metabolic syndrome is very common in patients with schizophrenia receiving long-term antipsychotic treatment (baseline prevalence of 40.9% in the CATIE trial), and it is generally believed that SGAs are more likely to be associated with this adverse condition.[24,25] In particular, clozapine and olanzapine are the SGAs thought to be associated with the highest rates of metabolic syndrome, while aripiprazole and ziprasidone are thought to have the lowest rates.[26] Regardless of antipsychotic treatment, all patients with schizophrenia require monitoring for weight gain, hypertension, dyslipidemia (eg, hypertriglyceridemia, low HDL cholesterol), and hyperglycemia on a regular basis.

TABLE 34-7 • Available Antipsychotics and Dosage Ranges

Generic Name	Trade Name	Starting Dose (mg/day)	Usual Dosage Range (mg/day)	Comments
First-Generation Antipsychotics				
Chlorpromazine	Thorazine	50-150	300-1000	Most weight gain among FGAs
Fluphenazine	Prolixin	5	5-20	
Haloperidol	Haldol	2-5	2-20	Higher dropout rate in first episode
Loxapine	Loxitane	20	50-150	
Loxapine inhaled	Adasuve	10	10	Maximum 10 mg per 24 hours Approved REMS program only
Perphenazine	Trilafon	4-24	16-64	
Thioridazine	Mellaril	50-150	100-800	Significant QTc prolongation
Thiothixene	Navane	4-10	4-50	
Trifluoperazine	Stelazine	2-5	5-40	
Second-Generation Antipsychotics				
Aripiprazole	Abilify	5-15	15-30	
Asenapine	Saphris	5	10-20	Sublingual only, no food or drink for 10 minutes after administration of the dose
Brexpiprazole	Rexulti	1	2-4	
Cariprazine	Vraylar	1.5	1.5-6	Because of long half-life, steady-state is not reached for several weeks
Clozapine	Clozaril	25	100-800	Check plasma level before exceeding 600 mg
Iloperidone	Fanapt	1-2	6-24	Care with dosing in CYP2D6 slow metabolizers
Lurasidone	Latuda	20-40	40-120	Take with food; ≥350 calories (≥1460 J)
Olanzapine	Zyprexa	5-10	10-20	Avoid in first episode because of weight gain
Paliperidone	Invega	3-6	3-12	Bioavailability increased when administered with food
Quetiapine	Seroquel	50	300-800	
Quetiapine XR	Seroquel XR	300 mg	400-800	
Risperidone	Risperdal	1-2	2-8	
Ziprasidone	Geodon	40	80-160	Take with food, ≥500 calories (≥2100 J)

Note: In first-episode patients, starting dose and target dose should generally be 50% of the usual dose range.

Source: Reproduced, with permission, from DiPiro JT, Talbert RL, Yee GC, Matzke GR, Wells BG, Posey L, eds. *Pharmacotherapy: A Pathophysiologic Approach.* 10th ed. New York, NY: McGraw-Hill; 2017.

Extrapyramidal side effects such as akathisia, dyskinesia, dystonia, and parkinsonism have been a concern of antipsychotic treatment since the availability of chlorpromazine, the first antipsychotic. The first-generation antipsychotics cause EPS to a greater extent than the second-generation antipsychotics, and the EPS caused by the SGAs are generally believed to be less severe. Antipsychotic-induced acute onset EPS (ie, akathisia, dystonia or parkinsonism) typically occurs shortly after the start of antipsychotic treatment or after a dose increase. These movement disorders are believed to be the result of blocking a substantial proportion of nigrostriatal dopamine D2 receptors. Patients may also have more than one type of EPS concurrently. Quetiapine and clozapine are the antipsychotics with the lowest rates of EPS.

Tardive dyskinesia (TD) has the potential to become an irreversible adverse effect of antipsychotic treatment. Therefore, all patients who are treated with antipsychotics need to be regularly monitored for the development of TD. This is done using a standardized clinical assessment such as the Abnormal Involuntary Movement Scale (AIMS) performed once every six months or as needed. MTM providers who perform an AIMS assessment with patients should be trained in the proper procedures and scoring of abnormal movements. The College of Psychiatric and Neurologic

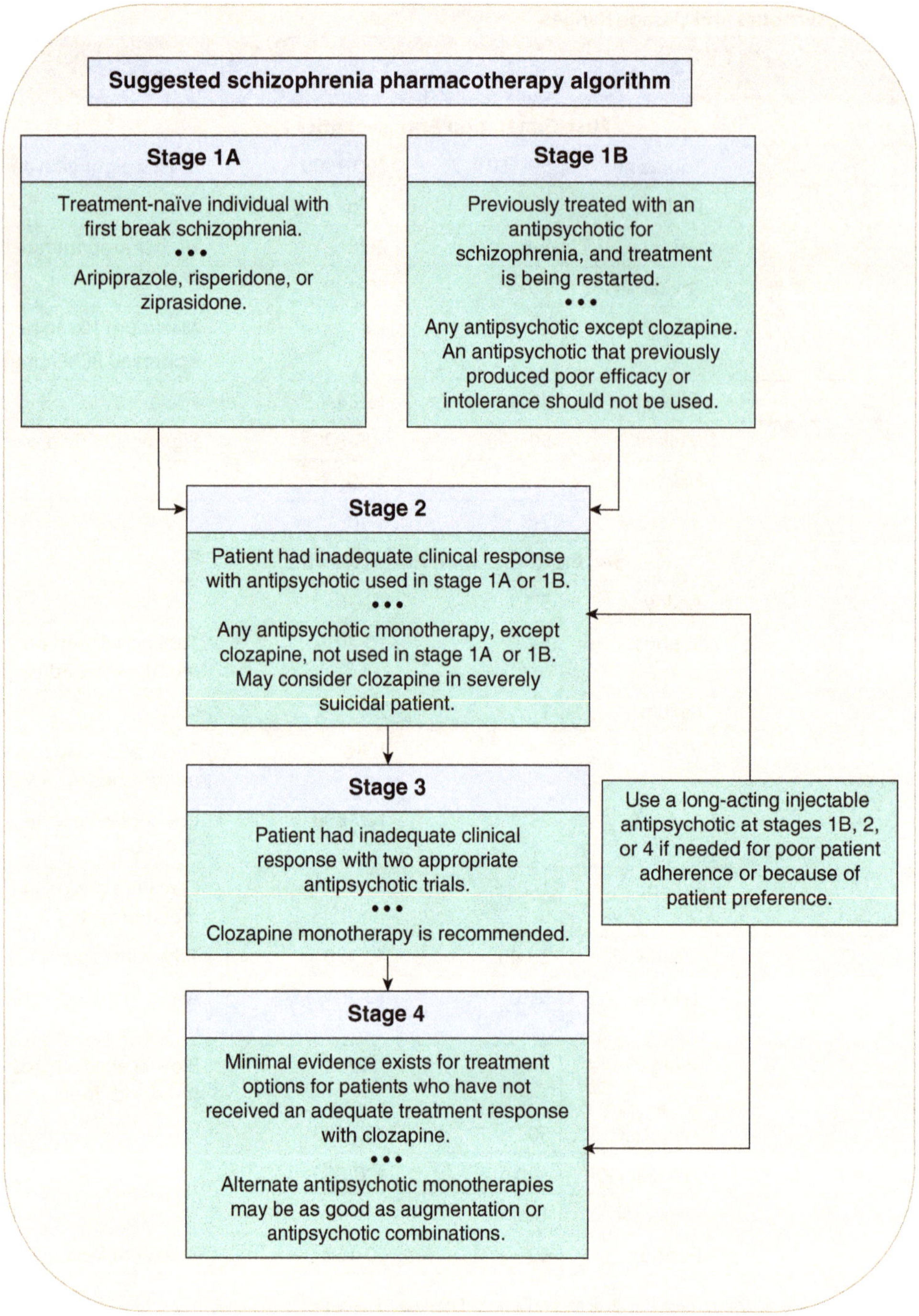

FIGURE 34-4 Algorithm for the pharmacotherapy of schizophrenia.

Note: Suggested pharmacotherapy algorithm for treatment of schizophrenia. Schizophrenia should be treated in the context of an interprofessional model that addresses the psychosocial needs of the patient, necessary psychiatric pharmacotherapy, psychiatric co-occurring mental disorders, treatment adherence, and any medical problems the patient may have.

Source: Reproduced, with permission, from DiPiro JT, Talbert RL, Yee GC, Matzke GR, Wells BG, Posey L, eds. *Pharmacotherapy: A Pathophysiologic Approach.* 10th ed. New York, NY: McGraw-Hill; 2017.

Pharmacists (www.cpnp.org) has developed an EPS training DVD that can assist pharmacists achieve this skill.

Hyperprolactinemia is a potential adverse effect of several antipsychotics with potent dopamine D2 receptor antagonism (eg, risperidone, paliperidone, perphenazine, haloperidol). Serum prolactin levels are measured when a patient is receiving an antipsychotic associated with hyperprolactinemia, and if they are also complaining of sexual dysfunction, breast enlargement, lactation, or menstrual cycle changes. Quetiapine has a warning about the development of cataracts. If this is a concern for the patient, then annual ophthalmologic assessments should be performed. QTc prolongation has been an issue with thioridazine and mesoridazine, and was reintroduced when ziprasidone was approved. Iloperidone also has specific QTc prolongation warnings in its labeling. Taken collectively, however, hyperprolactinemia, cataracts, and QTc prolongation, while not frequent

TABLE 34-8 • Relative Side-Effect Incidence of Commonly Used Antipsychotics[a,b]

	Sedation	EPS	Anticholinergic	Orthostasis	Weight Gain	Prolactin
Aripiprazole	+	+	+	+	+	+
Asenapine	+	++	±	++	+	+
Brexpiprazole	+	+	+	+	+	+
Chlorpromazine	++++	+++	+++	++++	++	+++
Clozapine	++++	+	++++	++++	++++	+
Fluphenazine	+	++++	+	+	+	++++
Haloperidol	+	++++	+	+	+	++++
Iloperidone	+	±	++	+++	++	+
Lurasidone	+	+	+	+	±	±
Olanzapine	++	++	++	++	++++	+
Paliperidone	+	++	+	++	++	++++
Perphenazine	++	++++	++	+	+	++++
Quetiapine	++	+	+	++	++	+
Risperidone	+	++	+	++	++	++++
Thioridazine	++++	+++	++++	++++	+	+++
Thiothixene	+	++++	+	+	+	++++
Ziprasidone	++	++	+	+	+	+

Relative side-effect risk: ± = negligible; + = low; ++ = moderate; +++ = moderately high; ++++ = high.

[a] Side effects shown are relative risk based on doses within the recommended therapeutic range.

[b] Individual patient risk varies depending on patient-specific factors.

Abbreviation: EPS = extrapyramidal side effects.

Source: Reproduced, with permission, from DiPiro JT, Talbert RL, Yee GC, Matzke GR, Wells BG, Posey L, eds. *Pharmacotherapy: A Pathophysiologic Approach.* 10th ed. New York, NY: McGraw-Hill; 2017.

TABLE 34-9 • Common Potential Drug Interactions with Antipsychotic Medications

Mechanism of Interaction	Examples of Interacting Drugs or Other Substances			Clinical Effect
	Pharmacodynamic Drug Interactions with Antipsychotics			
Muscarinic receptor blockade	*Anticholinergics* Benztropine Diphenhydramine Trihexyphenidyl			↑ Anticholinergic SE (Blurred vision, constipation, impaired cognition, and urinary retention)
Additive or synergistic sedation	*Sedatives* Benzodiazepines Concomitant AP Diphenhydramine Melatonin and melatonin agonists Mirtazapine Trazodone TCAs Hypnotics Opiates *Anticholinergics* Benztropine Diphenhydramine Trihexyphenidyl Mirtazapine			↑ sedation Lethargy Impaired cognition Impaired psychomotor activity ↑ Risk of accidents

(*Continued*)

TABLE 34-9 • Common Potential Drug Interactions with Antipsychotic Medications (*Continued*)

Mechanism of Interaction	Examples of Interacting Drugs or Other Substances			Clinical Effect
DA antagonist use for different indication	Metoclopramide			↑ EPS
		Cardiovascular Interactions		
QTc prolongation	Amitriptyline Clomipramine Imipramine Citalopram Fluoroquinolone antibiotics	Procainamide Quinidine		↑ Risk of ECG changes and dysrhythmias
Electrolyte changes	Diuretics			↑ Risk of ECG changes and dysrhythmias
Stimulation of presynaptic 5-HT receptors on DA neuron	SSRIs			↑ EPS
Sympatholytics: α-blockade-↓ NE release	Clonidine Methyldopa Prazosin Nitric oxide-containing products			↑ Hypotension
↑ DA receptor binding	Antipsychotics			↑ SEs, particularly EPS
		Pharmacokinetic Drug Interactions with Antipsychotics		
Substrate Antipsychotic and Mechanism of Action	**Inhibitor or Inducer**			**Clinical Effect**
Aripiprazole, brexipiprazole, cariprazine, and iloperidone				
Inhibition of AP metabolism (CYP2D6, CYP3A4)	*Antidepressants* Bupropion Clomipramine Doxepin Duloxetine Fluoxetine Fluvoxamine Paroxetine Sertraline *HIV protease inhibitors* Indinavir Nelfinavir Ritonavir	*Anti-infectives* Ciprofloxacin Clarithromycin Erythromycin Fluconazole Ketoconazole Itraconazole *Antipsychotics* Asenapine Chlorpromazine Haloperidol Perphenazine Thioridazine	*Miscellaneous* Chlorpheniramine Cimetidine Cocaine Diltiazem Diphenhydramine Grapefruit juice Hydroxyzine Methadone Quinidine Ticlopidine Verapamil	↑ AP effect ↑ SE
Induction of AP metabolism	*Antiepileptics* Carbamazepine Oxcarbazepine Phenobarbital Phenytoin	*Anti-infectives* Rifampin *Miscellaneous* Glucocorticoids Modafinil	*Herbals* St. John's wort	↓ AP effect
Asenapine Eating food or drinking liquids within 10 minutes of asenapine sublingual administration will decrease bioavailability.				
Inhibition of AP metabolism (CYP1A2)	*Antidepressants* Fluvoxamine	*Anti-infectives* Ciprofloxacin Fluoroquinolones	*Miscellaneous* Amiodarone Cimetidine	↑ AP effect ↑ SE

(*Continued*)

TABLE 34-9 • Common Potential Drug Interactions with Antipsychotic Medications (*Continued*)

Mechanism of Interaction	Examples of Interacting Drugs or Other Substances			Clinical Effect
Induction of AP metabolism	*Anti-infectives* Nafcillin	*Miscellaneous* Broccoli Brussels sprouts Chargrilled meat Smoking tobacco	*Miscellaneous* Insulin Modafinil Omeprazole	↓ AP effect
	Pharmacokinetic Drug Interactions with Antipsychotics			
Substrate Antipsychotic and Mechanism of Action	**Inhibitor or Inducer**			**Clinical Effect**
Brexpiprazole (see aripiprazole) Clozapine				
Inhibition of AP metabolism (CYP3A4, CYP1A2, CYP2C19)	*Antidepressants* Fluoxetine Fluvoxamine *HIV protease inhibitors* Indinavir Nelfinavir Ritonavir *Anticonvulsants* Felbamate Oxcarbazepine	*Anti-infectives* Ciprofloxacin Clarithromycin Erythromycin Fluconazole Fluoroquinolones Ketoconazole Itraconazole Nafcillin	*Miscellaneous* Amiodarone Diltiazem Cimetidine Grapefruit juice Haloperidol Modafinil Omeprazole Ticlopidine Topiramate Verapamil	↑ AP effect ↑ SE
Induction of AP metabolism	*Antiepileptics* Carbamazepine Phenobarbital Phenytoin	*Anti-infectives* Rifampin *Miscellaneous* Glucocorticoids Insulin Modafinil Omeprazole Smoking tobacco	*Herbals* St. John's wort	↓ AP effect
Haloperidol				
Inhibition of AP metabolism (CYP2D6, CYP3A4, CYP1A2)	*Antidepressants* Bupropion Doxepin Duloxetine Fluoxetine Fluvoxamine Paroxetine Sertraline *HIV protease inhibitors* Indinavir Nelfinavir Ritonavir Saquinavir	*Anti-infectives* Ciprofloxacin Clarithromycin Erythromycin Fluoconazole Fluoroquinolones Ketoconazole Itraconazole *Antipsychotics* Chlorpromazine Perphenazine	*Miscellaneous* Amiodarone Chlorpheniramine Cimetidine Diltiazem Diphenhydramine Grapefruit juice Hydroxyzine Methadone Quinidine Verapamil	↑ AP effect ↑ SE

(*Continued*)

TABLE 34-9 • Common Potential Drug Interactions with Antipsychotic Medications (*Continued*)

Mechanism of Interaction	Examples of Interacting Drugs or Other Substances			Clinical Effect
Induction of AP metabolism	*Anticonvulsants* Carbamazepine Oxcarbazepine Phenobarbital Phenytoin	*Anti-infectives* Nafcillin Rifampin *Miscellaneous* Broccoli Brussels sprouts Chargrilled meat Glucocorticoids Insulin Modafinil Omeprazole Tobacco smoking	*Herbals* St. John's wort	↓ AP effect
Iloperidone (see aripiprazole)				
Olanzapine				
Inhibition of AP metabolism (CYP3A4 and CYP1A2)	*Antidepressants* Fluoxetine (norfluoxetine) Fluvoxamine *HIV protease inhibitors* Indinavir Nelfinavir Ritonavir	*Anti-infectives* Ciprofloxacin Clarithromycin Erythromycin Fluconazole Fluoroquinolones Ketoconazole Itraconazole	*Miscellaneous* Amiodarone Cimetidine Diltiazem Grapefruit juice Verapamil	↑ AP effect ↑ SE
Induction of AP metabolism	*Antiepileptics* Carbamazepine Oxcarbazepine Phenobarbital Phenytoin *HIV non-nucleoside reverse transcriptase inhibitors* Efavirenz Nevirapine	*Anti-infectives* Nafcillin Rifampin *Miscellaneous* Broccoli Brussels sprouts Chargrilled meat Glucocorticoids Insulin Modafinil Omeprazole Smoking tobacco	*Herbals* St. John's wort	↓ AP effect
Paliperidone The bioavailability of paliperidone is significantly increased when it is taken with food. Although this could increase paliperidone effect, including adverse effects, the clinical significance is undetermined. Only potent CYP3A4 (eg, carbamazepine, rifampin, St. John's wort) inducers appear to increase paliperidone metabolism and affect dose requirements.				
Pharmacokinetic Drug Interactions with Antipsychotics				
Substrate Antipsychotic and Mechanism of Action	**Inhibitor or Inducer**			**Clinical Effect**
Lurasidone and quetiapine Inhibition of AP metabolism (CYP3A4)	*Antidepressants* Fluoxetine (norfluoxetine) Fluvoxamine Nefazodone *HIV protease inhibitors* Indinavir Nelfinavir Ritonavir Saquinavir	*Anti-infectives* Ciprofloxacin Clarithromycin Erythromycin Fluconazole Ketoconazole Itraconazole	*Miscellaneous* Amiodarone Cimetidine Diltiazem Grapefruit juice Verapamil	↑ AP effect ↑ SE

(*Continued*)

TABLE 34-9 • Common Potential Drug Interactions with Antipsychotic Medications (*Continued*)

Mechanism of Interaction	Examples of Interacting Drugs or Other Substances			Clinical Effect
Induction of AP metabolism	*Antiepileptics* Carbamazepine Oxcarbazepine Phenobarbital Phenytoin *HIV non-nucleoside reverse transcriptase inhibitors* Efavirenz Nevirapine	*Anti-infectives* Rifampin *Miscellaneous* Glucocorticoids Modafinil	*Herbals* St. John's wort	↓ AP effect
Lurasidone AUC and C_{max} increase by 2- and 3-fold when given with at least 350 calories (1460 J) of food regardless of fat content.				
Perphenazine and risperidone Note: Because risperidone's metabolite formed through CYP2D6 metabolism is active (paliperidone), the clinical significance of metabolic drug interactions with risperidone is unclear.				
Inhibition of AP metabolism (CYP2D6)	*Antidepressants* Bupropion Clomipramine Doxepin Duloxetine Fluoxetine Paroxetine Sertraline *Antipsychotics* Chlorpromazine Haloperidol (reduced haloperidol) Perphenazine	*Miscellaneous* Amiodarone Cimetidine Chlorpheniramine Cocaine Diphenhydramine Haloperidol Hydroxyzine Methadone Quinidine		↑ AP effect ↑ SE
Induction of AP metabolism (via CYP3A34, a minor pathway for risperidone)	Dexamethasone Rifampin			↓ AP effect
Ziprasidone The bioavailability of ziprasidone is increased 2-fold when it is taken with food. Consistent administration with food is recommended.				

Abbreviations: AP = antipsychotic; AUC = area under the curve; C_{max} = maximum plasma concentration; DA = dopamine; EPS = extrapyramidal symptoms; 5-HT = serotonin; NE = norepinephrine; SE = side effect; SSRI = serotonin selective reuptake inhibitor; TCAs = tricyclic antidepressants.

Source: Reproduced, with permission, from DiPiro JT, Talbert RL, Yee GC, Matzke GR, Wells BG, Posey L. eds. *Pharmacotherapy: A Pathophysiologic Approach.* 10th ed. New York, NY: McGraw-Hill; 2017.

adverse outcomes of antipsychotic treatment, still require active monitoring.

Referrals

MTM providers who work with individuals who have schizophrenia must have a sense of when they should refer the patient back to the mental health care provider, or to an emergency department. Situations that require referral many times center on either the possibility of a poor antipsychotic treatment outcome (where a new antipsychotic may be necessary), a new psychiatric diagnosis, or patient risk of harm to self or others. If the MTM provider detects a new or untreated mood component, this should prompt a referral back to the mental health care provider so that a proper diagnosis can be made and treatment initiated. If a patient endorses new or worsening suicidal thoughts, or does not feel safe, then this may be a situation where the MTM provider has the patient talk directly with a psychiatric assessment center affiliated with a hospital to determine if the patient meets criteria for a hospital admission. Alternatively, the MTM provider and patient may contact emergency medical transportation so that the patient can be brought to a local emergency department. Given the importance of ensuring that proper action is taken in these types of situations, it is highly important that the MTM provider develop a professional relationship with the patient's mental health care provider so that an understanding between the two professionals can be reached in advance of any key clinical situations.

TABLE 34-10 • Considerations in Individualizing Antipsychotic Therapy

Comorbid Condition	Preferred Drug Options
EPS (akathisia, dystonia, parkinsonism)	Quetiapine Clozapine
GERD	Select antipsychotics with low rates of weight gain and anticholinergic effects: eg, aripiprazole, lurasidone, risperidone/paliperidone, ziprasidone
History of recurrent aggression	clozapine
History of recurrent suicidality	clozapine
Hyperprolactinemia	aripiprazole, clozapine, quetiapine, ziprasidone
Metabolic syndrome/diabetes mellitus/ dyslipidemia	Select antipsychotic with low rates of weight gain: eg, aripiprazole, haloperidol, lurasidone, ziprasidone
Obstructive sleep apnea	Select antipsychotics with low rates of sedation and weight gain: eg, aripiprazole, lurasidone, risperidone/paliperidone, ziprasidone
QTc prolongation	AVOID: clozapine, iloperidone, thioridazine/mesoridazine, ziprasidone
Substance abuse	clozapine
Tardive dyskinesia	quetiapine clozapine
Treatment nonadherence	Long acting injectable antipsychotic: eg, fluphenazine, haloperidol, aripiprazole, olanzapine, risperidone/paliperidone

Abbreviations: EPS = extrapyramidal symptoms; GERD = gastroesophageal reflux disease.

CORE ELEMENT 5—DOCUMENTATION AND FOLLOW-UP

Clear and succinct documentation of MRPs and recommendations is a key component of the MTM service. Examples of potential MRPs in patients with schizophrenia are provided in Table 34-11. Sample communications and recommendations to providers to address medication-related issues are found in Figure 34-5. Recommendations should be written and may be communicated via fax, phone, or other means of secure electronic communication. The examples are only for illustrative purposes. Actual communications to providers should be individualized for the patient and based on

TABLE 34-11 • Medication-Related Problems (MRPs) in Patients with Schizophrenia

Category of MRP	Example Medication-Related Problem
Nonadherence	• Suboptimal control of positive symptoms (ie, auditory hallucinations, paranoia) because of nonadherence • Patient with residual negative symptoms (ie, amotivation, social withdrawal) • Patient with cognitive deficits (ie, poor working memory, difficulty with attention, slow processing speed) • Patient taking antipsychotic medication as needed • Patient not taking antipsychotic medication because of cost
Unnecessary medication	• Duplicate antipsychotic therapy in nonrefractory patient
Need for additional medication	• Current monotherapy for schizophrenia with suboptimal positive symptom control • Patient has received adequate clozapine treatment trial with prominent residual positive symptoms
Ineffective medication	• Adequate treatment trial of new antipsychotic without significant clinical response
Dosage too low	• Suboptimal control of positive symptoms
Dosage too high	• Patient with inner restlessness (possibly akathisia) on high-dose antipsychotic treatment • Patient with daytime sedation from dual antipsychotic treatment
Adverse drug event	• Orthostasis from antipsychotic • Metabolic syndrome risk • Tardive dyskinesia risk • Daytime sedation in a patient receiving a co-prescribed medication known to increase antipsychotic concentrations • Patient not taking antipsychotic because of sexual dysfunction (could also be classified under nonadherence)

Scenario: Patient given samples of lurasidone, but cannot afford Rx once samples are finished

MRP: Nonadherence

- **Assessment:**
  Patient with clear evidence of positive symptoms on lurasidone 80 mg. Lack of positive symptom control likely secondary to nonadherence because of high cost of lurasidone. Switching lurasidone to a generic atypical antipsychotic (eg, risperidone, olanzapine, ziprasidone) would provide more affordable antipsychotic treatment for the patient.
- **Plan:**
  Consider: (1) starting risperidone 1 mg twice daily with titration to 4-6 mg/day, and (2) taper and discontinue lurasidone.

Scenario: Opportunity to reduce antipsychotic pill burden

MRP: Unnecessary dual antipsychotic therapy resulting from stall in antipsychotic switch

- **Assessment:**
  Patient is currently receiving:
  - Lurasidone 80 mg daily
  - Risperidone 4 mg daily

  Patient was originally scheduled to switch from lurasidone to risperidone due to the high cost of lurasidone. Risperidone treatment was implemented and a target dose achieved, but patient did not discontinue lurasidone. Patient has been on above combination for 3 months and is exhibiting daytime somnolence and muscle stiffness.
- **Plan:**
  Consider tapering lurasidone dose by 20 mg every week to minimize risk of symptomatic rebound. Consider small risperidone dose increases of 0.5-1.0 mg to compensate for any increases in symptom severity that might be due to loss of therapeutic effect from lurasidone.

Scenario: Development of metabolic syndrome with olanzapine

MRP: Adverse drug event

- **Assessment:**
  Patient experiencing weight gain (current waist circumference = 45 in), increases in serum triglyceride (most recent = 315), reduction in HDL-cholesterol (most recent = 28) while receiving treatment with olanzapine 20 mg/day. Patient may benefit from switching olanzapine to an agent with a lower risk of metabolic syndrome such as ziprasidone or aripiprazole.
- **Plan:**
  Consider switch to aripiprazole (initial target dose = 15 mg/day) or ziprasidone (initial target dose = 120 mg/day).

Scenario: Development of tardive dyskinesia with risperidone

MRP: Adverse drug event

- **Assessment:**
  Patient experiencing peri-oral movements consistent with tardive dyskinesia; current AIMS score = 4. Current antipsychotic treatment risperidone 6 mg/day. Patient may benefit from switching risperidone to an agent with a lower risk of extrapyramidal side effects such as quetiapine.
- **Plan:**
  Consider switch to quetiapine (initial target dose = 300-400 mg/day), recommend adding quetiapine to risperidone first, and then slowly taper risperidone off by 1-2 mg every 1-2 weeks as tolerated. Anticipate movements to initially get worse once risperidone taper has been started.

FIGURE 34-5 Sample provider communications for schizophrenia.

the type of recommendation and the nature of the relationship with the provider.

Follow-up to assess mental status, effects of interventions, and potential adverse effects is important for patients with schizophrenia. The interval for follow-up will depend on specific characteristics of individual patients such as intensity of symptoms, level of functioning, and complexity of the intervention. In addition, patient characteristics such as age, level of support, and number of comorbidities may influence the capacity to return. Suggested intervals for follow-up are provided in Table 34-12.

TABLE 34-12 • Suggested Intervals for Follow-up in Patients with Schizophrenia

Follow-up and Monitoring in Patients with Schizophrenia
Antipsychotic response • One to two weeks after initiating or making changes in therapy. Be sure to assess the intensity of the patient's positive, negative, and cognitive symptoms; the capacity to function in everyday life should also be evaluated. • Once symptoms have stabilized, patients should be monitored every 1 to 6 months.
Tolerability • Monitor for adverse drug effects at each visit, especially onset of metabolic syndrome and onset of EPS or tardive dyskinesia. • AIMS evaluation needed every 6 months. • Metabolic syndrome monitoring (see Table 34-13). • Clozapine-treated patients require regular total WBC and ANC monitoring.

Abbreviations: AIMS = Abnormal Involuntary Movement Scale; ANC = absolute neutrophil count; EPS = extrapyramidal symptoms; WBC = white blood cell.

TABLE 34-13 • Recommended Metabolic Syndrome Monitoring for Patients Taking Atypical Antipsychotic Medications

Parameter	Baseline	4 Wk	8 Wk	12 Wk	Quarterly	Annually	Every 5 Yrs
Personal history	X					X	
Family history	X					X	
Weight (BMI)	X	X	X	X	X		
Waist circumference	X					X	
Blood pressure	X					X	
FPG	X					X	
FLP	X			X			X

Note: Additional or more frequent screening may be necessary based on a patient's individual risk or family history.

Abbreviations: BMI = body mass index; FPG = fasting plasma glucose; FLP = fasting lipid profile.

Source: Reproduced, with permission, from American Diabetes Association; American Psychiatric Association; American Association of Clinical Endocrinologists; North American Association for the Study of Obesity. Consensus development conference on antipsychotic drugs and obesity and diabetes. *Diabetes Care*. 2004;27(2):596-601.

REFERENCES

1. Crismon M, Kattura RS, Buckley PF. Schizophrenia. In: DiPiro JT, Talbert RL, Yee GC, Matzke GR, Wells BG, Posey L, eds. *Pharmacotherapy: A Pathophysiologic Approach*. 10th ed. New York, NY: McGraw-Hill; 2017. Available at http://accesspharmacy.mhmedical.com/content.aspx?bookid=1861&sectionid=146064659. Accessed May 19, 2017.
2. American Psychiatric Association. Schizophrenia spectrum and other psychotic disorders. In: *Diagnostic and Statistical Manual of Mental Disorders*. 5th ed. Washington, DC: American Psychiatric Association, 2013:87-122.
3. Castle DJ, Buckley PF. *Schizophrenia*. Oxford, UK: Oxford University Press; 2008.
4. McGorry PD. The next stage for diagnosis: validity through utility. *World Psychiatry*. 2013;12(3):213-214.
5. Saperstein AM, Kurtz MM. Current trends in the empirical study of cognitive remediation for schizophrenia. *Can J Psychiatry*. 2013;58(6):311-318.
6. Kay SR, Fiszbein A, Opler LA. The positive and negative syndrome scale (PANSS) for schizophrenia. *Schizophr Bull*. 1987;13(2):261-276.
7. Argo TR, Crismon ML, Miller AL, et al. *Schizophrenia Treatment Algorithms, Texas Medication Algorithm Project Procedural Manual*. Austin, TX: Texas Department of State Health Services, 2008. Available at http://www.dshs.state.tx.us/mhprograms. Accessed May 19, 2017.
8. Velligan DI, DiCocco M, Bow-Thomas C, et al. A brief cognitive assessment (BCA) for use with schizophrenia patients in a community clinic. *Schizophr Res*. 2004;71:273-283.
9. Velligan DI, Lopez L, Castillo DA, et al. Interrater reliability of using brief standardized outcome measures in a community mental health setting. *Psychiatr Serv*. 2011;62:558-560.
10. CMS. *Medicare Part D Medication Therapy Management Program Standardized Format*. Available at https://www.cms.gov/Medicare/Prescription-Drug-Coverage/PrescriptionDrugCovContra/Downloads/MTM-Program-Standardized-Format-English-and-Spanish-Instructions-Samples-v032712.pdf. Accessed May 19, 2017.
11. Kane JM, Robinson DG, Schooler NR, et al. Comprehensive versus usual community care for first-episode psychosis: 2-year outcomes from the NIMH RAISE early treatment program. *Am J Psychiatry*. 2015;173(4):362-372.
12. Kane JM, Schooler NR, Marcy P, et al. The RAISE early treatment program for first-episode psychosis: background, rationale, and study design. *J Clin Psychiatry*. 2015;76(3):240-246.
13. Kane J, Honigfeld G, Singer J, et al. Clozapine for the treatment resistant schizophrenic: a double-blind comparison with chlorpromazine. *Arch Gen Psychiatry*. 1988;45(9):789-796.
14. Citrome L. Iloperidone for schizophrenia: a review of the efficacy and safety profile for this newly commercialized second-generation antipsychotic. *Int J Clin Pract*. 2009;63(8):1237-1248.
15. Citrome L. Asenapine for schizophrenia and bipolar disorder: a review of the efficacy and safety profile for this newly approved sublingually absorbed second-generation antipsychotic. *Int J Clin Pract*. 2009;63(12):1762-1784.
16. McCormack PL. Cariprazine: first global approval. *Drugs*. 2015;75(17):2035-2043.
17. Prescribing information. Rexulti. Tokyo, Japan: Otsuka pharmaceutical Co, Ltd; July 2015.
18. Citrome L. Lurasidone for schizophrenia: a review of the efficacy and safety profile for this newly approved second-generation antipsychotic. *Int J Clin Pract*. 2011;65(2):189-210.
19. Clozapine FDA prescribing information. Teva Pharmaceuticals; revised November 2015.
20. Hasan A, Falkai P, Wobrock T, et al. World Federation of Societies of Biological Psychiatry (WFSBP) guidelines for the biological treatment of schizophrenia, part 1: update 2012 on the acute treatment of schizophrenia and the management of treatment resistance. *World J Biol Psychiatry*. 2012;13(5):318-378.
21. Buchanan RW, Kreyenbuhl J, Kelly DL, et al. The 2009 schizophrenia PORT psychopharmacological treatment recommendations and summary statements. *Schizophr Bull*. 2010;36(1):71-93.
22. Osser DN, Roudsari MJ, Manschreck T. The psychopharmacology algorithm project at the Harvard South Shore Program: an update on schizophrenia. *Harv Rev Psychiatry*. 2013;21(1):18-40.
23. Lieberman JA, Stroup S. The NIMH-CATIE schizophrenia study: what did we learn? *Am J Psychiatry*. 2011;168(8):770-775.
24. Lieberman JA, Stroup TS, McEvoy JP, et al. Effectiveness of antipsychotic drugs in patients with chronic schizophrenia. *N Engl J Med*. 2005;353:1209-1223.
25. McEvoy JP, Meyer JM, Goff Dc, et al. Prevalence of metabolic syndrome in patients with schizophrenia: baseline results from the Clinical Antipsychotic Trials of Intervention Effectiveness schizophrenia trial and comparison with national estimates from NHANES III. *Schizophr Res*. 2005;80(1):19-32.
26. Newcomer JW. Antipsychotic medications: metabolic and cardiovascular risk. *J Clin Psychiatry*. 2007;68 (suppl 4):8-13.
27. Citrome L. New second-generation long-acting injectable antipsychotics for the treatment of schizophrenia. *Expert Rev Neurother*. 2013;13(7):767-783.
28. Prescribing information. Zyprexa Relprevv. Indianapolis, IN: Lilly USA; December 2014.
29. Prescribing information. Invega Trinza. Titusville, NJ: Janssen Pharmaceuticals Inc; May 2015.
30. Prescribing information. Aristada. Waltham, MA: Alkermes Inc; October 2015.
31. Ereshefsky L, Saklad SR, Jann MW, et al. Future of depot neuroleptic therapy: pharmacokinetics and pharmacodynamic approaches. *J Clin Psychiatry*. 1984;45(5 pt 2):50-59.

32. Preskorn SH. Clinically important differences in the pharmacokinetics of the ten newer atypical antipsychotics: part 2. Metabolism and elimination. *J Psychiatr Pract.* 2012;18(3):361-368.

33. Hasan A, Falkai P, Wobrock T, et al. World Federation of Societies of Biological Psychiatry (WFSBP) guidelines for biological treatment of schizophrenia, part 2: update 2012 on the long-term treatment of schizophrenia and management of antipsychotic induced side effects. *World J Biol Psychiatry.* 2013;14(1):2-44.

34. Ereshefsky L. Drug–drug interactions with the use of psychotropic medications. *CNS Spectr* 2009;14(suppl 8):1-8.

35. Gaertner J, Ruberg K, Schlesiger G, Frechan S, Voltz R. Drug interactions in palliative care—it's more than cytochrome P450. *Palliat Med.* 2012;26(6): 813-825.

36. Kennedy WK, Jann MW, Kutscher EC. Clinically significant drug interactions with atypical antipsychotics. *CNS Drugs.* 2013;27(12):1021-1048.

37. American Diabetes Association; American Psychiatric Association; American Association of Clinical Endocrinologists; North American Association for the Study of Obesity. Consensus development conference on antipsychotic drugs and obesity and diabetes. *Diabetes Care.* 2004;27(2):596-601.

Review Questions

1. Which symptom is included in the diagnostic criteria for schizophrenia?
   a. Disorganized speech
   b. Cognitive deficits
   c. Depressed mood
   d. Illusions

2. Which action is most appropriate for the MTM provider when assessing a patient with schizophrenia?
   a. Anticipate cataracts as a common medical complication.
   b. Measure cognitive deficits using a brief clinical rating scale.
   c. Monitor for tardive dyskinesia only during first generation antipsychotic treatment.
   d. Interpret flat affect, poor speech productivity, and low energy as negative symptoms, not depression.

3. When measuring symptom severity of schizophrenia, what is the minimally accepted reduction in total scores that qualifies for a response and results from antipsychotic treatment?
   a. Remission
   b. 60%
   c. 40%
   d. 20%

4. Using living room language, how would an MTM provider describe one of the negative symptoms of schizophrenia?
   a. Hearing voices
   b. Inner restlessness
   c. Constant lack of motivation
   d. Always being suspicious of others

5. A patient with schizophrenia reports that symptoms have been bothersome for 3 days in a row. What information should be a part of the medication action plan?
   a. Tell the patient to call the psychiatrist and get changed to a new antipsychotic.
   b. Instruct the patient to double the dose of antipsychotic for a few days until the symptoms go away.
   c. Instruct the patient to disregard the symptoms.
   d. Instruct the patient to use coping skills when symptoms occur.

6. All of the following scenarios should result in the MTM provider referring the patient with schizophrenia back to the patient's psychiatrist **EXCEPT:**
   a. when the patient's schizophrenia symptoms worsen over time.
   b. when the patient's serum triglycerides increases over time.
   c. when the patient begins demonstrating evidence of abnormal, perioral movements.
   d. when the MTM provider identifies the patient as having a depressed mood and the patient is not being treated with an antidepressant.

7. A patient who has been receiving quetiapine 600 mg/day and haloperidol 10 mg/day concurrently for the past 4 months should have which medication-related problem categorized and explored?
   a. Ineffective medication
   b. Unnecessary medication
   c. Non-evidence-based medicine
   d. Dosage too high

8. A patient who has failed adequate treatment trials of risperidone and ziprasidone becomes eligible for consideration of which antipsychotic?
   a. Clozapine
   b. Quetiapine
   c. Olanzapine
   d. Aripiprazole

9. An MTM provider has a first encounter with a patient with schizophrenia who reports recently experiencing sedation, inner restlessness, dry mouth, constipation, and elevated triglycerides and glucose while receiving olanzapine 30 mg/day. Which antipsychotic causes the lowest rate of all these adverse effects?
   a. Clozapine
   b. Chlorpromazine
   c. Perphenazine
   d. Aripiprazole

10. Which statement about schizophrenia is correct?
    a. Schizophrenia is the one psychiatric illness that is not associated with substance abuse.
    b. Patients with schizophrenia can have poor memory and slowed processing speeds as part of their illness.
    c. Atypical antipsychotics improve severity of positive symptoms, negative symptoms, and cognitive deficits equally.
    d. The pathophysiology of the illness is best explained as first resulting from excessive dopamine activity in the limbic system, and then degeneration of the limbic system.

ANSWERS

1. a	2. b	3. d
4. c	5. d	6. b
7. b	8. a	9. d
10. b		

35

Stroke MTM Data Set

Katherine Vogel Anderson, PharmD, BCACP, and Sarah E. Honaker, PharmD

KEY POINTS

- Patients who have had a stroke or transient ischemic attack are at risk for recurrent stroke, myocardial infarction, and death.
- Smoking cessation, exercise, and weight management are beneficial lifestyle modifications for stroke survivors. Medication therapy management (MTM) providers should reinforce the importance of lifestyle modifications and incorporate these elements, as appropriate, into the medication action plan (MAP).
- Antihypertensives, statin therapy, antiplatelet agents, and anticoagulants are evidence-based therapies proven to reduce the risk of recurrent stroke. MTM providers should review the medication profile of stroke survivors to identify potential gaps in therapy.

INTRODUCTION TO STROKE

A leading cause of death and disability, stroke affects 800,000 Americans each year.[1,2] It is estimated that every 40 seconds, someone in the United States has a stroke, and every 4 minutes, someone dies as a result of a stroke. The majority of strokes are ischemic in nature. Figure 35-1 outlines a classification of stroke by mechanism.[2]

Risk factor modification is paramount for stroke prevention; risk factors for stroke are listed in Table 35-1. Patients who have a stroke or transient ischemic attack (TIA) are at risk for recurrent stroke, myocardial infarction, and death.[1] For patients who suffer a stroke, adherence to evidence-based treatment guidelines can prevent death, reduce disability, and improve outcomes. The acute management of stroke is beyond the scope of this chapter. Instead, this chapter will focus on secondary prevention of stroke in the outpatient setting.

Stroke Definitions

- **Stroke** – General term for abrupt onset neurological deficit lasting at least 24 hours
- **Ischemic stroke** – Occlusion of a cerebral artery caused by a thrombus or embolus
- **Hemorrhagic stroke** – Presence of blood in the brain that damages surrounding tissue (the management of hemorrhagic stroke is limited to the inpatient setting; treatment is not described in this chapter)
- **Cardioembolic stroke** – Emboli form in the heart, causing a stroke; usually a result of atrial fibrillation, valvular heart disease, and/or left ventricular thrombus
- **Transient ischemic attack (TIA)** – A transient episode of neurological dysfunction caused by focal brain, spinal cord, or retinal ischemia, without acute infarction, usually <24 hours in duration

TIA is a potent predictor of stroke. The distinction between stroke and TIA is less important, since many preventative treatment options are the same.[3]

Complications of Stroke

Stroke is a leading cause of disability. Among stroke survivors, 20% require institutional care after 3 months, and up to 30% of survivors remain permanently disabled.[4] In a study of Medicare patients discharged from the hospital following a stroke, only 45% of patients were able to return home; 24% of patients were discharged to inpatient rehabilitation centers, and 31% were discharged to skilled nursing facilities.[5] Table 35-2 provides an overview of disabilities after stroke. The location of the stroke is also important, as resulting damage affects specific areas of the body (Figure 35-2).[6]

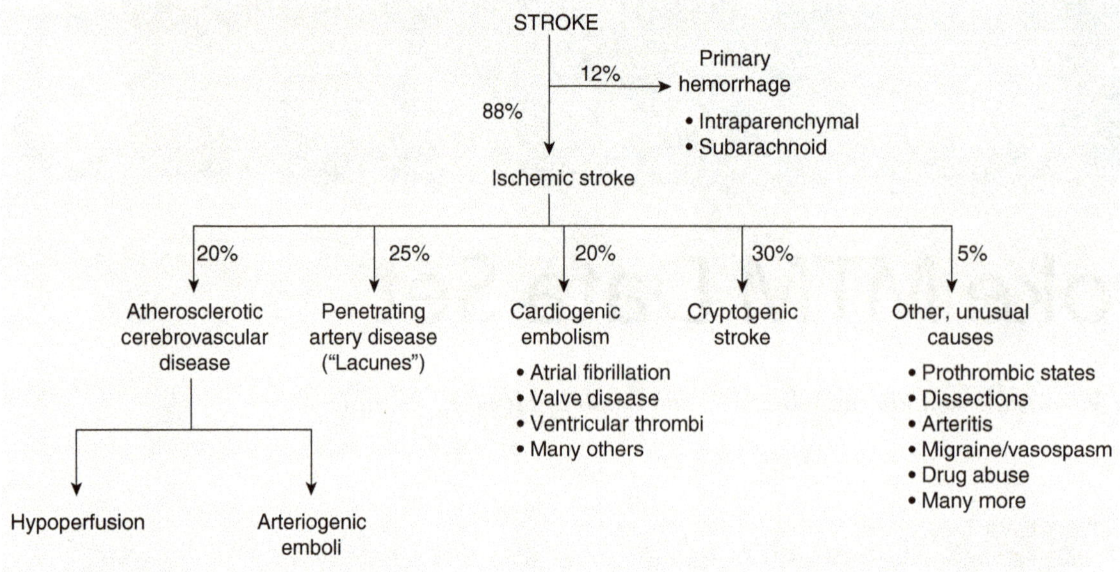

FIGURE 35-1 A classification of stroke by mechanism with estimates of the frequency of various categories of abnormalities. Approximately 30% of ischemic strokes are cryptogenic.

Source: Reproduced, with permission, from DiPiro JT, Talbert RL, Yee GC, Matzke GR, Wells BG, Posey L, eds. *Pharmacotherapy: A Pathophysiologic Approach.* 8th ed. New York, NY: McGraw-Hill; 2011.

TABLE 35-1 • Risk Factors for Ischemic Stroke

Nonmodifiable Risk Factors or Risk Markers
Age Low birth weight Race Genetic factors
Modifiable, Well Documented
Cigarette smoking Hypertension Diabetes Asymptomatic carotid stenosis Dyslipidemia Atrial fibrillation Sickle cell disease Poor diet Obesity Physical inactivity Other cardiac diseases (coronary heart disease, heart failure, PAD)
Potentially Modifiable, Less Well Documented
Migraine Metabolic syndrome Drug and alcohol abuse Inflammation and Infection Elevated Lp(a) Homocysteinemia Sleep-disordered breathing

Abbreviations: Lp(a)= lipoprotein(a); PAD= peripheral arterial disease.

Source: Reproduced, with permission, from DiPiro JT, Talbert RL, Yee GC, Matzke GR, Wells BG, Posey L, eds. *Pharmacotherapy: A Pathophysiologic Approach.* 10th ed. New York, NY: McGraw-Hill; 2017.

TABLE 35-2 • Stroke Complications—Incidence in Survivors

- Hemiparesis - 50%
- Inability to walk without assistance - 30%
- Cognitive deficit - 46%
- Depression - 35%
- Aphasia - 19%
- Dependence on others for activities of daily living - 26%

Source: References 6 and 7.

TABLE 35-3 • Therapeutic Goals for Secondary Stroke Prevention

Hypertension
- Elevated systolic and elevated diastolic blood pressures can increase risk of stroke
- Blood pressure reduction is recommended for all patients with ischemic stroke and TIA
- An absolute BP goal is uncertain; current guidelines suggest a systolic BP <140 mm Hg and a diastolic BP <90 mm Hg
- The risk of stroke is decreased more with larger decreases in BP
- Although the optimal drug therapy regimen is not known, data support diuretics +/- an angiotensin converting enzyme inhibitor

Diabetes
- Diabetes mellitus is a clear risk factor for stroke
- Adherence to current diabetes treatment guidelines for glucose control is necessary for stroke prevention (ie, achieving a hemoglobin A1c ≤7%)

Hyperlipidemia
- High-intensity statins are recommended to reduce the risk of stroke and cardiovascular events in patients with ischemic stroke/TIA of atherosclerotic origin with or without evidence for other ASCVD, and regardless of LDL-C (ie, > or <100 mg/dL)
- Patients with ischemic stroke/TIA and comorbid ASCVD should be managed according to current ACC/AHA cholesterol guidelines

Abbreviations: ACC/AHA = American College of Cardiology/American Heart Association; ASCVD = atherosclerotic cardiovascular disease; BP = blood pressure; LDL-C = low-density lipoprotein cholesterol; TIA = transient ischemic attack.

Source: References 3, 8, and 9.

> The most important modifiable risk factors for stroke are hypertension, diabetes, smoking, dyslipidemia, and atrial fibrillation

Therapeutic Goals for Stroke

Adherence to evidence-based therapies after a stroke reduces disability, prevents complications, decreases mortality, and prevents stroke recurrence. In addition to drug therapy, modification of risk factors is necessary to improve outcomes following a stroke. Table 35-3 provides an overview of secondary stroke prevention strategies.

Therapeutic Failures

Inability to afford medications, lack of transportation, lack of health insurance, lack of primary care provider, low income (< $20,000 annually), and out-of-pocket medical expenses of $2000.00 or more are all barriers to stroke care.[10] Compliance with blood pressure-lowering medications, statins, antiplatelet or anticoagulant therapies, diabetes medications, and improvements in lifestyle can certainly help prevent a second stroke—but not always. Unfortunately, data is limited for patients who are on the right medicine but have the misfortune of a recurrent stroke. For example:

1. A patient on aspirin has an ischemic stroke. There is no data to support increasing the dose of aspirin. There is no data to support switching from one antiplatelet agent to another (ie, aspirin to clopidogrel). While the addition of clopidogrel to aspirin may be indicated after a minor ischemic stroke or TIA, this combination should be continued for only 21 days. The combination of aspirin and clopidogrel is associated with an increased risk of bleeding and is therefore not recommended for long-term use.[3]
2. A patient on warfarin with a therapeutic INR has a stroke. There is no data to support adding aspirin or clopidogrel to warfarin therapy.[11] Only for patients with mechanical heart valves, who have a stroke while on therapeutic warfarin, is there evidence to support adding 75 to 325 mg of daily aspirin.[3,12]
3. For patients on aspirin who have a noncardioembolic stroke, data support the addition of dipyridamole.[13,14]

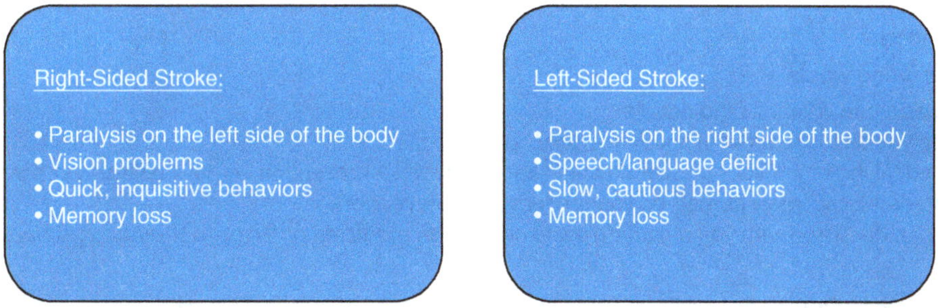

FIGURE 35-2 Complications of stroke by location.[6]

CORE ELEMENT 1—COMPREHENSIVE MEDICATION REVIEW FOR PATIENTS WITH STROKE

The following is a list of suggested questions to use when conducting a medication therapy review in a patient with stroke (Table 35-4). The number and types of questions will depend upon several factors, including the amount of time for the interview, number of concurrent medication-related problems (MRPs), urgency of MRPs, and the reliability of the patient in providing accurate information, among others. In time-limited interactions or in complex cases with multiple medical issues, the MTM provider may choose to target questions that help to identify or rule out issues of an urgent nature (see "Questions to Ask for Prevention/Assessment of Medical Emergencies" in Table 35-4). MTM providers should remember to use living room language during the interview (Figure 35-3) and be prepared for questions that patients may ask regarding stroke or stroke prevention therapy (Table 35-5).

CORE ELEMENT 2—PERSONAL MEDICATION LIST

The following is a sample personal medication list (PML) for a patient with stroke (Figure 35-4).[15] Additional medications for other disease states should be added and listed separately. MTM providers should remember to use plain language when creating the PML.

CORE ELEMENT 3—MEDICATION ACTION PLAN

The following is a sample medication action plan (MAP) for a patient with stroke (Figure 35-5).[15] This example is representative only of action steps for the patient with stroke. MAPs for other disease states or other MRPs should be added and listed separately. In general, only a few of the most important action steps should be listed so as not to overwhelm the patient. Other areas for patient self-management can be addressed at later visits. MTM providers should remember to use plain language when creating the MAP.

CORE ELEMENT 4—INTERVENTION AND/OR REFERRAL

Interventions for secondary prevention of stroke include lifestyle modifications and drug therapy. Table 35-6 summarizes lifestyle modifications, and Table 35-7 reviews nonpharmacologic therapies for stroke prevention. Medications should be selected on the basis of evidence and patient characteristics such as renal function, compelling disease states (eg, diabetes, cardiovascular disease), bleeding risk, and cost. All patients with a history of stroke should be on antihypertensive therapy and a statin (Table 35-3). Patients with a history of diabetes and stroke should be managed to achieve optimal glucose control. For patients with a history of noncardioembolic stroke, some type of antiplatelet therapy is required. Patients with a history of cardioembolic stroke—most often secondary to atrial fibrillation—should receive anticoagulation with a vitamin K antagonist, a direct thrombin inhibitor, or a factor Xa inhibitor. Table 35-8 provides details regarding drug therapy for stroke prevention, while Table 35-9 focuses on appropriate use of antithrombotic therapy after a stroke. Herbal supplements that have been used in stroke prevention are outlined in Table 35-10. Lastly, Figure 35-6 highlights emergency situations that require referral of stroke patients.

TABLE 35-4 • Questions to Ask When Conducting a Medication Review in a Patient with Stroke

Suggested Questions for the Patient With Stroke

• When did you have a stroke?
• How many stroke events have you had?
• Who else in your family has a history of stroke?
• What do you know about the health risks associated with stroke?
• What do you know about health conditions and lifestyle choices associated with increasing your risk of stroke?
• Have you ever experienced the following signs/symptoms of stroke?
  • Paralysis and/or numbness of face, arm, or leg on one side of body
  • Trouble walking
  • Dizziness
  • Severe, sudden headache
  • Trouble speaking, slurring words
  • Vision problems, blackened vision, seeing double
• What medications are you taking to prevent another stroke?
• Have you ever stopped taking any of your prescribed medications for stroke prevention without telling your physician? If so, why?
• What over-the-counter medications or herbals do you use for stroke prevention?
• What has your physician discussed with you regarding over-the-counter medications that you should avoid because they can increase your risk of stroke?

Questions to Ask for Prevention/Assessment of Medical Emergencies
• Crisis planning: What are the warning signs of a stroke, and what is your action plan? • Have you experienced sudden one-sided paralysis or numbness, severe headache, dizziness, trouble walking, speaking, or seeing? • Have you ever been hospitalized because of a stroke?

ACE inhibitor—a medicine used to help lower blood pressure; may also help prevent changes or damage to the heart and kidney.
Acute coronary syndrome—term used to cover any symptoms caused by decreased blood flow to the heart, such as a heart attack or chest pain.
Adverse event—something bad that happens, bad reaction, unexplained or unwanted effects.
Aldosterone antagonists—these medicines lower blood pressure by causing the body to absorb less salt.
Alpha blocker—a medicine used to lower blood pressure; it works by relaxing blood vessels.
Aneurysm—widening or ballooning of a portion of a blood vessel carrying blood away from the heart that happens because of weakness in the wall of the blood vessel.
Angioedema—a rare side effect of ACE and ARBs and a medical emergency with rapid swelling of lips, tongue, and throat that may affect breathing.
Angiotensin II—a compound in the blood that causes the blood vessels to narrow, which increases blood pressure; ACE inhibitors and ARBs decrease the effects of angiotensin II on blood pressure.
Anticoagulant—a medication used to prevent stroke by reducing the body's ability to make blood clots.
Antihypertensive medication—a medicine that lowers blood pressure.
Antiplatelet—a medication used to prevent stroke by reducing the action of platelets to decrease the formation of blood clots.
Aphasia—a language disorder resulting from a stroke that makes it hard for one to read, write, or speak.
ARB—a medicine used to help lower blood pressure; may also help prevent changes or damage to the heart and kidney.
Arrhythmia—irregular heartbeat, skipped heartbeat, heart problem; an example is atrial fibrillation.
Arteries—blood vessels that carry blood away from the heart.
Atherosclerosis—hardening or clogging of the arteries resulting from a buildup of fatty material; this could lead to decreased blood flow to important areas of the body and may cause a stroke.
Atrial fibrillation (a fib)—an irregular and often rapid heart rate that commonly causes poor blood flow to the body and is a risk factor for stroke.
β-blocker—a medicine used to help lower blood pressure and the rate the heart beats; works by decreasing the body's reaction to stress.
Blood glucose—blood sugar; since diabetes increases the risk of stroke, getting your glucose checked periodically is important.
BMI—body mass index; a measure of weight in relation to height that assigns people to a weight class of underweight, normal weight, overweight, or obese based on their amount of excess weight.
Bradycardia—a slow pace for the heart to beat, less than 60 times in a minute.
Calcium channel blocker—a medicine used to lower blood pressure or treat chest pain; works by decreasing the force of the heart pumping and relaxing blood vessels.
Cardiac—related to the heart.
Cardiologist—heart physician.
Chronic—constant, never ending, does not go away.
Chronic kidney disease—when the kidneys are not able to work well, which may cause high blood pressure and other serious health problems.
Coronary artery disease—narrowing and hardening of the small blood vessels that supply blood and oxygen to the heart because of a buildup of cholesterol, which may lead to a heart attack and is the leading cause of death worldwide.
Creatinine—a test that checks how well the kidneys are working; an increase means the kidneys are not working as well.
DASH diet—a diet high in fruits, vegetables, and low-fat dairy products, which is proven to lower blood pressure.
Diastolic—the bottom blood pressure number, smaller number; the pressure in the arteries when the heart relaxes.
Direct renin inhibitor—a medicine used to lower blood pressure by decreasing the activity of renin, which is a substance in the body that may lead to increases in blood pressure.
Direct vasodilator—a medicine used to lower blood pressure; it works by relaxing blood vessels.
Diuretic—water pill.
Edema—swelling because of the buildup of too much liquid.
EKG—a test that looks for any damage to or problems with your heart; measures the electrical activity of the heart.
Electrolytes—a type of necessary salt found in blood, such as salt, potassium, and calcium.
Elevate—raise, make higher.
Essential or primary hypertension—high blood pressure without a known cause.
Fasting lipid panel—a test of the fats in your blood taken after 8-12 hours without eating any food because the test results can change depending on what you eat.
Heart rate—how many times your heart beats each minute.
Hematocrit—a blood test looking at the amount of red blood cells you have; a very low amount could be a sign of anemia.
Hemiplegia—paralysis of one half of the body due to a stroke.
Hemorrhagic stroke—a stroke caused by a ruptured blood vessel.
Hyperkalemia—high potassium; very high potassium is a medical emergency and could cause a deadly change in the way your heart beats.
Hypertension—high blood pressure that increases the chance of heart attack, stroke, and kidney disease.
Hypertensive crisis—a combination of very high blood pressure and the shutdown of a major part of the body such as the brain, heart, or kidneys, which is a medical emergency.
Hypokalemia—low potassium, which may cause muscle weakness and cramping.
Hypotension—low blood pressure.
Ischemic stroke—a stroke caused by a clot or other blockage within blood vessels.
Lifestyle changes—recommended changes in lifestyle to lower your risk of stroke, which includes reaching a goal weight, decreasing the amount of alcohol you consume, exercising, or quitting smoking.
Low sodium diet—a diet with less than 2 grams (2000 milligrams) of salt each day, which may lower blood pressure and may be beneficial to people with heart problems or kidney disease.
Obese—having a body mass index (BMI) over 30, which increases your risk of having high blood pressure, diabetes, and cardiovascular disease.
Oral contraceptives—birth control medicine, may be a cause of stroke.
Orthostatic hypotension—dizziness or lightheadedness upon standing because of low blood pressure.
Overweight—having a body mass index (BMI) over 25, which increases your risk of having high blood pressure, diabetes, and heart disease.
Prehypertension—you may have high blood pressure in the future; the top number is 120-139 or the bottom number is 80-89.
Renin—a substance in the body that may lead to increases in blood pressure.
Serum potassium—a test to check the amount of potassium in your blood (see hyperkalemia and hypokalemia).
Smoking cessation—quitting smoking, which can lower your chance of heart disease.
Sodium—Salt, which can increase blood pressure if consumed.
Stage 1 hypertension—high blood pressure, where the top number is 140-159 or the bottom number is 90-99.
Stage 2 hypertension—very high blood pressure, where the top number is above 159 or the bottom number is above 99.
Stroke—a condition caused by bleeding or lack of blood in the brain, which may cause a loss of speech, memory, or other abilities.
Systolic—the top blood pressure number, the larger number; the pressure in the arteries when the heart contracts.
Tachycardia—a fast pace for the heart to beat, more than 100 times in a minute.
Topically—apply to the skin.
Transient ischemic attack (TIA)—similar symptoms to a stroke, but lasting less than 24 hours; often resolves within minutes and without permanent damage.
Veins—blood vessels that carry blood toward the heart.

FIGURE 35-3 Living room language for stroke.

TABLE 35-5 • Questions to Anticipate Regarding Stroke

- **What is a stroke?**
  A stroke is an incident in which the blood supply to the brain is reduced or blocked, resulting in damage to brain cells and reduction in certain functions for more than 24 hours.
- **What causes a stroke?**
  There are many factors that increase the risk of having a stroke. Risk factors that cannot be changed are age, African-American race, family history of stroke, male sex, and prior stroke, transient ischemic attack (TIA), or heart attack. Risk factors that can be changed or controlled are high blood pressure, cigarette smoking, diabetes, high cholesterol, sickle cell disease, carotid artery disease, coronary artery disease, peripheral artery disease, atrial fibrillation, heart failure, poor diet, obesity, and lack of physical activity.
- **What health problems are associated with stroke?**
  Left- or right-sided paralysis, vision problems, memory loss, speech problems, depression, pain, behavioral changes, and death may result from a stroke.
- **Why are stroke prevention medications so important?**
  It is important to control potential health problems that contribute to your risk of having a stroke. Medications can help reduce risks such as high blood pressure, diabetes, heart failure, atrial fibrillation, and other health conditions that can greatly increase your risk of stroke if left uncontrolled.
- **Can I just stop my medications if I feel okay?**
  Many medications that reduce risk of stroke may not have an effect that you can feel, but they are still doing their job. It is extremely important that you continue taking these medications to prevent future strokes.
- **When should I call my physician?**
  Seek immediate medical attention (Call 911) if you notice any signs or symptoms of a stroke, even if they are not constant or go away. Time is an important factor, and the longer a stroke goes untreated, the higher the chance of having permanent and severe brain damage and disability.
- **What should I do if I have a problem with my medications?**
  Never stop taking your stroke prevention medications without first talking to your physician. Speak with your physician and/or pharmacist to let them know about any problems you are having, and together you can make sure your medications are the right ones for you.

PERSONAL MEDICATION LIST FOR *<Insert Patient's name*, DOB: *mm/dd/yyyy>*	
Medication: Plavix (clopidogrel) 75 mg tablet	
How I use it: Take one tablet (75 mg) every morning	
Why I use it: To prevent stroke (anti-platelet/blood thinner)	**Prescriber:** Jones
Date I started using it: 10/27/2016	**Date I stopped using it:** *(Leave blank for patient's notes)*
Why I stopped using it: *(Leave blank for patient's notes)*	
Medication: Lozol (indapamide) 5 mg tablet	
How I use it: Take one tablet (5 mg) every morning	
Why I use it: Blood pressure/water pill; low blood pressure reduces risk of stroke	**Prescriber:** Jones
Date I started using it: 10/27/2016	**Date I stopped using it:** *(Leave blank for patient's notes)*
Why I stopped using it: *(Leave blank for patient's notes)*	

FIGURE 35-4 Example personal medication list for stroke medications.

<table>
<tr><td colspan="2" align="right">DATE PREPARED: <Insert date></td></tr>
<tr><td colspan="2">What we talked about:
You have a history of stroke. It is important to develop a stroke prevention plan consisting of medical treatment and lifestyle changes to reduce your chance of another stroke.</td></tr>
<tr><td>What I need to do:
Here are some things I can do to help reduce my risk of stroke:
• Speak with my providers about what risk factors I have for having another stroke.
• Develop a plan to control my risk factors with lifestyle changes and/or medications.
• Inform my family and friends to contact emergency medical services if I am experiencing symptoms of stroke and I am unable to do so.</td><td>What I did and when I did it:
(Leave blank for patient's notes)</td></tr>
<tr><td colspan="2"></td></tr>
<tr><td colspan="2">What we talked about:
It is important to recognize the signs and symptoms of stroke to know when to seek medical attention.</td></tr>
<tr><td>What I need to do:
• Learn to identify signs and symptoms of stroke, and inform my friends and family of the warning signs.
• Seek medical attention if I experience any of the following signs and symptoms:
  • Paralysis and/or numbness of face, arm, or leg on one side of body
  • Trouble walking
  • Dizziness
  • Severe, sudden headache
  • Trouble speaking, slurring words
  • Vision problems, blackened vision, seeing double</td><td>What I did and when I did it:
(Leave blank for patient's notes)</td></tr>
</table>

FIGURE 35-5 Example medication action plan for a patient with stroke.

TABLE 35-6 • Lifestyle Modifications for Management of Stroke

Modification	Recommendation
Cigarette smoking	Cigarette smoking and exposure to second hand smoke can increase stroke risk. Patients should be encouraged to quit smoking with counseling, nicotine replacement products, or prescription medications.
Nutrition	Consume a diet rich in fruits, vegetables, and low-fat dairy products with a reduction in dietary cholesterol, saturated fat, and total fat content. Dietary sodium should be reduced to ≤100 mmol per day (2.4 grams of sodium). Ideally, patients should consume <1.5 grams of salt per day. Routine supplementation with vitamins is not recommended.
Physical activity	Engage in regular aerobic physical activity (brisk walking) at least 30 minutes per day most days of the week. If there is disability present secondary to stroke, then supervised physical therapy or cardiac rehabilitation is recommended.
Alcohol consumption	Heavy drinking/alcoholism increases stroke risk. Limiting alcohol as follows is reasonable: Men: ≤2 drinks/day Women and lighter persons: ≤1 drink/day Of note, 1 drink equals 12 oz beer, 5 oz wine, or 1.5 oz of 80-proof whiskey.

Source: Reference 3.

TABLE 35-7 • Nonpharmacologic Considerations for Stroke

Rehabilitation	Physical therapy, occupational therapy, speech therapy, audiology, recreational therapy, psychiatric support, social work consultation, patient/family education programs, and patient/family support groups are all part of a comprehensive stroke rehabilitation program.
Surgery	Carotid endarterectomy—removal of atherosclerotic plaque from a blocked carotid artery Carotid stenting—use of balloon angioplasty or stents to open the carotid artery
Sleep apnea	A sleep study may be considered for patients with a history of stroke/TIA, given the high prevalence of sleep apnea in this population. Treatment of sleep apnea with continuous positive airway pressure (CPAP) is associated with improved outcomes.

Source: References 3 and 7.

TABLE 35-8 • Medications for Management of Stroke Prevention

Medication Class and Example Drugs	Common/Serious Side Effects[a]	Blackbox Warnings/ Contraindications	Pregnancy Category[b]
Aldosterone antagonists eplerenone spironolactone	Hyperkalemia Increase in SCr and liver enzymes Diarrhea Cough Fatigue Dizziness	• Anuria • Spironolactone: CrCl <10 mL/min • Eplerenone: CrCl <50 mL/min • Serum K >5.5 mEq/L • Type 2 diabetes with microalbuminuria	C
Angiotensin converting enzyme inhibitors (ACEI) benazepril enalapril fosinopril lisinopril ramipril	Angioedema Chronic dry cough Orthostatic hypotension Headache Hyperkalemia Hypotension Dizziness Fatigue	• Pregnancy • Angioedema • ACE inhibitor hypersensitivity	D
Angiotensin II receptor blockers (ARB) candesartan losartan valsartan	Dizziness Hypotension Diarrhea	• Pregnancy	D
β-blockers (BB) atenolol bisoprolol metoprolol propranolol	Mask hypoglycemia in diabetics May worsen insulin sensitivity, breathing disorders, and PVD Bradycardia Dizziness Exercise intolerance Fatigue Orthostatic hypotension (especially mixed α- and β-blockers)	• Abrupt discontinuation • Asthma (avoid nonselective BB) • AV block • Bradycardia • Cardiogenic shock • Heart failure (except bisoprolol, carvedilol, metoprolol succinate) • Hypotension • Pheochromocytoma (if not on α-blocker) • Sick sinus syndrome	D (atenolol) C (all others)
Calcium channel blockers (CCB)—dihydropyridines amlodipine felodipine nifedipine	Dizziness Flushing Gingival hyperplasia Headache Nausea Peripheral edema Postural hypotension Reflex tachycardia	• Dihydropyridine hypersensitivity • Avoid short-acting dihydropyridines to treat hypertension (ie, immediate-release nifedipine or nicardipine)	C
Calcium channel blockers (CCB)—nondihydropyridines diltiazem verapamil	Bradycardia Headache (diltiazem) Nausea (diltiazem) Constipation (verapamil)	• Acute MI • AV block • Cardiogenic shock • Hypotension • Heart failure/left ventricular systolic dysfunction • Sick sinus syndrome • Ventricular tachycardia • Wolff-Parkinson-White syndrome	C
Central alpha-2 agonists clonidine methyldopa	Bradycardia/AV block Dizziness Headache Sedation Somnolence Xerostomia	Clonidine: • Labor • Abrupt discontinuation Methyldopa: • Hepatic disease • Hepatitis • MAOI therapy	C

(Continued)

TABLE 35-8 • Medications for Management of Stroke Prevention (*Continued*)

Medication Class and Example Drugs	Common/Serious Side Effects[a]	Blackbox Warnings/ Contraindications	Pregnancy Category[b]
Combined α- and β-blockers carvedilol labetalol	Orthostatic hypotension Dizziness Bradycardia Exercise intolerance Fatigue	• Abrupt discontinuation • Acute heart failure • Asthma • AV block • Bradycardia • Cardiogenic shock • Severe hepatic disease • Sick sinus syndrome	C
Direct renin inhibitor aliskiren	Angioedema Cough Diarrhea Dizziness Headache Hyperkalemia Hypotension	• Pregnancy	D
Direct vasodilators hydralazine minoxidil	Headache Weakness Nausea Constipation Swelling of lower legs Tachycardia <u>Minoxidil</u>: excessive hair growth, fluid accumulation, atrial arrhythmias	Hydralazine: • Coronary artery disease • Rheumatic heart disease Minoxidil: • Angina • Cardiac tamponade • Pericardial effusion • Pheochromocytoma	C
Loop diuretics bumetanide furosemide torsemide	Hyperuricemia Hypomagnesemia Hypokalemia Hypocalcemia Hypochloremia Loss of appetite Bladder spasm Orthostatic hypotension Pancreatitis	• Anuria	C
Potassium-sparing diuretics amiloride triamterene	Hyperkalemia Hyperuricemia Nausea Vomiting Diarrhea Rash photosensitivity	• Hyperkalemia • Anuria • Renal failure • Severe liver disease	C
Thiazide diuretics chlorthalidone hydrocholorothiazide indapamide metolazone	Hypotension Hyperglycemia in diabetics Hypokalemia Hypercalcemia Hyponatremia Hypomagnesemia Hyperuricemia (at low doses) Azotemia (in renal disease)	• Anuria • Sulfonamide and thiazide diuretic hypersensitivity • CrCl <30 mL/min (except metolazone)	B
ADP receptor antagonist clopidogrel ticlopidine	Bleeding Fixed drug eruption Stevens-Johnson syndrome Colitis Gastrointestinal hemorrhage Agranulocytosis Aplastic anemia Pancytopenia Neutropenia Thrombotic thrombocytopenic purpura Hepatitis	Clopidogrel: • Poor metabolizers • Bleeding • GI bleeding • Intracranial bleeding Ticlopidine: • Anemia • Agranulocytosis • Neutropenia • Hematological disease	B

(*Continued*)

TABLE 35-8 • Medications for Management of Stroke Prevention (*Continued*)

Medication Class and Example Drugs	Common/Serious Side Effects[a]	Blackbox Warnings/ Contraindications	Pregnancy Category[b]
	Hepatotoxicity Liver failure Epidural hematoma Intracranial hemorrhage	• Thrombocytopenia • Thrombotic thrombocytopenic purpura	
ADP receptor antagonist clopidogrel ticlopidine	Intraocular hemorrhage Interstitial pneumonia Pulmonary edema Respiratory tract hemorrhage Drug withdrawal Rebound effect Rash Abdominal pain Diarrhea Indigestion Loss of appetite Nausea Dizziness	• Bleeding • Hepatic disease	
Antiplatelet salicylate aspirin	Gastrointestinal ulcer Bleeding Age-related macular degeneration Tinnitus Bronchospasm Angioedema Reye's syndrome	• Salicylate hypersensitivity	D
Antiplatelet salicylate/ vasodilator combination aspirin/extended-release dipyridamole	Abdominal pain Diarrhea Indigestion Bleeding Blood coagulation disorder Arthralgia Headache Stevens-Johnson syndrome Gastrointestinal hemorrhage Gastrointestinal perforation Gastrointestinal ulcer Intracranial hemorrhage Angioedema Reye's syndrome	• Reye's syndrome • Salicylate hypersensitivity • Viral infection	D
Factor Xa inhibitor fondaparinux	Injection site reaction Rash Fever Anemia Bleeding	• Epidural anesthesia • Lumbar puncture • Spinal anesthesia • Bleeding • Endocarditis • Renal failure • Thrombocytopenia	B
Low molecular weight heparin dalteparin enoxaparin	Diarrhea Hematoma Nausea Anemia Bleeding Thrombocytopenia Increased liver function tests Fever Eczematous drug eruption Skin necrosis Hemorrhage Intracranial hemorrhage Paraplegia Pneumonia	All: • Epidural anesthesia • Lumbar puncture • Spinal anesthesia • Bleeding • Heparin hypersensitivity • Porcine protein hypersensitivity Dalteparin: • Thrombocytopenia Enoxaparin: • Heparin-induced thrombocytopenia • Thrombocytopenia	B

(*Continued*)

TABLE 35-8 • Medications for Management of Stroke Prevention (*Continued*)

Medication Class and Example Drugs	Common/Serious Side Effects[a]	Blackbox Warnings/ Contraindications	Pregnancy Category[b]
Oral factor Xa inhibitor apixaban edoxaban rivaroxaban	Anemia Bleeding (gastrointestinal, vaginal, bruising) Hypersensitivity reaction Intracranial hemorrhage Intraocular hemorrhage Epidural hematoma	Apixaban: • Abrupt discontinuation • Bleeding • Epidural anesthesia • Lumbar puncture • Spinal anesthesia • Mechanical heart valves Edoxaban: • Abrupt discontinuation • Bleeding • Epidural anesthesia • Lumbar puncture • CrCL >95mL/min • Spinal anesthesia • Mechanical heart valves Rivaroxaban: • Bleeding • Abrupt discontinuation • Epidural anesthesia • Spinal anesthesia • Mechanical heart valves	B C C
Oral thrombin inhibitor dabigatran	Esophagitis Gastritis Gastroesophageal reflux disease Gastrointestinal hemorrhage Gastrointestinal ulcer Indigestion Bleeding Myocardial infarction Anaphylaxis Intracranial hemorrhage	• Bleeding • Mechanical heart valves	C
Vitamin K antagonist warfarin	Alopecia Cholesterol embolus syndrome Gangrenous disorder Tissue necrosis Hemorrhage Hypersensitivity reaction Compartment syndrome Intracranial hemorrhage Intraocular hemorrhage	• Bleeding • Alcoholism • Aneurysm • Aortic dissection • Dementia • Eclampsia • Endocarditis • Epidural anesthesia • GI bleeding • Head trauma • Hematological disease • Intracranial bleeding • Lumbar puncture • Pericardial effusion • Pericarditis • Preeclampsia • Pregnancy • Psychosis • Retinal bleeding • Spinal anesthesia • Stroke • Surgery	X

[a] This is a general list and does not include all side effects that can occur from these drugs. Consult a drug reference source for a more inclusive list before making any recommendations. MTM providers should also consult a comprehensive drug interaction database before making pharmacotherapy recommendations.

[b] Product labeling for all prescription drugs is being updated to reflect the new FDA Pregnancy Labeling and Lactation Rule. Please check individual product labeling for the most accurate and updated pregnancy information.

Abbreviations: AV = atrioventricular; CrCl = creatinine clearance; GI = gastrointestinal; K = potassium; MAOI = monoamine oxidase inhibitor; PVD = peripheral vascular disease; SCr = serum creatinine.

Source: Data compiled from reference 16.

TABLE 35-9 • Recommendations for Antithrombotic Therapy after a Stroke

Noncardioembolic Stroke
• Antiplatelet therapy is recommended over anticoagulant therapy • Four FDA-approved drugs are available: aspirin (ASA), aspirin + dipyridamole, clopidogrel, and ticlopidine • Because of issues with bone marrow toxicity, ticlopidine is rarely used • ASA 50-325 mg once daily, ASA 25 mg + dipyridamole 200 mg twice daily (Aggrenox®) or clopidogrel 75 mg once daily are all acceptable antiplatelet options • The combination of ASA and clopidogrel for secondary stroke prevention is not recommended because of increased risk of bleeding • Patients allergic to ASA can use clopidogrel instead
Cardioembolic Stroke
Atrial Fibrillation • Warfarin, dosed to achieve an INR between 2 and 3, apixaban 5 mg twice daily, dabigatran 150 mg twice daily, edoxaban 60 mg once daily, or rivaroxaban 20 mg once daily are all acceptable anticoagulant options • If patients are unable to tolerate warfarin, ASA may be used • The combination of ASA and clopidogrel is not recommended because of increased risk of bleeding **Valvular Disease** • Rheumatic mitral valve disease—warfarin dosed to achieve an INR between 2 and 3 • Nonrheumatic mitral valve disease or aortic valve disease – antiplatelet therapy **Prosthetic Heart Valves** • Aortic heart valves—warfarin treated to an INR between 2 and 3 • Mitral heart valves—warfarin treated to an INR between 2.5 and 3.5 **Left Ventricular Thrombus** • Warfarin treated to an INR between 2 and 3 for at least 3 months

Abbreviations: ASA = acetylsalicylic acid, ie, aspirin; FDA = Food and Drug Administration; INR = international normalized ratio.

Source: References 3, 11, 17, 18, 19, 20, 21, 22, 23, 24, and 25.

TABLE 35-10 • Herbal Supplements for Stroke

Supplement	Typical Dose	Action	Considerations	Grade[a]	Cost[b]
Betel nut	2.125 g orally (usually chewed)	Cholinergic activity and central nervous system stimulation → improved functional status after stroke	Purported to help with stroke recovery Abused as a recreational drug because of CNS stimulation Constituents are potentially carcinogenic Not safe for human use when used chronically at high doses	Insufficient evidence	$$
Black pepper	100 microliters by inhalation	Improves the ability to swallow after having a stroke	FDA recognizes black pepper as safe for use in food; however, when used in high concentrations black pepper can irritate the esophagus	Insufficient evidence	$
Citicoline	500-2000 mg once or twice daily x 6 weeks	Intermediate for the synthesis of phosphatidyl-choline; may also assist in choline synthesis → Allows for neuro-protection	Generally recognized as safe and effective by the FDA Approved in Europe and Japan for treatment of head trauma and stroke	Possibly effective	$$
Folic acid	Males older than 13 years: 400 micrograms per day; Females older than 13 years: 400-600 micrograms per day	Prevention of stroke by lowering homocysteine	Stroke mortality has decreased since the enrichment of grain products with folate, but more research is needed to make any conclusion	Insufficient evidence	$

[a] Level of evidence: "likely effective"—this product has a very high level of reliable clinical evidence supporting its use for a specific indication. Products rated "likely effective" are generally considered appropriate to recommend; "possibly effective"—this product has some clinical evidence supporting its use for a specific indication; however, the evidence is limited by quantity, quality, or contradictory findings. Products rated "possibly effective" might be beneficial, but do not have enough high-quality evidence to be recommended for most people; "insufficient evidence" indicates that there is insufficient reliable scientific evidence to provide an effectiveness rating.

[b] Cost: $ = $10/month supply in the recommended dosage; $$ = $11-$20/month.

Source: Data compiled from reference 27.

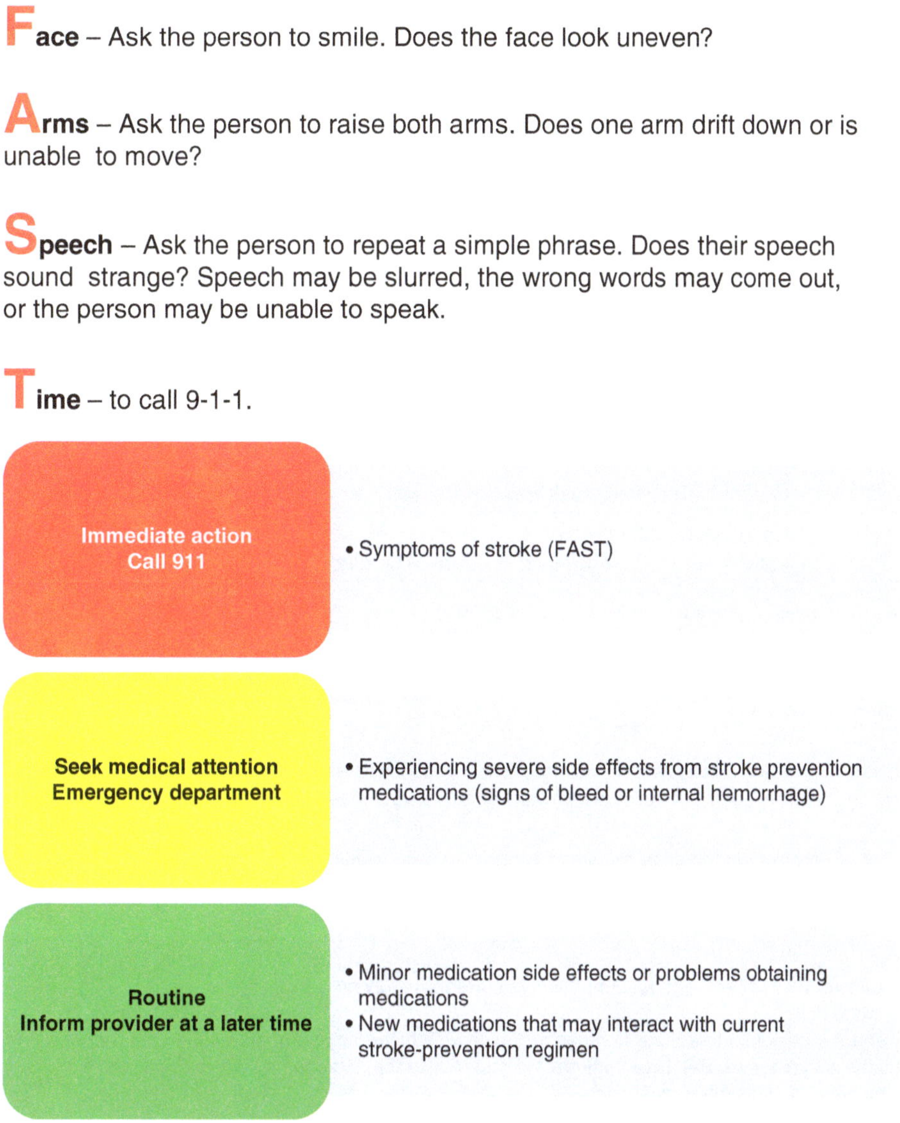

FIGURE 35-6 Warning signs of stroke (FAST) and referral for management of stroke.[28]

Providers often have the question of whether or not to hold antithrombotic medications for surgical procedures. Holding these medications in patients who are at high risk for another stroke is not recommended. For patients taking antiplatelet therapy, high-risk patients are those who have had a stroke within the last 3 to 6 months. For these patients, it is recommended to continue aspirin (or clopidogrel or Aggrenox) during the procedure, rather than stop antiplatelet therapy for 7 to 10 days prior to the procedure. (Note: If a patient is on both aspirin and clopidogrel because of placement of a coronary stent, then it is advised to hold off on any procedure until a later date or continue both agents during the procedure.) For patients taking warfarin, high-risk patients are those who have had a TIA or stroke within the last 3 months, have a CHA_2DS_2-VASc score of 5 or 6, or have a mechanical heart valve. For these patients, interruption of warfarin therapy could increase risk of stroke, so bridging with a low molecular weight heparin is recommended while off warfarin for the procedure.[26]

CORE ELEMENT 5—DOCUMENTATION AND FOLLOW-UP

Clear and succinct documentation of MRPs and recommendations is a key component of the MTM consult. Examples of potential MRPs in patients with stroke are provided in Table 35-11. Sample communications and recommendations to providers to address medication-related issues are found in Figure 35-7. Recommendations may be communicated via fax, phone, or other means of written or secure electronic communication. The examples are for illustrative purposes. Actual communications to providers should be individualized based on the type of recommendation, patient specific characteristics, and the nature of the relationship with the provider.

Follow-up to assess blood pressure, lipid panel, blood glucose, effects of interventions, and potential adverse effects is essential in patients with a history of stroke. The interval for follow-up will depend on a number of factors, including antithrombotic regimen, severity of stroke risk, type of intervention, and patient-specific factors such as age, comorbid conditions, and ability to return for follow-up. Suggested intervals for follow-up are provided in Table 35-12.

TABLE 35-11 • Medication-Related Problems (MRPs) in Patients with Stroke

Category of MRP	Example Medication-Related Problem
Nonadherence	• Suboptimal control of blood pressure because of nonadherence with lifestyle modifications (eg, restriction of salt, smoking cessation) • Suboptimal control of blood pressure because of patient missing doses of antihypertensive medication • Patient not taking antihypertensive, statin, diabetes, or antithrombotic medication because of cost
Unnecessary medication	• Duplicate therapy (eg, aspirin and clopidogrel without an approved indication for both)
Need for additional medication	• Monotherapy for hypertension with suboptimal blood pressure control • Patient with diabetes not at hemoglobin A1c goal • Patient with history of stroke not on antithrombotic therapy (ie, aspirin, clopidogrel or warfarin)
Ineffective medication	• Adequate trial of new antihypertensive without significant clinical response • Monotherapy with α-1 blocker, rather than evidence-based therapy
Dosage too low	• Suboptimal blood pressure control on low dose of antihypertensive agent • Low INR while on warfarin
Dosage too high	• Patient with elevated INR and nosebleeds
Adverse drug event	• Cough from ACE inhibitor • Patient not taking Aggrenox because of headache from dipyridamole

Abbreviations: ACE = angiotensin-converting enzyme; INR = international normalized ratio.

Scenario: Patient given prescription for Pradaxa but has stopped taking it because of upset stomach
MRP: Nonadherence, adverse drug event

• Assessment:
Patient with high risk for stroke on Pradaxa (dabigatran) 150 mg. Patient nonadherent with dabigatran because of adverse effects, particularly stomach upset. Switching dabigatran to another agent such as Xarelto (rivaroxaban) may decrease the likelihood of this adverse effect and increase compliance.

• Plan:
Consider discontinuation of Pradaxa and addition of Xarelto 20 mg daily with evening meal with follow-up to assess any adverse events.

Scenario: Patient with diabetes not at hemoglobin A1c goal
MRP: Need for additional medication

• Assessment:
Based on pharmacy claims and/or patient report, your patient is currently receiving:
  • Metformin 1000 mg twice daily
  Per patient record, at a high risk for stroke due to atrial fibrillation with diabetes and heart failure. Last reported A1c was 8.3%, above ADA goal of <7% for patients with diabetes. Because metformin is currently at the maximum effective dose, addition of a second medication such as a sulfonylurea may help bring patient to goal A1c.

• Plan:
If appropriate, please consider adding glipizide 5 mg daily and titrate based on serum glucose values to lower A1c to goal of <7%.

Scenario: Patient with elevated INR and nosebleeds
MRP: Dosage too high

• Assessment:
Patient is currently taking warfarin 7.5 mg daily for stroke prevention because of atrial fibrillation and CHA_2DS_2-VASc score of 3. INR has been between 3.5 and 3.9 at last three office visits (goal 2-3). Patient is complaining of nosebleeds. Because INR is elevated and patient is experiencing bleeding, a decrease in the dose of warfarin is warranted.

• Plan:
Consider decreasing total weekly warfarin dose by approximately 15% (7.5 mg) to bring INR to therapeutic range and decrease risk of bleeding events. Follow up with patient in 1 to 2 weeks to reassess INR and any complaints of bleeding.

Scenario: Patient with history of stroke not on antithrombotic therapy
MRP: Need for additional medication

• Assessment:
Patient reports having a stroke 2 years ago. Per pharmacy claims data, patient is not on an antithrombotic agent to decrease risk of another stroke. Addition of an antiplatelet agent such as aspirin or clopidogrel may decrease the risk of another stroke.

• Plan:
If appropriate, consider initiation of aspirin 81 mg daily to reduce risk of stroke in this patient. Monitor for signs and symptoms of bleeding events at follow-up visits.

FIGURE 35-7 Sample provider communications for stroke.

TABLE 35-12 • Suggested Intervals for Follow-up in Patients with Stroke

Anticoagulant monitoring
• Patients taking warfarin should have INR monitored every 1 to 2 weeks until within therapeutic range consistently. Follow-up time may be lengthened in well-controlled patients.
• No routine anticoagulation monitoring is necessary for the direct oral anticoagulants, although patients should follow up with providers at regular intervals for assessment of bleeding and compliance. Checking renal function and a complete blood count at least twice per year is reasonable.
Blood pressure response
• Measure 2 to 4 weeks after initiating or making changes in therapy.
• After blood pressure goal is met and blood pressure is stable, assuming no signs or symptoms of acute target-organ disease are present, patients should be monitored every 3 to 6 months.
• Patients with stage 2 hypertension, comorbid conditions, history of poor control, nonadherence, progressive target-organ damage, or symptoms of adverse drug effects should be followed more frequently.
Diabetes management
• Perform hemoglobin A1c test at least 2 times a year in patients who are meeting treatment goals (and who have stable glycemic control).
• Perform hemoglobin A1c test quarterly in patients whose therapy has changed or who are not meeting glycemic goals.
Dyslipidemia management
• Measure fasting lipid profile 4 to 12 weeks after statin initiation to determine adherence.
• Thereafter, lipid assessment may be repeated every 3 to 12 months as clinically indicated.
Toxicity
• Monitor for adverse drug effects 2 to 4 weeks after starting a new agent or dose increase. Monitor adverse bleeding events resulting from anticoagulants at each visit.
• Monitor adverse events every 6 to 12 months in stable patients.
• Serum potassium and creatinine should be monitored 1 to 2 times each year.

Abbreviation: INR = international normalized ratio.

Source: References 3, 8, and 9.

REFERENCES

1. Davis SM, Donnan GA. Secondary prevention after ischemic stroke or transient ischemic attack. *New Engl J Med.* 2012;366:1914-1922.
2. Benjamin EJ, Blaha MJ, Chiuve SE, et al. Heart disease and stroke statistics 2017 update: a report from the American Heart Association. *Circulation.* 2017;135(10):e229-e268.
3. Walter NK, Ovbiagele BO, Black HR, et al. Guidelines for the prevention of stroke in patients with stroke and transient ischemic attack: a guideline for healthcare professionals from the American Heart Association/American Stroke Association. *Stroke.* 2014;45(7):2160-2236.
4. Meschia JF, Bushnell CD, Boden-Albala B, Scaramucci A, D'Agostino RB, Wolf PA. Guidelines for the primary prevention of stroke: a statement for healthcare professionals from the American Heart Association/American Stroke Association. *Stroke.* 2014;45(12):3754-3832.
5. Buntin MB, Colla CH, Deb P, Sood N, Escarce JJ. Medicare spending and outcomes after postacute care for stroke and hip fracture. *Med Care.* 2010;48(9):776-784.
6. Kelly-Hayes M, Beiser A, Kase CS, Scaramucci A, D'Agostino RB, Wolf PA. The influence of gender and age on disability following ischemic stroke: The Framingham Study. *J Stroke Cerebrovasc Dis.* 2003;12(3):119-126.
7. Fagan SC, Hess DC. Stroke. In: DiPiro JT, Talbert RL, Yee GC, Matzke GR, Wells BG, Posey L, eds. *Pharmacotherapy: A Pathophysiologic Approach.* 10th ed. New York, NY: McGraw-Hill; 2017. http://accesspharmacy.mhmedical.com/content.aspx?bookid=1861&sectionid=132515962. Accessed May 08, 2017.
8. American Diabetes Association. Standards of medical care in diabetes—2017. *Diabetes Care.* 2017;40(suppl 1):S1-S135.
9. Stone NJ, Robinson JG, Lichtenstein AH, et al. 2013 ACC/AHA guideline on the treatment of blood cholesterol to reduce atherosclerotic cardiovascular risk in adults: a report of the American College of Cardiology/American Heart Association Task Force on practice guidelines. *Circulation.* 2014;129:S1-S45.
10. Wolf PA, Abbott RD, Kannel WB. Atrial fibrillation as an independent risk factor for stroke: the Framingham Study. *Stroke.* 1991;22(8):983-988.
11. You JJ, Stinger DE, Howard PA, et al. Antithrombotic therapy for atrial fibrillation; antithrombotic therapy and prevention of thrombosis, 9th ed. American College of Chest Physicians evidence-based clinical practice guidelines. *Chest.* 2012;141(2 suppl):e531S-e575S.
12. Turpie AGG, Gent M, Laupacis A, et al. Aspirin and warfarin after heart-valve replacement: a comparison of aspirin with placebo in patients treated with warfarin after heart-valve replacement. *New Engl J Med.* 1993;329(8):524-529.
13. Diener HC, Cunha L, Forbes C, Sivenius J, Smets P, Lowenthal A. European stroke prevention study 2: dipyridamole and acetylsalicylic acid in the secondary prevention of stroke. *J Neurol Sci.* 1996;143(1-2):1-13.
14. ESPRIT Study Group. Aspirin plus dipyridamole versus aspirin alone after cerebral ischaemia of arterial origin (ESPRIT): randomised controlled trial. *Lancet.* 2006;367(9523):1665-1673.
15. CMS. *Medicare Part D Medication Therapy Management Program Standardized Format.* Available at http://www.cms.gov/Medicare/Prescription-Drug-Coverage/PrescriptionDrugCovContra/Downloads/MTM-Program-Standardized-Format-Revisions-v071514-[ZIP-2MB].zip. Accessed May 7, 2017.
16. Clinical Pharmacology [database online]. Tampa, FL: Gold Standard, Inc.; 2017. Available at http://www.clinicalpharmacology.com. Accessed May 7, 2017.
17. Diener H-C, Bogousslavsky J, Brass LM, et al. Aspirin and clopidogrel compared with clopidogrel alone after ischemic stroke or transient ischemic attack in high-risk patients (MATCH): randomised, double-blind, placebo controlled trial. *Lancet.* 2004;364(9431):331-337.
18. Bhatt DL, Fox KAA, Hacke W, et al. [CHARISMA investigators] Clopidogrel and aspirin versus aspirin alone for the prevention of atherothrombotic events. *New Engl J Med.* 2006;354:1706-1717.
19. Kennedy J, Hill MD, Ryckborst KJ, et al. Fast assessment of stroke and transient ischaemic attack to prevent early recurrence (FASTER): a randomized controlled pilot trial. *Lancet Neurol.* 2007;6(11):961-969.
20. Connolly SJ, Ezekowitz MD, Yusuf S, et al. Dabigatran versus warfarin in patients with atrial fibrillation. *New Engl J Med.* 2009;361:1139-1151.

21. Patel MR, Mahaffey KW, Garg J, et al. Rivaroxaban versus warfarin in nonvalvular atrial fibrillation. *New Engl J Med.* 2011;365:883-891.
22. Granger CB, Alexander JH, McMurray JJV, et al. Apixaban versus warfarin in patients with atrial fibrillation. *New Engl J Med.* 2011;365:981-992.
23. Giugliano RP, Ruff CT, Braunwald E, et al. Edoxaban versus warfarin in patients with atrial fibrillation. *New Engl J Med.* 2013;369:2093-2104.
24. ACTIVE Writing Group of the ACTIVE Investigators; Connolly S, Pogue J, Hart R, et al. Clopidogrel plus aspirin versus oral anticoagulation for atrial fibrillation in the atrial fibrillation clopidogrel trial with irbesartan for prevention of vascular events (ACTIVE W): a randomised controlled trial. *Lancet.* 2006;367(9526):1903-1912.
25. Whitlock RP, Sun JC, Fremes SE, Rubens FD, Teoh KH. Antithrombotic and thrombolytic therapy for valvular disease: antithrombotic therapy and prevention of thrombosis, 9th ed: American College of Chest Physicians evidence-based clinical practice guidelines. *Chest.* 2012;141(2 suppl):e576S-e600S.
26. Eikelboom JW, Hirsh J, Spencer FA, Baglin TP, Weitz JI. Antiplatelet drugs: antithrombotic therapy and prevention of thrombosis, 9th ed: American College of Chest Physicians evidence-based clinical practice guidelines. *Chest.* 2012;141(2 suppl):e89S-e119S.
27. Natural Medicines [database online]. Somerville, MA: Therapeutic Research Center; 2017. Available at https://naturalmedicines.therapeuticresearch.com/. Accessed May 7, 2017.
28. American Heart Association. Heart attack or stroke? Call 911 first and fast. Available at http://www.heart.org/HEARTORG/Affiliate/Heart-Attack-or-Stroke-Call-911-First-And-Fast_UCM_435652_Article.jsp. Accessed May 7, 2017.

Review Questions

1. What is a modifiable risk factor for stroke?
   a. Age
   b. Gender
   c. Cigarette smoking
   d. Family history of stroke

2. A 70-year-old male patient has a history of stroke. Which factor would require intervention?
   a. A blood pressure reading of 130/80mmHg
   b. An LDL level of 150mg/dL
   c. Current weight equal to ideal body weight
   d. Two alcoholic beverages per week

3. A 75-year-old female is diagnosed with atrial fibrillation. She is prescribed warfarin for stroke prevention. Which range is most appropriate for the goal INR?
   a. 1.8-2.3
   b. 2.0-3.0
   c. 2.5-3.5
   d. 3.0-4.0

4. Using living room language, which definition best describes aphasia?
   a. The inability to perform communication skills effectively as the result of a previous stroke event.
   b. A disturbance of the comprehension and formulation of language caused by dysfunction in specific brain regions.
   c. A defect in the expression and comprehension of words caused by damage to the frontal and temporal lobes of the brain.
   d. A language disorder due to a stroke that makes it hard for one to read, write, or speak.

5. Which recommendation is appropriate to include in the MAP for a patient with history of stroke?
   a. Take aspirin every day.
   b. Inform your family and friends to contact emergency medical services if you are experiencing symptoms of stroke and are unable to do so.
   c. Lifestyle changes alone can reduce risk of stroke enough so that you do not have to take medications.
   d. The risk of having another stroke is greatly reduced after having a first stroke.

6. In which situation should a patient wait to inform his/her provider at the next office visit instead of seeking immediate action?
   a. Slurring speech or the inability to speak
   b. After raising both arms, one drifts down
   c. Receiving a new antibiotic that may interact with stroke-prevention medication
   d. Experiencing black, tarry stools and a stomach ache

7. Which medication-related problem is matched with the correct category of MRP?
   a. Nonadherence - patient with a history of stroke not on antithrombotic therapy
   b. Dosage too high - INR below goal while on warfarin
   c. Unnecessary medication - taking aspirin and clopidogrel without an approved indication for both
   d. Ineffective medication - patient on warfarin with INR above goal

8. Which statement is correct regarding lipid management in a patient who has a history of stroke?
   a. The goal LDL cholesterol is less than 70 mg/dL.
   b. High-intensity statins are indicated regardless of LDL cholesterol level.
   c. Niacin is indicated as first-line therapy.
   d. Statins are contraindicated during the first year after a stroke.

9. A patient who is taking aspirin has a noncardioembolic stroke. Which action is the most appropriate antiplatelet option for this patient?
   a. Switch to dipyridamole.
   b. Increase dose of aspirin.
   c. Add clopidogrel.
   d. Change to aspirin/dipyridamole.

10. A patient who was taking aspirin 81 mg daily had a minor stroke and is prescribed clopidogrel. The patient does not have atrial fibrillation. Which statement is correct regarding the combination of aspirin and clopidogrel in this patient?
    a. Clopidogrel should not be used with aspirin in this patient.
    b. Aspirin should be increased to 325 mg when clopidogrel is added.
    c. The combination of clopidogrel and aspirin may be used short term.
    d. Warfarin should be added to aspirin, rather than clopidogrel.

ANSWERS

1. c	2. b	3. b
4. d	5. b	6. c
7. c	8. b	9. d
10. c		

36

Thyroid Disorders MTM Data Set

Shannon A. Miller, PharmD, BCACP

KEY POINTS

- For patients with hypo- or hyperthyroidism, medication therapy management (MTM) providers should review the medication list for medications that may be contributing to thyroid dysfunction.
- MTM providers should be aware of and inquire about symptoms that may indicate under- or over-treatment of a thyroid condition. A thyroid function panel must confirm clinical suspicion.
- MTM providers should assess for conditions (eg, interacting medications or nonadherence) that may alter dosage requirements of thyroid medications.

INTRODUCTION TO THYROID DISORDERS

The thyroid normally synthesizes two thyroid hormones, thyroxine (T_4) and triiodothyronine (T_3), after glandular stimulation by thyroid-stimulating hormone (TSH).[1] Prior to this, thyrotropin-releasing hormone (TRH) produced by the hypothalamus stimulates the anterior pituitary to release TSH. This hypothalamic-pituitary-thyroid axis maintains thyroid hormone homeostasis through a negative feedback loop. That is, adequate thyroid hormone levels inhibit the release of TRH and TSH from the hypothalamus and pituitary, respectively (Figure 36-1).

Thyroid hormones regulate metabolism and affect essentially every organ system in the human body. T_4 is produced in greater amounts than T_3, but T_4 exhibits less biological activity. Production of T_3 occurs primarily through peripheral conversion of T_4 by deiodinase enzymes (80%), with approximately 20% of T_3 produced directly by the thyroid gland.[1]

Hyperthyroidism

Hyperthyroidism is a condition in which there is inappropriate synthesis and secretion of thyroid hormone (either T_3, T_4, or both) from the thyroid gland.[2,3,4] Thyroid hormone excess results either from overproduction (eg, Graves' disease, toxic multinodular goiter [TMNG], toxic adenoma) or, infrequently, thyroid inflammation (eg, thyroiditis). Graves' disease, an autoimmune disorder, accounts for 60% to 80% of cases of hyperthyroidism.

Other Terms Associated with Hyperthyroidism

- **Thyrotoxicosis** – a clinical state marked by inappropriately high thyroid hormone action in the peripheral tissues
  - Hyperthyroidism may cause thyrotoxicosis, but the terms are not synonymous
- **Thyroid storm** – a sudden and life-threatening condition with an increase in signs and symptoms of decompensated thyrotoxicosis, including fever greater than 102°F (38.8°C), tachycardia, tachypnea, nausea, vomiting, diarrhea, abdominal pain, and delirium
  - Usually precipitated by trauma, surgery, or infection
  - Arrhythmias, heart failure, ischemic heart disease, or coma may develop
  - Requires prompt treatment and hospitalization

Hypothyroidism

Hypothyroidism indicates a failure of the thyroid gland to produce or secrete adequate thyroid hormone to match the metabolic demands of the body.[5,6] Deficient thyroid hormone production

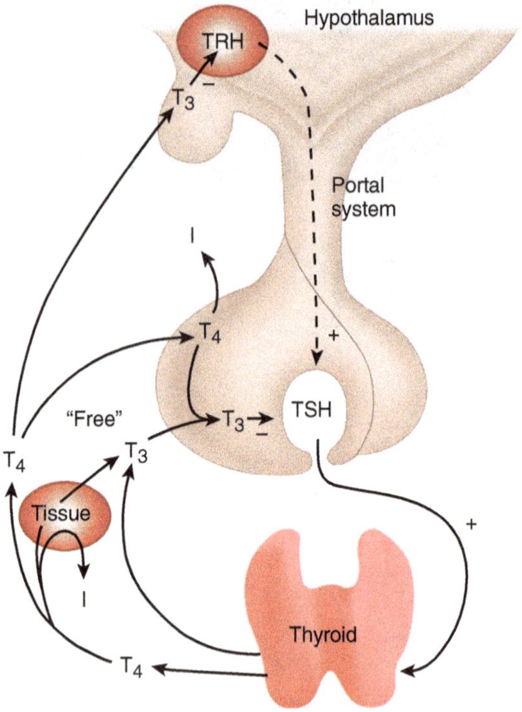

FIGURE 36-1 Hypothalamic-pituitary-thyroid hormone axis.
In both the hypothalamus and pituitary, 3,5′,3-triiodothyronine (T_3) is primarily responsible for inhibition of thyrotropin-releasing hormone (TRH) and thyroid-stimulating hormone (TSH) secretion.
Abbreviation: T_4 = thyroxine.
Source: Reproduced, with permission, from Brunicardi FC, Andersen DK, Billiar TR, et al. *Schwartz's Principles of Surgery.* 9th ed. New York: McGraw-Hill Publishing; 2010.

can be categorized as primary (an abnormality of the thyroid gland) or secondary (hypothalamic-pituitary dysfunction leading to insufficient stimulation of the thyroid gland). Chronic autoimmune thyroiditis (Hashimoto disease) is responsible for a majority of cases of primary disease, and it is the main etiology of hypothyroidism in the United States (Table 36-1). Secondary hypothyroidism is rare and accounts for approximately 1% of cases of hypothyroidism.

TABLE 36-1 • Causes of Hypothyroidism

Primary Hypothyroidism
Hashimoto disease
Iatrogenic hypothyroidism
Less Common
Iodine deficiency
Enzyme defects
Thyroid hypoplasia
Goitrogens
Secondary Hypothyroidism
Pituitary disease
Hypothalamic disease

Source: Reproduced, with permission, from DiPiro, JT, Talbert RL, Yee GC, Matzke GR, Wells BG, Posey LM, eds. *Pharmacotherapy: A Pathophysiologic Approach.* 10th ed. New York, NY: McGraw-Hill; 2017.

Complications of Thyroid Disorders

Hyperthyroidism. Excessive thyroid hormone levels can lead to cardiac problems (eg, atrial fibrillation, heart failure, myocardial infarction) or osteoporosis. Thyroid storm is a rare but serious condition that may develop in patients with hyperthyroidism.

Hypothyroidism. Left untreated, hypothyroidism may contribute to diastolic hypertension, hyperlipidemia, heart failure, infertility, cognitive impairment, and neuromuscular dysfunction. Rarely, myxedema coma may occur if hypothyroidism is inadequately treated. Myxedema coma is an extremely severe and potentially fatal manifestation of hypothyroidism characterized by mental status changes (eg, lethargy, cognitive dysfunction, psychosis), hypothermia, bradycardia, hypotension, hypoventilation, and hyponatremia.[1]

Diagnosis of Thyroid Disorders

Hyperthyroidism.[2,3,4] Patients with symptoms suggestive of hyperthyroidism (Table 36-2) should be referred for prompt evaluation of the serum TSH. Serum TSH will be low for patients with overt and subclinical hyperthyroidism, but a high free T_4 or free T_4 index (FT_4I) specifies overt disease (Table 36-3). If free T_4 or FT_4I are not elevated, a total or free T_3 test may be helpful because some patients with normal T_4 have elevated levels of T_3. Once the diagnosis of hyperthyroidism is confirmed, the etiology of the disease should be determined in order to guide treatment.

TABLE 36-2 • Clinical Signs and Symptoms of Thyroid Disorders

Hyperthyroidism	Hypothyroidism
Anxiety	Bradycardia
Diffuse or multinodular goiter	Coarse or thin hair
Difficulty sleeping	Cold intolerance
Dyspnea	Cold or dry skin
Emotional lability	Constipation
Exophthalmos (Graves' disease only)	Depression
Fatigue	Fatigue
Fine hair	Galactorrhea
Heat intolerance	Goiter
Hyperactive deep tendon reflexes	Hoarseness
Hyperdefecation	Menstrual irregularities
Menstrual irregularities	Muscle cramps
Nervousness	Myalgia
Palpitations	Peripheral edema
Proximal muscle weakness	Poor concentration
Sweating	Periorbital puffiness
Tachycardia	Slow relaxation of deep tendon reflexes
Weight loss (despite increased appetite)	Weakness
	Weight gain

Source: References 1, 3, and 6.

TABLE 36-3 • Thyroid Function Tests in Hyper- and Hypothyroidism

Category	TSH[a]	Free T_4[a]
Hyperthyroidism	low	high[b]
Subclinical hyperthyroidism	low	normal
Primary hypothyroidism	high	low
Secondary hypothyroidism	low-normal	low
Subclinical hypothyroidism	high	normal

[a] Reference ranges are specific to the laboratory where the assays are performed.

[b] Hyperthyroidism may be present if free T_4 is normal, but total or free T_3 is elevated.

Source: References 1, 2, 3, 4, 5, and 6.

Radioactive iodine uptake (RAIU) is most useful in differentiating between the major causes of thyrotoxicosis (Table 36-4); RAIU is increased when thyroid hormone is being overproduced, and RAIU is suppressed when thyrotoxicosis results from thyroid inflammation. Other diagnostic tests such as TSH-receptor antibodies (TRAb), thyroglobulin, and thyrotropin receptor antibodies may be helpful, particularly when radioisotope studies are contraindicated. Thyroid scans provide diagnostic value for thyroid nodular disease.

Patients with overt disease require treatment. Treatment is also appropriate for patients with TSH levels <0.1 mIU/L or those who are ≥65 years of age (or postmenopausal women not on estrogens or bisphosphonates). In addition, treatment is warranted for patients with cardiac risk factors, heart disease, osteoporosis, or hyperthyroid symptoms.

TABLE 36-4 • Differential Diagnosis of Thyrotoxicosis

Increased RAIU[a]	Decreased RAIU
TSH-induced hyperthyroidism	Inflammatory thyroid disease
TSH-secreting tumors	Subacute thyroiditis
Selective pituitary resistance to T_4	Painless thyroiditis
Thyroid stimulators other than TSH	Ectopic thyroid tissue
TSAb (Graves' disease)	Struma ovarii
hCG (trophoblastic diseases)	Metastatic follicular carcinoma
Thyroid autonomy	Exogenous sources of thyroid hormone
Toxic adenoma	Medications containing thyroid hormone or iodine
Multinodular goiter	Food sources containing thyroid gland

[a] The RAIU may be decreased if the patient has been recently exposed to excess iodine.

Abbreviations: hCG = human chorionic gonadotropin; RAIU = radioactive iodine uptake; TSAb = thyroid-stimulating antibodies; TSH = thyroid-stimulating hormone.

Source: Reproduced, with permission, from DiPiro, JT, Talbert RL, Yee GC, Matzke GR, Wells BG, Posey LM, eds. *Pharmacotherapy: A Pathophysiologic Approach.* 10th ed. New York, NY: McGraw-Hill; 2017.

Hypothyroidism. When symptoms suggest possible hypothyroidism (see Table 36-2), a serum TSH test should be ordered and, if elevated, should be followed by a serum free T_4 measurement.[5,6] An elevated TSH with a low serum free T_4 level indicates overt primary hypothyroidism. Free T_4 is within the reference range in patients with subclinical hypothyroidism (see Table 36-3). Measurement of antithyroid peroxidase antibodies (TPOAb) is helpful in patients with subclinical hypothyroidism because it predicts a higher risk of eventual progression to overt hypothyroidism. Treatment should be initiated in patients with serum TSH levels >10 mIU/L, regardless of symptoms, in order to avoid complications of the disease. Treatment may also be considered for patients with TSH levels between 5 and 10 mIU/L in addition to positive TPOAb, and patients with hypothyroid symptoms or evidence of atherosclerotic vascular disease or heart failure.

Table 36-5 provides an overview of medications that may alter thyroid status and necessitate increased monitoring or adjustment of thyroid medication. In a number of cases, the mechanisms behind alteration of thyroid hormone levels are unknown. For patients who are started on these medications, the MTM provider should monitor for signs or symptoms of thyroid disorders.

Goals of Treatment for Thyroid Disorders. The goal of therapy for all forms of thyroid disorders is restoration of the euthyroid state and elimination of symptoms. Treatment is necessary to reduce the risk of serious complications and improve quality of life for the patient.

CORE ELEMENT 1—COMPREHENSIVE MEDICATION REVIEW FOR PATIENTS WITH THYROID DISORDERS

The following is a list of suggested questions to ask a patient with hyper- or hypothyroidism during a medication therapy review (Table 36-6). MTM providers should use living room language

TABLE 36-5 • Medications that May Cause or Worsen Thyroid Disorders

Medication	Potential Effect
Amiodarone	Hypo- or hyperthyroidism
Bexarotene	Hypothyroidism
Ethionamide	Hypothyroidism
Interferon α	Hypo- or hyperthyroidism
Interleukin-2	Hypo- or hyperthyroidism
Iodine (including kelp supplements)	Hypo- or hyperthyroidism
Lithium	Hypo- or hyperthyroidism[a]
Thalidomide	Hypo- or hyperthyroidism
Tyrosine kinase inhibitors (sunitinib)	Hypo- or hyperthyroidism

[a] Hyperthyroidism is rare.

Source: References 2, 5, 7, and 8.

TABLE 36-6 • Questions to Ask When Conducting a Medication Review in a Patient with a Thyroid Disorder

Suggested Questions for the Patient with Hyperthyroidism	Suggested Questions for the Patient with Hypothyroidism

• How long have you had hyperthyroidism (overactive thyroid)?
• What medication(s) do you take for your thyroid condition?
  • How do you take the medication?
  • How long have you been taking your antithyroid medication? At the dose you are currently taking?
  • Do you take your antithyroid medication on an empty stomach or with food?
  • How often do you miss a dose of your antithyroid medication?
  • Have you ever stopped taking your prescribed antithyroid medication(s) without telling your physician? If so, why?
• Do you experience any of the following signs or symptoms of thyroid hormone levels still being too <u>*high*</u>?
  • feeling too hot and sweating a lot
  • having weak muscles
  • trembling
  • fast or uneven heartbeats
  • feeling tired or fatigued
  • losing weight even when you are eating normally
  • frequent bowel movements
  • trouble sleeping
• Have you ever experienced any of the following signs or symptoms of thyroid hormone levels being too <u>*low*</u>?
  • feeling too cold
  • gaining weight
  • being constipated
  • having dry skin and thin hair
  • feeling depressed, tired, or fatigued
  • having a hoarse voice
• What over-the-counter medications or herbals do you take?
• Do you have radioiodine therapy planned?
• When was the last time your physician did blood work to see how well the antithyroid medication was working?
  • How often does your physician normally check your blood work?
• Are you pregnant or planning on becoming pregnant?
	• How long have you had hypothyroidism (underactive thyroid)?
	• Have you ever had thyroid surgery (partial thyroidectomy)?
	• Have you ever been treated with radioiodine therapy?
	• What medication(s) do you take for your thyroid condition?
	  • How do you take the medication?
	  • What time of the day do you take the medication(s)?
	  • Do you take your thyroid medication(s) at the same time as other medications and/or vitamins?
	  • Do you take your thyroid medication(s) on an empty stomach or with food?
	  • How long have you been taking your thyroid medication? At the dose you are currently taking?
	  • What is the name of your thyroid medication (ie, generic or brand name product)?
	  • How often do you miss a dose of your thyroid medication?
	  • Have you ever stopped taking your prescribed thyroid medication(s) without telling your physician? If so, why?
	• Do you experience any of the following signs or symptoms of thyroid hormone levels still being too <u>*low*</u>?
	  • feeling too cold
	  • gaining weight
	  • being constipated
	  • having dry skin and thin hair
	  • feeling depressed, tired, or fatigued
	  • having a hoarse voice
	  • forgetfulness
	• Have you ever experienced any of the following signs or symptoms of thyroid hormone levels being too <u>*high*</u>?
	  • feeling too hot and sweating a lot
	  • having weak muscles
	  • trembling
	  • fast or uneven heartbeats
	  • feeling tired or fatigued
	  • losing weight even when you are eating normally
	  • frequent bowel movements
	  • trouble sleeping
	• What over-the-counter medications or herbals do you take?
	• When was the last time your physician did blood work to see how well the thyroid medication was working for you?
	  • How often does your physician normally check your blood work?
	• Have you recently lost weight or plan on losing weight?
	• Are you pregnant or planning on becoming pregnant?

Questions to Ask for Prevention/Assessment of Medical Emergencies	

• For patients taking a thionamide: Are you experiencing signs and symptoms of an infection like a fever ><u>100.5°F</u> (38°C) or a severe sore throat?
  • *Crisis planning*: What is your action plan if you have signs and symptoms of an infection?
• For patients taking a thionamide: Are you experiencing signs and symptoms of liver damage such as yellow skin or eyes (jaundice), dark urine, light-colored stool, severe fatigue, or abdominal pain?
  • *Crisis planning*: What is your action plan if you have signs and symptoms of liver damage?	

during the patient interview (Figure 36-2). In addition, MTM providers must be prepared to answer patient questions that may arise in regard to hyper- or hypothyroidism (Table 36-7).

CORE ELEMENT 2—PERSONAL MEDICATION LIST

The following is a sample personal medication list (PML) of thyroid medication for a patient with hyperthyroidism (Figure 36-3) and hypothyroidism (Figure 36-4).[9] Additional medications for other disease states should be added and listed separately. MTM providers should remember to use plain language when creating the PML.

CORE ELEMENT 3—MEDICATION ACTION PLAN

The following section shows sample medication action plans (MAPs) for patients with hyperthyroidism (Figure 36-5) and hypothyroidism (Figure 36-6).[9] The examples are representative

Adverse event—unwanted effect.

Agranulocytosis—a severe and life-threatening, but rare, side effect of antithyroid medications where the body does not make enough white blood cells; patients with agranulocytosis can get sick very easily.

Atrial fibrillation—an abnormally fast heartbeat that may mean you have too much thyroid hormone in your bloodstream.

β-Blockers—a class of medications that can help to control symptoms of overactive thyroid.

Endocrine—system of the body's glands that secrete hormones into the bloodstream.

Endocrinologist—physician who specializes in glands and hormones

Euthyroid—normal thyroid.

Exophthalmos—bulging of the eye out of the socket that sometimes occurs in people with Graves' disease.

Galactorrhea—milky nipple discharge unrelated to the normal milk production during breastfeeding that could potentially indicate not enough thyroid hormone.

Gland—an organ in your body that produces hormones.

Goiter—swelling of the thyroid gland that is a sign of thyroid disease.

Graves' disease—an autoimmune disorder where antibodies make the thyroid gland produce too much thyroid hormone.

Hashimoto disease—an autoimmune disorder where antibodies turn against the thyroid and gradually destroy the gland over months or years.

Hormone—a chemical substance produced by the body that sends out messages to other parts of the body.

Hyperthyroid—overactive thyroid.

Hypothalamus—an area of the brain that produces thyrotropin-releasing hormone (TRH), which signals the pituitary (see *Pituitary*).

Hypothermia—low body temperature that may be a sign of myxedema coma in patients with underactive thyroid (see *Myxedema coma*).

Hypothyroid—underactive thyroid.

Levothyroxine—man-made form of thyroxine.

Metabolism—how the body uses and stores energy.

Myalgia—muscle pain.

Myxedema coma—a life-threatening condition that occurs in patients with severe, undertreated hypothyroidism; causes a loss of consciousness and low body temperature; usually set off by infection, trauma, exposure to cold or certain medications.

Osteoporosis—bone loss that causes weak bones and may mean you have too much thyroid hormone in your bloodstream.

Palpitations—an abnormal heartbeat that may mean you have too much thyroid hormone in your bloodstream.

Pituitary—a gland located at the base of the brain that releases thyroid-stimulating hormone (TSH) to make the thyroid gland work harder.

Primary hypothyroidism—when something is wrong with the thyroid gland, not enough thyroid hormone is made.

Radioactive iodine uptake (RAIU)—a type of scan used to diagnose thyroid problems where a patient swallows a radioactive iodine capsule or fluid and the amount of iodine taken up by the thyroid gland is measured.

Radioiodine therapy—a capsule or liquid that has a small amount of radiation that you swallow to kill part of the thyroid gland; the amount of radiation does not increase the risk of getting cancer.

Secondary hypothyroidism—underactive thyroid that occurs when the hypothalamus or the pituitary gland are not working right to make the thyroid gland produce thyroid hormone.

Subclinical hypothyroidism—thyroid condition where thyroid function is only a little low; you may or may not have symptoms.

Synthetic—chemically produced or man-made.

T_3—(see *Triiodothyronine*).

T_4—(see *Thyroxine*).

Thionamide—medication that works to decrease the amount of thyroid hormone made by the thyroid gland.

Thyroid gland—a butterfly-shaped gland located at the base of the neck under the Adam's apple that produces thyroid hormone to signal the cells to make energy.

Thyroid hormone—hormones produced by the thyroid gland that control how the body uses and stores energy.

Thyroid storm—a life-threatening condition with rapid heartbeat, high fever, agitation, and hallucinations that can occur in patients with overactive thyroid; usually set off by an infection, injury, or trauma.

Thyroid-stimulating hormone (TSH)—a hormone produced by the pituitary gland that tells the thyroid gland to make more thyroid hormone; high TSH levels in the blood means that the body has a high need for thyroid hormone; low TSH levels means that the body has a low need for thyroid hormone.

Thyroidectomy—surgery to remove the thyroid gland.

Thyroiditis—inflammation of the thyroid gland.

Thyrotoxicosis—a condition of having too much thyroid hormone in the bloodstream, which may be because the body is making too much thyroid hormone or the thyroid gland has become inflamed.

Thyrotropin-releasing hormone (TRH)—a hormone produced by the hypothalamus that tells the pituitary gland to release thyroid-stimulating hormone (see *Thyroid-stimulating hormone*).

Thyroxine—the major thyroid hormone made by the thyroid gland.

Toxic multinodular goiter—having small growths or lumps in the thyroid gland that produce too much thyroid hormone.

Triiodothyronine—the active thyroid hormone that causes cells to make energy.

FIGURE 36-2 Living room language for thyroid disorders.

TABLE 36-7 • Questions to Anticipate Regarding Thyroid Disorders

General Questions Commonly Asked by Patients About Thyroid Disorders
• **What is the thyroid?** The thyroid is a butterfly-shaped gland located in your neck just below the Adam's apple that makes thyroid hormones. • **What do thyroid hormones do?** Thyroid hormones control the body's use and storage of energy (also known as metabolism).
Questions Commonly Asked by Patients About Hyperthyroidism
• **What causes too much thyroid hormone in the bloodstream?** Most patients with overactive thyroid have Graves' disease. In Graves' disease, the body's immune system makes an antibody that stimulates the thyroid to produce too much thyroid hormone. Less common causes of thyrotoxicosis (or having too much thyroid in the bloodstream) include: • noncancerous thyroid nodules (small growths or lumps in the thyroid gland) • taking too much thyroid hormone medication for underactive thyroid • thyroiditis (when the thyroid gland becomes inflamed and releases too much thyroid hormone into the bloodstream) • **How do I know if I have overactive thyroid or too much thyroid hormone in my bloodstream?** Patients who have too much thyroid hormone may experience some of the following symptoms: • feeling too hot and sweating a lot • having weak muscles • trembling • fast or uneven heartbeats • feeling tired or fatigued • losing weight even when you are eating normally • frequent bowel movements If you have these symptoms, you should talk to your physician about getting a blood test that might indicate that you have too much thyroid hormone in your blood. A blood test is the only way to tell for sure if a patient has an overactive thyroid. • **What health problems are associated with having too much thyroid hormone?** Since thyroid hormone drives the body's metabolism, having too much thyroid hormone results in a speeding up of the body. Left untreated, excessive thyroid hormone can result in weight loss, osteoporosis, and atrial fibrillation. • **What treatment alternatives are available for overactive thyroid?** Physicians may choose to treat patients with overactive thyroid with medications, radioactive iodine therapy, or surgery to remove the thyroid gland. The physician looks at many factors such as patient age, the severity and type of hyperthyroidism, and patient preference to choose which treatment is best. • **What types of medications are available for overactive thyroid?** There are two major categories of medications for overactive thyroid: • antithyroid medications reduce the amount of thyroid hormone made by the thyroid gland • β-Blockers help reduce the symptoms from hyperthyroidism until the thyroid imbalance is corrected • **Will I need to take medication after radioactive iodine therapy or surgery for my overactive thyroid?** Most patients who are treated with radioactive iodine or who have surgery will no longer produce enough thyroid hormone, so they will need to be treated with thyroid hormone supplements for the rest of their lives. • **How can I tell if my antithyroid medication is working?** A blood test is the only way to tell how well medication is working to treat your overactive thyroid. You will usually have blood tests 4 to 6 weeks after starting your antithyroid medication until thyroid levels are under control. Once you are off of antithyroid medications and in remission, you will have blood work at least once every 6 months to 1 year. • **How long do I have to take antithyroid medication?** Most patients are able to take antithyroid medication for 12 to 18 months before they are in remission. Some patients choose to take antithyroid medication at a low dose for a longer period of time, though, in order to lessen the risk that the overactive thyroid condition comes back. • **How likely is it that I will remain in remission for my overactive thyroid condition now that I have stopped medication?** About 20% to 30% of patients with Graves' disease who are treated with antithyroid drugs for a period of 12 to 18 months will have a prolonged remission of the disease. • **What should I do if I have a problem with my antithyroid medication?** Do not stop your thyroid medication without first talking to your physician and/or pharmacist. If you let them know the problems that you are having, they will work together with you to choose an alternative treatment for your overactive thyroid.

(Continued)

TABLE 36-7 • Questions to Anticipate Regarding Thyroid Disorders (*Continued*)

- **What should I do if I am pregnant or planning on becoming pregnant?**
  If you take antithyroid medication, you should talk to your physician before trying to get pregnant since you may need to take different medications at different times during your pregnancy. Also, you may need a dose adjustment of your medication. If you were treated with radioiodine, you should wait at least 6 months before trying to get pregnant, so your physician can make sure the thyroid is making enough hormone after treatment. Having a normal level of thyroid hormone in your body before pregnancy is important.

Questions Commonly Asked by Patients About Hypothyroidism

- **What causes underactive thyroid?**
  Underactive thyroid most commonly results from thyroid inflammation from an autoimmune disorder called Hashimoto thyroiditis. In this disease, the body's own antibodies turn against the thyroid and eventually destroy the thyroid gland. Other causes of underactive thyroid include:
  - treatment with radioactive iodine that destroys the thyroid gland
  - surgery to remove the thyroid gland
  - problems with the pituitary gland or hypothalamus, parts of the brain that influence secretion of thyroid hormone from the thyroid gland
- **How do I know if I have underactive thyroid?**
  Patients who have an underactive thyroid may experience some of the following symptoms:
  - feeling too cold
  - gaining weight
  - being constipated
  - having dry skin and thin hair
  - feeling depressed, tired, or fatigued
  - having a hoarse voice
  - forgetfulness

  If you have these symptoms, you should talk to your physician about getting a blood test to verify if you have the correct balance of thyroid hormone in your blood. A blood test is the only way to tell for sure if a patient has an underactive thyroid.
- **What health problems are associated with underactive thyroid?**
  Since thyroid hormone drives the body's metabolism, having an inadequate supply results in a slowdown in physical and mental functioning. Left untreated, underactive thyroid can result in increased blood pressure and cholesterol levels, and it can raise the risk of heart disease and chronic heart failure. For pregnant women, treatment of underactive thyroid is necessary for a healthy pregnancy and baby.
- **Why is it important to take my thyroid medication on an empty stomach?**
  Your body best absorbs thyroid medication when you have not eaten and you take the medication on an empty stomach.
- **Why is it important to separate my thyroid medication from certain medications and supplements?**
  Certain medications and supplements (eg, those with calcium and iron) bind to the thyroid medication. When this happens, your body cannot absorb the thyroid medication as well.
- **What do I do if I miss a dose of my thyroid replacement medication (levothyroxine)?**
  If you miss a dose of your levothyroxine, it is safe to take the missed dose the next day. If you frequently have trouble remembering to take your levothyroxine doses, contact your physician.
- **Is it okay to switch between brand and generic thyroid medication?**
  You should use the same brand of thyroid medication consistently throughout your treatment—this includes using the same generic formulation, too (ie, not switching from one generic to another). If the brand of your thyroid medication is changed, you will need to visit your physician and have blood tests done.
- **I have heard that some patients take T_3 together with T_4 (thyroxine). Is that recommended?**
  Some medicines, like natural formulations of thyroid hormone (Armour Thyroid), provide a mixture of T_3 and T_4. The majority of studies have not shown an advantage of combination therapy, and leading experts recommend avoiding this combination. The body naturally converts T_4 into T_3 as it needs it.
- **How can I tell if my thyroid replacement medication is working?**
  A blood test is the only way to tell how well medication is working to treat your underactive thyroid.
- **How often do I have to have blood work done to test my thyroid?**
  You will usually have blood tests 4 to 8 weeks after starting or changing the dose of your thyroid medication. Once you are on a stable dose of thyroid medication, you will have blood work at least once every year.
- **How long do I have to take thyroid replacement medication?**
  Having hypothyroidism (underactive thyroid) is usually a permanent condition that will require lifelong treatment with medication.

(*Continued*)

TABLE 36-7 • Questions to Anticipate Regarding Thyroid Disorders (*Continued*)

- **My thyroid hormone level is in the normal range because of my medication, but I continue not to feel right. What can I do about it?**
  If you continue to have fatigue, sleepiness, or forgetfulness, talk to your physician about whether other conditions, like sleep apnea or anemia, may be causing your symptoms. Also check with your physician about whether your thyroid treatment puts you within the normal TSH range of, roughly, 0.45 to 4.12 mIU/L. Many patients feel fine when their TSH is in the upper half of this range. Some endocrinologists recommend a TSH in the lower half of the range, below 2.5 mIU/L. If you are not below 2.5 mIU/L, you can talk to your physician about the possibility of trying a slightly increased thyroid hormone dose. Over-replacement of thyroid hormone can cause bad effects, so dose increases must be done with caution and with follow-up of your thyroid hormone levels.
- **What should I do if I have a problem with my thyroid medication?**
  Do not stop your thyroid medication without first talking to your physician and/or pharmacist. If you let them know the problems that you are having, they will work together with you to choose an alternative treatment for your underactive thyroid condition.
- **What should I do if I am pregnant or planning on becoming pregnant?**
  Many women with hypothyroidism have healthy pregnancies. Talk to your physician about your thyroid hormone levels since your body during pregnancy will require greater doses of thyroid hormone. You will need your thyroid hormone levels checked every 4 weeks.

only of action steps for patients with thyroid disorders. MAPs for other disease states or other medication-related problems (MRPs) should be added and listed separately. In general, only a few of the most important action steps should be listed, so as not to overwhelm the patient. Other areas for patient self-management can be addressed at later visits. MTM providers should remember to use plain language when creating the MAP.

CORE ELEMENT 4—INTERVENTION AND/OR REFERRAL

Interventions for Management of Thyroid Disorders

Hyperthyroidism. The severity and type of hyperthyroidism, patient age, and patient preference dictate treatment selection between the different interventions, which include antithyroid medications, radiation (^{131}I therapy), or thyroidectomy (Table 36-8).[2,3] Treatment for Graves' disease may involve any of these (Table 36-9). Medical therapy does not result in permanent remission for patients with nodular disease (ie, TMNG or toxic adenoma). Therefore, radioiodine therapy and thyroidectomy are preferable options for these patients. Antithyroid medications may be used to lower thyroid levels before definitive treatment. Low RAIU hyperthyroidism does not require antithyroid medication, radiation, or surgery because of its self-limiting nature and response to nonsteroidal anti-inflammatory drugs (NSAIDs), glucocorticoids, and β-blockers.

Ideally, treatment for hyperthyroidism produces remission of the thyroid disorder without inducing hypothyroidism. Doses of antithyroid medications can be titrated down to a maintenance level. The dose of antithyroid medications requires a careful balance. If the dose is too low, a euthyroid state may not occur. Conversely, excessive doses can precipitate hypothyroidism. In order to induce remission of Graves' disease and reduce risk of reoccurrence, patients should continue antithyroid therapy for an additional 12 to 18 months at the reduced dose. After this time, if TSH is normal, the antithyroid medication can be discontinued or tapered. Patients with normal TRAb levels at the end of treatment are more likely to achieve successful remission. Patients who do not achieve remission with pharmacological therapy may continue

PERSONAL MEDICATION LIST FOR *<Insert Patient's name*, DOB: *mm/dd/yyyy>*	
Medication: Methimazole 30 mg tablet	
How I use it: Take one tablet (30 mg) by mouth once daily	
Why I use it: Overactive thyroid	**Prescriber:** Dr. George Scott
Date I started using it: October 2017	**Date I stopped using it:** *(Leave blank for patient's notes)*
Why I stopped using it: *(Leave blank for patient's notes)*	
Medication: Propranolol 40 mg capsule	
How I use it: Take one capsule (40 mg) by mouth every 8 hours	
Why I use it: Overactive thyroid	**Prescriber:** Dr. George Scott
Date I started using it: October 2017	**Date I stopped using it:** *(Leave blank for patient's notes)*
Why I stopped using it: : *(Leave blank for patient's notes)*	

FIGURE 36-3 Example personal medication list for hyperthyroid medications.

PERSONAL MEDICATION LIST FOR *<Insert Patient's name*, DOB: *mm/dd/yyyy>*	
Medication: Levothyroxine 50 mcg tablet	
How I use it: Take one tablet (50 mcg) by mouth every morning	
Why I use it: Underactive thyroid	**Prescriber:** Dr. John Smith
Reminder: • Take this medication 30 minutes before breakfast on an empty stomach. • Do not take your multivitamin until 4 hours after taking this medication.	
Date I started using it: January 2013	**Date I stopped using it:** *(Leave blank for patient's notes)*
Why I stopped using it: *(Leave blank for patient's notes)*	

FIGURE 36-4 Example personal medication list for hypothyroid medications.

	DATE PREPARED: *<Insert date>*
What we talked about: • Potential serious side effects of methimazole and what to do if you experience them	
What I need to do: • Stop methimazole and call my physician right away if I develop signs of an infection like a bad sore throat or fever. • Stop methimazole and call my physician right away if I develop yellow eyes, dark urine, severe fatigue, or belly pain.	**What I did and when I did it:** *(Leave blank for patient's notes)*

FIGURE 36-5 Example medication action plan for a patient with hyperthyroidism.

a prolonged course of low-dose methimazole, but surgery or radioactive iodine are generally preferred.

Hypothyroidism. Several thyroid hormone replacement options exist for patients with hypothyroidism (Table 36-10), although levothyroxine (synthetic T_4) monotherapy is the mainstay of treatment.[5,6] Administration of T_4 mimics glandular thyroid hormone secretion, and peripheral tissues regulate conversion of synthetic T_4 to T_3. Animal-derived (porcine) desiccated thyroid, by contrast, has excessive amounts of T_3 relative to T_4, is not a pure preparation, and has stability concerns. Further, clinical studies have largely failed to show advantages of T_4/T_3 combination therapy on cognitive or mood outcomes versus T_4 alone.[12,13] The T_4/T_3 combination could potentially improve psychological well-being in patients with a specific polymorphism in type 2 deiodinase (DIO2), although this has not been confirmed and real-world genetic testing for a DIO2 polymorphism is impractical.[14] Of note, all thyroid replacement medications carry a blackbox warning against use as weight loss agents.[10]

The average daily dose for thyroid replacement with levothyroxine is 1.6 microgram per kilogram, but the initial dose should be based on weight, age, and cardiac status (Table 36-11). Patients preferably should take thyroid medication in the morning, between 30 and 60 minutes before breakfast, to improve absorption. Patients may alternatively choose to take thyroid medication 4 hours after the last meal of the day.[15] Patients who have difficulty adhering to a daily levothyroxine schedule can safely take the entire weekly levothyroxine dose 1 day per week.[5,16]

The MTM provider must be aware of the numerous medications, supplements, and dietary factors that can affect thyroid hormone dosing requirements (Table 36-12). The use of dietary supplements or herbal products to treat hypothyroidism is not recommended. This includes pharmacologic doses of iodine that may precipitate either hypothyroidism or thyrotoxicosis in patients with an intact thyroid gland. The potential for altered bioavailability among different formulations of levothyroxine makes switching products inadvisable.[17] Figure 36-7 lists criteria for referral for management of thyroid conditions.

	DATE PREPARED: *<Insert date>*
What we talked about: • Thyroid medication (levothyroxine) and calcium carbonate interaction; calcium carbonate can decrease how well the thyroid medication works	
What I need to do: • Take thyroid medication 30 minutes before breakfast on an empty stomach. • Take calcium carbonate at least 4 hours after the thyroid medication. • Take calcium carbonate by mouth with food every day at lunchtime and dinnertime. • Make an appointment with my physician to check my labs in 4 to 8 weeks.	**What I did and when I did it:** *(Leave blank for patient's notes)*

FIGURE 36-6 Example medication action plan for a patient with hypothyroidism.

CORE ELEMENT 5—DOCUMENTATION AND FOLLOW-UP

Clear and succinct documentation of MRPs and recommendations is a key component of the MTM consult. Examples of potential MRPs in patients with thyroid disorders are provided in Table 36-13.

Figures 36-8 and 36-9 provide samples of provider communications to address MRPs for hyperthyroidism and hypothyroidism, respectively. Recommendations may be communicated via fax, telephone, or other means of written or secure electronic communication. The examples provided are for illustrative purposes. Actual communications to providers should be individualized based on the type of recommendation, patient-specific characteristics, and the nature of the relationship with the provider.

Monitoring Patients with Thyroid Disorders

Regular follow-up with the patient to assess thyroid function tests, effectiveness of interventions, and potential adverse effects is crucial in the management of thyroid disorders.[1]

Hyperthyroidism. Patients with hyperthyroidism should be evaluated on an approximately monthly basis (every 4 to 6 weeks) from initiation of antithyroid therapy until a euthyroid state has been achieved.[2,3,12] Serum TSH is not an appropriate indicator of success early in treatment because levels may remain suppressed for many months. An elevated T_3 may be a sign of inadequate treatment, even with normal free T_4 levels. Clinical and laboratory evaluations should occur every 3 to 6 months during the maintenance therapy period and every 2 months for the first 6 months of remission. Thereafter, thyroid function monitoring every 6 to 12 months is appropriate.

TABLE 36-8 • Medications for Management of Hyperthyroidism

Drug Category	Dose	Adverse Reactions[a]	Notes
β-Adrenergic blockers		*Common*: bradycardia, light-headedness, masked signs of hypoglycemia, orthostatic hypotension, exercise intolerance, fatigue, worsened breathing disorders	• Appropriate for symptomatic relief for patients with hyperthyroidism of any cause, especially if HR >90 beats/minute • Used as primary therapy for thyroiditis • Usually used as adjunctive therapy for high RAIU hyperthyroidism • Contraindicated in acute decompensated heart failure; use caution in asthma and bronchospastic chronic obstructive lung disease • Abrupt discontinuation is a blackbox warning
propranolol[b]	10-40 mg TID-QID		• β-Blocker with the most experience for hyperthyroidism • May block T_4 to T_3 conversion at high doses • May also consider extended-release formulation
atenolol	25-100 mg daily or BID		• Relative β-1 selectivity
metoprolol[b]	25-50 mg BID-TID		• Relative β-1 selectivity • May also consider extended-release formulation
nadolol	40-160 mg daily		• May block T_4 to T_3 conversion at high doses
Thionamides			• Lower thyroid hormone levels in patients with Graves' disease, TMNG, toxic adenoma • Should be administered in relation to meals each day, either always with food or always between meals
methimazole	*Initial dose*: 5-30 mg daily (usually 15-30 mg daily) *Maintenance dose*: 5-10 mg daily *Maximum dose*: 120 mg daily	*Common*: rash, urticaria, arthralgia, gastrointestinal effects, elevated alkaline phosphatase *Serious*: dose-related agranulocytosis, aplasia cutis of the scalp in babies born to mothers taking methimazole	• Approximately 10 times more potent than PTU
propylthiouracil (PTU)	*Initial dose*: 50-300 mg TID-QID (usually 100 mg TID) *Maintenance dose*: 50 mg BID-TID *Maximum dose*: 1200 mg daily	*Common*: rash, urticaria, arthralgia, gastrointestinal effects, elevated ALT/AST *Serious*: vasculitis, non–dose-related agranulocytosis, severe liver damage with liver failure	• Methimazole is preferred over PTU except for cases of thyroid storm, methimazole allergy, or pregnancy in the first trimester
Radioactive iodine (^{131}I)		*Common*: hypothyroidism, exacerbation of Graves' orbitopathy, transient neck soreness, flushing, decreased taste *Serious*: none	• Contraindicated during pregnancy; women of childbearing age should have negative pregnancy test before treatment • May require pretreatment with antithyroid drugs in older or cardiac patients • Thyroid hormones may rise 1 to 2 weeks after treatment • Most patients become hypothyroid in 3 to 6 months (~100% in patients with Graves' disease vs 50%-75% with TMNG or toxic adenoma)

[a] This is a general list and does not include all side effects that can occur from these drugs. Consult a drug reference source for a more inclusive list before making any recommendations. MTM providers should also consult a comprehensive drug interaction database before making pharmacotherapy recommendations.

[b] Also available in once daily preparation.

Abbreviations: ALT = alanine aminotransferase; AST = aspartate aminotransferase; BID = twice daily; HR = heart rate; QID = 4 times daily; RAIU = radioactive iodine uptake; TID = 3 times daily; TMNG = toxic multinodular goiter.

Source: References 2, 3, 10, and 11.

TABLE 36-9 • Treatments for Hyperthyroidism Caused by Graves' Disease

Treatment	Advantages	Disadvantages	Comment
Methimazole (PTU second-line therapy)	Noninvasive Lower initial cost Low risk of permanent hypothyroidism Possible remission because of immune effects	Low cure rate (average 40%-50%) Adverse drug reactions Drug compliance	First-line treatment in children, adolescents, and in pregnancy Initial treatment in severe cases or preoperative preparation
Radioactive iodine (^{131}I)	Cure of hyperthyroidism Lowest cost, before adjustment for quality of life	Permanent hypothyroidism almost inevitable Might worsen ophthalmopathy Pregnancy must be deferred for 6-12 months; no breastfeeding Small potential risk of exacerbation of hyperthyroidism	Best treatment for toxic nodules and toxic multinodular goiter
Surgery	Rapid, effective treatment, especially in patients with large goiters	Most invasive Least costly in long term after quality-of-life adjustment Permanent hypothyroidism Pain, scar	Potential in pregnancy if major side-effect from antithyroid drugs Potential complications (recurrent laryngeal nerve damage, hypoparathyroidism) Useful when coexisting suspicious nodule present Option for patients who refuse radioiodine

Source: Reproduced, with permission, from DiPiro, JT, Talbert RL, Yee GC, Matzke GR, Wells BG, Posey LM, eds. *Pharmacotherapy: A Pathophysiologic Approach.* 10th ed. New York, NY: McGraw-Hill; 2017.

TABLE 36-10 • Thyroid Preparations Used in the Treatment of Hypothyroidism

Drug/Dosage Form	Content	Relative Dose	Comments/Equivalency
Thyroid USP Armour Thyroid, Nature-Throid, and Westhroid (T_4:T_3 ratio approximately 4.2:1); Armour, 1 grain = 60 mg; Nature-Throid and Westhroid, 1 grain = 65 mg. Doses include ¼-, ½- 1-, 2-, 3-, 4-, and 5-grain tablets	Desiccated beef or pork thyroid gland	1 grain (equivalent to 74 mcg [~60-100] mcg of T_4)	High T_3:T_4 ratio; inexpensive
Levothyroxine Synthroid, Levothroid, Levoxyl, Levo-T, Unithroid, and other generics 25, 50, 75, 88, 100, 112, 125, 137, 150, 175, 200, 300 mcg tablets; Tirosint 13-150 mcg liquid in gelatin capsule; 200 and 500 mcg per vial injection	Synthetic T_4	1000 mcg	Stable; predictable potency; generics may be bioequivalent; when switching from natural thyroid to l-thyroxine, lower dose by one half grain; variable absorption between products; half-life = 7 days, so daily dosing; considered to be drug of choice
Liothyronine Cytomel 5, 25, and 50 mcg tablets	Synthetic T_3	33 mcg (~equivalent to 100 mcg T_4)	Uniform absorption, rapid onset; half-life = 1.5 days, rapid peak and troughs
Liotrix Thyrolar ¼-, ½-, 1- 2-, and 3-grain tablets	Synthetic T_4: T_3 in 4:1 ratio	Thyrolar 1 = 50 mcg T_4 and 12.5 mcg T_3	Stable; predictable; expensive; risk of T_3 thyrotoxicosis because of high ratio of T_3 relative to T_4

Source: Reproduced, with permission, from DiPiro, JT, Talbert RL, Yee GC, Matzke GR, Wells BG, Posey LM, eds. *Pharmacotherapy: A Pathophysiologic Approach.* 10th ed. New York, NY: McGraw-Hill; 2017.

TABLE 36-11 • Dosing Guidelines for T_4 Replacement Therapy in Adults with Hypothyroidism

Population	Dosing
Nonpregnant patients <50 years old	1.6 mcg/kg/day initially[a] Adjust in increment changes of 12.5-25 mcg/day every 6 to 8 weeks
Patients ≥50 years of age	50 mcg/day initially
Patients with coronary artery disease[b]	12.5-25 mcg/day initially Monitor for the onset of anginal symptoms
Pregnant women[c]	For women already on thyroid replacement: • Add 2 additional doses per week of the current levothyroxine dose upon missed menstrual cycle or positive pregnancy test • Monitor serum TSH and total T_4 every 4 weeks during the first half of pregnancy and at least once between 26 and 32 weeks' gestation Goal TSH varies by trimester: • 0.1 to 2.5 mIU/L in the first trimester • 0.2 to 3.0 mIU/L in the second trimester • 0.3 to 3.0 mIU/L in the third trimester
Subclinical hypothyroidism	Choose initial dose based on TSH as follows: • 25 mcg for TSH 4.0 to 8.0 mIU/L • 50 mcg for TSH 8.0 to 12.0 mIU/L • 75 mcg for TSH >12.0 mIU/L

[a] Use ideal body weight to calculate thyroid replacement dose since lean mass is best predictive of daily thyroid requirements.

[b] Thyroid hormone increases heart rate and contractility leading to increased myocardial oxygen demand; higher starting doses may induce acute coronary syndromes or arrhythmias in patients with established ischemic heart disease.

[c] Pregnancy increases dose requirements by 25% to 50%; thyroid hormone should be reduced to prepregnancy dose immediately after giving birth, and thyroid function tests should be assessed after 6 weeks.

Abbreviation: TSH, thyroid stimulating hormone.

Source: References 5, 18, 19, 20, and 21.

From a toxicity standpoint, a complete blood cell count (CBC) with a differential white blood cell (WBC) count and a liver panel should be performed before starting antithyroid medication. The CBC with differential should be repeated if a patient complains of fever or pharyngitis. Likewise, a liver panel should be done for patients with signs and symptoms of liver injury.

Hypothyroidism. Measurements of TSH most reliably indicate treatment success in primary hypothyroidism, though controversy exists surrounding the most appropriate therapeutic endpoint for TSH.[5,6] Clinical treatment guidelines maintain that the upper limit of the TSH reference range for a given laboratory (approximately 4.12 mIU/L) is an adequate treatment goal. Proponents of a low-normal target (ie, 2.5 mIU/L) argue that more than 95% of rigorously screened normal euthyroid volunteers have serum values between 0.4 and 2.5 mIU/L.[25] Conversely, higher thyrotropin targets may be suitable for those aged >65 years. Serum TSH should not drop below the lower limit of normal for the reference range (approximately 0.45 mIU/L). TSH should be reassessed 4 to 8 weeks after initiating therapy or changing a dosage. Once the levothyroxine dose is stable, repeat TSH should be completed in 3 to 6 months and then annually thereafter.

In secondary hypothyroidism, assessment of free T_4, not TSH, guides treatment. Therapy should be adjusted to exceed the mid-normal value of the free T_4 reference range. In assessments of free T_4 for patients on levothyroxine, blood should be drawn before the daily dose is given. If not, the level will be transiently increased by 20% and, therefore, be inaccurate.[26]

The Role of the MTM Provider. The MTM provider should assess the most recent thyroid hormone panel to determine adequacy of treatment for patients with either hyper- or hypothyroidism. If levels are not available in a timely manner (as outlined previously), the MTM provider should recommend thyroid function testing. Furthermore, the MTM provider should evaluate the patient's symptoms to monitor for drug efficacy and toxicity. Screening for nonadherence and drug interactions with thyroid medications is another important role of the MTM provider.

TABLE 36-12 • Conditions that May Alter Thyroid Hormone Requirements

Patient misses doses of thyroid hormone (nonadherence)

Generic substitution for brand name product or vice versa, or substitution of a different generic product

Patient is pregnant or recently started or stopped estrogen-containing oral contraceptive or hormone replacement therapy[a]

Patient started taking sertraline[b]

Patient lost or gained weight

Decreased absorption of thyroid hormone

- Patient takes any of the following medications within 4 hours of thyroid hormone:
  - aluminum-containing antacids
  - bile acid sequestrants
  - calcium salts
  - ciprofloxacin
  - ferrous sulfate
  - fiber products
  - multivitamins (containing calcium carbonate or ferrous sulfate)
  - orlistat
  - proton-pump inhibitors/ H_2-receptor blocker famotidine
  - raloxifene
  - soy products
  - sucralfate
- Patient takes thyroid hormone with food
- Patient has malabsorption from gastrointestinal disorders
- Patients with extreme obesity (body mass index >40 kg/m^2)

Increased clearance of thyroid hormone

- Patient taking any of the following medications:
  - anticonvulsants (eg, carbamazepine, phenobarbital, phenytoin)
  - rifampin

[a] Estrogen and pregnancy increase T_4-binding globulin.

[b] Sertraline lowers serum thyroxine concentrations by an unknown mechanism.

Source: References 5, 22, 23, 24, and 25.

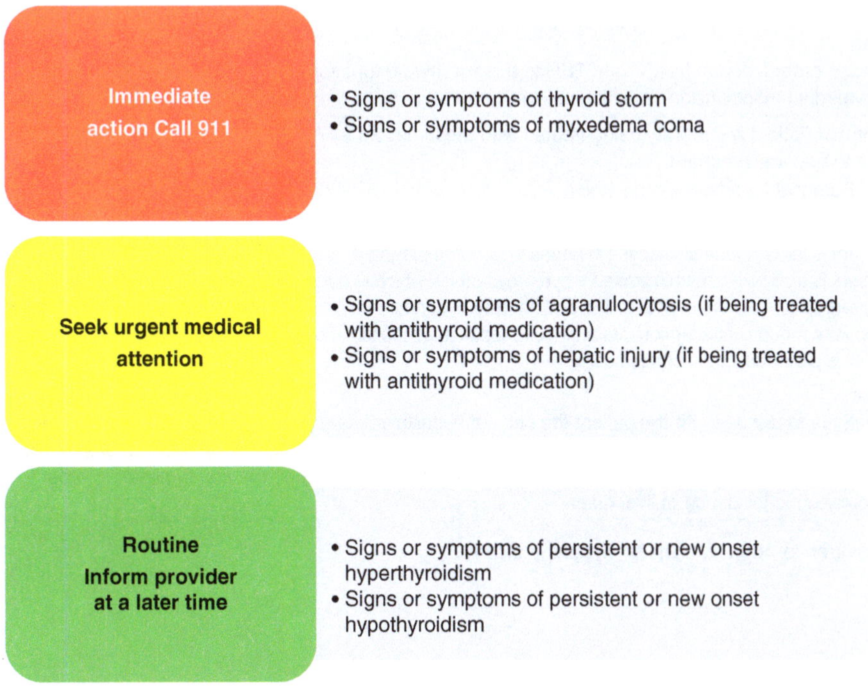

FIGURE 36-7 Referral for management of thyroid disease.

TABLE 36-13 • Medication-Related Problems (MRPs) in Patients with Thyroid Disorders

Category of MRP	Example Medication-Related Problem
Nonadherence	• Patient forgets to take levothyroxine in the morning • Patient takes levothyroxine with meals
Unnecessary medication	• T_3 replacement in addition to levothyroxine
Need for additional medication	• Patient was treated with radioiodine and now exhibits signs and symptoms of hypothyroidism
Ineffective medication	• Persistently elevated T_3 or T_4 after sufficient trial (eg, 12-18 months) of antithyroid medication
Dosage too low	• Elevated TSH despite thyroid replacement therapy • Elevated T_3 or T_4 despite antithyroid medication
Dosage too high	• Symptoms of hyperthyroidism on levothyroxine
Adverse drug event	• Agranulocytosis from antithyroid medication • Rash with methimazole use

Scenario: Patient has completed appropriate duration of therapy with methimazole
MRP: Inappropriate duration of therapy (or dosage too high)

- Assessment:
  Patient has been taking methimazole 30 mg daily for the past 24 months for Graves' disease. He was euthyroid per his thyroid function tests performed last week. Since patient has completed at least 12 to 18 months of maintenance therapy and TSH is within normal limits, drug discontinuation may be considered.
- Plan:
  Please consider stopping or tapering off methimazole therapy since recommended treatment duration of 12 to 18 months has elapsed and patient is euthyroid. It is advised to measure TRAb levels first, though, since normal levels indicate a greater chance of remission. Thyroid function testing (TSH ± free T_4) should occur every 6 to 12 months for the patient's life.

Scenario: Patient had radioiodine therapy 4 months ago and is now complaining of fatigue, weight gain, and cold intolerance
MRP: Need for additional medication

- Assessment:
  Patient complains of symptoms consistent with hypothyroidism (ie, fatigue, weight gain, cold intolerance). It is common for patients treated with radioiodine to become hypothyroid after treatment; patients will require lifelong thyroid supplementation.
- Plan:
  Please order a serum free T_4 and TSH to assess thyroid function. If free T_4 is suppressed or TSH is elevated, please consider initiation of levothyroxine.

Scenario: Patient is currently being treated with methimazole for hyperthyroidism and expresses desire to become pregnant
MRP: Potential for adverse drug event

- Assessment:
  Patient is taking prenatal vitamins in hopes to become pregnant.
  Patient is also taking methimazole for hyperthyroidism, which is not recommended for the first trimester of pregnancy. Counseled patient that optimal time to conceive is once euthyroid state has been reached. Recommended contraception use until the disease is controlled. If patient becomes pregnant, propylthiouracil is preferred for the first trimester.
- Plan:
  Continue to discuss with the patient the risks of hyperthyroidism and methimazole use for women during pregnancy. If patient becomes pregnant, recommend switching methimazole to propylthiouracil for the first trimester, and then switching back to methimazole after the first trimester in order to decrease the incidence of liver disease.

FIGURE 36-8 Sample provider communications for hyperthyroidism.[2]

Scenario: Patient recently switched from brand name Synthroid to generic levothyroxine **MRP:** Dosage too high/low
• Assessment: Patient's insurance no longer covers brand name Synthroid, and patient has been taking generic levothyroxine X 3 months. Potential bioavailability differences exist between different formulations, and small changes to levothyroxine dosing can cause significant changes in TSH. In general, TSH should be retested 6 weeks after any change in levothyroxine product. • Plan: Please consider ordering a serum TSH to assess patient's thyroid function with the current levothyroxine formulation. Titrate levothyroxine, as appropriate, to goal TSH 0.45-4.12 mIU/L.
Scenario: Patient has difficulty remembering to take levothyroxine 30 minutes before breakfast **MRP:** Nonadherence
• Assessment: Patient reports forgetting to take levothyroxine in the morning on an empty stomach several days out of the week, and she takes her dose with breakfast on days where she forgets. Taking levothyroxine with a meal reduces drug absorption. Alternative dosing strategies may be appropriate in order to improve compliance. After any change is made to thyroid hormone dosing, serum TSH should be reassessed in 4 to 8 weeks. • Plan: Recommend that patient take levothyroxine 4 hours after the last meal of the day to improve compliance. Check serum TSH within 4 to 8 weeks after making dosing adjustment to ensure TSH is within goal range of 0.45 to 4.12 mIU/L.
Scenario: Patient is on levothyroxine and is experiencing palpitations, nervousness, and anxiety **MRP:** Dosage too high
• Assessment: Patient complains of symptoms consistent with hyperthyroidism (ie, palpitations, nervousness, anxiety), which may indicate that his thyroid hormone replacement dose is too high. • Plan: Please order a serum TSH to assess thyroid function. If TSH is <0.45 mIU/L, please consider reducing levothyroxine dose.
Scenario: Patient on levothyroxine started taking calcium supplementation for osteoporosis **MRP:** Dosage too low (or ineffective medication)
• Assessment: Patient has been therapeutic on current levothyroxine dose for several years. Patient started taking OTC calcium carbonate supplementation last week for osteoporosis, which has the potential to decrease levothyroxine absorption. Recommended that patient avoid taking calcium tablets until at least 4 hours after levothyroxine dose. • Plan: Patient should continue to take levothyroxine 30 minutes daily before breakfast. She should take calcium carbonate at lunchtime and dinnertime.

FIGURE 36-9 Sample provider communications for hypothyroidism.
Source: References 5, 15, and 17.

REFERENCES

1. Jonklaas J, Kane MP. Thyroid Disorders. In: DiPiro, JT, Talbert RL, Yee GC, Matzke GR, Wells BG, Posey LM, eds. *Pharmacotherapy: A Pathophysiologic Approach*. 10th ed. New York, NY: McGraw-Hill; 2017.
2. Ross DS, Burch HB, Cooper DS, et al. 2016 American Thyroid Association Guidelines for diagnosis and management of hyperthyroidism and other causes of thyrotoxicosis. *Thyroid*. 2016;26(10):1343-1421.
3. McDermott MT. Hyperthyroidism. *Ann Intern Med*. 2012;157(1):ITC1-16.
4. Weetman AP. Graves' disease. *N Engl J Med*. 2000;343(17):1236-1248.
5. Jonklaas J, Bianco AC, Bauer AJ, et al. Guidelines for the treatment of hypothyroidism: prepared by the American Thyroid Association Task Force on Thyroid Hormone Replacement. *Thyroid*. 2014;24(12):1670-1751.
6. McDermott MT. In the clinic. Hypothyroidism. *Ann Intern Med*. 2009;151(11):ITC61.
7. Hamnvik OR, Larsen PR, Marqusee E. Thyroid dysfunction from antineoplastic agents. *J Natl Cancer Inst*. 2011;103(21):1572-1587.
8. Barbesino G. Drugs affecting thyroid function. *Thyroid*. 2010;20(7):763-770.
9. *Medicare Part D Medication Therapy Management Program Standardized Format*. Available at https://www.cms.gov/Medicare/Prescription-Drug-Coverage/PrescriptionDrugCovContra/Downloads/MTM-Program-Standardized-Format-English-and-Spanish-Instructions-Samples-v032712.pdf. Accessed April 24, 2017.
10. Clinical Pharmacology [database online]. Tampa, FL: Elsevier Gold Standard, Inc.; 2017. Available from: clinicalpharmacology-ip.com/default.aspx. Accessed April 24, 2017.
11. Cooper DS. Antithyroid drugs. *N Engl J Med*. 2005;352(9):902-917.
12. Escobar-Morreale HF, Botella-Carretero JI, Escobar del Rey F, et al. Review: treatment of hypothyroidism with combinations of levothyroxine plus liothyronine. *J Clin Endocrinol Metab*. 2005;90(8):4946-4954.
13. Grozinsky-Glasberg S, Fraser A, Nahshoni E, et al. Thyroxine-triiodothyronine combination therapy versus thyroxine monotherapy for clinical hypothyroidism: meta-analysis of randomized controlled trials. *J Clin Endocrinol Metab*. 2006;91(7):2592-2599.
14. Panicker V, Saravanan P, Vaidya B, et al. Common variation in the DIO2 gene predicts baseline psychological well-being and response to combination

thyroxine plus triiodothyronine therapy in hypothyroid patients. *Clin Endocrinol Metab.* 2009;94(5):1623-1629.

15. Bolk N, Visser TJ, Nijman J, et al. Effects of evening vs morning levothyroxine intake: a randomized double-blind crossover trial. *Arch Intern Med.* 2010;170(22):1996-2003.
16. Grebe SK, Cooke RR, Ford HC, et al. Treatment of hypothyroidism with once weekly thyroxine. *J Clin Endocrinol Metab.* 1997;82(3):870-875.
17. American Association of Clinical Endocrinologists, The Endocrine Society, American Thyroid Association. AACE, TES, and ATA Joint Position Statement on the Use and Interchangeability of Thyroxine Products. American Association of Clinical Endocrinologists website. December 8, 2004. www.aace.com/pub/pdf/guidelines/AACE-TES-ATA-ThyroxineProducts.pdf. Accessed April 24, 2017.
18. Roos A, Linn-Rasker SP, van Domburg RT, et al. The starting dose of levothyroxine in primary hypothyroidism treatment: a prospective, randomized, double-blind trial. *Arch Intern Med.* 2005;165(15):1714-1720.
19. Stagnaro-Green A, Abalovich M, Alexander E, et al. Guidelines of the American Thyroid Association for the diagnosis and management of thyroid disease during pregnancy and postpartum. *Thyroid.* 2011;21(10):1081-1125.
20. Yassa L, Marqusee E, Fawcett R, et al. Thyroid hormone early adjustment in pregnancy (the THERAPY) trial. *J Clin Endocrinol Metab.* 2010;95(7):3234-3241.
21. Teixeira PF, Reuters VS, Ferreira MM, et al. Treatment of subclinical hypothyroidism reduces atherogenic lipid levels in a placebo-controlled double-blind clinical trial. *Horm Metab Res.* 2008;40:50-55.
22. Sachmechi I, Reich DM, Aninyei M, et al. Effect of proton pump inhibitors on serum thyroid-stimulating hormone level in euthyroid patients treated with levothyroxine for hypothyroidism. *Endocr Pract.* 2007;13(4):345-349.
23. Centanni M, Gargano L, Canettieri G, et al. Thyroxine in goiter, Helicobacter pylori infection, and chronic gastritis. *N Engl J Med.* 2006;354(17):1787-1795.
24. McCowen KC, Garber JR, Spark R. Elevated serum thyrotropin in thyroxine-treated patients with hypothyroidism given sertraline. *N Engl J Med.* 1997;337(14):1010-1011.
25. Baloch Z, Carayon P, Conte-Devolx B, et al. Laboratory medicine practice guidelines. Laboratory support for the diagnosis and monitoring of thyroid disease. *Thyroid.* 2003;13(1):3-126.
26. Ain KB, Pucino F, Shiver TM, et al. Thyroid hormone levels affected by time of blood sampling in thyroxine-treated patients. *Thyroid.* 1993;3(2):81-85.

Review Questions

1. Which statement correctly describes a step in the hypothalamic-pituitary-thyroid axis?
   a. TSH stimulates the pituitary to release TRH.
   b. T_4 stimulates the thyroid gland to produce TSH.
   c. T_3 is converted to T_4 by deiodinase enzymes.
   d. T_3 inhibits TRH through negative feedback.

2. A patient is taking thyroid replacement for hypothyroidism. Which question is LEAST appropriate to ask this patient?
   a. Do you take your thyroid medication on an empty stomach?
   b. Do you take your thyroid medication at the same time as other medications and/or vitamins?
   c. Do you remain in an upright position for 30 minutes after taking your thyroid medication?
   d. What is the name of your thyroid medication (ie, generic or brand name product)?

3. All of the following therapeutic goals are appropriate for a patient with hypothyroidism **EXCEPT:**
   a. Eliminate symptoms of cold intolerance and fatigue.
   b. Avoid overtreatment and symptoms of tachycardia and weight loss.
   c. Attain a TSH level of <4.12 mIU/L but >0.45 mIU/L.
   d. Achieve remission by continuing thyroid hormone supplementation for 12 to 18 months.

4. All of the following are appropriate definitions for thyroid-related terms using living room language **EXCEPT**:
   a. exophthalmos—eye appears to bulge out of the socket.
   b. myxedema coma—having very high thyroid hormone levels; similar to thyrotoxicosis.
   c. galactorrhea—discharge of milk-like substance from the nipple.
   d. goiter—enlargement of the thyroid gland.

5. A 33-year-old female patient takes methimazole for Graves' disease. Which recommendation is the LEAST appropriate for the medication action plan?
   a. Tell the physician if you are pregnant or thinking about becoming pregnant.
   b. Go to a physician regularly for blood tests to check your thyroid.
   c. Tell your physician immediately if you have yellow skin or eyes, light-colored stool, or dark urine.
   d. Stop medication immediately if you feel depressed, gain weight, or have constipation.

6. A patient reports feeling "under the weather" with a sore throat and a fever and has a past medical history significant for diabetes, hyperthyroidism, and hyperlipidemia. Currently, the patient is currently taking metformin, glipizide, methimazole, and atorvastatin. What is the most appropriate management of this patient at the present time?
   a. No referral is necessary since symptoms will likely resolve spontaneously.
   b. The MTM provider should refer the patient to the primary care physician.
   c. The MTM provider should suggest the patient seek urgent medical attention.
   d. The MTM provider should call 911.

7. A patient underwent radioactive iodine therapy for toxic adenoma several months ago. Today, the patient reports having fatigue, weight gain, constipation, and muscle cramps. What is the correct categorization for this patient's medication-related problem?
   a. Need for additional therapy
   b. Ineffective medication
   c. Drug dosage too high
   d. Nonadherence

8. What is the standard of treatment for a patient with Hashimoto disease?
   a. Levothyroxine
   b. Combination T_4/T_3 therapy
   c. Antithyroid medication
   d. Radioactive iodine

9. Which test is the most appropriate to assess severity of disease and effectiveness of treatment in patients with hypothyroidism?
   a. Free T_4 levels
   b. Total T_4 levels
   c. Free T_3 levels
   d. TSH levels

10. A 72-year-old male has a history of hypertension, atrial fibrillation, gastroesophageal reflux disease, and depression. Current medications include metoprolol tartrate, amiodarone, warfarin, pantoprazole, and sertraline. His TSH is elevated, and serum free T_4 levels are subtherapeutic. Which of his medications is most likely contributing to this patient's laboratory results?
    a. Metoprolol tartrate
    b. Amiodarone
    c. Omeprazole
    d. Sertraline

ANSWERS

1. d	2. c	3. d
4. b	5. d	6. c
7. a	8. a	9. d
10. b		

Index

Page references followed by *f* indicate figures; those followed by *t* indicate tables.

D

O

www.ingramcontent.com/pod-product-compliance
Lightning Source LLC
Chambersburg PA
CBHW080138231125
35696CB00003B/7
9781260108453